Davis's
NCLEX-RN REVIEW

Patricia Gauntlett Beare, RN, PhD
Professor
Louisiana State University Medical Center
School of Nursing
New Orleans, Louisiana

Davis's NCLEX-RN REVIEW

THIRD EDITION

F. A. Davis Company • Philadelphia

F. A. Davis Company
1915 Arch Street
Philadelphia, PA 19103

Printed in the United States of America

Last digit indicates print number: 10 9 8 7 6 5 4 3 2 1

Acquisitions Editor: Alan Sorkowitz
Developmental Editor: Ann Houska
Production Editor: Elena Coler
Designer: William T. Donnelley
Cover Designer: Louis J. Forgione
Cover Photograph: Doug Rickards

As new scientific information becomes available through basic and clinical research, recommended treatments and drug therapies undergo changes. The author(s) and publisher have done everything possible to make this book accurate, up to date, and in accord with accepted standards at the time of publication. The authors, editors, and publisher are not responsible for errors or omissions or for consequences from application of the book, and make no warranty, expressed or implied, in regard to the contents of the book. Any practice described in this book should be applied by the reader in accordance with professional standards of care used in regard to the unique circumstances that may apply in each situation. The reader is advised always to check product information (package inserts) for changes and new information regarding dose and contraindications before administering any drug. Caution is especially urged when using new or infrequently ordered drugs.

Library of Congress Cataloging in Publication Data
Davis's NCLEX-RN review/[edited by] Patricia Gauntlett Beare.—3rd ed.
    p.;cm
    Includes bibliographical references and index.
    ISBN 0-8036-0577-3 (pbk.:alk. paper)
    1. Nursing—Examinations, questions, etc. 2. Nursing—Outlines, syllabi, etc.
    [DNLM: 1. Nursing—Examination Questions. 2. Nursing—Outlines. 3. Licensure, Nursing—
Examination Questions. 4. Licensure, Nursing—Outlines. WY 18.2 D265 2001] I. Title: NCLEX-
RN review. II. Beare, Patricia Gauntlett.
RT55.D38 2001
610.73'076—dc21

00-031473

FOREWORD TO THE CANDIDATE FOR REGISTERED NURSE LICENSURE

As you begin to study for the National Council Licensing Examination (NCLEX), remember that *you are a winner*. You have succeeded in learning the content and skills necessary for you to graduate from your nursing program. Your teachers believe you will practice safe, competent nursing. Now you must review the essential content to successfully pass the examination that will enable you to practice as a registered nurse.

Experts in nursing have identified the essentials for nursing practice and presented them to you in outline form in this text. Practice tests have been formulated by nurse/teachers from diploma, associate degree, baccalaureate degree, and nursing service programs to help you apply your nursing knowledge through simulated clinical practice test questions.

All that remains is for you to set up a study schedule to thoroughly review this content and take the practice tests. The practice tests will provide rationale and answers to help you "think through" the underlying principles behind the right answer. Your study skills should serve as the basis for your review. As you review, you will develop the confidence in your nursing skills and decrease your fears of not passing this examination.

Remember, you are a winner! You will pass this test!

Patricia Gauntlett Beare, RN, PhD

PREFACE

The purpose of this book is to provide the candidate for registered nurse licensure with a concise review of the information needed to pass the NCLEX-RN licensing exam and with the opportunity to apply this information in answering test questions that simulate clinical situations. Since the publication of the first edition, the NCLEX-RN has been converted to an electronic exam employing computer-adaptive testing (CAT). To help the candidate become familiar and comfortable with this new testing scheme, this third edition includes a computer practice disk with more than 652 questions not found in the book. This disk helps the student simulate the NCLEX-RN CAT testing environment, and its scoresheet functions provide valuable feedback that allows the student to target study to specific subject areas.

The book's first unit explains the NCLEX-RN test process, offers tips on how to study for the exam, and provides additional knowledge and application of content through critical thinking when answering test questions. The five chapters in Unit II address, respectively, maternity, pediatric, medical-surgical, gerontological, and psychiatric nursing. The content reviews in these chapters are written by noted experts in each subject area, several of whom are the authors of major textbooks in the field. In addition to content reviews, each of these chapters also contains test questions in the subject area. Unit III includes a content review and test on nursing leadership and management, subjects getting increased coverage on the NCLEX, as well as tests on growth and development, nutrition, and calculation of dosages. Unit IV consists of 11 integrated practice tests that, like the NCLEX itself, combine all the subject areas into each test. These tests are written by nurse clinicians and educators who have previously written test questions for the NCLEX and who represent schools or hospitals throughout the United States. Finally, two appendices provide a list of abbreviations commonly used in nursing practice and contact information for state boards of nursing. With 1731 test questions in the book, and another 652 on the enclosed practice disk, the third edition offers more than 2300 test questions in addition to comprehensive, outline-style content reviews of the core subject areas in nursing. The addition of a management chapter and test questions to the text as well as to the disk helps students apply this new content to the clinical area.

All test questions, in both the book and the disk, are coded according to the NCLEX test plan for the subject area and client needs category that they address. Rationales are provided for both correct and incorrect answer choices to help the student learn not just the right answer but *why* it is the right answer.

The content presented in this book will enable the NCLEX-RN candidate to review essential nursing knowledge and apply this knowledge to test questions in the examination.

Through careful study, candidates will no longer fear the unknown as they review and master the knowledge, skills, and abilities to be successful in passing the examination and embarking on their careers as registered nurses.

ACKNOWLEDGMENTS

Many people, too numerous to mention, have helped make this third edition a reality.

To Alan Sorkowitz, Nursing Editor at F. A. Davis, who supervised the production of the text, special thanks for his patience.

To the many special contributors, who shared their expertise and generated many new ideas for student preparation for the NCLEX-RN licensure examination.

To Sam Rondinelli, Production Manager, who adroitly guided this book through the production process, special thanks and gratitude.

To the reviewers who, through their constructive critiques, greatly enhanced the quality of this unique NCLEX-RN review book.

A very special acknowledgment to all our students, personal friends, and colleagues for their support.

CONTRIBUTORS

Carol G. Allen, RN, MSN
Associate Professor and Associate Director for
  Undergraduate Studies in Nursing
Northwestern State University of Louisiana
Shreveport, Louisiana

Ola Burns Allen, RNC, DNSc
Professor and Associate Dean for Academic Affairs
University of Mississippi Medical Center
School of Nursing
Jackson, Mississippi

Claudia P. Barone, RN, MSN
Professor and Associate Dean for Academic Affairs
Instructor of Adult Health Nursing
University of Arkansas for Medical Sciences
Little Rock, Arkansas

Linda Bass, RN, PhD
Assistant Professor
Texas Tech University Health Sciences Center
Lubbock, Texas

Cecily Betz, PhD, RN
University of California–Los Angeles
Los Angeles, California

Billie E. Bitowski, RN, MSN
Associate Professor
Northwestern State University of Louisiana
Shreveport, Louisiana

Carolyn Elston Bond, RN, MSN
Assistant Professor
Northwestern State University of Louisiana
Shreveport, Louisiana

Mollie K. Bradley, RN, EdD
Assistant Professor
University of South Alabama
College of Nursing
Mobile, Alabama

Linda Calhoun, RN, MNSc, NNP
Clinical Instructor
University of Arkansas for Medical Sciences
Little Rock, Arkansas

Barbara Camune, RN, MSN
University of Texas Medical Branch
Galveston, Texas

Lizabeth L. Carlson, MSN, RNC, DNSc
Assistant Professor
Delta State College of Nursing
Cleveland, Mississippi

Robin Webb Corbett, RNC, MSN
Clinical Assistant Professor
Department of Parent Child Nursing
East Carolina University
School of Nursing
Greenville, North Carolina

Sharon Pierce Corbin, RN, MS
Professor
Harford Community College
New Freedom, Pennsylvania

Sharon Decker, RN, CS, MSN, CCRN
Associate Professor of Clinical Nursing
Director of Clinical Simulation
Texas Tech University Health Sciences Center
Lubbock, Texas

Lou Everett, RN, EdD
Associate Professor
Department of Community and Mental Health
  Nursing and Nursing Services Administration
East Carolina University
Greenville, North Carolina

Carol Farley-Toombs, MS, RN, CS
University of Rochester
College of Nursing
Rochester, New York

Nazie Sue L. Fontenot, MSN, CNS
Assistant Professor
McNeese State University
College of Nursing
Lake Charles, Louisiana

Diane B. Graham, RN, MSN
Associate Director of Non-Traditional Programs in Nursing
Northwestern State University of Louisiana
Shreveport, Louisiana

Diane B. Hamilton, PhD, RN
Professor
Western Michigan University
School of Nursing
Kalamazoo, Michigan

Marie L. Hart, RNC, MSN, PhD
Instructor
Texas Tech University Health Sciences Center
Lubbock, Texas

Loretta C. Henry, MS, BS
Assistant Professor
McNeese State University
College of Nursing
Lake Charles, Louisiana

Ellen Holmgren, RN, MSN
Joliet Junior College–Nursing Education
Joliet, Illinois

Judith M. Kachel, EdD, RN
Nursing Instructor
Joliet Junior College–Nursing Education
Joliet, Illinois

Eileen Keefe, RN, MSN, C
Louisiana State University
New Orleans, Louisiana

Colleen Kestel-Branchaw, RN, MSN
Joliet Junior College–Nursing Education
Joliet, Illinois

Christine Krol, RN, MSN
Nursing Instructor
Joliet Junior College–Nursing Education
Joliet, Illinois

Dottie W. Kubricht, RN, MN
Southeastern Louisiana University
Hammond, Louisiana

JoAnn Langford, RN, MSN
Delgado Community College
Charity School of Nursing
New Orleans, Louisiana

Pauline S. Lea, RN, MN, CS
Baton Rouge General Medical Center
School of Nursing
Baton Rouge, Louisiana

Bonnie Juvé Meeker, DNS, RN
Southeastern Louisiana University
Hammond, Louisiana

Mary Alice Middlebrooks, RN, MSN
Assistant Professor in Nursing
Northwestern State University of Louisiana
Shreveport, Louisiana

Tommie L. Norris, RN, DNSc
Assistant Professor
University of Memphis
Memphis, Tennessee

Benni Ogden, RN, MSE
Assistant Professor
University of Arkansas for Medical Sciences
Little Rock, Arkansas

Sally B. Olds, MSN, RNC
Associate Professor
Chair, Department of Holistic Nursing
Beth El College of Nursing
Colorado Springs, Colorado

Louise Plaisance, RN, C, DNS
Our Lady of the Lake
Baton Rouge, Louisiana

Demetrius J. Porsche, RN, CCRN, DNS
Associate Professor
LSUMC School of Nursing
New Orleans, Louisiana

Susan K. Pryor, RN, MN, DNS
Faculty
Southeastern Louisiana University
Hammond, Louisiana

Helen Ptak, PhD, RN
Professor
University of Mississippi at Hattiesburg
Hattiesburg, Mississippi

Donita T. Qualey, RN, MN
Delgado Community College
Charity School of Nursing
New Orleans, Louisiana

Lona Ratcliffe, RN, MN
Associate Professor
Department of Parent Child Nursing
East Carolina University
Greenville, North Carolina

Gloria Rauch, RN, MSN
Professor
University of Arkansas for Medical Sciences
Little Rock, Arkansas

Susan Ray, MSN, DNSc
Louisiana State University
School of Nursing
New Orleans, Louisiana

M. Evonne Robinson, RN, MN
Assistant Professor
Department of Nursing
Nicholls State University
Thibodaux, Louisiana

Virginia Kay Rogers, RN, C, MS, MED
Doctoral Student
LSUMC
New Orleans, Louisiana

Jacqueline Schexnayder, RN, MN
Delgado Community College
Charity School of Nursing
New Orleans, Louisiana

Kara Schmitt, PhD
Director of Testing Services
Department of Licensing and Regulation
Lansing, Michigan

Sandra S. Swick, RNC, MSN
Assistant Professor of Nursing
Texas Tech University Health Sciences Center
Lubbock, Texas

Lee Ann Thomas, RN, MN
Baton Rouge General Medical Center
School of Nursing
Baton Rouge, Louisiana

Patricia E. Thompson, EdD, RN
Associate Professor
Parent-Child Department Chair
College of Nursing
University of Arkansas for Medical Sciences
Little Rock, Arkansas

Golden Tradewell, MSN, RN
Associate Professor
McNeese State University
College of Nursing
Lake Charles, Louisiana

Janetta Tradup, RN, CS, MSN
Associate Professor of Nursing
Texas Tech University Health Sciences Center
Lubbock, Texas

Doris Tucker, RN, EdD
Instructor
University of Arkansas for Medical Sciences
Little Rock, Arkansas

Kathy A. Viator, RN, MSN, DNS
Southeastern Louisiana University
University Station Box 781
Hammond, Louisiana

Ann T. Warner, MS, BSN
Instructor
McNeese State University
College of Nursing
Lake Charles, Louisiana

Lucille F. Whaley, EdD, RN
Specialist, Parent Child Nursing
Sunnyvale, California

Susan Williams, RN, DNS
Assistant Professor
East Carolina University
Greenville, North Carolina

Emily Zabrocki, RN, PhD
Faculty
Joliet Junior Collete–Nursing Education
Joliet, Illinois

Consultants

Carolyn Mosley, RN, PhD
Associate Professor
Department Chair
Louisiana State University
New Orleans, Louisiana

Patricia E. Thompson, EdD, RN
Associate Professor
Interim Associate Dean for Service
University of Arkansas for Medical Sciences
Little Rock, Arkansas

Golden Tradewell, MSN, RN
Associate Professor
McNeese State University
College of Nursing
Lake Charles, Louisiana

CONTENTS

APPENDICES 663

UNIT I

What You Need to Know About the NCLEX-RN

CHAPTER 1

Development, Administration, and Scoring of the NCLEX-RN™*

Kara Schmitt, PhD

The National Council Licensure Examination for Registered Nurses (NCLEX-RN), developed by the National Council of State Boards of Nursing (NCSBN), is designed to measure a licensing candidate's knowledge of the nursing process and client health needs considered necessary for public protection. Using the test plan, each examination reflects the knowledge, skills, and abilities essential to meet the needs of clients with commonly occurring health problems. The examination is used to determine whether a candidate can appropriately react and respond to various problems commonly associated with a registered nurse's (RN's) responsibilities in typical clinical settings. The examination content is structured in such a manner that jurisdictional Boards of Nursing can be reasonably assured that individuals who pass the examination are minimally competent to practice entry-level RN nursing and to protect the health, safety, and welfare of its citizens.

Applying to Take the NCLEX-RN

In April 1994, RN licensure candidates began taking the NCLEX-RN on computers at many conveniently located sites throughout the United States and its territories. In order to sit for the examination, you, as an RN candidate, need to submit certain documentation and fees to both the Board of Nursing in the jurisdiction in which you wish to be licensed and to The Chauncey Group International, Ltd. (Chauncey). Generally, two separate submissions of documents and fees are required, although some jurisdictions may ask that both the licensure application and fee and the examination application and fee be sent directly to them.

The Board of Nursing in which you wish to be licensed requires a licensure application along with verification of educa-

tion such as a certificate of completion or an official transcript from an approved school of nursing. Depending on the jurisdiction, you may also have to submit a licensure fee, application fee, and/or temporary license fee. All relevant documents and fees must be submitted to the appropriate Board office before you will be allowed to take the examination.

Because each jurisdiction has different requirements, it is essential that you be thoroughly familiar with the specifications associated with the jurisdiction in which you wish to be licensed. In most instances, faculty from the nursing program that you attended can instruct you as to the necessary forms and fees to submit. Typically, your program also has the necessary licensure and examination applications for you to complete. If your program does not furnish you with these instructions and forms, or if you wish to be licensed in a jurisdiction other than the one in which you received your education, it is your responsibility to contact the specific Board office for these forms and/or information, including the NCLEX™ Candidate Bulletin. Appendix B includes a listing of all Boards, their addresses, and phone numbers. It is essential that you complete the licensure application accurately, enclose the correct fee, and ensure that all additional documentation is forwarded to the Board as soon as possible. Remember, you will not be allowed to take the examination until the appropriate Board has determined that you are eligible.

Candidates with a physical disability should contact the licensing jurisdiction as early as possible to arrange for special accommodations. Information will be provided as to how to request the required accommodations as well as what type of documentation is necessary to initiate the process.

Foreign-educated candidates should recognize that additional documentation of education and proof of English-language competency may be required when submitting the licensure application. For this reason, if you were educated outside of the United States, you should contact the appropriate Board to ascertain what specific documentation and/or

---

examination results are required. In addition, you may want to contact the Commission on Graduates of Foreign Nursing Schools (CGFNS) for various requirements that you may have to fulfill. The address and phone number for CGFNS is:

Commission on Graduates of Foreign Nursing Schools
3624 Market Street
Philadelphia, PA 19104
(215) 349-8767

In addition to applying for a license, you need to apply to sit for the examination either through Chauncey or through the jurisdiction in which you wish to be licensed. Examination applications can be obtained through your school of nursing or the desired licensing jurisdiction. The examination application, along with the fee of $88, may be submitted to Chauncey at any time, even before completing your education or being deemed eligible to take the test.

If you have a credit card, you can call Chauncey using their toll-free number (1-800-551-1912, Monday through Friday, 8:00 AM–8:00 PM Eastern Time) to register for the examination. An additional fee ($9.25) is charged for this service. If you wish to phone in your registration, you will be asked for your credit card number, its expiration date, and the exact name that appears on your card, in addition to the examination application information. The money placed on credit card registration is not refundable.

Once the jurisdiction in which you wish to be licensed has determined your eligibility and communicates this to Chauncey, you are sent an *Authorization to Test*. This document is required to schedule an appointment and must be presented at the test site in order for you to take the exam. As soon as you receive this document, verify that the spelling of your name is correct and that it matches exactly the name included on the official signed photographic identification you will be using for admission to the examination. If the two names do not match, call Chauncey immediately. If your *Authorization to Test* and identification do not match, you may be denied admission to the examination.

Scheduling an Appointment

Once you receive the *Authorization to Test,* you may call any of the Sylvan Prometric (Sylvan) Technology Centers where you wish to be tested or the Sylvan toll-free number (1-800-800-1123) to schedule an appointment. Be sure to have your *Authorization to Test* available when you call because you will be asked for your authorization number, identification number, and expiration date for testing (determined by the appropriate Board of Nursing), as well as your name and phone number. Sylvan personnel will verify your name and address as shown in the computer.

If you are a first-time candidate, you will be scheduled within 30 days of calling, if you desire. If you are a repeat candidate, you will be scheduled within 45 days, if you desire. You do not need to call for an appointment as soon as you receive the *Authorization to Test*. Even if you do call immediately, you do not need to schedule an appointment within the 30 or 45 days. You may schedule your examination appointment at a time convenient for you, but you **must** schedule an appointment before the expiration date shown on the *Authorization to Test.*

Because you have the opportunity to make a specific appointment, be sure to select a time that is convenient for you.

Do not schedule your test at the same time as another critical event. Schedule the examination when you will be able to devote 100% of your mental energies to the examination. If, however, you have scheduled your examination and later learn that it will not be convenient, you can reschedule the appointment by calling the Sylvan Technology Center where you are scheduled or the central toll-free number at least 3 days before the appointment date. You will first have to cancel the original appointment and then make another one.

Once you have called for an appointment, be sure to write the location, date, and time somewhere so that you will remember the information. You will also be given directions for finding the site. You might want to put all of this on your *Authorization to Test* because you will need to bring it with you to the examination.

If you lose your *Authorization to Test*, call Chauncey to request another. If you discover it missing immediately before your examination, you should still call Chauncey so that the Sylvan Center can be alerted that you do not have the document. You will probably still be allowed to test provided you have sufficient identification.

Basis for the Examination Content

The purpose of the NCLEX-RN is to help Boards of Nursing determine whether licensure candidates are *minimally competent* to practice entry-level nursing, thus protecting the public. In order to accomplish this purpose, it is necessary for the NCSBN to know what an entering nurse actually does *on the job*. Once this is known (based on a job analysis), an accurate evaluation instrument (examination) can be created to measure a candidate's knowledge, skills, and abilities relative to these activities.

The primary purpose of a job analysis is to ascertain the frequency with which certain tasks are performed by entering nurses, as well as the criticality of these tasks (i.e., which tasks, if performed incorrectly, could do serious or critical harm to the patient). Some tasks, such as performing cardiopulmonary resuscitation, may not be done on a regular or daily basis; however, if they are not done immediately and correctly, the patient could die. Although it is important to know both the frequency of performance and the criticality of incorrect performance, the criticality is the more important factor. Accordingly, the criticality of a task is given greater weight in the development of a test plan.

The July 1988 NCLEX-RN was the first administration of the examination using the results of a job analysis completed in 1986. Since then, a new job analysis has been conducted every three years to ensure that the examination reflects tasks performed on the job. The most recent job analysis was completed in 1996.

Examination Content (Test Plan)

The examination is not designed to merely measure your ability to recall or recognize certain facts. Its primary purpose is to assess how well you can apply the facts learned in school to common nursing situations. Accordingly, most items in the examination relate to your ability to (1) apply information or knowledge acquired in one situation and correctly transfer that knowledge to a similar situation; or (2) analyze a complex relationship by breaking it into simpler components, making comparisons, or identifying the relationships between or among certain pieces of information. Remember, the examination is designed to measure how well you will respond in typical, real-life clinical settings. The examination content is based on the following premise:

> Upon entry into nursing practice, the registered nurse is expected to care for the client and/or to assist the client's significant others in the provision of care. The registered nurse is expected to identify the health needs and/or problems of clients throughout their life cycle and in a variety of settings, to plan and to initiate appropriate action based upon nursing diagnoses derived from these assessments, and to evaluate the extent to which expected outcomes of the plan of care are achieved.[1]

Based on this premise, and the results of the job analysis, the test plan[2] (specifications for constructing each form of the examination) consists of four categories of **client needs** that are further subdivided to define the content associated with each client need. The percentage of questions allocated to each client need subcategory is shown in Table 1–1.

A safe, effective care environment is achieved by (1) providing integrated, cost-effective care to clients by coordinating, supervising, and/or collaborating with members of the multidisciplinary health care team; and (2) protecting clients and health care personnel from environmental hazards.

Health promotion and maintenance of the client is obtained by (3) assisting the client and significant others through the normal expected stages of growth and development from conception through advanced age; and (4) managing and providing care for clients in need of prevention and early detection of health problems.

Psychosocial integrity is achieved by (5) promoting the client's ability to cope with, adapt to, and/or problem solve situations related to illnesses or stressful events; and (6) managing and providing care for clients with acute or chronic mental illnesses.

Physiological integrity focuses on (7) providing comfort and assistance in the performance of activities of daily living; (8) managing and providing care related to the administration of medications and parenteral therapies; (9) reducing the likelihood that clients will develop complications or health problems related to existing conditions, treatments or procedures;

and (10) managing and providing care to clients with acute, chronic, or life-threatening physical health conditions.

Computerized Adaptive Testing

In April 1994, the NCLEX-RN examination underwent a significant change by converting from a paper-and-pencil administered test to a computerized adaptive test (CAT). Since then, the examination has been administered by computer at a convenient location on a day convenient for the candidate with only a small number of candidates being tested at the same time. Results are available to the candidate's licensure jurisdiction within 48 hours of taking the test.

With CAT, there is still a maximum amount of time allowed (5 hours) and a maximum number of items presented (265), but each candidate receives an examination that is tailor-made to fit the ability level of that individual. It is very unlikely that any two candidates would receive exactly the same set of items, as no two candidates have exactly the same ability. The selection of items presented, as well as the number of items, is based on how well a candidate answers the preceding items (a determination of his or her ability).

A *minimum* of 75 items, of which 15 are experimental items (unscored items used solely to determine how well they work and their difficulty) are presented. Because the experimental items are not identified, candidates should answer *all* items as if they were scored. The *maximum* number of items presented is 265, including the 15 experimental items. The number of items presented does not, however, automatically indicate whether a candidate has passed or failed.

All items have a known difficulty level; that is, an item is either easy or difficult for the candidate population to answer correctly. This information is obtained by analyzing the experimental items given to a large number of candidates. If every candidate answers an item correctly, it would be considered easy. If only a few candidates answer an item correctly, it would be considered difficult.

At the start of the examination, you will be presented with an item that has a low or moderate difficulty level. If you answer the item correctly, you will be given a slightly more difficult item. If you answer the initial item incorrectly, you will

Table 1–1. NCLEX-RN Test Plan	
Categories	Percentage of Test Questions
A. Safe, Effective Care Environment	
1. Management of Care	7–13
2. Safety and Infection Control	5–11
B. Health Promotion and Maintenance	
3. Growth and Development Through the Life Span	7–13
4. Prevention and Early Detection of Disease	5–11
C. Physosocial Integrity	
5. Coping and Adaptation	5–11
6. Psychosocial Adaptation	5–11
D. Physiological Integrity	
7. Basic Care and Comfort	7–13
8. Pharmacological and Parenteral Therapies	5–11
9. Reduction of Risk Potential	12–18
10. Physiological Adaptation	12–18

be given a slightly easier item. The computer continues selecting items based on how well you responded to previous items. If you miss an item, the next item will be slightly easier. If you answer the next item correctly, the following item will be slightly more difficult. Throughout the examination, you will be presented with items that are targeted to your ability level; they will be neither too easy nor too difficult for *you*. The computer is programmed to stop presenting items when one of the following conditions has occurred:

1. Your measure of competence is known to be *above* or *below* the passing standard and at least 75 items have been answered
2. You have taken the maximum number of items (265)
3. You have tested for the maximum number of hours (5)

Before the computer stops the test, all candidates are presented with a sufficient number of items covering the test plan to determine accurately whether they possess the necessary knowledge, skills, and abilities to practice competently. Regardless of your level of competence, you will be tested on *every* aspect of the test plan.

Passing Standard

The minimum passing level was determined by the National Council's Board of Directors, based on input from a panel of nurses who evaluated a typical examination. The panel was instructed thoroughly in the definition of "minimally competent" and what this term means in real life. After there was consensus as to the meaning of this term, the members were asked to individually evaluate each item in terms of "the percentage of 100 minimally competent RN candidates who would answer the item correctly." If an item was considered relatively easy, a greater percentage of candidates would be likely to answer the item correctly. If an item was considered more difficult, a smaller percentage of candidates would answer the item correctly. Individual decision making was done for each of the items presented. Based on the statistical data and definition of minimal competence, a passing score could be established. With this methodology, there is no percentage of items that must be answered correctly, nor is there a predetermined percentage of candidates who will pass.

Item Format

The examination consists of a number of multiple-choice items involving a clinical setting (situation) on which a question is based, or an individual statement or question relating to a client and/or family members. Following each situation or introductory statement, you are required to select which of four choices *best* responds to the question being asked. Because the examination is designed to measure an individual's competence to practice safely in the work setting, the items generally relate to various "real-life" situations in which nursing intervention and decision making are required. Although you must possess basic nursing knowledge (i.e., facts about the human body and the way it operates), the primary focus is on whether you are able to correctly apply these concepts in a variety of typical clinical settings.

Each item includes an introductory statement, problem or question (*stem*) to which the candidate must respond. Following the stem are four choices (*options*). Only one of these options is correct (*key*); the other three are known as *distractors*.

Distractors are created in such a way that they may seem correct to someone who is unfamiliar with or uncertain about nursing terminology, procedures, or general practice. The items are not designed to "trick" candidates. Rather, they are constructed in such a manner that it is possible to discriminate between candidates who are minimally competent (qualified to enter the profession) and those who are not.

Examination Administration

The following points highlight what you should expect on your test day:

1. Try to arrive at the site one half hour before your appointment so that you will have ample time to check in.
2. Bring your *Authorization to Test* and two pieces of identification, one of which must be an official identification that includes your photograph and signature. The name on this identification MUST MATCH the name on your *Authorization to Test*. If it doesn't, you may not be permitted to test.
3. Once your identification has been confirmed, you will be asked to sign a log book, provide a thumbprint, and be photographed.
4. At this time, you will be given basic instructions regarding the computer operation and administration procedures. If you have any questions regarding the information, be sure to ask for clarification.
5. Before entering the testing room, you will be required to place *all* of your personal belongings in a locker and will be given a key to the locker. The lockers are small, so do not bring anything large into the center. The *only* item that you can bring into the testing room is your primary piece of identification.
6. You will be shown to a pre-assigned computer. Before you begin testing, you and the test administrator will confirm that the photograph that appears on the computer screen is the one taken during sign-in and that it is a photo of yourself.
7. During the examination, you will be monitored by the test administrator and a videotape will be made of everyone in the testing room. An audio monitor inside the room will permit the administrator to hear any noise being made by those being tested.
8. If you have any questions during the examination or if you wish to take an unscheduled break, raise your hand and the test administrator will assist you.
9. Before the actual examination, you will be given a practice test so that you can be familiar with the two keys that are needed to answer an item.
10. Based on each response given, the computer will select the next appropriate item for you. Because the correctness of each answer that you select determines the difficulty of the next item, you will not be allowed to return to a previously shown item, nor will you be able to skip an item. You must respond to every item presented and then go on to the next item. The computer will stop automatically when (1) a decision regarding your competency can be made and you have answered the minimum number of items, (2) the maximum number of items have been delivered, or (3) the maximum testing time has occurred.

11. Each item presented, as well as your response, is stored immediately. Therefore, if your computer stops working for any reason (e.g., a power failure), when it is restarted you will be able to resume testing at exactly the same place.
12. After 2 hours, the computer will stop automatically and you will be required to take a 10-minute break. You must leave the testing room, but you do not have to leave the Sylvan area. After 10 minutes, you can resume testing. An hour and a half later, you will be permitted to take an optional break. Any breaks taken, other than the mandatory break, will count against your total testing time.
13. Neither the number of items you answer nor the amount of time you spend testing is indicative of your pass/fail status.
14. Immediately following the conclusion of your examination, your responses are transmitted to a central location for processing. Within 48 hours, your results are electronically transmitted to the jurisdiction in which you wish to be licensed. A paper copy of your results is also mailed to that jurisdiction.

Examination Results

Each jurisdiction must complete its own processing of the results. In general, you should receive your results 2–3 weeks following the examination.

Candidates who pass the examination will receive a notification of pass; no score will be provided. Depending on the jurisdiction's procedures, you may or may not receive your license with your test results.

Candidates who do not pass the examination will receive a notice of fail. No numeric score will be provided. You will, however, be sent a Diagnostic Profile that shows your personal areas of strength and weakness on the NCLEX test. You should use the information provided to help you prepare for the reexamination.

A failing notice will also include information on how often you can repeat the examination and how soon you can reapply for a re-examination. The NCSBN has established a retake policy of no more than four administrations per year and no more frequently than once in any 3 months. Jurisdictions have the authority to impose other restrictions provided that their retake policy is no more lenient than the one established by the NCSBN.

You cannot overcome these restrictions by applying to another state for licensure, changing your name, or applying to take the examination in another state. The computerized registration system continues to track candidates after they have first applied to take the examination. Once you register, you are assigned a permanent, unique identification number that is used every time you apply to take the examination.

Examination Review

If you fail the examination, you can request an examination review, but hand scoring will not be available. The reason is that there is nothing to hand score. The answers you selected were automatically entered and stored in the computer. Accordingly, there is no possibility that your answers were "misread."

An examination review is feasible because the exact items presented to you, along with your responses, were retained by the computer. If you wish to review your test and your licensing jurisdiction permits it, you will need to submit a written request and fee to the jurisdiction. Once your request is approved, your test and answers will be transmitted to the Sylvan Technology Center chosen by the jurisdiction. This location may not necessarily be the one in which you took the examination. Although you can take the examination outside of the licensing jurisdiction, you will be required to review the examination within the licensing jurisdiction at the specified site.

You will be shown only the items you answered incorrectly. The answer you selected as well as the correct answer will be presented. If you wish to challenge an item, you will be asked to prepare documentation as to why you should be given credit for the item.

In all of the years that the NCLEX-RN has been administered, there have been very few challenges to the examination items, and none of the challenges has resulted in a score change. The reason for this is that before including an item on an examination, it has been reviewed numerous times by many individuals involved in the nursing profession, and has been included in an examination as a try-out item so that adequate statistics have been obtained. All items have been scrutinized thoroughly before they are actually presented to candidates and scored.

Summary

Although CAT may be a new experience for you, you should not be unduly worried or anxious about the format of the examination. It is still a multiple-choice test. The main differences are that the items are displayed on a computer screen instead of on paper and you use two computer keys instead of a pencil. These are minor differences compared with the many advantages associated with CAT:

1. Quicker administration of the examination after you have been determined eligible by the licensing jurisdiction
2. Taking the examination whenever and wherever you want
3. Taking the examination in pleasant, uncrowded conditions
4. Answering 265 or fewer items
5. Completing the examination in 5 hours or less
6. Receiving results in less time
7. Being able to start work as a licensed RN sooner

REFERENCES

1. National Council of State Boards of Nursing: Test Plan for the National Council of Licensure Examination for Registered Nurses. National Council of State Boards of Nursing, Chicago, 1989.
2. Steele, Donna and Wendt, Anne: National Council Detailed Test Plan for the NCLEX-RN® Examination. National Council of State Boards of Nursing, Chicago, 1997.

CHAPTER 2

Preparing for and Taking the NCLEX-RN

Kara Schmitt, PhD
Bonnie Juvé Meeker, DNS, RN

Performing well on exams is important in our society, and even as young children we learn that high scores on school exams denote success and lead to confidence and rewards. As you know, the most challenging exam you will face after graduating from nursing school is the National Council Licensing Examination (NCLEX-RN). If you succeed in passing this exam, you will be licensed to practice nursing.

While preparing for and taking the NCLEX-RN, you must constantly remember that you have the ability to pass the examination. Although the manner in which you will be responding to items may be different (computer instead of paper and pencil), and there may be more items than included in previous tests, the examination is still just an examination. As you study for the examination, remember that *confidence, like success, is a result of hard work and preparation.* In order to do well, you must be both psychologically and intellectually prepared.

Test Anxiety

Although stress and anxiety do *not* have exactly the same definition, these terms are used interchangeably in this chapter. Stress and anxiety are normal reactions to preparing for and taking a major test like the NCLEX-RN. If you ask friends who have already passed the examination if they were anxious before and during the examination, they will certainly say "Yes!" In fact, some amount of anxiety is actually *good* and has been found to improve test-taking ability. On the other hand, uncontrollable anxiety will hurt your ability to do well. It has been said that stress is "the spice of life or the kiss of death—depending on how we cope with it."[1] By learning how to recognize and deal with stress effectively, you can use it to your advantage.

The ability to recognize and respond to stress or anxiety varies from person to person. No single method will work for everyone; therefore, this chapter is intended merely to give you some methods you might use to reduce seemingly uncontrollable and incapacitating stress.

The best way to deal with stress is to take specific steps to cope with the stress-producing situation and to reduce stress. Proper study behavior and thorough preparation are the best ways to reduce the stress experienced before and during an examination.

An inappropriate approach, which in the end will increase the stress, is to deny the importance of the task (examination) that you must accomplish. Statements such as "The exam is filled with trick questions anyway, so why bother studying" or "If I don't do well, it means I just wasn't lucky" are inappropriate and will not help you. Instead, you need to concentrate your efforts on proper studying and positive thinking.

Some of the characteristics frequently associated with test anxiety include:

1. Feeling insecure about your performance
2. Worrying a great deal about things not under your control
3. Thinking about how much brighter or better others are
4. Thinking about what will happen if you fail
5. Feeling that you are not as prepared as you could or should be (assuming that you really did prepare)
6. Worrying about not having enough time to finish the test
7. Feeling that you will be letting yourself and others down
8. Feeling that you could and should have done better.[2]

These eight feelings can be categorized into four major symptoms of anxiety,[3] which can and must be handled in order to overcome the anxiety-producing situation. Each of these four symptoms is discussed briefly.

Anxiety-Producing Mental Activities. Worrying about nonspecific problems or situations and fretting over everything that could go wrong are associated with this symptom.

Self-criticism, self-blame, and general negative self-talk lead to low self-confidence and disorganized problem solving. Telling yourself that you cannot do something or that you are stupid will lead to failure. Another trait associated with this symptom is false thinking about yourself and the world around you—the "Everyone is so much better than I am" syndrome.

Misdirected Attention. Instead of focusing on the task at hand, such as studying for or taking an examination, you focus on internal and external distractors. These could include watching other people study, looking at the clock, or daydreaming. If you focus on the wrong thing, you will be less efficient and more likely to become emotionally upset.

Physiological Distress. When you are anxious, your body reacts both physiologically and psychologically. Some of the physiological symptoms include sweating, increased heart rate, nervous stomach, or headache. If you focus on the physiological symptoms to a significant degree, you will be less able to focus on your studies or the examination.

Inappropriate Behavior. This symptom is exhibited by avoiding the task that needs to be done (procrastination), by withdrawing prematurely from the task, or by doing something else when you should be focusing on the task at hand (for example, talking to your neighbor instead of studying). Other aspects of inappropriate behavior include rushing through the examination or study material without focusing on the information or, at the opposite extreme, being excessively compulsive and rereading everything more than is necessary. A final element is trying to push yourself to keep going when you are tense rather than taking the time to relax.

In order to reduce stress to a manageable level, you need to determine what symptoms or behaviors you are exhibiting. One way to learn more about your individual expression of stress is to find a comfortable, relaxing environment; close your eyes; and really imagine and concentrate on how you feel or what you do when you study. How are you going to feel when it is 1 week before the examination? When it is 1 day before the examination? When it is the day of the examination? When you are sitting at the computer taking the examination? Try to think carefully about these events and how you will really feel. If you are honest in the evaluation of these situations and your feelings, you will be better equipped to change the way you handle stress.

Another way to learn more about your own coping ability is to reflect on and make note of what you actually do while studying. Do you watch other people? Do you daydream? Do you begin worrying about the test? Do you stop studying because you think it will do no good? You will probably need to keep a log of your behaviors following several study periods in order to obtain an accurate picture of your behaviors.

After you have recorded all of your distractors, make a list of what you can do to reduce your level of anxiety. For instance, telling yourself that you can never learn the material is self-defeating. Instead, remind yourself that you learned the material in the past and did well in school. After all, you are ready to graduate or have graduated, so you must have learned what was necessary to reach this stage in your pursuit of a nursing career.

Another aid to learning more about yourself and your reaction to stress is to respond "true" or "false" to each of the following statements in terms of what you do or how you respond during periods of stress.

True or False

1. I constantly bite my nails, fidget with my hair, tap my fingers, or perform other similar behaviors.
2. I smoke or drink more frequently.
3. I tend to eat more or eat less, or I eat less healthy foods.
4. I avoid doing what I should be doing.
5. I feel like there is too much to do in too short a time.
6. I worry about everything—the examination, my health, my family, my work, etc.
7. I seem to have more physical or health-related problems.
8. I become irritated or lose my temper more quickly over trivial matters.
9. I seem to have less energy and seem to want to sleep more.
10. I have trouble falling asleep or sleeping for my normal amount of time.
11. I am more critical of myself or think of myself as worthless.
12. I seem to forget more day-to-day activities or responsibilities, such as forgetting to get groceries, forgetting an appointment, or forgetting to return a phone call.
13. I have trouble relaxing and enjoying myself even when at a social event or with people I like.
14. I tend to daydream more.

Items 1 through 3 may be viewed as bad habits, which simply become more prevalent during times of stress or anxiety. The key to deciding whether these three behaviors are detrimental to successful completion of the required task is to determine whether you are doing them more than usual during times of stress. If you answered "true," they could be negatively influencing your effectiveness in preparing for and taking the examination. At the same time, if you try to become "perfect" and eliminate normal bad habits during a stressful situation, you may actually increase your level of stress. It is not necessary for you to eliminate all bad habits at this time, but you should keep them under control.

Items 4 through 14 focus on symptoms of anxiety. If you responded "true" to most of these items, it is time for you to reevaluate your thoughts about yourself and the future examination. You need to focus less on what is going on around you or inside you and more on understanding and solving the problem that is causing the anxiety. Begin to view the examination as a problem to be solved or a challenge you must meet. Do not view it as something that is a punishment or a catastrophic event.

Begin to view the test realistically. It is not a measure of your self-worth, your ability to be successful, or your future happiness. It is merely a single measure of what you know.

Develop a positive attitude toward the test. Eliminate the negative thoughts and feelings you have about it, and do not think about how poorly you might perform on the examination.

Choose to take the test. The examination is not being forced on you; rather, you chose to take it. If you view the examination as something you want to do, you are in control and the examination is no longer controlling you. Because you chose to take the test, you must also choose to study for it.

Concentrate on what you can and must do *now*. Do not think about what you should have studied yesterday (the past) or what your NCLEX-RN results will be (the future). Direct your attention on the present and expend your energy on the current task. Right now, you need to concentrate on studying for the examination. On the day of the examination, your energy must be focused on understanding the questions and responding correctly.

As stated previously, *some* test anxiety is actually good for you. Too much, however, will hinder your performance, and you will not be able to demonstrate adequately the knowledge you actually possess. People who are anxious about taking tests can help themselves by:

1. Learning to be less demanding of themselves
2. Revising their expectations about the consequences of failure and viewing the task as less alarming
3. Strengthening their study skills
4. Gaining more self-control over their worry and emotionality[4]

If anxiety is handled in a positive manner, it can assist in "promoting survival, healthy adaptation and development. In its nonadaptive modes, it can promote incompetence and extreme and lasting misery."[5]

In any situation, if you convince yourself that you are going to fail, you will. Instead of being negative about yourself, trying to decide what others will think of you if you fail, or deciding that you will do poorly on the examination, think *positively*. Negative statements made to yourself or others can significantly reduce the effectiveness of your preparation. Think positively and you will feel positive.

Read the examples of typical negative and positive statements shown in Table 2–1. Are you guilty of making any of the negative statements? If so, begin using and believing in the statements shown in the right (positive) column.

Avoid *why*, *if only*, and *what if* types of questions or statements, such as "Why did I ever think I could be a nurse?" or "If only I had more time, I could do better," or "What if I don't do well on the examination?" These expressions tend to reinforce feelings of helplessness, frustration, and anger.

Eliminate them from your internal thoughts and external statements.

Stress and anxiety can and will be reduced if you take *positive* action and think *positive* thoughts about yourself and your abilities. At the same time, recognize that it is natural for you to feel some anxiety about the examination. The statement "don't worry" is ridiculous advice because all of us worry about the unknown to some extent. You must, however, worry in a constructive manner and must be prepared for the examination.

Study Environment

Not only is what you study important, but the conditions under which you study are also important influences on your ability to learn and remember. Both internal (daydreaming) and external (noise) distractions will interfere with your ability to concentrate and learn.

Think about where and how you generally study. Are you studying in an optimal place and manner? You want to be comfortable and relaxed while studying, yet at the same time you need to be able to focus all of your attention and energy on the material you are reading, reviewing, and learning.

The following questions should assist you in your evaluation of whether the location and manner in which you study are the most conducive to learning.

1. When I begin studying, do I have all necessary books,

Table 2–1. Changing Negative Self-Talk to Positive Self-Talk

Negative Statements

"I have to get a perfect score."
"I always get upset during a test."
"I'm a failure because I didn't remember . . ."
"If the test has questions on . . . topic, I'll just die."
"What if I fail the exam?"
"I'll let my family down if I don't pass this test."
"I'm too stupid to be a nurse."
"The test is designed to trick candidates, so it doesn't matter if I study."
"I'll never be able to understand all of this material."
"Thank heavens I made it through this study session!"
"I just know I'll be scared during the exam."
"Everyone expects me to do poorly, so why bother trying to do otherwise?"
"I don't know why I have to take this test. I got good grades in school and that should be enough."

Positive Statements

"I want to do well, but I don't have to get every item correct."
"If I feel myself getting tense during the test, I know how to relax."
"Just because I forgot about . . . doesn't mean that I'm a failure. I remembered lots of the other material."
"Since I'm not real comfortable with . . . topic, I'd better study it more."
"I don't expect to fail, but if I do, I'll just have to study harder and do better the next time."
"Sure, my family wants me to do well, but they'll still accept me if I don't pass."
"I made it through school, and I can make it through the exam."
"If I study, I can do well; it's my responsibility to prepare."
"Just relax and try rereading this section. I know I can figure it out."
"Wow, I really learned a lot while studying today. I hope tomorrow goes as well."
"I know I'll do well on the exam because I'm capable and I studied."
"I don't care what others think about my chance of passing the exam; I know I can do it."
"I want to take this test simply because it will confirm that I really did learn while I was in school."

paper, pencils and pens, and study materials with me so that I do not waste time finding them?

2. Do I schedule a block of time (1–2 hours) for studying?
3. Do I take short breaks (10–15 minutes) while studying for long periods of time and then return to work immediately?
4. Do I spread out my studying over a period of time rather than trying to do all of it at the last minute?
5. If I study with friends, do they have good study habits and do we really study?
6. Do I have a plan for studying and stick to it?
7. Do I feel rested when I study?
8. If I begin to feel tense or tired, do I stop studying for a while and try to relax?
9. If I begin to daydream or worry, do I take a few minutes to permit myself to daydream or worry rather than let these activities interfere with my studying?
10. Do I concentrate on the material that I am studying rather than thinking about other things?
11. Have I included some time in my schedule for social activities and exercise?
12. When I am done studying for the day, do I feel I have accomplished something?
13. Am I able to remove myself mentally from my environment; that is, can I block out potential distractions?
14. Is the area in which I study relaxing and comfortable, but not to such an extent that I fall asleep?
15. Is the area in which I study quiet and basically free from interruptions?
16. Is my desk (study area) neat and well organized so that I have enough room to study effectively?
17. Is the lighting sufficient and nonglaring?
18. When it is time to study, do I do so immediately and eagerly?
19. Do I reward myself when I feel I have done an exceptionally good job of studying?

If you answered "yes" to each of these questions, you are studying in an appropriate atmosphere and with the proper frame of mind. If you answered "no" to some questions, try to determine what you need to do to improve the conditions. Remember: how, when, and where you study does make a difference in your ability to concentrate and learn.

Preparing for the NCLEX-RN

One of your first tasks is to learn all you can about the actual examination—how it is constructed, the type of questions included, how long you have to complete the test, and so on. The information in Chapter 1 is a good starting point, but you should also read the material provided by the National Council of State Boards of Nursing and ask your instructors about the test. The better informed you are about the examination, the better you can prepare for it.

You also need to keep in mind that everything you did during your education to become a nurse—attending classes, applying good listening skills, taking clear and concise notes, doing your homework, reading all assignments, and taking course examinations—has helped you to prepare for the NCLEX-RN. Draw on these experiences as you prepare to take the final step in the learning process.

The suggestions in this section are provided to help you learn to study more aggressively and actively. Underlining or highlighting key words or passages is a good start, but that is passive learning and is not as effective for long-term memory. You need to develop active learning skills to improve your chances for remembering the material.[6,7]

Relate the material you have just read to information you learned in the past. Does the new material relate to something that you already know? Does this knowledge help you understand how to deal with any specific nursing situation? Is there a relationship among various facts that you have already learned? If so, what is that relationship? **Think, do not just memorize!**

Ask yourself questions about the material you have just read. Try to predict how the material might be worded in the examination.

Form study groups to review information and ask each other questions. This is an excellent way to share your knowledge while you benefit from the knowledge of others. When you form a study group, keep the following points in mind.[8]

1. Study with others who are at your ability level or slightly above. If you were an average student in school, do not study with those who always got As. They may skip over material that is necessary for you to review. On the other hand, if you consistently got As, do not study with students who received Cs. They will want to study and review material that you don't need to study. Remember, the members of the study group should assist each other.
2. Keep sufficient time available for you to study on your own. Do not plan to spend all of your study time with the group.
3. Keep the group serious. Although there will be times when you "get off the subject," you should keep this to a minimum. Always keep in mind the real purpose for being together, and do not become distracted with trivial matters.
4. Keep the group small. If there are more than five people working together, there is a greater tendency to become distracted.
5. Do not meet too often. A few short meetings will provide the intensity and seriousness needed to get the work done. Also, you need time between meetings to prepare on your own.
6. Come to the meetings prepared with questions about areas you do not understand. Prepare mock test items to share with the others.

Above all, all members of the study group need to be actively involved in the process, must be willing to devote sufficient time to prepare for the meetings, and must contribute positively to the group.

Make notes of key concepts that are important to remember. Also, take notes on areas in which you feel less certain and use them as a reminder that you need to continue learning more about those topics.

Develop flash cards to help you remember dates, facts, formulas, and other factual material. Use 3 × 5 index cards to write short, factual questions on one side (What is the normal blood pressure for an adult?) and the answer on the reverse side. Add to the set of cards as you continue studying; review the cards on a weekly basis. At first you may want to read the questions and answers together to help you learn. Later you should ask yourself the questions and respond out loud. Check to see if you are correct. You can also have someone else read the questions to you. If you do not know the answer to a question, put that card back into the stack and ask the question again. If you know the material, you should be able to answer each question in a few seconds.

Be interested in the material. Just because you have wanted to be a registered nurse (RN) for a number of years, this does not mean that everything you studied in school was personally of interest to you. Regardless of your interest in a subject or the profession, there were undoubtedly some topics that you found boring, uninteresting, or irrelevant. As you prepare, however, you need to become interested in the total field in order to learn better. Convince yourself that the "boring" topics are really critical, and try to relate them to topics that interest you.

Use prepared test questions such as those in this book to help you study. Take a general, comprehensive RN-related examination as a practice test to help you determine your strengths and weaknesses. Use this information as a basis for preparing your study schedule. The better you do on the practice test, the less time you may need to devote to studying. Be sure to be honest with your appraisal of your performance and the areas that you need to study. Start with the areas of weakness first, so you can devote more time to studying them. After you have reviewed the weak areas, take the same test or another one to see what improvements you have made. Use various sources of test items to become familiar with different ways in which the same information can appear on the test.

As you respond to each item, read the stem and options carefully, select the option you think is correct, and go on to the next item. Do not leave items blank, and do not return to items after you have made your selection. Because you must answer each item presented in CAT before going on to the next, now is the time for you to get into the habit of, and feel comfortable with, responding to a single item and moving forward.

Set specific goals for yourself. A broad goal of "I need to learn about nursing" or "I need to know enough to pass the test" will not help you. Instead, choose which nursing components you will learn during the week and then during each day. Have specific, concrete goals for each study period.

Establish a schedule for each day's studying and reviewing. Remain flexible, however, so that should you wish to go to an unplanned party or go out to dinner when you have scheduled a study period, you can do so without feeling guilty. At the same time, too much flexibility can lead to procrastination and can cause you to become tense and stressed when you realize that instead of studying 10 hours during the week, you have only studied 2 hours. When you establish a weekly schedule, plan for the "unplanned" event to occur. If you do this, you will not feel guilty or stressed when something you want to do becomes available. Also, remember that if you do forfeit some study time on one day, you need to make up that time on another day.

Write summaries of what you have read. Rephrase information so that you can understand it better. Use mnemonics or silly phrases to remember certain facts. Use word associations. In other words, writing out the information either in your own words or with the help of a clever saying can help you remember the material better.

If information is not clear in one book, read another to see if the same material is explained any better. Although the same material may be included in a number of books, the manner in which it is explained and the way it is presented (with or without drawings, charts, and so forth) can make a

difference in how well you understand the information. You should also rely on your instructors and peers for clarification of material that may be difficult for you to grasp.

Visualize the information you have just read. Mentally try to see how what you have read would actually look or work. Try to visualize a patient with certain conditions or symptoms. What would you be observing? Try to visualize yourself performing a certain procedure. How would you perform it?

Overlearn the material. Everyone forgets information regardless of how much studying is done. You should not expect to remember all of the material you were taught during your nursing education. However, you can improve the likelihood of remembering more if you continue to review and relearn the material even after you think you know it. The more active (visualizing, rephrasing, verbalizing) your learning, the greater your probability of remembering it.

At the conclusion of each study period, take a few minutes to **outline the key material you have just studied and learned.** These outlines can then serve as future review materials. Some key elements of a good outline include:

1. Using underlining or symbols to identify key points
2. Using sufficient space to allow for clarification or expansion based on later studying
3. Recording all formulas, equations, and rules exactly
4. Writing legibly on one side of the paper
5. Writing your own ideas or questions as well as facts
6. Using your own words to help reinforce a concept
7. Using personal nursing care experiences to clarify points

Now that you have learned what you should be doing to become a more active learner, you need to put these activities into place. During the next few study periods, do not try to study any differently than you normally would. Instead, at the end of each study period, take the assessment test shown in Table 2–2. Use the questions to evaluate how you need to change your studying behavior.

Whenever you answered "no," keep those points in mind the next time you study. Do not feel frustrated if you find that you have not included all of the steps in your studying; just keep trying to improve. The overused phrase "Rome wasn't built in a day" is applicable in this instance as well as in your overall preparation for the examination. It might take you some time and effort to learn how to study more effectively and actively.

Test Question Analysis and Test-Taking Techniques

Test taking can be very stressful. Certain strategies can be used to make test taking less stressful and help you make the right decision when answering questions. These strategies are called "testwise" and can maximize application of the information you already possess from effective study habits or previous knowledge about the subject being tested. Before taking the NCLEX-RN, or any other exam, you can learn certain test-taking techniques in order to be successful on the exam. You can accomplish this through a course directed by an instructor or through self-directed preparation, such as study outlines, books of questions, or computerized exams.

The NCLEX-RN exam consists entirely of multiple-choice questions, which are familiar to you because they were commonly used in your nursing school curriculum to evaluate

Table 2–2. **Study Approach Checklist Questions: Answer Yes or No**

1. Did you make a note of the material you were unsure of in order to restudy it later?
2. Did you look over the topic headings as well as any study questions at the end of the chapter before beginning to read the entire section?
3. When you finished the initial reading, reciting, and reviewing, did you look over your notes and check your memory of the major headings and subpoints under each heading?
4. Did you carefully determine the most important topics to be learned (or the topics you know the least about) and determine your time frame for learning them?
5. Did you take clear and concise notes while you studied?
6. Did you read the material and try to answer questions you developed that covered the key information?
7. After reading a section or chapter, did you answer correctly the questions included at the end, and did you try to develop examples of nursing situations in which this knowledge might be useful?
8. Did you vary your speed of reading according to the difficulty and familiarity of the material as well as according to your purpose for reviewing the material?
9. Did you pause after reading each section to underline or jot down the important points, and did you make notes on material you did not understand completely?
10. Did you go back to the material that you were unsure of and review it again (in the same book or in a different book)?

student progress. Multiple-choice questions are used because they are objective and can comprehensively assess complex subject matter. However, these tests are composed of questions geared to a national body of test takers and have been carefully written to avoid local bias, hints, or "give-aways" in the stems or answers.

Multiple-Choice Tests

There is a right way and a wrong way to answer multiple-choice items. Although you have probably answered thousands of them during your course of study, you may find it advantageous to review the following suggestions. Part of doing well on any examination is being *testwise*, that is, knowing how to figure out the correct answer even if you are not 100% certain. You may have a wealth of knowledge and be one of the smartest in your class, but if you do not know how to respond to multiple-choice questions, you will be unable to prove this knowledge. For better or worse, part of the score you receive on any examination depends on your test-taking ability.

Budget your time and pace yourself accordingly. Even with CAT, in which the number of questions and actual time spent on the test will vary, you know that you will have a maximum of 5 hours and a maximum of 265 items. This works out to slightly over **1 minute per item.** You should keep this time frame in mind as you are presented with each item. Although you might need to spend more than 1 minute for certain items, your overall goal should be 1 minute per item.

Keep moving at a steady pace. If a question is difficult and

you are spending too much time on it, make an educated guess and move on to the next item. Remember, in CAT, if you select an incorrect option you will be given the opportunity to demonstrate your competence with a slightly easier item. If you get the next one correct, you will be given a slightly more difficult item. One or two incorrect responses will not result in failure!

Read each question thoroughly but quickly. Do not keep reading the same question over and over. Select your response and move on. In general, your first reaction to a question is the correct one. Do not try to second-guess what might be intended or try to figure out if there is a "trick" to the question. As a rule, the items are straightforward, basic, and designed to determine if you are *minimally* competent. Read each of the stems and all of the options carefully and then make your selection.

Concentrate on one item at a time. Do not worry about how many more items will be presented to you, how many of the candidates have already left the testing room, or how much time remains. Focus only on the item on the screen in front of you at that time.

Do not stop trying. Even if there are several items in a row that seem unfamiliar to you, do not start worrying about the examination as a whole. Just answer the items to the best of your ability and move forward.

Focus on key words in the stem. Mentally highlight these words or phrases and keep them in mind as you read the options. You might even want to jot down some key words on scratch paper to help you remember them as you read the options.

If a question requires calculations, **talk yourself through each step of the process.** At the same time, do not try to do the calculations in your head. Use the scratch paper provided at your workstation. Double-check your computations to be certain that you have not made some minor arithmetical error. Generally, the incorrect options included in computational questions are based on mistakes typically made in the calculations (for instance, dividing instead of multiplying). This means that one of the answers provided could match yours and still be wrong.

Break down complex stems into smaller, more manageable sections. Make certain that the response you select is correct for each of the separate components within the stem. If an option works for one segment of the question, but not another, then the option is probably incorrect.

Reword a difficult stem and see if that helps you to better understand the intent of the item. Use your own words to ask the question included in the stem.

Try answering the question before you have read the options provided. The stem should provide sufficient information so that you know the direction of the question and the general response being sought. Start thinking about what you should be looking for as you read the options. This process will help you save time even if the answer you initially think is correct is not one of the options provided. At least you will be thinking about what to look for.

Read all options before selecting the one you think is correct. A well-constructed test will have four plausible responses, and it is your responsibility to select the *best*. Too often candidates read the first few options and decide that one of them is correct without reading all of the options. While one of those options may be *good*, it may not be the *best*.

Eliminate the distractors that are obviously wrong, and then pick among the remaining ones by using a rational thought process. At the same time, do not eliminate an option unless you are absolutely certain you understand every word in the phrase or sentence.

Use logic and common sense to figure out the correct response. The items are based on situations that an entering nurse would encounter. The items do not include exotic or unique situations or problems that only an experienced nurse would be able to understand. If the situation presented is one that you have not personally experienced, try to recall a similar situation and how you handled it. Then look at the options to see if you can apply any of them to a situation you are familiar with.

Relate each option to the stem. Make sure that the answer you selected fits the intent of the stem and is grammatically correct.

Try to figure out the meaning of unfamiliar words in the stem and options in terms of the context of the sentences. You might also be able to figure out the meaning of words by dividing them into prefixes and suffixes that you know.

Use cues in the stem and in the distractors to help you figure out the correct response.

If you must guess, use logic. After you have eliminated the options that you know are wrong, see if there are any test construction flaws that might help you figure out the intended answer. Given the extensive editing done before assembling the NCLEX-RN, it is doubtful that any errors will be found, but you might as well look for them. Some of the more common test construction flaws are:

Length: Select the longest response if all other options are approximately equal in length.

Location: The correct response is more likely to be in the middle unless the options are ordered in terms of length.

Grammar: Incorrect options may not always fit the stem grammatically.

Language: Unusual or highly technical language typically indicates that the particular option is not correct.

Qualification: If one option includes qualifiers such as "generally," "tends to," or "usually," and the other options do not, select the option that includes the qualification.

Generalizability: The correct option will tend to have greater applicability and flexibility.

Specifics: Options that include the words "always" or "never" are typically not correct. There are very few instances in life that "always" occur.

A Guide to Specific Test-Taking Techniques

The following information describes how to analyze test questions and pick the correct answer. Various test-taking strategies can be used to determine what the question is really asking. One such technique is breaking the question down into parts. The following section describes how you can master this technique.

Elements of the Multiple-Choice Question with Examples

The Scenario

This is a concise description of the client, and information about the client's problem and/or case. It is also called the

"stem," and asks the question. The stem can be presented in a complete or incomplete sentence. In addition to sentence structure, you must decide if the stem is positive or negative. This is referred to as polarity. Positive polarity indicates what is true about the situation while negative polarity indicates what is false. Focus on whether the item is asking for a positive or negative response. Negative words (*not, except*) are usually emphasized in the stem to help you recognize that you must reverse your thought process. When you respond to a negatively worded item, read each of the options and decide whether it is a true or false statement. If the item asks you to select the procedure that you would *not* follow, the false option is the correct response.

Example: Question Stem That Is a Complete Sentence with Negative Polarity

---

A 21-month-old child is admitted to the pediatric unit with a fractured left femur and is placed in Bryant's traction. Which assessment by the nurse indicates that the traction is improperly applied?
A. The child's buttocks are raised slightly off the mattress.
B. The weights hang freely at the foot of the bed.
C. Pulses are present and equal in both feet.
D. The left hip is raised slightly off the mattress and the right hip is on the mattress.

What does the question ask? The question asks which assessment indicates that the traction is improperly applied. The key word here is "improperly," which indicates negative polarity.

(A) indicates the correct traction position.

(B) and (C) are both correct statements for a client in Bryant's traction.

(D) is the correct answer because it is the only incorrect response.

What is important here is that you have to look for key words that indicate negative polarity, which means false information about the problem. Other key words that indicate negative polarity include: "not," "except," "contraindicated," "least," "avoid," and "never." NCLEX-RN does not use these negative words, but some nursing examinations use these types of questions.

Example: Question Stem That Is a Complete Sentence with Positive Polarity

---

What symptom would a client with pyrexia most likely exhibit?
A. Elevated blood pressure
B. Tachycardia
C. Dyspnea
D. Precordial pain

What does the question ask? The question asks what is the most likely symptom of pyrexia. The key words are "most likely," which indicates positive polarity.

(A) is incorrect. Blood pressure is not necessarily elevated with fever.

(B) is correct. The pulse increases to meet increased tissue demands for oxygen during the febrile state.

(C) is incorrect. Fever may not cause difficulty in breathing.

(D) is incorrect. Pain is not related to fever.

Other key words that indicate positive polarity include: "always," "most," and "usually." Positive polarity indicates the truth about what the question is asking and determines if you are able to understand, extrapolate, or apply correct information.

Incomplete Sentence Items

This is a group of words that forms the beginning of the stem and becomes complete when combined with one of the answer choices. These types of items are often used on exams and can be developed to elicit true or false information, which identifies positive or negative polarity.

Example: Incomplete Sentence Item with Positive Polarity

The most important electrolyte of intracellular fluid is:
A. Potassium
B. Sodium
C. Calcium
D. Chloride

(A) is correct. The concentration of potassium is greater inside the cell and is extremely important in establishing a membrane potential, a critical factor in the cell's ability to function.

(B) is incorrect. Sodium is the most abundant cation of the extracellular compartment.

(C) is incorrect. Calcium is the most abundant electrolyte in the body and is concentrated in the teeth and bones, not intracellularly.

(D) is incorrect. Chloride is an extracellular anion.

Key words in this stem are "most important," which indicate truth about what the stem is asking to complete the sentence.

Example: Incomplete Sentence with Negative Polarity

The nurse understands that a pulmonary embolism is an unlikely complication during the postoperative period following:
A. A saphenous vein ligation
B. A hysterectomy
C. A prostatectomy
D. An appendectomy

(A) is incorrect. After the diseased varicose vein is removed, this places stress on the deep venous system and increases the risk of thrombi.

(B) is incorrect. Even though ambulation is generally done soon after surgery, pelvic surgery increases risk of thrombus formation.

(C) is incorrect. The client may or may not be out of bed the same day, depending on the surgical approach. Mobility may be hampered by discomfort and a continuous bladder irrigation Foley.

(D) is correct. The client is usually out of bed the same day, and with mobility, there is less risk of developing venous stasis that could lead to thrombus formation.

The key word is "unlikely," which indicates false information about the subject.

Distractors

Distractors are incorrect but reasonable and tempting choices that are designed to distract you from the correct answer.

Example: Question with Distractor

During the administration of an enema, the client complains of intestinal cramps. The nurse should:
A. Discontinue the procedure
B. Stop until the cramps have subsided
C. Lower the height of the container and continue
D. Give it at a slower rate

(A) is a distractor. Cramps are not a reason to discontinue the enema entirely. Temporary clamping of the tubing usually relieves the cramps and the enema can be continued.

(B) is correct. Administration of additional fluid when a client complains of abdominal cramps increases discomfort because of additional pressure. By clamping the tubing for a few minutes, the cramps are allowed to subside and the enema can be continued.

(C) is a distractor. This will reduce the flow of the solution, which will decrease pressure, but not reduce it entirely.

(D) is a distractor. Slowing the rate decreases pressure but does not reduce it entirely. This is similar to the previous answer.

Example: Question with Distractor

The chief complaint of a client with Vincent's angina is:
A. Chest pain
B. Dyspnea
C. Shoulder discomfort
D. Bleeding oral ulcerations

(A), (B), and (C) are distractors and are symptoms related to angina pectoris, in which there is insufficient oxygenation to the heart muscle (myocardium).

(D) is correct. You have know that Vincent's angina (trenchmouth) is an infection of the mouth resulting in bleeding gums, pain when swallowing and talking, and fever. It has nothing to do with the heart.

Key Concepts in the Question

The most important skill you must develop and use is the ability to read the question carefully and determine key concepts in the question. Each question is carefully constructed with key concepts that relate to the client, the problem, and specific aspects of the problem.

Client: Information about age, gender, and marital status is usually relevant. When a child's age is given, it can be an important link to the answer, because the question may be asking developmental information. Also, vital signs and preoperative teaching methods vary with age.

Problem or Behavior: This is usually a disease process, a symptom, or a behavior that identifies a client problem.

Problem Circumstances: Is the question asking for nursing interventions, client symptoms, or family responses? Which aspect of the nursing process is the question referring to, for example, assessment, planning, implementation, or evaluation? Does the question ask information relevant to a specific problem or symptom exhibited by the client? Are there additional details about the client or the problem that seem to be important?

Test Item Analysis

The following sample questions show you how to analyze test items and how to successfully choose the correct answer to each question.

Sample Question #1

An adult male client is receiving radiation therapy for the treatment of prostate cancer. The nurse assesses for side effects from the radiation therapy. Which assessment measure is indicated?
A. Assessment of deep tendon reflexes
B. Palpation of lymph nodes
C. Monitoring of blood pressure and pulse
D. Careful observation of the skin

What does the question ask? The question asks, what is the assessment measure for side effects of radiation therapy? In order to correctly answer the question, you have to know that skin damage is a major side effect of radiation therapy.

(A) Deep tendon reflex changes are not a direct result of radiation therapy.

(B) Lymph node changes may indicate therapeutic effects of radiation therapy, but not side effects as the question asked.

(C) Blood pressure and pulse changes are not a direct result of radiation therapy.

(D) is correct. The question asked for an assessment measure related to a side effect of radiation therapy.

Sample Question #2

An adult male client is receiving radiation therapy for prostate cancer. Which statement made by the client indicates a need for further teaching about prevention of complications while receiving radiation therapy?
A. "After I leave therapy today, I will go to the park and sit in the sun and breathe the fresh air."
B. "I will rent a movie instead of going out to the movie theater."
C. "I will eat a light breakfast before my radiation therapy."
D. "I like to use body powder and lotion, but I will avoid it until all radiation treatments are finished."

What does the question ask? The question asks which statement indicates that the client does not understand and needs further instruction about preventing complications of radiation therapy.

(A) is the correct choice because a person receiving radiation therapy should avoid the sun since it causes skin reactions that are aggravated by sun exposure.

(B), (C), and (D) are all good actions for the client to take to help prevent complications of radiation therapy; therefore, they are not correct answers to this question.

Sample Question #3

The nurse enters the room to administer a preoperative medication to a 55-year-old man scheduled for a colon re-

section. What action is most appropriate for the nurse to take immediately before administering the medication?
A. Administer the ordered enema.
B. Discuss postoperative care.
C. Teach coughing and deep-breathing techniques.
D. Ask the client to void.

It is important to recognize that this is a **time frame** question. How do you know that? In the question stem you see the clues of "preoperative" and "immediately before administering the medication."

What does the question ask? It asks for the most appropriate action immediately before giving the preoperative medication. All of the options are nursing care activities the nurse should do at some point in the preoperative care of this client. The question asks for the most appropriate action immediately before administering the preoperative medication. The time frame words, as mentioned previously, are the key to answering the question correctly.

(A) If an enema is ordered before a colon resection, this prep would have been done the evening before or several hours before the procedure. This would ensure adequate evacuation of the bowel. An enema would not be appropriate immediately before the preoperative medication because the procedure will start within about 1 hour.

(B) Discussing postoperative care with the client is not the most appropriate immediately before administering preoperative medication. Postoperative teaching is done hours to days before the procedure.

(C) is incorrect for the same reason as (A) and (B). Coughing and deep-breathing techniques should be done several hours or the evening before the procedure.

(D) This is correct. Asking the client to void immediately before administering the preoperative medication is most appropriate and follows preoperative preparation protocol.

Sample Question #4

The nurse is caring for a client who vomits upon returning to the nursing unit following an uneventful stay in the post-anesthesia care unit. Which potential complication from vomiting is the client most at risk to develop?
A. Aspiration pneumonia
B. Incisional pain
C. Wound dehiscence and evisceration
D. Electrolyte imbalance

What does the question ask? The question asks what complication of vomiting the client is most at risk to develop.

(A) is correct. Aspiration and the possibility of pneumonia development is the most likely complication to occur in the immediate postoperative period.

(B) Vomiting could cause incisional pain. This, however, is not the most likely complication, and the stem does not state that the client has an incision.

(C) Dehiscence and evisceration could occur following violent vomiting. The question did not indicate that the vomiting was violent or that the client had an incision. Dehiscence and evisceration usually take a few days to develop and are not as common as other complications.

(D) Electrolyte imbalance can occur following prolonged

vomiting but is not the most likely complication to occur in the immediate postoperative period. The client scenario includes information indicating that it is shortly after the surgery was performed.

Additional Testwise Techniques

A few other test-taking techniques will be useful to you during an exam. These include: **priority setting, initial assessment, essential safety, odd man wins, same answer, umbrella answer, opposites,** and **repeated words.**

Priority Setting

Many questions on an exam ask the nurse to set priorities. This can be asked in different ways such as:
What should the nurse do initially?
Which action takes priority?
What should the nurse do first?
What is essential for the nurse to do?

Example: Priority Setting

A 58-year-old man is admitted with a cerebral vascular accident (CVA). Which goal is of highest priority in the early part of hospitalization? The client('s):
A. Will maintain skin integrity.
B. Will be continent of urine.
C. Lungs will be clear upon auscultation.
D. Will maintain joint mobility.

CLIENT: A 58-year-old man.
PROBLEM/BEHAVIOR: Cerebral vascular accident.
DETAILS: Early part of hospitalization.

What does the question ask? The question asks for the highest priority goal during the early part of hospitalization.
(A) is incorrect. Skin breakdown and contractures will take some time to develop.
(B) is incorrect. Urinary continence is definitely a long-term goal. It is not the priority.
(C) is correct. The nurse will work to accomplish all of the goals listed, but atelectasis can develop very quickly.
(D) is incorrect. Maintaining joint mobility is a long-term goal.

Initial Assessment

Remember, the first step in the nursing process is assessment. When the stem of a question asks for the initial nursing action, always look to see if there is a relevant assessment answer. The nurse will take an action only when there is enough data to act upon. You would call the physician only when there is not a nursing action that should be taken first. Look for an assessment answer or emergency nursing action.

Example: Initial Assessment

A 52-year-old man had knee surgery. Postoperative orders include Demerol 50 mg IM every 3–4 hours as needed for pain. Soon after he returns to the postoperative nursing unit, he asks for pain medication. His medical records in-

dicate he was medicated 3 hours ago. Which of the following actions would be most appropriate for the nurse to take initially?
A. Assess the location and degree of pain.
B. Reposition the client and check on him in 20 minutes.
C. Refill and replace the ice bag ordered for the knee.
D. Administer the prescribed narcotic analgesic.

CLIENT: A 52-year-old man who had knee surgery.
PROBLEM/BEHAVIOR: The client asks for pain medication soon after he returns to the postoperative nursing unit.
DETAILS: He has Demerol 50 mg IM ordered every 3–4 hours PRN for pain. He was last medicated 3 hours ago.

What does the question ask? The question asks for the most appropriate initial action for the nurse to take. This means, "Look for an assessment answer."
(A) is correct. This is an assessment answer. The question does not say anything about pain except that the client requests pain medication. Before giving pain medication, the nurse should determine that the pain the client has is postoperative pain for which the medication was ordered.
(B), (C), and (D) are nursing interventions and are done after assessment.

Essential Safety

When the stem of the question asks what is essential for the nurse to do, think safety. Many test questions will be safety questions, because being a safe practitioner is an important aspect of nursing.

Example: Essential Safety

A 54-year-old client is admitted for a bronchoscopy. When he returns to his room on the postoperative nursing unit, what is essential for the nurse to do?
A. Explain that he cannot have anything to eat or drink for several hours.
B. Administer oxygen to the client at 4 L/min.
C. Position the client in a semiprone position.
D. Have a tracheostomy set at the bedside.

CLIENT: A 54-year-old man.
PROBLEM/BEHAVIOR: Client had a bronchoscopy.
DETAILS: Client has returned to his room after the procedure.

What does the question ask? The question asks about essential nursing care. Since the key word is "essential," you must think *safety.*
(A) is essential. To prevent aspiration, the client must remain NPO until the gag and cough reflexes have returned. Because the client had local anesthetic and is awake, he can understand that he needs to comply with NPO status. Local anesthetic is lidocaine to numb the gag reflex.
(B) and (D) are incorrect because oxygen is usually not needed nor is a tracheostomy set indicated.
(C) is incorrect because a bronchoscopy is performed under local anesthesia and therefore a semiprone position is not indicated. The appropriate position for the client would be semi-Fowler's.

Odd Man Wins

This means that the answer that is different from the others is very likely the correct answer. It may be the longest or the shortest or simply very different in content or style.

Example 1: Odd Man Wins

Suppose you read the test question and you recognize what it is asking. Your answer choices include:
A. Cupcake
B. Birthday cake
C. Robin
D. Wedding cake

(C) is the correct answer because it is the one that is different or odd. The others are all cakes and (C) is a type of bird.

Example 2: Odd Man Wins

Suppose your answer choices include:
A. Horse
B. Fish
C. Cow
D. Dog

(B) is correct because it is different from the others. All others are four-legged animals. When using this technique, you must realize that the answer that is different must make sense and must relate to what the question is asking.

Example 3: Odd Man Wins in Nursing Care

The nurse is caring for a 46-year-old woman with thyroid disease and must observe for thyroid crisis. Which nursing observations would be most suggestive of thyroid crisis?
A. Decreased temperature
B. Rapid pulse
C. Decreased respirations
D. Lethargy

CLIENT: A 46-year-old woman.
PROBLEM/BEHAVIOR: Thyroid disease.
DETAILS: Observing for thyroid crisis. You are not told what type of thyroid disease the client has.

What does the question ask? The question asks for observations that are most suggestive of a thyroid crisis. You may not remember whether that is hypo- or hyperthyroid function. First, look at the answer choices.

(A), (C), and (D) all indicate lowered metabolism.

(B) is correct, because it is the only answer that indicates hyperfunction. Even if you do not recall whether thyroid crisis is hypo- or hyperfunction of the thyroid, you can answer the question by recognizing that three answers relate to hypofunction and only one relates to hyperfunction. This is how the Odd Man Wins technique can be successfully used to choose the correct answer to a challenging question.

Same Answer

If two or more answers say the same thing in different words, then none of those choices are correct.

Example: Same Answer

A 35-year-old woman has been diagnosed with hypertension. The nurse is teaching the client about her diagnosis. The client asks the nurse why she should not smoke. Which statement best describes why a person with hypertension should not smoke?
A. Smoking causes the arteries to constrict.
B. The tars in smoke cause changes in lung tissue.
C. The lungs are damaged by smoking.
D. Smoking residues build up in the bladder.

CLIENT: A 35-year-old female.
PROBLEM/BEHAVIOR: Hypertension.
DETAILS: Client asks why she should not smoke.

What does the question ask? The question asks why someone with hypertension should not smoke.

Answers (B) and (C) say the same thing. Even if you are unsure of the correct answer, you can eliminate those two answers because they are too similar. Note that all of the choices are true, but only (A) answers the question that was asked in the stem, so it is the correct answer. (B) and (C) relate to lung disease and (D) relates to bladder cancer.

Umbrella Answer

This refers to one answer that includes all of the others. This answer is better than all the others because it includes them. How does that work? The umbrella answer includes and describes steps in the nursing process, such as: problem solving through critical thinking, assessing signs and symptoms, determining the nursing diagnosis, planning and carrying out nursing care, and evaluating the outcome criteria.

Example: Umbrella Answer

The nurse is caring for a postoperative client who is in pain. The therapeutic goal is to:
A. Administer pain medication.
B. Change the client's position.
C. Divert the client's attention.
D. Promote an optimal comfort level.

CLIENT: A postoperative client.
PROBLEM/BEHAVIOR: Postoperative pain.
DETAILS: None.

What does the question ask? The question asks for the therapeutic goal for this patient. All answers are actions that the nurse may take. The stem asks for the therapeutic goal.

(A), (B), and (C) are actions that will help achieve the goal of (D), which is promoting optimal comfort for the client.

(D) is the correct answer because it includes all the others.

Opposites

When two answers are opposite, such as "turn on the right side" and "turn on the left side," or "high blood pressure" and "low blood pressure," the answer is usually one of the two.

Example: Opposites

What nursing intervention is most appropriate to decrease joint pain in a person in sickle cell crisis?
A. Immobilize the joint and apply ice packs.
B. Administer aspirin and apply cool compresses.
C. Perform passive range-of-motion exercises and apply warm compresses.
D. Elevate the extremity and avoid movement of the joint.

CLIENT: Person with sickle cell crisis.
PROBLEM/BEHAVIOR: Sickle cell crisis.
DETAILS: Joint pain.

What does the question ask? The question asks for a nursing intervention to decrease joint pain.

Note the two opposite answers, (A) and (C). The answer will be one of these two, and in this case the correct answer is (C). It would be helpful to recognize that the client is in sickle cell crisis, in which there is red blood cell clumping and obstruction of circulation. Heat is a vasodilator and will increase circulation. Therefore, passive range-of-motion exercises will keep the joint from developing a contracture.

(A) and (B) are incorrect because you would apply heat, not ice packs or cool compresses, to dilate vessels, and aspirin is contraindicated because of the acid load which causes sickling.

(D) is incorrect because elevation the extremity and immobilizing it are not the best ways to decrease joint pain in someone with sickle cell crisis.

Repeated Words

In this type of question, words from the question are repeated in the answer. Frequently the same word or a synonym will be in both the question and the answer.

Example: Repeated Words

A client who is obviously upset says to the nurse, "I want to talk to the head nurse—no, make that the director of nursing and the owner of this hospital. I am upset!" The best initial response for the nurse to make is:
A. "Whom do you wish to see first?"
B. "You seem upset."
C. "Why do you want to talk with them?"
D. "Don't be angry."

CLIENT: A person who is obviously upset.
PROBLEM/BEHAVIOR: Upset/anger.
DETAILS: Asking to see individuals in authority.

What does the question ask? The question asks for the best initial response for the nurse to make. Note that the client is described as obviously upset.

(A) does not deal with the client's feelings.

(B) is correct. It repeats the word "upset," and it is the only answer that focuses on feelings. The nurse shares her observations with the client.

(C) asks the client why he wants to talk to the persons he requested. "Why" questions can make the person more defensive and escalate the anger.

(D) tells the client not to be angry. He is clearly angry. It is inappropriate for the nurse to tell him how to feel, and an angry person would not listen to that anyway.

Students' Comments Regarding Test Taking

Students were surveyed to find out what strategies they used to successfully choose right answers on an exam and pass. In addition to the previously mention strategies, students said they used the following methods to guide their decisions:

"I read each question and each multiple-choice answer thoroughly. After reading each answer, I decide which one does not apply and choose what I feel is the best answer."

"I read the question once, then I re-read it slowly to make sure I understand what is being asked. I then look at the answers and pick the best one. If I am unsure what answer is correct, I look at each choice and think about why it may be right or wrong. I also stop and think about what information I know related to the question."

"I read the question and cover the answers. After understanding the question, I try to answer it without looking at the choices. If that doesn't work, I can always pull out two choices that sound right. Then, I review the facts pertaining to those two choices and make my decision."

"I narrow it down to the two likely answers and then use my knowledge to choose the best answer."

"I choose answers to test questions by applying learned knowledge with confidence, or if I'm not sure, I use an educated guess."

"When I take a test, I read the entire question and I then try to think of the answer before looking at the choices. If I see that my answer is one of the choices, then I immediately pick it and move on to the next question. I do not look at the other choices because I may start debating about changing my answer. If my answer is not a choice, then I re-read the question and choose the best choice by process of elimination."

"I choose answers by looking at the stem for what is specifically asked for or for a "clue." Also, if I can narrow down the possible choices, I go with my first response. With this technique, hopefully I won't come back and change my answer unless I get a "clue" further along in the exam."

"I read all of the answers and if I know the right one for sure, I pick it. If there are two or more answers that sound right, then I choose the most logical answer or guess. I eliminate answers that I know cannot possibly be correct."

Another student commented:

"My method of test taking includes reading the question and answering it on my own and choosing the corresponding multiple-choice answer. This prevents me from being confused by the other answers. If I don't know the answer immediately, I read the answer options and hope one answer will stand out as the correct choice based on my understanding of the topic. Then, if I am still unsure of the answer, I begin eliminating choices I know are wrong. I do this by using knowledge I have on the subject and by critically thinking to find a relationship between the question and the answer. If I still can't decide on an answer, I guess from among the answers that I have not eliminated and hope I guess correctly. My advice for taking an exam is to remain calm and think through the questions. Also, I remember that the correct answer is right there in front of me; I just have to recognize it."

These comments from students have a common theme of "process of elimination." In other words, delete choices that are untrue and that do not apply, and use basic knowledge to choose from among the other choices.

When these same students were asked what factors helped them choose the correct answer, they commonly mentioned:

Knowledge gained from lecture, class activities, text readings, and clinical experiences.

Study habits: reading and becoming familiar with the material.

Focusing on what the question is asking so that you do not miss the point and get it wrong.

Looking for answers you have heard before. If you have never heard of an answer choice, it is probably wrong (a distractor).

Looking for key words such as "always," "never," etc.

Asking these questions: Is the choice logical? Does it fit the scenario/situation? Does what I know about the subject relate to the choices?

Common Themes Summary

Overall, you can learn to recognize the importance of the circumstances within the question stem or scenario. By using knowledge gained through reading textbook assignments, reviewing case studies with practice questions, and then synthesizing the information, you can learn to choose the correct answer. Also, you can learn to identify the correct answer to a question as a result of direct patient care in the clinical area.

You can focus on the best answer by eliminating false or distractor items, which usually leaves two reasonable choices. If you use previous knowledge about the subject to identify important concepts and themes, you can then use critical thinking to choose the correct answer.

Scheduling Your Study Time Effectively

At some point during your education, you probably stayed up all night studying for an examination, took the examination, and returned to your room and slept. How much of the material did you remember later that day? Probably not much! Remember this, and keep in mind that cramming has no long-term benefit. You may remember the material for a few hours after you have studied, but probably not for the duration of the examination. Therefore, if you want to do well on the examination and in your career, you have to begin preparing early and *not* try to cram all the information into a few nights or hours of studying.

The following schedule will help you prepare for the NCLEX-RN without trying to learn and remember everything at the last minute. Not only should the studying you do prepare you for the examination, it should also provide an additional benefit—help you become a better nurse as you start your career.

Even though you do not know the exact day on which you will take the examination, you should be able to make a reasonable estimate that it will take place 4–6 weeks after you graduate, assuming that all of the required applications and fees have been submitted on time. You can certainly schedule the examination later if a different time would fit your work and personal schedules better. With an estimate of when you will likely take the test in mind, count backwards from that date 2–3 *months* and start doing the following activities:

1. Begin organizing your textbooks and class notes in a meaningful manner.
2. Begin making notes of the nursing subjects with which you feel least comfortable.
3. Begin learning more about the format and content of the examination as well as what will be expected of you. Review the first two chapters in this book as well as other material that describes the test; look at the format of items presented in this book and others; and talk to your instructors or friends who may have already taken the examination. Gain a thorough understanding of all facets of the NCLEX-RN.
4. Take a practice test that includes items similar to those likely to be on the actual NCLEX-RN to see how well you do and to assess your strengths and weaknesses.
5. Establish a study schedule that includes adequate time to prepare but also recognizes the need for flexibility, social activities, family or personal responsibilities, and so forth. You might consider developing a 3-month calendar on which you write down all known events or activities as well as reasonable study times (4–5 days per week with 1–3 hours of study per day). The number of times you study per week as well as the amount of time spent each day should be based on how well you did on the practice test, how confident you feel, and the number of weeks before the test that you start studying.

Starting *4–8 weeks before the examination,* you should:

1. Begin reviewing the areas of weakness first so that you will have time to review these areas again before the exam.
2. Develop, organize, and maintain your own notes in each subject for a final review before the examination.
3. Form a study group that meets once a week. Prepare specific topics and questions for discussion before each meeting.
4. Take at least one review test every few weeks to help you become more familiar with the type of items that might be asked as well as to reassess your performance.
5. After a month of studying, take the original pretest to see how well you are now doing. Have you improved in the areas that you were initially weak in? Have you maintained your knowledge in the areas you were initially strong in? Review the results and adjust your study schedule accordingly.
6. Develop your own situational questions as a technique for reviewing.
7. *As soon as you know your test date,* make reservations at a hotel or motel close to the site, preferably within walking distance, for the night before the examination. This

should particularly be done if you live more than 1 hour from the site and your examination is scheduled for the morning. Even if you have an afternoon administration, you should consider staying close to the site so that you are not rushed in the morning. Car problems, traffic, road repairs, and other delays can and do occur. Even if these events do not make you late for the examination, they will definitely increase your anxiety level.

8. Maintain sufficient time for eating, sleeping, exercising, socializing, and working. Do *not* become a study hermit!

One week before the examination, you need to:

1. Begin a concentrated *review* of the material.
2. Take the pretest for the last time and evaluate your performance.
3. Recite key ideas to yourself. Make sure you have memorized and understand all essential formulas, equations, and procedural steps.
4. Rest, eat well, and do not dwell on the test during your nonstudy times.
5. Make certain you have all documents required for admission to the examination. If you have any questions, call the Sylvan Technology Center where you will be taking the examination, Educational Testing Service, or your Board of Nursing office (see Appendix B). If you have doubts, take the time to obtain the correct information.

On the day before the examination:

1. Whether you are staying at a hotel or your own home, drive to the site to make certain you know exactly how to get there, how long the drive will take, and whether there is any road construction that might delay your travel.
2. Do something you enjoy during the day. Have a nice quiet dinner and relax that evening. Do not keep thinking about the test and whether or not you will do well.
3. If you are with colleagues who are taking the test, refrain from discussing it with them.
4. If you feel you absolutely have to review your notes, do so once and then not again. Do *not* keep returning to them.
5. Get sufficient sleep. You need to be both physically and mentally alert the next day.
6. Double-check to make certain you have all required documents for the next day.

Coping with the Actual Examination Administration

The examination day has finally arrived, and although you may be anxious or worried, you know you have prepared adequately, and you know how to maintain a helpful level of anxiety. Be confident as you start the day and try to follow these recommendations:

1. Get up early enough so that you are not rushed and can have a good breakfast. As a nurse, you have studied enough nutrition to know that breakfast is the most important meal of the day.
2. Wear comfortable clothes, preferably layered so that you can be comfortable regardless of the room temperature.
3. Make certain you have everything you need—your *Authorization to Test*, an official signed photographic iden-

tification as well as another piece of identification, money, directions to the site, something to do while waiting for the start of the examination, etc.

4. Arrive at the examination site on time, and preferably early. If you are driving, start at least one half to one hour *earlier* than you think is necessary in case an unexpected problem occurs. It is better to arrive early than late! If you are early, do not just sit and wait. Do something that will take your mind off the examination—read a book, do a crossword puzzle, or work on a craft.
5. Avoid discussing the examination with others who are waiting to take the examination. Leave your review notes and books at home or at the hotel.
6. Listen carefully to the instructions given before entering the testing room. If you have any questions, ask them now.

Most researchers have found that the greatest level of anxiety in a testing situation occurs while you wait for the test to begin or during the first few minutes of the examination. If you find this happening to you at the start of the test, or any time during the test, some rapid relaxation may be helpful. You should use this technique as soon as you are aware of feelings of anxiety. If you wait, these feelings may become heightened and more difficult to reduce.

One recommended method for rapid relaxation is:[9]

1. Close your eyes. As you sit in your chair, tense all your muscles. Really try to "scrunch up" as many muscles as you can.
2. Once you have tensed the muscles, take a deep breath (inhale through your nostrils) and hold your breath for a count of five, keeping your muscles tensed all the time.
3. After reaching the count of five, simultaneously exhale rapidly through your lips and quickly let go of your muscle tightness by silently telling yourself to *relax*.
4. With your eyes still closed, go as limp in the chair as you possibly can after relaxing.
5. Now, with your muscles relaxed, take a second deep breath through your nostrils. Hold your breath for a couple of seconds. Then *slowly* exhale through your lips.
6. As you exhale, repeat the word "calm" to yourself. You will probably repeat the word 7–10 times while slowly exhaling.
7. Repeat these steps once or twice to achieve greater relaxation. Each time through the steps will take approximately 30 seconds.

In addition to this relaxation technique, a number of other steps will help you remain calm during the examination:

1. As soon as the examination starts, jot down formulas or ideas that you think you might forget during the examination on the scratch paper provided.
2. Develop an *assertive* yet realistic attitude. Approach the test determined that you will do your best, but also accept the limits of what you know. Use everything you know to do well, but do not get angry with yourself if you are uncertain about the answer to a particular item.
3. Remember the guidelines on how to take multiple-choice tests.
4. Do not spend too much time thinking about alternative responses once you have selected the one you think is correct. At the same time, before striking the enter key a second time, quickly double-check your answer and the other options just to make certain you do not make a careless mistake.

5. Concentrate on the critical task—doing well on the examination—and give it your complete attention. Do not waste time worrying, doubting yourself, or wondering how others are doing. Do not become concerned if one or more candidates leave the testing room before you do. Do not worry about what you should have done; instead, concentrate on what you are doing now. Your only concern should be how well one person is doing and that person is *you.*

6. Budget your time. Although sufficient time has been allocated for the examination, you need to be aware of the time constraints. Wear a watch (turn off the alarm if you have one on your watch) and refer to it periodically, but do not be ruled by it. The watch should not become a distraction to your ability to concentrate. The computer screen will also display the time, but a watch is a better way to keep track of the time.

7. Do not permit lapses of memory to create unhealthy anxiety or fear; you are not expected to remember everything you learned in school.

8. Do not waste time with emotional reactions to the items. If you do not know the answer to an item, that is fine. Select the option that seems the most reasonable and proceed to the next item.

9. Above all, *remain confident* and resolve to work at top efficiency throughout the entire examination. Remain positive and convinced that you will do well.

At the conclusion of the examination, you should be pleased with your performance. Whether you took 1 hour or 5 hours to complete the examination is unimportant and not an indicator of how well you did. If you did well in school and prepared for the examination, you should have had no major problems with the questions asked. Now is not the time to worry about your performance because there is nothing you can do about the results except wait. Fortunately, the wait should not be very long, and within a few weeks you will know the actual outcome of your performance.

REFERENCES

1. Fiore, N and Pescar, SC: Conquering Test Anxiety. Werner Books, New York, 1987, p 43.
2. Sarason, IG (ed): Test Anxiety: Theory, Research and Application. Laurence Erlbaum Associates, Hillsdale, NJ, 1980, p 112.
3. Ottens, AJ: Coping with Academic Anxiety. The Rosen Publishing Group, New York, 1984, p 4.
4. Sarason, op cit.
5. Sarason, op cit, p 18
6. Sherman, TM and Wildman, TM: Proven Strategies for Successful Test Taking. Charles E. Merrill Publishing, Columbus, OH, 1982.
7. Kesselman-Turkel, J and Peterson, F: Test Taking Strategies. Contemporary Books, Chicago, 1981.
8. Fry, R: "Ace" Any Test. Career House, Hawthorne, NJ, 1992.
9. Ottens, op cit, p 91.

Clinical Specialties: Content Reviews and Tests

CHAPTER 3

Maternity Nursing: Content Review and Test

Sally B. Olds, MSN, RNC
Lizabeth L. Carlson, MSN, RNC, DNSc

The childbearing experience is a time of enormous change. The pregnant woman's body responds to the altered hormone levels even before the growing uterus is apparent. The expectant family changes and reorganizes as the couple plans for the addition of a new family member. The maternal-child nurse has an opportunity to provide teaching and support during this unique process that links us together, one generation to another.

Conception and the Maternal-Fetal Environment

Fertilization

1. **Gametogenesis** is a process in which germ cells are produced. The female gamete (ovum) is produced in the graafian follicle during oogenesis. The male gamete is produced in the seminiferous tubules of the testes during spermatogenesis.
2. **Meiosis** is a special process of cell division in gametes that reduces the number of chromosomes in each gamete to half of the normal 46 to 23. Therefore, each fertilized ovum will have half of its genetic material from the mother, and half from the father. Of the 23 chromosomes, one is a sex chromosome. The sex chromosome from the mother will always be an X chromosome. The sex chromosome from the father can be either an X or a Y chromosome.
3. Ovulation occurs 14 days before the beginning of the next menstrual cycle—day 14 of a 28-day cycle and day 20 of a 34-day cycle.
4. Conception occurs when the ovum and sperm unite in the outer one third of the fallopian tube. The fertilized ovum contains a total of 46 chromosomes (22 pairs of matched chromosomes and 2 sex chromosomes).

5. The fertilized ovum is called a **zygote**.
6. A female zygote is created if a sperm carrying an X chromosome fertilizes the ovum, which results in the zygote having the female sex chromosomes of XX; a male zygote occurs when the ovum is fertilized by a sperm carrying a Y chromosome, which results in the zygote having the male sex chromosomes of XY.
7. The zygote is transported through the fallopian tube by a fluid current.
8. The zygote changes through a process called **cleavage**.
9. The early cellular changes result in cells called the **morula, blastomere,** and **blastocyst**.
10. The developing fetus is called a **pre-embryo** for the first 2 weeks of gestation, an **embryo** from week 3 through week 8, and a **fetus** until the time of birth (Table 3–1).

Embryonic Membranes and Amniotic Fluid

1. The embryonic membranes, called the **amnion** and **chorion**, are formed at the time of implantation.
2. The membranes surrounding the growing embryo and fetus contain amniotic fluid, which is slightly alkaline in nature; its volume ranges from 500–1000 mL after 20 weeks of gestation. The fluid is constantly replaced.
3. The fetus swallows approximately 400–500 mL/day.
4. The fetus also "breathes" amniotic fluid in and out of the lungs.
5. Substances contained in the amniotic fluid include albumin, bilirubin, creatinine, fat, enzymes, epithelial cells, lecithin, and sphingomyelin.
6. The functions of the amniotic fluid are to:
   A. Provide a fluid cushion to prevent trauma
   B. Allow the fetus to move with ease
   C. Maintain the fetus at a uniform temperature
   D. Promote development of fetal lung tissue

		Table 3–1. **Fetal Development**		
Week of Gestation	Length	Weight	Appearance	Organ Development
1 wk		Free-floating blastocyst		
2–3 wk	2 mm crown to rump	Groove is formed along middle of back	Beginning of blood circulation Tubular heart	
4 wk	4–6 mm crown to rump	0.4 g	Noticeable limb buds	Tubular heart is beating
8 wk	3 cm crown to rump	2 g	Clearly resembles a human being	Eyelids begin to fuse. Circulatory system through umbilical cord is well established
12 wk	8 cm (3.2 inch)	45 g	Face well formed; limbs long and slender	Kidneys begin to form urine Spontaneous movements occur
16 wk	14 cm (5.9 inch)	200 g	Active movements present; fetal skin appears transparent	Skeletal ossification, lanugo hair develops. Sex of fetus can be determined visually
20 wk	19 cm (8 inch)	465 g	Lanugo covers entire body; skin less transparent	Has nails on fingers and toes; muscles well developed. Heartbeat can be detected by fetoscope. Woman can feel baby more
24 wk	28 cm crown to rump	780 g	Hair on head well formed; skin covering body is reddish and wrinkled	Reflex hand grasp; vernix caseosa covers entire body
28 wk	38 cm crown to heel	1200 g	Limbs well flexed	Brain develops rapidly; eyelids open and close; lungs still, physiologically immature. Eyes reopen
32 wk	30 cm	2000 g	Bones are fully developed but are soft and flexible	Lungs are not fully mature. Fetus begins storing iron, calcium, and phosphorus
36 wk	42–48 cm	2500 g	Body and extremities are "filling out." Fetus looks less wrinkled	Nails reach end of fingertips. Vernix continues to cover most of body
40 wk	48–52 cm	3000–3600 g	Skin is pinkish and smooth. Lanugo present on upper arms and shoulders	Vernix caseosa in creases and folds of skin. Fingernails extend beyond fingertips

Adapted from Olds, SB, London, ML, and Ladewig, PL: Maternal-Newborn Nursing: A Family Centered Approach, ed 3. Addison-Wesley, Menlo Park, CA, 1988; with permission.

E. Provide fluid for the fetus to swallow
F. Protect the fetal head during labor

Placenta

1. The placenta is an organ that provides metabolic and nutrient exchange between the maternal and fetal systems.
2. Placental development and circulation begin about 3 weeks after conception. The placenta is fully formed and functioning at 3 months of gestation.
3. At 40 weeks' gestation, the placenta contains 15–20 subdivisions called **cotyledons**, is about 6–8 inches in diameter, 1–1.2 inches thick, and weighs about one sixth the weight of the fetus.
4. The maternal surface of the placenta is red and fleshlike; the fetal surface is shiny and smooth.
5. The placenta produces four hormones:
   A. Progesterone
      (1) Is essential for pregnancy
      (2) Stimulates development of decidua
      (3) Decreases contractility of the uterus
   B. Estrogen or estriol
      (1) Stimulates proliferation of breast tissue and enlargement of the uterus

     (2) Stimulates uterine contractility
     (3) Depends on essential precursors from fetal adrenal glands for its production
   C. Human placental lactogen (HPL)
      (1) Is also called **human chorionic somatomammotropin**
      (2) Enhances maternal metabolism
   D. Human chorionic gonadotropin (HCG)
      (1) Stimulates corpus luteum to secrete estrogen and progesterone (corpus luteum functions to about the 11th week of pregnancy)
      (2) Exerts an effect on interstitial cells of testes to produce testosterone in the male fetus

Umbilical Cord

1. Cord attaches the fetus to the placenta.
2. It contains two arteries and one vein.
3. Umbilical vessels are surrounded by Wharton's jelly, which protects the cord from pressure and kinking.
4. Cord is approximately 50–55 cm in length.
5. It attaches to the center of the fetal side of the placenta. Occasionally the cord attaches to the edge of the placenta; this is called a **Battledore insertion.**

Fetal Circulation

1. Fetal circulation contains five unique structures (Fig. 3–1):
   A. **Umbilical vein:** carries oxygen and nutrients to the fetus
   B. **Two umbilical arteries:** carry deoxygenated blood and waste products from the fetus
   C. **Ductus venosus:** shunts the umbilical vein to the inferior vena cava, bypassing the liver and organs of digestion
   D. **Foramen ovale:** shunts blood from right atria to left atria, bypassing the ventricles and lungs
   E. **Ductus arteriosus:** shunts blood from pulmonary artery to aorta, bypassing the lungs

2. Fetal heart rate (FHR) is 110–160 bpm, or approximately twice the maternal heart rate.

Maternal Physiological Adaptations to Pregnancy

Cardiovascular System

1. Blood volume increases progressively during pregnancy until it is about 45% above prepregnant levels.
2. A 30%–50% increase in blood volume is due to increases in both plasma and red blood cells (RBCs).

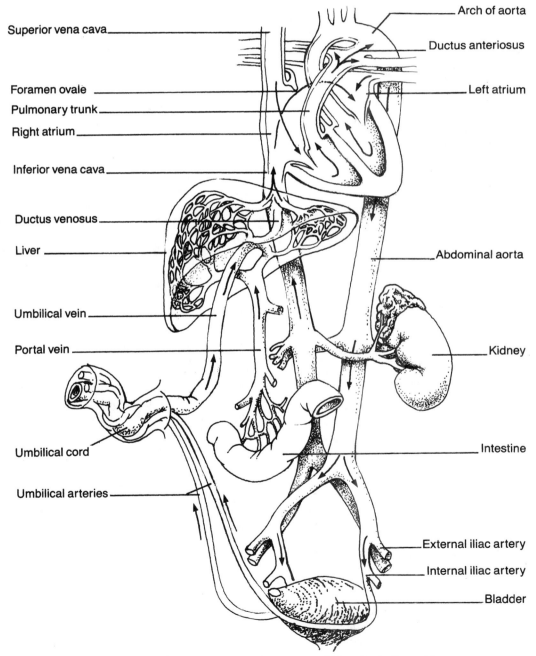

Figure 3–1. Diagram of the fetal circulation. The course of blood is indicated by arrows.

3. Pulse may increase about 10 bpm.
4. Blood pressure is lowered in second trimester, and then gradually increases in third trimester, but should not exceed prepregnant levels.
5. Total RBC volume increases by 20%.
6. Cardiac output increases by 20%–30%.
7. Hematocrit (HCT) remains above 35 mg/dL.
8. Hemoglobin may decrease to 10.5 g/dL because of hemodilution. This is called physiologic anemia. Iron supplementation is not necessary unless the hemoglobin falls below this level.
9. White blood cell (WBC) production increases as blood volume increases. Average WBC count is 10,000–11,000 WBC/mm^3 during pregnancy, with a peak of 25,000 WBC/mm^3 during labor.
10. Fibrin level of blood increases by about 40%.
11. Peripheral resistance increases.
12. Heart is pushed upward and to the left because of displacement of the diaphragm as the uterus enlarges.
13. The cerebrospinal fluid space decreases secondary to enlargement of the vessels surrounding the spinal cord.

Respiratory System

1. Pregnancy induces a small degree of hyperventilation, which causes a mild respiratory alkalosis.
2. O$_2$ consumption increases by about 15%–20% between the 16th and 40th week of gestation.
3. Vital capacity increases slightly.
4. Respiratory rate is essentially unchanged.
5. Diaphragm is elevated secondary to encroachment of the enlarging uterus. This can cause shortness of breath.

Gastrointestinal System

1. Gastrointestinal (GI) symptoms of nausea and vomiting are common in the first trimester because of secretion of HCG.
2. Alterations in taste and smell are common for many women.
3. Gum tissue may become soft, swollen, and bleed easily. The gum changes are estrogen related.
4. Gastric emptying time and intestinal mobility is delayed, which leads to bloating and constipation.
5. Hemorrhoids may occur later in pregnancy secondary to increased venous pressure.
6. Appendix is displaced upward and to the right, away from McBurney's point. This makes diagnosis of appendicitis difficult.

Urinary Tract

1. Urinary frequency occurs in first trimester secondary to pressure of enlarging uterus on the bladder. Near the end of the pregnancy, the weight of the uterus once again causes pressure on the bladder, resulting in urinary frequency.
2. Dilation of the kidneys, renal pelvis, and ureters may occur, especially on the right side, because of the elevated progesterone levels, and pressure of the enlarging uterus.
3. Glomerular filtration rate and renal plasma flow increase early in pregnancy.
4. Glycosuria may occur because of increased glomerular filtration.

5. Clearance of creatinine and urea increases secondary to increased renal function.
6. Side-lying position of mother increases excretion of H$_2$O and Na$^+$.

Endocrine System

1. Thyroid gland has increased vascularity and hyperplasia, which is associated with increased circulating estrogens.
2. Basal metabolic rate rises to +25% in late pregnancy. The increase is associated with the increased demands of fetus and uterus and with increased oxygen consumption.
3. Size of parathyroids increases. The increase parallels fetal calcium needs.
4. Pituitary gland enlarges slightly.
5. Circulating cortisol levels are increased because of increased estrogen levels. The cortisol levels regulate carbohydrate and protein metabolism.

Reproductive System

Uterus

1. Uterus enlarges primarily as a result of an increase in size of myometrial cells.
2. Uterus changes from a prepregnant size of 7.5 × 5 × 2.5 cm, a weight of 60 g (2 oz), and a capacity of 10 mL, to 28 × 24 × 21 cm, a weight of 1000 g (2.2 lb), and a capacity of 5000 mL.
3. The size and number of the blood vessels and lymphatics increase greatly during the pregnancy.
4. Irregular contractions (called **Braxton Hicks sign**) occur throughout pregnancy, but may not be noticed by the pregnant woman until the third trimester. These contractions must be differentiated from regular (true) contractions, which result in cervical dilation.

Cervix

1. Endocervical glands secrete a thick, tenacious mucus plug. The plug is expelled from the endocervical canal when cervical dilation begins.
2. Increased vascularization causes softening of the cervix, which is called **Goodell's sign**. This softening also causes easy flexion of the uterus against the cervix called **McDonald's sign**. The cervix takes on a blue-purple coloration, also caused by increased vascularization, which is called **Chadwick's sign**.

Ovaries

1. Ovaries cease ovum production.
2. Corpus luteum persists until the 10th–12th week of pregnancy.

Vagina and Labia

1. Hypertrophy of vaginal epithelium occurs.
2. Increased vascularization and hyperplasia occur.
3. Vaginal secretions, which are thick, white, and acidic, increase.
4. Vaginal cells contain higher levels of glycogen, which predisposes the pregnant woman to vaginal yeast infections.
5. Increase in blood flow results in blue-purple color in labia and vagina (**Chadwick's sign**).

Breasts

1. Breast size increases.
2. Superficial veins become prominent.
3. Nipples become more erectile.
4. Hypertrophy of Montgomery's tubercules occurs.
5. Colostrum may leak from breasts in last trimester of the pregnancy.

Skin

Increased levels of melanocyte-stimulating hormone stimulate pigmentation changes.

1. Pigmentation of skin may increase in areola, the nipples, the vulva, the perineal area, and the linea alba. The increase in pigmentation of the line from the umbilicus to the pubis is called the linea nigra.
2. Seventy percent of women develop pigmentation over the forehead, cheeks, and nose. This is called **chloasma,** or mask of pregnancy.
3. Striae (reddish purple stretch marks) may occur on the abdomen, breasts, thighs, and upper arms.
4. Vascular spider nevi may develop on neck, chest, face, arms, and legs.
5. Hair growth rate may decrease due to estrogen effects.

Skeletal System

1. Relaxation of the joints of the pelvis is caused by relaxin, a hormone secreted during pregnancy.
2. Woman's center of gravity changes during pregnancy.
3. Posture changes and lordosis occur as pregnancy advances.

Metabolism

1. Most metabolic functions accelerate during the pregnancy.
2. If a woman is at a normal weight for her height, the recommended weight gain is 25–35 lb (3.5 lb in first trimester and a little less than a pound a week in the second and third trimesters) (Table 3–2).
3. Increased levels of estrogen, lowered serum protein, and increased intracapillary pressure and permeability cause water retention.
4. Fats are more completely absorbed.
5. Nitrogen retention is increased early in pregnancy and continues to increase in the second and third trimesters.
6. Iron demand is increased because of the increase in RBCs, hemoglobin, blood volume, and increased tissue needs.
7. Iron transfer through the placenta is toward the fetus. Five sixths of iron stored in fetal liver is accumulated after the 26th week of pregnancy.

Table 3–2. **Distribution of Total Weight Gain**	
Fetus	7.5 lb
Placenta and membranes	1.5 lb
Amniotic fluid	2 lb
Uterus	2.5 lb
Breasts	3 lb
Increased blood volume	3–4 lb
Extravascular fluid and fat reserves	5.5–14.5 lb
Total	25–35 lb

8. Calcium is progressively absorbed and retained throughout pregnancy.

Maternal Psychological Adaptation to Pregnancy

1. Pregnancy is viewed as a developmental stage.
2. The woman's response varies according to her own emotional makeup, her sociocultural background, her support system, and her acceptance or rejection of the pregnancy.
3. Psychological responses include ambivalence, acceptance, introversion, mood swings, and body image changes.
   A. **Ambivalence:** This feeling occurs early in the pregnancy and is common even when the pregnancy is planned.
   B. **Acceptance:** When a woman accepts the pregnancy, she tends to display happiness and pleasure and experiences fewer physical discomforts.
   C. **Introversion:** A turning inward is common to pregnant women as they attend to planning for and adjusting to the new baby.
   D. **Mood swings:** The extent of mood swings ranges from ecstasy to great despair. Mood swings are more prevalent in early pregnancy as hormone levels increase.
   E. **Body image changes:** Pregnancy is associated with marked changes in a woman's body. These physical changes affect how a woman views herself as well as how she perceives others to view her.
4. **Maternal role transition:** the steps a woman takes toward becoming a mother.
   A. The first step is **mimicry,** where the woman observes and copies behaviors of pregnant women and mothers. Mimicry often starts in the first trimester.
   B. **Role-play** is when the woman acts out mothering behaviors. She may ask to hold another woman's baby. The pregnant woman is very sensitive to the responses of others as she role-plays.
   C. **Fantasy** is daydreaming about how she will act as a mother with her own child. They may be pleasant or unpleasant.
   D. **Looking for a role fit** occurs after the pregnant woman has developed role expectations of a "good" mother for herself. She then compares her self-expectations to behaviors she observes in other mothers and either accepts or rejects those behaviors.
   E. Finally, **Grief work** is the process of the woman giving up certain roles and images of herself that will permanently change once she has her baby. This step is necessary so she can take on her new identity as a mother.
5. **Maternal tasks of pregnancy:** There are four maternal tasks of pregnancy as the pregnant woman forms a relationship with her fetus, and rearranges family relationships.
   A. **Seeking safe passage** is the most important task for the woman. It is the process of ensuring the safety of herself and her fetus through pregnancy and birth by obtaining prenatal care, and following the traditional practices of her culture as they relate to pregnancy, birth, and the postpartum period.
   B. **Securing acceptance** of the pregnancy and baby from other family members includes reworking family relationships so that the woman's new role as a mother and the new baby is welcomed as a family member.
   C. **Learning to give of self** is a task that must be learned

by a pregnant woman. The process starts when the woman learns she is pregnant and allows the embryo/fetus to grow and develop within her body. Pregnant women learn to give by both giving and receiving. Baby showers are an important way for the pregnant woman to validate pleasure in giving and receiving.

D. **Committing herself to the unborn child.** This maternal task of pregnancy is also known as developing attachment to the fetus. It is the only maternal task that starts in the first trimester and does not end until the end of the newborn period. This task is also called "binding in" to the pregnancy. Events that make the fetus more real, such as seeing the fetus on sonogram, feeling fetal movement, or hearing the fetal heart beat, result in the woman feeling surges of love for the fetus. The woman feels protective of her fetus, and has increased feelings of vulnerability. The woman starts to take pleasure in thinking about her new role as a mother.

The Antepartal Period

Nursing Process in the First Trimester (Months 1–3)

Assessment

Nursing History

1. Current history
   A. First day of last normal menstrual period
   B. Whether complications such as bleeding or cramping are present
   C. Woman's feelings about the pregnancy
2. Past pregnancy history
   A. Number of pregnancies, abortions, and stillbirths
   B. Course of previous pregnancies
   C. Woman's blood type and Rh factor
3. Family medical history
   A. Presence of chronic disease such as diabetes, cardiovascular disease, pulmonary disease, and/or pregnancy-induced hypertension (PIH)
   B. Family history of multiple births
4. Past medical history
   A. Childhood diseases/immunizations
   B. Previous illnesses or hospitalizations
5. Current medical history
   A. Current weight, prepregnant weight
   B. Medications currently being taken
   C. Current intake of caffeine and alcohol; tobacco use
   D. Substance use/abuse
   E. Presence of any disease conditions

Signs and Symptoms of Pregnancy

SUBJECTIVE (PRESUMPTIVE)

1. Amenorrhea
2. Nausea and vomiting
3. Urinary frequency
4. Breast tenderness
5. Quickening

OBJECTIVE (PROBABLE)

1. Changes in pelvic organs—Goodell's sign, Chadwick's sign, Hegar's sign, uterine enlargement
2. Enlargement of abdomen
3. Braxton Hicks contractions
4. Uterine souffle
5. Pigmentation of the skin
6. Abdominal striae
7. Ballottement

DIAGNOSTIC TESTS/METHODS (FOR POSITIVE SIGNS)

1. Fetal heartbeat by Doppler at 10–12 weeks and by fetoscope at 18–20 weeks (normal rate ranges between 110–160 bpm).
2. Fetal movement felt by trained examiner
3. Fetal electrocardiogram
4. Ultrasound exam that visualizes gestational sac, fetal heart, or fetal parts

Psychosocial, Developmental, and Cultural Assessment

1. Parents may experience disbelief regarding pregnancy.
2. Mother may display emotional lability—unexplained crying, anger, depression, ambivalent feelings.
3. Partner may have increased energy as virility is confirmed by wife's pregnancy.
4. Father may suffer physiological symptoms with mother; this is called **couvade.** Symptoms include nausea, vomiting, and fatigue.
5. Some view pregnancy as an illness.
6. Mother may become dependent and introspective.

Planning

1. Safe, effective care environment
   A. Provide education regarding environmental safety.
2. Physiological integrity
   A. Promote maternal-fetal well-being.
3. Psychosocial integrity
   A. Promote psychosocial adaptation.
4. Health promotion and maintenance
   A. Promote self-care activities.

Implementation

1. Obtain complete health history.
2. Determine gravidity (number of pregnancies) and parity (number of pregnancies that progressed past 20 weeks' gestation).
   A. **Nulligravida:** a woman who has never been pregnant
   B. **Primigravida:** a woman who is pregnant for the first time
   C. **Multigravida:** a woman in at least her second pregnancy
3. Determine parity (number of births past 20 weeks' gestation, whether the fetus was born alive or not).
   A. **Nullipara:** a woman who has not had a birth at more than 20 weeks of gestation
   B. **Primipara:** a woman who has had one birth that occurred after the 20th week of gestation
   D. **Multipara:** a woman who has had more than one birth after 20 weeks of gestation
4. Record obstetrical history using GTPAL method (G = gravida; T = term birth, i.e., 38–42 weeks of gestation;

P = preterm birth, i.e., after 20 weeks and before 37 completed weeks of gestation; A = abortions, spontaneous and therapeutic; L = living children).

Example

A pregnant woman has had three prior term pregnancies. One of these pregnancies was twins, with one twin dead at the time of birth.

G = 4 (current pregnancy and 3 others)

T = 3 (twins count for 1 pregnancy, and 2 other pregnancies)

P = 0 (no birth occurred prior to 37 weeks)

A = 0 (no abortions reported)

L = 3 (2 living children from singleton births, 1 living child from the twin pregnancy). The stillborn child is not counted.

The above example could also be recorded as Gravida and Para: G_4, P_3.

5. Calculate expected date of birth (EDB) using Nägele's rule. Historically, this term was called expected date of confinement (EDC). Or it may be referred to as the estimated date of delivery (EDD). Be sure to calculate the EDB from the last *normal* menses. Some women may have light spotting or bleeding for a few days approximately 3 weeks after their previous normal menses. This is probably when implantation occurred. Nägele's rule: subtract 3 months from the first day of the last normal menstrual period, add 7 days, change the year (if necessary).

Example

A woman is currently pregnant. The 1st day of her last normal menstrual period (LMP) was September 2.

September −	(9th month) 3 months	2 days	of the current year
June +	(6th month)	7 days	of the current year
June		9 (EDB)	of the next year

---

6. Complete physical assessment
   A. Obtain weight.
   B. Check blood pressure, pulse, respirations.
   C. Examine breasts by inspection and palpation.
   D. Examine abdomen by inspection, auscultation, percussion, and palpation.
   E. Examine external genitalia.
   F. Perform speculum examination.
      (1) Inspect cervix.
      (2) Obtain Pap smear.
      (3) Inspect vaginal mucosa.
   G. Perform bimanual abdominovaginal palpation.
      (1) Palpate uterus and cervix.
      (2) Assess cul-de-sac and the adnexal area.
   H. Obtain smears for gonorrhea.
7. Assist in obtaining laboratory specimens.
   A. Collect urine for urinalysis, and also assess for glycosuria and proteinuria.
   B. Collect blood specimen for Venereal Disease Research Laboratory (VDRL) (syphilis test), complete blood count (CBC), HCT, blood type and Rh, and rubella titer (>1:10 indicates immunity).

8. Assess fundal height (Fig. 3–2).
9. Auscultate fetal heart. May hear with Doppler as early as 10–12 weeks.
10. Determine whether expectant woman is in high-risk category or is at risk for preterm labor (Tables 3–3 and 3–4).
11. Provide nutritional teaching:
    A. Assess current 24-hour intake.
    B. Assess current knowledge of nutrition and needs during pregnancy.
    C. Provide teaching based on identified needs. Include information on need for eating foods from the food pyramid daily, on increasing caloric intake 300 cal/day, on increasing protein intake to 60 g/day, and on minimum weight gain of 3–4 lb in the first trimester and 21–22 lb in the second and third trimesters.
    D. Vitamin intake should be increased, especially folic acid. Sources of folic acid include legumes, green leafy vegetables, eggs, milk, and whole-grain breads (Table 3–5).
12. Provide information regarding exercise. Advise that high-impact exercise and use of hot tubs or saunas are not recommended during pregnancy.
13. Provide counseling regarding work. Work can usually continue unless it involves heavy lifting or exposure to environmental dangers.

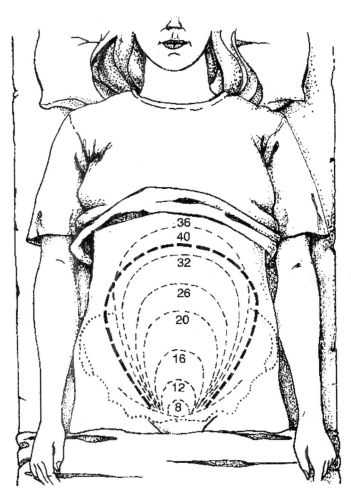

Figure 3–2. Approximate height of the fundus at various weeks of pregnancy. (Adapted from Olds, SB, London, ML, and Ladewig, PL: Maternal Newborn Nursing: A Family Centered Approach, ed 4. Addison-Wesley, Redwood City, CA, 1992, p 300.)

Table 3-3. Factors That Place the Pregnancy at Risk

Elevated blood pressure
Cardiac problems or presence of kidney or respiratory diseases
Beginning the pregnancy at a weight > 200 lb or < 100 lb
Age younger than 16 or older than 35
Consumption of alcohol on frequent basis or use of drugs
Smoking one pack of cigarettes a day or more
Malnutrition

Table 3-4. Factors That Increase the Risk of Preterm Birth

Age younger than 18 or older than 40
Previous abortions
Work outside the home, especially if it is heavy or stressful
Weight gain of < 5 kg (11 lb) by 32 weeks of gestation
Presence of a multiple pregnancy
Previous preterm birth

14. Provide information regarding danger signs of pregnancy (Table 3–6).
15. Provide information regarding common discomforts of pregnancy and self-care measures (Table 3–7).
16. Advise that prenatal visits will usually be scheduled:
    Every 4 weeks for first 28 weeks of gestation
    Every 2–3 weeks from 28–36 weeks
    Thereafter, every week until birth
17. Provide information regarding possible first-trimester testing (Table 3–8).
18. Provide counseling related to childbirth education.
    A. Classes provide information related to changes of pregnancy, the course of labor and birth; exercises to prepare the body for birth; methods of relaxation, focusing, and controlled breathing to use during labor and birth.
    B. The most common childbirth preparation techniques are those of the American Society for Psychoprophylaxis in Obstetrics (Lamaze); Bradley, and Kitzenger methods.

19. Provide counseling regarding substances.
    A. Do not take any medications unless prescribed or approved by the health care provider. This includes over-the-counter preparations.
    B. If mother or those close around her smoke, encourage them to attend a smoking cessation program. If smoking continues, encourage woman and others to cut down number of cigarettes per day and to avoid smoking in enclosed areas (the house, a car, etc.). This will prevent the pregnant woman from inhaling secondhand smoke and its harmful substances.
20. Provide counseling and support regarding sexuality and pregnancy.
    A. Sexual activity may continue in low-risk pregnancies.
    B. The woman's sexual desires may increase (especially in the second trimester), or decrease as hormone levels change, genital tissues become engorged, and common discomforts are experienced.

Evaluation

Ensure that:
1. The expectant woman and her partner verbalize understanding of environmental risks.
2. The expectant woman and her fetus are within normal limits during first trimester.
3. The expectant family is accepting of the pregnancy.
4. The expectant woman is knowledgeable regarding self-care activities.

Nursing Process in the Second Trimester (Months 4–6)

Assessment

Physical Assessment

Assess for signs that pregnancy is progressing normally:
1. Weight gain has been 3–4 lb in first trimester and averages 4 lb/mo in second trimester. Weight gain should not exceed 1 lb/wk.

Table 3-5. Maternal Nutrition of Pregnancy and Lactation

	While Pregnant		While Breast-Feeding	Food Source
	15–18 yr	*19+ yr*		
Calories	2400 (300 cal more than calorie intake before pregnancy)	2300 (300 cal more than calorie intake before pregnancy)	+500 cal above prepregnant levels	
Protein	46 g	44 g		Meat, poultry, fish, eggs, legumes, milk, tofu
Calcium	1600 mg	1200 mg	+400 mg above prepregnant levels	Milk, legumes, seafood, tofu, dark-green leafy vegetables
Iron	18 mg+	18 mg+	Cannot be met by diet intake; must be supplemented with 30–60 mg supplemental iron	Lean meats, dark-green leafy vegetables, eggs and whole-grain breads, cereals, dried fruits
Folic acid	400 μg	400 μg	400 μg. Cannot be met by diet alone. All women should eat a diet that includes foods high in folic acid and take a supplement containing 400 μg of folic acid daily.	Liver, dark-green leafy vegetables

Table 3–6. Danger Signs of Pregnancy

Danger Signs	Conditions That May Be Indicated
Sudden gush of clear fluid from vagina	Premature rupture of the amniotic membranes
Bleeding from the vagina	Abruptio placentae, placenta previa Cervical lesions "Bloody show"
Persistent vomiting	Hyperemesis gravidarum
Severe headache and/or blurring of vision, or spots before the eyes	Hypertension, pre-eclampsia
Abdominal pain	Premature labor, abruptio placentae
Oral temperature greater than 101°F (38.3°C)	Infection
Swelling of lower legs, hands, and face	PIH
Absence of fetal movement	Fetal death

2. Blood pressure is lower than prepregnant levels.
3. Nausea and vomiting have ceased.
4. Breast tenderness is noted.
5. Urinary frequency is abnormal in the second trimester.
6. Fundus reaches level of umbilicus at approximately 20 weeks' gestation.

7. Primiparous woman feels fetal movement (quickening) at 18–20 weeks. A multiparous woman may feel quickening as early as 16 weeks.
8. FHR is auscultated by fetoscope at 18–20 weeks. Rate remains between 110–160 bpm.

Psychosocial and Cultural Assessment

1. Pregnancy is validated through maternal description of positive signs (enlarging uterus, quickening, etc.).
2. Woman announces pregnancy by verbal report and/or wearing maternity clothes.
3. Woman becomes reflective and introspective as she continues to progress in maternal role transition.

Planning

1. Safe, effective care environment
   A. Provide counseling regarding environmental safety for the expectant woman and a safe intrauterine environment for the fetus.
2. Physiological integrity
   A. Promote maternal-fetal well-being.
3. Psychosocial integrity
   A. Promote maternal psychosocial adaptation.
4. Health promotion and maintenance
   A. Encourage self-care activities.

Table 3–7. Common Discomforts of Pregnancy

Common Discomfort	Trimester When it Usually Occurs	Cause	Self-Care Measure
Nausea and vomiting	1st	Presence of HCG; altered carbohydrate levels	Eat crackers before arising; eat small frequent meals; avoid spicy or greasy foods.
Urinary frequency	1st and 3rd	Mechanical compression of bladder	Drink 2 qt fluid per day.
Fatigue	1st and 3rd	Absence of relaxing, stress of pregnancy on body	Arrange frequent rest periods during the day.
Tenderness of breasts	1st through 3rd	Presence of increased estrogen, increased progesterone, increased breast size	Wear supportive bra.
Tender, swollen gums	1st through 3rd	Increased estrogen level, dental hygienic practices	Use soft toothbrush, brush 2–3×/day; floss daily; maintain good nutrition.
Clear vaginal mucus discharge	1st through 3rd	Increased estrogen levels, increased vascularity of cervix and vagina, increased cervical mucus	Avoid douching; bathe frequently; wear cotton-crotch underwear.
Nasal stuffiness	1st through 3rd	Increased estrogen; swelling of nasal tissues, dryness	Use humidifier in house; avoid use of nasal sprays or antihistamines.
Heartburn	2nd and 3rd	Increased progesterone, decreased GI motility, displacement of stomach by enlarging uterus	Eat small frequent meals; sit upright for 30 min following a meal; avoid fatty, greasy, spicy foods.
Varicose veins	2nd and 3rd	Venous congestion, vasodilation	Elevate legs frequently during the day; wear supportive hose; avoid crossing the legs while sitting.
Ankle edema	2nd and 3rd	Increased capillary permeability, vasodilation, increased venous pressure below uterus	Elevate feet during the day; wear supportive stockings; avoid cuts or abrasions to legs and feet.
Hemorrhoids	2nd and 3rd	Constipation, venous engorgement	Increase exercise (for instance, walking); maintain fluid intake at 2–3 L/day; increase fiber in diet.
Constipation	2nd and 3rd	Increased progesterone levels, decreased intestinal motility	As listed above.
Backache	2nd and 3rd	Increased curvature of back as pregnancy advances	Wear low-heeled shoes; do pelvic lift exercises every day; practice good body mechanics.
Leg cramps	2nd and 3rd	Altered calcium-phosphorus balance	Do not use milk as only source of calcium; release cramp by dorsiflexion.

Table 3–8. Testing During First Trimester

	Sonogram	Chorionic Villus Sampling
Description	Ultrasound visualization of the fetus, uterus, placenta	Aspiration of tissue from the placenta site
Purpose	1. Validate pregnancy. 2. Determine fetal viability. 3. Ascertain fetal age, position. 4. Determine placental position.	To collect fetal cells for chromosomal observation
Nursing plan and intervention	1. Explain procedure. 2. Provide preprocedure fluids; encourage bladder fullness for improved visualization. 3. Assure that procedure is painless. 4. Encourage partner to be present. 5. Provide photograph of fetus, if possible. 6. Explain that there are no postprocedure problems or treatment.	1. Explain procedure. 2. Validate that informed consent has been signed. 3. Provide reassurance during procedure. 4. Monitor maternal vital signs every 5 min for at least 30 min. Monitor FHR. 5. Provide postprocedure instructions. —Rest for 12–24 hr. —Report uterine cramping. —Report vaginal bleeding and elevated temperature.

Implementation

1. Document expected changes in pregnancy, and report abnormalities to physician.
2. Auscultate FHR. Note funic souffle (blowing sound created by blood coursing through umbilical vessels in umbilical cord) and uterine souffle (blowing sound created by blood coursing through placental vessels). Funic souffle is the same as the FHR; uterine souffle is the same rate as the maternal pulse.
3. Determine fundal height.
4. Determine need for further teaching and counseling.
5. Review prenatal exercises such as Kegel, squatting, tailor sitting, and pelvic rock.
6. Provide opportunity for questions.
7. Provide counseling and support.

Evaluation

Ensure that:
1. The expectant woman verbalizes understanding of environmental risks to herself and her baby.
2. The expectant woman and her fetus is within normal limits during second trimester.
3. The expectant woman validates the pregnancy and becomes introspective.
4. The expectant woman is using self-care measures to promote health and relieve common discomforts.

Nursing Process in the Third Trimester (Months 7–9)

Assessment

Physical Assessment

Assess for signs that pregnancy is progressing normally:
1. Weight gain has been approximately 16 lb by the beginning of the 7th month.
2. Weight continues at about 3.5–4 lb/mo or approximately 1 lb/wk.
3. FHR continues at 110–160 bpm.
4. Fundal height increases at appropriately 1 cm per week of gestation.
5. Expectant woman monitors fetal activity.
6. Urinary frequency returns late in third trimester.
7. Vaginal secretions remain clear and watery.
8. Blood pressure may rise slightly but does not exceed +30 mm Hg systolic or 90 mm Hg diastolic.
9. No proteinuria or glycosuria.
10. Only slight edema of feet and ankles, which is relieved by elevation.

Psychosocial and Cultural Assessment

1. Woman has increased anxiety related to fear of body mutilation, fear of labor and birth process, and her ability to cope successfully.
2. Woman verbalizes wish to end the pregnancy.
3. Expectant father may be anxious regarding his ability to cope with labor and fears of losing his partner.
4. Woman prepares place for infant within the home.

Planning

1. Safe, effective care environment
   A. Provide opportunities for expectant couple to tour birthing facilities.
   B. Discuss progress of couple in childbirth education program.
2. Physiological integrity
   A. Discuss changes in third trimester and during birth process.
   B. Demonstrate methods of assessing fetal activity.
3. Psychosocial integrity
   A. Provide opportunities for counseling and discussion of psychosocial aspects.
4. Health promotion and maintenance
   A. Review self-care activities.
   B. Provide opportunities to discuss parenting activities that will promote infant health.

Implementation

1. Document expected changes in pregnancy, and report abnormalities to physician.
2. Auscultate FHR.
3. Determine fundal height.
4. Determine fetal presentation and position (Fig. 3–3).
5. Determine need for further teaching and counseling.
6. Provide time to discuss parental wishes regarding labor and birth.
7. Provide counseling and support.
8. Teach method of monitoring fetal activity. To increase the woman's understanding, demonstrate the method and how to fill out the record. During subsequent visits, review the record with the expectant woman, and provide opportunities for questions and discussion.

9. Provide information regarding:
   A. Signs of pregnancy complications
   B. Signs of labor
   C. When to go to the birthing area
   D. When to contact the physician or certified nurse-midwife
   E. Concerns of siblings
10. Review tests that may be done in late pregnancy (Table 3–9).

Evaluation

Ensure that the expectant woman and/or her partner:
1. Tours birthing facilities and feels acquainted with surroundings.

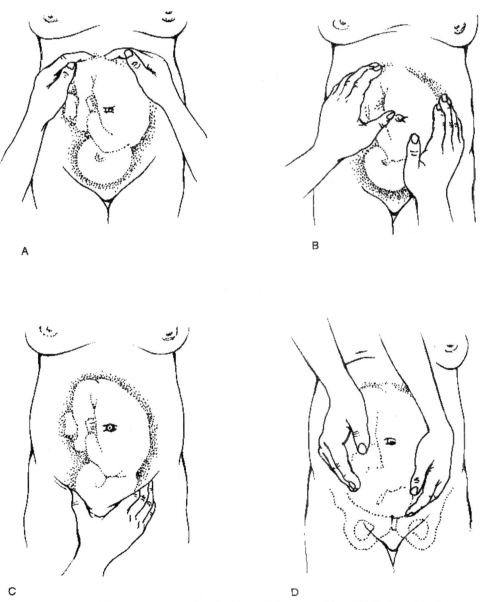

A   B   C   D

Figure 3–3. Leopold's maneuvers of palpation of fetal position. (*A*) Determine fetal part in fundus. (*B*) Determine whether back is on the right or the left side. (*C*) Determine fetal part in the pelvic inlet. (*D*) Estimate degree of descent.

Table 3–9. Testing During Third Trimester	
Test	Purpose
Sonogram	To assess fetal size, monitor growth, or determine positions To assess internal structures such as kidneys, bladder To locate the placenta prior to other procedures or to determine the presence of a problem such as placenta previa To locate a pocket of amniotic fluid, to assess amount of fluid, and to enable physician to "tap" fluid by amniocentesis for further testing To assess placental maturity
Amniocentesis	To aspirate fluid from uterus in order to do further testing for fetal lung maturity, such as L/S ratio, presence of P6, creatinine level

2. Attends childbirth education program.
3. Can list signs/symptoms of pregnancy complications
4. Can verbalize expected changes in third trimester and during birth.
5. Maintains fetal activity records.
6. Has opportunity to ask questions and receive support.
7. Is practicing self-care activities.
8. Begins to speak of parental–infant-care activities.

Assessment Techniques for High-Risk Pregnancy

Maternal Assessment of Fetal Activity

Description

This is a method of assessing the number of fetal movements for a specified amount of time each day. It is based on the knowledge that fetal activity occurs frequently throughout the day and that a sudden change in activity may signal distress in the fetus.

Nursing Care

1. Teach a method of assessing fetal activity.
2. Ask for return demonstration in method of assessment and completing the record.
3. Discuss record at each visit.

Doppler Blood-Flow Studies (Umbilical Velocimetry)

Description

An ultrasound beam is directed at the umbilical artery and/or a maternal vessel such as the arcuate. The resulting picture shows a waveform that can be interpreted.

Findings

To interpret the waveforms, the systolic (S) peak (the highest peak) is divided by the end diastolic (D) component (the lowest component). Normal systolic-to-diastolic (S/D) ratio is 2.8

at 20 weeks' gestation, with a slow decline to 2.2 at term (38–42 weeks).

An abnormal S/D ratio is considered to be 3.0 and above. This higher ratio is caused by narrowing of the vessels and reflects decreased uteroplacental perfusion.

Nursing Care

1. Explain test and possible results.
2. Carefully administer the test.

   NOTE: Test is performed by nurse with advanced skills.

3. Evaluate results.
4. Communicate results to parents.

Nonstress Test

Description

The nonstress test (NST) is based on the knowledge that fetal activity results in an acceleration of the FHR in a normal fetus. Acceleration of the FHR suggests that the fetus has an intact central and autonomic nervous system that is not affected by intrauterine hypoxia. NST is frequently done in the last 8 weeks of pregnancy (Table 3–10).

Findings

Reactive test: At least two accelerations that are at least 15 bpm above the baseline fetal heart rate, and last at least 15 seconds, are present in a ten-minute time period.
Nonreactive test: Accelerations are not present, or do not meet the criteria for reactivity.

Nursing Care

1. Explain test procedure and possible findings.
2. Complete test.
3. Evaluate findings.
4. Communicate test results to woman.

Biophysical Profile

Description

The biophysical profile is an assessment of five biophysical variables: fetal breathing movement, fetal movements of body or limbs, amniotic fluid volume, and reactive FHR (accelerations with fetal movement). Each variable is assigned a score of 0, 1, or 2, and the maximum score is 10.

Findings

Ten of 10 or 8 of 10 with normal amniotic fluid volume: No intervention is needed.

Eight of 10 with abnormal amniotic fluid volume: If fetal renal function is normal and amniotic membranes are intact, delivery is indicated.

Six of 10 with normal amniotic fluid volume: If fetus is mature, then delivery is indicated; if fetus is immature, repeat test in 24 hours. If score at that time is 6 of 10 or below, deliver fetus.

Four of 10, 2 of 10, or 1 of 10: Deliver fetus.

Table 3–10. Fetal Evaluation Techniques		
	Nonstress Testing (NST)	**Contraction/Stress Test (CST)**
Description	Fetal response to active and passive states is recorded for 10-min period.	Fetal response is induced. Uterine activity is recorded for a 90–120 min period.
Purpose	Determines fetal response to cyclical periods of rest and activity. Normally, fetal movement will accelerate the FHR by ≥ 15 bpm, lasting ≥ 15 sec.	Determines the presence of uteroplacental or fetal pathology. A negative (normal) response is the absence of late deceleration of FHR with uterine contractions. A positive (abnormal) response is the presence of late deceleration with uterine contractions.
Nursing plan and intervention	1. Explain procedure. 2. Apply external fetal and maternal monitoring devices to maternal abdomen. 3. Place mother in semi-Fowler's position, turned slightly to left. 4. Monitor maternal blood pressure every 5–10 min. 5. Ensure the adequate recording of FHR and/or uterine activity. 6. Inform parents of findings.	1. Explain procedure. 2. Apply external fetal and maternal monitoring devices to maternal abdomen. 3. Place mother in semi-Fowler's position, turned slightly to left. 4. Monitor maternal blood pressure and contractions every 15 min or with each increase of IV oxytocin (Pitocin). 5. Administer oxytocin IV drip as ordered. Follow agency protocol. 6. Ensure adequate recording of uterine activity and FHR. 7. Inform parents of findings.

Nursing Care

1. Explain test and possible results.
2. Carefully administer test.

    NOTE: Nurses with advanced skills should perform test.

3. Provide support to parents during testing.
4. Explain test results.

Contraction Stress Test

Description

The contraction stress test (CST) is a means of evaluating the fetus's ability to withstand the stress of uterine contractions. When fetal or placental problems exist, late decelerations occur with contractions. The test may be accomplished by a breast self-stimulation test or oxytocin challenge test (OCT). A contraction pattern of three contractions with a duration of at least 40 seconds in 10 minutes is desired for this test.

Findings

Negative: Late decelerations do not occur with contractions.
Positive: Late decelerations occur with 50% or more contractions.
Equivocal: Late decelerations occur with <50% of contractions.

Nursing Care

1. Explain test and possible results.
2. Carefully administer test.
3. Monitor FHR continuously.
4. Evaluate results.
5. Communicate results to woman or couple.

Tests to Evaluate Fetal Maturity

See Tables 3–11 and 3–12.

The Intrapartal Period

The intrapartal period is a time of rapid change. The woman's body is drawn into the birth process as each body system becomes involved in the labor and birth. The expectant couple will now be able to use the tools they have learned during the prenatal period. The nurse in the birthing area has an opportunity to use assessment skills and to support the couple during their birth experience.

Characteristics of Birth

Theories regarding initiation of labor include the following:
1. **Oxytocin stimulation theory:** Although the mechanism is unknown, the uterus becomes increasingly sensitive to oxytocin as the pregnancy progresses.
2. **Progesterone withdrawal theory:** A decrease in progesterone production may stimulate prostaglandin (PG) synthesis and enhance the effect of estrogen, which has a stimulating effect on uterine muscles.
3. **Estrogen stimulation theory:** Estrogen stimulates irritability of uterine muscles and enhances uterine contractions.
4. **Fetal cortisol theory:** Cortisol may affect maternal estrogen levels.
5. **Fetal membrane phospholipid–arachidonic acid–prostaglandin theory:** The synthesis of PG is affected by levels

Table 3–11. Evaluation of Fetal Maturity by Testing Amniotic Fluid	
Test	**Result**
L/S ratio	2:1 ratio is present after 35 weeks' gestation (3:1 ratio in diabetic women)
Prosphatidylglycerol	Present after 35 weeks' gestation
Creatinine	2 mg/dL correlates with ≥ 37 weeks of gestation

Table 3–12. **Fetal Blood Sampling and Estriol Level Determination**		
	Fetal Blood Sampling	Estriol Level Determination
Description	The analysis of a fetal blood sample obtained generally during labor when fetal distress is apparent. This invasive procedure requires rupture of the membrane and cervical dilation of 3–4 cm.	An analysis of urine and/or serum to determine the placenta's ability to synthesize fetal steroid precursors into estriol.
Purpose	Determine the presence of fetal hypoxia by analyzing fetal pH, PO_2, PCO_2.	Determine the adequacy of placental function. A sudden or consistent drop in estriol levels is associated with fetal distress.
Nursing plan and intervention	1. Explain procedure. 2. Place mother in lithotomy position. 3. Secure FHR monitor. 4. Assist with visualization of the presenting part and securing of blood specimen. 5. Postprocedure, observe for maternal bleeding and fetal tachycardia.	1. Explain procedure. 2. Facilitate the obtaining of serial blood samples as ordered. 3. Instruct mother in obtaining a 24-hr urine sample.

of estrogen and progesterone. PG stimulates smooth muscle to contract.
6. Labor is likely initiated by a combination of all of the above mechanisms.

Premonitory Signs of Labor

1. Lightening occurs as fetus settles or descends into pelvic inlet.
2. Braxton Hicks contractions increase in frequency and may become uncomfortable.
3. Softening of the cervix (also called "ripening").
4. "Bloody show"—a pink-tinged mucus that is expelled from the vagina. The pinkish tint is from small amounts of blood from capillaries in the cervix.
5. Rupture of amniotic membranes.
6. Many women experience a sudden burst of energy.
7. Some women experience diarrhea.

Stages of Labor and Birth

First Stage

1. The first stage begins with true labor contractions and ends with complete dilation of the cervix (Table 3–13).
2. The length of the first stage ranges from 6–18 hours in a primigravida and 3–10 hours in a multigravida.
3. The first stage is divided into three phases: latent, active, and transition.
   A. **Latent phase** begins with the start of true labor until 4 cm of cervical dilation:
      (1) Contractions range from every 15–30 minutes and last 15–30 seconds. The intensity begins as mild and progresses to moderate.
      (2) Woman may feel anticipation and excitement.
      (3) Her focus is outward.
   B. **Active phase** is from 4–7 cm.
      (1) Contractions are every 3–5 minutes and last about 60 seconds. Intensity is moderate.

      (2) Woman becomes more serious, and it takes greater concentration to maintain breathing pattern.
      (3) The woman focuses more inward.
   C. **Transition phase** is from 8–10 cm.
      (1) Contractions are every 2–3 minutes and last 45–90 seconds. Intensity is strong.
      (2) Woman feels overwhelmed and may lose control.
      (3) The woman's focus is now totally introspective.
      (4) Women frequently vomit during transition.

Second Stage

1. The second stage begins with complete cervical dilation and ends with birth of the baby.
2. Average length of second stage ranges from 0.5–2 hours for primigravida and 10–60 minutes for multigravida.
3. Woman is involved in pushing efforts.

Third Stage

1. The third stage begins with birth of the baby and ends with birth of the placenta.
2. Length of third stage ranges from 5–30 minutes.
3. Woman begins attachment with newborn and may feel exhilarated.

Table 3–13. **Characteristics of True and False Labor**	
True Labor	False Labor
Contractions are regular.	Contractions are irregular.
Contractions increase in frequency and duration.	Contractions stay the same.
Discomfort is felt in back and radiates around to abdomen.	Discomfort is felt in abdomen.
Walking usually increases the contraction pattern.	Contractions usually decrease with walking.

Fourth Stage

1. The fourth stage begins with birth of the placenta and ends 1–4 hours after birth.
2. Woman may feel exhilarated and/or exhausted. She may want to interact with the newborn or may need to rest.
3. The woman is often ravenous.

Mechanisms of Labor

1. **Engagement:** Point when biparietal diameter of fetal head passes the pelvic inlet.
2. **Descent:** Downward movement of the fetal head into the birth canal.
3. **Flexion:** Flexion of the fetal chin down onto the fetal chest.
4. **Internal rotation:** Rotation of the fetal head to pass through the ischial spines.
5. **Extension:** As fetal head passes under symphysis pubis, fetal head extends.
6. **External rotation:** Rotation of the fetal head to allow shoulders to pass through ischial spines.

Maternal Physiological Adaptations to Labor and Birth

Cardiovascular System

1. Supine hypotension occurs in approximately 10%–15% of women. It is caused by occlusion of the vena cava by the heavy uterus when the pregnant woman lies on her back. Symptoms include decreased blood pressure, increased pulse, dizziness, pallor, and cool clammy skin. Immediate treatment includes turning woman to left side, starting O_2 at 7–10 L/min by face mask, and monitoring maternal vital signs and fetal heart rate. Recovery is usually rapid.
2. Cardiac output increases by 10%–15% in the resting phase between contractions and by 30%–50% during uterine contractions. This causes an increase in the blood pressure during contractions, especially the systolic blood pressure.
3. Immediately after birth, cardiac output is approximately 80% above prelabor values.

Respiratory System

1. O_2 consumption increases 40% in the first stage of labor and another 100% during the second stage of labor.

Hemopoietic System

1. Leukocytosis may reach 25,000 WBC/mm^3 or more during labor. This increase in the WBCs does not indicate infection unless there are also other signs/symptoms that indicate infection.
2. There is an increase in plasma fibrinogen and a decrease in blood coagulation time.

Pain During Labor

1. Pain during the first stage is associated with dilation of the cervix, hypoxia of uterine muscle cells during contractions, and stretching of the lower uterine segment. The pain is felt in the uterus, over the lower abdominal wall, and over the lower lumbar and sacral areas.
2. Second-stage pain is associated with hypoxia of the muscle cells in the uterus during contractions, distention of the vagina and perineum, and pressure on adjacent structures. The pain is felt in the lower portion of the uterus, around the upper margin of the legs, and in the perineal area.
3. Pain during the third stage is associated with uterine contractions and cervical dilation during the birth of the placenta.
4. The woman's ability to tolerate labor and birth pain is affected by her knowledge of labor and birth, coping abilities, fatigue level, presence of anxiety, and cultural factors.

Fetal Physiological Adaptations to Labor

1. FHR is maintained at 110–160 bpm.
2. As pressure is exerted on the fetal head during contractions, there may be a decrease in FHR called an **early deceleration.**

Nursing Process During the First Stage

Assessment

Nursing History (on Admission)

1. Name and age
2. Attending physician or certified nurse-midwife
3. Personal data: blood type, Rh, current weight and amount of weight gain, allergies to medications and other substances
4. Data regarding this pregnancy: gravida, para.
5. Status of labor: characteristics of contractions and whether membranes have ruptured
6. The woman's birth plan.

Physical Assessment

1. Assess maternal vital signs.
2. Assess uterine contractions. Determine frequency, duration, and intensity (Table 3–14).
3. Assess contractions either by palpation or by an electronic monitor.
4. Assess cervical dilation and effacement.
5. Assess fetal station presentation and position by Leopold's maneuvers and/or vaginal examination (Figs. 3–4 and 3–5).
6. Assess FHR.
   A. May use ultrasound Doppler, fetoscope, or electronic fetal monitor (EFM).
   B. When auscultating, listen for 30–60 seconds between contractions to establish a baseline rate, then listen through the contraction and for 15–30 seconds after the contraction. Auscultation should be done at least hourly during the latent phase, every 30 minutes during the active phase, and every 15 minutes during the second stage of labor.
7. Evaluate FHR pattern.
   A. Normal pattern is baseline rate of 110–160 bpm, with average variability and the absence of late or variable decelerations. Early decelerations may be present (Fig. 3–6).
   B. Variability of FHR
      (1) Cause: result of the interplay between the parasympathetic and sympathetic system

Table 3–14. Description of Intrapartal Terms

Term	Description	Medical Record Documentation
Effacement	Shortening, thinning of cervix.	Percent of effacement (0%–100%)
Dilation	Opening of the cervix.	<10 cm (10 cm is also called "complete")
Lightening	Settling of fetal presenting part into pelvic inlet. Occurs 2–3 wk prior to labor in primigravida and at onset of labor in multigravida.	Lightening
Engagement	Fetal presenting part in superior pelvic strait or inlet.	Engaged
Station	Relationship of fetal presenting part to the level of the ischial spines (Fig. 3–4).	Above spines: −3, −2, −1 At spines: 0 Below spines: +1, +2, +3 On perineum: +4
Fetal presentation	Fetal part that first enters the pelvis (Fig. 3–5).	
Types	Cephalic—any part of fetal head (occurs 97% of the time)	Cephalic
	• Occiput, vertex	O
	• Brow	B
	• Face	M (mentrum or chin)
	Breech—buttocks and/or feet (sacrum)	S (sacrum)
	• Complete—buttocks and feet present	Complete breech
	• Footling—one or both feet present	Footling breech (single or double)
	• Frank—buttocks only present	Frank breech
Position	Relationship of fetal presenting part (O, B, M, S) to the maternal pelvis (right, left, anterior, posterior).	Examples: LOA, ROA, LSP (The middle letter is the baby's presenting part; the outer letters are the mother's right or left pelvis, anterior or posterior pelvis.)
Show	Vaginal discharge of mucus, fluid, and increasing amounts of blood.	Amount is scant, moderate, or copious.
Membranes	Amniotic membranes that encase the fetus and amniotic fluids. The membranes rupture spontaneously or artificially.	SROM or AROM (spontaneous rupture of membranes or artificial rupture of membranes)
Contractions	The tightening of the uterine muscle during the labor process.	
Frequency	From beginning of one contraction to beginning of next one.	Minutes
Duration	From beginning of one contraction until it relaxes.	Seconds
Intensity	Strength or dentability of uterus.	Mild, moderate, or strong
Rest period	Time between contractions.	Minutes
Rhythm	Regularity with which contractions occur.	Irregular or regular

(2) Short-term (beat to beat) or long-term (3–5 cycles or fluctuations per minute)

(3) Clinical significance: indicates fetus can respond to environment (a reassuring pattern)

C. Acceleration
(1) Cause: response of FHR to movement or other stimulus
(2) Clinical significance: indicates fetal well-being (a reassuring pattern)
(3) Nursing interventions: none needed. Fetal movement or contractions can cause accelerations

D. Early deceleration
(1) Cause: compression of fetal head associated with contractions and pressure of head on cervix
(2) Shape: is uniform, inversely mirrors uterine contraction, starts and ends with contraction.
(3) Clinical significance: considered a reassuring pattern
(4) Nursing interventions: none needed

E. Late deceleration
(1) Cause: uteroplacental insufficiency.
(2) Shape: is smooth and inversely mirrors contraction,

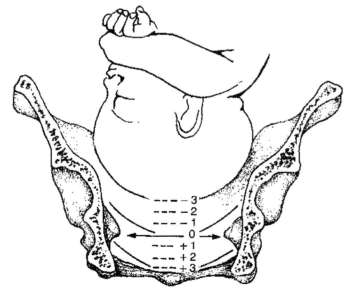

Figure 3–4. Stations of the fetal head.

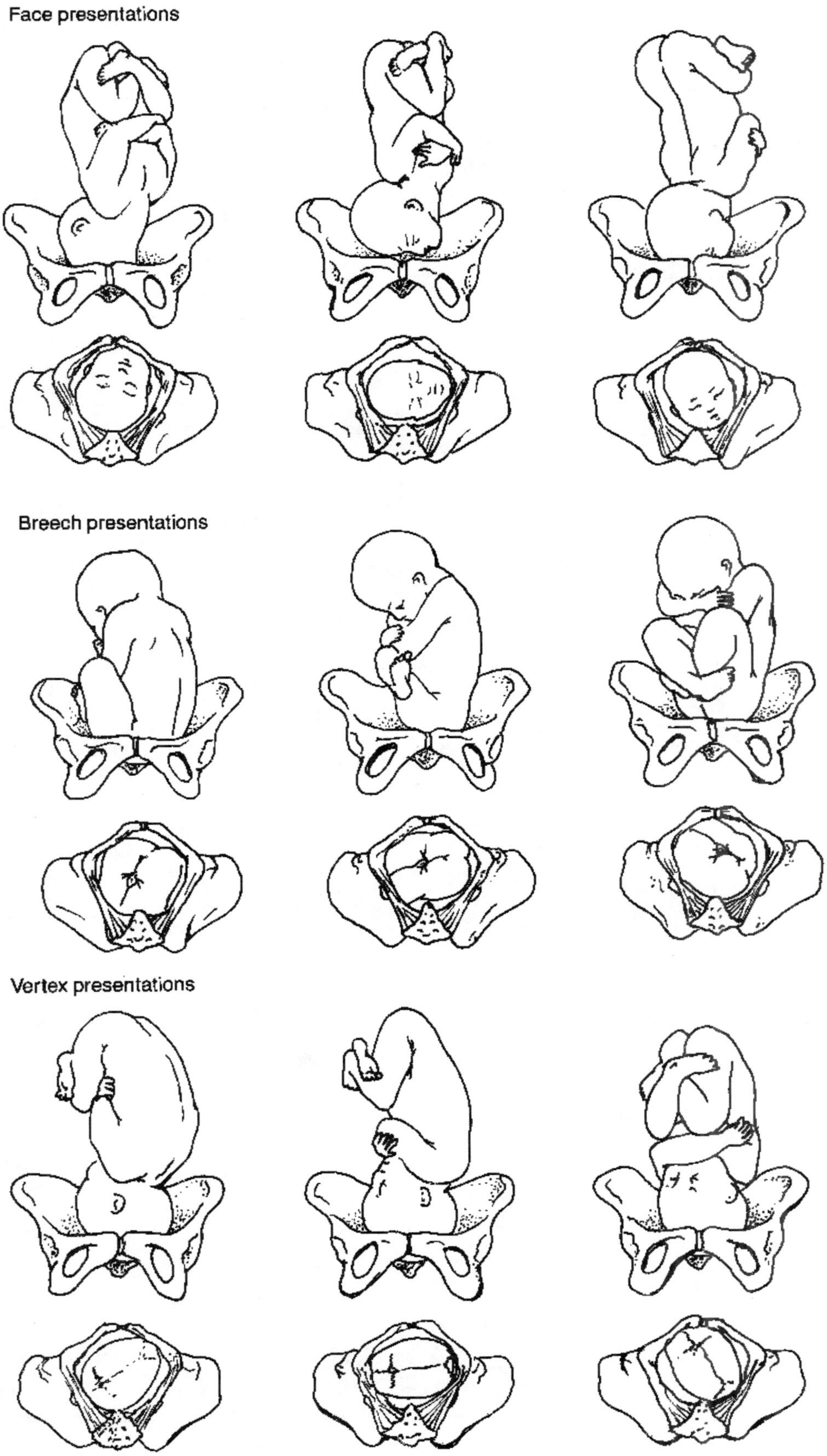

Face presentations

Breech presentations

Vertex presentations

Figure 3–5. Fetal presentations. (Adapted from Benson, RC: Handbook of Obstetrics and Gynecology, ed 7. Lange Medical Publications, Los Altos, CA, 1980.)

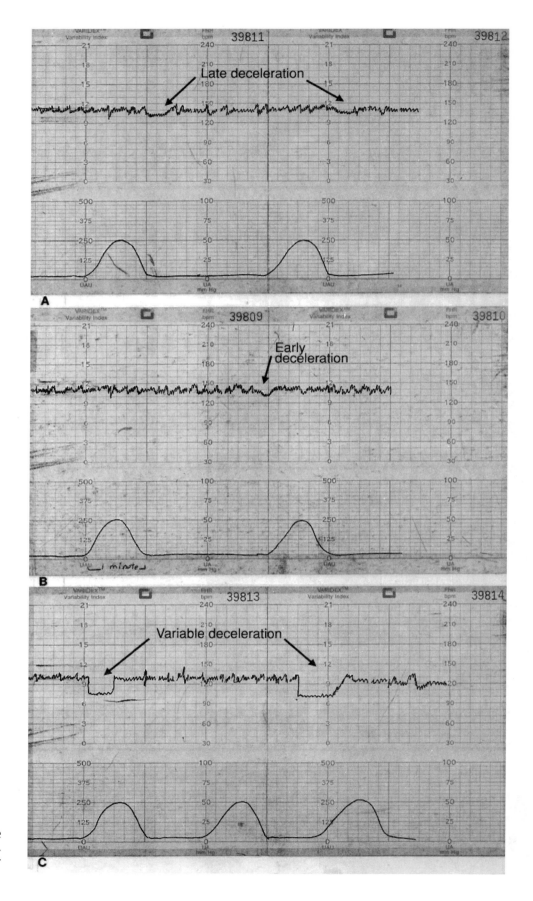

Figure 3–6. Fetal heart rate patterns. (*A*) Late deceleration. (*B*) Early deceleration. (*C*) Variable deceleration.

it starts anytime during the contraction, but does not end until after the contraction ends.

    (3) Clinical significance: may indicate fetal distress.

    (4) Nursing interventions: maximize uteroplacental perfusion by turning mother to left side, administering O_2 at 7–10 L/min by face mask, increasing IV fluids to treat hypotension and to decrease intensity of contractions (discontinue IV oxytocin [Pitocin] if it is being used). Maintain continuous fetal monitoring tracing.

  F. Variable decelerations

    (1) Cause: umbilical cord compression

    (2) Shape: varies in onset, occurrence, and waveform

    (3) Clinical significance: indicates compression of umbilical cord; may be associated with fetal distress

    (4) Nursing interventions: change maternal position. If pattern is severe, administer O_2 at 7–10 L/min via face mask. Nurse needs to be suspicious of a prolapsed cord with this deceleration pattern.

  G. Decreased variability

    (1) Cause: anoxia, medications that depress the central nervous system (CNS), fetal sleep

    (2) Clinical significance: is short-term if associated with fetal sleep or with medications; may be ominous if pattern persists more than 30 minutes or variability continues to decrease

    (3) Nursing interventions: carefully evaluate pattern, maintain continuous FHR tracing.

  H. Fetal blood sampling

    (1) It may be done when fetal distress is indicated.

    (2) Method of obtaining: physician places endoscope against fetal presenting part, and then a blood sample is obtained from the fetal scalp.

    (3) Results: normal $\geq$ 7.25 pH; pre-acidotic = 7.20–7.24; acidotic status is indicated by pH < 7.20.

Psychosocial and Cultural Assessment

1. Assess coping skills, level of anxiety, and response to labor.
2. Assess couple's interaction and support system.

Planning

1. Safe, effective care environment
  A. Orient couple to surroundings.
  B. Promote physical safety.
2. Physiological integrity
  A. Promote maternal-fetal well-being during the birth process.
3. Psychosocial integrity
  A. Provide support and counseling to couple during labor.
4. Health promotion and maintenance
  A. Encourage self-care activities and support measures during labor and birth.
  B. Monitor woman and fetus

Implementation

1. Complete maternal-fetal physical assessments.
  A. In latent and active phase of labor, assess maternal blood pressure, pulse, and respirations every 60 minutes as long as findings remain in normal range. In transition phase, increase assessments to every 30 minutes.
  B. Monitor oral temperature every 4 hours if membranes are intact, every 2 hours for ruptured membranes.
  C. Determine if membranes are ruptured by checking with nitrazine test tape.
  D. Assess FHR: In the latent phase, assess FHR every 60 minutes for low-risk women and every 30 minutes for high-risk women if normal characteristics are present (average variability, baseline 110–160 bpm range, absence of late or variable decelerations). In active and transition phases, assess FHR every 30 minutes for low-risk women and every 15 minutes for high-risk women if normal characteristics are present.
2. Evaluate uterine contractions every 30 minutes and each time FHR is evaluated.
3. Evaluate progression of cervical dilation, effacement, and fetal descent.
4. Provide support measures for expectant woman and coach (Table 3–15).
5. Maintain comfort measures.
6. Support breathing methods.
7. Provide teaching and associated nursing care for regional blocks, if used (Table 3–16).
8. Administer analgesics as needed.
9. Use EFM for the following indications:
  A. Decreased fetal movement
  B. Abnormalities in FHR
  C. Meconium-stained fluid
  D. Abnormal presentation and position
  E. Intrauterine growth retardation (IUGR) or postdate
  F. Presence of maternal complication such as PIH, diabetes
  G. Maternal fever
  H. Oxytocin augmentation or induction
  I. Bleeding
10. Encourage woman to empty her bladder every 2 hours.
11. Provide ice chips to moisten mouth. Maintain intake of clear fluids only.
12. Monitor labor for signs of fetal distress such as:
  A. Meconium staining of amniotic fluid
  B. Fetal hyperactivity or lack of activity
  C. FHR baseline changes such as tachycardia or bradycardia
  D. Loss of FHR baseline variability
  E. Presence of late or variable decelerations

Evaluation

Ensure that:
1. The childbearing couple is knowledgeable regarding surroundings.
2. The childbearing couple understands and practices safety measures.
3. The childbearing woman and her fetus experience a safe labor and birth and their physiological parameters remain within normal limits.
4. The childbearing couple acknowledges that support was received during labor and birth.
5. The childbearing couple uses self-care and support measures.

Table 3–15. Normal Progress, Psychological Characteristics, and Nursing Support During First and Second Stages of Labor

Phase	Cervical Dilation	Uterine Contractions	Woman's Response	Support Measures
Stage 1 Latent phase (Friedman: latent phase)	1–4 cm	Every 15–30 min, 15–30 sec duration Mild intensity	Usually happy, talkative, and eager to be in labor. Exhibits need for independence by taking care of own bodily needs and seeking information.	Establish rapport on admission and continue to build during care. Assess information base and learning needs. Be available to consult regarding breathing technique if needed; teach breathing technique if needed and in early labor. Orient family to room, equipment, monitors, and procedures. Encourage woman and partner to participate in care as desired. Provide needed information. Assist woman into position of comfort, encourage frequent change of position, and encourage ambulation during early labor. Offer fluids or ice chips. Keep couple informed of progress. Encourage woman to void every 1–2 hr. Assess need for, and interest in, using visualization to enhance relaxation and teach if appropriate.
Active phase (Friedman: active phase–acceleration phase and phase of maximum slope)	4–7 cm	Every 3–5 min, 30–60 sec duration Moderate intensity	May experience feelings of helplessness; exhibits increased fatigue and may begin to feel restless and anxious as contractions become stronger; expresses fear of abandonment. Becomes more dependent as she is less able to meet her needs.	Encourage woman to maintain breathing patterns; provide quiet environment to reduce external stimuli. Provide reassurance, encouragement, support; keep couple informed of progress. Promote comfort by giving back rubs, sacral pressure, cool cloth on forehead, assistance with position changes, support with pillows, effleurage. Provide ice chips, ointment for dry mouth and lips. Encourage to void every 1–2 hr.
Transition (Friedman: active phase–deceleration phase)	8–10 cm	Every 2–3 min, 45–90 sec duration Strong intensity	Tires and may exhibit increased restlessness and irritability; may feel she cannot keep up with labor process and is out of control. Physical discomforts; fear of being left alone; may fear tearing open or splitting apart with contractions.	Encourage woman to rest between contractions; if she sleeps between contractions, wake her at beginning of contraction so she can begin breathing pattern (increases feeling of control). Provide support, encouragement, and praise for efforts. Keep couple informed of progress; encourage continued participation of support persons. Promote comfort as listed above but recognize many women do not want to be touched when in transition. Provide privacy. Provide ice chips, ointment for lips. Encourage to void every 1–2 hr.
Stage 2	Complete		May feel out of control, helpless, panicky.	Assist woman in pushing efforts. Encourage woman to assume position of comfort. Provide encouragement and praise for efforts. Keep couple informed of progress. Provide ice chips. Maintain privacy as woman desires.

From Olds, SB, London, ML, and Ladewig, PL: Maternal-Newborn Nursing: A Family Centered Approach, ed 4. Addison-Wesley, Redwood City, CA, 1992, p 668, with permission.

Table 3–16. **Regional Anesthesia**				
Type of Block	Injection Site	Time of Administration	Characteristic of the Block	Nursing Considerations
Epidural	Epidural space at L3-4. Catheter may be left in place.	First stage of labor after 5–6 cm dilation. May use repeated doses. May be given in second stage.	May cause hypotension. Relieves pain from contractions and numbs vagina and perineum. Does not cause headache, as dura is not penetrated.	Assess blood pressure. Maintain side-lying position. Maintain IV fluids; increase fluids if hypotension occurs. Provide support during block.
Spinal	Spinal subarachnoid space at L3-5.	Just before birth of the baby.	Relieves pain from contractions; numbs vagina, perineum, and lower extremities. May cause hypotension. May cause postpartum headache.	Assess blood pressure. Place rolled blanket under (R) hip to displace uterus from vena cava. Maintain IV fluids. Provide support during block.
Pudendal	Pudendal nerve through a transvaginal route.	Just before birth of the baby.	Relieves perineal discomfort and numbs area for episiotomy.	Provide support during block.
Local	Perineum.	Just before birth of the baby.	Numbs perineum for episiotomy and repair.	Provide support during block.

Nursing Process During the Second Stage

Assessment

Physical Assessment

1. Assess maternal blood pressure, pulse, and respirations every 5–15 minutes.
2. Assess FHR every 15 minutes for low-risk women and every 5 minutes for high-risk women.
3. Assess labor progress.
   A. Labor has been progressive, with cervical dilation of approximately 1 cm/hr for primigravidas and 1.5 cm/hr for multigravidas.
   B. Fetal descent is occurring and is demonstrated by change in fetal station. By the end of the first stage, the fetus is usually +2 station.
   C. Uterine contractions are every 2–3 minutes and last 60–75 seconds. Intensity is strong.
   D. The amount of bloody show increases.
   E. The woman feels the urge to bear down.

Psychosocial and Cultural Assessment

1. Assess woman's response to labor.
   A. Woman may show intense concentration on the pushing effort.
   B. Woman may be eager to participate or may have difficulty.
2. Assess coping pattern.

Planning

1. Safe, effective care environment
   A. Promote a quiet, focused environment to enhance pushing efforts.
2. Physiological integrity
   A. Monitor maternal and fetal status.
3. Psychosocial integrity
   A. Provide encouragement for pushing efforts.

4. Health promotion and maintenance
   A. Support ongoing comfort measures and pushing efforts.

Implementation

1. Continue assessments of maternal blood pressure, FHR, and uterine contractions every 5 minutes.
2. Assist laboring woman into a position that promotes comfort and assists pushing efforts. Woman may choose lithotomy, semisitting, kneeling, side-lying, hands and knees, or squatting position.
3. Observe for signs of approaching birth such as:
   A. Perineal bulging
   B. Appearance of the fetal head
4. Provide comfort measures such as:
   A. Offering ice chips to moisten mouth
   B. Placing cool washcloth on forehead
   C. Supporting woman's body and/or extremities during pushing
5. Prepare for the birth.
6. Complete perineal cleansing or perineal scrub.

Evaluation

Ensure that:
1. The laboring woman is able to remain focused on pushing.
2. The laboring woman and her fetus maintain physical parameters within normal limits.
3. The laboring woman feels encouragement during this stage.
4. The laboring woman feels comfortable.

Nursing Process During the Third Stage

Assessment

Physical Assessment

1. Determine that normal third-stage progress is occurring.
   A. Rhythmic contractions occur until the placenta is born.

	Score		
Sign	0	1	2
Appearance (color)	Pale	Body pink, extremities blue*	Pink
Pulse (heart rate)	Absent	Below 100	Above 100*
Grimace (reflex irritability)	Absent	Grimace	Vigorous cry*
Activity (muscle tone)	Limp	Some flexion of extremities	Active motion*
Respiration (respiratory effort)	Absent	Slow, irregular	Crying*

Table 3–17. **Apgar Scoring Chart**

*Normal

B. Birth of placenta occurs 5–30 minutes after birth of the baby.
C. Signs of placental separation
  (1) Fundus rises slightly in abdomen.
  (2) Uterus changes shape.
  (3) Umbilical cord lengthens.
  (4) Slight gush of blood from vagina is noted.
D. Placental expulsion
  (1) Schultze's mechanism (center portion of placenta separates first and shiny fetal surface emerges from the vagina).
  (2) Duncan's mechanism (margin of placenta separates and dull, red, rough maternal surface emerges from vagina first). Duncan's mechanism is associated with retained placental fragments.
E. Following birth of the placenta, the uterine fundus remains firm and is located 2 fingerbreadths (FB) below the umbilicus.
F. New mother may experience shivering or chills.

2. Assess maternal blood pressure following birth of the baby.
3. Assess status of the uterus. Contractions will continue until birth of the placenta.
4. Assess the newborn's Apgar score (Table 3–17), and complete initial newborn assessment (Table 3–18).
5. Examine placenta to document that all cotyledons and membranes are present.

Psychosocial and Cultural Assessment

1. Assess need for parental support following birth.
2. Assess parents' readiness to interact with their newborn.

Planning

1. Safe, effective care environment
  A. Complete initial assessment of the newborn to assure airway patency.

Table 3–18. **Initial Newborn Evaluation**

Assess	Normal Findings
Respirations	Rate 30–60, irregular
	No retractions, no grunting
Apical pulse	Rate 110–160 and somewhat irregular
Temperature	Skin temperature 97.8°F (36.5°C)
Skin color	Body pink with bluish extremities
Umbilical cord	Two arteries and one vein
Gestational age	Should be 38–42 wk to remain with parents for extended time
Sole creases	Sole creases that involve the heel

In general, expect: scant amount of vernix on upper back, axilla, groin; lanugo only on upper back; ears with incurving of upper ⅔ of pinnae and thin cartilage that springs back from folding; male genitalia—testes palpated in upper or lower scrotum; female genitalia—labia majora larger; clitoris nearly covered

In the following situations, newborns should generally be stabilized rather than remaining with parents in the birth area for an extended period of time:

Apgar score is < 8 at 1 min and < 9 at 5 min, or a baby requires resuscitation measures (other than whiffs of O_2).

Respirations are below 30 or above 60, with retractions and/or grunting.

Apical pulse is below 110 or above 160 with marked irregularities.

Skin temperature is below 97.8°F (36.5°C).

Skin color is pale blue, or there is circumoral pallor.

Baby is < 38 or > 42 weeks' gestation.

Baby is very small or very large for gestational age.

There are congenital anomalies involving open areas in the skin (meningomyelocele).

From Olds, SB, London, ML, and Ladewig, PL: Maternal-Newborn Nursing: A Family Centered Approach, ed 4. Addison-Wesley, Redwood City, CA, 1992, p 680, with permission.

2. Physiological integrity
   A. Monitor maternal and newborn status.
3. Psychosocial integrity
   A. Provide support in parental-newborn interactions.
4. Health promotion and maintenance
   A. Provide support and comfort measures during the third stage.

Implementation

1. Observe and record birth of the placenta.
2. Monitor maternal blood pressure.
3. Dry the baby completely.
4. Complete initial newborn assessments.
5. Provide initial newborn care.
   A. Provide warmth.
   B. Prevent infection.
   C. Promote parental-newborn attachment.
6. Administer oxytocic drug as per physician's order.

Evaluation

1. See that newborn establishes and maintains adequate respiratory pattern.
2. Be sure that mother and newborn maintain normal physical parameters.
3. Monitor new parents to be sure they are able to interact with newborn as desired.
4. Make sure mother feels comfortable and supported during the third stage.

Nursing Process During the Fourth Stage

Assessment

Physical Assessment

1. Determine that fourth stage is progressing within normal limits.
   A. Blood pressure returns to prelabor level.
   B. Pulse is slightly lower than in labor.
   C. Fundus remains contracted, in the midline, and is located 1–2 FB below the umbilicus.
   D. Lochia is scant to moderate in amount and is red (rubra).
   E. Bladder is nonpalpable.
   F. The perineum is intact.

Psychosocial and Cultural Assessment

1. Assess mother's emotional state. May vary from exhaustion to euphoria.
2. Understand that some mothers may wish to interact with their baby, and others may wish to rest at this time.

Planning

1. Safe, effective care environment
   A. Complete frequent assessments to monitor maternal birth recovery.
2. Physiological integrity
   A. Monitor maternal status.

3. Psychosocial integrity
   A. Enhance maternal-newborn attachment.
4. Health promotion and maintenance
   A. Teach self-care measures to prevent bleeding and enhance comfort.

Implementation

1. Complete maternal assessments every 15 minutes for 1 hour, then every 30 minutes for 1 hour, and then hourly for 2 hours.
2. Provide comfort measures.
   A. Provide warmed blankets and/or hot drinks for shivering or chilling.
   B. Place ice pack on perineum to decrease swelling and increase comfort.
   C. Offer sponge bath.
   D. Provide clean linens (especially if woman has used bed for labor and birth).
3. Massage fundus, if needed.

Evaluation

Ensure that the mother:
1. Has her physical parameters monitored at frequent intervals.
2. Has uneventful recovery period and does not develop complications.
3. Has opportunity to interact with newborn as desired.
4. Can demonstrate fundal massage and practice comfort measures.

Obstetrical Procedures

Amniotomy

1. Amniotomy is the artificial rupture of membranes (AROM).
2. Purpose: to stimulate labor.
3. Advantages
   A. Amniotomy stimulates contractions.
   B. Amniotic fluid can be evaluated.
4. Disadvantages
   A. Once amniotomy is done, birth must occur within 24 hours (may necessitate cesarean birth).
   B. Increased risk of prolapsed cord.
   C. Risk of infection.
5. Nursing care
   A. Auscultate FHR before and after AROM.
   B. Record time of AROM, FHR, and characteristics of fluid (amount, color, odor).
   C. Instruct woman to remain in bed unless fetal presenting part is well engaged (to prevent prolapse of umbilical cord).

Induction

1. Elective induction may be accomplished by oxytocin infusion.
2. Purpose: to stimulate labor.
3. Advantages
   A. IV oxytocin induction is usually successful when labor readiness has been established (fetal maturity is established and Bishop score is 9 or more).
   B. Maternal and fetal status can be closely monitored.

4. Disadvantages
    A. Is an invasive procedure
    B. Carries risk of hypertonic labor, fetal distress, alterations in blood pressure, ruptured uterus
5. Indications: postmaturity; premature rupture of membranes (PROM); PIH; presence of maternal disease such as diabetes mellitus; fetal demise
6. Contraindications: grand multiparity, placental abnormalities, previous uterine surgery, fetal distress, preterm fetus, positive CST, abnormal fetal presentation, presenting part above inlet, cephalopelvic disproportion (CPD).
7. Nursing care
    A. Obtain baseline tracing of uterine contractions (if present) and FHR for at least 20 minutes.
    B. Follow established protocols.
    C. Increase IV dosage only after assessing contractions, FHR, and maternal blood pressure and pulse.
    D. Do not increase rate once desired contraction pattern is obtained (contraction frequency 2–3 minutes, lasting 60 seconds).
    E. Discontinue oxytocin if contraction frequency is less than 2 minutes or duration is more than 90 seconds, or if fetal distress is noted.

Forceps Birth

1. Forceps may be used as low or outlet forceps or for mid-forceps procedures.
2. Purpose: to provide traction or to assist in rotation of the fetus.
3. Advantages
    A. Can provide assistance when laboring woman is exhausted, or pushing efforts have been diminished by administration of a regional block
    B. May decrease need for cesarean birth
4. Disadvantages
    A. May cause maternal complications such as vaginal and perineal lacerations and postpartal hemorrhage
    B. May cause neonatal complications such as facial bruising, edema, cerebral trauma
5. Nursing care
    A. Explain procedure to woman.
    B. Encourage her to relax perineum and breathe during forceps application.
    C. Advise physician when contraction is present.
    D. Assess newborn for facial bruising or edema.

Episiotomy

1. Episiotomy is a surgical incision of the perineal body. It may be in the midline or mediolateral aspect of the perineum.
2. Purpose: to minimize stretching of perineal tissues, decrease chance of perineal lacerations, decrease trauma to the fetal head, and shorten the length of the second stage.
3. Advantage: may prevent perineal trauma and pressure on fetal head
4. Disadvantages: may extend into a longer incision (laceration); takes longer to heal, may become infected, increased pain
5. Nursing care
    A. Place ice pack against perineum after birth.

    B. Assess for redness, edema, ecchymoses, drainage, and approximation of skin edges (**REEDA**).

Cesarean Birth

1. Cesarean birth is the birth of the infant through an abdominal incision.
2. Indications for a cesarean include breech presentation, preterm birth, fetal distress, dysfunctional labor, CPD, prolapsed cord, abruptio placentae, placenta previa, active herpes, transverse lie, and previous cesarean section with "classic" uterine incision.
3. Associated complications include maternal infection, hemorrhage, blood clots, and injury to bladder. The major neonatal complication is inadvertent preterm birth. The major newborn side effect is transient tachypnea of the newborn (TTN).
4. Nursing care
    A. Provide teaching regarding need for cesarean. Answer questions. Facilitate informed consent process by explaining the prep and procedure, and indication(s) for cesarean.
    B. Complete preoperative preparation.
    C. Obtain maternal heart rate vs. FHR.
    D. Provide ongoing assessments in recovery period.

Vaginal Birth After Cesarean

1. Vaginal birth after cesarean (VBAC) is increasing in incidence. It is possible when previous uterine incision was a transverse low incision and contraindications are not present.
2. Contraindications include CPD, placenta previa, abruptio placentae, multiple gestation, previous cesarean section with "classic" uterine incision, inability to perform cesarean in 30 minutes if needed.
3. Nursing care
    A. Monitor labor progress, maternal and fetal status.
    B. Provide support and counseling.
    C. Be alert for fetal distress, dysfunctional labor, and signs of uterine rupture.

The Postpartal Period

The postpartal period extends for 6 weeks after birth and is a time of physical and psychological readjustment after childbirth.

Nursing Process During the Postpartal Period

Assessment

Physical Assessment

Assess for the following manifestations:
1. Vital signs
    A. In first 24 hours, the temperature may normally elevate to 100.4°F (38°C).
    B. On day 2 through day 10, a temperature of 100.4°F or higher may indicate infection, especially if other symptoms of infection are present.

C. Blood pressure remains stable after birth.

D. Bradycardia of 50–70 bpm is common for first 6–10 days.

2. Breasts are soft for first 2 days; then engorgement may occur if not breast feeding.

3. Abdomen is soft and appears loose. Diastasis recti (separation of rectus abdominis) may be apparent.

4. GI system
   A. Hunger following birth is common.
   B. Woman is frequently thirsty.
   C. Bowel may be sluggish.

5. Uterus
   A. Immediately after birth, fundus is located in the midline and 2 FB below the umbilicus.
   B. Within 12 hours after birth, the fundus rises to the level of the umbilicus or 1 FB above.
   C. Fundus remains firm. A firm uterus controls bleeding by clamping off uterine blood vessels. A boggy (soft) uterus should be gently massaged until it is firm. At times, oxytocic medication (such as methylergonovine maleate [Methergine]) may need to be given postoperative in order to maintain uterine firmness.
   D. Fundal height descends 1 FB/day. Process is called **involution.** Fundus is no longer palpable above symphysis pubis after about 9 days.
   E. Afterpains are common in first 2–3 days following birth, especially for multiparas and breast-feeding mothers.

6. **Lochia** is the vaginal discharge from the uterus.
   A. Lochia rubra—lasts 2–3 days and is composed of blood, mucus, and particles of decidua. It is red in color.
   B. Lochia serosa—lasts from 3rd–10th day and is composed of serous, watery discharges. It is pinkish or brownish in color.
   C. Lochia alba—lasts from 10th–21st day. It is whitish-yellow in color.
   D. Foul-smelling lochia may be indicative of a uterine infection.
   E. Small clots (the size of the fingernail on the little finger) may be present in the lochia rubra. Large clots should not be present. Lochia may pool in the vagina while the woman lies down and feel like a gush when the woman stands up.

7. Urinary output
   A. Diuresis occurs in first 24 hours. The woman voids large amounts (1 liter or more) at frequent intervals, and is so diaphoretic she will have to change her gown. Linens may also have to be changed.
   B. Bladder emptying may be a problem because of swelling and bruising of tissues around the urethra and decreased sensation of bladder filling due to regional anesthesia.
   C. The woman should void within the first 6–8 hours after birth. A full bladder pushes the uterus upward and keeps it from firmly contracting. It will also usually be deviated to the right side.

Psychosocial and Cultural Assessment

See Table 3–19.

Planning

1. Safe, effective care environment
   A. Create environment conducive to parental-infant interaction and taking on the parental role.
2. Physiological integrity
   A. Promote maternal-neonatal well-being.
3. Psychosocial integrity
   A. Provide support and counseling for new parents.
4. Health promotion and maintenance
   A. Provide teaching regarding postpartal self-care measures and infant care.

Implementation

1. Complete postpartum assessment every 4–8 hours. Include the following areas:
   A. Take and record vital signs.
   B. Palpate breasts. Note firmness and complaints of breast tenderness. Assess nipples for tenderness/soreness, blisters, and cracking in breast-feeding mothers.

Table 3–19. Psychological Responses to Childbearing

Phase	Characteristics	Nursing Plan and Intervention
Taking in	First 2–3 days, mother is reflective, dependent. She ponders new roles, pregnancy, and birth experiences. She has a sense of wonder about the baby. She needs sleep, food, fluids, quiet.	Initiate actions; indicate expectations about self-care; promote rest. Compliment on successful delivery. Provide anticipatory guidance regarding mothering skills and family bonding. Interpret events for meaningfulness.
Taking hold	At 3–4 days, the mother begins to initiate action. She provides self-care and is impatient with physical discomforts. She is interested in the infant, organized, and eager to learn. This period lasts up to 2 wk.	Praise mothering behaviors. Provide instructions as requested. Facilitate independent functioning.
Letting go: "postpartum blues"	At 3–4 wk, the mother may feel a great loss and grieve for the absent in utero infant. She may be tearful, irritable, confused, unable to make a decision, exhausted.	Indicate that behaviors are normal. Listen, provide support to all family members. Ensure infant safety and care.

C. Palpate abdomen. Note any distention and diastasis recti.
D. Palpate fundus. Note height, position (midline or to the side), and firmness. If fundal descent is not as expected, palpate bladder for distention and assess lochia for amount.
E. Inspect perineum for bruising, edema. Inspect episiotomy for approximation of skin edges, bruising, areas of firmness that might indicate a hematoma. Note presence of hemorrhoids.
F. Inquire about areas of tenderness of legs. Note reddened, tender areas. Check Homan's sign.
G. Inquire about urinary and bowel elimination.
H. Assess comfort level and need for pain relief.
2. After initial recovery period, assess vital signs every 8 hours.
3. Promote urinary and bowel function.
   A. Urine elimination
      (1) Encourage urinary elimination within 6–8 hours. Catheterization may be necessary to relieve bladder distention.
      (2) Measure urine output for first few voidings (usually at least three voids).
      (3) Note frequent voiding of small amount (≤100 mL), which may indicate retention with overflow.
      (4) Teaching regarding urinary system
         (a) Maintain adequate fluids.
         (b) Empty bladder on regular basis.
         (c) Wipe from front to back.
   B. Feces elimination
      (1) Encourage adequate fluid intake.
      (2) Administer stool softeners as needed and desired.
      (3) Ask about measures the woman usually uses to assist with feces elimination. Use the measures if possible.
      (4) Teaching regarding feces elimination
         (a) Maintain adequate fluids.
         (b) Exercise daily.
         (c) Include fiber and roughage in diet.
4. Promote perineal healing and teach self-care measures.
   A. Apply ice packs for first 6–12 hours.
   B. Cleanse perineum by using warm water rinse.
   C. Offer sitz baths 2–4 times a day.
   D. Use local anesthetic spray or witch hazel pads (Tucks).
   E. Apply pads from front to back and change frequently (could be changed with each voiding).
   F. Instruct woman to report blood clots, foul-smelling lochia, or a change from lochia alba or serosa back to lochia rubra.
5. Provide breast care and teach self-care measures.
   A. Breast-feeding mothers should:
      (1) Cleanse breasts with warm water (no soap).
      (2) Wear a supportive bra.
      (3) Apply Lansoloh cream or breast milk/colostrum for nipple soreness.
      (4) Be taught breast massage.
      (5) Be assisted with breast-feeding technique (see Breast-feeding, below).
   B. Non–breast-feeding mothers should:
      (1) Wear a supportive bra.
      (2) Use a breast binder if desired.
      (3) Avoid breast stimulation.
      (4) Be offered cold/ice packs to decrease swelling and inflammation from engorgement.

6. Teach abdominal and pelvic strengthening exercises.
   A. Modified sit-ups should be included.
   B. Kegel exercises should also be used.
   C. Woman should be advised that increase in vaginal flow or return to lochia rubra may occur if activity has been excessive.
7. Provide information regarding sexual activity.
   A. Couples are advised to resume sexual activity in about 3–6 weeks postbirth. At this time, discharge of lochia alba has ended, and the perineal tissues and episiotomy have healed.
   B. Ovulation may occur, so contraceptive measures are needed to prevent pregnancy.
   C. The woman may experience a decrease in vaginal secretions for a few months. The couple may need to use K-Y jelly or some other type of vaginal lubricant.
8. Provide infant-care teaching.
   A. Common variations in infants
      (1) Milia are small white sebaceous cysts, usually over the nose. They need to be left alone and will disappear in a few weeks.
      (2) Telangiectatic nevi ("stork bites") are reddish areas located between the eyes and on the nape of the neck. They blanch with pressure and darken when the infant cries. They will disappear spontaneously by the second birthday.
      (3) Newborn rash, also called erythema neonatorum toxicum, is raised and looks somewhat like mosquito bites. This rash disappears spontaneously in a few hours or days.
      (4) Mongolian spot is a bluish pigmented area over the lower back and sacrum. It disappears by the time the child is 5 or 6 years of age. It is more common in babies of Mediterranean, African, Asian, or Native American descent.
   B. Cord care
      (1) Cord will dry and fall off by itself in 7–10 days.
      (2) Cleanse the cord 3–4 times a day with alcohol wipes or a cotton ball dipped in 70% isopropyl alcohol. Do not let alcohol run over abdomen. Alcohol is a cleaning and drying agent. If newborn cries during cleansing, it is because the alcohol is cold, not because it hurts.
      (3) Fold diaper below cord until it falls off.
      (4) Sponge bathe the baby, do not immerse baby in water until the cord has come off.
      (5) Watch for redness around cord and oozing of yellowish discharge. If any of these are present, call healthcare provider.
   C. Circumcision care
      (1) After a Plastibell circumcision, a small plastic ring is left on the penis. The ring falls off in about 5–7 days. If it has not come off spontaneously by the 8th day, call the healthcare provider.
         (a) Do not use A & D ointment on the penis, because it may cause the ring to slip off prematurely.
         (b) Cleanse penis by drizzling warm water over it. Do not rub with washcloth.
      (2) After Hogan circumcision with a Gomco clamp, the penis will appear reddened with raw edges around it. It is important to apply A & D ointment to the penis a minimum of 4–6 times a day or with each diaper change to provide comfort and keep the penis from adhering to the diaper.

(3) Check penis for bleeding. Small spotting of blood in diaper may occur in the first few hours to 24 hours.
D. Elimination
  (1) Expect six to eight wet diapers per day.
  (2) Feces elimination will vary for each newborn.
  (3) Perineal area and buttocks need to be cleansed with each diaper change.
  (4) A diaper change is recommended before and after each feeding.
E. Diapers
  (1) Discuss cloth vs. disposable diapers.
F. Feeding pattern
  (1) Bottle-fed infant usually eats every 3–4 hours.
  (2) Breast-fed infant should be fed on demand, usually about every 2–4 hours.
  (3) Mother should hold infant for feeding.
  (4) Mother should burp infant after every 0.5–1 oz, or if breast-feeding, between breasts.
G. Phenylketonuria (PKU)
  (1) PKU testing is required by law. A test is completed before leaving the birth setting and is repeated in 7–14 days.
H. Temperature
  (1) Infant's temperature may be taken by axillary or tympanic route, rarely the rectal route.
      (a) For axillary route, shake down thermometer to below 96°F (35.5°C), place thermometer in axilla, hold arm firmly down over the thermometer for 3–5 minutes.
      (b) For rectal route, shake thermometer down to below 96°F (35.5°C), lubricate end of thermometer, and insert 0.5 inch into the rectum for 3–5 minutes. The thermometer must be held continuously.
I. Signs of illness should be reported to healthcare provider
  (1) Temperature greater than 101°F (38.4°C) or below 97.6°F (36.3°C)
  (2) Prolonged irritability and crying
  (3) Projectile vomiting
  (4) Lethargy
J. Car seat
  (1) Approved car seat is required by law.
  (2) Car seat should face the back of the car for newborns.
K. Newborn bath
  (1) Gather supplies prior to bath.
  (2) Place small towel or washcloth in bottom of tub. Fill with about 2–3 inches of lukewarm 100°–102°F (37.7°–38.8°C) water.
  (3) Use nonperfumed soap and lotions.
  (4) Wash face first. Do not use soap. Cleanse eyes one at a time from inner to outer canthus.
  (5) Shampoo hair. Use soft brush to massage scalp.
  (6) Wash body and extremeties and rinse with hands or place infant in tub (after cord falls off).
  (7) Cleanse perineal area.
  (8) Apply alcohol to cord.
  (9) Dry and redress infant.
L. Formula preparation and feeding
  (1) Mother should use formula recommended by pediatrician or pediatric nurse practitioner unless parents have own wishes. Then discussion is needed.
  (2) Types of preparation vary from powder that is mixed, to a concentrate that is diluted, ready-to-feed-formula.
  (3) Sterilization is no longer used if parents have a city water supply.
M. Breast-feeding
  (1) Cleanse nipple and areola with plain water after each feeding and allow nipples to air-dry.
  (2) Avoid soap on nipples; soap dries out tissues.
  (3) If breast pads are used, remove any plastic from them. The plastic causes moisture to be held against the nipple, leading to tissue breakdown.
  (4) Hold infant in a variety of positions to ensure adequate emptying of the breast.
  (5) Nurse baby for as long as the baby wants, about 20 minutes on each side.
  (6) Break suction by inserting little finger into side of infant's mouth.
  (7) When baby has finished nursing on one breast, burp the baby before nursing on second breast.
  (8) Begin nursing on side that the baby finished on during the last feeding. Some mothers place a safety pin on their bra to help remember which side to begin on.
  (9) Breast-feeding should be initiated as soon as possible after birth. If breast-feeding is interrupted, a good manual pump or electric pump should be used on a regular schedule. The breast milk may be saved and frozen for later use. Expressed milk may be stored in the refrigerator for up to 24 hours and may be frozen in sealed plastic bags for up to 6 months. The bag should be in the back of the freezer. The milk is thawed by placing the plastic bag in a bowl of lukewarm water. *Do not microwave* the milk.
  (10) Breast-feeding mothers should consume 500 cal more than their prepregnant caloric level and at least four 8-oz glasses of noncaffeinated fluids per day.

Evaluation

1. Be sure parents have opportunities for interaction with their baby.
2. Ensure that mother and baby remain within normal physiological parameters.
3. Provide parents with support and counseling.
4. Confirm that mother is able to demonstrate self-care measures and infant care.

The Neonatal Period

Nursing Process During the Neonatal Period

Assessment

Physical Assessment

Assess for the following manifestations:
1. Vital signs
   A. Temperature is normally between 97.6°F (36.4°C) and 98.8°F (37.1°C).

B. Apical pulse is assessed for 60 seconds and is between 120–160 bpm.

C. Respirations are counted by listening with a stethoscope for 60 seconds. The rate is normally 30–60 breaths/min.

2. Measurements
   A. Length averages 18–20.5 inches (45.8–52.3 cm).
   B. Head circumference averages 13–14 inches (33–35 cm).
   C. Chest circumference averages 12.5 inches (32 cm).

3. Head
   A. Appearance: round or molded. Size is approximately 25% of infant's body. Caput succedaneum or cephalohematoma may be present. **Caput succedaneum** is localized swelling over the presenting part. It does cross suture lines. **Cephalohematoma** is a collection of blood between the skull bone and the periosteum. It does *not* cross suture lines.
   B. Posterior fontanelle: triangle-shaped, nonpulsating, 1–2 cm. Closes at 8–12 weeks.
   C. Anterior fontanelle: open, soft, flat, pulsating, diamond-shaped, 3–4 cm long, 2–3 cm wide; closes at 18 months. Fontanelles feel soft to the touch; depression of fontanelle indicates dehydration and bulging indicates increased intracranial pressure.
   D. Face: puffy, round.
   E. Eyes: puffy, slate blue or gray, blink reflex present, sclera has bluish tint. Permanent eye color is established by 3–12 months of age.
   F. Ears: symmetrical. Top of ears should be even with or above an imaginary line drawn from the inner to outer canthus of the eye.
   G. Nose: pug, patent nares. Infant is obligatory nose breather for first 4–5 months of life. Must keep nares clear. Neonate sneezes to remove obstruction.
   H. Mouth: symmetrical grimace, strong sucking reflex, rooting reflex, hard and soft palates present, frenulum allows tongue extension. Epstein's pearls may be present on gums and/or hard palate.

4. Neck: short, creased with skin folds.

5. Chest: circumference 1–2 cm smaller than head.
   A. Sternum: 5 cm long.
   B. Appearance: symmetrical; breast engorgement may occur from maternal hormones. Extra nipples (supernumerary) may be located below the true nipples.
   C. Heart apex (point of maximum intensity) at fourth intercostal space, left of the midclavicular line; S_1 louder than S_2.
   D. Resonance on percussion, clear bilateral breath sounds, and respiratory rhythm irregular.

6. Abdomen: circumference same as chest.
   A. Appearance: cylindrical with slight protrusion.
   B. Umbilicus: translucent, bluish, moist, three vessels, covered with Wharton's jelly.
   C. Bowel sounds present 2–3 hours after birth.

7. Anogenital area: patent anus, first meconium stool and urine within 24 hours (if no voiding at birth).
   A. Female genitalia: may have hymeneal tag and a milky vaginal discharge tinged with mucus and/or blood; labia minora large.
   B. Male genitalia: has slender penis, descended testes, foreskin may not retract easily. Rugae present on scrotum.

8. Extremities: appear short, symmetrical in shape and movement. All digits are present. **Polydactyly** is more than five digits on an extremity; **syndactyly** is the fusing of two or more digits.

9. Back: straight, C-shaped. Sacral dimpling may be present. Tuft of hair present over sacrum is frequently associated with spina bifida.

10. Skin
    A. **Acrocyanosis** is cyanosis of hands and feet that occurs just after birth. It is due to inadequate circulation as neonatal circulation becomes established.
    B. **Milia** (clogged sebaceous glands) may be present over nose.
    C. **Lanugo** (fine downy hair) may be present on shoulders.
    D. **Vernix caseosa** (white cheeselike substance) may be present in skin creases.
    E. **Telangiectatic nevi** (flat, reddish marks) may be present on eyelids, between eyes, and on nape of neck.
    F. **Erythema neonatorum toxicum** (maculopapular rash) may be present over body.

11. Reflexes

12. Laboratory findings
    A. Blood volume is approximately 80–85 mL/kg.
    B. Hemoglobin is 15 to 20 g/mL.
    C. HCT is 43%–61%.
    D. Blood glucose is >45 mg/dL.

13. Periods of reactivity
    A. First period of reactivity lasts about 30–60 minutes after birth. Newborn is awake and may be interested in breast-feeding. Respiratory and heart rates are increased.
    B. Sleep phase lasts approximately 2–4 hours. Pulse and respiratory rate return to baseline.
    C. Second period of reactivity lasts from 4–6 hours. Pulse and respiratory rates increase again.

Psychosocial and Cultural Assessment

1. Mother and father state they are pleased with their newborn.
2. The parent holds the infant close to his or her body.
3. Parents verbalize that the infant is normal and healthy.
4. Parent holds the infant so that eye contact is possible and demonstrates comfort being alone with the baby.
5. Parents perceive the baby as attractive or beautiful.
6. The parents talk about the baby and are tolerant when the infant cries.
7. Parents hold the infant during feeding.
8. Infant takes ½–2 oz per feeding from bottle or breast and advances to 4 oz.
9. The infant sleeps 15–17 hours a day, waking during the night for feeding.

Planning

1. Safe, effective care environment
   A. Provide safe environment for neonatal adaptation.
2. Physiological integrity
   A. Monitor neonatal well-being.
3. Psychosocial integrity
   A. Provide opportunities for support of neonate and parental-infant interactions.

4. Health promotion and maintenance
   A. Provide infant-care teaching for parents.

Implementation

1. Complete gestational age and admission assessments.
2. Maintain respirations. Suction neonate as needed. Observe for grunting, nasal flaring, and retractions.
3. Assess gestational age.
4. Obtain blood glucose and HCT levels.
5. Place prophylactic eye treatment in eyes for treatment of *Neisseria gonorrhoeae*. Common medications are erythromycin (Ilotycin) and silver nitrate (1%).
6. Administer phytonadione—vitamin K$_1$ (Aqua-MEPHYTON)—to prevent a transient deficiency of factors II, VII, IX, X.
7. Maintain body temperature. Place baby under radiant heaters. Check axillary temperature every 2 hours. Bathe infant at 4–6 hours if temperature is stable.

Ongoing Care

1. Complete physical assessment every 8 hours.
2. Monitor respirations, pulse, and temperature.
3. Prevent infection.
   A. Wash hands prior to handling each infant.
   B. Apply cleansing and drying agent to umbilical cord.
4. Weigh infant daily. Infant may lose up to 10% of birthweight. Usually regains weight by 7th–10th day of life.
5. Maintain nutrition and GI function.
   A. Offer first feeding of glucose water at 4–6 hours of life if infant formula feeding; observe for choking and cyanosis. Breast-feeding infants should receive their mother's colostrum for the first feeding, as it is a physiologic substance and less harmful to the lungs if aspirated than glucose water.
   B. Feed thereafter at breast or with bottle on demand; anticipate "spitting up" as the baby learns to coordinate sucking and swallowing and evacuates excessive mucus.
   C. Anticipate that infant will consume ½–2 oz of milk, increasing to 2–4 oz on subsequent day.
   D. Facilitate infant's consumption of the initial breast milk (colostrum), which is high in fat, protein, vitamin K, and immune factors.
   F. Encourage breast-feeding by suggesting a comfortable side-lying or sitting position for the mother, stroking the infant's cheek so the infant will turn, allowing nipple to be placed into a wide open mouth.
6. Observe for the first meconium (dark green to black) stool passed in the first 24 hours of life, followed by dark greenish brown transitional stools; breast-fed babies will have 3–4 golden yellow seedy stools a day, and bottle-fed babies will have 1–2 yellowish white stools a day.
7. Observe circumcised site for bleeding.
8. Administer Heptavac per physician's order.
9. Facilitate parenting skills and family bonding.
   A. Reassure parents regarding their abilities to parent.
   B. Inform the parents regarding:
      (1) Meaning of the infant's crying
      (2) Reducing or adding auditory, visual, and tactile stimuli
      (3) Position the infant likes best

      (4) Feeding and bathing techniques
      (5) Importance of observations and recordkeeping
   C. Encourage limited or unlimited rooming-in.
   D. Promote care participation by siblings and grandparents.
10. Instruct parents in safety practices.
    A. Never leave infant alone in bathtub or parked car.
    B. Keep plastic bags away from infant.
    C. Place infant in a prone position after feeding.
    D. Check temperature of warmed formula.
    E. Keep diaper pins closed and away from infant.
    F. Do not tie pacifier or necklace around infant's neck.

Evaluation

1. Ensure that the neonate exhibits normal adaptation to extrauterine life.
2. Maintain neonatal respirations, temperature, nutrition, and general well-being.
3. Ensure that neonate and parents are interacting on a frequent basis.
4. Ensure that parents have received infant-care teaching.

Disorders During Pregnancy
Disorders During the Antepartal Period

Bleeding Disorders: Abortion or Miscarriage

Description

Abortion is the spontaneous termination of a pregnancy before the 20th week of gestation. It may be described as:
1. **Spontaneous:** Occurs naturally during 2nd or 3rd month.
2. **Habitual:** Spontaneous loss of three or more pregnancies.
3. **Complete:** All related tissues and the fetus are expelled.
4. **Incomplete:** Some but not all of the parts of conception are expelled.
5. **Threatened:** Bleeding and/or cramping, but no cervical dilation or rupture of membranes, possible loss of the pregnancy.
6. **Missed:** The fetus dies, but the products of conception are retained in the uterus. Induction may be necessary if the pregnancy is not spontaneously expelled after several weeks or months. There is an increased risk for maternal DIC if the pregnancy is retained for a prolonged period of time.
7. **Inevitable:** Bleeding and cramping with cervical dilation. Loss of pregnancy.

Assessment

PHYSICAL ASSESSMENT

Assess for the following clinical manifestations:
1. Vaginal bleeding, spotting or hemorrhage, clots
2. Low abdominal cramping
3. Passing of tissue through the vagina
4. Shock

PSYCHOSOCIAL AND CULTURAL ASSESSMENT

1. Expectant woman and partner verbalize fear and disappointment.

2. Couple may express feelings of guilt; expectant parents may feel that they did something to cause the spontaneous abortion.

Planning for Imminent or Incomplete Abortion

1. Safe, effective care environment
   A. Provide information regarding treatment plan.
2. Physiological integrity
   A. Promote maternal physical well-being.
3. Psychosocial integrity
   A. Provide opportunities for counseling and support.
4. Health promotion and maintenance
   A. Provide teaching related to self-care measures.

Implementation

1. Observe for vaginal bleeding and cramping.
2. Save expelled tissue and clots for examination.
3. Monitor vital signs every 5 minutes to 4 hours depending on maternal status.
4. Maintain woman on bed rest.
5. Observe for signs of shock, and institute treatment measures.
6. Prepare for dilatation and curettage, if appropriate.
7. Provide support, but avoid offering false assurance.

Evaluation

Ensure that the woman:
1. Is free from anemia and/or infection.
2. Is free of vaginal bleeding, or her physiological status has returned to normal following the abortion.
3. Verbalizes feelings regarding the event and the outcome, as does significant other.
4. Understands self-care measures.

Hydatidiform Mole

Description

A hydatidiform mole is a developmental anomaly of the placenta that results in changing chorionic villi into a mass of clear vesicles. The edematous grapelike cluster may be benign or may develop into choriocarcinoma (cancer).

Assessment

PHYSICAL ASSESSMENT

1. Vaginal bleeding may be intermittent, bright red or dark brown, slightly or profuse in amount. Bleeding usually occurs by the 12th week.
2. Hyperemesis is common and may be caused by high levels of HCG.
3. Fundal height is greater than expected for dates.
4. HCG levels are elevated.
5. Ultrasonography reveals characteristic "snow storm" pattern, and no FHR is detectable.
6. FHR is not detectable by auscultation.
7. Symptoms of PIH may be present before the 20th week (elevated blood pressure, edema, and proteinuria).

PSYCHOSOCIAL AND CULTURAL ASSESSMENT

1. Incidence is low in America but high in the Far East, especially Taiwan.
2. Condition occurs more frequently with increased maternal age.
3. Diminished self-esteem may result.
4. Woman may experience fear of pregnancy.
5. Fear for own life may occur owing to possibility of choriocarcinoma.

Planning

1. Safe, effective care environment
   A. Provide information regarding treatment plan.
2. Physiological integrity
   A. Promote maternal physical well-being.
3. Psychosocial integrity
   A. Provide opportunities for counseling and support.
4. Health promotion and maintenance
   A. Provide teaching related to self-care.

Implementation

1. Coordinate diagnostic testing.
2. Prepare woman for uterine evacuation, induced abortion. Hysterectomy may be necessary.
3. Observe for postprocedure hemorrhage and infection.
4. Instruct and facilitate follow-up care.
   A. Monitor HCG levels for 1 year.
   B. Instruct regarding birth control measures so that pregnancy can be prevented during the 1-year follow-up.
   C. For women diagnosed with choriocarcinoma, chemotherapeutic agent, such as methotrexate, may be given.
5. Provide support during family's grieving period.

Evaluation

Ensure that the woman:
1. Has rapidly decreasing HCG titers.
2. Recovers physically after evacuation of the molar pregnancy.
3. Verbalizes a positive self-image.
4. Avoids conception during the treatment period.
5. Voices understanding regarding need to avoid pregnancy as per her physician's recommendations.

Ectopic Pregnancy

Description

An ectopic pregnancy results from implantation of the fertilized ovum outside the uterus, generally in the fallopian tube. The fallopian tube may be constricted as the result of acute or chronic pelvic infections or developmental defects.

Nursing Assessment

PHYSICAL ASSESSMENT

Assess for the following clinical manifestations:
1. Sharp, localized pain in lower abdomen, which is caused by expansion and possible rupture of the tube. May have syncope and referred shoulder pain.
2. Irregular vaginal bleeding.

3. Abdominal rigidity, distention.
4. Shock—decreased blood pressure, increased heart rate.
5. Palpable mass in the cul-de-sac or adnexa.
6. HCG titers may be lower than normal.

PSYCHOSOCIAL AND CULTURAL ASSESSMENT

1. Severe pain may contribute to disorientation, lack of cooperation.
2. Unawareness of pregnancy may lead to fears.
3. Parents grieve over loss of the pregnancy.

Planning

1. Safe, effective care environment
   A. Woman is able to participate in decision making regarding treatment plan.
2. Physiological integrity
   A. Provide pain relief measures and monitor for shock.
3. Psychosocial integrity
   A. Provide opportunities for counseling and support.
4. Health promotion and maintenance
   A. Provide teaching related to self-care.

Implementation

1. Provide pain relief.
2. Manage shock.
   A. Administer O_2, IV fluids.
   B. Type and cross-match blood.
3. Prepare for surgery, laparotomy with removal of the ectopic pregnancy, and perhaps the affected fallopian tube (salpingectomy).
4. Provide postoperative care.
   A. Give routine postoperative care.
   B. Assess vaginal bleeding.
   C. Offer emotional support.

Evaluation

Ensure that the woman:
1. Has participated in decision making.
2. Is free of pain and normotensive.
3. Acknowledges support through the treatment process.
4. Demonstrates knowledge of self-care measures.

Placenta Previa

Description

In placenta previa, the placenta is implanted near or over the maternal cervical os (Figure 3–7). The placement is described as:
1. **Complete or central:** The center of the placenta lies directly over the cervical os.
2. **Incomplete or partial:** A portion of the placenta covers the cervical os.
3. **Marginal or low implantation:** The outer edge of the placenta lies on or near the cervical os.

Assessment

PHYSICAL ASSESSMENT

Assess for the following clinical manifestations:
1. Painless unexplained uterine bleeding after the 20th week (usually around week 27); each succeeding vaginal bleed is greater than the last.
2. Bleeding generally occurs in intermittent gushes.
3. Sonogram of the uterus validates placental placement.
4. Profuse hemorrhaging can occur in the third trimester as the os gradually dilates, pulling away from the placenta and causing profuse bleeding.

PSYCHOSOCIAL AND CULTURAL ASSESSMENT

1. Incident of placenta previa increases with fetal development defects, twin gestation, or previous infertility.
2. Apprehension regarding maternal and infant safety will follow first bleeding episode.
3. Three out of four women with placenta previa are multigravidas.

Planning

1. Safe, effective care environment
   A. Monitor for bleeding episodes.
2. Physiological integrity
   A. Monitor maternal-fetal status.
3. Psychosocial integrity
   A. Provide opportunities for support and counseling.
4. Health promotion and maintenance
   A. Provide education for self-care.

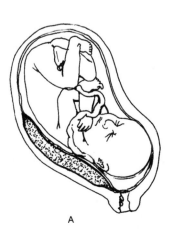
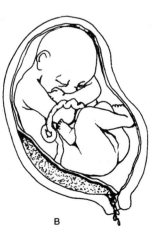
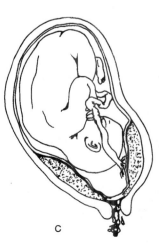

A   B   C

Figure 3–7. Placenta previa. (*A*) Low implantation. (*B*) Partial placenta previa. (*C*) Central (total) placenta previa.

Implementation

1. Do not perform vaginal or rectal exams or give enemas.
2. Prepare patient for diagnostic testing: sonogram to monitor fetal heart tones (FHT).
3. Facilitate "double setup" vaginal examination by obstetrician.
   A. Preparation for cesarean section is completed before vaginal examination.
   B. Examination is done in operating room.
   C. Type and cross-match for possible blood transfusion.
4. Manage bleeding episodes.
   A. Keep woman NPO.
   B. Monitor vital signs, FHR (by continuous EFM).
   C. Maintain woman on absolute bed rest.
   D. Start and/or maintain IV.
   E. Maintain perineal pad count to estimate amount of bleeding (1 g of weight is approximately 1 mL).
   F. Prepare for cesarean birth.
   G. Maintain meticulous sterile techniques.
5. Support parents, encourage them to verbalize feelings.
6. Instruct parents regarding nature of problem.
7. Prepare for a cesarean birth care, if necessary.
8. Prepare woman for vaginal birth—if pregnancy is near term, the cervix is favorable, and marginal placental placement is identified.

Evaluation

Ensure that expectant woman:
1. Exhibits self-limiting bleeding episodes with no harm to infant or mother.
2. Demonstrates normal vital signs, HCT, and hemoglobin; FHR should be between 110–160 bpm with average variability and no late or variable decelerations.
3. Verbalizes apprehension she feels.
4. Verbalizes self-care measures related to rest and monitoring bleeding.

Incompetent Cervix

Description

Cervical incompetence is the premature dilation of the cervix. The dilation usually occurs in the fourth or fifth month of pregnancy. It may be associated with cervical trauma as a result of previous surgery or birth. Cervical incompetence is treated surgically with a Shirodkar-Barter or McDonald procedure.

Assessment

PHYSICAL ASSESSMENT

Assess for the following clinical manifestations:
1. Vaginal bleeding at 18–28 weeks of gestation.
2. Recurrent painless, spontaneous, early third-trimester abortion or premature labor.
3. Fetal membranes may be visible through cervix.

PSYCHOSOCIAL AND CULTURAL ASSESSMENT

1. Recurrent spontaneous abortions may contribute to anxiety and discouragement.
2. Guilt may be experienced.

Planning/Goals

1. Safe, effective environment
   A. Provide teaching regarding the surgical treatment procedure.
2. Physiological integrity
   A. Monitor expectant woman for signs of contractions or for rupture of membranes.
   B. Ensure that pregnancy is carried to term.
3. Psychosocial integrity
   A. Provide opportunities for parents to talk about their feelings.
4. Health promotion and maintenance
   A. Teach expectant woman the signs that should be reported to the physician.

Implementation

1. Obtain accurate obstetrical history, especially of relatively painless second-trimester pregnancy losses.
2. Maintain woman on bed rest.
3. Monitor FHR.
4. Prepare for surgery: McDonald procedure (purse string around cervix) can be removed for a vaginal delivery, or Shirodkar-Barter (cerclage) is left in place (delivery must be cesarean).
5. Observe for possible postoperative complications.
   A. Rupture of the membranes, which will require that the cervical suture be removed and pregnancy terminated.
   B. Contractions of the uterus, which the physician will attempt to control.
6. Instruct client in postprocedure care.
   A. Maintain bed rest for 24 hours.
   B. Report vaginal bleeding immediately.
   C. Report increased uterine cramping immediately.

Evaluation

Ensure that the expectant woman:
1. Understands the surgical procedure that was done.
2. Does not have contractions.
3. Carries the pregnancy to term.
4. Feels positive about the chances of maintaining the pregnancy, as does significant other.
5. Verbalizes that she will report to the physician if she experiences uterine contractions or rupture of membranes.

Hyperemesis

Description

Hyperemesis is pernicious vomiting in pregnancy.

Assessment

PHYSICAL ASSESSMENT

Assess for the following clinical manifestations:
1. Intractable vomiting at any time
2. Weight loss of 25% or more
3. Ketosis, ketonuria (alkalosis)
4. Dehydration—poor skin turgor, dry tongue
5. Epigastric pain
6. Drowsiness and confusion

7. Uncoordinated movements, jerking
8. Jaundice
9. Coma

PSYCHOSOCIAL AND CULTURAL ASSESSMENT

1. Uncertainty regarding the pregnancy
2. Inordinate stress present in couple's life

Planning

1. Safe, effective care environment
    A. Expectant woman establishes normal fluid and electrolyte balance.
2. Physiological integrity
    A. Provide IV and/or oral fluids to re-establish fluid and electrolyte balance.
3. Psychosocial integrity
    A. Create opportunities to explore woman's feelings about the pregnancy and coping abilities.
4. Health promotion and maintenance
    A. Provide teaching related to need for fluids.

Implementation

1. Facilitate hospital admission, if required.
2. Administer parenteral fluids, vitamins, sedatives, as prescribed.
3. Monitor intake, output, and daily weight.
4. Assess state of hydration.
5. Begin oral feedings slowly with fluids. Progress to six small feedings a day.
6. Obtain psychiatric consultation, if indicated.

Evaluation

Ensure that the woman:
1. Is well hydrated.
2. Has normal electrolyte values.
3. Verbalizes feelings and ability to cope with the pregnancy.
4. Verbalizes knowledge of need for fluid.

Pre-Existing Conditions

Diabetes Mellitus

Description

Diabetes mellitus is insufficiency or lack of insulin production and secretion by the pancreas, which is amplified by pregnancy. Predisposing factors include family history of diabetes, obesity, stress, and pancreatic tumor.

There are two methods of classifying diabetes mellitus. White's classification is the oldest method. In 1979, a new classification was developed by the National Diabetes Group of the National Institutes of Health and is currently used by most physicians.

WHITE'S CLASSIFICATION (REFLECTIVE OF ONSET AND PATHOLOGY)

Class A: Gestational diabetes controlled by diet
Class B: Onset after age 20, duration up to 9 years, no vascular changes

Class C: Onset at age 10 to 19, duration of 10 to 19 years, no vascular changes
Class D: Onset before age 10, duration of 20 or more years, retinal and vascular changes
Class E: Pelvic vessels calcified
Class F: Kidney changes

NATIONAL DIABETES GROUP OF NATIONAL INSTITUTES OF HEALTH CLASSIFICATION

1. Diabetes mellitus
    A. Type I: insulin-dependent (IDDM)
    B. Type II: non–insulin-dependent (NIDDM)
       (1) Nonobese NIDDM
       (2) Obese NIDDM
    C. Type III (gestational diabetes)

Assessment

PHYSICAL ASSESSMENT

Assess for the following clinical manifestations:
1. Hyperemesis during early pregnancy
2. Glycosuria, ketonuria
3. Elevated blood glucose, glucose tolerance test (GTT)
4. Polydipsia, polyphagia, polyuria
5. Rapid weight gain
6. Previous large babies weighing 4000 g or more.

PSYCHOSOCIAL AND CULTURAL ASSESSMENT

1. Anxiety is associated with fears of fetal harm or demise.
2. Uncertainty regarding appropriate method of delivery may stress parents.
3. Stress may be felt from coping with a disease process as well as the pregnancy.

Planning

1. Safe, effective care environment
    A. Test regularly for glucose levels.
    B. Implement insulin and dietary regulation as needed.
2. Physiological integrity
    A. Observe for signs of hypoglycemia and hyperglycemia.
3. Psychosocial integrity
    A. Provide counseling and support.
4. Health promotion and maintenance
    A. Assess knowledge level of woman relative to disease and provide teaching.

Implementation

1. Obtain accurate obstetrical and diet history.
2. Assess health status and report abnormalities to physician.
    A. Hydramnios
    B. Large infant size
    C. FHR
    D. Weight, blood pressure
3. Facilitate and instruct regarding insulin injections.
    A. Blood-sugar levels are used to determine insulin requirements.
    B. Testing blood 4 times daily.
    C. Teaching home use of blood-monitoring device.
    D. Regular or NPH insulin or a combination of both will be used.

E. Ketoacidosis and hypoglycemia must be treated promptly.

F. Insulin requirements are highest in the third trimester and drop precipitously after birth.

G. Oral hypoglycemics are to be avoided. They cross the placenta and are teratogenic.

4. Encourage regular exercise for weight and blood-sugar control.

5. Provide diet instruction.
   A. Avoid calorie restrictions.
   B. Provide 2200–2400 kcal/day.
   C. Carbohydrate intake should be 45% of caloric intake.
   D. Protein—20%.
   E. Fat—35% (polyunsaturated).
   F. Eat at regularly scheduled times (three meals and two to four snacks daily).
   G. Observe for hypoglycemia.

6. Monitor for urinary and vaginal tract infection.

7. Anticipate and prepare for birth.
   A. Fetal maturity determined by lecithin/sphingomyelin (L/S) ratio. Need 3:1 ratio and presence of PG.
   B. Vaginal birth is preferable to cesarean birth.

8. Observe for the following complications:
   A. Hydramnios
   B. Preeclampsia, eclampsia
   C. Stillbirth
   D. Neonatal respiratory distress syndrome (RDS), congenital anomalies, hyperbilirubinemia, hypoglycemia
   E. Postpartum hemorrhage, infection

9. Provide parental support during childbearing experience.

10. Breast-feeding decreases insulin requirements and should be encouraged.

11. Provide postpartum contraceptive information.
    A. Avoid oral contraceptives because diabetes causes vascular changes and may increase the risk for DVTs.
    B. Use barrier contraceptives, natural family planning.

Evaluation

Ensure that expectant woman:
1. Remains normoglycemic.
2. Shows no signs or symptoms of hypoglycemia or hyperglycemia.
3. Verbalizes support.
4. Verbalizes understanding of her disease and the implications of diabetes for pregnancy.

Cardiac Disease

Description

Cardiac decompensation can occur with the normal cardiac changes of pregnancy in combination with maternal cardiac pathology: mitral stenosis or regurgitation, aortic valve stenosis, or regurgitation. The most common problem is congestive heart failure due to increased cardiac demands and blood volume associated with normal pregnancy.

Assessment

PHYSICAL ASSESSMENT

Assess for the following clinical manifestations:
1. Pedal edema, progressive generalized edema
2. Exertional dyspnea, basilar rales
3. Moist cough
4. Tachycardia, irregular pulse
5. Increasing fatigue
6. Cyanosis of lips and nail beds
7. Heart murmurs
8. Severe/persistent fungal infections (Candida, etc.).

PSYCHOSOCIAL AND CULTURAL ASSESSMENT

1. Frustration may occur as activity level is curtailed.
2. Anxiety is associated with fear of fetal and maternal demise.

Planning

1. Safe, effective care environment
   A. Protect from infection.
2. Physiological integrity
   A. Promote graded activity and periods of rest.
3. Psychosocial integrity
   A. Promote client acceptance of need for activity restriction.
4. Health promotion and maintenance
   A. Provide education for self-care.

Implementation

See Table 3–20.

Evaluation

Ensure that expectant woman:
1. Remains free of infection.
2. Follows activity and rest recommendations.
3. Monitors her physical response to activity.
4. Participates in self-care activities.

Acquired Immunodeficiency Syndrome

Description

Acquired immunodeficiency syndrome (AIDS) is caused by the human immunodeficiency virus (HIV). It may be contracted through contamination with blood or body fluids, blood products (contaminated IV needles), heterosexual sexual activity, or passed to the fetus.

Assessment

PHYSICAL ASSESSMENT

Assess for the following clinical manifestations:
1. History of IV drug use and/or prostitution
2. Malaise
3. Progressive weight loss
4. Lymphadenopathy
5. Diarrhea
6. Evidence of opportunistic infection
7. Fever
8. Evidence of Kaposi's sarcoma (purplish, reddish brown lesions)

PSYCHOSOCIAL AND CULTURAL ASSESSMENT

1. AIDS occurs most frequently in women with a history of IV drug use.
2. Anxiety about future of self and child.

Planning

1. Safe, effective care environment
   A. Protect from infection.

Table 3–20. Classification and Nursing Management of Pregnant Woman with Cardiac Disease

Classification	Client Symptoms	Nursing Plan and Intervention
I	No symptoms even with physical activity	1. Obtain additional evening rest. 2. Prevent and/or obtain early treatment of infections. 3. Anticipate vaginal delivery with regional block and forceps.
II	Comfortable at rest with symptoms during ordinary physical activity	1. Avoid strenuous exercise. 2. Administer prophylactic penicillin, digitalis, diuretics. 3. Obtain frequent rest periods. 4. Anticipate vaginal delivery with regional block, oxygen, forceps.
III	Comfortable at rest with symptoms during less than ordinary physical activity	1. Reduce physical activity. 2. Avoid emotional stress. 3. Administer penicillin, digitalis, diuretics. 4. Facilitate early hospitalization and delivery. 5. Anticipate recommendation of early therapeutic abortion.
IV	Symptoms at rest	1. Anticipate recommendation of early therapeutic abortion; 50% mortality associated with delivery. 2. Administer penicillin, digitalis, diuretics, rotating tourniquets. 3. Prepare for vaginal delivery.

2. Physiological integrity
   A. Maintain isolation precautions.
3. Psychosocial integrity
   A. Provide opportunities for counseling.
4. Health promotion and maintenance
   A. Provide education for self-care regarding isolation precautions and prevention of infection.

Implementation

1. Observe blood and body-secretion precautions, and teach precautions to client.
2. Maintain isolation to protect client from other organisms.
3. Follow blood and secretion precautions during all contact with expectant woman (antepartal, intrapartal, postpartal) and for the newborn infant.
4. Provide education regarding disease process and greatly decreased risk of transmission to the newborn if treated with Zidovidine in the last trimester of pregnancy.

Evaluation

Ensure that the expectant woman:
1. Is protected from further infection.
2. Participates in maintaining blood and body-secretion isolation.
3. Is able to verbalize her feelings about her condition.
4. Verbalizes knowledge of disease condition and implications for the future.

Hypertension

Description

Hypertension is elevated blood pressure occurring during the second trimester in the absence of preeclamptic symptomatology. This is regarded as essential hypertension unmasked by pregnancy and is generally permanent.

Assessment

PHYSICAL ASSESSMENT

Assess for the following clinical manifestations:
1. Blood pressure elevation to 140/90 if no preexisting hypertension.
2. Retinal changes demonstrate arterial-venous nicking.

PSYCHOSOCIAL AND CULTURAL ASSESSMENT

1. Hypertension occurs more frequently in older multipara.
2. American black women experience a higher incidence.
3. Woman may grieve about the lifelong nature of hypertension.

Planning

1. Safe, effective environment
   A. Monitor blood pressure on routine basis.
2. Physiological integrity
   A. Promote maternal-fetal well-being.
3. Psychosocial integrity
   A. Provide counseling and support
4. Health promotion and maintenance
   A. Provide education for self-care.

Implementation

1. Assess blood pressure every 2 weeks for the first 2 trimesters, then weekly until birth.
2. Assess weight; test urine for protein, indicating preeclampsia; report abnormalities to physician.
3. Administer and instruct regarding drug therapy.
   A. Antihypertensive drugs: methyldopa (Aldomet)
   B. Avoid diuretics unless the benefits outweigh the risks.
4. Instruct regarding nature, progress of disease.
5. Encourage frequent rest periods.
6. Counsel to avoid undue stress.

7. Provide diet instruction.
   A. No added salt diet
   B. High protein
   C. Maintain fluid intake.
   D. Routine prenatal nutrition
8. Anticipate early vaginal or cesarean birth.

Evaluation

Ensure that expectant woman:
1. Remains normotensive.
2. Progresses to birth with no further complications, as does the fetus.
3. Verbalizes support.
4. Verbalizes knowledge of self-care measures, treatment regimen, balanced activity and rest, and information regarding her medication.

Disorders That Develop During Pregnancy

Pregnancy-Induced Hypertension

Description

Pregnancy-induced hypertension is a set of symptoms occurring during pregnancy, which include edema, hypertension, proteinuria, convulsions, and coma. Eclampsia occurs at the point of convulsions. Etiology is unclear but appears to be associated with reduced uteroplacental blood flow.

Assessment

PHYSICAL ASSESSMENT

Assess for clinical manifestations (Table 3–21).

PSYCHOSOCIAL AND CULTURAL ASSESSMENT

1. American blacks have a higher incidence of PIH for age, parity, and familial incidence.
2. PIH occurs more frequently in young primiparous women and multiparous women older than the age of 35.
3. Predisposing factors include inadequate protein intake, multiple pregnancy, hydatidiform mole, and chronic renal and vascular disease.

Planning

1. Safe, effective care environment
   A. Prevent progression of PIH to convulsions.

2. Physiological integrity
   A. Monitor maternal and fetal well-being.
3. Psychosocial integrity
   A. Provide counseling and support.
4. Health promotion and maintenance
   A. Provide teaching related to self-care measures.

Implementation

1. Facilitate early prenatal assessment, especially among high-risk groups.
2. Assess physical parameters.
   A. Blood pressure.
   B. Weight.
   C. Urine for protein.
   D. Edema of face, hands, pretibial area.
   E. Check reflexes for hyperreflexia.
3. Provide diet instruction and assess compliance.
   A. Adequate Na; avoid added salt and high sodium foods.
   B. Maintain fluid intake.
   C. Ensure high protein intake (1 g/kg per day).
   D. Maintain good prenatal nutrition.
4. Instruct regarding medications.
   A. Antihypertensive drugs: Aldomet, Apresoline
   B. Sedation: phenobarbital; avoid Valium as it is associated with an increased risk of aspiration if seizures occur.
5. Facilitate hospitalization, if required.
6. Promote bed rest, rest on left side, quiet environment.
7. Prevent convulsions.
   A. Administer magnesium sulfate ($MgSO_4$) loading dose (4–6 g) and maintain at 1–2 g/hr (given IV by infused pump).
   B. Obtain $MgSO_4$ blood levels at least every 4 hours.
   C. Use fetal monitor for continuous FHR tracing.
   D. Assess urine output, proteinuria, vital signs, reflexes, and respiratory effort hourly.
   E. Administer calcium gluconate for $MgSO_4$ overdose.
   F. Prepare for labor induction or cesarean birth.
   G. Continue $MgSO_4$ for 24 hours after birth.

Evaluation

Ensure that expectant woman:
1. Complies with treatment regimen and does not develop eclampsia.
2. Progresses to birth without further complications, as does her baby.
3. Verbalizes support and increased coping ability.
4. Verbalizes self-care measures.

Table 3–21. Symptomatology of Preeclampsia and Eclampsia

Symptom	Preeclampsia	Eclampsia
Edema	Mild to moderate, pretibial area	Severe in face, hands, pretibial area
Proteinuria	Trace, 1+ to 2+*	Copious, 3+ to 4+
Weight gain	2–2.5 lb/wk*	Sudden large increase
Blood pressure	Systolic is ≥30 mm Hg; diastolic is ≥15 mm Hg above baseline, 140/90 to 160/110*	Systolic > 160 Diastolic > 110
Other	Headache, blurred vision, pulmonary edema, epigastric pain, oliguria, hyperreflexia tremors, twitching	Tonic-clonic seizures, cyanosis, fetal distress

*Two of three symptoms must be present to constitute preeclampsia.

Hydramnios

Description

Hydramnios is an excess of amniotic fluid ≥2000 mL. Predisposing factors include the following:
1. Maternal diabetes mellitus
2. Preeclampsia, eclampsia
3. ABO, Rh incompatibilities
4. Multiple pregnancies

Assessment

PHYSICAL ASSESSMENT

Assess for the following clinical manifestations:
1. Ballottement results in fluid waves.
2. Fundal height excessive for gestation.
3. Fetus difficult to outline with palpation.
4. Supine hypotension.
5. Sonogram for fetal abnormalities of the central nervous system or GI tract

PSYCHOSOCIAL AND CULTURAL ASSESSMENT

1. Is frustrated regarding easy fatigability.
2. Communicates concerns, loss of comfort.

Planning

1. Safe, effective care environment
   A. Promote maternal comfort.
2. Physiological integrity
   A. Promote maternal-fetal well-being.
3. Psychosocial integrity
   A. Provide opportunities for counseling and support.
4. Health promotion and maintenance
   A. Provide education related to self-care measures to increase comfort.

Implementation

1. Facilitate testing: amniocentesis, sonogram (see Table 3–9).
2. Assess FHR with rupture of membrane.
3. Anticipate premature labor, postpartum hemorrhage, caused by overdistention of uterine muscle tissue.
4. Instruct and explain the following:
   A. Nature of problem
   B. Need to obtain immediate medical attention for problem
   C. Need to observe for preeclampsia

Evaluation

Ensure that expectant mother:
1. Verbalizes increased comfort.
2. Progresses to uneventful birth, as does her baby.
3. Verbalizes support.
4. Verbalizes self-care measures.

Intrauterine Fetal Death

Description

Intrauterine fetal death results from unknown or various other possible causes: chromosomal aberration, spontaneous abortion, ectopic pregnancy, or maternal or fetal illness.

Assessment

PHYSICAL ASSESSMENT

Assess for the following clinical manifestations:
1. Vaginal bleeding, uterine cramping.
2. Cessation of FHR, no fetal movement.
3. Weight gain and fundal height not consistent with gestation.
4. Estriol level decreased.
5. Sonogram may confirm fetal demise.

PSYCHOSOCIAL AND CULTURAL ASSESSMENT

1. Mother may skip appointments because she is aware of fetal death.
2. Verbalization may reflect guilt as the mother articulates what she could or could not have done to prevent death of fetus.

Planning

1. Safe, effective care environment
   A. Provide information regarding the birth procedure.
2. Physiological integrity
   A. Monitor maternal physical status during the birth.
3. Psychosocial integrity
   A. Provide opportunities for parents to work through grief process.
4. Health promotion and maintenance
   A. Provide education for self-care following birth.

Implementation

1. Review fetal activity records with the woman.
2. Contact expectant women who have missed appointments.
3. Provide information to clarify misconceptions.
4. Provide information related to diagnostic techniques to determine fetal death.
5. Assist with induction.
6. Remain with woman continuously.
7. Provide time for parents to be close with infant after delivery if parents desire.
8. Assist parents in working through grief process.

Evaluation

Ensure that the woman:
1. Is knowledgeable about the birth procedure.
2. Has vital signs and coagulation factors that remain within normal limits.
3. Is working through the grief process with significant other.
4. Verbalizes postpartal self-care measures.

Disorders During the Intrapartal Period

Premature Labor

Description

Premature labor is labor that occurs between 20 and 37 completed weeks of gestation. In 20%–30% of the cases, preterm premature rupture of membranes (PPROM) precedes premature labor. In the other 70%–80% of the cases, its cause is unknown.

Assessment

PHYSICAL ASSESSMENT

Assess for the following clinical manifestations:
1. Onset of labor is spontaneous.
2. Membranes may rupture.
3. Uterine contractions are palpable:
   ≤10 minutes apart
   ≤30 seconds in duration
4. Cervix is effaced and dilated.

PSYCHOSOCIAL AND CULTURAL ASSESSMENT

1. Woman may express fear regarding outcome for the baby.
2. Woman may express feelings of guilt.
3. Coping abilities are stressed because of hospitalization, intense attention directed to the gestation, and worry regarding ability to afford the medical care.

Planning

1. Safe, effective care environment
   A. Provide information regarding treatment plans.
2. Physiological integrity
   A. Administer treatment to arrest labor and monitor maternal-fetal status.
3. Psychosocial integrity
   A. Provide opportunities for parents to talk about their feelings.
4. Health promotion and maintenance
   A. Provide education regarding self-care measures.

Implementation

1. Assist in assessment of fetal age: sonography, estriol levels, L/S ratio, etc.
2. Anticipate progression of labor if:
   A. Gestation is ≤37 weeks.
   B. Membranes are ruptured.
   C. Maternal complications occur.
   D. Fetal complications occur.
   E. Labor advances; cervix dilates to 4 cm and is 80% effaced.
3. Maintain woman on bed rest in left lateral position.
4. Administer IV fluids. May hydrate with 500 mL before beginning any other therapy.
5. Carry out prescribed procedure to assist labor as appropriate.
   A. Administer sympathomimetic agents (ritodrine, terbutaline) or MgSO$_4$
   B. Observe for maternal hypotension, tachycardia, arrhythmia; have antidote propranolol available if using sympathomimetic and calcium gluconate if using MgSO$_4$ as tocolytic agent.
   C. Monitor maternal vital signs, breath sounds.
   D. Monitor FHR, contractions continuously.
6. Administer glucocorticoid therapy (betamethasone) as ordered to hasten fetal lung maturity if birth can be delayed 48 hours.
7. Avoid narcotic analgesics; mild analgesics may be necessary during labor and birth.
8. Inform and support parents through labor arrest and/or birth.
9. Provide premature infant care (see Disorders of the Neonate, below).

Evaluation

Ensure that expectant woman:
1. Verbalizes knowledge of treatment plan.
2. Has labor arrested and that maternal-fetal status is within normal limits.
3. Verbalizes fears and concerns.
4. Verbalizes signs and symptoms of preterm labor, need for resting during day, nutritional and fluid needs, recognition of warning signs and understands how to take her medication.

Dysfunctional Labor

Description

Contractile problems occur when uterine contractions are ineffective; their cause is unknown. The contractions may be either hypertonic or hypotonic in character.

Assessment

PHYSICAL ASSESSMENT

1. Hyperactive pattern—uterine contractions occurring approximately every 2 minutes. Intensity increases, resting tone increases. Pain is out of proportion to labor progress. Occurs in latent phase.
2. Hypoactive pattern—uterine contractions occurring approximately every 5–10 minutes. Intensity decreases. Pattern develops after regular contractions have progressed labor to the active phase.
3. Cervical dilation slows with both patterns.
4. Fetal descent slows or stops with both patterns.
5. Expectant mother becomes exhausted and dehydrated with both patterns.

PSYCHOSOCIAL AND CULTURAL ASSESSMENT

1. Hypertonic pattern occurs more frequently in primigravida.
2. Fatigue and discouragement are common.
3. Lack of cooperation, confusion may accompany exhaustion.

Planning

1. Safe, effective care environment
   A. Explain the treatment plans.
2. Physiological integrity
   A. Assess maternal-fetal status.
3. Psychosocial integrity
   A. Provide support and facilitate expression of feelings.
4. Health promotion and maintenance
   A. Administer comfort measures.

Implementation

HYPERTONIC PATTERN

1. Promote relaxation.
2. Encourage breathing pattern during contractions.
3. Use visualizations, muscle, touch, etc., to enhance rest and comfort.
4. Administer analgesic and/or sedation as ordered.
5. Monitor hydration status.

6. Provide support and encouragement.
7. May administer a tocolotic to decrease the high uterine resting tone and improve placental circulation.
8. May administer a sedative to promote rest.

HYPOTONIC PATTERN

1. Assist with x-ray pelvimetry to diagnose CPD.
2. Promote rest, reduce environmental stimuli.
3. Assess for hydration, exhaustion. IV may be prescribed to maintain hydration and electrolyte balance.
4. Provide support and encouragement.
5. Anticipate oxytocin augmentation if CPD is ruled out.
   A. Mainline IV of lactated Ringer's solution.
   B. Secondary bottle with 10 U oxytocin in 1000 mL lactated Ringer's solution. Administer by infusion pump and established augmentation protocol.
6. May deliver via cesarean if the above measures are ineffective.

Evaluation

Ensure that the expectant woman:
1. Verbalizes understanding of treatment plan, as does significant other.
2. Remains within normal limits, as does the fetus.
3. Verbalizes feelings and asks questions freely, as does significant other.
4. Maintains comfort.

Prolapsed Cord

Description

A prolapsed umbilical cord is displaced between the presenting part and the amnion or else protrudes through the cervix. The resulting danger is compression of the cord, thereby compromising fetal circulation.

Nursing Assessment

Assess for the following clinical manifestations:
1. The umbilical cord is seen or palpated.
2. FHR is irregular and slow.
3. Fetal heart monitor will display deep variable deceleration.
4. Fetal pH may be acidotic.
5. If fetal hypoxia is severe, violent fetal activity may occur and then cease.
6. Predisposing factors may be present.
   A. Transverse or breech position
   B. Prematurity
   C. Multiple birth
   D. Hydramnios
   E. CPD

Psychosocial and Cultural Assessment

1. Mother may not be aware there is a problem.
2. Confusion and fear may result when mother is informed.

Planning

1. Safe, effective care environment
   A. Relieve pressure on umbilical cord.

2. Physiological integrity
   A. Monitor FHR continuously.
3. Psychosocial integrity
   A. Provide support and encouragement.
4. Health promotion and maintenance
   A. Provide information regarding treatment.

Implementation

1. Assess mothers with predisposing factors carefully.
2. Monitor FHR after membranes have ruptured.
3. Relieve cord pressure immediately.
   A. Place mother in knee-chest or deep Trendelenburg position.
   B. Elevate fetal presenting part that is lying on the cord with a sterile, gloved hand. Do not attempt to push cord into the uterus. Call for help!
4. Administer O_2 by face mask to mother at 7–10 L/min.
5. Monitor FHR continuously.
6. Inform and support mother.
7. Prepare for emergency cesarean birth.
8. Anticipate a large surgical incision with rapid birth of fetus.
9. Assess infant for hypoxia.
10. Assist with cesarean birth.

Evaluation

1. Ensure that FHR remains in range of 110–160 bpm, without variable deceleration pattern.
2. Ensure that FHR is continuously monitored until birth.
3. Ensure that couple verbalizes feelings of support and decreased anxiety.
4. Ensure that couple verbalizes understanding of treatment plan.

Ruptured Uterus

Description

A ruptured uterus involves complete or incomplete separation of the uterine tissue due to unknown causes, uterine scars, or oxytocic agents. Fetal death frequently occurs, with guarded maternal prognosis because of hemorrhaging.

Assessment

PHYSICAL ASSESSMENT

Assess for the following clinical manifestations:
1. Mother complains of pain representative of a complete uterine rupture. Pain may be:
   A. Shearing or tearing
   B. Excruciating
   C. Diffuse or localized
2. Contractions may cease and/or fail to progress.
3. Relaxation between contractions is incomplete.
4. Abdomen is rigid.
5. Signs of maternal shock may be noted: rapid weak pulse, cold and clammy skin, pale-to-cyanotic color.
6. FHR is slow or absent. Fetus is easily palpated.
7. Fetal activity is violent, then absent.
8. Fetal outline can be felt outside of the uterus

9. Signs of incomplete rupture include:
   A. Abdominal pain that occurs during and between contractions.
   B. Contractions continue but cervix fails to dilate.
   C. Slight vaginal bleeding.
   D. FHR cannot be detected.

PSYCHOSOCIAL AND CULTURAL ASSESSMENT

1. Mother is anxious, restless, confused, weak.

Planning

1. Safe, effective care environment
   A. Monitor for presence of pre-existing conditions.
2. Physiological integrity
   A. Assess maternal-fetal status and initiate emergency care.
3. Psychosocial integrity
   A. Provide encouragement and support.
4. Health promotion and maintenance
   A. Administer measures to treat shock and blood loss.

Implementation

1. Assess maternal and infant vital signs carefully.
2. Discontinue oxytocic agent immediately if being administered.
3. Treat shock symptoms.
   A. Assess vital signs every 5–15 minutes.
   B. Administer O_2 by face mask at 7–10 L/min.
   C. Increase IV flow rate.
   D. Place mother in Trendelenburg position.
   E. Administer blood.
   F. Monitor urine output.
   G. Continuously monitor FHR.
4. Prepare for cesarean section or histotomy with hysterectomy.
5. Inform and support family members.
6. Provide postoperative care appropriate for procedure.

Evaluation

1. Assess laboring woman for pre-existing conditions.
2. Ensure that baby is born by emergency cesarean section with no signs of hypoxia.
3. Ensure that couple verbalizes feelings of support once emergency is over.
4. Ensure that mother is normotensive with hemoglobin and HCT levels are within normal values.

Abruptio Placentae

Description

Abruptio placentae is premature separation of the placenta from uterine wall. The separation may be complete or partial. Central placenta separation will cause concealed bleeding, making the uterus tender and firm; marginal separation will result in external bleeding. Shock may result in either case.

Assessment

PHYSICAL ASSESSMENT

Assess for the following clinical manifestations:
1. Vaginal bleeding may be scant or profuse.

2. Uterine irritability, tenderness, uneven tone, and rigidity. This is known as **Couvelaire uterus.**
3. Abdominal pain is continuous or intermittent.
4. Signs of maternal shock occur: hypotension, rapid pulse, dyspnea.
5. Violent fetal activity occurs followed by inactivity.
6. FHR is slow to absent.
7. Late deceleration is noted in FHR.
8. May have blood stained amniotic fluid (**port wine stained**).

PSYCHOSOCIAL AND CULTURAL ASSESSMENT

1. Excruciating pain and shock contribute to confusion.
2. Mother may be restless, anxious, and weak.

Planning

1. Safe, effective care environment
   A. Provide teaching regarding treatment measures.
2. Physiological integrity
   A. Monitor maternal-fetal status.
3. Psychosocial integrity
   A. Allay apprehension through support.
4. Health promotion and maintenance
   A. Administer measures to treat shock and blood loss.

Implementation

1. Respond to symptoms.
2. Treat shock symptoms.
   A. Administer O_2 by tight face mask at 7–10 L/min.
   B. Increase IV flow rate.
   C. Administer blood.
   D. Place mother in Trendelenburg position.
   E. Assess vital signs every 5–15 minutes.
   F. Monitor urine output.
   G. Continuously monitor FHR.
3. Observe for signs and symptoms of coagulation problems.
4. Measure abdominal girth.
5. Remain with woman.
6. Monitor labor pattern continuously if labor is allowed to continue, or prepare for cesarean birth.

Evaluation

Ensure that:
1. The woman and her partner understand treatment plan.
2. The woman and fetus' physiologic status remains within normal limits.
3. The woman and her partner verbalize decrease of anxiety and feelings of support once emergency is over.
4. The woman remains normotensive; hemoglobin and HCT levels are within normal limits.

Disorders of the Postpartum Period

Puerperal Fever and Postpartum Infection

Description

An infection of the reproductive tract may occur within the first 10 days after birth or abortion. The infection may extend through the circulatory system and lymphatics and develop into peritonitis and pelvic cellulitis. The most common causative organisms are group B β-hemolytic streptococci and *Escherichia coli*.

Assessment

PHYSICAL ASSESSMENT

Assess for the following clinical manifestations:
1. Elevated temperature ≥ 101°F (38.3°C), chills
2. Foul-smelling lochia
3. Abdominal tenderness, pelvic pain
4. Dysuria, burning on urination
5. Tachycardia
6. Increased WBC
7. Presence of predisposing
    A. Traumatic birth
    B. Prolonged difficult labor
    C. Dehydration
    D. Excessive vaginal discharge
    E. PROM
    F. Anemia
    G. Retained placental fragment
    H. Hemorrhage

PSYCHOSOCIAL AND CULTURAL ASSESSMENT

1. Mother experiences frustration associated with extreme fatigue.
2. May appear uncooperative, uninterested.

Planning

1. Safe, effective environment
    A. Provide teaching regarding hygienic measures.
2. Physiological integrity
    A. Administer treatment specific to infection.
3. Psychosocial integrity
    A. Provide opportunities for mother to express her feelings.
4. Health promotion and maintenance
    A. Provide education for self-care.

Implementation

1. Assess vital signs every 2–4 hours. Obtain cultures, blood and urine samples as ordered if temperature is elevated.
2. Evaluate pain and lochia.
3. Administer IV antibiotics, fluids, analgesics as prescribed.
4. Provide routine postpartum care. Use meticulous hand-washing techniques. Teach hand washing to mother.
5. Provide warm sitz baths and compresses or heat lamp.
6. Provide reassurance and support.
7. Isolate woman as indicated.

Evaluation

Ensure that the woman:
1. Demonstrates hand washing and verbalizes understanding of hygienic measures.
2. Continues ordered medication to full recovery.
3. Verbalizes feelings and increased ability to cope.

4. Verbalizes understanding of self-care measures to treat infection, prevent infection, and increase comfort.

Mastitis

Description

Mastitis is inflammation of breast tissue, generally caused by staphylococcus organisms at 2–4 weeks after birth

Assessment

PHYSICAL ASSESSMENT

Assess for the following clinical manifestations:
1. Nipple fissures, cracked nipples, bleeding from nipple
2. Breast pain, engorgement, redness
3. Fever, chills, tachycardia
4. Noninfected blocked milk ducts with milk stasis
    A. Breasts are hard, red, warm, and tender.
    B. Outer upper quadrant of breast is generally involved.
    C. Breasts are not completely emptied.

PSYCHOSOCIAL AND CULTURAL ASSESSMENT

1. Anxiety and feelings of inadequacy associated with interruption in breast-feeding

Planning

1. Safe, effective environment
    A. Provide hygienic teaching.
2. Physiological integrity
    A. Administer treatment as indicated.
3. Psychosocial integrity
    A. Provide support and encouragement.
4. Health promotion and maintenance
    A. Provide education for self-care.

Implementation

1. Administer antibiotic as prescribed.
2. Facilitate breast comfort.
    A. Provide a support bra with wide, adjustable straps.
    B. Apply local heat or cold.
    C. Administer pain medication.
3. Enhance lactation in breast-feeding mothers.
    A. Encourage nursing of infant unless otherwise ordered.
    B. Empty breast with manual expression or pump.
4. Teach techniques in breast care and feeding.
5. Reassure mother that condition will subside and normal lactation will resume.
6. Observe for breast abscess.
7. Teach hand washing and cleansing of breasts.

Evaluation

Ensure that the woman:
1. Demonstrates hand-washing and hygienic measures.
2. Is free of breast pain and symptoms of infection, has normal temperature.
3. Verbalizes support and feels encouragement to continue breast-feeding.
4. Continues breast-feeding with no further problems.

Postpartum Hemorrhage

Description

Postpartum hemorrhage is classified as early or late. Early postpartum hemorrhage occurs when the blood loss is more than 500 mL in the first 24 hours after birth. Late postpartal hemorrhage occurs after the first 24 hours.

Assessment

PHYSICAL ASSESSMENT

Assess for the following clinical manifestations:
1. Observe for predisposing factors.
   A. Early postpartal hemorrhage
      (1) Uterine atony
      (2) Lacerations of cervix, vagina, and perineum
      (3) Retained placenta or placental fragments
      (4) Overdistended uterus in labor (hydramnios, multiple gestation, large fetus)
      (5) Use of forceps at birth
   B. Late postpartal hemorrhage
      (1) Retained placental fragments are more likely with Duncan mechanism of placental separation.
2. Palpate fundus and massage if not firm.
3. Palpate bladder.
4. Assess amount of lochia.

Planning

1. Safe, effective care environment
   A. Assess abnormal bleeding.
2. Physiological integrity
   A. Evaluate maternal status and restore to normal.
3. Psychosocial integrity
   A. Provide opportunities for verbalization.
4. Health promotion and maintenance
   A. Promote education for self-care.

Implementation

1. Palpate fundus; massage if not firm.
2. Assess amount of bleeding.
3. Facilitate bladder emptying.
4. Assess lochia and measure amount of blood loss.
5. Monitor HCT and hemoglobin levels.
6. Administer blood as ordered.
7. Treat shock.
   A. Administer O_2 by face mask at 7–10 L/min.
   B. Administer IV fluids.
   C. Monitor vital signs.

Evaluation

Ensure that the woman:
1. Has normal amount of lochia flow.
2. Has vital signs within normal limits; hemoglobin and HCT levels within normal range.
3. Verbalizes feelings regarding the hemorrhage.
4. Understands self-care related to assessing fundus and lochia, hand washing, and need for rest and graded activity.

Disorders of the Neonate

Preterm Infant

Description

A preterm infant is one born before 38 weeks' gestation. The major problem of a preterm infant is immaturity of all systems, most notable respiratory and gastrointestinal.

Assessment

PHYSICAL ASSESSMENT

Assess for the following clinical manifestations:
1. Gestational age is $\leq$ 37 weeks.
2. Extremities are thin, with minimal creasing on soles and palms.
3. Lanugo is present on skin. Hair on head is present in woolly patches.
4. Skin is thin, with visible blood vessels and minimal pads of fat. Skin may appear jaundiced.
5. Testes are undescended in male infant; labia majora are narrow in female infant.
6. Respirations are irregular, with periodic apnea.
7. Bowel sounds are diminished, with tympany on percussion, abdominal distention, and infrequent stools.
8. Infant temperature is below normal (97.8°F, 36.5°C).
9. Blood studies reveal hypoglycemia (blood sugar is <45 mg/100 mL) and polycythemia.
10. Infant has difficulty in sucking and swallowing.
11. Infant extends extremities and does not maintain flexion.

PSYCHOSOCIAL AND CULTURAL ASSESSMENT

1. Parents demonstrate disbelief, shock, impaired perceptions, inability to understand, guilt.
2. Parents fear holding the baby, being alone with the baby, and leaving the hospital.
3. Parents lament the loss of a "perfect" baby.
4. Parents may be concerned about financial responsibility for infant.
5. Parents fear for newborn's life.

Planning

1. Safe, effective care environment
   A. Assess preterm infant at frequent intervals.
2. Physiological integrity
   A. Maintain infant's respiratory and nutritional status and temperature within normal limits.
3. Psychosocial integrity
   A. Provide comfort and touch for infant.
   B. Provide opportunities for parents to verbalize feelings.
4. Health promotion and maintenance
   A. Educate parents regarding the newborn's care.

Implementation

1. Administer antibiotics as prescribed (ampicillin, kanamycin, gentamicin).
2. Maintain fluid and electrolyte balance.
   A. Administer replacement electrolytes as prescribed (HCO_3 and Ca), and monitor heart rhythm during administration.

B. Administer IV fluid therapy.
3. Maintain cardiopulmonary function.
   A. Administer O_2 and humidification by cannula, hood, continuous positive airway pressure, or mechanical ventilation.
   B. Facilitate chest physiotherapy with gentle tapping over chest.
   C. Coordinate diagnostic procedures: x-ray, blood work, pulmonary function studies.
   D. Take axillary temperature, apical pulse, and respiration every 2–4 hours.
   E. Secure temperature probe on infant's abdomen, and check temperature inside warming unit.
   F. Handle infant carefully; position infant every 1–2 hours.
   G. Monitor intake, output, and weight daily.
   H. Apply gentle tactile stimulation for periodic apnea; suction as necessary.
4. Avoid exposing infant to infection.
5. Provide developmental care with 'nesting' and 'kangaroo care' (with stable preterm infants).
6. Bathe infant daily using mild cleansing agents and gentle stroking over small areas at a time.
7. Gavage-feed with Nos. 8 to 5 tubes; bottle-feed with a premature nipple every 2–3 hours.
8. Freeze breast milk that will not be used within 24 hours.
9. Provide psychosocial support to parents and infant.
   A. Talk with parents, and assist them to understand and deal with each other's feelings.
   B. Share information regarding the infant—weight gain, quality of sucking, oral intake.
   C. Reinforce positive caring behaviors.
   D. Coordinate services for financial support.
   E. Provide infant with colorful objects, music box, and gentle rocking.
   F. Share caregiving responsibilities with parents.

Evaluation

1. Assess preterm infant frequently to detect stability or development of abnormal patterns.
2. Ensure that preterm infant has physiological parameters within normal limits: respirations are 30–50/min without retraction or grunting; temperature is maintained; infant is progressively gaining weight.
3. Provide opportunities for the preterm infant to be held and cuddled.
4. Ensure that parents understand how to care for their infant.

Post-term Infant

Description

A post-term infant is one born after 42 weeks of gestation.

Assessment

PHYSICAL ASSESSMENT

Assess for the following clinical manifestations:
1. Observe for complications related to post-term infants:
   A. Hypoglycemia
   B. Meconium aspiration
   C. Polycythemia
   D. Seizure activity
   E. Cold stress
2. Appears wide-eyed and alert.
3. Parchment-like skin, no lanugo or vernix. Skin is dry and cracked.
4. Fingernails are long and extended over ends of fingers.
5. Scalp hair is profuse.
6. Body appears long and thin. Extremities show wasting of fat and muscle.
7. Meconium staining may be present on nails and umbilical cord.

PSYCHOSOCIAL AND CULTURAL ASSESSMENT

1. Baby may be irritable.
2. Parents are concerned for their infant.

Planning

1. Safe, effective care environment
   A. Assess post-term infant for development of complications.
2. Physiological integrity
   A. Maintain infant's physiological status.
3. Psychosocial integrity
   A. Provide cuddling for infant.
   B. Provide opportunities for parents to verbalize feelings.
4. Health promotion and maintenance
   A. Provide education for parents regarding their infant's care.

Implementation

1. Provide normal newborn care.
2. Be alert for signs of complications.
3. Maintain infant's temperature.
4. Provide education for parents.

Evaluation

1. Ensure that post-term infant is free of complications.
2. Ensure that post-term infant's physiological status is maintained—temperature and respiratory rate are within normal limits.
3. Provide opportunities for post-term infant to be held and cuddled.
4. Ensure that parents have verbalized feelings regarding their infant.
5. Ensure that parents demonstrate infant-care practices.

Small for Gestational Age and Large for Gestational Age

Respiratory Distress

Description

Neonatal respiratory difficulty due to one of the following:
1. **Respiratory distress syndrome** (hyaline membrane disease): Surfactant is absent, deficient, or altered in the alveolar lining. Symptoms occur within 6–12 hours of birth.
2. **Aspiration syndromes:** Fluid and/or meconium are aspirated, diminishing pulmonary perfusion. Severity of the

problem is related to the amount and depth of aspirate. Infant is symptomatic at birth.

3. **Apnea due to prematurity:** Apnea episodes lasting more than 20 seconds, accompanied by cyanosis, hypotonia, and/or metabolic acidosis.
4. **Pneumonia:** Congenital or infectious lung infiltrate apparent 2–5 days after birth.
5. **Transient tachypnea of the newborn (also called wet lung syndrome):** Excessive pulmonary fluid found in infants who do not undergo vaginal birth or who do so very rapidly (Table 3–22).

Assessment

PHYSICAL ASSESSMENT

Assess for the following clinical manifestations:
1. Presence of predisposing factors such as prematurity, maternal diabetes or bleeding, cesarean section, low Apgar score
2. Extremities flaccid and edematous.
3. Hypothermia, hypotension.
4. Skin pale and/or cyanotic.
5. Respirations—grunting or whining, sternal and/or intercostal retracting, nasal flaring, cyanosis, tachypnea, diminished breath sounds, abnormal x-ray findings. Arterial blood gases reveal hypoxemia, hypercarbia, and respiratory acidosis.
   A. Assess respirations—rate, rhythm, cyanosis, struggling with respirator, decreased breath sounds, noisy respiration, retracting.

Psychosocial and Cultural Assessment

1. Parental anxiety is immense and may be demonstrated as anger, hostility, shock, disbelief, withdrawal.
2. Parents express fear of permanent brain and lung damage.
3. Onset of symptoms may occur at home if the delivery was at home or if the hospital stay was short.

Planning

1. Safe, effective care environment
   A. Assess infant for predisposing factors.

2. Physiological integrity
   A. Assess infant's respiratory status frequently.
3. Psychosocial integrity
   A. Provide parents with an opportunity to verbalize fears.
4. Health promotion and maintenance
   A. Promote infant-care teaching for parents.

Implementation

1. Provide pharmacotherapy and IV therapy.
   A. Administer antibiotics (ampicillin, kanamycin).
   B. Assess umbilical artery catheter for infection, hemorrhage, thromboembolism.
   C. Administer IV fluids.
   D. Administer IV bicarbonate 1–2 mEq/kg of body weight, slowly, as ordered, to correct acidosis.
   E. Prepare for administration of exogenous surfactant
2. Monitor and enhance respiratory function.
   A. Obtain arterial blood gas sample every 4 hours by umbilical artery catheter.
   B. Administer O_2 by hood, continuous positive airway pressure, or volume ventilation. Warm and humidify oxygen.
   C. Prevent infant fatigue by spacing activities, handling and stimulating infant as little as possible.
   D. Suction as needed, usually hourly if infant has an endotracheal tube and is on a mechanical ventilator; hyperoxygenate prior to suctioning.
   E. Facilitate chest physiotherapy 30–45 minutes after meals; gently percuss for 1–2 minutes in each position. Suction prior to position change.
   F. Position with neck slightly hyperextended, and change position every 1–2 hours.
   G. Lower environmental O_2 very slowly as indicated by blood gases and TCMs as infant improves; this avoids "flip-flop," which is characterized by severe cyanosis and respiratory collapse.
3. Monitor vital signs.
   A. Maintain body temperature between 86°F (30°C) and 93°F (34°C) with incubator or radiant warmer.
4. Provide pharmacotherapy and IV therapy.
   A. Administer antibiotics (ampicillin, kanamycin).

Table 3–22. **Characteristics of SGA and LGA Infants**		
	SGA	LGA
Definition	Below 10th percentile.	Above 90th percentile.
Associated problems	Congenital problems, fetal distress, hypoglycemia, polycythemia, congenital infection, aspiration of meconium.	Birth trauma, IDM, hypoglycemia, RDS, hypotension, sepsis.
Nursing care	Maintain airway. Maintain temperature. Observe for signs of respiratory distress. Monitor glucose levels. Observe for signs of hypoglycemia. Provide neutral thermal zone (NTZ). Minimize heat loss. Initiate feedings. Evaluate hematocrit. Observe for signs of sepsis. Provide touch, cuddling. Support parents. Teach parents about their baby.	Maintain respirations. Monitor temperature. Monitor glucose levels. Observe for signs of hypoglycemia. Minimize heat loss. Initiate early feeding. Prevent sepsis. Provide touch and cuddling for infant. Support parents. Provide teaching for parents.

B. Assess umbilical artery catheter for infection, hemorrhage, thromboembolism.
C. Administer IV fluids.
D. Administer IV bicarbonate 1–2 mEq/kg of body weight, slowly, as ordered, to correct acidosis.
5. Monitor and enhance respiratory function.
  A. Obtain arterial blood gas sample every 4 hours by umbilical artery catheter.
  B. Administer O_2 by hood, continuous positive airway pressure, volume ventilation, or pediatric liquid ventilation. Warm and humidify oxygen with 'dry' methods of oxygenation.

Evaluation

1. Assess infant quickly and begin supportive therapy.
2. Maintain infant's normal respiratory rate and rhythm in a non–oxygen-enriched environment.
3. Ensure that infant maintains normal skin color and blood gas levels.
4. Give parents opportunity to verbalize feelings.
5. Ensure that parents verbalize understanding of infant care.

Hypoglycemia

Description

Hypoglycemia is indicated by blood glucose below 30 mg/dL in the first 72 hours after birth and below 40 mg/dL after the first 3 days. It may also be defined as a glucose test strip result below 45 mg/dL. Hypoglycemia is secondary to high maternal prenatal blood-sugar levels that overstimulated fetal insulin production. Insulin production remains high compared to circulating glucose. This condition is usually found in infants of diabetic mothers.

Assessment

PHYSICAL ASSESSMENT

Assess for the following clinical manifestations:
1. Predisposing factors
  A. Preterm birth, prematurity
  B. Unusually large for gestational age
  C. Maternal diabetes, hypertension
  D. Infant stress
2. Jitteriness, twitching, seizures
3. Poor feeding, weak sucking reflex
4. Irregular respiration, with possible cyanotic attacks, and respiratory distress
5. Edema, resulting in bloated appearance
6. Weak, high-pitched cry
7. Poor muscle tone
8. Low blood sugar and low serum calcium levels (hypocalcemia)

PSYCHOSOCIAL AND CULTURAL ASSESSMENT

1. Parents may be unaware of or misunderstand problem.
2. Mother may experience feelings of guilt.

Planning

1. Safe, effective environment
  A. Assess signs of hypoglycemia.
2. Physiological integrity

A. Maintain normal glucose levels.
3. Psychosocial integrity
  A. Provide opportunities for parents to ask questions.
4. Health promotion and maintenance
  A. Provide education regarding infant care.

Implementation

1. Assess vital signs and blood chemistry frequently. Watch for seizures.
2. Monitor infant blood-sugar levels every 30 minutes to 6 hours as ordered.
3. Administer 5%–10% glucose IV or po as ordered. Always follow with a protein feeding (formula or breast-feeding), to prevent the low blood glucose levels that follow glucose administration.
4. Facilitate early full feedings to maintain normal blood sugar.
5. Prevent infection.

Evaluation

1. Detect infant's episode of hypoglycemia quickly.
2. Ensure that infant maintains normal blood glucose level at 45–100 mg/dL.
3. Encourage parents to ask questions freely and share concerns.
4. Ensure that parents verbalize understanding of infant's special care needs.

Infections of the Neonate (Diarrhea, Pneumonia, Septicemia)

Description

The infant may contract a bacterial infection, usually caused by a streptococcus organism or *E. coli*. Predispositions include prematurity, PROM, prolonged labor, multiple procedures on neonate.

Assessment

PHYSICAL ASSESSMENT

Assess for the following clinical manifestations:
1. Onset of symptoms—2 days to 4 weeks of life
2. Lethargic, irritable, high-pitched cry, poor skin turgor
3. Abdomen—distended, tympany on percussion, active bowel sounds, diarrhea, vomiting, poor feeding and sucking ability
4. Respiration—irregular and rapid with periods of apnea
5. Temperature instability, usually unable to maintain body temperature (hypothermia).
6. Leukocytosis or leukopenia

PSYCHOSOCIAL AND CULTURAL ASSESSMENT

1. Parents may be anxious and concerned for infant.

Planning

1. Safe, effective care environment
  A. Monitor infant for signs of infection.
2. Physiological integrity
  A. Maintain normal body temperature.

3. Psychosocial integrity
   A. Provide support for parents.
4. Health promotion and maintenance
   A. Educate parents regarding special care for their infant.

Implementation

1. Assist in monitoring and controlling infection.
   A. Administer antibiotics (ampicillin, kanamycin, gentamicin).
   B. Maintain strict isolation techniques.
   C. Obtain culture specimen as ordered—throat, urine, blood, cord stump, circumcision, stool, sputum, chest x-ray, serology studies.
2. Provide O_2 and fluid therapy as prescribed.
   A. Administer O_2 and humidification by hood, continuous positive airway pressure, or mechanical ventilation.
   B. Assess hydration—skin turgor, moistness of mucous membranes, fullness of eyeballs and fontanelles, alertness, fluid output.
   C. Maintain NPO with decompression of stomach with feeding tube.
   D. Administer IV fluids.
3. Take axillary temperature, apical pulse; assess respiratory rate every 2 hours. Maintain temperature at 98.8°F (36.5°C).
4. Monitor intake and output, daily weight.
5. Suction as necessary.
6. Attend to feeding needs.
   A. Provide a pacifier for the NPO infant for non-nutritive sucking.
   B. Start feedings via feeding tube. Give the infant a pacifier for nonnutritive sucking with tube feedings.
   C. Resume fluid intake with small amounts of water and advance to diluted proprietary formula or breast milk.
7. Provide skin care.
   A. Expose buttocks to air in the event of diaper rash.
   B. Reposition infant every 2–3 hours.
8. Support parents.
   A. Talk with parents, and assist them to verbalize their feelings.
   B. Provide reassurance with calm words and manner.
   C. Share information regarding the infant—procedures, temperature, etc.
   D. Provide infant with colorful objects and a music box.

Evaluation

1. Recognize infant's infectious process quickly and begin therapy.
2. Check infant's temperature to ensure that it is within normal limits.
3. Let parents verbalize feelings and ask questions as needed.
4. Have parents verbalize understanding of infant care.

Hyperbilirubinemia

Description

Hyperbilirubinemia is elevated bilirubin as the result of one of the following:
1. **Physiological jaundice:** At 3–5 days of life the infant has increased bilirubin production and decreased conjugation, resulting in elevated serum bilirubin.

2. **Prematurity:** Infant's liver is not mature enough to metabolize bilirubin.
3. **ABO, Rh incompatibilities:** Mother produces antibodies that cross the placenta and cause infant red-cell hemolysis.
4. **Breast milk:** Produces a hormone (pregnanediol), which reduces the excretion rate of bilirubin.
5. **Extravascular hemolysis:** Bruises, cephalohematoma, petechiae, rapid hemolysis of blood.
6. **Others:** Polycythemia, glucose-6-phosphate-dehydrogenase deficiency, certain drugs, hypoglycemia, hypoxia, chemicals such as phenol.

Assessment

PHYSICAL ASSESSMENT

1. Bilirubin (total cord) <2 mg/dL; 0–1 days <6–8 mg/dL; 1–2 days <8–12 mg/dL; 3–5 days <12–16 mg/dL. Bilirubin (direct) 0–1 mg/dL
2. Moderately severe cases—palpable spleen, enlarged liver, poor feeding, edema, vomiting, fever, dark urine
3. Kernicterus—diminished Moro's reflex, poor sucking ability, difficulty feeding, high-pitched cry, "setting sun" eyes, irritability, opisthotonos, seizures

PSYCHOSOCIAL AND CULTURAL ASSESSMENT

1. Parents are anxious and fearful, either asking many questions or remaining silent.
2. Far Eastern, Mediterranean, and Middle Eastern persons have a higher incidence of glucose-6-phosphate dehydrogenase deficiency.
3. Parent may have used phenol or phenol-containing substance to clean the nursery.

Planning

1. Safe, effective care environment
   A. Recognize signs of jaundice.
2. Physiological integrity
   A. Maintain treatment for jaundice.
3. Psychosocial integrity
   A. Provide support and counseling for parents.
4. Health promotion and maintenance
   A. Provide teaching for parents regarding care of jaundiced infant.

Implementation

1. Provide care during phototherapy. (Phototherapy is the use of intense fluorescent lights to reduce serum bilirubin by photo-oxidation.)
   A. Keep infant fully undressed while under the lights, and shield the infant's eyes.
   B. Monitor temperature every 2 hours.
   C. Offer fluids every 2 hours to avoid dehydration, alternating formula and water.
   D. Change infant's position every 6 hours.
   E. Weigh every 12 hours; monitor intake and output; assess hydration.
   F. Shield the infant's eyes from light; every 12 hours turn off light, remove shield, and allow parents to view and/or hold infant; check for evidence of conjunctivitis; recover eyes with a clean shield.

G. Anticipate and observe for frequent dark green stools, dark urine, and possible tanning or so-called bronze baby syndrome.

H. Place a Plexiglas shield between the infant and the light.

I. Maintain a record of the number of hours each bulb is used, to ensure consistent quality of light emission.

J. Monitor bilirubin levels every 6–8 hours or as needed.

K. May use a fiber optic blanket–facilitates the attachment process because the infant can be held by parents, and eye contact can be made because the eye shield is unnecessary.

2. Management of exchange transfusion

A. Maintain NPO.

B. Aspirate stomach contents, and suction airway prior to procedure.

C. Confirm that informed consent has been signed by parents.

D. Check blood for appropriate typing.

E. Restrain infant.

F. Place infant under radiant warmer for procedure.

G. Record incremental amounts of blood withdrawn and infused.

H. Monitor vital signs every 5–15 minutes.

I. Monitor glucose and calcium levels.

J. Monitor follow-up bilirubin levels every 6–8 hours.

K. Assess abdomen hydration, Moro's reflex.

3. Encourage parents to visit infant at nursery window.

4. Share information with parents regarding infant's condition—bilirubin levels, weight.

5. Provide auditory stimulation for infant with a music box or humming.

6. Anticipate normal direct bilirubin levels.

Evaluation

1. Treat infant promptly.

2. Monitor infant's serum bilirubin level until returns to normal.

3. Have parents verbalize understanding of jaundice and treatment plan.

4. Have parents demonstrate infant-care techniques.

1. A 20-year-old woman who is $G_1 P_0$ comes to the prenatal clinic for her initial exam. She is 10 weeks pregnant. She asks why the baby needs amniotic fluid. The nurse would explain that amniotic fluid:

   A. Keeps the fetus's skin moist
   B. Provides a cushion for trauma and facilitates movement
   C. Contains the blood vessels that oxygenate the fetus
   D. Provides an acidic medium for the fetus to swallow

2. The nurse discusses with a client a prenatal test to screen for spinal anomalies done between 16 and 20 weeks' gestation, which is called the:

   A. Enzyme-linked immunosorbent assay (ELISA)
   B. VDRL
   C. BHCG
   D. α-Fetoprotein (AFP)

3. A female client wants to know how she can be positively sure she is pregnant. The nurse answers:

   A. Breast tenderness with pigment changes
   B. Enlargement of the abdomen
   C. FHR by Doppler at 10–12 weeks
   D. Amenorrhea

4. In taking a client's history at her first visit to the prenatal clinic, the nurse would determine the following information:

   A. The first day of the last normal menstrual period
   B. The partner's physiological symptoms of pregnancy
   C. The number of pregnancies the client's mother had
   D. The energy level of the client

5. In screening for factors that place the pregnancy at risk, the nurse would assess a client at her first prenatal visit for:

   A. Emotional lability
   B. Nausea and vomiting
   C. Changes in bowel habits
   D. Vaginal bleeding and cramping

6. A client has missed two menstrual periods and has a positive pregnancy test and exam. After counseling, she decides to have an elective abortion. The nurse should explain that the procedure used for termination in early pregnancy is:

   A. PG suppository
   B. Saline infusion
   C. Dilation and suction
   D. Laminaria

7. The nurse instructs a client in signs of postabortion complications requiring her return to the physician. Which statement by the client indicates she needs additional teaching?

   A. "I should take Tylenol if I have abdominal pain and tenderness."
   B. "I may have feelings of sadness after the abortion."
   C. "My vaginal bleeding should be scant for 2 weeks."
   D. "I should call the physician if my temperature is 98.6°F (37°C)."

8. A 40-year-old primigravida is scheduled for an amniocentesis at 16 weeks' gestation. The nurse explains that the purpose of the procedure is to:

   A. Evaluate the sex of the fetus
   B. Perform genetic studies
   C. Assess L/S ratio
   D. Monitor the bilirubin level

9. Following an amniocentesis, a client will be monitored 1 hour by the nurse for:

   A. Temperature elevation
   B. Bladder spasms
   C. Spontaneous rupture of the membranes
   D. Increased fetal activity

10. A client who is $G_2 P_1$ arrives for her 28-week appointment. She is complaining of hemorrhoids and constipation. A nursing recommendation would include:

    A. Decrease daily exercise.
    B. Take laxatives at bedtime.
    C. Take prenatal vitamins every other day.
    D. Increase daily water and fiber intake.

11. At her 28-week appointment, a client is to receive a RhoGam injection. The nurse explains this is to:

    A. Prevent 3-day measles
    B. Protect the fetus from isoimmunization
    C. Prevent neonatal jaundice
    D. Protect the mother from fetal bacteria

12. At the clinic, the nurse would perform the following procedure to determine the position of the fetus:

    A. Leopold's
    B. Valsalva's
    C. Ritgen's
    D. Credé's

13. A client reports lack of fetal movement at her scheduled antepartum visit. No FHTs are auscultated and ultrasound confirms intrauterine fetal demise. The nurse would expect the client to exhibit the following behavior, initially, after hearing the news.

    A. Bargaining
    B. Acceptance
    C. Anger
    D. Denial

14. A client and her husband arrive at the hospital for induction of labor postfetal demise. Because she is 28 weeks pregnant, her cervix is unripe. The nurse expects which of the following will be used to soften and efface her cervix?

    A. Pitocin IV
    B. Laminaria

C. Amniotomy

D. Normal saline solution

15. PG gel is ordered for induction of labor postfetal demise in a 28-week gestational pregnancy. The nurse explains that side effects might include:

A. Dysuria

B. Muscle weakness

C. Nausea, vomiting, and diarrhea

D. Headaches

16. When planning care for a client postfetal demise, a physiological complication of intrauterine fetal demise that can be serious is:

A. Heart murmurs

B. Disseminated intravascular coagulation (DIC)

C. Pyelonephritis

D. Endometriosis

17. A couple expresses uncertainty about seeing and holding the baby after postfetal demise delivery. Based on the theories of grief, the nurse responds:

A. "That is a difficult decision to make, but I will support you."

B. "Perhaps only your husband should see the baby."

C. "Many parents have nightmares afterwards."

D. "It is only good to see normal babies."

18. A couple who have just undergone postfetal demise delivery want to visit a friend down the hall who just delivered a beautiful baby girl. The nurse's best response is to:

A. Discourage this visit; it will increase their depression

B. Discourage walking; it is too strenuous

C. State, "It will make your friend feel guilty; don't go"

D. Agree to accompany them to the room

19. A woman who is $G_1 P_0$ is attending the prenatal clinic for her 37th-week exam. She asks many questions about complications and labor signs. She asks the nurse when it is appropriate to go to the labor and delivery unit. The nurse responds:

A. "When you pass the mucus plug"

B. "If you feel pressure over your bladder"

C. "When you have a large gush of fluid from your vagina"

D. "If you have nausea and vomiting"

20. An obese 28-year-old client is seen for the first time at the clinic. The nurse is assessing her for PIH. The sign(s) that indicate possible PIH is (are):

A. Swollen hands, face, and feet

B. Abdominal cramping

C. Headache relieved by acetaminophen

D. Clear nipple discharge

21. A rapid plasma reagin (RPR) test is ordered on a client at her 37th-week prenatal visit. The nurse explains that it screens for:

A. Chlamydia

B. Syphilis

C. Human papilloma virus (HPV)

D. Gonorrhea

22. The nurse arranges for a client who is 37 weeks pregnant to have a NST. The nurse explains to her that the purpose of this test is to:

A. Determine readiness for labor

B. Evaluate diabetic control

C. Measure the age of the placenta

D. Evaluate the condition of the fetal CNS

23. A client has class I cardiac disease. She is 37 weeks pregnant. The nurse would instruct her to:

A. Reduce physical activity

B. Avoid emotional stress

C. Plan for a vaginal delivery with a regional block

D. Anticipate cesarean delivery

24. A woman who is $G_1 P_0$ arrives at the hospital with questionable ruptured membranes. In order to confirm ruptured membranes, the following test will be done:

A. Sterile vaginal exam

B. Gram's stain of the fluid

C. Sterile speculum exam testing with nitrazine paper

D. Ultrasound

25. A sample of a client's vaginal fluid is evaluated under the microscope. The nurse would report positive ruptured membranes if:

A. The fluid has a fern shape

B. Yeast buds are present

C. The odor is fishy

D. There are many WBCs

26. A client is at 26 weeks' gestation with prematurely ruptured membranes. In order to help mature the fetus' lungs in utero, the nurse would anticipate the physician would order:

A. $MgSO_4$

B. Betamethasone

C. Exosurf

D. Ritodrine

27. Nursing care for effective management of preterm PROM includes:

A. Administering narcotics

B. Reassuring the mother that the "baby will be fine"

C. Encouraging ambulation

D. Monitoring for signs of infection

28. A client delivers a 26-week-old baby boy by cesarean section. Immediate nursing care of the infant includes:

A. Apgar scoring

B. Dubowitz assessment

C. Weighing and measuring

D. Gavage feeding

29. Complications of preterm birth for the newborn can be serious. The nurse must observe for:

A. Undescended testicles

B. Sole creases and lanugo

C. Changes in respiratory status
D. Hyperglycemia

30. In the immediate postpartum period, a common complication of cesarean birth that the nurse must assess for is:

    A. Full bladder
    B. Hemorrhage due to uterine atony
    C. Shivering
    D. Elevated temperature

31. The nurse might expect a family's reaction to a preterm birth to be:

    A. Lack of interest
    B. Realistic expectations
    C. Happiness about a "perfect baby"
    D. Impaired perceptions of the baby's status

32. A client is in active labor. She desires to have epidural anesthesia for the pain. While assisting with administration of the epidural block, the nurse's role is to:

    A. Position the client
    B. Scrub the client's back
    C. Inject the medication
    D. Encourage breath-holding during the procedure

33. The nurse must remain alert for signs of dangerous complications following epidural administration for the woman in labor, which include:

    A. Drowsiness
    B. Severe headaches
    C. Hypotension
    D. Numbness in legs and feet

34. A nursing intervention that a woman in labor needs during the time an epidural block is in effect includes:

    A. Decreasing IV fluids
    B. Dipsticking urine for protein
    C. Range of motion in lower extremities
    D. Catheterizing her bladder

35. A client has a postpartum hemorrhage. Nursing action for this problem is to:

    A. Insert vaginal packing
    B. Massage the uterus
    C. Apply ice to the perineum
    D. Administer a blood transfusion

36. A 15-year-old woman who is $G_1 P_0$ is preeclamptic. The nurse caring for the client will be administering $MgSO_4$. The primary reason the nurse administers $MgSO_4$ is to:

    A. Prevent seizures
    B. Lower blood pressure
    C. Promote uterine relaxation
    D. Decrease urine output

37. During an assessment of a client, who is receiving $MgSO_4$ for preeclampsia, the nurse recognizes the following as a dangerous sign:

    A. Systolic heart murmur
    B. BP 110/80

C. Urine output of 10 mL/hr
D. Decreased deep tendon reflexes (DTRs)

38. The antidote the nurse would administer for a client with an overdose of $MgSO_4$ is:

    A. Calcium gluconate
    B. Sodium bicarbonate
    C. Calcium carbonate
    D. Folic acid

39. A diabetic client is 10 weeks pregnant. She takes regular and NPH insulin twice a day. The nurse should warn her that in the first trimester, she should watch for:

    A. Hypoglycemia episodes
    B. Rapid weight gain
    C. Vision changes
    D. Hypertension

40. Immediately after birth of a baby, the nurse plans for a diabetic woman's change in insulin requirements:

    A. Remain the same
    B. Increase
    C. Drop precipitously
    D. Decrease slightly

41. Nursing care of the infant of a diabetic mother (IDM) includes assessment for:

    A. Low blood pressure
    B. Edema
    C. Change in muscle tone
    D. Hypoglycemia

42. A client who is 3 days old is slightly jaundiced. He was born at 38 weeks' gestation. The nursery nurse is aware that this jaundice is related to:

    A. Prematurity
    B. ABO incompatibility
    C. Physiological jaundice
    D. Extravascular hemolysis

43. Nursing care of the infant with hyperbilirubinemia who is under bilirubin lights includes:

    A. Daily bath
    B. Shielding infant's eyes while under the lights
    C. Bottle-feeding only
    D. Observing for bloody, mucous stools

44. When teaching a mother whose baby has hyperbilirubinemia, predisposing factors for hyperbilirubinemia include:

    A. Rh isoimmunization
    B. Postmaturity
    C. Cesarean birth
    D. Teenage mother

45. A client is 35 weeks pregnant. At her scheduled appointment, she is having heavy, painful bleeding. The nurse knows that this is a sign of:

    A. Placenta previa
    B. Normal bloody show

C. Passage of the mucus plug
D. Abruptio placentae

46. At the hospital, a client is attached to the fetal monitor for abruptio placentae. A common pattern of decelerations often seen with this condition is:

A. Late decelerations
B. Early decelerations
C. Variable decelerations
D. Mid-decelerations

47. A client has abruptio placentae and labor is precipitous. Fetal heart tones should be monitored by the nurse every:

A. minute
B. 5 minutes
C. 10 minutes
D. 15 minutes

48. A client receives a midline episiotomy. A priority of nursing care is to:

A. Promote healing of sutures
B. Prevent bladder distention
C. Prevent swelling of the perineum
D. Reduce hemorrhoids

49. A client is diagnosed with mastitis 10 days after delivery. The nurse assesses the client for a sign of this problem:

A. Lack of milk production
B. Nipple burning with breast-feeding
C. Hard, reddened, tender breasts
D. Dimpled skin on breasts

50. A client who is at 42 weeks' gestation is scheduled for a CST. She is admitted for evaluation and possible induction of labor. The nurse explains to her that the purpose of this antepartum test is to evaluate:

A. Cervical dilation
B. Readiness for induction
C. Braxton Hicks contractions
D. Respiratory function of the placenta

51. A client is scheduled for an ultrasound. The nurse explains to the client that the primary use of ultrasound in post-term pregnancy is to:

A. Determine sex of the fetus
B. Evaluate placental age
C. Confirm fetal presentation
D. Assess for fetal abnormalities

52. A client who is at 42 weeks' gestation is scheduled for induction. Her physician performs an amniotomy. The nurse's role in this procedure is to:

A. Listen to FHTs
B. Give fundal pressure
C. Have the client empty bladder
D. Perform vaginal exam to evaluate for prolapsed cord

53. A client at 38 weeks' gestation has irregular contractions. Her physician orders Pitocin induction. The safest way to administer Pitocin is:

A. IM for comfort

B. Mainline IV
C. IV piggyback as a secondary solution
D. Orally

54. A client still has irregular contractions. Her physician orders Pitocin. She expresses concern about induction, and the nurse replies:

A. "Pitocin is a dangerous drug."
B. "The hospital can handle any emergency."
C. "Tell me more about your fears; maybe I can alleviate them."
D. "You will be monitored closely, to look for complications."

55. During Pitocin administration, the nurse recognizes a tetanic contraction and fetal bradycardia. The nurse's first intervention would be to:

A. Reposition in Trendelenburg
B. Administer O$_2$ by face mask
C. Hydrate with primary fluids
D. Turn off the Pitocin IV

56. A G$_4$ P$_3$ client arrives at the hospital in active labor. She has been scheduled for her fourth cesarean section. A major complication the nurse would be concerned about is:

A. Precipitous labor
B. Placenta previa
C. Ruptured uterus
D. Dysfunctional labor

57. A client would be cleared for a VBAC if:

A. The uterine incision was transverse
B. Her deliveries were for breech babies
C. Her other cesareans were for CPD
D. There were twins in this pregnancy

58. Suddenly, a client who is in active labor screams out in pain and then quiets down. She has had three previous cesarean sections. The nurse's first priority is to:

A. Put on sterile gloves for delivery
B. Call the physician
C. Speed up her IV fluids
D. Check the contraction pattern

59. A client has had a rupture of her uterus during labor. Recognizing this situation as serious, the nurse would prepare to:

A. Turn the client to her left side
B. Resuscitate the baby
C. Start the 10-minute abdominal scrub
D. Hold the fetal head off the cord

60. A baby has just been delivered by low forceps. He is a term infant with a cord around the neck one time. The nurse in delivery would focus primarily on assessing the baby's:

A. Tissue perfusion
B. Sucking reflex
C. Respiratory effort
D. Meconium passage

61. During the initial exam, the nurse notices a bluish black area on the newborn's sacrum. This is called:

    A. Erythema neonatorum toxicum
    B. Stork bite
    C. Milia
    D. Mongolian spot

62. A mother is breast-feeding. The nurse explains that the amount of time needed to completely empty each breast is:

    A. 5 minutes
    B. 7 minutes
    C. 10–15 minutes
    D. 20–30 minutes

63. A 2-day-old baby is ready to be discharged from the hospital. What should the nurse include when teaching about cord care?

    A. Use peroxide on the base of cord after diaper change.
    B. Do not immerse the infant while bathing until cord falls off.
    C. It is normal to have yellow drainage from the cord.
    D. The cord dries and falls off in 7 days.

64. A client has not voided since the delivery of her baby 6 hours ago. The nurse knows that:

    A. It is common to delay voiding for 12 hours
    B. Diuresis occurs 48 hours after delivery
    C. Bladder emptying may be problematic due to swelling
    D. She is dehydrated and does not need to void

65. A client's abdomen is loose and soft after delivery. The nurse will assess for a common herniation that appears after delivery, which is:

    A. Umbilical hernia
    B. Diastasis recti
    C. Inguinal hernia
    D. Hiatal hernia

66. A new mother is afraid of her new role as mother. She is reliving her delivery experience and has a sense of wonder about the baby. The nurse knows that this is Rubin's phase of:

    A. Taking hold
    B. Taking in
    C. Letting go
    D. Attachment

67. A $G_3 P_1$ client is expecting twins. A primary goal of her prenatal care will be to:

    A. Prevent preterm delivery
    B. Limit weight gain to 40 lb
    C. Equalize the size of the twins
    D. Prevent stretch marks

68. In educating a woman in labor about timing contractions, the nurse defines "frequency" as the interval from the:

    A. End of one contraction to the start of the next
    B. Beginning of one contraction to end of that contraction
    C. End of one contraction to end of the next contraction
    D. Beginning of one contraction to the beginning of the next

69. The nurse is explaining tests to assess the growth of twins during pregnancy. Which of the following would the nurse explain to the client?

    A. Amniocentesis
    B. NST
    C. Ultrasound
    D. GTT

70. The delivery nurse is prepared for this common complication with twin deliveries:

    A. Retained placental fragments
    B. Prolapsed cord
    C. Meconium-stained fluid
    D. Placenta previa

71. During recovery after delivery of twins, a client begins to hemorrhage. The nurse recognizes this as usually related to:

    A. Urinary tract infection (UTI)
    B. Hemorrhoids
    C. Uterine atony
    D. Inability to breast-feed at delivery

72. A client is 14 weeks pregnant. She complains of 3 days of bleeding since her LMP. The nurse recognizes that first-trimester bleeding puts the client at risk for:

    A. Ectopic pregnancy
    B. Spontaneous rupture of membranes
    C. Threatened abortion
    D. Incompetent cervix

73. A client who is 14 weeks pregnant has a history of pelvic inflammatory disease (PID) and lower left quadrant pain. This would increase the risk of:

    A. Ectopic pregnancy
    B. Molar pregnancy
    C. Placenta previa
    D. Spontaneous abortion

74. A woman who is $G_5 P_2$ is concerned about fetal loss because of an incompetent cervical os. She is scheduled for a cerclage. The nurse explains to her that a cerclage is used to:

    A. Reduce risk of PROM
    B. Prevent preterm dilation of the cervix
    C. Prevent trauma in case of precipitous delivery
    D. Protect mother from abnormal Pap smears

75. When a client goes into labor after a cerclage has been performed, the nurse will assist with:

    A. Mechanical dilation of the cervix
    B. A Pap smear
    C. Removal of the suture
    D. Cultures of the cervix

76. A woman who is $G_1 P_0$ complains of fatigue during an antepartum visit. She is 10 weeks pregnant. The nurse explains that fatigue is caused by:

    A. Low blood pressure
    B. Increased blood volume
    C. Decreased appetite
    D. Hormone changes

77. A client's hemoglobin is below normal during an antepartum visit. She is placed on iron therapy. The nurse teaches that iron is absorbed when it is taken with:

   A. Milk
   B. Meals
   C. Orange juice
   D. Water

78. A client asks about physical activity during pregnancy. The nurse should reply:

   A. "Start an aerobic exercise regimen today."
   B. "Don't exercise at all; it will hurt your baby."
   C. "Running is encouraged during pregnancy."
   D. "Maintain your normal activities."

79. A client complains of leg cramps at night while she is pregnant. Part of the nurse's education includes recommending that she eat foods rich in:

   A. Calcium
   B. Vitamin E
   C. Folic acid
   D. Beta carotene

80. A client is 4–5 cm dilated at 40 weeks. She is complaining of severe backache with contractions. The nurse will administer an analgesic IV when:

   A. The contraction is at its peak
   B. The contraction starts to its peak
   C. The uterus is at rest
   D. The contraction ends

81. A client becomes anxious and restless and is losing control during labor. The nurse recognizes this as:

   A. Late phase
   B. Active labor
   C. Transition
   D. Complete dilation

82. The physician decides to perform a pudendal block during labor in a client. The nurse explains that this:

   A. Numbs the perineum
   B. Stops the pressure feeling
   C. Paralyzes the lower extremities
   D. Is given in the lumbar area

83. At the time of a baby's delivery, the nurse watches for the sign of placental separation, which includes:

   A. A sharp abdominal pain
   B. A large gush of blood
   C. An urge to void
   D. The umbilical cord lengthening

84. In order to assess for thrombophlebitis on a client postdelivery, the nurse would evaluate:

   A. Babinski's reflex
   B. Homans' sign
   C. Psoas sign
   D. Moro's reflex

85. A client has just delivered a 6-lb 2-oz boy. She is concerned about the way he looks. The delivery nurse reassures the mother that a pink body with purple feet and hands is a normal condition called:

   A. Acrocyanosis
   B. Mongolian condition
   C. Sternal retractions
   D. Patent ductus arteriosus

86. A baby's chin is quivering and he is trembling a little postdelivery. The nurse replies to the mother that this is probably due to a:

   A. High sugar level
   B. Very cold temperature
   C. Startle reflex
   D. Immature nervous system

87. A mother is unsure about breast-feeding her newborn. The nurse's best response would be:

   A. "I'll tell the nursery nurse that you want a bottle."
   B. "You have to decide immediately."
   C. "Let's feed him by breast-feeding initially; I'll help you."
   D. "Breast-feeding is best; don't even consider bottle-feeding."

88. A mother took tetracycline during pregnancy for an acne condition. She asks if there could be a problem with the baby. The nurse responds that the baby could:

   A. Be deaf
   B. Have discolored teeth
   C. Be a slow learner
   D. Have webbed fingers and toes

89. A couple comes to the clinic very excited because the woman missed her period 5 weeks ago. She is experiencing early morning nausea, urinary frequency, and fatigue. In anticipating questions about pregnancy, the nurse would need to be aware that these are:

   A. Positive signs of pregnancy
   B. Probable signs of pregnancy
   C. Presumptive signs of pregnancy
   D. Signs that also could indicate bladder infection

90. When a client comes for her prenatal visit, the nurse measures her abdomen for growth and size of the fetus. Her fundal height is measured at 20 cm. What landmark could the nurse use to verify this measurement with the client's gestational date?

   A. Her symphysis
   B. Her hip bones
   C. Her sternum
   D. Her umbilicus

91. A client phones the clinic because she has discovered a brown discoloration line on the midline of her abdomen. She is 18 weeks pregnant and wants to know if this will hurt her baby. How should the nurse at the clinic respond?

   A. Ask her to come in for skin cancer assessment.
   B. Reassure her that this is a linea nigra and common in pregnancy.
   C. Ask what foods she has been eating recently.
   D. Tell her this is a stretch mark and not to worry.

92. A client calls the labor and delivery unit at 2 AM. His wife is 10 weeks pregnant and has been crying for an hour. He does not know what to do. How should the nurse respond?

    A. "She must be very upset; what did you do?"
    B. "Bring her to the emergency room for an anxiety evaluation."
    C. "Excess hormones can cause pregnant women to cry without reason."
    D. "Probably she will need counseling; here are some referral agencies."

93. At her first prenatal visit, a pregnant woman is being interviewed by the nurse for her health history. She is pregnant for the fourth time, has had one baby at 38 weeks' gestation, premature twins at 35 weeks, and a spontaneous abortion. How would the nurse communicate this information to the healthcare team?

    A. Gravida 4, para 3, a_1
    B. Gravida 4, para 2, T_1, P_2, A_1, L_3
    C. Gravida 4, para 3, T_1, P_2, A_1, L_3
    D. Gravida 4, para 2, T_1, P_1, A_1, L_3

94. As part of a health history for pregnancy, a client tells the nurse that she is unsure of her blood type and Rh factor. She had a spontaneous abortion at 10 weeks and did not seek medical attention. After lab work, she is found to have type O, Rh-negative blood. What high-risk factor should the nurse identify for the health team?

    A. The client may be at high risk for spontaneous abortion.
    B. The client may have become Rh sensitized during her first pregnancy.
    C. The client's fetus may have CNS malformations due to Rh incompatibility.
    D. The client is at risk for noncompliance with prenatal appointments.

95. A client arrives via wheelchair in the labor and delivery unit. She has bright red blood running down her legs. Her husband explains that this started 20 minutes ago and that she has been in "horrible pain" since then. The nurse begins to assess the client. Which of the following assessment skills would she avoid?

    A. External FHR monitoring
    B. Vital sign determination
    C. Palpation of abdomen
    D. Vaginal exam

96. When a 41-year-old client comes for a second-trimester prenatal visit, she complains that she feels her stomach fluttering and thinks she has the flu. What information can the nurse provide to reassure her?

    A. "Many pregnant ladies get mild GI upset."
    B. "This is the baby moving and will become easier to recognize later on."
    C. "Take some tea and crackers to settle it."
    D. "Rest, drink fluids, and take Tylenol to get over it."

97. A client who is 32 weeks pregnant complains of vaginal itching and thick, curdy, white discharge. The nurse knows that this is a common condition of pregnancy caused by:

    A. Yeast overgrowth
    B. Gonorrhea
    C. Trichomonas
    D. Herpes

98. A client comes to the clinic for her first prenatal visit. Her LMP was June 10th. In order to determine her estimated delivery date, what tool would the nurse use?

    A. Nägele's rule
    B. McDonald's rule
    C. Hegar's sign
    D. Quickening

99. A client has not felt the baby move for about 6 hours. She is anxious and crying when she arrives in the labor and delivery unit for an NST. After applying the external fetal monitor, the nurse can reassure her by showing her a reactive NST, which is characterized by:

    A. FHR between 110–160 bpm
    B. Variable decelerations lasting 10–20 seconds and decreasing 20 bpm
    C. Three accelerations in 10 minutes lasting 10–15 seconds at 10 beats above the baseline
    D. One acceleration in 10 minutes lasting 10–15 seconds at 10 beats above the baseline

100. A client is 41 weeks pregnant and not dilated at all. She comes to the labor and delivery unit for an antenatal fetal test. The nurse will run Pitocin to produce contractions, which will help the nurse to evaluate placental circulation and fetal well-being. What does the nurse call this test?

    A. Nipple stimulation test
    B. NST
    C. Oxytocin challenge test (OCT)
    D. CST

101. A client is about 3 weeks larger in uterine size than her dates indicate. The physician orders an ultrasound to diagnose multiple fetuses. What information should the nurse give the client in preparation for the test?

    A. "Do not eat or drink after midnight."
    B. "Drink several glasses of water 1 hour before, and do not urinate."
    C. "Empty your bladder immediately before the test."
    D. "Give yourself an enema prior to the test."

102. A client at 35 weeks' gestation is in labor with a diagnosis of abruptio placenta. What pattern on the fetal monitor should the nurse anticipate?

    A. Late decelerations
    B. Early decelerations
    C. Variable decelerations
    D. Accelerations with fetal movement

103. A labor and delivery nurse is watching the fetal monitor strip on a client whose fetus has been at −3 station. Suddenly the FHR drops from 150 to 90 bpm and stays there. What is the first thing the nurse should do to help the fetus?

    A. Check for ruptured membranes.
    B. Call for the physician.
    C. Turn client to left side or knee-chest position.
    D. Prepare for cesarean section.

104. A client has been making steady progress in labor. When she is starting to push, she lets out a blood-curdling scream and contractions stop. What sign would the nurse recognize as life threatening in this situation?

    A. Decrease in FHTs to 120 bpm
    B. Inability to push baby out
    C. Client anxious and restless
    D. Palpation of fetal parts through abdominal wall

105. A client is being induced into labor with IV Pitocin because she is 2 weeks late. Her contractions have been 2–3 minutes apart, lasting 60 seconds, moderately firm. The nurse is palpating her contractions. One lasts 2½ minutes. What should the nurse do?

    A. Turn up the Pitocin IV.
    B. Empty the client's bladder.
    C. Turn off the Pitocin IV.
    D. Administer terbutaline.

106. A client arrives in the labor and delivery unit with a perineal pad on, stating that she "thinks she ruptured her bag of water." One way the nurse can assess if the bag is really ruptured is to:

    A. Perform a ferning test
    B. Feel the perineal pad for moisture
    C. Check at the vaginal opening with nitrazene paper
    D. Do a vaginal examination

107. The labor and delivery nurse is coaching a client and her partner in Lamaze breathing techniques. She is using pant-and-blow breathing patterns. By this the nurse could assess that the client is in what stage of labor?

    A. Latent phase
    B. Transition
    C. Active phase
    D. Pushing

108. A client just ruptured her membranes spontaneously when she went to the bathroom to urinate. As soon as she gets back to bed, what is the first assessment the nurse should make?

    A. Check color and quantity of the fluid.
    B. Perform vaginal examination for dilation.
    C. Instruct the client to remain in bed the remainder of labor.
    D. Listen to FHTs.

109. A client is in labor and dilated 2 cm. Her contractions are 6 minutes apart, lasting 30 seconds, and moderate in intensity. She has a backache and is talking throughout contractions. The nurse should recognize this as what stage of labor?

    A. Early latent phase
    B. Late active phase
    C. Transition
    D. Second stage

110. At delivery the nurse is responsible for care of the neonate. What test is used to assess the adaptation to extrauterine life?

    A. Silverman score
    B. Apgar score

C. Denver Developmental Screening Test
    D. Dextrostick determination

111. A 1-hour-old neonate is being examined in the newborn nursery. On examination the nurse elicits a positive Ortolani's sign. The nurse should recognize that the cause of this is:

    A. Syndactyly
    B. Startle reflex
    C. Congenital hip dislocation
    D. Babinski's reflex

112. A 24-hour-old neonate has been breast-fed 4 times and has just passed his first stool. The nursery nurse should know that this stool would be:

    A. Yellow, puttylike
    B. Yellow, curdy, with a foul odor
    C. Brown, mushy, no odor
    D. Blackish, green, thick and sticky

113. A newborn is diagnosed with Down syndrome. His parents did not hold him in delivery and wish to see him now. What should the nurse observe as a sign of positive bonding with this baby?

    A. Avoidance of eye contact
    B. Holding baby at an arm's length from body
    C. Eye contact, stroking, cuddling
    D. Eye contact, refusal to hold

114. On the 2nd postpartum day, a client starts complaining of pain in her right calf. What assessment techniques would the nurse use to evaluate the problem?

    A. Vital signs, inspection, DTRs
    B. Palpation of femoral pulses, observation of ambulatory pattern
    C. Homans' sign, inspection, palpation
    D. Assessment of pedal edema, DTRs, blood pressure on the leg

115. At 6 hours postdelivery, a client calls the nurse because her perineum is painful and throbbing. When the nurse inspects the episiotomy site, her left perineum is 6 cm longer than the right side, hard, purple, and very tender. The nurse should recognize that this is caused by:

    A. A ruptured blood vessel
    B. A misplaced suture
    C. An abscess
    D. Normal swelling after delivery

116. A client has a postpartum hematoma on her right perineum. Based on this diagnosis, what nursing intervention is appropriate?

    A. An analgesic
    B. Benzocaine (Americaine) spray
    C. Hot pack
    D. Ice pack

117. A client is breast-feeding for the first time. She complains to the nurse that her nipples are sore. The nurse observes the next feeding and is able to offer the following suggestion:

    A. Let the baby suck only on the tip of the nipples.
    B. Place the whole areola and nipple in the baby's mouth.

C. Use a pacifier to teach the baby to suck.
D. Change to bottle-feeding; the baby's mouth is too small for the breast.

118. A client had an epidural for delivery. She is 4 hours postdelivery and bleeding heavily. When the nurse massages her fundus, it is very firm and located under her right rib cage. What is the first intervention the nurse can do to alleviate this problem?

A. Give oxytocic drugs as ordered.
B. Empty the client's bladder.
C. Have client breast-feed the baby.
D. Massage client's uterus for 15 minutes.

119. A client arrives at the antepartum unit with severe backache, urinary frequency, dysuria, fever, and chills. She began feeling "bad" this morning and went to see her obstetrician. She is 14 weeks pregnant. What IV antibiotic is effective against pyelonephritis and safe during this stage of pregnancy?

A. Tetracycline
B. Kanamycin
C. Ampicillin
D. Erythromycin

120. A client delivered a 10-lb 4-oz baby 6 hours ago. She received a perineal laceration into the rectal mucosa with delivery. Her physician has ordered docusate sodium (Colace) twice daily. In giving anticipatory discharge planning, what should the nurse include about this drug?

A. Limit fluid intake.
B. Continue to use this for at least 1 month.
C. It will cause frequent, loose stools.
D. It is used to soften the first stool after delivery.

121. A client is in labor and dilated to 4 cm. Her physician orders meperidine (Demerol) IV push for pain. What information should the labor and delivery nurse know about administering this drug to a laboring woman?

A. Rapid administration is best.
B. It cannot be given directly into a vein but needs dilution.
C. It causes FHR tachycardia.
D. It increases FHR variability.

122. A client enters the emergency department with extreme abdominal pain on the right side. Her LMP was 10 weeks earlier. She is diagnosed with an ectopic pregnancy. The nurse obtained a blood specimen for pregnancy testing. What hormone does the nurse know will be elevated?

A. Estrogen
B. Progesterone
C. Human growth hormone
D. HCG

123. A woman who is gravida 1 para 0 has been receiving $MgSO_4$ for 12 hours for her PIH. The nurse recognizes a sign of potential drug toxicity and turns off the $MgSO_4$. What sign does the nurse recognize as dangerous?

A. Respiratory rate under 12 breaths/min
B. Urine output of 35 mL/hr

C. DTRs of 2+, no clonus
D. Normal blood pressure after prolonged elevated blood pressure

124. A client is 12 hours postpartum, and she is being discharged in the morning. Because she pushed for 3 hours and delivered an 11-lb boy, she has a cluster of hemorrhoids. Which of the following beliefs expressed by the client indicates a need for further teaching for the client?

A. Stool softeners will make defecation easier.
B. Sitz baths will relieve the pain.
C. Hydrocortisone creams will relieve the swelling.
D. Frequent enemas will relieve constipation.

125. A physician prescribes a narcotic IV push for the laboring client. What is the most important thing for the nurse to know about narcotic administration during labor?

A. Give it rapidly through one contraction.
B. Give it slowly, from the beginning to the peak of the contraction.
C. Give it during the entire contraction.
D. Give it between contractions only.

126. In the delivery room, a client is preparing to crown the baby's head. She has not had any anesthesia and is requesting some now. What medication does the nurse prepare for local anesthesia?

A. Nitrous oxide
B. Tetracaine (Pontocaine)
C. Lidocaine (Xylocaine)
D. Benzocaine spray

127. An obese woman who is gravida 3 para 2 is at 22 weeks' gestation. She has had medical problems with elevated blood pressure since her first pregnancy. Her physician does not want her to take diuretics during her pregnancy. He prescribed hydralazine (Apresoline) four times a day. What does the office nurse need to teach her about this medication?

A. It lessens the normal postural hypotension of pregnancy.
B. Bioavailability of the drug is increased by taking it with food.
C. If a dose is missed, take two to catch up.
D. Dependent edema is normal and does not need to be reported.

128. When the nurse begins the induction for fetal demise, the nurse will be using dinoprostone (Prostin E_2) suppositories. In order to make the client more comfortable during this procedure, what medications should the nurse have available?

A. Antibiotics
B. Antihistamines
C. Aspirin
D. Antiemetics and antidiarrheals

129. A 24-year-old woman who is gravida 1 para 0 is admitted to the labor and delivery unit because she has had a fetal demise at 18 weeks. Her physician wants to

induce her to deliver the fetal remains before septic conditions develop. What medication will the nurse use to induce her labor?

A. Dinoprostone suppository
B. Pitocin IV
C. Syntocinon nasal spray
D. Laminaria

130. An 18-year-old mother contracted chickenpox 8 days ago. She delivered the baby by cesarean section. The baby does not have any skin lesions, but the incubation period is 10 days to 3 weeks. The pediatrician wants to prevent or at least minimize this disease for the newborn. What medication would the nurse administer?

A. Vitamin B_{12}
B. Varicella vaccination
C. Varicella-zoster immune globulin
D. Acyclovir IV

131. The clinic nurse discussed common discomforts of pregnancy in the first trimester with a primiparous client at 7 weeks' gestation. The nurse realizes client teaching has been effective when the client makes which of the following statements?

A. "Some women are more interested in sex during this stage of pregnancy."
B. "I can expect to have some shortness of breath during this pregnancy stage."
C. "My breasts may become tender and larger during this pregnancy stage."
D. "I may wake up with leg cramps at night during this stage of pregnancy."

132. A client at 26 weeks' gestation with sickle cell disease was admitted to the obstetric unit with a diagnosis of sickle cell crisis. Which of the following nursing orders would be most appropriate for this client?

A. Support joints with pillows.
B. Maintain strict bed rest.
C. Administer oxygen via face mask.
D. Provide active range-of-motion exercises.

133. A client at term is in the active phase of labor. She complains of abdominal pain between contractions. The nurse notes an increase in the uterine baseline tone and repetitive drops in the fetal heart rate that mirror contractions but do not return to the baseline until well after contractions end. Dark red vaginal bleeding and abdominal rigidity are noted on further assessment. Based on this information, the nurse should initiate client teaching about which of the following procedures?

A. Amniocentesis
B. Oxytocin augmentation
C. Amnioinfusion
D. Cesarean delivery

134. A client in transition requested pain medication and received butorphanol (Stadol) 1 mg IVP 2 hours ago. Delivery is now imminent. Which of the following actions by the nursery nurse would have priority?

A. Prepare to suction the oropharynx.
B. Prepare to calculate newborn Apgars.
C. Prepare infant and maternal ID bands.
D. Prepare to administer naloxone (Narcan).

135. A 19-year-old postpartum client is preparing to be discharged home with her term newborn. She is a college student and wishes to defer another pregnancy for at least 3 years. She smokes a pack a day of cigarettes. Which of the following contraceptive methods would be most appropriate for this client?

A. Natural family planning
B. Condoms and foam
C. Depo-Provera injection
D. Oral contraceptives

136. The nursery nurse is caring for a newborn who is pale and jittery and has a high-pitched cry. Which of the following nursing actions would be most appropriate?

A. Check newborn serum glucose levels.
B. Review maternal history for substance use.
C. Check newborn axillary temperature.
D. Review newborn white blood cell count.

137. A client is 12 hours postpartum. A routine nursing assessment reveals the fundus 2 cm above the umbilicus, deviated to one side, and slightly boggy. Lochial flow is moderate to heavy. The client reports she has been voiding small, frequent amounts. Considering these assessment findings, which of the following nursing actions should be performed first?

A. Massage the uterine fundus.
B. Document these normal findings.
C. Check for bladder distention.
D. Notify the healthcare provider.

138. A client at term is in the second stage of labor and has pushed for approximately 30 minutes. The nurse notes perineal bulging and calls the healthcare provider for delivery. Before the healthcare provider arrives, the woman shouts, "The baby is coming!" Delivery is imminent. Which of the following nursing actions would be most appropriate?

A. Don sterile gloves and apply firm pressure to the presenting part.
B. Call for help and instruct the client to cross her legs.
C. Call for help and quickly complete the perineal prep.
D. Don sterile gloves and apply gentle pressure to the perineum.

139. A client at 28 weeks' gestation had a 1-hour glucose tolerance test (GTT) result of 144 g/dL. The nurse realizes that client teaching regarding this screening test was effective when the client makes which of the following statements?

A. "This means I'll need further testing of my blood sugar."
B. "I'll have to control my blood sugars with diet and exercise."
C. "Now I'll have to learn how to give myself insulin."
D. "This is a normal blood sugar result for pregnancy."

140. A 20-year-old client weighed 130 lb before she became pregnant, which was an appropriate prepregnant weight for her height. Now at 24 weeks' gestation she expressed concern to the OB clinic nurse about her current weight of 144 lb. Which of the following responses by the nurse best indicates an understanding of the nutritional requirements of pregnancy?

    A. "You are gaining too much weight. You need to decrease calories."
    B. "This is an appropriate amount of weight for you to have gained."
    C. "Your baby may be born too small. You need to gain more weight."
    D. "Try to eliminate fatty foods from your diet so you gain less."

141. The clinic nurse has just finished teaching a class on sexuality during pregnancy. She knows teaching has been effective when a participant makes which of the following comments?

    A. "I should avoid intercourse during the time I would normally have had my period."
    B. "Sexual intercourse should be avoided during the last trimester of pregnancy."
    C. "My sexual desire will most likely stay the same throughout my pregnancy."
    D. "I will probably enjoy sexual activity more than usual in the second trimester."

142. A primiparous client in the first trimester of pregnancy tells the clinic nurse that she has substituted hot tea for coffee at breakfast. Her hemoglobin level was 10 g/dL today, and she reports taking her iron supplements twice daily, with breakfast and supper. Which of the following responses by the nurse to the client would be most appropriate?

    A. "That's a good start! Tea has much less caffeine than coffee."
    B. "Add a little lemon to your tea so your iron pill is better absorbed."
    C. "Your iron levels are low, so you'll have to eliminate all caffeine."
    D. "It's OK to drink coffee or tea; caffeine doesn't affect the fetus."

143. A client at her first prenatal visit has received teaching about methods of increasing her hemoglobin through iron intake. The nurse recognizes that teaching has been effective when the client makes which of the following statements?

    A. "I'll have a citrus drink when I eat red meat."
    B. "I'll take my iron pill with my meals."
    C. "I'll take my iron pill between meals."
    D. "I'll eat a raw spinach salad every day."

144. A client at 34 weeks' gestation arrives on the OB unit for a non-stress test (NST). To best find the location of the strongest fetal heart tones, the nurse should take which of the following actions?

    A. Ask the client where the fetal heart tones are normally found.
    B. Perform Leopold's maneuvers for fetal position and presentation.

    C. Locate the top of the uterine fundus for tocotransducer placement.
    D. Measure from the pubis to the top of the uterine fundus.

145. An oxytocin stress test (OCT) was ordered for a diabetic client at 32 weeks' gestation. The nurse notes an increase in the fetal heart rate of 15 bpm with each contraction. The nurse interprets this finding as:

    A. Negative
    B. Positive
    C. Reactive
    D. Nonreactive

146. A client at term was admitted to the obstetric unit with contractions of 60-second duration every 3–4 minutes. Vaginal exam revealed that the cervix was dilated 4 cm and 90% effaced. Membranes were intact and fetal station was −1. Two hours later, no further labor progress had been made. The uterine contractions were now every 7–8 minutes with a duration of 30–45 seconds. The fetal heart pattern was reassuring. Which of the following nursing actions would be most appropriate in this situation?

    A. Prepare for amnioinfusion.
    B. Encourage the client to ambulate.
    C. Prepare for tocolysis.
    D. Discharge the client home.

147. A client at term was admitted to the obstetric unit with complaints of constant uterine cramping. Vaginal exam revealed that the cervix was dilated to 2 cm and 50% effaced. The fetal station was at −3. Electronic fetal and contraction monitoring was started. The monitoring strip revealed a high uterine resting tone and irregular, short contractions. The fetal heart pattern was reassuring. Which of the following nursing interventions would be most appropriate for this client?

    A. Prepare for an amniotomy.
    B. Prepare for oxytocin augmentation.
    C. Obtain an order for analgesia.
    D. Encourage the client to ambulate.

148. A client was admitted to the obstetric unit in active labor and frank rupture of membranes. A fetal scalp electrode and intrauterine pressure catheter were inserted. The client had progressed to 8-cm dilation when the nurse noted abrupt decreases in the fetal heart rate of 15–20 bpm with a quick return to baseline. These rate changes occurred both with and without contractions. The nurse should prepare to initiate patient teaching regarding which of the following procedures?

    A. Cesarean birth
    B. High forceps delivery
    C. Oxytocin induction
    D. Amnioinfusion

149. A client has been in the second stage of labor for 2 hours. The nurse assesses the fetal station and position and finds the presenting part at −1 station and occiput

posterior (OP). Which of the following nursing actions would be most appropriate in this situation?

A. Assist the client to a hands and knees position.
B. Assist the client to flex her knees against her abdomen.
C. Assist the client to a squatting position for pushing.
D. Assist the client to ambulate in the unit halls.

150. A client was discharged home with her term newborn 48 hours after delivery. The OB nurse made a home visit 1 day later. The following assessment findings on the mother were noted. Breasts firming with lactation and leaking of thin, whitish fluid from the nipples. Firm fundus 3 cm below the umbilicus, lochial stain 3–5 cm on the perineal pad and brownish-red in color. The perineum was intact with slight swelling. Which of the following nursing actions would be indicated?

A. Document these normal findings.
B. Discuss perineal hygiene with the client.
C. Notify the healthcare provider of abnormal findings.
D. Instruct the client to seek medical attention immediately.

151. A multiparous client in the forth stage of labor tells the nurse, "I want to breast-feed but my breasts got so engorged last time, I could hardly stand it. Do I have to go through that again?" Which of the following replies by the nurse would be best?

A. "If you keep the baby on a strict 4-hour schedule, the milk will come in slower and there will be less engorgement."
B. "You should feed your baby formula until your milk comes in so there is less breast stimulation, which will prevent engorgement."
C. "We can give you some pills called Parlodil to keep your milk from coming in and causing breast engorgement."
D. "I will bring your baby out to nurse now. Be sure and feed the baby often. This will prevent engorgement the most effectively."

152. An adolescent client is admitted to the recovery area after delivery of a 7-lb infant. One of the nursing diagnoses formulated for her plan of care is "High risk for impaired bonding related to young maternal age and lack of support." Which of the following nursing interventions would be most appropriate to address this diagnosis?

A. Encourage the client to breast-feed her infant.
B. Discuss the positive features of the baby with her.
C. Bring the baby to her after the first period of reactivity.
D. Encourage the client to room-in with her baby.

153. The nurse is preparing a client at 16 weeks' gestation for an amniocentesis. Which of the following nursing actions has priority?

A. Ensure the client has a full bladder.
B. Ensure that lab results are on the chart.
C. Ensure that the client empties her bladder.
D. Ensure that the client has remained NPO.

154. A client at 18 weeks' gestation is seen at the clinic for maternal serum alpha fetal protein (MSAFP) results. The results were low. The nurse realizes that the client understands this finding when she makes which of the following statements?

A. "This test result means that everything is fine."
B. "My baby will probably have a neural tube defect."
C. "This result means my baby will be retarded."
D. "More testing will be needed to see if my baby is OK."

155. A client at 28 weeks' gestation was seen for a routine clinic appointment. She complained about frequent heartburn. She asked the clinic nurse why this occurs. Which of the following replies by the nurse is most accurate?

A. "Heartburn means your baby has a lot of hair."
B. "Heartburn means you are carrying a boy."
C. "Heartburn is caused by pregnancy hormones."
D. "Heartburn is caused by carrying your baby high."

ANSWERS

1. **(B)** Client need: physiological integrity; subcategory: physiological adaptation; content area: maternity

   RATIONALE
   (A) Vernix keeps the skin moist, not the fluid. (B) The amniotic fluid has five functions: provides a cushion to prevent trauma, allows fetal ease of movement, maintains a uniform fetal temperature, provides fluid for swallowing, and protects the fetal head during labor. (C) Amniotic fluid does not contain blood vessels. (D) Amniotic fluid is an alkaline, not an acid.

2. **(D)** Client need: physiological integrity; subcategory: reduction of risk potential; content area: maternity

   RATIONALE
   (A) ELISA is used for HIV screening. (B) VDRL is used for syphilis screening. (C) BHCG is used to determine pregnancy, especially ectopic pregnancy. (D) Elevated levels of AFP in amniotic fluid or maternal serum have been found to reflect open neural tube defects.

3. **(C)** Client need: physiological integrity; subcategory: physiological adaptation; content area: maternity

   RATIONALE
   (A) Breast tenderness can be due to hormonal changes other than pregnancy. (B) Enlargement can be related to gas, weight gain, and abdominal conditions other than pregnancy. (C) The positive signs of pregnancy include FHR by Doppler at 10–12 weeks and by fetoscope at 18–20 weeks; fetal movement perceived by trained examiner; fetal ECG; ultrasound visualization of fetal parts. (D) Amenorrhea is influenced by endocrine, metabolic, psychological changes and systemic disease.

4. **(A)** Client need: psychosocial integrity; subcategory: coping and adaptation; content area: maternity

   RATIONALE
   (A) The LMP is useful in calculating the EDC. Mothers need to know this information to master the tasks of pregnancy. (B) A partner's physiological symptoms are not part of the medical record. (C) The parity of the client's mother is not important; however, the number of multiple gestations can be influential in treatment. (D) Most pregnant women are tired in the first trimester; this is not crucial information.

5. **(D)** Client need: physiological integrity; subcategory: reduction of risk potential; content area: maternity

   RATIONALE
   (A) Emotional lability may last through the pregnancy, but it generally is not pathological. (B) Unless nausea and vomiting cause severe dehydration and electrolyte imbalance, the pregnancy is not at risk. (C) Bowel changes are affected by the progesterone levels of pregnancy; constipation is expected. (D) Danger signs of pregnancy include bleeding from the vagina, sudden gush of clear fluid from the vagina; fever and chills, severe headaches with blurred vision; abdominal pain; generalized swelling of the face and limbs; and absence of fetal movement.

6. **(C)** Client need: safe, effective care environment; subcategory: safety and infection control; content area: maternity

   RATIONALE
   (A) PG suppositories are used for second-trimester fetal demise. (B) Saline infusion is unsafe and should no longer be used. (C) The method of choice for first-trimester elective abortion is suction curettage because it is safe and can be done at minimal expense. (D) Laminaria is used to soften and efface a cervix prior to induction of labor.

7. **(A)** Client need: health promotion and maintenance; subcategory: prevention and early detection of disease; content area: maternity

   RATIONALE
   (A) Abdominal tenderness and pain can be signs of uterine infection and should be reported to a physician. (B) Sadness after abortion is normal, even if the termination is elective. (C) Bleeding after termination can last up to a month. (D) Fever is indicated by a temperature of 101°F (38.3°C) in women postabortion.

8. **(B)** Client need: psychosocial integrity; subcategory: coping and adaptation; content area: maternity

   RATIONALE
   (A) Fetal sex cannot be determined until after 20 weeks. (B) Amniocentesis performed at this point in pregnancy would be for genetic purposes. The woman's age places her at risk for a Down syndrome baby. (C) L/S ratio is used to determine the lung maturity of the fetus during the third trimester. (D) Bilirubin levels are drawn from the fluid to monitor fetuses compromised by isoimmunization.

9. **(C)** Client need: physiological integrity; subcategory: reduction of risk potential; content area: maternity

   RATIONALE
   (A) Temperature elevation related to the procedure would not occur for at least 24 hours. (B) Bladder spasms are uncommon. (C) Rupture of the membranes is a potential complication of amniocentesis. (D) FHR patterns are monitored, not fetal activity.

10. **(D)** Client need: physiological integrity; subcategory: basic care and comfort; content area: maternity

    RATIONALE
    (A) Increased daily activity is recommended. (B) Stool softeners are used in pregnancy after all other measures have failed. (C) Prenatal vitamins do not cause constipation and should be taken daily. (D) Increased fluid intake, adequate roughage or bulk in diet, regular bowel habits, and adequate daily exercise can often maintain good bowel function in women who have not had a previous problem.

11. **(B)** Client need: safe, effective care environment; subcategory: safety and infection control; content area: maternity

    RATIONALE
    (A) Rubella vaccine prevents 3-day measles, but it cannot be administered until after delivery. (B) An Rh-negative woman who delivers an Rh-positive, ABO-compatible infant has a 16% risk of being sensitized as a result of her pregnancy. RhoGam prevents this. (C) RhoGam will not prevent neonatal jaundice unless it is caused solely from isoimmunization. (D) The mother cannot be infected from the fetus, and RhoGam is not bacteriocidal.

12. **(A)** Client need: physiological integrity; subcategory: reduction of risk potential; content area: maternity

    RATIONALE
    (A) Leopold's maneuvers are four maneuvers of abdominal palpation used to assess fetal lie and position. (B) Valsalva's maneuver is the act of holding one's breath and pushing on the perineum. (C) Ritgen maneuver is used to support the fetal head on the perineum at delivery. (D) Credé's maneuver is a method of external bladder massage that is no longer used in obstetrics.

13. **(D)** Client need: psychosocial integrity; subcategory: coping and adaptation; content area: maternity

    RATIONALE
    (A) Bargaining is the third stage of grieving. This may or may not be present, depending on the couple's preparation for the death

of the fetus. (B) The final stage is acceptance, which may take months for resolution. (C) Anger is the second stage, resulting from feelings of loneliness, loss, and maybe guilt. (D) The first stage is denial of the death of the fetus. Even when the initial healthcare provider suspects fetal demise, the couple is hoping that a second opinion will be different.

14. **(B)** Client need: physiological integrity; subcategory: pharmacological and parenteral therapies, content area: maternity

RATIONALE

(A) IV Pitocin is used to induce contractions, not soften the cervix, especially prior to the third trimester. (B) Laminaria (dehydrated seaweed) may be inserted into the cervical canal. The secretions of the cervix are absorbed, and the laminaria expands to aid with effacement and dilation. (C) Amniotomy will aid in descent of the fetal head once labor is established, but in fetal demise, it is not effective in effacing the cervix. (D) Normal saline solution is no longer used for midtrimester abortions.

15. **(C)** Client need: physiological integrity; subcategory: pharmacological and parenteral therapies, content area: maternity

RATIONALE

(A) Dysuria may be caused by a UTI or a cervicovaginal infection. (B) Muscle weakness may be caused by grief. (C) Prostaglandin E$_2$ suppositories or gel are used extensively in the management of intrauterine fetal demise in the second trimester of pregnancy. GI side effects are caused by smooth-muscle stimulation. (D) Headaches may be caused by intense crying, elevated blood pressure, or electrolyte imbalance, not PGs.

16. **(B)** Client need: physiological integrity; subcategory: reduction of risk potential, content area: maternity

RATIONALE

(A) Mitral valve prolapse may be caused by untreated streptococcal infections, not fetal demise. (B) Prolonged retention of the dead fetus may lead to the development of DIC. (C) Pyelonephritis is not associated with fetal demise. (D) Endometriosis is a cause of infertility, not fetal demise.

17. **(A)** Client need: psychosocial integrity; subcategory: coping and adaptation; content area: maternity

RATIONALE

(A) Some couples may not be convinced of the death until they view and hold the stillborn. If they choose to see the stillborn, prepare the couple for what they will be seeing: "the baby is bruised" and other appropriate statements. (B) It is therapeutic for the couple to view the baby together. (C) Seeing the actual baby is less traumatic than imagining a horribly disfigured baby. (D) It helps parents to see fetal anomalies as well as normal baby features, so that grief can eventually be resolved.

18. **(D)** Client need: psychosocial integrity; subcategory: coping and adaptation; content area: maternity

RATIONALE

(A) Facing reality and other children is difficult, but it may help the couple acknowledge their grief. (B) Ambulation is encouraged after delivery to prevent thrombophlebitis. (C) A close friend may be a source of support to the grieving couple. (D) Seeing healthy babies is a necessary step in acceptance. Support from people will make it easier.

19. **(C)** Client need: safe, effective care environment; subcategory: safety and infection control; content area: maternity

RATIONALE

(A) The mucus plug can be passed several weeks prior to the onset of labor. (B) When the fetus settles into the pelvis, the mother will probably experience bladder pressure and frequency. (C) When membranes rupture, the amniotic fluid may be expelled in large amounts. If engagement has not occurred, the danger of the umbilical cord washing out with the fluid exists. (D) Nausea and vomiting can be prodromal signs of labor, but they are not indicative of actual labor.

20. **(A)** Client need: physiological integrity; subcategory: reduction of risk potential; content area: maternity

RATIONALE

(A) A BP of 150/100 is sometimes designated as moderate preeclampsia. Generalized edema, seen as puffy face, hands, and dependent areas such as ankles and lower legs, may be present. (B) Abdominal cramping may be a sign of early labor, but not PIH. (C) Severe headaches with photophobia that are not relieved by medication can be caused by PIH. (D) Clear nipple discharge is early milk letdown, not PIH.

21. **(B)** Client need: physiological integrity; subcategory: reduction of risk potential; content area: maternity

RATIONALE

(A) Chlamidiazyme is the test for chlamydia. (B) Diagnosis for syphilis is made by dark-field microscopy for spirochetes. Blood tests such as the VDRL, RPR, and more specific fluorescent treponemal antibody absorption tests are commonly done. (C) The Pap smear is currently the most common screening test for HPV. (D) A gonorrhea culture, or gonozyme test, is diagnostic for gonorrhea.

22. **(D)** Client need: physiological integrity; subcategory: reduction of risk potential; content area: maternity

RATIONALE

(A) Readiness for labor is determined by a Bishop score. (B) Diabetic control is evaluated by blood glucose monitoring. (C) Placental age is determined by ultrasound. (D) Accelerations of the FHR imply an intact central and autonomic nervous system that is not being affected by intrauterine hypoxia.

23. **(C)** Client need: health promotion and maintenance; subcategory: prevention and early detection of disease; content area: maternity

RATIONALE

(A) Physical activity can be continued throughout pregnancy with a class I cardiac condition. (B) Emotional stress should not adversely affect the client's condition. (C) Use of low forceps provides the safest method of birth, with lumbar epidural anesthesia to reduce the stress of pushing. (D) Surgery is a stress on the cardiovascular system and can cause complications in women with cardiac disease.

24. **(C)** Client need: physiological integrity; subcategory: reduction of risk potential; content area: maternity

RATIONALE

(A) Vaginal examination is only done if the client is in labor and is deferred if membranes are ruptured. (B) Gram's stain is performed to look for infection. (C) Amniotic fluid is alkaline, and an alkaline fluid turns the nitrazine test tape a dark blue. (D) Ultrasound can be used to visualize pockets of amniotic fluid, but it is not routinely used to determine ruptured membranes.

25. **(A)** Client need: physiological integrity; subcategory: reduction of risk potential; content area: maternity

RATIONALE

(A) A small amount of fluid can be placed on a glass slide, allowed to dry, and then looked at under a microscope. A ferning pattern confirms the presence of amniotic fluid. (B) Yeast buds are present with *Monilia*. (C) Fishy odor is caused by bacterial vaginosis. (D) Many WBCs are indicative of inflammation.

26. **(B)** Client need: physiological integrity; subcategory: pharmacological and parenteral therapies; content area: maternity

RATIONALE

(A) MgSO$_4$ is used to stop preterm labor or to control seizure activity in PIH. (B) Betamethasone is a glucocorticoid that acts to accelerate fetal lung maturation and prevent hyaline membrane disease. (C) Exosurf is lung surfactant given after preterm delivery to help mature the lungs. (D) Ritodrine is used to stop preterm labor.

27. **(D)** Client need: safe, effective care environment; subcategory: safety and infection control; content area: maternity

    RATIONALE

    (A) Narcotics are not used because they could neurologically depress the fetus. (B) If the baby is prematurely delivered, it is unrealistic to give false reassurance. (C) Bed rest with bathroom privileges is the usual treatment. (D) The nurse observes the woman for signs and symptoms of infection by frequently monitoring vital signs (especially temperature and pulse), describing the character of the amniotic fluid, and reporting elevated WBC to the physician or nurse-midwife.

28. **(A)** Client need: physiological integrity; subcategory: reduction of risk potential; content area: maternity

    RATIONALE

    (A) The purpose of the Apgar score is to evaluate the physical condition of the newborn at birth and the immediate need for resuscitation. (B) Dubowitz scoring is done 4–6 hours after birth. (C) Weighing and measuring is done in the nursery, not at the delivery. (D) Gavage feeding is postponed until the baby is stabilized; in premature infants it may be several weeks.

29. **(C)** Client need: physiological integrity; subcategory: reduction of risk potential; content area: maternity

    RATIONALE

    (A) Undescended testicles in the preterm male newborn is expected—with maturity they should descend normally. (B) Sole creases will be absent; lanugo will be present on all preterm babies. (C) All preterm newborns and especially IDMs are at risk for RDS. (D) Very small babies are at risk for hypoglycemia, not hyperglycemia.

30. **(B)** Client need: safe, effective care environment; subcategory: safety and infection control; content area: maternity

    RATIONALE

    (A) The bladder stays empty with a Foley catheter. (B) The dressing and perineal pad must be checked every 15 minutes for at least an hour, and the fundus should be gently palpated to determine whether it is remaining firm. (C) Shivering is a side effect of anesthetic withdrawal, and not a complication. (D) Hypothermia is common immediately following delivery, not fever.

31. **(D)** Client need: psychosocial integrity; subcategory: coping and adaptation; content area: maternity

    RATIONALE

    (A) Families are extremely nervous and interested in the well-being of the preterm baby. (B) Often unrealistic expectations of the growth and development of the preterm baby are held by the family. (C) Many of the premies have anomalies. Preterm babies do not look like the "perfect" baby of the magazines. (D) Denial is the first stage normally experienced in the grieving process. The parents need careful and complete explanations and the opportunity to take part in the decision making.

32. **(A)** Client need: safe, effective care environment; subcategory: management of care; content area: maternity

    RATIONALE

    (A) The woman is positioned on her left side with her shoulders parallel and her legs slightly flexed. (B) The anesthesia provider cleans the client's back prior to injection of anesthetic. (C) Medication initially is injected by the person administering the anesthesia. (D) Regular, slow chest breathing is encouraged during epidural administration.

33. **(C)** Client need: safe, effective care environment; subcategory: safety and infection control; content area: maternity

    RATIONALE

    (A) Relaxation may cause drowsiness, which is welcomed. (B) Severe headaches are a complication of spinal anesthesia. (C) If hypotension occurs, the nurse assists with corrective measures. The nurse takes the woman's blood pressure and pulse every 1–2 minutes during the first 15 minutes after injection. (D) Numbness in legs and feet is a sign of effective anesthesia.

34. **(D)** Client need: physiological integrity; subcategory: reduction of risk potential; content area: maternity

    RATIONALE

    (A) IV fluids need to be increased during epidural administration to prevent cardiovascular collapse. (B) Urine protein is used for PIH and pyelonephritis. (C) Motor and sensory neurons for the lower extremities are often blocked by the epidural anesthesia. (D) The bladder should be assessed at frequent intervals because the epidural block lessens the urge to urinate. Catheterization may be necessary because most women are unable to void.

35. **(B)** Client need: safe, effective care environment; subcategory: safety and infection control; content area: maternity

    RATIONALE

    (A) Vaginal packing is performed by a physician. (B) Fundal massage should be performed until the uterus contracts. (C) Perineal ice will not affect the uterine tone. (D) Blood transfusions are given on physician's orders only.

36. **(A)** Client need: physiological integrity; subcategory: pharmacological and parenteral therapies; content area: maternity

    RATIONALE

    (A) The purpose of $MgSO_4$ is to depress the CNS and avert maternal seizures and fetal hypoxia. (B) Initially the blood pressure may drop, but it will return to hypertensive levels. (C) Uterine relaxation may be a side effect of $MgSO_4$, but higher dosages of the medication are given to stop preterm labor than for PIH. (D) Decreased urine output may be caused by $MgSO_4$, but that is not the purpose of administration.

37. **(C)** Client need: physiological integrity; subcategory: reduction of risk potential; content area: maternity

    RATIONALE

    (A) Systolic heart murmur is frequently heard during the stress of labor. (B) A BP < 140/90 is considered normal when $MgSO_4$ is run via IV. (C) Hourly output can be assessed. Output should be 700 mL in 24 hours or at least 30 mL/hr. (D) Decreased DTRs are the desired effect of the drug.

38. **(A)** Client need: safe, effective care environment; subcategory: safety and infection control; content area: maternity

    RATIONALE

    (A) Calcium gluconate is the antidote for $MgSO_4$. (B) Sodium bicarbonate is used to neutralize acidosis. (C) Calcium carbonate is used for epigastric distress. (D) Folic acid is used for normal neurological development of the fetus.

39. **(A)** Client need: physiological integrity; subcategory: reduction of risk potential; content area: maternity

    RATIONALE

    (A) Rapid treatment of hypoglycemia is essential to prevent brain damage, because the brain requires glucose to function. (B) Weight loss is common in the first trimester. (C) Increased estrogen levels cause vision changes. (D) Hypertension will not show up until the late second trimester or early third trimester.

40. **(C)** Client need: physiological integrity; subcategory: physiological adaptation; content area: maternity

RATIONALE

(A) Three months prior to pregnancy, insulin levels should remain steady. (B) Insulin levels increase steadily during pregnancy. (C) Postpartum maternal insulin requirements fall significantly. This occurs because levels of HPL, progesterone, and estrogen fall after placental separation and their anti-insulin effect ceases. (D) Insulin levels decrease significantly.

41. **(D)** Client need: physiological integrity; subcategory: reduction of risk potential; content area: maternity

RATIONALE

(A) Blood pressure should be normal. (B) Edema of the eyelids is common. (C) Poor muscle tone of a limb may signify birth injury, especially after shoulder dystocia. (D) After birth the most common problem of the IDM is hypoglycemia.

42. **(C)** Client need: physiological integrity; subcategory: physiological adaptation; content area: maternity

RATIONALE

(A) Thirty-eight weeks is considered term. (B) ABO incompatibility will show up within the first 24 hours. (C) About 50% of full-term neonates and 80% of preterm neonates exhibit physiological jaundice on about the second or third day after birth. (D) Extravascular hemolysis results from bruising at delivery.

43. **(B)** Client need: safe, effective care environment; subcategory: safety and infection control; content area: maternity

RATIONALE

(A) A daily bath is not given to preserve natural skin lubrication. (B) Because it is not known if phototherapy injures the delicate eye structures, particularly the retina, the nurse applies eye patches over the newborn's closed eyes during exposure. (C) Babies can still be breast-fed during phototherapy. (D) Observe stools for meconium or other brownish black heme being passed. Bloody stools should not be found.

44. **(A)** Client need: physiological integrity; subcategory: physiological adaptation; content area: maternity

RATIONALE

(A) A primary cause of hyperbilirubinemia is hemolytic disease of the newborn secondary to Rh incompatibility. (B) Prematurity predisposes the infant to jaundice, not postmaturity. (C) Cesarean delivery has no effect on jaundice. (D) A mother's age has no influence on jaundice.

45. **(D)** Client need: safe, effective care environment; subcategory: safety and infection control; content area: maternity

RATIONALE

(A) Placenta previa is painless bleeding, which may be scant to heavy. (B) Normal show is combined with mucus and is usually small to moderate in amount. (C) A mucus plug is clear without blood. (D) Signs of abruptio placentae include severe and steady pain, sudden onset, external bleeding, dark venous blood.

46. **(A)** Client need: safe, effective care environment; subcategory: safety and infection control; content area: maternity

RATIONALE

(A) If fetal hypoxia progresses unchecked, irreversible brain damage or fetal demise may result. If fetal hypoxia occurs because of a decrease in uteroplacental blood flow, late decelerations generally occur. (B) Early decelerations are benign patterns associated with fetal head compression. (C) Variable decelerations are related to cord compression. (D) A mid-deceleration is not distinguishable from a variable deceleration.

47. **(B)** Client need: safe, effective care environment; subcategory: management of care; content area: maternity

RATIONALE

(A) Nurses cannot do this without a continuous fetal monitor, and then charting every 1 minute would not make sense. (B) As this more rapid pattern is identified, the need for more frequent assessments will be apparent. During the second stage of labor, some protocols recommend charting FHTs after each contraction. (C) Standards say that FHTs should be charted no more often than every 5 minutes close to delivery. (D) A precipitous delivery would probably end before 15 minutes were up.

48. **(C)** Client need: physiological integrity; subcategory: reduction of risk potential; content area: maternity

RATIONALE

(A) Check the healing of the perineum; sutures cannot be seen. (B) An empty bladder will not affect the perineum. (C) Apply ice glove or ice pack the first 24 hours. (D) Hemorrhoids will shrink with perineal care and medication, and they are not manually reduced after delivery.

49. **(C)** Client need: physiological integrity; subcategory: reduction of risk potential; content area: maternity

RATIONALE

(A) Milk production starts 3–4 days postpartum. (B) Nipple burning is related to positioning at the breast and initiation of feeding. (C) Erythema and swelling are present in the upper, outer quadrant of the breast. Axillary lymph nodes are enlarged and tender. (D) Dimpled skin is a sign of breast cancer.

50. **(D)** Client need: safe, effective care environment; subcategory: safety and infection control; content area: maternity

RATIONALE

(A) Cervical dilation is evaluated by vaginal exam. (B) Bishop score is used for inducibility. (C) True labor is evaluated by cervical change with contractions. Braxton Hicks contractions do not cause dilation. (D) It is a means of evaluating the O_2 and CO_2 exchange of the placenta.

51. **(B)** Client need: physiological integrity; subcategory: reduction of risk potential; content area: maternity

RATIONALE

(A) Ultrasound is never done for sex determination unless it involves genetic studies. (B) Assessment of placental age in a post-term pregnancy provides a gauge of placental functioning and risk to the fetus of continuing the pregnancy. (C) Fetal presentation can be determined by Leopold's maneuvers. (D) Visualization to identify anomalies is poorer at term.

52. **(A)** Client need: safe, effective care environment; subcategory: management of care; content area: maternity

RATIONALE

(A) It is imperative that the FHT be auscultated before and immediately after the procedure so that any changes from the previous FHT pattern can be noted. (B) Fundal pressure should not be used with amniotomy. (C) Bladder status does not affect amniotomy. (D) The physician who performs the amniotomy checks for prolapsed cord, not the nurse.

53. **(C)** Client need: safe, effective care environment; subcategory: safety and infection control; content area: maternity

RATIONALE

(A) Pitocin may be ordered IM after delivery. (B) Pitocin is never given mainline during labor. (C) After the infusion is started, the oxytocin solution is piggybacked into the primary tubing part closest to the catheter insertion. (D) Buccal Pitocin was taken off the market in the early 1980s because absorption was sporadic.

54. **(C)** Client need: psychosocial integrity; subcategory: coping and adaptation; content area: maternity

    RATIONALE

    (A) A healthy respect for Pitocin should be developed. (B) "Emergency" implies danger when administering the drug. (C) Additional information about the client's fears needs to be gathered before any explanations are appropriate. (D) Mentioning "complications" implies that some are expected.

55. **(D)** Client need: safe, effective care environment; subcategory: safety and infection control; content area: maternity

    RATIONALE

    (A) Side positioning is helpful to increase oxygenation to the fetus; Trendelenberg is used for prolapsed cord. (B) O_2 will not help much during a tetanic contraction, but it should be started. (C) Hydration to correct hypotension should be started. (D) When there is evidence of possible fetal distress, treatment is centered on relieving the hypoxia and minimizing the effects of anoxia on the fetus. If oxytocin is in use, it should be discontinued.

56. **(C)** Client need: safe, effective care environment; subcategory: safety and infection control; content area: maternity

    RATIONALE

    (A) Precipitous labor would probably have a good outcome if the baby was smaller than the other three. (B) Placenta previa would present with bleeding. (C) A ruptured uterus involves the tearing of previously intact uterine muscle or of an old uterine scar. (D) Dysfunctional labor is not common with a history of previous cesarean sections.

57. **(A)** Client need: safe, effective care environment; subcategory: safety and infection control; content area: maternity

    RATIONALE

    (A) No maternal death in association with VBAC in a client with a previous lower-segment incision has been reported for decades in industrialized countries. (B) Breech presentation is frequently associated with a specific pelvic shape and will recur in subsequent pregnancies. (C) Previous CPD is a contraindication for VBAC. (D) Multiple gestation following a previous cesarean section is an indication for a repeated cesarean section.

58. **(C)** Client need: physiological integrity; subcategory: reduction of risk potential; content area: maternity

    RATIONALE

    (A) The nurse cannot perform the delivery, because the client will not be able to push with a ruptured uterus. (B) The nurse should stabilize the client first, then call the physician. (C) Sudden searing abdominal pain is indicative of uterine rupture. The IV rate should be increased in anticipation of severe hemorrhage and shock prior to transfer to the operating room. (D) Contraction pattern will no longer show up.

59. **(B)** Client need: physiological integrity; subcategory: physiological adaptation; content area: maternity

    RATIONALE

    (A) Turning on the side would decrease BP, which is contraindicated with ruptured uterus. (B) When blood supply to the uterus is interrupted, about 80% of fetuses demonstrate fetal distress. Preparation is needed to resuscitate the infant. (C) In an emergency, povidone-iodine is poured over the abdomen and formal scrub is bypassed. (D) Usually a prolapsed cord does not coincide with a ruptured uterus.

60. **(C)** Client need: physiological integrity; subcategory: physiological adaptation; content area: maternity

    RATIONALE

    (A) All newborns have some acrocyanosis at delivery. (B) A sucking reflex is necessary for breast-feeding after delivery, but it is not the priority. (C) The first breath of life—the gasp in response to mechanical, chemical, thermal, and sensory and physical changes associated with birth—initiates the serial opening of the alveoli. (D) Meconium passage can happen in the first 24 hours of life and signifies a patent intestinal tract.

61. **(D)** Client need: physiological integrity; subcategory: basic care and comfort; content area: maternity

    RATIONALE

    (A) Erythema neonatorum toxicum is a newborn rash that normally appears in the first 2 days of life. (B) Stork bites are hemangiomas. (C) Milia are small white pimples on the face resulting from mother's hormones. (D) Mongolian spots are macular areas of bluish black pigmentation found on the dorsal area and the buttocks.

62. **(C)** Client need: psychosocial integrity; subcategory; coping and adaptation; content area: maternity

    RATIONALE

    (A) Five minutes is too short. (B) Seven minutes is too short. (C) Total feeding time is usually no longer than 10–15 minutes at each breast. (D) After 10–15 minutes, the baby uses the breast as a pacifier.

63. **(B)** Client need: health promotion and maintenance; subcategory: prevention and early detection of disease; content area: maternity

    RATIONALE

    (A) Peroxide does not dry the cord. (B) The infant may be put in a tub after the cord has fallen off and the circumcision site is healed (approximately 2 weeks). (C) Pus from the cord is a sign of infection. (D) The cord dries in about 2 weeks.

64. **(C)** Client need: physiological integrity; subcategory; reduction of risk potential; content area: maternity

    RATIONALE

    (A) The bladder fills rapidly after delivery and may need to be emptied several times during the first 12 hours. (B) Diuresis occurs in the first 12–24 hours postpartum. (C) A careful monitoring of intake and output should be maintained, and the bladder should be assessed for distention until the woman demonstrates complete emptying of the bladder with each voiding. (D) Dehydration is common, but diuresis occurs anyway.

65. **(B)** Client need: physiological integrity; subcategory: reduction of risk potential; content area: maternity

    RATIONALE

    (A) The umbilicus may pop outward during pregnancy and returns to normal after delivery. (B) Often pressure of the enlarging uterus on the abdominal muscles causes the rectus abdominis muscle to separate, producing diastasis recti. (C) Inguinal hernia is not caused by pregnancy. (D) Hiatal hernia may be caused by pregnancy, but it is not visible in the abdomen.

66. **(B)** Client need: psychosocial integrity; subcategory: psychosocial adaptation; content area: maternity

    RATIONALE

    (A) Taking hold occurs on the 2nd–3rd day postpartum and involves becoming proficient in caring for the baby. (B) During the first day or two following birth, the woman tends to be passive and somewhat dependent. She may have a great need to talk about her perceptions of her labor and birth. In Rubin's early work (1961), she labeled this the "taking-in" phase. (C) Letting go has to do with grief, not attachment. (D) Attachment is the general term for the bonding that takes place between mother and child.

67. **(A)** Client need: health promotion and maintenance; subcategory: prevention and early detection of disease; content area: maternity

RATIONALE

(A) The incidence of preterm birth is 12 times that of single births, and only 5% of twins reach 40 weeks' gestation. (B) Weight gain is based on the body size and height of the pregnant woman as well as on the number of fetuses she is carrying. (C) It is not possible to ensure fetuses of equal growth. (D) Prevention of striae has to do with the elasticity of the skin, not prenatal care.

68. **(D)** Client need: physiological integrity; subcategory: physiological adaptation; content area: maternity

RATIONALE

(A) "Rest period" begins at the end of one contraction to the start of the next. (B) "Duration" is the time that the contraction lasts. (C) Peak-to-peak timing is incorrect, because this varies with the duration and strength of the contraction. (D) The correct way to time frequency of contractions is from the beginning of one contraction to the beginning of the next contraction. The interval from the beginning to the end of a single contraction is the duration.

69. **(C)** Client need: physiological integrity; subcategory: reduction of risk potential; content area: maternity

RATIONALE

(A) Amniocentesis may determine if the twins are identical or fraternal. (B) NST can determine the well-being of both the fetuses, but not the size or growth. (C) Serial ultrasounds are done to assess the growth of each fetus and to provide early recognition of IUGR. (D) GTT is used to diagnose diabetes mellitus, not fetal growth.

70. **(B)** Client need: physiological Integrity; subcategory: reduction of risk potential; content area: maternity

RATIONALE

(A) A manual exploration of the uterus is commonly done with twin deliveries so that fragments are not left. (B) In some instances the second twin may need to be born by cesarean section. Complications that would require this include profound fetal distress, prolapse of the cord, and contractions of the uterus that trap the second twin. (C) Meconium fluid is found in twin deliveries with the same frequency as single deliveries. (D) Placenta previa will be diagnosed prior to delivery.

71. **(C)** Client need: physiological integrity; subcategory: physiological adaptation; content area: maternity

RATIONALE

(A) Pain and cramping are related to UTI, not hemorrhage. (B) Hemorrhoids do not bleed after delivery. (C) Uterine atony can frequently be anticipated in the presence of overdistention of the uterus; dysfunctional labor, when the uterus does not contract properly; oxytocin use in labor; and use of anesthesia that produces uterine relaxation. (D) Breast-feeding does help to prevent uterine atony, but overdistention of the uterus is the usual cause following twin delivery.

72. **(C)** Client need: physiological integrity; subcategory: physiological adaptation; content area: maternity

RATIONALE

(A) Lack of uterine enlargement and FHTs are signs of ectopic pregnancy. (B) Bleeding in spontaneous rupture of membranes has no relationship to bleeding in the first trimester. (C) Unexplained bleeding, cramping, and backache jeopardize the fetus. (D) Incompetent cervix does not cause uterine bleeding.

73. **(A)** Client need: physiological integrity; subcategory: reduction of risk potential; content area: maternity

RATIONALE

(A) Ectopic pregnancy may result from a number of different causes, including tubal damage caused by PID, previous pelvic or tubal surgery, etc. (B) Molar pregnancy causes early PIH and rapid uterine enlargement, not pain. (C) Placenta previa involves painless bleeding. (D) Scarring of the tubes and uterus can cause difficulty with implantation, but not spontaneous abortion once pregnancy is established.

74. **(B)** Client need: psychosocial integrity; subcategory: coping and adaptation; content area: maternity

RATIONALE

(A) PROM can occur with a cerclage in place. (B) The treatment most commonly used is the Shirodkar-Barter operation (cerclage). Once the suture is in place, a cesarean birth may be planned. The success rate of carrying a pregnancy to term is 80%–90%. (C) If a cerclage is in place during delivery, the cervix can be torn or a cesarean section may be necessary. (D) Cerclage does not have anything to do with Pap smears.

75. **(C)** Client need: safe, effective care environment; subcategory: management of care; content area: maternity

RATIONALE

(A) A cervix is only mechanically dilated with a dilatation and curettage. (B) Pap smears are done postpartum. (C) The suture may be released at term and vaginal birth permitted. (D) Cultures are only done if the client is symptomatic for infection.

76. **(D)** Client need: physiological integrity; subcategory: physiological adaptation; content area: maternity

RATIONALE

(A) Low blood pressure should not cause fatigue. (B) Increased blood volume carries more RBCs; therefore anemia is not the cause of fatigue. (C) Increased appetite with increased intake should cause more energy. (D) Excessive fatigue may be noted within a few weeks after the first menstrual period and may persist throughout the first trimester. Most of the hormones produced during pregnancy are initially from the corpus luteum.

77. **(C)** Client need: physiological Integrity; subcategory: basic care and comfort; content area: maternity

RATIONALE

(A) Milk may hinder absorption. (B) Meals contain a wide variety of nutrients that may inhibit absorption. (C) Absorption of iron from nonmeat sources may be enhanced by combining them with a good vitamin C source. (D) Water is not helpful for absorption, and stomach upset may occur.

78. **(D)** Client need: health promotion and maintenance; subcategory: growth and development though the life span; content area: maternity

RATIONALE

(A) Aerobic exercises should not be started during pregnancy, but they may be continued. (B) Exercise will not hurt the baby. (C) Walking is encouraged during pregnancy. (D) Normal participation in exercise can continue throughout an uncomplicated pregnancy. Pregnancy is not the time to learn a new or strenuous sport.

79. **(A)** Client need: health promotion and maintenance; subcategory: prevention and early detection of disease; content area: maternity

RATIONALE

(A) Proposed contributing factors for leg cramps include an inadequate calcium intake, an imbalance in calcium and phosphorus, and enlarged uterus pressing on pelvic nerves. (B) Vitamin E helps with placental development. (C) Folic acid prevents neural tube defects. (D) Beta carotene is needed for fetal growth.

80. **(B)** Client need: safe, effective care environment; subcategory: safety and infection control; content area: maternity

RATIONALE

(A) Contraction at the peak does not give enough time for first pass to the mother before the fetus receives the drug. (B) It has been suggested that the IV injection be given with the onset of a contraction, when the blood flow to the uterus and the fetus is decreased. (C) When the uterus is at rest, the mother and fetus share initial circulation of the drug. (D) At contraction's end, full placental circulation is in effect.

81. **(C)** Client need: psychosocial integrity; subcategory: coping and adaptation; content area: maternity

    RATIONALE

    (A) Latent phase begins with the onset of regular contractions and should not exceed 20 hours. (B) Active phase includes dilatation of the cervix from 3–8 cm and progressive fetal descent. (C) The nurse should be alert for signs of the transition phase, including behavioral changes (such as increasing irritability) and a decrease in coping mechanisms. (D) Complete dilatation is accompanied by a strong urge to push.

82. **(A)** Client need: physiological integrity; subcategory: pharmacological and parenteral therapies; content area: maternity

    RATIONALE

    (A) The pudendal block provides perineal anesthesia for the second stage of labor, birth, and episiotomy repair. It anesthetizes the perineal, dorsal, and inferior hemorrhoidal nerves. (B) Pressure will only be blocked by regional anesthesia. (C) Only the perineum is numbed by a pudendal block. (D) A pudendal block is given through the vagina into the pudendal nerve.

83. **(D)** Client need: physiological integrity; subcategory: physiological adaptation; content area: maternity

    RATIONALE

    (A) Contraction pain (cramping) is felt with placental separation. (B) A trickle of blood usually precedes separation. (C) During delivery there is no urge to void, because the pressure is removed from the bladder. (D) Signs of placental separation usually appear around 5 minutes after the birth of the infant. These signs are globular-shaped uterus, a rise of the fundus in the abdomen, a gush of blood, and further protrusion of the umbilical cord out of the vagina.

84. **(B)** Client need: physiological integrity; subcategory: reduction of risk potential; content area: maternity

    RATIONALE

    (A) Babinski's reflex is used for neurological assessment. (B) Pain in the foot or leg is a positive Homans' sign, with dorsiflexion of the client's foot. A positive Homans' sign suggests thrombus. (C) Psoas sign is used for appendicitis. (D) Moro's reflex is the startle reflex found in newborns.

85. **(A)** Client need: psychosocial integrity; subcategory: coping and adaptation; content area: maternity

    RATIONALE

    (A) Acrocyanosis (bluish discoloration of the hands and feet) may be present in the first 2–6 hours after birth. This condition is due to poor peripheral circulation, especially when the baby is exposed to cold. (B) Mongolian spots are normal pigmented areas of purple-blue seen in black and Asian people. (C) Sternal retractions are seen in the rib cage. (D) A patent ductus arteriosus is failure to adapt from fetal circulation to external circulation and is found in the chest.

86. **(D)** Client need: psychosocial integrity; subcategory: coping and adaptation; content area: maternity

    RATIONALE

    (A) Babies get jittery when they have hypoglycemia. (B) Babies mottle when they are cold; they cannot shiver. (C) A startle reflex involves the arms, not the face. (D) Neonatal tremors are common in the full-term newborn. The CNS is immature and newborn's movements are uncoordinated.

87. **(C)** Client need: psychosocial integrity; subcategory: coping and adaptation; content area: maternity

    RATIONALE

    (A) Giving pros and cons of both feeding methods is appropriate teaching. (B) Mothers can consider this up to the time that the milk comes in. (C) The nurse caring for the breast-feeding mother should help the woman to achieve independence and success in her feeding efforts. (D) Breast-feeding is best for infants, but not for every situation.

88. **(B)** Client need: psychosocial integrity; subcategory: coping and adaptation; content area: maternity

    RATIONALE

    (A) Tetracycline does not cause deafness. (B) Permanent, gray-brown discoloration of tooth enamel occurs in the fetus following maternal ingestion of tetracycline during pregnancy. (C) Antibiotics do not affect the CNS. (D) Webbed fingers and toes are a genetic trait.

89. **(C)** Client need: physiological integrity; subcategory; physiological adaptation; content area: maternity

    RATIONALE

    (A) Positive signs include FHTs, fetal movements, and visualization of the fetus by ultrasound. (B) Probable signs include objective changes in the uterus, enlargement of the abdomen, and skin pigmentation patterns. (C) These are the most common signs and symptoms of pregnancy but can be caused by other conditions; that is why they are called presumptive. (D) Nausea and fatigue are not common signs of a bladder infection.

90. **(D)** Client need: physiological integrity; subcategory: reduction of risk potential; content area: maternity

    RATIONALE

    (A) Symphysis will not help measure fundal height. (B) Hip bones will not help measure fundal height. (C) At about 36 weeks' gestation with a single fetus, the fundus may reach the sternum. (D) At 20 weeks' gestation and about 20 cm the umbilicus is a perfect landmark, because it is midway in the abdomen.

91. **(B)** Client need: physiological integrity; subcategory: physiological adaptation; content area: maternity

    RATIONALE

    (A) There is no reason to suspect cancer. (B) The darker pigmentation is caused by increased hormones and will lighten or disappear after pregnancy. From her description, it can only be a linea nigra. (C) Foods do not affect pigmentation of the abdomen unless it is hives. (D) Stretch marks occur where the skin is stretched from weight gain. Initially they are dark red, then silver colored.

92. **(C)** Client need: physiological integrity; subcategory: physiological adaptation; content area: maternity

    RATIONALE

    (A, B, D) This answer is inappropriate because she is not pathological, and it is not caused by the husband's actions. It would close the door to communication if the nurse accused the husband. (C) Men frequently do not understand why a pregnant woman cries seemingly without a cause. This is especially true if she has been very stable before pregnancy. Often the woman cannot express in words why she is crying. It is best to try and be supportive even if she is not understood.

93. **(D)** Client need: physiological integrity; subcategory: reduction of risk potential; content area: maternity

    RATIONALE

    (A, B, C, D) Gravida indicates the number of times a person has been pregnant, including this pregnancy. Para indicates the number of deliveries after 20 weeks' gestation. Multiple fetuses are counted as one pregnancy, one delivery. T is the number of term deliveries after 37 weeks. P is the number of preterm deliveries before 37 weeks. Ab is the number of spontaneous or induced abortions prior to 20 weeks. L is the number of living children. (Here each baby is counted as one.) The only answer accurately describing the woman's history is D.

94. **(B)** Client need: physiological integrity; subcategory: reduction of risk potential; content area: maternity

    RATIONALE

    (A) Although multiple abortions put a person at risk, one abortion is not considered significant. (B) The client may have become Rh sensitized, especially if she did not receive RhoGam after delivery. This can cause isoimmunization of the fetus. (C) There are no known CNS malformations caused by Rh incompatibility. (D) Even though she did not seek medical help after her abortion, there is no reason to believe the client will not show up for prenatal visits.

95. **(D)** Client need: physiological integrity; subcategory: reduction of risk potential; content area: maternity

    RATIONALE

    (A) The nurse needs to immediately listen to FHTs, preferably with an external fetal monitor. (B) Blood pressure and pulse are needed to determine safety from shock for mother and fetus. (C) Palpation of the abdomen will give the nurse information about contractions, rigidity of the uterus, and tenderness of the abdomen to determine cause of bleeding. (D) A vaginal exam should never be done in the presence of vaginal bleeding unless the client is in a room equipped with the personnel and team to do an emergency cesarean section. This should never be performed by a nurse.

96. **(B)** Client need: physiological integrity; subcategory: reduction of risk potential; content area: maternity

    RATIONALE

    (A) Stomach fluttering during the second trimester is not a symptom of GI upset. (B) Many women mistake "quickening" or movement of the baby for the flu. Multigravidas usually recognize the fetal activity earlier and more accurately than primigravidas. The nurse can reassure the client that this is a positive, happy sensation and that she will not start feeling bad. This is usually felt between 16 and 22 weeks. (C) Tea and crackers may be effective for GI upset, but they are not appropriate for fetal activity. (D) This answer is not appropriate for fetal movement.

97. **(A)** Client need: physiological integrity; subcategory: reduction of risk potential; content area: maternity

    RATIONALE

    (A) Yeast "infection," monilia candidiasis, is influenced by a change in the vaginal pH due to pregnancy hormones. (B) Gonorrhea is a sexually transmitted bacterial infection that requires antibiotic therapy. The discharge is usually green. (C) Trichomonas is caused by a flagellated trichomonad and has a very foul-smelling, yellow discharge. (D) Pain and a fluid-filled vesicle, usually on the perineum, characterizes herpes.

98. **(A)** Client need: physiological integrity; subcategory: reduction of risk potential; content area: maternity

    RATIONALE

    (A) Nägele's rule: Count back 3 months and add 7 days. (B) McDonald's rule is for determining fundal height, not EDC. (C) Hegar's sign is the softening and compressibility of the lower uterine segment at about 7 weeks' gestation. (D) Quickening is the feeling of fetal activity, usually between 16–20 weeks. Because it varies, it is helpful, but not very specific, in pointing the exact EDC.

99. **(C)** Client need: physiological integrity; subcategory: physiological adaptation; content area: maternity

    RATIONALE

    (A) An FHR within normal range for baseline does not tell how the fetus is tolerating stress or its neurological integrity. (B) Variable decelerations are common, not reassuring, and not criteria in NST assessment. (C, D) Unless the fetus has three or more accelerations in a specified time frame, the NST is nonreactive. The acceleration must also be at least 10 beats above baseline and last 10–15 seconds.

100. **(C)** Client need: physiological integrity; subcategory: pharmacological and parenteral therapies; content area: maternity

    RATIONALE

    (A) A nipple stimulation test can cause hypertonic contractions that skew the test. (B) A NST does not involve contractions. (C) Oxytocin is the generic name for Pitocin and causes contractions. (D) A contraction stress test implies that the person was having spontaneous contractions and did not need stimulation.

101. **(B)** Client need: physiological integrity; subcategory: reduction of risk potential; content area: maternity

    RATIONALE

    (A) It is not necessary to fast from food or drink prior to test. (B, C) In order to visualize the uterus, the bladder must be full. (D) An enema is not necessary as intestinal tract visualization does not interfere with uterine ultrasound.

102. **(A)** Client need: physiological integrity; subcategory: reduction of risk potential; content area: maternity

    RATIONALE

    (A) Abruptio placentae involves separation of the placenta from the uterus; this in turn causes decreased placental oxygenation leading to late decelerations. (B) Early decelerations are caused by head compression. (C) Variable decelerations are caused by cord compression. (D) Accelerations with fetal movements are a reassuring sign of fetal well-being not usually found with bleeding problems during pregnancy.

103. **(C)** Client need: physiological integrity; subcategory: reduction of risk potential; content area: maternity

    RATIONALE

    (A) Ruptured membranes may be important for prolapsed cord, but this is assessed after turning. (B) Whether the FHR returns or not, the physician needs to be notified, but time is wasted if the nurse calls before intervening. (C) It is possible that the cord got compressed as the head descended. Change in position can alleviate the compression. (D) Because an FHR of 90 bpm is not ominous, a cesarean may not be indicated, depending on outcome. To start preparing for surgery is not the first intervention.

104. **(D)** Client need: physiological integrity; subcategory; reduction of risk potential; content area: maternity

    RATIONALE

    (A) If it is a low-segment rupture, heart tones may drop but the fetus should be born alive. (B) Inability to push is not an important issue. (C) Client may be restless and anxious owing to stage of labor, becoming "shocky" or worrying about the baby. This may be an indication of beginning shock but in itself is not diagnostic of life-threatening problems during the second stage of labor. (D) The client most probably ruptured her uterus. If rupture is high, fetal parts will be palpable through the abdominal wall. There is a high mortality rate for both mother and fetus if this happens. The physician can elect to do emergency cesarean section or forceps delivery.

105. **(C)** Client need: physiological integrity; subcategory: reduction of risk potential; content area: maternity

     RATIONALE

     (A) Turning up the Pitocin IV may cause fetal distress or rupture the uterus. (B) Emptying the client's bladder may relieve pain with contractions but will not shorten their duration. (C) The nurse should turn off the Pitocin IV to decrease the hyperstimulation. (D) If only one contraction is long, terbutaline is not indicated. If a pattern of hyperstimulation continues, terbutaline is indicated.

106. **(C)** Client need: physiological integrity; subcategory: reduction of risk potential; content area: maternity

     RATIONALE

     (A) A ferning test is not possible unless a physician has collected some fluid on a slide after sterile speculum examination. (B) Feeling for moisture is nonspecific because vaginal mucus and urine can also leak. (C) Nitrazene paper is a test to check for amniotic fluid leakage. Amniotic fluid is alkaline and will turn the paper dark blue. (D) The nurse should not perform a vaginal examination unless the client is in active labor, because the nurse can introduce bacteria into the vagina through examination.

107. **(C)** Client need: physiological integrity; subcategory: reduction of risk potential; content area: maternity

     RATIONALE

     (A) The type of breathing used in latent phase is slow chest pattern. (B) During active phase a pant-and-blow pattern prevents hyperventilation. (C) During transition, shallow panting helps to prevent premature pushing. (D) During pushing, the client is instructed to "hold your breath and bear down."

108. **(D)** Client need: physiological integrity; subcategory: reduction of risk potential; content area: maternity

     RATIONALE

     (A) Color and quantity of fluid are indicators of fetal status but are less reliable than FHR. (B) Performing a vaginal examination may or may not be appropriate, depending on the circumstances. Vaginal dilation does not affect fetal well-being. (C) Rupture of membranes does not preclude getting up to the bathroom if the fetal head is engaged. (D) It is most important to know that FHR is within normal range.

109. **(A)** Client need: physiological integrity; subcategory: physiological adaptation; content area: maternity

     RATIONALE

     (A) The latent phase usually ends by the time the client has dilated to 3–4 cm. It is characterized by short contractions of mild to moderate intensity closer than 10 minutes apart. The client is relatively comfortable, although she may complain of backache, pressure, leg cramps, and the need to void frequently. (B, C, D) This stage is much more advanced than the client's situation.

110. **(B)** Client need: physiological integrity; subcategory: physiological adaptation; content area: maternity

     RATIONALE

     (A) The Silverman score is used to assess respiratory problems. (B) The Apgar score is used to assess muscle tone, color, respiration, cry, and heart rate. (C) The Denver Developmental Screening Test is used when the child is about 6 months old to assess neurological integrity. (D) Dextrosticks are used to assess hypoglycemia in the newborn.

111. **(C)** Client need: physiological integrity; subcategory: reduction of risk potential; content area: maternity

     RATIONALE

     (A) Syndactyly is fusion of the toes or fingers to cause webbing. (B) Moro's reflex is the normal startle reflex. (C) Ortolani's sign is produced by a click or thud as the head of the femur is dislocated from the acetabulum. (D) Babinski's reflex is elicited as a normal neurological sign when stimulus is applied to the sole of a newborn's foot.

112. **(D)** Client need: physiological integrity; subcategory: basic care and comfort; content area: maternity

     RATIONALE

     (A) A yellow, puttylike stool is consistent with bottle-feeding. (B) A yellow, curdy stool usually follows as a transition stool after meconium. It should not have an odor. (C) Infants' stools change to brown color 4 to 7 days after birth. (D) The meconium stool is the first bowel movement. This contains bile and amniotic components and is very thick and sticky. Sometimes this type of stool lasts 1 to 2 days.

113. **(C)** Client need: psychosocial integrity; subcategory: coping and adaptation; content area: maternity

     RATIONALE

     (A) Avoidance of eye contact is a negative sign. (B, D) Refusing to hold the baby or keeping him at an arm's length is a way of avoiding attachment. (C) Eye contact and close handling and touching are very positive signs of bonding. Eye contact alone is not enough.

114. **(C)** Client need: physiological integrity; subcategory: reduction of risk potential; content area: maternity

     RATIONALE

     (A) Taking vital signs will not indicate anything specific to calf. DTRs are unaffected by blood clots. (B) Ambulation is contraindicated if phlebitis is suspected. (C) The nurse would need to inspect for redness, edema, circulatory changes (mottling). Palpation would include assessing for tenderness on touch, capillary refill of both extremities, feeling of heat at site, evaluation of size of area. Homans' sign is used daily to assess pain in calves of postpartum clients. (D) Pedal edema may or may not be pres-ent. Taking blood pressure on the affected leg may move a clot.

115. **(A)** Client need: physiological integrity; subcategory: reduction of risk potential; content area: maternity

     RATIONALE

     (A) The hematoma is a large blood blister caused by a ruptured blood vessel at delivery. (B) A misplaced suture would be visible and not cause the edema. (C) It is too soon after delivery for an abscess to form. (D) Normal edema is not hard and purple, and it is bilateral.

116. **(D)** Client need: physiological integrity; subcategory: reduction of risk potential; content area: maternity

     RATIONALE

     (A) An analgesic will help with the discomfort but not address the problem. (B) Benzocaine will give local relief only. (C) Hot packs are contraindicated because heat will increase circulation and bleeding into the tissue will be more rapid. (D) An ice pack will reduce the swelling and pain and slow the circulation so that the blood from the ruptured vessel will not continue to seep into the tissue.

117. **(B)** Client need: physiological integrity; subcategory: reduction of risk potential; content area: maternity

     RATIONALE

     (A) If the baby sucks only on the tips, they will get blood blisters from the suction. (B) By putting more than the nipple tip in the baby's mouth, milk will let down faster and easier, and nipples will be less sore. (C) The baby already sucks well; otherwise her nipples would not be sore. (D) A baby can learn to open the mouth wide enough to accommodate the breast.

118. **(B)** Client need: physiological integrity; subcategory; reduction of risk potential; content area: maternity

     RATIONALE

     (A, D) Addition of oxytocic drugs or uterine massage when the uterus is already firm could cause rupture. (B) If the client had epidural anesthesia, she probably does not have the urge to urinate. A misplaced bladder can cause heavy bleeding. If the client cannot void, catheterization is required. (C) Breast-feeding helps to reduce bleeding and augment involution, but the uterus cannot clamp down if the full bladder keeps it displaced.

119. **(C)** Client need: safe, effective care environment; subcategory: safety and infection control; content area: maternity

     RATIONALE

     (A) Tetracycline is not given in pregnancy, because it causes gray discoloration of the fetal teeth. (B) Kanamycin is not recommended in pregnancy, because of its ototoxic and nephrotoxic properties. It crosses the placenta. (C) Ampicillin is the drug of choice for IV use for renal infections. (D) Erythromycin is safe during pregnancy, but it is ineffective against UTIs.

120. **(D)** Client need: physiological integrity; subcategory: pharmacological and parenteral therapies; content area: maternity

     RATIONALE

     (A) After delivery an adequate fluid intake (eight glasses per day) is necessary. Fluids are encouraged, not restricted. (B) Limited use of docusate sodium (usually 1 week) is advised. (C) Docusate sodium increases secretion of intestinal fluid to soften stool but does not cause diarrhea or increased frequency. The first defecation after delivery can be painful and feared by mothers with fresh episiotomies. (D) Generally, docusate sodium is given to prevent straining the fresh suture line during defecation with hard, dry stool.

121. **(B)** Client need: physiological integrity; subcategory: pharmacological and parenteral therapies; content area: maternity

     RATIONALE

     (A) It is given slowly over several minutes to avoid nausea, vomiting, and respiratory depression. (B) Meperidine can cause vein irritation, redness up the arm, marked increase in heart rate, and syncope if given undiluted. (C, D) Effects on the fetus include decreased FHR variability (long and short term) and a mild decrease in FHR. These side effects are minimized if meperidine is administered from the beginning to the peak of the contraction when blood flow to the placenta is minimal.

122. **(D)** Client need: physiological integrity; subcategory: physiological adaptation; content area: maternity

     RATIONALE

     (A, B) Estrogen and progesterone may be elevated for many reasons and are not used as predictors of pregnancy. (C) Growth hormone is not a predictor of pregnancy and is normally found in children and adolescents. (D) HCG is the hormone tested for in both urine and serum for pregnancy.

123. **(A)** Client need: safe, effective care environment; subcategory: safety and infection control; content area: maternity

     RATIONALE

     (A) A respiratory rate of 12 breaths/min is life threatening, because it indicates that the magnesium has affected the respiratory musculature and respiratory center in the brain. Calcium gluconate would be administered by IV push to counteract the respiratory depression. (B) Normal minimal urine output is 30 mL/hr. (C) DTRs are expected to become normal or decreased. (D) A normal blood pressure would be a welcomed sign.

124. **(D)** Client need: health promotion and maintenance; subcategory; prevention and early detection of disease; content area: maternity

RATIONALE

(A) Hemorrhoids are a common sequel of long second-stage labor and large babies. Mothers are started on stool softeners after delivery to help relieve the anxiety and pain associated with first defecation. (B) Sitz baths will relieve the pain. (C) Hydrocortisone cream will help shrink the size and relieve the pain. Many physicians also order a lidocaine topical spray and/or witch hazel pads (Tucks) to alleviate pain. (D) Frequent enemas will aggravate the hemorrhoids.

125. **(B)** Client need: safe, effective care environment; subcategory: safety and infection control; content area: maternity

     RATIONALE

     (A) Narcotics have side effects of nausea and vomiting if given too rapidly. They must be given over several minutes. (B, C) Because placental blood flow to the fetus is very diminished during the contraction, especially from start to peak, it is important to administer the narcotic then. This prevents the fetus from receiving the full effect of the medication. (D) Narcotics are not to be given by IV push between contractions because the fetus will become depressed.

126. **(C)** Client need: physiological integrity; subcategory: pharmacological and parenteral therapies; content area: maternity

     RATIONALE

     (A) Nitrous oxide is a general anesthetic. (B) Tetracaine has a very slow onset, narrow spread, and highly toxic nature. It is only used for subarachnoid blocks. (C) Lidocaine is the drug of choice for local anesthesia because it is versatile, has rapid onset, moderate duration, and excellent spread. (D) Benzocaine spray is a topical foam that is effective for analgesia in episiotomies, but not useful for anesthesia.

127. **(B)** Client need: physiological integrity; subcategory: pharmacological and parenteral therapies; content area: maternity

     RATIONALE

     (A) Hydralazine accentuates the normal postural hypotension of pregnancy, and the client needs to change position slowly. (B) Food keeps the drug from being absorbed too rapidly. (C) Never double blood pressure medication unless directed by the physician. (D) Mild dependent edema is common in the late third trimester; the client is in mid-second trimester. Edema needs to be reported promptly to her physician.

128. **(D)** Client need: safe, effective care environment; subcategory: management of care; content area: maternity

     RATIONALE

     (A) Antibiotics are not necessary unless there are signs of sepsis. (B) Antihistamines may cause drowsiness but are usually not used in this procedure. (C) Aspirin works as an antiprostaglandin and is contraindicated. (D) Because dinoprostone causes diarrhea, nausea, and vomiting, both an antiemetic and antidiarrheal should be used concomitantly.

129. **(A)** Client need: physiological integrity; subcategory: pharmacological and parenteral therapies; content area: maternity

     RATIONALE

     (A) Dinoprostone is used in suppository form or gel to soften the cervix and produce uterine contractions for missed abortions and fetal death prior to 28 weeks' gestation. (B) Pitocin is ineffective this early in pregnancy. (C) Syntocinon nasal spray is only used for milk letdown in postpartum clients. (D) Laminaria, a genus of kelp or seaweed that, when dried, has the ability to absorb water and expand with considerable force, is used to soften the cervix prior to induction of abortion, but it will not produce contractions.

130. **(C)** Client need: physiological integrity; subcategory: pharmacological and parenteral therapies; content area: maternity

    RATIONALE

    (A) Vitamin B_{12} is sometimes used for recurrent adult herpes simplex outbreaks, but not for outbreaks in babies. (B) Variola (smallpox) vaccination is no longer given to anyone and would be ineffective in this case. (C) VZIG is the γ-globulin for chickenpox. It is frequently given as soon as possible after delivery to augment the baby's immunity and to prevent serious sequalae. (D) Acyclovir is given to adults and, occasionally as a last resort, to babies with fulminating herpes-varicella infections.

131. **(C)** Client need: health promotion and maintenance; subcategory: growth and development through the life span; content area: maternity

    RATIONALE

    (A) The nausea and vomiting, breast discomfort, and emotional lability generally cause the pregnant woman to have decreased interest in sexual activity during the first trimester. (B) Shortness of breath in the absence of cardiac disease is associated with the third trimester, when the enlarged uterus encroaches on the diaphragm. (C) Breast enlargement and tenderness are common presumptive signs of pregnancy in the first trimester. (D) Nocturnal leg cramps are associated with an imbalance of calcium and phosphorus and generally do not start until the middle to end of the second trimester.

132. **(A)** Client need: physiological integrity; subcategory: basic care and comfort; content area: maternity

    RATIONALE

    (A) Signs of sickle cell crisis include abdominal, joint, chest, vertebral, and/or extremity pain. Nurses must provide comfort measures such as repositioning, supporting joints with pillows, and abdominal splinting when the client coughs. (B) Strict bed rest may cause joint immobility and pain. The client should be assisted with movement in bed and ambulation as ordered. (C) Oxygen administration requires a medical order. (D) Sickled cells tend to clump together and occlude small arteries and capillaries. This occlusion causes tissue ischemia. Care must be taken to avoid further damage to the joints during a sickle cell crisis.

133. **(D)** Client need: physiological integrity; subcategory: reduction of risk potential; content area: maternity

    RATIONALE

    (A) Amniocentesis is indicated for genetic testing during the second trimester, or when a client is in preterm labor, to determine fetal lung maturity. This client is at term and there are no maternal conditions (such as maternal diabetes) that would indicate a problem with fetal lung maturity. (B) Oxytocin causes uterine contractions, can cause uterine tetany, and can lead to or cause uteroplacental insufficiency. The fetal heart rate pattern shows late decelerations, a condition caused by uteroplacental insufficiency. (C) Amnioinfusion is indicated when there is thick meconium-stained fluid (to dilute the fluid and decrease the risk of fetal aspiration), and when there is evidence of cord compression (variable decelerations). (D) This client has symptoms of a placental abruption. This is a medical emergency for both the client and fetus. Since a vaginal delivery cannot be rapidly accomplished (active phase of labor is from 4–7 cm dilation), cesarean birth is indicated.

134. **(D)** Client need: safe, effective care environment; subcategory: safety and infection control; content area: maternity

    RATIONALE

    (A) The oropharynx is suctioned on the perineum by the health care provider. Further suctioning can stimulate the vagal response and bradycardia. (B) Newborn Apgars are calculated at 1 and 5 minutes after birth. (C) Maternal and infant IDs should already be prepared and are not a priority action for this fetus. (D) Stadol is a respiratory depressant that has a peak action in 30 minutes and duration of 3 hours. When an expectant mother receives narcotic analgesia shortly before delivery, the infant may be too depressed at birth for spontaneous respirations. Narcan will immediately reverse the respiratory depressant effects of the Stadol.

135. **(B)** Client need: health promotion and maintenance; subcategory: prevention and early detection of disease; content area: maternity.

    RATIONALE

    (A) Natural family planning requires a great deal of planning sexual intercourse around the menstrual cycle and signs of ovulation. It can be an effective method of birth control for motivated, mature adults. It is not likely to be an effective method of birth control for an older adolescent. (B) The combination of condoms and contraceptive foam has a high success rate (93%–97%) in preventing pregnancy. It is easily obtained and is low cost (free if obtained from the public health department). (C) This client smokes a pack a day of cigarettes. Hormonal contraception is not recommended for women who smoke 10 or more cigarettes daily. (D) Hormonal contraception is not recommended for women who smoke more than 10 cigarettes daily because of the increased risk of clotting and stroke.

136. **(A)** Client need: physiological integrity; subcategory: reduction of risk potential; content area: maternity

    RATIONALE

    (A) Newborn infants with a blood glucose level below 45 g/dL will exhibit signs of hypoglycemia such as a high-pitched cry, irritability, paleness, jitteriness, and diaphoresis. (B) Newborn symptoms of maternal substance abuse are tremors, a prolonged high-pitched cry, irritability, inconsolability, muscular rigidity, restlessness, and an exaggerated startle reflex. (C) Signs of cold stress are a decreased temperature, tachypnea, respiratory distress, and tachycardia. Signs of hyperthermia are skin flushing, tachypnea, and tachycardia. (D) Signs of newborn sepsis are temperature instability, rash, tachypnea and/or apnea, cyanosis, mottling, tachycardia, vomiting, diarrhea, lethargy, irritability, and decreased muscle tone.

137. **(C)** Client need: physiological integrity; subcategory: reduction of risk potential; content area: maternity

    RATIONALE

    (A) Massage of the uterine fundus is appropriate when the fundus is at or below 1 cm above the umbilicus (where the fundus should be for 12 hours postpartum). This fundus is high and deviated to the side, requiring further nursing assessment to determine the cause. (B) The fundus should be at the umbilicus or no more than 1 cm above the umbilicus, firmly contracted, and in the midline for a client 12 hours postpartum. (C) A full bladder will push the uterus upward and to one side (usually the right side) and prevent it from firmly contracting down. The fundus will not return to its expected position and state until the bladder is emptied. (D) Medical intervention is not required in this situation.

138. **(D)** Client need: physiological integrity; subcategory: reduction of risk potential; content area: maternity

    RATIONALE

    (A) Applying pressure to the presenting part will delay delivery and can cause fetal hypoxia and brain damage. (B) Having the client cross her legs will also delay delivery and cause fetal damage. (C) The perineal prep is not essential when delivery is imminent; the nurse needs to prepare to deliver the baby. (D) The nurse should don sterile gloves to protect the fetus, mother, and herself from infectious organisms. Application of gentle pressure to the perineum will support the perineal tissues and help prevent tearing.

139. **(A)** Client need: health promotion and maintenance; subcategory: prevention and early detection of disease; content area: maternity

RATIONALE

(A) The 1-hour GTT is a screening test for gestational diabetes. A result equal to or above 140 requires follow-up testing with a 3-hour GTT. (B) The 1-hour GTT is a screening test, not diagnostic. If the client is determined to have gestational diabetes via the 3-hour GTT, then she may be able to control blood glucose levels with diet and exercise. (C) Insulin is not always required for control of gestational diabetes. (D) Serum glucose levels in pregnancy should range from <105 (fasting) to <120 (after meals).

140. **(B)** Client need: health promotion and maintenance; subcategory: growth and development through the life span; content area: maternity

RATIONALE

(A–D) Women who start pregnancy at an appropriate weight for their height should gain 3–4 lb the first 12 weeks and then slightly less than 1 lb (0.90) per week for each additional week of pregnancy. A weight gain of 3–4 lb plus 10.8 lb is an appropriate gain of 13.8–14.8 lb.

141. **(D)** Client need: physiological integrity; subcategory: physiological adaptation; content area: maternity

RATIONALE

(A) A woman is no more likely to abort during the time she would normally have had her menses than at any other time during pregnancy. In the absence of other risk factors (preterm labor, incompetent cervix), intercourse should not harm the pregnancy. (B) Sexual intercourse is not contraindicated in the third trimester unless risk factors for preterm labor, or placenta previa, are present. (C) Many women have different levels of sexual desire at different stages of pregnancy, depending on their general sense of well being and the presence of physical discomforts. (D) The second trimester of pregnancy is one of general well being for most women. The discomforts of early pregnancy (nausea and vomiting, breast tenderness) are largely gone, the enlarging uterus is not yet interfering with comfort and rest, and the pelvic organs are congested with blood, creating more interest in sexual activities.

142. **(B)** Client need: health promotion and maintenance; subcategory: prevention and early detection of disease; content area: maternity

RATIONALE

(A) Tea does have less caffeine than coffee; however, the tannin in tea decreases the absorption of iron. (B) Lemon juice is high in vitamin C. The presence of vitamin C seems to cancel the inhibitory effect of tannin on iron absorption. (C) There is no evidence that caffeine affects the absorption of iron. (D) The consumption of large amounts of caffeine in pregnancy may increase the risk of spontaneous abortion, preterm birth, and small-for-gestational-age newborns. It also affects the absorption and excretion of calcium and zinc.

143. **(C)** Client need: health promotion and maintenance; subcategory: prevention and early detection of disease; content area: maternity

RATIONALE

(A) Vitamin C only increases the absorption of non-heme iron. Red meat is heme iron. (B) Iron absorption is inhibited when taken with food. (C) Iron supplements are best absorbed on an empty stomach. (D) The oxalates in certain raw dark leafy greens such as spinach and collard greens inhibit the absorption of iron. Cooking the greens neutralizes the oxalates.

144. **(B)** Client need: physiological integrity; subcategory: reduction of risk potential; content area: maternity

RATIONALE

(A) A fetus at 34 weeks' gestation can still move relatively freely. Asking the client where fetal heart tones are usually found is not the best method of locating the strongest point of fetal heart tones. (B) Fetal heart tones are heard best over the fetal back. Performance of Leopold's maneuvers allows the nurse to identify fetal landmarks and determine the location of the fetal back. (C) The top of the uterine fundus is the optimal location for the tocodynamometer to monitor uterine activity. (D) Measuring from the pubis to the top of the uterine fundus is done to determine the size of the uterus, which should be analogous to fetal gestational age.

145. **(A)** Client need: physiological integrity; subcategory: physiological adaptation; content area: maternity

RATIONALE

(A) The presence of fetal heart rate accelerations with contractions is a reassuring finding regarding fetal well-being. A reassuring finding is reported as negative on an oxytocin stress test. (B) Late decelerations in the fetal heart rate with 50% or more uterine contractions are a non-reassuring finding in an oxytocin stress test. Nonreassuring findings with an OCT are reported as positive. (C) The presence of two or more accelerations upon fetal movement/stimulation, or 15 bpm lasting 15 or more seconds in a 10-minute time period, is the criteria for a reactive nonstress test (NST). (D) The absence of accelerations with fetal movement, or accelerations that do not meet the criteria for reactivity, constitute a nonreactive NST.

146. **(B)** Client need: physiological integrity; subcategory: physiological adaptation; content area: maternity

RATIONALE

(A) Amnioinfusion is indicated for diluting thick meconium-stained fluid and to relieve pressure on the fetal umbilical cord when membranes are ruptured and severe variable decelerations in the fetal heart rate are present. (B) With hypotonic labor dysfunction, uterine contractions decrease in strength, frequency, and duration, and labor ceases to progress. The onset of hypotonic labor dysfunction occurs in the active phase of labor. Treatment is targeted toward increasing the strength and effectiveness of contractions. Oxytocin augmentation, amniotomy, and ambulation are used to achieve this goal. (C) The purpose of tocolysis is to decrease/stop uterine contractions to the point that they do not cause cervical change. (D) Exhaustion is one side effect of hypotonic uterine dysfunction. The client is still having contractions, even though they are ineffective. The client needs her labor to advance to delivery.

147. **(C)** Client need: physiological integrity; subcategory: physiological adaptation; content area: maternity

RATIONALE

(A) Amniotomy should not be performed unless the fetal presenting part is well engaged to prevent cord prolapse. A −3 station is not well engaged. In addition, amniotomy decreases the size of the uterine cavity and causes increased uterine irritability. Increased uterine irritability can compromise uteroplacental perfusion and fetal well being. (B) Administration of an oxytocic agent causes uterine contractions and is effective for labor induction and augmentation of ineffective uterine contraction in hypotonic labor dysfunction. (C) Signs/symptoms of hypertonic labor dysfunction are uncoordinated and irregular uterine contractions that are ineffective, with constant crampy pain, and a high uterine resting tone. Hypertonic dysfunction typically occurs during the latent phase of labor. The high uterine tone decreases blood supply to the uterus and the fetus. The primary intervention for hypertonic labor dysfunction is pain relief to promote a normal labor pattern. The almost constant pain the woman experiences can cause her to lose confidence in her ability to cope with labor and birth. Frustration and anxiety reduce her pain tolerance and further decrease contraction effectiveness. (D) A woman quickly becomes exhausted with the constant pain of hypertonic labor dysfunction. Pain relief, sedation, and perhaps tocolysis are used to promote relaxation and rest. Rest and relaxation will often facilitate development of a normal labor pattern and labor progression.

148. **(D)** Client need: safe, effective care environment; subcategory: management of care; content area: maternity

RATIONALE

(A) The fetal heart rate findings describe variable decelerations, which are caused by cord compression. If cord compression can be relieved and the baseline heart rate is reassuring, immediate delivery is not indicated. (B) ACOG defines appropriate forceps deliveries as outlet (the presenting part is on the perineum, with the scalp visible at the vaginal opening), low (the leading edge of the fetal skull is at station +2), and midforceps (the leading edge of the fetal skull is between 0 and +2 stations). A high forceps delivery is contraindicated because it is associated with fetal and maternal tissue damage. (C) Oxytocin infusion could cause increased pressure on the umbilical cord. It is also not indicated when there is adequate labor progress. (D) Amnioinfusion is the infusion of a warmed isotonic solution into the uterine cavity through the IUPC to dilute thick meconium staining of the amniotic fluid, or when there is evidence of cord compression with ruptured membranes. The fluid infusion cushions the cord and relieves pressure.

149. **(A)** Client need: physiological integrity; subcategory: reduction of risk potential; content area: maternity

RATIONALE

(A) Assisting the client to a hands and knees position enlists the help of gravity to rotate the fetal head from OP to OA so that the smallest diameter of the fetal head is leading through the birth canal and fetal descent is facilitated. (B) McRobert's maneuver straightens the pelvic curve and increases the AP diameter of the pelvic inlet. McRobert's maneuver is used to relieve shoulder dystocia. (C) A squatting position will not rotate the fetal head. Continued pushing will only exhaust the client. (D) Ambulation will assist fetal descent when the fetal position is OA.

150. **(A)** Client need: physiological integrity; subcategory: physiological adaptation; content area: maternity

RATIONALE

(A–D) Breast milk usually comes in approximately 72 hours after delivery. Firm, leaking breasts are an expected finding. The uterine fundus is found approximately 1 cm above the umbilicus 12 hours after delivery. It then decreases in size by approximately 1 cm per 24 hours. Lochia is rubra (bright to dark red) and moderate to heavy (6–10 cm in size) in amount the first 2 days postpartum. It then changes to lochia serosa (brown to pink) and small to moderate (4–6 cm in size) in amount for the next 7 days. Lochia alba (yellow/white) is found from days 10 to 21 and is scant (2–4 cm in size) to small in amount. Perineal edema and discomfort is at its peak 72 hours postpartum, and then rapidly subsides. These are expected, normal findings.

151. **(D)** Client need: health promotion and maintenance; subcategory: prevention and early detection of disease; content area: maternity

RATIONALE

(A) Adherence to a strict schedule increases the risk of breast engorgement. (B) Emptying the breasts less often by formula feeding increases the risk of engorgement. (C) Parlodil dries up breast milk and was prescribed for formula feeding mothers only. In addition, it had serious side effects, including stroke, when administered to postpartum women, and its use is no longer recommended. (D) Immediate and frequent breast-feeding dramatically decreases the risk of breast engorgement in breast-feeding women.

152. **(D)** Client need: psychosocial integrity; subcategory: coping and adaptation; content area: maternity

RATIONALE

(A) Breast-feeding encourages maternal/infant contact and interaction, but is not the most effective method of promoting bonding/attachment. (B) Pointing out the positive features of the newborn while the mother holds him/her is another method of promoting bonding, but is less effective than other methods. Discussing positive features of the baby without the baby there is even less helpful. (C) The optimal time for parental/newborn interaction is during the first period of reactivity. Both the parents and the infant are in a state of heightened awareness and eager for interaction. The baby is asleep for several hours after the first period of reactivity and interaction is hindered. (D) Rooming-in is the single most effective method of facilitating the bonding/attachment process because of the many opportunities for interaction and learning infant cues and personality.

153. **(C)** Client need: safe, effective care environment; subcategory: safety and infection control; content area: maternity

RATIONALE

(A) A full bladder acts as a window for ultrasound evaluation of the fetus. Ultrasound is used to guide the needle for amniocentesis, but there is a risk for bladder damage from the needle if it is full. (B) It is important to ensure all laboratory results are filed in the chart, but this is not a priority nursing action. (C) The bladder must be empty to avoid inadvertent puncture of the bladder wall by the amniocentesis needle during the procedure. (D) It is not necessary for the client to be NPO for this procedure. There is little risk of vomiting and aspiration.

154. **(D)** Client need: health promotion and maintenance; subcategory: prevention and early detection of disease; content area: maternity

RATIONALE

(A) MSAFP is a screening test. High or low results do not necessarily mean the pregnancy is normal. They are also not diagnostic of abnormalities. (B) High MSAFP results may indicate a neural tube defect. (C) Low MSAFP results are associated with possible Down syndrome. (D) MSAFP is a screening test that is performed to determine if further testing (repeat MSAFP, targeted ultrasound, amniocentesis) is needed to rule out fetal abnormalities.

155. **(C)** Client need: health promotion and maintenance; subcategory: growth and development through the life span; content area: maternity

RATIONALE

(A) This is an old wives' tale. Heartburn is not caused by fetal hair. (B) This is an untrue statement even when considering old wives' tales. In folklore, male gender is associated with a fetal heart rate in the low ranges of normal, not with heartburn. (C) Progesterone decreases the muscle tone of the esophagus and allows reflux of stomach contents into the esophagus. The resulting sensation is what we call heartburn. (D) The enlarging uterus crowds the stomach and decreases its capacity, especially in multifetal pregnancies, which can increase heartburn, but carrying a fetus "high" does not cause heartburn.

Pediatric Nursing: Content Review and Test

Lucille F. Whaley, EdD, RN
Cecily Betz, PhD, RN
Susan Ray, MSN, DNSc

The Ill or Hospitalized Child

Nursing Care of the Ill Child

Meaning of Illness to Child

1. Infant
   A. Change in familiar routine and surroundings
   B. Separation from love object
2. Toddler
   A. Fear of separation, desertion; separation anxiety highest in this age group
   B. Cause of illness perceived as a concrete condition, circumstance, or behavior
3. Preschool
   A. Fear of bodily harm or mutilation, castration
   B. Fear of intrusive procedures
   C. Separation anxiety less intense than for toddler
   D. Causation same as for toddler; often considers own role in causation (i.e., illness as punishment for wrongdoing)
4. School-age
   A. Fear of physical nature of illness
   B. Concern regarding separation from peers and ability to maintain position in group
   C. Cause of illness perceived as external, although located in body
5. Adolescent
   A. Anxious regarding loss of independence, control, identity
   B. Concern about privacy
   C. Malfunctioning organ or process perceived as cause of illness
   D. Ability to explain illness

Response to Separation

1. Greatest impact between ages 1 and 3
2. Three phases identified:
   A. Protest: crying for parents, refusing attention of anyone else, inconsolable in grief.
   B. Despair: crying ceases, depression evident (quiet, withdrawn, apathetic, and sense of hopelessness), intense grieving.
   C. Detachment (denial): superficial appearance of adjustment. Child detaches from parent in effort to escape emotional pain. Child appears interested in environment, and forms relationship with caregiver. Child may ignore parents when they return.

Signs and Symptoms of Separation Anxiety

1. **Protest:** lasts from hours to days. Child:
   A. Cries and screams
   B. Searches with eyes for parent(s)
   C. Clings to parent when present
   D. Avoids and rejects contact with strangers
   E. Displays anger. Attacks strangers verbally and physically
   F. Attempts to physically prevent parent(s) from leaving
2. **Despair:** duration varies. Child:
   A. Is quiet/withdrawn
   B. Shows limited interaction
   C. Is depressed, sad
   D. Is uninterested in environment
   E. Is noncommunicative
   F. Regresses to earlier behaviors (e.g., thumb-sucking, bed-wetting, use of bottle)
   G. Frequently refuses to eat

3. **Detachment:** rarely seen in acute setting. Seen in prolonged separation or long-term care setting. Child:
   A. Shows increased interest in surroundings
   B. Interacts with strangers or familiar caregivers
   C. Forms new but superficial relationships
   D. Appears happy
   E. Shows only passive or superficial interest in parents

Response to Pain

1. Young infant
   A. Generalized body response: sometimes local reflex withdrawal on stimulation
   B. Loud crying
   C. Facial expression reflects pain
   D. Body movements: squirming, writhing, jerking, and flailing
2. Older infant
   A. Localized body response, deliberate withdrawal on stimulation
   B. Loud crying
   C. Facial expression reflects pain
   D. Physical resistance, attempt to push stimulus away after applied
   E. Uncooperative: refuses to be still, attempts escaping
   F. Nonresponsive to distraction and anticipatory preparation for procedures
3. Young child
   A. Loud crying, screaming
   B. Verbal expressions
   C. Thrashing of extremities
   D. Physical resistance before and during application of stimulus
   E. Requires physical restraint for painful procedures
   F. Clings to family member, soliciting emotional support
   G. Restless and irritable with continuing pain
   H. May strike out at someone, attempt of blaming another for pain
4. School-age child
   A. Girls express fear of pain more than boys.
   B. Concerned with physical disability more than pain.
   C. Fears being told something is wrong with them.
   D. Can verbally communicate pain: location, intensity, and description.
   E. Passive behaviors for dealing with pain: rigidity, clenching fist or teeth, acting brave.
   F. Overt behaviors of pain: biting, kicking, escaping, crying, pulling away, bargaining. If exhibit these behaviors may deny later to prevent embarrassment to peers.
   G. May request help with controlling their pain. Example: "Will you hold my hand?"
   H. May mask fear of pain and appear composed: calmness. Verbal cues to watch for are: facial expression, silence, lack of activity, false sense of "I'm okay."
5. Adolescent
   A. Fear of pain associated with body image and being different from peers.
   B. Pain responses include: numerous questions, withdrawing, rejecting others, questioning the competency of others, fear of losing control, projected confidence or conceited attitude. Also, increased muscle tension and body control, and quiet.

C. Physical restraint and aggression uncommon unless an unexpected procedure develops or child was unprepared for a procedure.

Nursing Care of the Hospitalized Child

Assessment

1. Perform routine physical assessment.
2. Acquire baseline data related to condition for later comparison.
3. Perform pain assessment, if indicated.
4. Determine developmental level of child.
5. Obtain health history and history of hospitalization.
6. Perform psychosocial assessment.
7. Assist with diagnostic procedures.

Planning

1. Safe, effective care environment
   A. Reduce or eliminate environmental hazards.
   B. Transport, restrain, and position child safely.
   C. Ensure safety during procedures, including surgery.
2. Physiological integrity
   A. Carry out procedures with minimum distress to child.
   B. Prevent or minimize bodily injury and/or pain.
3. Psychosocial integrity
   A. Prevent or minimize effects of separation.
   B. Support and educate child and family.
   C. Help child maintain control.
   D. Prepare child and family for procedures and surgery.
   E. Use play as diversion and for stress reduction.
4. Health promotion and maintenance
   A. Promote optimum health.
   B. Promote nutrition and hydration.
   C. Prepare family for home care.
   D. Promote growth and development

Implementation

1. Keep harmful items out of reach of child.
2. Keep side rails up for infants and young children.
3. Allow freedom on unit within defined and enforced limits.
4. Restrain child if necessary for safety, but limit use.
5. Explain hospital routines, items, procedures, and events in language appropriate to child's age.
6. Use terms familiar to the child (e.g., those for bodily functions).
7. Maintain a routine similar to what the child is accustomed to at home, whenever possible.
8. Provide consistency of personnel as much as possible.
9. Promote family interaction; encourage child and family contact and rooming-in whenever possible.
10. Encourage parents to participate in care.
11. Maintain contact with family; talk to child about family; encourage child to talk about home.
12. Allow sibling visitation if possible.
13. Provide an atmosphere that allows free expression of feelings.
14. Allow child choices whenever possible.

15. Explain procedures to the child; what he will experience, and what he can do to help; explain at his level of understanding; relate unfamiliar things and events to those familiar to the child; clarify terms.
16. Convey an attitude of confidence and one that indicates cooperation is expected.
17. Allow child to see and handle strange and possibly frightening items.
18. Be honest with child.
19. Be consistent in behaviors toward child.
20. Communicate disapproval of undesired behavior, not disapproval of child.
21. Accept regressive behaviors.
22. Praise child for cooperation.
23. Allow ample time for play.
24. Encourage play activities and diversion appropriate to child's age, condition, and interests.
25. Employ play as a nursing tool.
26. Encourage interaction with other children when appropriate.
27. Help family support child emotionally.
28. Interpret child's behavior and appearance (e.g., protesting and regressive behaviors, appearance of equipment, incisions, etc.).
29. Teach family skills and procedures needed for home care.

Evaluation

Ensure that child:
1. Has consistent caregivers.
2. Exhibits no evidence of discomfort.
3. Verbalizes or plays out feelings and concerns.
4. Discusses home and family.
5. Exhibits an understanding of information presented.
6. Cooperates in care and participates in care activities.
7. Is visited frequently or constantly by parents.
8. Is cared for with the cooperation of parents.

Ensure that family:
1. Demonstrates an understanding of child's behavior, becomes familiar with therapies.
2. Demonstrates the ability to provide home care.

Nursing Care of the Child with a Chronic Illness or Disability

Assessment

1. Perform routine physical assessment.
2. Emphasize special observations related to suspected or determined diagnosis.
3. Identify family stresses.
4. Assess family's coping skills, abilities, and resources.
5. Assist with diagnostic procedures.
6. Be alert for evidence of overprotection or neglect.

Planning

See Nursing Care of the Ill Child, pp. 97–98.
1. Safe, effective care environment
   A. Promote safe environment according to needs of individual child.

2. Physiological integrity
   A. Promote compliance with therapeutic plan of care.
   B. Prevent complications.
3. Psychosocial integrity
   A. Assist through grief process.
   B. Promote a positive self-image in child.
   C. Support and educate child and family as needed.
   D. Prepare child and family for diagnostic procedures, surgery.
4. Health promotion and maintenance
   A. Promote optimum health.
   B. Prepare family for care.

Implementation

1. Support child and family at time of diagnosis and throughout the course of the disease or condition
   A. Project an attitude that conveys acceptance of child and family.
   B. Allow for expression of feelings and concerns.
   C. Assist family and older child through grief process.
   D. Explore child's and family's reactions to the disorder.
   E. Emphasize positive aspects of prognosis, expected capabilities of child.
2. Explain or reinforce explanation of condition or disease and therapies.
3. Help family distinguish between reality and fantasy regarding disease or disability.
4. Help family develop a thorough plan of care with emphasis on long-term needs.
5. Encourage participation in care of hospitalized child.
6. Be available to family as listener, resource.
7. Interpret child's and family's behavior to each other.
8. Help child and family identify strengths and support systems.
9. Promote constructive thinking in child and family.
10. Encourage social activity for both child and family.
11. Promote normalizing activities and peer contact for child.
12. Emphasize child's abilities.
13. Promote attainment of developmental skills and tasks.
14. Assist with improving appearance and grooming.
15. Encourage self-care appropriate to capabilities and as much independence as condition allows.
16. Encourage activities appropriate for developmental level.
17. Help child and family set realistic goals for current and future activities.
18. Refer to community agencies and resources (i.e., parent and/or child support groups, specific disease-related agencies, mental health services).
19. Teach family skills and procedures needed to access educational and supportive services and resources.

Evaluation

Ensure that:
1. Family and child (where appropriate) demonstrate an understanding of the disease or condition.
2. Family and child verbalize feelings and concerns.
3. Family and child identify strengths and support systems.
4. Child and family develop realistic short- and long-term plans.
5. Family members display an attitude of confidence in ability to cope.

6. Child engages in activities appropriate to developmental level, interests, and capabilities.
7. Child exhibits no evidence of overprotection or neglect.
8. Child is clean, well groomed, attractively dressed.
9. Child and family contact appropriate agencies and services.
10. Child and family adhere to therapeutic plan.

Newborn Disorders

The Preterm Infant

Description

A preterm infant is one born before completion of 37 weeks' gestation, regardless of birth weight.

1. **Low-birth-weight infant:** infant whose birth weight is less than 2500 g regardless of gestational age.
2. **Very-low-birth-weight infant:** infant whose weight is less than 1500 g.
3. **Small-for-gestational-age infant:** infant whose birth weight is not appropriate for age.
4. **Intrauterine growth retardation:** infant whose intrauterine growth is retarded.

Pathophysiology

1. Factors related to prematurity
   A. Multiple pregnancies
   B. Maternal disease (e.g., eclampsia, uncontrolled diabetes)
   C. Placenta abruptio or previa
   D. Previous premature labor
   E. Maternal age under 20 or above 35 years
2. Outlook largely related to state of physiological and anatomical maturity of various organs and systems at time of birth
3. Fetal anomalies
4. Maternal psychosocial factors (e.g., poverty)

Signs and Symptoms

1. Very small, scrawny appearance
2. Skin: red to pink with visible veins
3. Fine, feathery hair; lanugo on back and face
4. Little or no evidence of subcutaneous fat
5. Head large in relation to body
6. Sucking pads prominent
7. Lying in "relaxed attitude"
8. Limbs extended
9. Ear cartilages poorly developed
10. Few fine wrinkles on palms and soles
11. Clitoris prominent in female
12. Scrotum underdeveloped, nonpendulous, with minimal rugae, undescended testicles in male
13. Lax, easily manipulated joints
14. Absent, weak, or ineffectual grasping, sucking, and swallowing reflexes
15. Other neurological signs are absent or diminished
16. Inability to maintain body temperature
17. Dilute urine
18. Pliable thorax
19. Periodic breathing, hypoventilation
20. Frequent episodes of apnea, irregular respirations

Therapeutic Management

1. Determine by status of infant, especially in relation to:
   A. Cardiopulmonary support
   B. Thermoregulation
   C. Nutritional needs, hydration status
   D. Susceptibility to infection
   E. Activity intolerance
2. Prevent complications

Nursing Care

ASSESSMENT

1. Perform routine newborn assessment.
2. Perform gestational age assessment.
3. Assist with diagnostic procedure.
4. Perform ongoing systematic assessment of functioning.
   A. Weighing 2–3 times daily
   B. Respiratory assessment
      (1) Rate and regularity
      (2) Use of any accessory muscles
      (3) Presence of any retractions, nasal flaring
      (4) Breath sounds, secretions
   C. Cardiovascular assessment
      (1) Heart rate and rhythm
      (2) Heart sounds, including suspected murmurs
      (3) Point of maximum intensity
      (4) Blood pressure
   D. Gastrointestinal (GI) assessment
      (1) Presence of any abdominal distention, increase in circumference, shiny skin
      (2) Feeding behavior
      (3) Regurgitation or emesis
      (4) Bowel sounds
   E. Genitourinary assessment
      (1) Abnormalities, if any
      (2) Urinary output: amount, color, specific gravity
   F. Neurological and musculoskeletal assessment
      (1) Movements: random, jittery, twitching, spontaneous, elicited
      (2) Position or attitude at rest
      (3) Presence of reflexes
      (4) Level of response
      (5) Changes in head circumference
      (6) Pupillary responses
   G. Temperature assessment
      (1) Axillary
      (2) Relationship to ambient temperature
   H. Skin assessment
      (1) Color: cyanosis can be cardiovascular or respiratory
      (2) Discolored areas
      (3) Texture, turgor, characteristics (dry, flaky, peeling)
      (4) Skin lesion(s), rash

PLANNING

1. Safe, effective care environment
   A. Provide routine care of the newborn infant.
   B. Provide external warmth.
   C. Protect from infection.
2. Physiological integrity
   A. Facilitate respiratory efforts.
   B. Conserve energy.
   C. Prevent complications.

3. Psychosocial integrity
   A. Provide sensory stimulation.
   B. Promote parent-infant relationships.
   C. Support and educate family.
   D. Prepare family for procedures.
4. Health promotion and maintenance
   A. Promote optimum health.
   B. Achieve and maintain optimum hydration and nutrition.
   C. Prepare family for home care.
   D. Promote growth and development.

IMPLEMENTATION

1. Position for maximum respiration: head of crib slightly elevated.
2. Provide and monitor supplemental oxygen and/or assisted ventilation as prescribed.
3. Provide external warmth according to infant's condition and toleration.
   A. Well wrapped in open crib.
   B. Warm heating pad or mattress.
   C. Thermoregulated closed crib (Isolette).
   D. Overhead warming unit.
   E. Position away from windows or drafts to prevent radiant or convective heat loss.
   F. Humidified atmosphere to reduce evaporative heat loss.
   G. Knitted cap for infant.
   H. Use of radiant heat source or heat shield when removing infant from Isolette.
4. Reduce energy expenditure.
   A. Ease respiratory efforts.
   B. Maintain neutral thermal environment.
   C. Implement gavage feeding if infant becomes tired with conventional feeding methods.
   D. Organize nursing activities and assessments to minimize disturbance.
   E. Promote rest: reduce environmental distractions (e.g., dim lights or cover crib with blanket, eliminate or reduce noise, etc.).
5. Implement institutional policies for prevention of spread of infection; teach precautions to family.
6. Administer supplemental fluids as prescribed. Monitor IV infusion carefully, and monitor output, daily weights.
7. Provide nutrition.
   A. Nipple-feed with soft nipple that supplies nourishment without exertion (expressed mother's milk, banked breast milk, special formula).
   B. Assist with breast-feeding (for families who indicate desire).
   C. Gavage-feed.
   D. Assess for signs of dehydration or overhydration.
8. Prevent skin breakdown.
   A. Clean with clear water or mild, nonalkaline cleanser 2–3 times/wk.
   B. Assess any topical applications for possible toxic effects.
   C. Rinse skin well following use of alcohol or povidone-iodine solutions.
   D. Avoid damage to delicate skin (e.g., removing tape, careful use of scissors for removal of bandages).
9. Use infection-control procedures to prevent spread of infection.

10. Implement appropriate infant stimulation when infant can tolerate, and recognize signs of overstimulation.
11. Explain or reinforce explanation of condition and therapies to family.
12. Encourage parents to express feelings and concerns.
13. Encourage family to become involved in infant's care.
14. Teach family skills needed for home care.

EVALUATION

Ensure that infant:
1. Has regular, unlabored breathing within normal limits.
2. Has temperature within desirable limits (97.7°F or 36.5°C).
3. Exhibits no evidence of dehydration.
4. Consumes appropriate amount of nourishment without difficulty.
5. Exhibits a steady weight gain.
6. Is free of complications.
7. Responds to appropriate stimuli.
8. Is cared for by family and is bonding with them.
9. Is able to be cared for at home by family, who demonstrate an understanding of the infant's condition.

Hyperbilirubinemia

Description

Hyperbilirubinemia is excessive accumulation of bilirubin in the blood.

Classification

1. Nonconjugated hyperbilirubinemia
   A. Direct reacting
   B. Implies impaired liver function
   C. Type most commonly observed in newborns
2. Conjugated hyperbilirubinemia
   A. Indirect reacting
   B. Implies functioning liver
   C. Usually caused by obstruction or absence of bile duct
   D. Rare in newborns

Pathophysiology

1. Breakdown of red blood cells into heme and globin
2. Heme portion converted to bilirubin in presence of enzyme glucuronyl transferase
3. Deficiency of glucuronyl transferase or increase in red blood cell breakdown
4. Increased levels of unconjugated bilirubin in the blood
5. Types of unconjugated hyperbilirubinemia:
   A. Physiological jaundice (icterus neonatorum)
      (1) Immature hepatic function plus increased bilirubin load from red blood cell hemolysis
      (2) Appears after 24 hours, peaks at 2–3 days of age
   B. Breast-feeding jaundice
      (1) Cause unknown
      (2) Early: 3–4 days of age
      (3) Late: 4–5 days of age
   C. Hemolytic disease
      (1) Blood antigen incompatibility (isoimmunization) causes hemolysis of large numbers of red blood cells.

(2) Liver unable to conjugate and excrete excess bilirubin.

(3) Appears during first 24 hours following birth.

Signs and Symptoms

1. Jaundice: yellowish discoloration of skin
   A. Bright yellow or orange skin (unconjugated)
   B. Greenish, muddy yellow skin (conjugated)
   C. Intensity unrelated to degree of bilirubinemia

Therapeutic Management

1. Prevent kernicterus (bilirubin encephalopathy).
2. Remove excess bilirubin.
   A. Phototherapy to alter bilirubin into a more soluble form.
   B. Exchange transfusion to replace infant's sensitized red blood cells and bilirubin; correct anemia; treatment of choice for isoimmunization.
   C. Prevent blood incompatibility by administration of Rh_o immune globulin to all unsensitized Rh-negative mothers after delivery.

Nursing Care

ASSESSMENT

1. Perform routine physical assessment.
2. Assist with diagnostic procedures: serum bilirubin levels, Coombs' test (infants of Rh-negative mothers).

PLANNING

1. Safe, effective care environment
   A. Perform routine care for the newborn.
2. Physiological integrity
   A. Assist with measures to reduce serum bilirubin levels.
   B. Prevent complications from therapy.
3. Psychosocial integrity
   A. Support and educate family.
   B. Prepare family for procedures.
4. Health promotion and maintenance
   A. Promote optimum health.
   B. Prepare family for home care.

IMPLEMENTATION

1. Explain or reinforce explanation of condition and therapies.
2. Place infant under fluorescent light.
3. Turn frequently to expose all body surface areas to light; assess skin for rashes and burns.
4. Shield infant's eyes with opaque mask of proper size.
   A. Close eyes before application.
   B. Position to prevent occlusion of nares.
   C. Check several times per day for evidence of discharge, excessive pressures on lids, corneal irritation.
5. Avoid oily lubricants or lotions on skin.
6. Promote adequate fluid intake.
7. Observe for evidence of dehydration and drying skin.
8. Monitor temperature closely to detect early signs of hyperthermia.
9. Teach family skills and procedures needed for home care, including home phototherapy.
10. Assist with exchange transfusion.

A. Keep umbilicus moist in case site is needed for transfusion.
B. Assist with procedure.
C. Keep accurate records of blood volumes exchanged.
D. Monitor infant's condition: vital signs, thermoregulation.
E. Dress umbilicus as prescribed and observe periodically for evidence of bleeding.

EVALUATION

Ensure that infant:
1. Exhibits no evidence of jaundice.
2. Has serum bilirubin level within normal limits.
3. Remains well hydrated and free of complications.
4. Is able to be cared for by the family, who demonstrates an understanding of the child's condition.

Respiratory Distress Syndrome

Description

Respiratory distress syndrome refers to respiratory dysfunction in neonates, primarily related to developmental delay in lung maturation.

Pathophysiology

1. Decreased surfactant production
   A. Unequal inflation of alveoli on inspiration
   B. Collapse of alveoli on end-expiration
2. Flexible, soft rib cage impeding lung expansion
3. Diminished O_2 to tissues and inability to excrete excess carbon dioxide
   A. Anaerobic metabolism and formation of lactic acid
4. With each breath, increased energy expenditure to reinflate
5. Decreased lung expansion, with fewer inflated alveoli

Signs and Symptoms

1. Dyspnea
2. Tachypnea (up to 80–120 breaths/min)
3. Pronounced substernal retractions
4. Fine inspiratory rales (crackles) heard over both lungs
5. Audible expiratory grunt
6. Flaring of external nares
7. Cyanosis
8. Peripheral edema
9. Systemic hypotension
10. Progressive disease
    A. Flaccidity
    B. Inertness
    C. Unresponsiveness
    D. Frequent apneic episodes
    E. Diminished breath sounds

Therapeutic Management

1. Provide O_2.
   A. Increase ambient O_2 concentration in Isolette or by oxygen hood.
   B. Institute assisted ventilation: continuous positive airway pressure.
2. Correct acidosis with IV sodium bicarbonate.

3. Administer artificial surfactant.
4. Oxygenate blood by extracorporeal membrane oxygenation (ECMO).
5. Maintain neutral thermal environment to conserve energy and oxygen utilization.
6. Conserve energy by minimal handling, IV, or gavage feeding.

Nursing Care

ASSESSMENT

1. Perform general assessment of premature infant.
2. Perform thorough respiratory assessment.
    A. Determine respiratory rate and regularity.
    B. Describe use of accessory muscles; substernal, intercostal, or subclavicular retractions; nasal flaring.
    C. Describe breath sounds: rales (crackles), wheezing, wet diminished sounds, areas of absence of sound, grunting.
    D. Describe secretions.
    E. Determine whether suctioning is needed.
    F. Describe cry.
    G. Describe ambient O_2 and method of delivery; if intubated, describe size of tube, type of ventilator, and settings.
3. Assist with diagnostic procedures: radiography, blood gas measurements.

PLANNING

1. Safe, effective care environment
    A. Protect from injury and infection.
    B. Provide warmth.
2. Physiological integrity
    A. Promote respiratory efforts.
    B. Conserve energy.
    C. Prevent complications.
3. Psychosocial integrity
    A. Support and educate family.
    B. Prepare family for procedures.
4. Health promotion and maintenance
    A. Promote optimum health.
    B. Achieve and maintain optimum hydration and nutrition.
    C. Prepare family for care.
    D. Promote growth and development.

IMPLEMENTATION

1. Place infant in Isolette or crib with overhead warmer.
2. Maintain a neutral thermal environment.
3. Maintain O_2 as prescribed.
4. Remove secretions from airway as needed.
5. Apply chest physiotherapy, if prescribed.
6. Position for maximum respiratory excursion and minimal effort.
    A. Position on side with head supported on small folded towel.
    B. Keep head aligned with body and neck slightly extended.
7. Monitor O_2 administration, including ventilator if used.
8. Assist with administration of surfactant.
9. Assist with ECMO if employed.
10. Provide nutrition.
    A. Feed via gavage to conserve energy and provide sufficient calories, or

B. Nipple-feed with soft nipple, allowing sufficient time for rest.
11. Employ careful skin care to prevent breakdown or injury.
12. Wean from respirator and/or O_2 therapy as prescribed.
13. Explain or reinforce explanation of condition and therapies to family.
14. Teach family skills needed for care (e.g., cardiopulmonary resuscitation).

EVALUATION

Ensure that infant:
1. Breathes without effort.
2. Maintains optimum blood gas measurements without ventilatory assistance.
3. Remains free of complications.
4. Is able to be cared for by the family, who understand the child's condition.

Neonatal Sepsis (Septicemia)

Description

Neonatal sepsis (septicemia) is generalized bacterial disease in the bloodstream.

Pathophysiology

1. Acquired
2. Prenatal: infected amniotic fluid, across placenta from maternal bloodstream
3. Birth: from contact with maternal tissues
4. Postnatal: cross-contamination from other infants, personnel, or objects in environment
5. More frequent occurrence in high-risk infants (e.g., preterm infants and those born after a difficult or traumatic delivery)

Signs and Symptoms

1. Subtle, vague, and nonspecific signs
    A. Failure to thrive
    B. Does not "look well"
2. Respiratory distress
    A. Apnea
    B. Irregular, grunting respirations
    C. Retractions
3. Gastric distress
    A. Vomiting
    B. Diarrhea
    C. Abdominal distention
    D. Absent stools (from paralytic ileus)
    E. Poor sucking and feeding
4. Skin manifestations
    A. Cyanosis
    B. Pallor
    C. Mottling
    D. Jaundice
    E. Lesions associated with specific organisms
5. Central nervous system (CNS) involvement
    A. Irritability
    B. Apathy
    C. Tremors
    D. Seizures

E. Coma

F. Signs of increased intracranial pressure (meningitis)

6. Fever frequently absent

Therapeutic Management

1. Aggressive administration of IV antibiotics
2. Supportive therapy (e.g., O_2 administration)
3. Careful regulation of fluid and electrolytes
4. Temporary discontinuation of oral feedings
5. Transfusions of polymorphonuclear leukocytes

Nursing Care

ASSESSMENT

1. Perform routine physical assessment: special attention to potential sources of infection (e.g., umbilicus, nasopharyngeal cavity, ear canals, skin lesions).
2. Assist with diagnostic procedures: examination of blood, spinal fluid, urine, stool, and any skin-lesion examinations.
3. Observe for side effects of antibiotics.

PLANNING

1. Safe, effective care environment
   A. Prevent spread of infection.
2. Physiological integrity
   A. Help eliminate infective organisms.
   B. Prevent complications.
3. Psychosocial integrity
   A. Support family.
4. Health promotion and maintenance
   A. Promote optimum health.
   B. Achieve and maintain optimum hydration and nutrition.
   C. Promote growth and development.

IMPLEMENTATION

1. Provide external warmth.
2. Reduce energy expenditure.
3. Implement institutional policies to prevent spread of infection.
4. Monitor IV infusion.
5. Administer antibiotics as prescribed.
6. Monitor O_2 administration and infant's response.
7. Explain or reinforce explanation to family of condition and therapies.
8. Encourage family to express feelings.
9. Teach family skills needed for care.

EVALUATION

Ensure that infant:

1. Exhibits no evidence of infection.
2. Remains free of complications.
3. Is able to be cared for by family members, who demonstrate understanding of child's condition.

Respiratory Disorders

Laryngotracheobronchitis (Croup)

Description

Laryngotracheobronchitis (croup) is inflammation of the larynx, trachea, and bronchi.

Pathophysiology

1. Edema of the respiratory mucosa produces a narrowing of the air passages, causing variable degrees of airway obstruction.
2. It is usually preceded by an upper respiratory infection and begins at night.
3. Most common in children ages 3 months to 3 years.
4. Usually of viral etiology, particularly the parainfluenza viruses.
5. Males are at higher risk.
6. Usually occurs in winter months.

Signs and Symptoms

1. Irritability
2. Restlessness
3. Hoarseness
4. "Brassy" or "barking" cough
5. Inspiratory stridor
6. Respiratory distress
7. Rhinorrhea with low-grade fever
8. Anorexia
9. Nausea and vomiting (often)
10. Diarrhea (sometimes)
11. Crackles (rales), wheezing, or rhonchi heard on auscultation
12. Respiratory failure (potential complication)
13. Accessory muscles used during breathing
14. Cyanosis
15. Symptoms worse at night

Therapeutic Management

1. Mild disease can be treated at home
   A. Careful observation for symptoms of respiratory obstruction (stridor at rest, cyanosis, severe agitation/fatigue, retractions, inability to drink fluids)
   B. Bed rest
   C. Cool, humidified atmosphere
   D. Fluids
   E. Reduction of temperature (if elevated)
   F. Avoid crying episodes and agitation
   G. Immediately take to emergency department for respiratory obstruction.
2. Severe disease requires hospitalization
   A. All of the above
   B. High-humidity environment
   C. O_2
   D. Parenteral fluids
   E. Racemic epinephrine for transient relief
   F. Corticosteroids may be used to reduce inflammation
   G. Acetaminophen for fever.
   H. Keep endotracheal intubation equipment available

Nursing Care

ASSESSMENT

1. Perform routine physical assessment.
2. Perform in-depth assessment for:
   A. Rate, depth, and rhythm of respirations.

B. Presence of flaring nares; grunting; and substernal, intracostal, or suprasternal retractions.

C. Pallor, cyanosis.

D. Association of dyspnea with pain, rest, or exertion.

E. Evidence of infection.

F. Type, frequency, and intensity of cough.

G. Presence of rales, wheezing, and/or stridor.

H. Evidence of and character of any sputum.

3. Assist with diagnostic procedures: chest radiography, serum electrolytes, blood gas measurements.

PLANNING

1. Safe, effective care environment
   A. See Nursing Care of the Ill Child, pp. 97–98.
   B. Prevent spread of primary infection to others.
2. Physiological integrity
   A. Facilitate respiratory efforts.
   B. Promote rest.
   C. Promote comfort.
   D. Reduce temperature (significant elevation).
   E. Administer pharmacologic agents.
3. Psychosocial integrity
   A. Promote coping of child and family.
   B. Support child and family during adaptation.
4. Health promotion and maintenance
   A. Prevent dehydration.
   B. Provide nourishment.
   C. Prevent complications.
   D. Prepare family for home care.

IMPLEMENTATION

1. Administer humidified O_2 as prescribed (mist tent, nasal, hood).
2. Position for optimum ventilation: head of bed elevated.
3. Monitor respiratory status regularly; monitor effects of O_2 therapy in cases of respiratory failure, ventilator assistance.
4. Administer nose drops; suction nasal passages to facilitate breathing.
5. Administer decongestants, bronchodilators, and expectorants as prescribed.
6. Administer antipyretics as prescribed.
7. Support child and family.
8. Encourage presence of family.
9. Provide constant attendance during acute illness.
10. Encourage intake of cool fluids, such as fruit juices, soft drinks, gelatin.
11. Monitor parenteral fluid administration, if prescribed.
12. Have emergency endotracheal or tracheostomy equipment available.
13. Implement measures to prevent spread of infection to others.
14. Administer antibiotics as prescribed.
15. Administer chest physiotherapy, if prescribed.
16. Teach family procedures needed for care, including expected results of medications, their possible side effects, and infection control.

EVALUATION

Ensure that child:

1. Is free of respiratory distress.
2. Rests comfortably and plays quietly.
3. Complies with medical regimen, as does the family.

Epiglottitis

Description

Epiglottitis is inflammation of the epiglottis and surrounding areas (supraglottic area and aryepiglottic folds).

Pathophysiology

1. Inflammation of the glottis, usually caused by Haemophilus influenzae type B.
2. Rapid progression of disease can result in complete airway obstruction in a few hours.
3. Most often seen in children 3–7 years of age.
4. Incidence is equal among males and females.

Signs and Symptoms

1. Abrupt onset
2. Rapidly progressive to severe respiratory distress
3. Elevated temperature
4. Toxic appearance
5. Characteristic posture: insists on sitting upright, leaning forward with chin thrust out, mouth open, and tongue protruding
6. Irritability
7. Anxious, apprehensive, frightened expression
8. Thick, muffled voice and croaking "froglike" sound on inspiration
9. Throat red and inflamed with distinctive large, cherry red, edematous epiglottis (seldom observed except by qualified examiner, as described below)
10. Pallor progressing to cyanosis
11. Four Ds of epiglottis (drooling, dysphagia, dysphonia, and distressed inspiratory efforts)
12. Tachycardia
13. Elevated WBC

Therapeutic Management

1. Examine throat with extreme care in a place where facilities are available for emergency endotracheal intubation or tracheostomy.
2. Maintain patent airway. Intubation may be necessary.
3. Close monitoring of oxygenation status.
4. Administer humidified oxygen.
5. Administer antibiotics to eradicate organisms.
6. Administer antipyretics.
7. Mechanical ventilation may be required.

Nursing Care

ASSESSMENT

1. Same as for laryngotracheobronchitis.
2. If epiglottitis is suspected, do not attempt to visualize epiglottis.

PLANNING

1. Prevent respiratory obstruction.
2. See Laryngotracheobronchitis, pp. 104–105.

IMPLEMENTATION

1. Refer to physician immediately.
2. See Laryngotracheobronchitis, pp. 104–105.

EVALUATION

1. See Laryngotracheobronchitis, pp. 104–105.

Tonsillitis

Description

Tonsillitis is inflammation of the tonsillar structures in the oropharynx.

Pathophysiology

1. Bacterial or viral invasion of tonsillar tissues with inflammation, swelling, and erythema (sometimes exudate).
2. Infection usually occurs in association with pharyngitis.
3. Enlargement causes discomfort and difficulty in swallowing.
4. Cause can be viral or bacterial.
5. Most common bacterial cause is Group A β-hemolytic streptococci.

Signs and Symptoms

1. Difficulty swallowing and breathing
2. Nasal, muffled voice
3. Persistent cough
4. Often associated with otitis media and hearing difficulty
5. Enlargement visible on throat examination, may be red or covered with white exudate.
6. Recurrent sore throat
7. Fever

Therapeutic Management

1. Medical
   A. Symptomatic treatment
   B. Antibiotics (for throat culture positive for group A β-hemolytic streptococcus)
2. Surgical
   A. Tonsillectomy (removal of the palatine tonsils)
   B. Usually with adenoidectomy (removal of adenoids)
3. Pre-operatively
   A. WBC with differentials, and bleeding and clotting profiles
   B. Urinalysis

Nursing Care (Tonsillectomy)

ASSESSMENT

1. Preoperatively
   A. Perform routine assessment.
   B. Assist with diagnostic procedures: bleeding and clotting times.
2. Postoperatively
   A. Take pulse and respirations frequently.
   B. Observe for signs of bleeding.
      (1) Rapid pulse
      (2) Restlessness
      (3) Frequent swallowing, clearing of throat
      (4) Nausea and vomiting
   C. Inspect throat for evidence of oozing or hemorrhage.
   D. Inspect vomitus for evidence of fresh bleeding.

PLANNING

1. Safe, effective care environment
   A. See Nursing Care of the Ill Child, pp. 97–98.
2. Physiological integrity
   A. Promote hydration and nutrition.
   B. Relieve discomfort.
   C. Facilitate drainage.
   D. Prevent complications.
3. Psychosocial integrity
   A. Support child and family.
   B. Prepare child and family for surgery.
   C. Promote coping and adaptation.
4. Health promotion and maintenance
   A. Prepare family for posthospital care.

IMPLEMENTATION

1. Offer cool fluids and liquid diet first 12–24 hours post-surgery (avoid red liquids that give appearance of blood).
2. Apply ice collar.
3. Offer soft diet after 24 hours; then advance to regular diet for age.
4. Administer analgesics as needed for discomfort.
5. Position on side or stomach while sleeping.
6. Discourage child from swallowing mucus secretions.
7. Discourage child from coughing frequently, clearing throat, or blowing nose.
8. Avoid acidic fluids or foods (e.g., orange or tomato juice) until healing takes place; do not use straw.
9. Reassure child and family about what to expect (e.g., expectoration of blood-tinged mucus, temporary alteration in voice).
10. Support child and family.
11. Prepare family for posthospital care.

EVALUATION

Ensure that child:
1. Recovers from surgery uneventfully.
   A. No evidence of bleeding

Acute Otitis Media

Description

Acute otitis media is infection/blockage of the middle ear.

Pathophysiology

1. Infection usually follows an upper respiratory infection.
2. It is primarily the result of a blocked eustachian tube, which prevents normal drainage of middle-ear secretions.
3. Microorganisms proliferate in this warm, fertile environment.
4. Common organisms causing infection: *Streptococcus pneumoniae, Haemophilus influenzae,* and *Moraxella catarrhalis.*

Signs and Symptoms

1. General
   A. Earache (otalgia)
   B. Fever
   C. Possible purulent drainage
   D. Loss of appetite
   E. Irritability

F. Complaints of pain (older children)

G. Evidence of hearing loss in affected ear

2. Infants
   A. Crying
   B. Restless and difficult to comfort
   C. Rolling of head from side to side
   D. Tendency to rub, hold, or pull affected ear
   E. Diarrhea

3. Otoscopic examination reveals:
   A. Bright red or opaque, bulging or retracting tympanic membrane with diminished mobility
   B. Possibly no visible bony landmarks or light reflex
   C. Drainage: yellowish-green, purulent, and foul odor (indicates perforation of tympanic membrane)

4. Effusion
   A. Tinnitus, popping sounds
   B. Hearing loss, if prolonged delays in speech development
   C. Balance disturbances

Therapeutic Management

1. Medical
   A. Antibiotics to eradicate organisms
   B. Analgesics to control discomfort
   C. Acetaminophen for high fever
   D. Decongestants (of questionable value)

2. Surgical
   A. May require myringotomy (surgical incision of eardrum)

Nursing Care

ASSESSMENT

1. Perform routine physical assessment.
2. Assess for evidence of generalized infection.
3. Examine external auditory canal for evidence of inflammation.
4. Assess child for evidence of hearing loss in affected ear.
5. Perform or assist with diagnostic procedures: audiography, tympanometry, pneumatic otoscopy, acoustic reflectometry.

PLANNING

1. Safe, effective care environment
   A. See Nursing Care of the Ill Child, pp. 97–98.
2. Physiological integrity
   A. Assist in eradication of organism.
   B. Relieve discomfort.
3. Psychosocial integrity
   A. Support child and family.
   B. See Nursing Care of the Ill Child, pp. 97–98.
4. Health promotion and maintenance
   A. Prevent complications.
   B. Educate family for home care.

IMPLEMENTATION

1. Administer antibiotics as prescribed.
2. Administer analgesics as prescribed.
3. Administer decongestants, if prescribed.
4. Apply local heat: have child lie (affected ear down) on a heating pad wrapped in a towel.
5. Cleanse external ear with sterile cotton swabs or pledgets soaked in saline.

6. Cleanse any drainage from ear, and keep area dry to prevent excoriation.
7. Encourage fluid intake.
8. Prepare family for surgical intervention, if appropriate.
   A. Myringotomy
   B. Placement of pressure-equalizing tubes
9. Emphasize the importance of following a full course of antibiotics.
10. Prepare family for care, including possible side effects of medication, and for complications, e.g., chronic otitis media (unusual if treated).
11. Emphasize the importance of follow-up care.

EVALUATION

Ensure that child:
1. Appears comfortable.
2. Has ear canal and surrounding skin free of drainage and irritation.
3. Has family who adheres to medical directives.
4. Develops no complications.

Bronchial Asthma

Description

Bronchial asthma is a reactive lower airway disorder characterized by smooth muscle constriction (bronchospasm), increased viscid secretions, and mucosal edema, usually in response to an allergen.

Pathophysiology

1. Symptoms may be precipitated by allergic response to an allergen (pollens, dust, animal dander), exercise, certain foods, smoke or other irritants, rapid changes in environmental temperature, upper respiratory infection, or emotional stress.
2. Bronchospasm.
3. Increased mucus secretion and viscosity.
4. Edema.
5. Reduced diameter of air passage.
6. Hyperactivity of small and large airways.
7. Air trapping causing prolonged expiration.
8. Inadequate oxygenation of blood.
9. Air hunger.

Signs and Symptoms

1. Hacking, paroxysmal, irritative, nonproductive cough.
2. Shortness of breath, flaring nares.
3. Elevated pulse diaphoresis.
4. Prolonged expiratory phase of respiration.
5. Audible wheeze.
6. Restlessness and apprehension, accompanied by an anxious facial expression.
7. Child speaks with short, panting, broken phrases.
8. Older children may sit in the upright position, hunched over, with hands on bed or chair, and arms braced.
9. Chest auscultation reveals coarse, loud breath sounds; sonorous rales; coarse rhonchi; and generalized expiratory wheezing, which becomes increasingly high pitched.
10. Chest hyperresonant on percussion.
11. Cyanosis of nail beds, circumoral cyanosis.

12. Substernal, suprasternal, intercostal retractions.
13. Abdominal pain.
14. With repeated episodes, child develops barrel chest and elevated shoulders, and uses accessory muscles of respiration.

Therapeutic Management

1. Eliminate or avoid proved or suspected irritants and allergens.
2. Prevent attacks: avoid precipitating factors; administer cromolyn sodium.
3. Relieve or minimize symptoms.
   A. Bronchodilators to relax bronchiole musculature
   B. Adrenergics to relax bronchial muscle
   C. Corticosteroids to reduce edema and modify immune response
4. Treat acute attacks promptly.
5. Educate child and family regarding short- and long-range management.
6. Treat status asthmaticus.
   A. Hospitalization with intensive nursing care
   B. IV fluids
   C. Continuous respiratory and cardiac monitoring
   D. Bronchodilators (IV)
   E. Adrenergics
   F. Antibiotics
   G. Corticosteroids (IV)
   H. Humidified O_2 therapy

Nursing Care

ASSESSMENT

1. See Signs and Symptoms, pp. 107–108.
2. Obtain history to determine possible precipitating factors.
3. Assess environment for presence of possible allergens.
4. Assist with diagnostic procedures: chest radiography, sputum examination, immunological blood tests, skin tests, pulmonary function tests, challenge tests.
5. Assess family interpersonal relationships for evidence of dissension, overprotection, or manipulation.
6. Acute Care
   A. Monitor IV fluids and output.
   B. Monitor vital signs frequently.
   C. Auscultate lung fields.

PLANNING

1. Safe, effective care environment
   A. Remove allergenic materials from environment.
   B. Avoid exposure to infection.
   C. Prevent situations that precipitate an attack, e.g., extremes of weather, air pollutants (especially smoke), and infections.
2. Physiological integrity
   A. Relieve symptoms (e.g., bronchospasm).
   B. Adhere to therapeutic regimen (e.g., medications, breathing exercises).
   C. Prevent complications.
3. Psychosocial integrity
   A. Promote normal activities.
   B. Discourage overprotection by family.
   C. Promote short- and long-term adaptation to the disease.

4. Health promotion and maintenance
   A. Maintain optimum health with good nutrition, adequate rest, and appropriate exercise.
   B. Avoid exposure to infections.
   C. Manage minor illnesses at onset.
   D. Prepare child and family for home care.
   E. Promote self-care management.
   F. Promote growth and development.

IMPLEMENTATION

1. Acute attack
   A. Administer bronchodilators, adrenergics, corticosteroids, and antibiotics as prescribed, and monitor child's response.
   B. Position in high Fowler position for optimum ventilation.
   C. Provide humidified oxygen as prescribed, and monitor child's response.
   D. Administer mucolytic agents as prescribed, and monitor child's response.
   E. Monitor child's hydration status.
2. Long-term supervision and support
   A. Teach preventive management, avoidance of precipitating factors, appropriate exercise, sound health maintenance.
   B. Explain expected results of medications and their possible side effects.

EVALUATION

Ensure that child:
1. Exhibits normal respiratory rate, rhythm, and quality.
2. Adheres to prescribed regimen, as does the family.
3. Engages in activities appropriate to age and interests.
4. Maintains optimum health practices, as does the family.
5. Copes with life stresses appropriately as does the family.

Cystic Fibrosis

Description

Cystic fibrosis is a multisystem disorder primarily affecting the exocrine (mucus-producing) glands.

Pathophysiology

1. Instead of thin, freely flowing secretions, mucous glands produce a thick mucus.
2. Mucus accumulates, dilating and eventually obstructing small ducts and passages.
3. Blockage of pancreatic ducts
   A. Prevents enzymes from reaching the duodenum
   B. Markedly impairs digestion and absorption of nutrients
   C. Produces cystic dilation, degeneration, and eventual fibrosis of the acini (small gland lobes)
4. Blockage of respiratory tract bronchioles and bronchi
   A. Patchy atelectasis and hyperinflation
5. Male clients usually azospermic.
6. Sweat glands fail to reabsorb sodium.
7. Abnormally high levels of sodium and chloride in the sweat.
8. Disease may lead to sodium depletion.
9. Disease is inherited as an autosomal-recessive trait.

Signs and Symptoms

1. Meconium ileus in newborn period (earliest sign)
   A. Abdominal distention
   B. Vomiting
   C. Failure to pass stools
2. GI
   A. Large, bulky, loose, frothy, extremely foul-smelling stools
   B. Weight loss
   C. Marked tissue wasting
   D. Failure to grow
   E. Distended abdomen
   F. Thin extremities
   G. Decreased or absent pancreatic enzymes, especially trypsin, in stools
3. Pulmonary
   A. Frequent upper respiratory infections
   B. Chronic cough, which becomes paroxysmal
   C. Thick, tenacious mucus
   D. Eventual barrel chest, dyspnea, clubbing of fingers and toes
   E. Radiographic evidence of patchy areas of atelectasis and obstructive emphysema
4. Biochemical
   A. Sweat chloride concentrations. 60 mEq/L is diagnostic.
   B. Salty taste to sweat (often reported by parents).
5. Delayed puberty

Therapeutic Management

1. Remove obstruction (meconium ileus).
2. Facilitate lung clearance.
3. Prevent and treat pulmonary infections.
4. Replace pancreatic enzymes.
5. Facilitate growth.
6. Prevent complications.

Nursing Care

ASSESSMENT

1. Perform or assist with diagnostic tests: chest radiography, sweat electrolytes, pulmonary function, tests for pancreatic enzymes, fat-absorption tests.
2. Assess family's interpersonal relationships with child and response to the disease.

PLANNING

1. Safe, effective care environment
   A. See Nursing Care of the Ill Child, pp. 97–98.
   B. Avoid exposure to infections.
2. Physiological integrity
   A. Improve aeration.
   B. Facilitate bronchial clearance.
   C. Promote growth.
3. Psychosocial integrity
   A. Explore feelings regarding an inherited disease.
   B. Explore family's feelings regarding a child with a chronic illness with a shortened life expectancy.
   C. Encourage genetic counseling.
   D. Provide long-term support and follow-up care.
4. Health promotion and maintenance
   A. Maintain optimum health.
   B. Prevent complications.
   C. Prepare family for home care.
   D. Encourage as normal a lifestyle as possible.

IMPLEMENTATION

1. Assist with diagnostic procedures (perform sweat chloride test as prescribed).
2. Provide and/or supervise respiratory therapy as prescribed.
   A. Nebulization
   B. Chest physiotherapy
   C. Breathing exercises
3. Administer antibiotics, mucolytics, and expectorants as prescribed.
4. Provide nutritious, attractive meals and snacks.
5. Encourage extra intake of fluids.
6. Monitor IV infusion, if prescribed.
7. Administer pancreatic enzymes as prescribed.
8. Provide conscientious skin care (salt accumulation may be irritating).
9. Implement and maintain appropriate infection-control measures.
10. Teach family administration of medications, including expected results and possible side effects.
11. Teach family use of equipment, respiratory management.
12. Promote compliance with prescribed therapies.
13. Encourage and promote self-care.
14. Encourage as normal a lifestyle as possible (e.g., engaging in activities within capabilities, attending school, peer relationships).
15. Support child and family.
16. Refer to genetic counseling services.
17. Refer to agencies providing special services (e.g., Cystic Fibrosis Foundation).

EVALUATION

Ensure that child:
1. Breathes easily.
2. Manages bronchial secretions with minimal stress.
3. Appears well nourished and gains weight appropriate to developmental stage.
4. Displays no evidence of complications, especially upper respiratory infection.
5. Engages in activities appropriate to developmental level, capabilities, and interests.

Ensure that family:
1. Seeks appropriate counseling.
2. Complies with therapeutic regimen.

Gastrointestinal Disorders

Cleft Lip and/or Palate

Description

Cleft lip is a congenital malformation consisting of one or more clefts in the upper lip. Cleft palate is a congenital defect characterized by a fissure in the midline of the palate.

Pathophysiology

1. Cleft lip: failure of the maxillary and median nasal processes to fuse during embryonic development (6–8 weeks' gestation). Can be unilateral or bilateral.
   A. Defect may range from a notch in the vermilion border of the lip to complete separation extending to the floor of the nose.

2. Cleft palate: failure of the two sides of the palate to fuse during embryonic development (7–12 weeks' gestation).
   A. Defect may occur in isolation or in association with cleft lip.

Signs and Symptoms

Cleft Lip
1. Notched vermilion border, sizes vary.
2. Dental anomalies can occur.

Cleft Palate
1. Nasal distortion
2. Midline or bilateral cleft, extending uvula and soft/hard palate
3. Nasal cavity exposure

Therapeutic Management

1. Surgical closure of the defects at the optimum age (repair of cleft lip precedes repair of palate).
2. Prevent complications.
3. Facilitate normal growth and development of the child.
4. Rehabilitate for optimum speech and hearing within limitations of residual impairment, if any.

Nursing Care

ASSESSMENT

1. Perform routine assessment of newborn.
2. Monitor weight gain and ability to feed (preoperatively).
3. Assess family's acceptance of infant's condition and adherence to treatment regimen.

PLANNING

1. Safe, effective care environment
   A. Perform routine assessment of newborn.
2. Physiological integrity
   A. Facilitate healing of operative site.
   B. Prevent complications.
3. Psychosocial integrity
   A. Facilitate family's adjustment to a child with a facial defect.
   B. Promote normal lifestyle for child.
4. Health promotion and maintenance
   A. Implement a feeding method appropriate to extent of the defect, parental preference, and ease of management.
   B. Prepare family for home care.

IMPLEMENTATION

1. Use special nipple or appliance when feeding (e.g., lamb's nipple, flanged nipple, gravity-flow nipple, rubber-tipped syringe, or specially designed feeding appliance); modify standard nipple with small single slit or cross cut at end.
2. Feed with infant's head held in upright position.
3. Provide soft diet postoperatively for older children until healing takes place.
4. Teach breast-feeding mothers positioning of infant as for formula feeding and placing nipple in the infant's mouth; lip cleft can be filled by molding breast to fill gap or with mother's thumb.
5. Bubble frequently during feeding.

6. Convey an attitude of acceptance of infant and family; promote effective family coping.
7. Protect operative site (cleft lip).
   A. Avoid positioning on stomach.
   B. Apply elbow restraints (if able to turn on side use jacket restraint).
   C. Maintain metal appliance (if applied in the operating room).
   D. Cleanse operative site, as prescribed, after feeding and as indicated.
   E. Prevent sucking: use medicine dropper or Asepto syringe; do not use pacifier until healing has occurred; prevent excessive crying.
8. Protect operative site (cleft palate).
   A. Avoid placing objects in child's mouth, e.g., standard spoon (use only wide-bowled spoon), tongue depressor, thermometer.
   B. Restrain arms.
   C. Rinse mouth with water after feeding.
9. Provide analgesic medication and nonpharmacologic comfort measures for pain.
10. Support and educate family regarding home care.
11. Teach family to observe for signs of speech or hearing impairment.
12. Refer family to appropriate community resources (e.g., Cleft Palate Foundation).

EVALUATION

Ensure that child:
1. Takes feedings well and displays appropriate weight gain.
2. Is an accepted and loved member of the household as exhibited by the family.
3. Has clean surgical site that is free of trauma and infection.
4. Develops normal patterns of speech articulation and intonation.
5. Hears without difficulty.
6. Is supported by family members, who use community resources appropriately.

Tracheoesophageal Fistula, Esophageal Atresia

Description

Tracheoesophageal fistula or esophageal atresia is a congenital malformation resulting from failure of the esophagus to develop a continuous passage; the esophagus may or may not form a connection to the trachea.

Pathophysiology

The anomaly appears in one of the following ways:
1. Proximal esophageal segment terminates in a blind pouch; distal segment is connected to the trachea or primary bronchus by a short fistula at or near the bifurcation (most common anomaly).
2. Blind pouches at end of the proximal and the distal esophagus, which are widely separated and with no communication to the trachea.
3. Otherwise normal trachea and esophagus connected by a common fistula.
4. Fistula from the trachea to the upper esophageal segment or to both the upper and lower segments (rare).

Signs and Symptoms

1. Excessive salivation and drooling.
2. Coughing.
3. Choking or regurgitation with feeding.
4. Cyanosis with feeding.
5. Child may stop breathing.
6. Catheter gently passed into the esophagus meets resistance if the lumen is blocked.
7. Diagnosis established by radiographic demonstration of anomaly.
8. Abdominal distention noted with crying.
9. Recurrent episodes of pneumonia during the first few months of life.

Therapeutic Management

1. Prevent pneumonia.
   A. Feed by gastrostomy.
   B. Drain oral secretions via tube inserted into proximal blind pouch or cervical esophagostomy.
2. Perform surgical repair of defect (time of repair depends on the type of defect and condition of the infant).
3. Promote adequate nutrition.

Nursing Care

ASSESSMENT

1. Perform routine newborn assessment.
2. Observe for evidence of anomaly, primarily the "3 Cs": coughing, choking, and cyanosis (especially following ingestion of fluid).
3. Assist with diagnostic procedures: bronchoscopy with telescopic endoscopy, chest radiography.

PLANNING

1. Safe, effective care environment
   A. Perform routine care of the newborn.
2. Physiological integrity
   A. Prevent aspiration of fluid and secretions into trachea.
   B. Feed via gastrostomy as prescribed.
   C. Provide conscientious postoperative care at time of surgical correction.
3. Psychosocial integrity
   A. Meet oral needs of infant.
   B. Facilitate family's adjustment to an infant with a physical defect.
4. Health promotion and maintenance
   A. Provide health supervision as appropriate.
   B. Prepare family for home care.
   C. Promote growth and development.

IMPLEMENTATION

1. Recognize defect as soon after birth as evident.
2. Position for optimum drainage of secretions: usually supine, with head elevated at 45–60 degrees.
3. Suction oropharynx as needed.
4. Aspirate secretions from proximal blind pouch, manually or by intermittent or continuous suction.
5. Feed prescribed formula via gastrostomy tube.
6. Provide for infant's sucking needs with pacifier, especially during gastrostomy feedings.

7. Observe postoperatively for ability to swallow without choking and for satisfactory eating behavior.
8. Change position from back to side every 2 hours postoperatively.
9. Percussion and postural drainage 2–3 days postoperatively.
10. Prepare family for appearance of child (e.g., presence of chest tubes).
11. Assist family in coping with the infant and his or her needs and therapies.
12. Teach family skills needed for home care.

EVALUATION

Ensure that infant:
1. Is free of respiratory distress.
2. Has clear lungs.
3. Retains feedings, exhibits appropriate weight gain.
4. Has family members who exhibit appropriate behavior with infant.
5. Has family members who demonstrate the ability to provide care for the infant at home.

Hypertrophic Pyloric Stenosis

Description

Hypertrophic pyloric stenosis is hypertrophy and hyperplasia of the circular muscle of the pylorus resulting in obstruction of pyloric sphincter.

Pathophysiology

1. Gross enlargement of the circular pyloric musculature produces severe narrowing of the pyloric canal, causing partial or complete obstruction at the stomach outlet.

Signs and Symptoms

1. Vomiting
   A. Progresses to projectile in character.
   B. Occurs shortly after a feeding.
   C. May follow each meal or appear intermittently.
   D. Vomitus contains no bile, may be blood tinged.
2. Infant hungry, avid eater; accepts second feeding after vomiting.
3. No evidence of pain or discomfort.
4. Weight loss.
5. Signs of dehydration.
6. Distended upper abdomen.
7. Palpable olive-shaped tumor in right upper quadrant of abdomen.
8. Visible gastric peristalsis.
9. Narrow, elongated pyloric canal and delayed emptying are visible on radiographic examination.
10. Hypochloremic acidosis develops with excessive loss of gastric juices.

Therapeutic Management

1. Correct any dehydration and electrolyte imbalance.
2. Provide surgical relief of obstruction by pyloromyotomy (Ramstedt-Fredet-Weber procedure).

Nursing Care

ASSESSMENT

1. Perform routine infant assessment.
2. Observe infant's eating behaviors, especially vomiting pattern.
3. Assess for dehydration.
4. Assist with diagnostic procedures: upper GI series, ultrasound, laboratory assessment of electrolyte status.

PLANNING

1. Safe, effective care environment
   A. See Nursing Care of the Ill Child, pp. 97–98.
2. Physiological integrity
   A. Provide nutrition.
   B. Prevent vomiting.
   C. Prevent complications.
3. Psychosocial integrity
   A. Meet infant's sucking needs.
   B. Support family and prepare for surgery.
   C. Promote healthy parent-child relationships.
4. Health promotion and maintenance
   A. Provide health supervision.
   B. Prepare family for home care.

IMPLEMENTATION

1. Monitor IV infusion as prescribed.
2. Monitor intake and output.
3. Monitor nasogastric suction, if present.
4. If feeding orally, employ techniques to minimize vomiting.
   A. Feed slowly; use firm nipple with small hole (prevent too rapid ingestion of formula).
   B. Hold infant in semiupright position.
   C. Bubble frequently.
   D. Place on right side after feeding.
   E. Handle minimally after feeding.
   F. Avoid overfeeding postoperatively.
   G. Observe and record infant's response to feedings.
5. Institute pharmacologic and nonpharmacologic methods to relieve postoperative pain.
6. Teach family skills needed for home care.

EVALUATION

Ensure that infant:
1. Takes and retains feedings.
2. Exhibits a satisfactory weight gain.
3. Has parents who demonstrate the ability to manage infant's care.

Imperforate Anus

Description

Imperforate anus is a congenital malformation in which the rectum has no outside opening.

Pathophysiology

1. Defects vary from those with normal internal and external sphincters and separated from the outside by an anal membrane, to a rectum that ends above the puborectalis muscle with absence of internal and external sphincters.

The latter is usually associated with fistulae, rectourethral in the male or rectovaginal in the female patient.
2. Anus may be patent but stenosed.

Signs and Symptoms

1. Absence of an anus, dimple present.
2. Increasing abdominal distention.
3. Failure to pass meconium.
4. Passage of stool through inappropriate opening.
5. Stenosis produces difficult defecation and a ribbonlike stool.
6. Digital and endoscopic examination identifies blind pouch.
7. Radiographic examination provides evidence of anorectal anomaly.

Therapeutic Management

1. Anal stenosis: manual dilation
2. Imperforate anus: one or more of the following:
   A. Anoplasty
   B. Surgical reconstruction by abdominal-perineal pull-through procedure
   C. Temporary colostomy during neonatal period followed by rectal and anal reconstruction at about 1 year of age
   D. Permanent colostomy

Nursing Care

ASSESSMENT

1. Perform routine physical assessment of the newborn.
2. Observe for passage of meconium.
3. Assist with diagnostic procedures: endoscopy, radiography (with child inverted), retrograde urethrocystogram confirms presence of rectourethral fistula.

PLANNING

1. Safe, effective care environment
   A. Perform routine care of the newborn.
2. Physiological integrity
   A. Promote wound healing.
   B. Promote normal excretory function.
   C. Prevent infection and trauma.
3. Psychosocial integrity
   A. Support family.
   B. Prepare family for surgical procedure.
   C. Promote bonding/attachment.
4. Health promotion and maintenance
   A. Provide appropriate hydration and nutrition.
   B. Prepare family for home care.

IMPLEMENTATION

1. Avoid taking temperature rectally.
2. Monitor IV fluids and/or hyperalimentation as prescribed.
3. Monitor intake and output; weigh daily.
4. Maintain nasogastric suction, if prescribed.
5. Offer pacifier to satisfy non-nutritive sucking needs.
6. Maintain scrupulous anal and perineal care.
7. Observe stool pattern.
8. Position infant in side-lying or prone position with hips elevated.

9. Provide pharmacologic and nonpharmacologic comfort measures to relieve postoperative pain.
10. Provide formula or diet for age as soon as peristalsis is detected.
11. Support family and teach care needed for home management (e.g., rectal dilation, wound care, colostomy care).

EVALUATION

Ensure that infant:
1. Is well hydrated and well nourished.
2. Displays normal stool pattern.
3. Has operative site free of infection.
4. Can be cared for by family members, who show ability to carry out prescribed care.

Hirschsprung's Disease (Megacolon)

Description

Hirschsprung's disease (megacolon) is mechanical obstruction caused by inadequate motility in part of the large intestine.

Pathophysiology

1. Absence of parasympathetic ganglion cells in a segment of colon.
2. Lack of peristaltic movements.
3. Accumulation of intestinal contents.
4. Distention of the bowel proximal to the defect.
5. Evaluation of solids, liquids, and gases does not occur.

Signs and Symptoms

1. Absence of meconium stool in the newborn period
2. Reluctance to ingest fluids
3. Bile-stained vomitus
4. Abdominal distention
5. Constipation and/or overflow diarrhea (older infants)
6. Ribbonlike stool
7. Palpable fecal mass
8. Failure to thrive

Therapeutic Management

1. Surgical removal of aganglionic portion of the bowel, a three-stage procedure
   A. Temporary colostomy
   B. Complete correction with bowel anastomosis (usually at 1 year of age)
   C. Colostomy closure

Nursing Care (Operative)

ASSESSMENT

1. Perform routine assessment.
2. Observe bowel pattern.
3. Assess general hydration and nutritional status.
4. Assist with diagnostic procedures: radiography, rectal biopsy, anorectal manometry.

PLANNING

1. Safe, effective care environment
   A. See Nursing Care of the Ill Child, pp. 97–98.

2. Physiological integrity
   A. Provide nutrition and hydration.
   B. Facilitate bowel evacuation.
3. Psychosocial integrity
   A. Foster healthy parent-child relationships.
   B. Prepare child and family for surgical procedure and postoperative colostomy care.
4. Health promotion and maintenance
   A. Prevent complications.
   B. Prepare family for home care, including postoperative colostomy care.

IMPLEMENTATION

1. Preoperative
   A. Maintain nasogastric suction.
   B. NPO.
   C. Monitor IV therapy.
   D. Administer enemas, laxatives as prescribed.
   E. Administer antibiotics as prescribed.
   F. Measure abdominal circumference, and monitor elimination pattern.
   G. Reinforce and clarify explanations to family regarding surgical procedure and its ramifications.
2. Postoperative
   A. Maintain nasogastric suction.
   B. Avoid taking temperature rectally.
   C. Monitor progress, including vital signs, abdominal girth measurements, frequency and nature of stools.
   D. Monitor IV therapy.
   E. Provide colostomy care as prescribed.
   F. Provide diet as prescribed.
   G. Support family and teach colostomy and/or wound care as indicated.

EVALUATION

Ensure that child:
1. Exhibits a normal bowel elimination pattern.
2. Is well nourished and well hydrated.
3. Remains free of infection.
4. Is able to be cared for at home by family.

Celiac Disease

Description

Celiac disease is a malabsorption disease characterized by hypersensitivity to gluten.

Pathophysiology

1. Affected individuals are unable to hydrolize peptides contained in the gluten faction of wheat, barley, rye, and oats.
2. Toxic substances accumulate in the gut.
3. Inflammation and ulceration of intestinal mucosa results.

Signs and Symptoms

1. Age of onset 9–18 months.
2. Failure to thrive.
3. Muscle wasting, especially of buttocks and extremities.
4. Diarrhea and vomiting.
5. Bulky, foul-smelling stools (steatorrhea).

6. Anemia; bruises and bleeds easily.
7. Irritability, uncooperativeness, apathy.
8. Celiac crisis.
   A. Precipitated by infection
   B. Prolonged fluid and electrolyte depletion
   C. Emotional disturbance
   D. Alteration in diet
9. Behavioral changes may include irritability, apathy, lack of cooperation.

Therapeutic Management

1. Dietary elimination of gluten
2. Supplemental vitamins and minerals

Nursing Care

ASSESSMENT

1. Perform routine physical assessment.
2. Particular attention to bowel elimination.
3. Assist with diagnostic procedures (e.g., stool collection, intestinal biopsy, gluten challenge).

PLANNING

1. Safe, effective care environment
   A. See Nursing Care of the Ill Child, pp. 97–98.
2. Physiological integrity
   A. Implement and maintain gluten-free diet.
3. Psychosocial integrity
   A. See Nursing Care of the Ill Child, pp. 97–98.
4. Health promotion and maintenance
   A. Promote good health practices.
   B. Prepare family for home care.

IMPLEMENTATION

1. Provide special gluten-free diet: eliminate barley, wheat, oats, rye.
2. Substitute offending grains with other grains: corn, rice, soybeans.
3. Administer vitamin and mineral supplements as prescribed.
4. Teach family about the disease and its management.
5. Teach family diet planning.
   A. Appropriate grain products
   B. How to read food labels for hidden presence of gluten, including gravies, "hydrogenated vegetable protein," and "vegetable protein added"
6. Teach family signs of celiac crisis.
7. Reinforce explanations of the disease and therapies.
8. Encourage child to assume responsibility for diet adherence as early as possible.
9. Stress that gluten restriction is usually a lifelong necessity.

EVALUATION

Ensure that child:
1. Receives prescribed diet, which is adhered to by the family.
2. Achieves age-appropriate weight and height.

Intussusception

Description

Intussusception is an invaginating, or telescoping, of a portion of the intestine into an adjacent distal portion of the intestine.

Pathophysiology

1. Most common site is the ileocecal valve.
2. The ileum invaginates into the cecum and colon.
3. Intussusception obstructs passage of intestinal contents beyond the defect.
4. The two walls of the intestine press against each other.
5. Inflammation, edema, and decreased blood flow.
6. Fecal material contains primarily blood and mucus: the characteristic "currant-jelly" stool.

Signs and Symptoms

1. Sudden intermittent, severe abdominal pain
   A. Child screams and draws knees onto chest.
   B. Child appears comfortable between pain episodes.
2. Vomiting
3. Extreme restlessness
4. Passage of red currant-jellylike stools
5. Tender, distended, boardlike abdomen
6. Palpable sausage-shaped mass in upper right quadrant
7. Shock/sepsis can occur if obstructed for > 12 hours

Therapeutic Management

1. Nonsurgical hydrostatic reduction by barium enema
2. Surgical correction: direct manual reduction, resection of nonviable intestine

Nursing Care

ASSESSMENT

1. Perform routine physical assessment.
2. Listen carefully to family's description of symptoms.
3. Observe stooling.
4. Observe behavior.
5. Assist with diagnostic procedure: barium enema.

PLANNING

1. Safe, effective care environment
   A. See Nursing Care of the Ill Child, pp. 97–98.
2. Physiological integrity
   A. Prepare child for emergency therapeutic procedure(s).
   B. Observe child for complications (e.g., fever, dehydration, peritonitis).
3. Psychosocial integrity
   A. Support child and family.
   B. Prepare child and family for procedures.
4. Health promotion and maintenance
   A. Promote and maintain optimum hydration and nutrition.
   B. Prepare family for home care.

IMPLEMENTATION

1. Monitor stooling pattern and behavior: report passage of brown stools immediately (may indicate reduction of intussusception).
2. Monitor vital signs and IV infusion.
3. Maintain nasogastric suction, if used.
4. Provide conscientious postoperative care.
5. Observe child for evidence of recurrence (sometimes follows nonsurgical reduction).
6. Explain or reinforce explanations of condition and therapy.

EVALUATION

Ensure that child:
1. Exhibits normal stooling pattern.
2. Is free of discomfort.
3. Is able to be cared for at home by family.

Diarrhea

Description

Diarrhea is a noticeable or sudden increase in the number of stools. The consistency of the stools is reduced and the fluid content is increased. The stools tend to be greenish in color. Diarrhea can involve any part of the GI tract and be a symptom of gastroenteritis, enteritis, enterocolitis, or colitis.

Pathophysiology

1. Variable etiology
   A. Acute diarrhea
      (1) Infection in the GI tract
      (2) Toxic reaction to poisons
      (3) Dietary indiscretions (e.g., hyperosmolar formula, green apples)
      (4) Infectious process outside the GI tract (e.g., upper respiratory tract infection, communicable disease, emotional tension)
   B. Chronic diarrhea
      (1) Malabsorption disorder
      (2) Anatomical defect
      (3) Abnormal gastric motility
      (4) Hypersensitivity (allergic) reaction
      (5) Inflammatory response
   C. Any or all of the following:
      (1) Increased secretion of water and electrolytes
      (2) Diminished absorption of solutes
      (3) Osmotic gradient—unabsorbed solutes in bowel lumen draw fluids from bowel surfaces
      (4) Reduced absorptive surface
2. Loss of water and electrolytes causes:
   A. Dehydration
   B. Electrolyte imbalances

Signs and Symptoms

1. Mild diarrhea: a few loose stools daily but no other symptoms
2. Moderate diarrhea: several loose or watery stools daily
3. Severe diarrhea: numerous stools to continuous stooling
4. Accompanying signs appear in varying degrees depending on state of toxicity and dehydration
   A. Subnormal to elevated temperature
   B. Vomiting
   C. Fretfulness and irritability to lethargy, moribundity, coma
   D. Cry lacks vigor
   E. Drawn, flaccid expressions
   F. Weight loss mild (5%) to marked (15%)
   G. Color pale to gray or mottled
   H. Decreased to poor skin turgor
   I. Dry to parched mucous membranes
   J. Decreased urine output to marked oliguria
   K. Pulse normal to rapid and thready
   L. Rapid respirations
   M. Sunken fontanelle
   N. Absent tearing and salivation
   O. Sunken eyeballs
5. Electrolyte and acid-base alterations

Therapeutic Management

1. Provide fluid therapy.
   A. Meet ongoing physiological fluid needs.
   B. Replace previous fluid losses.
   C. Replace ongoing normal and abnormal fluid losses.
2. Correct electrolyte and acid-base imbalances.
3. Eliminate and/or correct cause of diarrhea.
4. Prevent spread of infection.
5. Prevent complications.

Nursing Care

ASSESSMENT

1. Perform routine physical assessment.
2. Observe stool pattern and consistency, vomiting.
3. Assess (on admission and throughout care) weight, state of hydration, signs and symptoms of electrolyte imbalances, neurological status, sensory responses, behavior.
4. Take history for information regarding possible etiological agent.
5. Assist with diagnostic procedures: laboratory tests of fluid and electrolyte status, acid-base balance; stool examination.
6. Test stools for pH, glucose, blood (guaiac), if prescribed.

PLANNING

1. Safe, effective care environment
   A. See Nursing Care of the Ill Child, pp. 97–98.
   B. Prevent spread of diarrhea to others.
2. Physiological integrity
   A. Promote rehydration and hydration.
   B. Re-establish nutrition appropriate to age and condition.
   C. Relieve associated symptoms.
   D. Prevent complications.
3. Psychosocial integrity
   A. See Nursing Care of the Ill Child, pp. 97–98.
   B. Support and educate child and family.
   C. Prepare child and family for procedures.
4. Health promotion/maintenance
   A. Promote optimum health.
   B. Prepare family for home care.

IMPLEMENTATION

1. Monitor IV fluid administration, if prescribed; monitor for signs and symptoms of electrolyte imbalance.
   A. Restrain extremities as needed to maintain IV infusion.
2. Feed oral rehydration fluids as prescribed.
3. Gradually reintroduce diet for age as indicated.
4. Implement and carry out appropriate isolation precautions. Instruct family and others in their use.
5. Administer antibiotics as prescribed.
6. Keep accurate intake and output records.
7. Take and record weight, specific gravity measurements.
8. Avoid rectal temperature measurements.

9. Provide meticulous skin care, especially of anal, perineal, and buttock areas.
10. Provide special mouth care, especially if child is NPO.
11. Provide for sucking needs with pacifier if child is NPO or on limited oral fluids.
12. Provide comfort measures appropriate to developmental level.
13. Explain or reinforce explanation to family of condition and therapies.
14. Teach family skills and procedures needed for home care.

EVALUATION

Ensure that child:
1. Takes and retains prescribed oral fluids.
2. Exhibits evidence of good hydration and satisfactory weight for age.
3. Has vital signs within normal range for age.
4. Consumes adequate diet for age.
5. Has skin free of discoloration or irritation.
6. Has moist and clean mucous membranes.
7. Can be cared for by family who demonstrates an understanding of child's care and management.
8. Does not spread diarrhea to others.

Enterobiasis (Pinworms)

Description

Enterobiasis (pinworms) involves intestinal infestation with the nematode *Enterobius vermicularis,* the common pinworm.

Pathophysiology

1. Eggs ingested or inhaled.
2. Eggs hatch in upper intestine and mature.
3. Worms migrate to cecal area and mate.
4. Female worms proceed to anal area and lay eggs.
5. Movement of worms on skin and mucous membrane surfaces causes intense itching.
6. Eggs deposited on hands and under fingernails during scratching.
7. Period of communicability is 2–3 weeks.

Signs and Symptoms

1. Intense perianal itching
2. Perianal dermatitis and excoriation secondary to scratching
3. Evidence of itching in young children
   A. General restlessness and irritability
   B. Poor sleep
   C. Bed-wetting
   D. Distractibility and short attention span
4. Recurrence common

Therapeutic Management

1. Administration of antihelmintics, such as mebendazole, pyrantel pamoate, piperazine citrate, pyrvinium pamoate

Nursing Care

ASSESSMENT

1. Perform routine physical assessment.
2. Assist with diagnostic procedures: identify parasite.

PLANNING

1. Safe, effective care environment
   A. Prevent spread of infestation.
2. Physiological integrity
   A. Help eradicate organisms.
3. Psychosocial integrity
   A. Support and educate child and family.
   B. Prepare child and family for collecting specimens and administration of medication.
4. Health promotion and maintenance
   A. Promote optimum health.

IMPLEMENTATION

1. Explain or reinforce explanation of condition and therapies.
2. Teach family how to collect specimens for examination.
   A. Construct tape with loop of transparent tape, sticky side out, placed around the end of a tongue depressor.
   B. Apply to perianal region in morning as soon as child awakens and before a bowel movement or bath.
   C. Place in jar or plastic bag loosely.
3. Teach family to administer medication: single dose, followed in 2 weeks with a second dose.
4. Teach child and family preventive measures.
   A. Wash hands after toileting and before eating.
   B. Keep child's fingernails short.
   C. Bathe or shower daily.
   D. Discourage child from biting nails, placing fingers in mouth, and scratching anal area.

EVALUATION

1. Ensure that family demonstrates an understanding of the condition and the ability to carry out instructions.
2. Ensure that neither the child nor others exhibit evidence of infestation.

Giardiasis

Description

Giardiasis is an inflammatory intestinal infestation with the protozoan *Giardia lamblia.*

Pathophysiology

1. Transmitted by person-to-person contact, contaminated water (especially mountain lakes, streams, pools), food, and animals (especially puppies).
2. Infestation begins with ingestion of the cysts, the nonmotile stage of the organism.
3. Pathogenic mechanism unknown.
4. Communicable as long as infected person excretes cysts.
5. Incubation period is 1–4 weeks.

Signs and Symptoms

1. Infants and young children
   A. Diarrhea
   B. Vomiting
   C. Anorexia
   D. Failure to thrive
   E. Anemia

2. Older children
   A. Abdominal cramps
   B. Intermittent loose stools
   C. Constipation
   D. Stools often malodorous, watery, pale, and greasy

Therapeutic Management

1. Eliminate organism with administration of furazolidone, quinacrine, or metronidazole.
2. Enteric precautions for duration of disease.

Nursing Care

ASSESSMENT

1. Perform routine physical assessment.
2. Assist with diagnostic procedures: collect multiple stool specimens (difficult to diagnose) for identification of organisms and/or cysts, and perform counterimmunoelectrophoresis and enzyme-linked immunosorbent assay tests.

PLANNING

1. Safe, effective care environment
   A. Prevent spread of infestation.
2. Physiological integrity
   A. Help eliminate organisms.
3. Psychosocial integrity
   A. Support and educate child and family.
   B. Prepare child and family for administration of medication.
4. Health promotion and maintenance
   A. Promote optimum health.

IMPLEMENTATION

1. Explain or reinforce explanation of disease and therapies.
2. Teach family to administer medication.
   A. Administer with or after meals.
3. Teach preventive measures.
   A. Careful hand washing before eating, handling food, and after toileting.
   B. Change infant's diapers as soon as soiled, and dispose in plastic bag in closed receptacle.
   C. Disinfect diaper changing areas and toilet seats.
   D. Drink water that is specially treated, especially when camping.
   E. Wash all raw fruits and vegetables.
   F. Teach children to defecate only in toilet.
   G. Keep animals away from playgrounds and sandboxes.

EVALUATION

1. Ensure that family demonstrates an understanding of the disease and the ability to provide home care.
2. Ensure that neither the child nor others exhibit evidence of infestation.

Cardiovascular Disorders

Congenital Heart Disease

Description

Congenital heart disease is a structural defect resulting from developmental arrest or deviation.

Pathophysiology

1. Defects with increased pulmonary blood flow
   A. Increased pulmonary blood flow with decreased systemic blood flow
   B. Left-to-right shunting of blood through an abnormal opening
   C. Demonstrate signs and symptoms of congestive heart failure
2. Defects with decreased pulmonary blood flow
   A. Desaturated blood mixes with saturated blood in the systemic circulation.
   B. Right-to-left shunting of blood through an abnormal opening and obstruction to pulmonary blood flow.
   C. Cyanosis present.
3. Obstructive defects
   A. Anatomical narrowing of vessel causes obstruction of blood flow exiting the heart.
   B. Signs of congestive heart failure (more severe defects).
   C. Patent ductus arteriosus: failure of fetal ductus arteriosus to completely close after birth increasing pulmonary circulation.
   D. Coarctation of aorta: localized narrowing of the aorta causing decreased circulation.
   E. Atrial septal defect: abnormal opening between the right and left atria.
   F. Ventricular septal defect: abnormal opening between the right and left ventricles; defect can vary in size from pinhole to complete absence of septum.
   G. Pulmonary stenosis: narrowing or stricture at the entrance to the pulmonary artery.
   H. Aortic stenosis: narrowing or stricture of the aortic valve or the entrance to the aorta.
4. Mixed defects
   A. Desaturated pulmonary blood flow mixes with saturated systemic blood flow: survival in the postnatal period depends on mixing of saturated and desaturated blood within heart.
   B. Pulmonary congestion due to increased pulmonary blood flow (results in differences between pulmonary artery pressure and aortic pressure).
   C. Decreased cardiac output.
   D. Cyanosis may be present; signs of congestive heart failure.
5. Classic defects
   A. Tetralogy of Fallot: classic form consists of four defects:
      (1) Ventricular septal defect
      (2) Pulmonic stenosis
      (3) Overriding aorta
      (4) Right ventricular hypertrophy
   B. Transposition of the great arteries: pulmonary artery leaves the left ventricle and the aorta exits from the right ventricle, with no communication between systemic and pulmonary circulations
   C. Truncus arteriosus: failure of normal septation and division of the embryonic bulbar trunk into the pulmonary artery and aorta, resulting in a single vessel that overrides both ventricles
   D. Tricuspid atresia: failure of the tricuspid valve to develop, resulting in no communication between the right atrium and right ventricle
6. Characteristics
   A. Defects with increased pulmonary blood flow
      (1) Patent ductus arteriosus

(2) Atrial septal defect
(3) Ventricular septal defect
B. Defects with decreased pulmonary blood flow
(1) Tetralogy of Fallot
(2) Tricuspid atresia
C. Obstructive defects
(1) Coarctation of aorta
(2) Pulmonary stenosis
(3) Aortic stenosis
D. Mixed defects
(1) Transpartition of the great arteries
(2) Truncus arteriosus

Signs and Symptoms

1. Infants
   A. Generalized cyanosis
   B. Cyanosis during exertion, especially crying, feeding, straining
   C. Dyspnea, especially following physical effort
   D. Fatigue
   E. Failure to thrive
   F. Hypotonia
   G. Feeding difficulties
   H. Paroxysmal hypercyanotic attacks (some defects)
   I. Heart failure
   J. Recurrent infections
   K. Diaphoresis
   L. Pulmonary edema
2. Older children
   A. Impaired growth and development
   B. Delicate, frail body
   C. Fatigue
   D. Dyspnea on exertion
   E. Orthopnea
   F. Digital clubbing (cyanotic defects)
   G. Squatting for relief of dyspnea (cyanotic defects)
   H. Headache
3. Other possible observations
   A. Bounding pulse
   B. Murmur
   C. Thrill
   D. Tachycardia
   E. Difference in pulse between upper and lower extremities (coarctation of the aorta)
   F. Polycythemia (cyanotic defects)

Therapeutic Management

1. Medical
   A. Improve circulatory efficiency.
      (1) Digitalis administration
      (2) Prostaglandin E administration (some defects)
   B. Remove and prevent excess fluid accumulation.
      (1) Low-sodium diet (formula)
      (2) Diuretic administration
   C. Prevent complications.
      (1) Supplemental vitamin administration
      (2) Supplemental iron administration
      (3) Potassium chloride administration
      (4) Acid-base imbalance

2. Surgical
   A. Cardiac catheterization to establish diagnosis
   B. Surgical correction appropriate to the specific defect at optimum age
   C. Palliation to relieve symptoms until surgical correction can be accomplished
   D. Monitoring to detect postoperative complications (e.g., respiratory failure, congestive heart failure, cardiac arrhythmias).

Nursing Care

ASSESSMENT

1. Perform routine physical assessment with particular attention to the following:
   A. Assess rate and quality of pulses.
   B. Take blood pressure (intra-arterial and intracardiac monitoring following open heart surgery).
   C. Palpate for evidence of hepatic or splenic enlargement, thrills.
   D. Observe for evidence of cardiopulmonary impairment (e.g., cyanosis, dyspnea, clubbing of fingers and toes), sweating (infants).
   E. Auscultate chest to detect abnormal heart sounds (e.g., murmurs, dysrhythmias, gallops, friction rubs).
2. Take careful health history, especially relative to:
   A. Weight gain
   B. Feeding behavior
   C. Exercise intolerance
   D. Frequency of infection
   E. Unusual posturing (squatting; assuming knee-chest position)
   F. Achieving appropriate developmental milestones
3. Assist with diagnostic procedures: electrocardiography (ECG), radiography, sonography, echocardiography, cardiac catheterization.

PLANNING

1. Safe, effective care environment
   A. See Nursing Care of the Ill Child, pp. 97–98.
2. Physiological integrity
   A. Decrease energy expenditure.
   B. Improve circulatory efficiency.
   C. Prevent complications (e.g., excess fluid accumulation, congestive heart failure, upper respiratory infection).
3. Psychosocial integrity
   A. See Nursing Care of the Ill Child, pp. 97–98.
   B. Assist child and family in coping with the condition and its manifestations.
   C. Support and educate child and family.
   D. Prepare child and family for procedures and surgery.
   E. Help family maintain as normal a lifestyle as possible.
4. Health promotion and maintenance
   A. Promote optimum health.
   B. Achieve and maintain optimum hydration and nutrition.
   C. Prepare family for home care.
   D. Promote growth and development.

IMPLEMENTATION

1. Position for optimum cardiopulmonary efficiency.
2. Feed slowly.

3. Allow for frequent rest periods; schedule nursing activities to minimize disturbance of rest.
4. Help child and family select activities appropriate to the condition.
5. Monitor intake and output.
6. Avoid extremes of temperature.
7. Administer drugs as prescribed: digoxin (Lanoxin), iron preparation, diuretic, potassium chloride.
8. Administer O_2 as prescribed, and monitor child's response; suction as needed; monitor chest tube drainage.
9. Administer oral and IV fluids as prescribed.
10. Provide analgesics as needed for pain.
11. Monitor for complications.
12. Feed low-salt formula, if prescribed.
13. Protect child from contact with persons with infections.
14. Explain or reinforce explanation of condition and therapies.
15. Help family distinguish between realistic and unfounded fears.
16. Help family to cope with the physical effects of the condition (e.g., cyanotic spells, poor feeding, exercise intolerance).
17. Teach family skills and procedures needed for home care, including expected results of medications and their possible side effects.
18. See Nursing Care of the Ill Child, pp. 97–98.
19. Refer family for genetic counseling.
20. Instruct parents on need for antibiotic prophylaxis.

EVALUATION

Ensure that child:
1. Rests quietly and breathes easily.
2. Has vital signs within acceptable limits.
3. Consumes sufficient fluid and food for age.
4. Achieves normal growth and development for age.
5. Is free of infection.
6. Has parents who demonstrate an understanding of the child's condition and therapies.
7. Has parents who demonstrate the ability to provide optimum care for the child.

Rheumatic Fever

Description

Rheumatic fever is an inflammatory disease affecting the heart, blood vessels, joints, central nervous system, and subcutaneous tissues.

Pathophysiology

1. Occurs as a delayed sequela of infections with group A β-hemolytic streptococcus
2. Believed to occur as an autoimmune process
3. Inflammatory reaction in connective tissues of heart, joints, and skin
4. Edema of involved tissues
5. Scarring and permanent damage to involved tissue can occur.

Signs and Symptoms

1. Diagnosis based on Jones's criteria
2. Major manifestations:
   A. Carditis: tachycardia, cardiomegaly, murmur, precordial friction rub, precordial pain
   B. Polyarthritis: migratory swollen, hot, red, painful joint(s)
   C. Sydenham's chorea: sudden aimless, irregular movements of extremities; involuntary facial grimaces; speech disturbances; emotional lability
   D. Subcutaneous nodes: nontender swelling located over bony prominences
   E. Erythema marginatum: transitory, nonpruritic erythematous disc-shaped macules with well-demarcated border
3. Minor manifestations:
   A. Fever: low-grade, usually spiking in the afternoon
   B. Arthralgia without arthritic changes
   C. History of previous rheumatic fever or rheumatic heart disease
   D. Increased erythrocyte sedimentation rate
   E. C-reactive protein
   F. Leukocytosis
   G. Anemia
   H. Prolonged PR interval on ECG
   I. Scarlatiniform rash

Therapeutic Management

1. Eradicate group A β-hemolytic streptococci with penicillin.
2. Prevent permanent cardiac damage.
   A. Bed rest during acute phase
   B. Corticosteroids to suppress severe myocardial inflammation
3. Palliate other symptoms.
   A. Anti-inflammatory agents to suppress joint inflammation
   B. Mild sedation to alleviate anxiety and restlessness caused by chorea
   C. Acetaminophen to relieve discomfort
4. Prevent recurrence with long-term administration of penicillin.

Nursing Care

ASSESSMENT

1. Perform routine physical assessment.
2. Take history for evidence of antecedent streptococcus infection.
3. Assist with diagnostic procedures: ECG, laboratory tests.

PLANNING

1. Safe, effective care environment
   A. See Nursing Care of the Ill Child, pp. 97–98.
2. Physiological integrity
   A. Help eradicate organisms.
   B. Alleviate symptoms.
   C. Prevent complications.
3. Psychosocial integrity
   A. See Nursing Care of the Ill Child, pp. 97–98.
   B. Support and educate child and family.
   C. Prepare child and family for procedures, surgery.
4. Health promotion and maintenance
   A. Maintain and promote optimum health.
   B. Prepare family for home care.

IMPLEMENTATION

1. Administer penicillin or other antibiotic as prescribed (both therapeutic and prophylactic) and monitor for signs of improvement and untoward effects.
2. Administer corticosteroids, anti-inflammatory drugs, analgesics, sedation as prescribed, and monitor for signs of improvement and untoward effects.
3. Help family cope with child's enforced limited activity, if prescribed.
4. Provide pharmacologic and nonpharmacologic pain relief measures.
5. Use safety precautions (chorea and muscle weakness).
6. Promote and maintain nutritional status.
7. Explain or reinforce explanation of disease.
8. Teach family skills and procedures needed for home care, including possible side effects of medication.
9. Emphasize importance of prophylactic penicillin.

EVALUATION

Ensure that child:
1. Exhibits no evidence of cardiac dysfunction.
2. Exhibits no rash or nodes, moves joints without pain.
3. Displays no evidence of streptococcal infection.
4. Resumes former activities.

Schönlein-Henoch Purpura

Description

Schönlein-Henoch purpura is a self-limited hypersensitivity vasculitis.

Pathophysiology

1. This form of purpura occurs in children aged 6 months to 16 years, most frequently between ages 2 and 8 years.
2. It often follows an upper respiratory infection.
3. It may be an allergic response or evidence of drug sensitivity.
4. Inflammation of small blood vessels, especially capillaries, occurs.
5. Extravasation of blood into skin produces characteristic petechial skin lesions.
6. Hemorrhages also occur in GI tract, synovia, glomeruli, and CNS.

Signs and Symptoms

1. Malaise
2. Purpura: symmetrical; most commonly on buttocks, legs; may include extensor surfaces of arms
3. Edema (often): scalp, eyelids, lips, ears, dorsal surfaces of hands and feet
4. Arthritis: asymptomatic swelling around a single joint or painful swelling of several joints, especially knees and ankles
5. GI: recurrent colicky midabdominal pain, nausea and vomiting (often), stools containing blood (gross or occult)
6. Renal: hematuria, casts, proteinuria

Therapeutic Management

1. Primarily supportive
2. Acetaminophen for discomfort
3. Corticosteroids for severe edema, arthralgia, abdominal pain

4. Observe for and manage GI and renal involvement.

Nursing Care

ASSESSMENT

1. Perform routine physical assessment.
2. Describe skin manifestations.
3. Observe for GI or renal symptoms.
4. Assist with diagnostic procedures: laboratory tests.

PLANNING

1. Safe, effective care environment
   A. See Nursing Care of the Ill Child, pp. 97–98.
2. Physiological integrity
   A. Relieve discomfort.
   B. Prevent complications.
3. Psychosocial integrity
   A. See Nursing Care of the Ill Child, pp. 97–98.
   B. Support and educate child and family.
   C. Prepare child and family for procedures, surgery.
4. Health promotion and maintenance
   A. Maintain and promote optimum health.
   B. Achieve and maintain optimum hydration and nutrition.
   C. Prepare family for home care.

IMPLEMENTATION

1. See Nursing Care of the Ill Child, pp. 97–98.
2. Administer acetaminophen and corticosteroids as prescribed.
3. Explain or reinforce explanation of condition and therapies.
4. Teach family skills and procedures needed for home care.

EVALUATION

Ensure that child:
1. Appears comfortable.
2. Exhibits no rash.
3. Exhibits no evidence of GI or renal involvement.
4. Can be cared for at home by the family, who demonstrates an understanding of the child's condition.

Kawasaki's Disease

Description

Kawasaki's disease is acute febrile vasculitis, affecting primarily the cardiovascular system.

Pathophysiology

1. Disease occurs primarily in children younger than 5 years of age.
2. Extensive inflammation of the arterioles, venules, and capillaries, which later progresses to include the main coronary arteries, heart, and larger veins.
3. Disease occurs in three phases: acute, subacute, and convalescent.

Signs and Symptoms

1. Acute phase (10–14 days): diagnosis is made if child exhibits 5 of 6 manifestations, including fever:
   A. Abrupt onset of fever persisting for more than 5 days, not responsive to antibiotics

B. Bilateral congestion of the ocular conjunctiva without exudation lasting 3–5 weeks
C. Changes in the mucous membranes of the mouth
(1) Erythema and fissuring of the lips
(2) Diffuse reddening of the oropharynx (strawberry tongue)
D. Changes in peripheral extremities
(1) Pronounced reddening of hands and feet
(2) Edema of hands and feet
(3) Membranous desquamation of fingertips and toes
E. Erythematous rash, affecting primarily the trunk
F. Swelling of cervical lymph nodes
2. Subacute phase (10–25 days)
A. Arthritis
B. Arthralgia
C. Anorexia
D. Irritability
E. Desquamation of digits, palms, soles
F. Panvasculitis of coronary and arteries, formation of aneurysms
3. Convalescent phase (25–60 days)
A. Signs of illness no longer evident
B. Bow's lines

Therapeutic Management

1. Control fever and symptoms of inflammation with aspirin.
2. Prevent dehydration with ample oral and/or IV fluids.
3. Minimize possible cardiac complications with administration of γ-globulin.
4. Monitor cardiac status.

Nursing Care

ASSESSMENT

1. Perform routine physical assessment.
2. Pay particular attention to mucocutaneous assessment, vital signs, cardiac status.
3. Assist with diagnostic procedures: baseline cardiac studies (e.g., ECG, chest radiography, echocardiography).

PLANNING

1. Safe, effective care environment
A. See Nursing Care of the Ill Child, pp. 97–98.
2. Physiological integrity
A. Relieve discomfort.
B. Prevent complications.
3. Psychosocial integrity
A. See Nursing Care of the Ill Child, pp. 97–98.
B. Support and educate child and family.
C. Prepare child and family for procedures and surgery.
4. Health promotion and maintenance
A. Maintain and promote optimum health.
B. Prepare family for home care.
C. Promote growth and development.

IMPLEMENTATION

1. Administer aspirin and γ-globulin as prescribed.
2. Initiate measures to lower fever (e.g., tepid sponge baths, fluids).
3. Provide comfort measures to relieve pain.
4. Monitor cardiovascular status.
5. Provide meticulous mouth and skin care.
6. Provide fluids and nourishment as prescribed.
7. Explain or reinforce explanation of disease and therapies.
8. Teach family skills and procedures needed for home care.

EVALUATION

1. Ensure that child is comfortable.
2. Detect evidence of any cardiovascular complication early and implement appropriate intervention.
3. Ensure that family demonstrates an understanding of the disease and the ability to provide home care.

Hematopoietic Disorders

Leukemia

Description

Leukemia is cancer of the blood-forming tissues.

Pathophysiology

1. Unrestricted proliferation of immature white blood cells depresses production of formed elements of the blood in bone marrow.
2. Infiltration and replacement of tissue with nonfunctioning cells produce clinical manifestations described below.
3. Intense metabolic needs of proliferating leukemic cells deprive body cells of nutrients.

Signs and Symptoms

1. Decreased red blood cells
A. Pallor and fatigue
B. Anemia
2. Neutropenia
A. Susceptibility to infection
B. Fever
3. Decreased platelet production
A. Bruising, bleeding, petechiae
4. Infiltration of bone marrow
A. Susceptibility to fractures
B. Bone pain
5. Infiltration of reticuloendothelial system
A. Enlarged liver, spleen, lymph glands
6. Increased intracranial pressure and ventricular enlargement
A. Severe headache
B. Vomiting
C. Irritability
D. Papilledema
7. Meningeal irritation
A. Pain
B. Stiff neck
8. Hypermetabolism
A. Muscle wasting
B. Weight loss
C. Anorexia
D. Fatigue

Therapeutic Management

1. Achieve and maintain remission.
2. Administer chemotherapy as directed by treatment protocol.

3. Provide CNS therapy to prevent complications of myelo-suppression (from chemotherapeutic agents).
   A. Prevent infection with protective isolation or other appropriate precautions.
4. Replace blood elements.
5. Relieve pain.

Nursing Care

ASSESSMENT

1. Perform routine physical assessment.
2. Assist with diagnostic tests (e.g., blood counts, lumbar puncture, bone marrow aspiration, biopsy).
3. Observe for signs of complications (e.g., bleeding, ulceration, CNS symptoms).
4. Assess family's coping capabilities and support systems.

PLANNING

1. Safe, effective care environment
   A. See Nursing Care of the Ill Child, pp. 97–98.
   B. Prevent transfer of infection to the child.
   C. Prevent trauma that might precipitate bleeding.
2. Physiological integrity
   A. Help achieve a remission.
   B. Relieve pain.
   C. Alleviate symptoms.
3. Psychosocial integrity
   A. See Nursing Care of the Ill Child, pp. 97–98.
   B. Educate child and family.
   C. Help child and family cope with effects of the disease and its therapies.
   D. Prepare child and family for procedures, therapies.
   E. Help family face the uncertainty of child's prognosis and course of disease.
4. Health promotion and maintenance
   A. Promote optimum health.
   B. Achieve and maintain optimum hydration and nutrition.
   C. Prepare family for home care.

IMPLEMENTATION

1. Implement and maintain protective isolation.
2. Administer chemotherapeutic agents as prescribed; monitor for toxic effects.
3. Administer blood products as prescribed.
4. Administer analgesics as prescribed.
5. Position for optimal comfort.
6. Use minimal and gentle physical manipulation.
7. Avoid taking rectal temperatures.
8. Administer antiemetic for nausea as prescribed.
9. Provide meticulous, nontraumatic skin and mouth care.
10. Change position frequently.
11. Promote rest; encourage frequent rest periods.
12. Stimulate appetite with attractive, enticing meals and foods of child's choice; provide nutritious supplements.
13. Explain or reinforce explanation of disease, therapies, and their expected and toxic effects.
14. Encourage family to express their feelings and concerns.
15. Arrange for additional support sources (e.g., spiritual agencies, parent groups).
16. Teach family skills and procedures needed for home care.

EVALUATION

Ensure that child:
1. Attains and maintains a remission.
2. Appears comfortable and verbalizes no complaints of pain.
3. Consumes an adequate amount of appropriate foods.
4. Exhibits no evidence of infection, bleeding, or other complications.
5. Appears rested and engages in appropriate activities.
6. Copes with effects of therapies, as does the family.
7. Can be cared for at home by the family, which demonstrates an understanding of the disease and the consequences of therapies.
8. Has family that is open to counseling and verbalizes feelings and concerns.
9. Has family that avails itself of outside support groups and agencies.

Sickle Cell Disease

Description

Sickle cell disease is a genetically transmitted disease in which normal adult hemoglobin (HbA) is partly or completely replaced by hemoglobin S (HbS).

Pathophysiology

1. HbS is transmitted as an autosomal dominant gene but displays an autosomal recessive inheritance pattern.
   A. Homozygote produces sickle cell disease.
   B. Heterozygote produces sickle cell trait.
2. Occurs primarily in persons of black or Mediterranean ancestry.
3. Decreased O_2 concentration in the blood causes HbS to change structure, causing red blood cells to assume a rigid crescent or sickle shape.
4. Sickle cells become entangled and enmeshed with one another, increasing blood viscosity.
5. Circulation slows, causing circulatory stasis, obstruction of small vessels, and thrombosis.
6. Eventual tissue ischemia and necrosis occur.

Signs and Symptoms

1. Growth retardation and delayed puberty
2. Chronic anemia
3. Marked susceptibility to sepsis
4. Vaso-occlusive crisis (sickle cell crisis)
   A. Effects of ischemia related to areas of involvement
      (1) Pain in involved areas
      (2) Extremities: painful swelling of hands, feet (dactylitis), joints; ulceration
      (3) Abdomen: severe abdominal pain, vomiting, anorexia
      (4) Cerebrum: symptoms of stroke, visual disturbances
      (5) Chest: pain, pulmonary disease
      (6) Liver: jaundice, hepatomegaly
      (7) Kidney: hematuria
      (8) Penis: priapism
5. Laboratory evidence of disease
   A. Positive Sickledex.

B. Hemoglobin electrophoresis identifies type and extent of abnormal hemoglobin.

Therapeutic Management

1. Identify presence of HbS.
2. Prevent sickling phenomenon: promote adequate oxygenation, maintain hemodilution, avoid cold and vasoconstriction.
3. Treat sickle cell crisis.
   A. Bed rest to minimize O_2 use
   B. Oral or IV fluids
   C. Electrolyte replacement
   D. Administration of analgesics for pain relief
   E. Blood replacement for anemia, exchange transfusion in selected cases
   F. Antibiotics to treat existing infections
   G. Short-term O_2 therapy for severe anoxia
4. Splenectomy for recurrent pooling of blood in the organ (sequestration).

Nursing Care

ASSESSMENT

1. Perform routine physical assessment.
2. Perform or assist with screening and/or diagnostic tests: Sickledex, electrophoresis, blood count.
3. Assist in diagnostic tests to assess effects of complications: radiography, tomography, renal function tests, liver function tests.

PLANNING

1. Safe, effective care environment
   A. See Nursing Care of the Ill Child, pp. 97–98.
2. Physiological integrity
   A. Relieve pain (crisis).
   B. Promote adequate hydration.
   C. Prevent complications.
3. Psychosocial integrity
   A. See Nursing Care of the Ill Child, pp. 97–98.
   B. Support and educate child and family.
   C. Prepare child and family for procedures, surgery.
4. Health promotion and maintenance
   A. Prevent sickling crisis.
   B. Promote optimum health.
   C. Prepare family for home care.
   D. Promote growth and development.

IMPLEMENTATION

1. Administer O_2 if ordered.
2. Administer analgesics as prescribed for pain.
3. Provide warmth to affected areas.
4. Encourage ample oral fluids; force fluids if needed; monitor for electrolyte imbalances; monitor IV infusion.
5. Monitor for signs and symptoms of complications.
6. Monitor for reactions to transfusions.
7. Explain or reinforce explanation of condition and therapies.
8. Teach family skills and procedures needed for home care, including ways to avoid situations that cause increased use of O_2 (e.g., strenuous physical activity, emotional stress, environments of low O_2 tension, known sources of infection).

9. Emphasize need for medical attention for infections.
10. Direct family to genetic counseling services and organizations that provide support and services.

EVALUATION

Ensure that child:
1. Does not suffer a sickle cell crisis (e.g., is free of pain or other symptoms).
2. Is well hydrated.
3. Remains free of infection.
4. Can be cared for at home by family members, who demonstrate an understanding of the disease.
5. Is supported by family members, who seek genetic counseling.

Hemophilia

Description

Hemophilia refers to a group of bleeding disorders in which there is a deficiency of one of the factors needed for coagulation of blood.
1. Hemophilia A: deficiency of factor VIII (antihemophilic factor; antihemophilic globulin)
2. Hemophilia B (Christmas disease): deficiency of factor IX

Pathophysiology

1. Disorder is transmitted by X-linked recessive inheritance pattern.
2. Deficiency of factor VIII prevents formation of thromboplastin.
3. Blood is unable to coagulate.
4. Bleeding into tissues can occur anywhere.
   A. Joints: crippling, disabling deformities
   B. Neck, mouth, thorax: airway obstruction
   C. GI tract: obstruction
   D. Spinal cord: paralysis
   E. Brain: stroke
   F. Muscles: nerve compression and muscle fibrosis

Signs and Symptoms

1. Prolonged bleeding anywhere from or in the body
2. Prolonged bleeding from trauma (e.g., umbilical cord, circumcision, cuts, loss of deciduous teeth, epistaxis, injection)
3. Excessive bruising, even from slight injury
4. Hemarthrosis (bleeding into joint cavities), especially of knees, ankles, elbows, shoulders and hips
5. Hematoma formation
6. Bleeding into muscle, especially the iliopsoas, the gastrocnemius, and the forearm flexor
7. Spontaneous hematuria

Therapeutic Management

1. Replace missing blood factor with one of the following:
   A. Factor VIII concentrate
   B. Cryoprecipitate
   C. Fresh frozen plasma
2. Prevent chronic crippling effects of joint bleeding.
   A. Corticosteroids and/or nonsteroidal anti-inflammatory agents, to reduce inflammation
   B. Cold compresses to joint

3. Administer ibuprofen for discomfort as prescribed.
4. Identify persons at risk for the disorder.

Nursing Care

ASSESSMENT

1. Perform routine physical assessment, assessing site of involvement and extent of impairment.
2. Take careful histories.
   A. Health history for evidence of previous bleeding episodes, circumstances of current episode
   B. Family history for evidence of other affected members

PLANNING

1. Safe, effective care environment
   A. See Nursing Care of the Ill Child, pp. 97–98.
   B. Prevent trauma.
2. Physiological integrity
   A. Relieve discomfort.
   B. Prevent and control bleeding episodes.
   C. Prevent crippling effects of bleeding.
3. Psychosocial integrity
   A. See Nursing Care of the Ill Child, pp. 97–98.
   B. Support and educate child and family.
   C. Prepare child and family for procedures, surgery.
4. Health promotion and maintenance
   A. Maintain and promote optimum health.
   B. Prepare family for home care.
   C. Promote self-management of therapies.
   D. Promote growth and development.

IMPLEMENTATION

1. Administer and monitor child's reaction to clotting factor as prescribed, both prophylactic and therapeutic.
2. Administer ibuprofen as prescribed for pain.
3. Prevent trauma.
   A. Set limits on behavior to prevent falling and impact injuries.
   B. Encourage noncontact sports participation.
   C. Reduce strain on lower joints by maintaining ideal weight for age.
   D. Alter environment to reduce injury, especially in toddlers (carpeted floors, padded furniture).
   E. Encourage use of soft toothbrush.
   F. Caution regarding use of sharp instruments, including razor for adolescent boys.
4. Control or decrease local bleeding.
   A. Immobilize and elevate affected part.
   B. Apply pressure for 10–15 minutes.
   C. Apply cold to promote vasoconstriction.
5. Prevent crippling effects.
   A. Apply splints as prescribed.
   B. Encourage or perform passive range-of-motion exercises.
6. Explain or reinforce explanation of disease and therapies.
7. Teach family (including the child) skills and procedures needed for home care, especially administration of clotting factor.
8. Encourage child to assume responsibility for own care.
9. Encourage genetic counseling for the family.
10. Encourage parents and child to express feelings and make appropriate decisions regarding everyday activities and future plans.

EVALUATION

Ensure that child:
1. Exhibits no evidence of bleeding.
2. Exhibits no evidence of tissue damage.
3. Can be cared for at home by family members, who demonstrate an understanding of the disease.
4. Is supported by family members, who seek genetic counseling.
5. Achieves developmental milestones.

Idiopathic Thrombocytopenic Purpura

Description

Idiopathic thrombocytopenic purpura is an acquired hemorrhagic disorder characterized by a marked decrease in the number of platelets.

Pathophysiology

1. Results in excessive destruction of platelets and/or decrease in production of platelets
2. Interferes with blood clotting
3. Causes easy bleeding, particularly noted beneath the skin
4. Believed to be an autoimmune process
5. May occur as a reaction to some drugs or to blood transfusion
6. Occurs in three types of idiopathic thrombocytopenic purpura (ITP): acute, chronic, and recurrent

Signs and Symptoms

1. Occurrence in children 2–8 years of age. Peak occurrence between 2 and 4 years.
2. Most common after a febrile, viral illness
3. Easy bruising: evidenced as petechiae (usually in mucous membranes and sclera), ecchymoses
4. Bleeding from mucous membranes
   A. Epistaxis
   B. Bleeding gums
   C. Hematuria
   D. Hematemesis
   E. Melena (rare)
   F. Hemarthrosis
   G. Menorrhagia

Therapeutic Management

1. Restriction of child's activity at onset and if bleeding is active
2. Corticosteroids for children with highest risk for serious bleeding
3. Administration of packed red cells for blood loss
4. Administration of γ-globulin to increase platelet count (in chronic ITP)
5. Splenectomy in selected cases

Nursing Care

ASSESSMENT

1. Perform routine physical assessment; identify sites of bleeding, purpuric areas.
2. Assist with diagnostic tests.

PLANNING

1. Safe, effective care environment
   A. See Nursing Care of the Ill Child, pp. 97–98.
2. Physiological integrity
   A. Prevent and/or control bleeding.
   B. Prevent complications.
3. Psychosocial integrity
   A. See Nursing Care of the Ill Child, pp. 97–98.
   B. Support and educate child and family.
   C. Prepare child and family for procedures, surgery.
4. Health promotion and maintenance
   A. Promote optimum health.
   B. Prepare family for home care.
   C. Promote growth and development.

IMPLEMENTATION

1. Administer and monitor child's response to medications (e.g., corticosteroids, antibiotics) as prescribed.
2. Implement measures to prevent bleeding (see Hemophilia, pp. 123–124).
3. Monitor for signs of infection.
4. Promote rest.
5. Administer lateral preparations for discomfort. Do not administer aspirin or nonsteroidal anti-inflammatory drugs.
6. Explain or reinforce explanation of condition and therapies.
7. Teach family skills and procedures needed for home care.

EVALUATION

Ensure that:
1. Child exhibits no evidence of bleeding.
2. Family demonstrates an understanding of the condition and the ability to provide home care.

Endocrine Disorders

Diabetes Mellitus

Description

Diabetes mellitus is a disease of metabolism characterized by a deficiency (relative or absolute) of pancreatic insulin.
1. Insulin-dependent, or type I: onset typically in childhood and adolescence
2. Non-insulin-dependent, or type II: onset usually after age 40
3. Maturity-onset diabetes of youth: transmitted as an autosomal-dominant disorder

Pathophysiology

Essential abnormality is related to absolute insulin deficiency due to failure of the β-cells of the pancreas to secrete insulin.

Signs and Symptoms

1. "Three polys"
   A. Polyphagia
   B. Polyuria
   C. Polydipsia
2. Weight loss
3. Irritability; child "not himself or herself"
4. Shortened attention span
5. Lowered frustration tolerance
6. Fatigue
7. Hyperglycemia
8. Possibly diabetic ketoacidosis
   A. Ketones as well as glucose in urine
   B. Dehydration
   C. Vomiting
   D. Electrolyte imbalance
   E. Metabolic acidosis
   F. Abdominal pain
   G. Kussmaul's respirations
   H. Fruity acetone breath
   I. Drowsiness progressing to coma

Therapeutic Management

1. Insulin replacement
2. Exercise
3. Nutritional intake that:
   A. Provides sufficient calories to balance daily expenditure for energy
   B. Satisfies requirements for growth and development
   C. Restricts complex sugars
4. Management of hypoglycemia, illnesses, ketoacidosis
5. Promote adherence to regimen and self-management of disease.
6. Prepare parents/child for possible honeymoon phase.

Considerations Related to the Child's Age

1. Birth to 3 years
   A. Consistency with diet can be difficult during this age group
   B. Toddlers are finicky eaters. Meals may become a control issue.
   C. Diluted doses of insulin may be required.
   D. Establishing rituals may make adjustment easier.
   E. Allow child to participate in management (selecting snack for self from appropriate choices, identifying finger to stick during glucose testing).
2. Four to six years
   A. Offer simple explanations of disease process and management. Important for the child to understand that its not his/her fault.
   B. Allow the child to make decisions regarding foods to eat, both during mealtime and for snacks.
   C. Use names the child can understand to identify feelings of hypoglycemia. This will help to recognize hypoglycemia earlier.
   D. Allow the child to be active in insulin administration (cleaning the injection site).
3. Seven to twelve years of age
   A. The child may be embarrassed about having diabetes. This could interfere with compliance at school; therefore, it is very important to handle diabetic management carefully, and not embarrass the child in front of school friends.
   B. School personnel should be taught s/sx of hypoglycemia, blood glucose monitoring, and how to treat hypoglycemic episodes.
   C. Promote the involvement of the child in the management (puncturing finger for glucose testing, choosing injection sites. The older school-age child can give injections and perform fingersticks).

4. Adolescents
   A. Peer acceptance is important for this age group. For peer acceptance the adolescent might omit some routines of care for diabetes in order to fit in with the crowd.
   B. It is important to know how to motivate the adolescent, to promote adherence.
   C. Promote involvement in the management (Keeping own record of glucose readings and insulin doses, choosing appropriate food plans, administering correct doses of insulin under supervision).

Nursing Care

ASSESSMENT

1. Signs and symptoms of disease.
2. Assist with diagnostic test
3. Family's present knowledge of disease process
4. Family's financial resources
5. Family's coping and support systems

PLANNING

1. Safe, effective care environment
   A. See Nursing Care of the Ill Child, pp. 97–98.
   B. Prevent injury from hypoglycemic/hyperglycemic episodes.
2. Physiological integrity
   A. Teach parents/child disease process and management.
   B. Prevent hypoglycemic/hyperglycemic episodes.
   C. Prevent complications of disease.
   D. Promote the child's involvement in the management of disease.
3. Psychosocial integrity
   A. See Nursing Care of the Ill Child, pp. 97–98.
   B. Promote self-esteem.
   C. Refer to support groups for juvenile diabetes.
   D. Create positive learning environment for child and family.
4. Health promotion and maintenance
   A. Prepare child/family for home maintenance.
   B. Promote optimum health.
   C. Promote growth and development.

EVALUATION

Ensure that:
1. Child/family understand responsibilities of diabetes management.
2. Child/family can recognize and treat hypoglycemia and hyperglycemia.
3. Child/family are able to cope with the disease and management.
4. Child/family access support for the child and the management of diabetes.
5. Child maintains peer relationships.

Lymphocytic Thyroiditis (Hashimoto's Disease)

Description

Lymphocytic thyroiditis (Hashimoto's disease) is an autoimmune thyroid disorder.

Pathophysiology

1. Marked hereditary susceptibility
2. Production of antibodies in response to thyroid antigens

3. Lymphocytic infiltration of thyroid gland, inflammation, and replacement of normal thyroid structures with fibrous tissues

Signs and Symptoms

1. Enlarged thyroid gland: firm, freely movable, nontender
2. Tracheal compression: sense of fullness, hoarseness, dysphagia

Therapeutic Management

1. Administration of thyroid hormone to depress secretion of thyroid-stimulating hormone

Nursing Care

ASSESSMENT

1. Perform routine physical assessment.
2. Assist with diagnostic procedures: laboratory tests for thyroid hormone.

PLANNING

1. Safe, effective care environment
   A. See Nursing Care of the Ill Child, pp. 97–98.
2. Physiological integrity
   A. Relieve symptoms of disease.
   B. Prevent complications.
3. Psychosocial integrity
   A. See Nursing Care of the Ill Child, pp. 97–98.
   B. Support and educate child and family.
4. Health promotion and maintenance
   A. Prepare family for home care.

IMPLEMENTATION

1. Administer thyroid hormone as prescribed.
2. Explain or reinforce explanation of condition and treatment.
3. Teach family skills needed for home care.

EVALUATION

1. Ensure that child's thyroid gland diminishes in size.
2. Ensure that family demonstrates an understanding of the condition and the ability to provide home care.
3. See also Nursing Care of the Adult Client with Hyperthyroidism, p. 287.

Hypothyroidism (Congenital)

Description

Hypothyroidism is a deficiency in secretion of thyroid hormones.

Pathophysiology

Deficiency of thyroid hormone causes various alterations in growth and development.

Signs and Symptoms

1. Infancy
   A. Cool, dry, mottled skin
   B. Coarse, sparse hair
   C. Enlarged tongue
   D. Hoarse cry

E. Lethargy
F. Difficulty feeding
G. Prolonged physiological jaundice
H. Constipation
I. Hypotonia, sluggish reflexes
2. Childhood
   A. See Nursing Care of the Adult Client with Hypothyroidism, p. 289.

Therapeutic Management

1. Administer levothyroxine.

Nursing Care

ASSESSMENT

1. Perform routine physical assessment.
2. Assist with diagnostic procedures: thyroid function tests.

PLANNING

1. Safe, effective care environment
   A. See Nursing Care of the Ill Child, pp. 97–98.
2. Physiological integrity
   A. Prevent complications.
3. Psychosocial integrity
   A. See Nursing Care of the Ill Child, pp. 97–98.
   B. Support and educate child and family.
   C. Prepare child and family for procedures, surgery.
4. Health promotion and maintenance
   A. Promote optimum health.
   B. Prepare family for home care.

IMPLEMENTATION

1. Explain or reinforce explanation of condition and treatment.
2. Teach family administration and monitoring of untoward effects of levothyroxine.

EVALUATION

1. Ensure that child displays normal growth and development.
2. Ensure that family demonstrates an understanding of the disease and the ability to provide home care.

Genitourinary Disorders

Urinary Tract Infection

Description

Urinary tract infection is infection of any portion of the urinary tract: urethritis, cystitis, ureteritis, pyelonephritis.

Pathophysiology

Bacterial invasion of urinary structures, usually confined to the bladder but may ascend to upper collecting system and kidney where it produces inflammatory changes, with scarring and loss of renal tissue.

Signs and Symptoms

1. In children younger than 2 years:
   A. Failure to thrive (FTT)
   B. Poor feeding
   C. Vomiting
   D. Diarrhea
   E. Abdominal distention
   F. Frequent or infrequent voiding
   G. Constant squirming
   H. Strong-smelling urine
   I. Abnormal stream
   J. Persistent diaper rash
   K. Irritability
   L. Lethargy
   M. Unexplained jaundice
2. In children older than 2 years:
   A. Enuresis
   B. Daytime incontinence (toilet-trained child)
   C. Fever
   D. Strong or foul-smelling urine
   E. Increased frequency of urination
   F. Dysuria
   G. Urgency
   H. Abdominal pain
   I. Flank pain
   J. Hematuria
   K. Vomiting (preschool children)

Therapeutic Management

1. Eliminate organisms with antibacterial preparations: systemic penicillins, sulfonamides.
2. Detect or correct functional or anatomical abnormalities.
3. Prevent recurrences.
4. Preserve renal function.

Nursing Care

ASSESSMENT

1. Perform routine physical assessment.
2. Observe elimination behaviors: amount and character of urine output.
3. Assist with diagnostic procedure: urinalysis, intravenous pyelography, cystoscopy, voiding, cysto-urethrography, ultrasonography.

PLANNING

1. Safe, effective care environment
   A. See Nursing Care of the Ill Child, pp. 97–98.
2. Physiological integrity
   A. Assist in eradicating organisms.
   B. Prevent complications.
3. Psychosocial integrity
   A. See Nursing Care of the Ill Child, pp. 97–98.
   B. Support and educate child and family.
   C. Prepare child and family for procedures.
4. Health promotion and maintenance
   A. Promote optimum health.
   B. Achieve and maintain optimum hydration.
   C. Prevent recurrence.
   D. Prepare family for home care.

IMPLEMENTATION

1. Administer antimicrobials as prescribed.
2. Teach child and family preventive hygienic habits (e.g., wipe genitals from front to back, avoid tight-fitting clothing in genital area).

3. Encourage adequate fluid intake and regular bladder emptying.
4. Explain or reinforce explanation of condition and treatment.
5. Explain procedures needed for diagnosis and evaluation.
6. Teach family skills and procedures needed for home care, including expected results of medications, their possible side effects, and signs and symptoms of recurrent infections.

EVALUATION

Ensure that child:
1. Is free of infection.
2. Demonstrates good hygienic practices, as does the family.

Ensure that family:
1. Demonstrates an understanding of the condition and the ability to provide home care.

Nephrotic Syndrome

Description

Nephrotic syndrome is the clinical manifestation of any of the various glomerular disorders in which increased glomerular permeability to plasma protein results in massive urinary loss of protein.

Pathophysiology

1. Increased glomerular permeability to protein (especially albumin), which causes protein to leak through membrane into urine (hyperproteinuria).
2. Decreased colloidal osmotic pressure in capillaries.
3. Tissue hydrostatic pressure exceeds pull of osmotic pressure, which causes fluid to accumulate in interstitial spaces (edema, ascites).
4. Reduced intravascular volume (hypovolemia), including renal blood flow.
5. Increased reabsorption of sodium and water in response to decreased blood volume.
6. Increased secretion of antidiuretic hormone and aldosterone.

Signs and Symptoms

1. Weight gain
2. Edema
   A. Puffiness around eyes
   B. Abdominal swelling
   C. Labial or scrotal swelling
3. Diarrhea
4. Anorexia
5. Normal or slightly decreased blood pressure
6. Increased susceptibility to infection
7. Lethargy
8. Easily fatigued
9. Urine
   A. Decreased
   B. Frothy
   C. Darkly opalescent

Therapeutic Management

1. Activity as tolerated
2. Salt restriction (during edematous stage)
3. Fluid restriction, if severe edema
4. Corticosteroids; prednisone
5. Immunosuppressive agents in severe cases: cyclophosphamide
6. Prevention of infection with prophylactic antibiotics (sometimes)

Nursing Care

ASSESSMENT

1. Perform routine physical assessment.
2. Observe amount and character of urine.
3. Assess edema: measure intake, output, and specific gravity of urine; weight; abdominal girth.
4. Assess intravascular volume: take pulse, blood pressure.
5. Assist with diagnostic procedures: urinalysis, serum protein measurements, renal biopsy (sometimes).

PLANNING

1. Safe, effective care environment
   A. See Nursing Care of the Ill Child, pp. 97–98.
   B. Prevent infection.
2. Physiological integrity
   A. Facilitate reduction in secretion of urinary protein and maintain a protein-free urine.
   B. Prevent complications.
   C. Conserve energy.
3. Psychosocial integrity
   A. See Nursing Care of the Ill Child, pp. 97–98.
   B. Support and educate child and family.
   C. Prepare child and family for procedures, surgery.
4. Health promotion and maintenance
   A. Promote optimum health.
   B. Achieve and maintain optimum hydration and nutrition.
   C. Prepare family for home care.

IMPLEMENTATION

1. Place in room with children without infections.
2. Practice careful medical asepsis.
3. Avoid contact with infected persons or items.
4. Administer corticosteroids, immunosuppressive agents, and antibiotics as prescribed; monitor for side effects of medications.
5. Provide meticulous skin care, especially in skin folds of edematous areas.
6. Change child's position frequently.
7. Promote quiet activities.
8. Provide appropriate diet for age, with attractive presentation and snacks to encourage eating.
   A. Provide no added salt and discourage salty foods (e.g., potato chips).
9. Explain or reinforce explanation of condition and treatment.
10. Teach family skills and procedures needed for home care, including expected results of medications and their possible side effects.

EVALUATION

Ensure that child:
1. Exhibits no evidence of fluid accumulation.
2. Achieves normal urinary output.

3. Exhibits no evidence of infection or skin breakdown.
4. Engages in activities appropriate to age and condition.

Ensure that family:

1. Demonstrates understanding of the condition and ability to provide home care.

Acute Poststreptococcal Glomerulonephritis

Description

Acute poststreptococcal glomerulonephritis is a diffuse inflammation of the renal glomeruli following a streptococcal infection of the throat or skin.

Pathophysiology

1. Antigen-antibody reaction of renal tissues to group A β-hemolytic streptococci
2. Swelling and inflammation of glomerular capillary loops
3. Decreased filtration of plasma
4. Excessive accumulation of water and sodium retention
5. Expanded plasma and interstitial fluid volume
6. Circulatory congestion and edema
7. Reduced urine output

Signs and Symptoms

1. Edema, especially periorbital
2. Hematuria
3. Low-grade fever
4. Anorexia
5. Malaise
6. Pallor
7. Irritability
8. Lethargy
9. Ill-appearing child
10. Headache
11. Abdominal or flank pain
12. Dysuria
13. Vomiting
14. Mild to moderately elevated blood pressure
15. Urine
    A. Severely reduced volume
    B. Cloudy
    C. Smoky brown color
16. Hematological tests
    A. Elevated antistreptolysin-O titer, erythrocyte sedimentation rate, C-reactive protein

Therapeutic Management

1. Restricted activity during acute phase
2. Regular diet with sodium restricted according to severity of symptoms
3. Dietary potassium restricted during periods of oliguria
4. Antibiotics
5. Antihypertensives (if diastolic pressure elevated for dye)

Nursing Care

ASSESSMENT

1. Perform routine physical assessment.
2. Take health history for evidence of recent streptococcal infection.
3. Monitor vital signs, weight.
4. Assess for signs of hypertension, circulatory overload.
5. Carefully measure intake and output.
6. Observe character of urine.
7. Assist with diagnostic procedures: urinalysis, blood count, throat culture, serological tests (e.g., erythrocyte sedimentation rate, C-reactive protein), measures of serum complement activity.

PLANNING

1. Safe, effective care environment
   A. See Nursing Care of the Ill Child, pp. 97–98.
   B. Promote rest.
2. Physiological integrity
   A. Provide appropriate diet and promote appetite.
   B. Prevent and observe for complications.
3. Psychosocial integrity
   A. See Nursing Care of the Ill Child, pp. 97–98.
   B. Support and educate child and family.
   C. Prepare child and family for procedures, surgery.
4. Health promotion and maintenance
   A. Promote optimum health.
   B. Prepare family for home care.

IMPLEMENTATION

1. Encourage frequent rest periods.
2. Provide and encourage quiet activities.
3. Administer antibiotics and antihypertensives as prescribed, and monitor their effects.
4. Monitor for electrolyte imbalances: hyperkalemia.
5. Delete extra salt from meals; discourage highly salted foods (e.g., potato chips, salted nuts).
6. Provide low-potassium diet, if prescribed.
7. Explain or reinforce explanation of condition and treatment.
8. Teach family skills and procedures needed for home care, including expected results of medication and possible side effects.

EVALUATION

Ensure that child:

1. Plays quietly and rests as needed.
2. Consumes a sufficient amount of appropriate foods.
3. Displays no evidence of complications.

Ensure that family:

1. Demonstrates an understanding of the condition and the ability to provide home care.

Cryptorchidism (Cryptorchism)

Description

Cryptorchidism (cryptorchism) is failure of one or both testes to descend normally through the inguinal canal into the scrotal sac.

Pathophysiology

1. Normally canal atrophies and closes after descent.
2. Descent can be arrested at any point along the inguinal canal.
3. Usual course is spontaneous descent within a year.

Signs and Symptoms

1. Rarely a cause of discomfort
2. Empty scrotum: unilateral or bilateral
3. Testes palpable if within the inguinal canal

Therapeutic Management

1. Medical: human gonadotropin administration (limited to older children)
2. Surgical: orchiopexy before age 3 years

Nursing Care

ASSESSMENT

1. Perform routine physical assessment.

PLANNING

1. Safe, effective care environment
   A. See Nursing Care of the Ill Child, pp. 97–98.
2. Physiological integrity
   A. Prevent complications.
3. Psychosocial integrity
   A. See Nursing Care of the Ill Child, pp. 97–98.
   B. Reduce castration anxiety and promote positive body image.
   C. Support and educate child and family.
   D. Prepare child and family for surgery.
4. Health promotion and maintenance
   A. Promote optimum health.
   B. Prepare family for home care.
   C. Promote growth and development.

IMPLEMENTATION

1. Provide meticulous wound care.
2. Explain or reinforce explanation of condition and treatment.
3. Encourage early repair of the defect.
4. Present positive feedback to child and family.
5. Teach family skills and procedures needed for home care.

EVALUATION

Ensure that child:
1. Exhibits no evidence of infection.
2. Displays a positive body image.
Ensure that family:
1. Seeks early evaluation and therapy.
2. Demonstrates an understanding of the condition and the ability to provide home care.

Wilms' Tumor

Description

Wilms' tumor is a malignant neoplasm of the kidney.

Pathophysiology

1. Probably arises from a malignant, undifferentiated cluster of primordial cells capable of initiating regeneration of an abnormal structure.
2. Tumor tends to remain encapsulated for an extended period of time; rupture of capsule results in spread (seeding) of tumor cells into abdomen.

A. Stage I: limited to kidney; completely resectable
B. Stage II: extends beyond kidney; completely resectable
C. Stage III: confined to abdomen; tumor is not completely resectable
D. Stage IV: hematogenous metastases to lung, liver, bone, brain
E. Stage V: bilateral renal involvement present at diagnosis

Signs and Symptoms

1. Abdominal enlargement
2. Firm, nontender abdominal mass
3. Symptoms related to pressure of local or metastasized tumor on tissues
4. Gross hematuria
5. Malaise
6. Fever
7. Hypertension

Therapeutic Management

1. Surgical removal of tumor
2. Radiation and chemotherapy

Nursing Care

ASSESSMENT

1. Perform routine physical assessment.
2. Assist with diagnostic procedures (e.g., abdominal ultrasound, abdominal computed tomography (CT) scan or magnetic resonance imaging (MRI), chest x-ray, chest CT scan, biochemical and hematological studies, urinalysis).

PLANNING

1. Safe, effective care environment
   A. See Nursing Care of the Ill Child, pp. 97–98.
2. Physiological integrity
   A. Prevent tumor spread.
   B. Prevent complications.
3. Psychosocial integrity
   A. See Nursing Care of the Ill Child, pp. 97–98.
   B. Support and educate child and family.
   C. Prepare child and family for procedures, surgery.
4. Health promotion and maintenance
   A. Promote optimum health.
   B. Prepare family for home care.

IMPLEMENTATION

1. Avoid palpating abdomen after diagnosis is suspected or confirmed.
2. Explain or reinforce explanation of condition and treatment.
3. Administer chemotherapy prescribed.
4. Provide support to family and encourage expression of feelings regarding a child with a life-threatening disorder.
5. Teach family skills and procedures needed for home care.
6. Educate family regarding observations for symptoms of side effects of chemotherapy or radiotherapy.

EVALUATION

Ensure that child:
1. Has uneventful recovery from surgery.

2. Displays no ill effects of treatment.
3. Does not exhibit signs of metastases.

Ensure that family:

1. Expresses feelings and concerns.
2. Demonstrates an understanding of the condition and the ability to provide home care.

Neurological Disorders

Myelomeningocele (Infant)

Description

1. Myelodysplasia is abnormal development of any part of the spinal cord in embryonic life (between 24 and 28 days' gestation).
2. Spina bifida is a defect in closure of vertebral arches, with varying degrees of tissue protrusion through body cleft.
3. Spina bifida occulta is incomplete fusion of posterior vertebral arches, without accompanying herniation of spinal cord or meninges.
4. Meningocele is a hernial protrusion of a saclike cyst of meninges containing spinal fluid.
5. Myelomeningocele is a hernial protrusion of a saclike cyst containing meninges, spinal fluid, and a portion of the spinal cord with its nerves.

Pathophysiology

1. Degree of neurological dysfunction is directly related to the anatomical level of the defect.
2. Sensory disturbances usually parallel motor dysfunction (see Signs and Symptoms, below).

Signs and Symptoms

1. Neurological impairment
   A. Below second lumbar vertebra
      (1) Flaccid, areflexic paralysis of lower extremities
      (2) Sensory deficit
      (3) Incontinence with constant dribbling of urine
      (4) Lack of bowel control
      (5) Joint deformities (e.g., talipes valgus or varus, contractures, kyphosis, lumbosacral scoliosis, hip dislocations)
   B. Below third sacral vertebra
      (1) No motor impairment
      (2) Saddle anesthesia with bladder and anal sphincter paralysis (often)

Therapeutic Management

1. Surgical skin coverage and closure of lesion
2. Treatment complications: meningitis, UTI, hydrocephalus, decubiti
3. Correction of any associated orthopedic deformities

Nursing Care

ASSESSMENT

1. Perform routine assessment.
2. Assess functional abilities including motor performance and sensory deficits.

3. Assist with diagnostic procedures: transillumination, hip and spinal roentgenographs, renal ultrasound.
4. Observe pressure areas for signs of skin breakdown.
5. Assess for evidence of complications (e.g., enlarging head, dislocated hip, urinary tract infection meningitis).

PLANNING

1. Safe, effective care environment
   A. See Nursing Care of the Ill Child, pp. 97–98.
2. Physiological integrity
   A. Prevent trauma to the myelomeningocele sac (preoperative).
   B. Prevent complications.
3. Psychosocial integrity
   A. See Nursing Care of the Ill Child, pp. 97–98.
   B. Support and educate child and family.
   C. Prepare child and family for procedures and/or surgery.
4. Health promotion and maintenance
   A. Promote optimum health.
   B. Achieve and maintain optimum hydration and nutrition.
   C. Prepare family for home care.
   D. Assist family in accessing community services and support (i.e., school, physical therapy, occupational therapy, recreational).

IMPLEMENTATION

1. Apply sterile, moist, nonadherent dressing over sac and moisten with saline or antimicrobial solution as prescribed; avoid sac contamination by stool and urine.
2. Use care in cleaning soiled sac.
3. Position infant on stomach or side.
4. Place infant on fleece pad to reduce pressure on knees and ankles.
5. Maintain legs in abduction with pad between knees and roll beneath ankles.
6. Avoid diapering; place infant on diaper or pad and change as needed.
7. Employ meticulous skin care, especially in genital area because of leaking urine and stool.
8. Monitor for signs and symptoms of meningitis: irritability, fever, seizures, and feeding intolerance.
9. Provide gentle range-of-motion exercises to paralyzed extremities as prescribed.
10. Explain or reinforce explanation of condition and treatment.
11. Teach family skills needed for home care, including signs of increased intracranial pressure—hydrocephalus is a frequent complication of myelomeningocele.

EVALUATION

1. Ensure that evidence of complications is recognized early and that appropriate interventions are implemented.

Ensure that infant:

1. Remains clean and intact, with no evidence of infection or breakdown.
2. Does not exhibit evidence of infection.

Ensure that family:

1. Demonstrates an understanding of the condition and the ability to provide home care.
2. Demonstrates acceptance of child's condition.

Hydrocephalus

Description

Hydrocephalus is a condition caused by an imbalance in the production and absorption of cerebrospinal fluid (CSF) in the ventricular system

1. Communicating: CSF flows freely through the ventricular system to the subarachnoid space.
2. Noncommunicating: Obstruction to flow of CSF occurs within the ventricular system.
3. Acquired: This form occurs secondarily to another condition such as tumors, vascular malformations, intracranial bleeding meningitis.
4. Congenital: This form includes congenital malformations such as Chiari II malformations, congenital atresia of the foramina of Luschka and Magendie.

Pathophysiology

1. Increased accumulation of CSF in the ventricles.
2. Ventricles become dilated.
3. Brain substance is compressed against the surrounding rigid bony cranium.
4. Destruction of brain tissue.

Signs and Symptoms

1. Infancy
   A. Irritability
   B. Lethargy
   C. Crying when picked up, which quiets when allowed to rest
   D. Possible changes in level of consciousness
   E. Opisthotonos
   F. Feeding difficulties
   G. Brief, shrill, high-pitched cry
   H. Abnormal increase in head circumference
   I. Full or bulging fontanelle
   J. "Sunset" appearance of eyes
2. Early infancy
   A. Abnormally rapid head growth
   B. Bulging, tense, nonpulsatile fontanelles
   C. Dilated scalp veins
   D. Separated cranial sutures
   E. Macewen's sign ("cracked pot" sound) on head percussion
   F. High-pitched cry
   G. Developmental delays
3. Later infancy
   A. Enlarging frontal bones ("bossing")
   B. Depressed eyes
   C. Sclera visible above iris ("setting sun" sign)
   D. Sluggish pupil response
   E. Developmental delays
4. Childhood
   A. Headache on awakening, with improvement following emesis or assuming upright position
   B. Papilledema
   C. Diplopia
   D. Extrapyramidal tract signs
   E. Irritability
   F. Lethargy

G. Apathy
H. Confusion
I. Later stages: bradycardia and/or altered respirations and seizures (life threatening if not attended to)

Therapeutic Management

1. Surgical
   A. Remove obstruction (e.g., tumor cyst).
   B. Relieve intracranial pressure via lumbar puncture or ventricular tap during preoperative period.
   C. Shunt CSF from ventricle to extracranial compartment (usually the peritoneum) to relieve intracranial pressure.
   D. Revise shunt as needed during growth.
2. Medical
   A. Treat complications: infection, shunt malfunction.

Nursing Care

ASSESSMENT

1. Perform routine physical assessment.
2. Measure head circumference routinely: daily on children with myelomeningocele repair and those with cranial infections.
3. Perform neurological examination; observe for signs of increasing intracranial pressure.
4. Observe for signs of infection preoperatively and postoperatively.
5. Assist with diagnostic procedures: echoencephalography, tomography.

PLANNING

1. Safe, effective care environment
   A. See Nursing Care of the Ill Child, pp. 97–98.
2. Physiological integrity
   A. Prevent complications of the disorder or the corrective surgery.
3. Psychosocial integrity
   A. See Nursing Care of the Ill Child, pp. 97–98.
   B. Support and educate child and family.
   C. Prepare child and family for procedures, surgery.
4. Health promotion and maintenance
   A. Promote optimum health.
   B. Prepare family for home care.

IMPLEMENTATION

1. Support head to prevent strain on neck; turn frequently to avoid pressure injury (preoperatively).
2. Position on unoperated side to prevent pressure on subcutaneous shunt valve and other pressure areas.
3. Keep flat to prevent too rapid reduction of intracranial fluid, if ordered.
4. Place on waterbed or sheepskin mat.
5. Pump valve mechanism as directed, if prescribed.
6. Monitor intake and output, including IV, to prevent fluid overload.
7. Provide meticulous skin care, especially in pressure areas.
8. Provide pharmacologic and nonpharmacologic comfort measures for pain relief.
9. Monitor for signs of infection (increased temperature).

10. Explain or reinforce explanation of condition and treatment.
11. Teach family skills needed for long-term home care.

EVALUATION

1. Ensure that child exhibits no evidence of infection or increased intracranial pressure.
2. Ensure that family demonstrates understanding of condition and ability to provide long-term home care.

Bacterial Meningitis

Description

Bacterial meningitis is infection of the meninges.

Pathophysiology

1. Usual organisms: *H. influenzae* (type B), *Neisseria meningitidis* (meningococcal meningitis), *Streptococcus pneumoniae* (pneumococcal meningitis)
2. Most commonly a result of vascular dissemination from a focus of infection elsewhere in the body
3. Infective process: inflammation, exudation, white blood cell accumulation, varying degrees of tissue damage

Signs and Symptoms

1. General
   A. Fever
   B. Vomiting
   C. Irritability
   D. Seizures
   E. Nuchal rigidity; may progress to opisthotonos
2. Neonates
   A. Poor suck/feeding
   B. Diarrhea
   C. Poor cry
   D. Poor muscle tone
   E. Hypothermia
   F. Apnea
3. Infants and young children
   A. Bulging fontanelle (infants)
   B. High-pitched cry
   C. Anorexia
4. Children and adolescents
   A. Headache
   B. Alterations in sensorium
   C. Positive Kernig's and Brudzinski's signs
   D. May develop delirium, aggressive or maniacal behavior, drowsiness, stupor, coma

Therapeutic Management

1. Prevent spread of infection.
2. Administer antimicrobials.
3. Maintain optimum hydration.
4. Maintain ventilation.
5. Reduce intracranial pressure.
6. Manage shock.
7. Control seizures.
8. Control extremes of body temperature.
9. Treat complications: cerebral edema; hydrocephalus; subdural effusion, empyema.

Nursing Care

ASSESSMENT

1. Perform routine physical assessment.
2. Perform regular neurological assessment.
3. Observe for signs of increased intracranial pressure, shock, respiratory distress.
4. Assist with diagnostic procedures: lumbar puncture, CT or MRI, cultures (CSF, blood), CBC, other laboratory tests.

PLANNING

1. Safe, effective care environment
   A. See Nursing Care of the Ill Child, pp. 97–98.
   B. Prevent or reduce environmental stimulation.
   C. Prevent transmission of disease to others.
2. Physiological integrity
   A. Help eradicate organisms.
   B. Prevent complications.
3. Psychosocial integrity
   A. See Nursing Care of the Ill Child, pp. 97–98.
   B. Support and educate child and family.
   C. Prepare child and family for procedures, surgery.
4. Health promotion and maintenance
   A. Promote optimum health.
   B. Achieve and maintain optimum hydration and nutrition.
   C. Prepare family for home care.

IMPLEMENTATION

1. Implement appropriate isolation precautions and maintain as needed.
2. Teach family proper protective procedures.
3. Administer antimicrobials as prescribed.
4. Monitor and maintain IV infusion.
5. Keep environmental stimuli at a minimum (e.g., quiet, dimly lit room; avoiding noisy activities and excessive handling of child).
6. Implement pain relief measures (analgesics).
7. Implement seizure precautions.
8. Position for comfort: head of bed slightly elevated, side-lying position; no pillow to reduce neck stretching.
9. Observe and record any seizure activity.
10. Administer anticonvulsive medication, if ordered.
11. Monitor for potential complications: intracranial pressure, fever, seizures, and hearing loss.
12. Explain or reinforce explanation of disease and treatment.
13. Teach family skills needed for home care, including expected results of medication and possible side effects.

EVALUATION

Ensure that signs of complications:
1. Are detected early and appropriate interventions implemented.
Ensure that child:
1. Appears comfortable, alert, and oriented.
2. Is seizure-free.
Ensure that family:
1. Demonstrates an understanding of the condition and the ability to provide home care.
Ensure that others:
1. Remain free of infection.

Seizure Disorders

Description

A seizure disorder is a symptom complex reflecting abnormal discharge of cortical neurons and characterized by recurrent, paroxysmal attacks of unconsciousness or impaired consciousness and accompanied by a succession of muscular contractions or abnormal behavior.

1. Partial seizures
   A. Simple: Seizures are characterized by localized motor symptoms; somatosensory, psychic, or autonomic symptoms; or a combination of these with no loss of consciousness.
   B. Complex: Manifestations vary widely and include gaping, lip smacking, chewing, purposeless behaviors; characterized by period of altered behavior, amnesia for behavior, inability to respond to environment, possible decrease or loss of consciousness.
2. Generalized seizures
   A. Tonic-clonic seizures (traditionally known as "grand mal"): Tonic phase is characterized by contraction of skeletal muscles, apnea, cyanosis, bowel and bladder incontinence. Clonic phase that follows is characterized by violent jerking caused by rhythmic contraction and relaxation of muscles. This is followed by a postictal phase, characterized by sleep and confusion.
   B. Absence seizures: These are characterized by brief loss of consciousness, with little or no alteration in muscle tone.
   C. Atonic and akinetic seizures: These are characterized by sudden, momentary loss of muscle tone and postural control.
   D. Myoclonic seizures: These are characterized by sudden, brief contractures of a muscle or group of muscles involving head, arm, or trunk.
   E. Infantile spasms: These are characterized by sudden dropping forward of the head and neck, with trunk flexed forward and knees drawn up.

Pathophysiology

1. Spontaneous electric discharge initiated by a group of hyperexcitable cells (epileptogenic focus).
2. Partial seizures: Discharges from foci are limited to a more or less circumscribed region of the cerebral cortex.
3. Generalized seizures: Discharges arise in the reticular formation and involve both hemispheres. Discharge spreads to brain stem.

Signs and Symptoms

1. Absence seizures
   A. Brief loss of consciousness
   B. Abrupt onset; several to hundreds of brief episodes per day
   C. Minimal or no alteration in muscle tone
   D. Often mistaken for inattentiveness or day-dreaming
   E. Onset between 3 and 8 years of age
2. Tonic-clonic seizures
   A. Seizures occur without warning.
   B. Tonic phase: lasts about 10–20 seconds.
      (1) Immediate loss of consciousness
      (2) Falls to floor, if standing

(3) Eyes roll upward
(4) Stiffening in generalized, symmetrical tonic contraction of entire body
(5) Arms usually flexed
(6) Legs, head, and neck extended
(7) Increased salivation
(8) Possible peculiar piercing cry
(9) Apneic; may become cyanotic
(10) Bowel and bladder incontinence
   C. Clonic phase: lasts about 1–2 minutes or longer.
      (1) Violent jerking movements as the trunk and extremities undergo rhythmic contraction and relaxation.
      (2) Client may foam at the mouth.
      (3) Client may be incontinent of urine and feces.
   D. As attack ends, movements become less intense, occur at longer intervals, then cease entirely.
   E. Postictal phase: sleep and confusion.

Therapeutic Management

1. Control seizures or reduce their frequency with anticonvulsants.
2. Discover and correct cause when possible.
3. Help child live as normal a life as possible.
4. Epilepsy surgery may be indicated in children with intractable, uncontrolled seizures who have not responded to various antiepileptic drugs.

Nursing Care

ASSESSMENT

1. Perform routine physical assessment.
2. Take family history for evidence of seizures or other paroxysmal disorders.
3. Take careful history of the seizure.
   A. Age at onset of seizures
   B. Time of day seizures occur
   C. Detailed description of seizure
   D. Any precipitating factors: environmental, physical
   E. Sensory phenomena associated with seizure
   F. Duration and progression of seizure
   G. Feelings and behavior following seizure
4. Observe seizure.
   A. Behavior at onset of seizure
      (1) Change in facial expression
      (2) Cry or other sound
      (3) Stereotyped or automatous movements
      (4) Random activity
      (5) Position of head, body, extremities
      (6) Time of onset
   B. Movement
      (1) Change of position, if any
      (2) Site of commencement
      (3) Tonic phase: length, parts of body involved
      (4) Clonic phase: twitching or jerking, parts of body involved, sequence of parts involved, any change in character of movements
      (5) Face
         (a) Color change: pallor, cyanosis, flushing
         (b) Perspiration
         (c) Mouth position, teeth clenched, frothing, tongue bitten

(6) Eyes
    (a) Position: straight ahead, deviation
    (b) Pupils (if able to assess): change in size, equality, reaction to light, and accommodation
(7) Respiratory effort
    (a) Presence and length of apnea
    (b) Any cyanosis
    (c) Presence of stertor
(8) Other: involuntary urination or defecation
C. Behavior following seizure
  (1) State of consciousness
  (2) Orientation
  (3) Motor ability
  (4) Speech
  (5) Sensations
D. Side effects of antiepileptic drugs
E. Psychosocial data on child and family coping
5. Assist with diagnostic procedures: electroencephalogram, skull radiography, tomography, blood studies.

PLANNING

1. Safe, effective care environment
  A. See Nursing Care of the Ill Child, pp. 97–98.
  B. Prevent injury to child during seizure.
2. Physiological integrity
  A. Prevent seizures if possible.
3. Psychosocial integrity
  A. See Nursing Care of the Ill Child, pp. 97–98.
  B. Support child and family.
  C. Educate child and family.
  D. Prepare child and family for procedures.
  E. Promote positive self-image in child.
4. Health promotion and maintenance
  A. Promote optimum health.
  B. Prepare family for long-term home care.

IMPLEMENTATION

1. Administer anticonvulsants as prescribed.
2. Protect child from injury during seizure.
  A. Do not attempt to restrain child or use force.
  B. Ease child down to prevent falling if child is standing or sitting.
  C. Avoid placing anything in child's mouth.
  D. Loosen restrictive clothing.
  E. Prevent from hitting hard or sharp objects during uncontrolled movements.
  F. Move furniture or other objects out of way.
  G. Do not attempt to move child, unless in danger.
3. Advise child subject to frequent seizures to wear protective helmet.
4. Maintain side rails on bed; cover hard surfaces.
5. Advise child subject to daily seizures not to engage in activities in which he might be injured.
6. Explain or reinforce explanation of condition and treatment.
7. Dispel myths and fears about the disease to child and family.
8. Help child and family deal with problems related to the disorder.
9. Teach family skills needed for home care, including monitoring for possible side effects of medication.
10. Emphasize need for adherence to medical regimen.

11. Help child and family determine activities appropriate to child's condition, interests, and developmental level; avoid contact sports, climbing trees, or apparatus from which child might fall.

EVALUATION

Ensure that child:
1. Exhibits no evidence of physical injury.
2. Remains seizure-free.
3. Expresses feelings and concerns regarding disease and its ramifications.

Ensure that family:
1. Demonstrates an understanding of the condition and the ability to provide home care.
2. Adheres to home-care instructions and accesses community services for long-term support.
3. Treats child as any other child in the family.

Reye's Syndrome

Description

Reye's syndrome is toxic encephalopathy associated with other organ involvement and characterized by fever, profoundly impaired consciousness, and disordered hepatic function.

Pathophysiology

1. Inflammation of brain causes edema and increased intracranial pressure.
2. Liver appears yellow or reddish with considerable amount of fat distributed in small droplets throughout.
3. Reduction in enzymes that convert ammonia to urea, resulting in hyperammonemia.

Signs and Symptoms

1. Prodromal symptoms may include:
  A. Malaise
  B. Cough
  C. Rhinorrhea
  D. Sore throat
  E. History of viral illness 4–7 days prior to onset
2. Stage I
  A. Vomiting, lethargy, drowsiness
  B. Ability to follow commands
  C. Brisk pupillary reaction
  D. Appropriate response to painful stimuli
3. Stage II
  A. Disorientation, combativeness, delirium
  B. Hyperventilation
  C. Hyperactive reflexes
  D. Appropriate responses to painful stimuli
  E. Pupillary reaction sluggish
4. Stage III
  A. Obtunded, coma
  B. Hyperventilation
  C. Decorticate posturing
  D. Preservation of pupillary light reaction and oculo-vestibular reflexes (although sluggish)
5. Stage IV
  A. Deepening coma, seizures
  B. Decerebrate posturing

C. Loss of oculocephalic reflexes, large fixed pupils, loss of cortical reflexes
6. Stage V
   A. Coma, flaccid paralysis
   B. Loss of deep tendon reflexes
   C. Respiratory arrest
   D. Flaccidity

Therapeutic Management

1. Restore blood sugar level with hypertonic IV glucose and insulin.
2. Control cerebral edema by preventing fluid overload: fluid restriction, hypertonic IV solutions.
3. Osmotherapy (e.g., mannitol to induce cerebral dehydration).
4. Correct acid-base disturbances.
5. Produce muscle relaxation with pancuronium, barbiturates.
6. Eliminate factors known to increase intracranial pressure.
7. Decrease CO_2 levels with controlled ventilation.
8. Reduce O_2 demand by curarization and sedation.

Nursing Care

ASSESSMENT

1. Perform routine physical assessment.
2. Assess vital signs, neurological status, and central venous pressure frequently; monitor intracranial pressure.
3. Assess level of consciousness.
4. Observe for signs of overhydration.
5. Assist with diagnostic procedures: laboratory studies (e.g., liver enzyme studies, liver-dependent clotting factors, ammonia levels, liver biopsy, lumbar puncture [if done]).

PLANNING

1. Safe, effective care environment
   A. See Nursing Care of the Ill Child, pp. 97–98.
   B. Prevent physical injury.
2. Physiological integrity
   A. Maintain respiratory integrity.
   B. Prevent increased intracranial pressure.
   C. Reduce cerebral edema.
   D. Provide basic needs.
   E. Prevent complications.
3. Psychosocial integrity
   A. See Nursing Care of the Ill Child, pp. 97–98.
   B. Support family.
   C. Prepare family for procedures.
4. Health promotion and maintenance
   A. Promote optimum health.
   B. Achieve and maintain optimum hydration and nutrition.
   C. Prepare family for home care.

IMPLEMENTATION

1. Provide intensive care nursing.
2. Maintain patent airway; monitor ventilation.
3. Insert Foley catheter and nasogastric tube; monitor intake and output.
4. Position to prevent increased intracranial pressure.
   A. Elevate head of bed as prescribed (usually 15–30 degrees).

B. Avoid activities that increase intrathoracic or intra-abdominal pressure.
   C. Avoid neck vein compression.
   D. Avoid activities that cause pain, emotional stress, crying.
5. Administer mannitol as prescribed.
6. Administer barbiturates and muscle relaxants as prescribed.
7. Place on alternating pressure, egg-crate mattress, or sheepskin to reduce pressure on bony prominences.
8. Provide nutrition via nasogastric or gastrostomy tube, if ordered.
9. Provide hygienic care as tolerated by child.
10. Explain or reinforce explanation of condition and treatment.
11. Support family.
12. Teach family skills needed for home care.

EVALUATION

Ensure that child:
1. Regains consciousness and normal neurological function.
2. Assumes preillness activities.
Ensure that family:
1. Demonstrates an understanding of the condition and treatment and the ability to provide home care.

Musculoskeletal Disorders

Clubfoot

Description

A congenital anomaly in which the foot is twisted out of its normal shape or position
1. Talipes: deformity involving the ankle
2. Pes: indicating involvement of the foot

Pathophysiology

The cause is unknown. The cause has been attributed to abnormal position and restriction during uterine growth. Others attribute the defect to arrested uterine growth.
   See Signs and Symptoms, below.

Signs and Symptoms

1. Some positional deformities are:
   A. Talipes varus: inversion or bending inward
   B. Talipes valgus: eversion or bending outward
   C. Talipes equinus: plantar flexion in which toes are lower than heel
   D. Talipes calcaneus: dorsiflexion in which toes are higher than heel
2. Most common deformity is:
   A. Talipes equinovarus: foot pointed downward and inward in various degrees of anomaly

Therapeutic Management

1. Correct anomaly by application of successive casts.
2. Maintain correction until normal muscle balance is attained.
3. Surgery done when serial casting has reached plateau.
4. Follow-up observation to avert possible recurrence.

Nursing Care

ASSESSMENT

1. Perform routine physical assessment.

PLANNING

1. Safe, effective care environment
   A. See Nursing Care of the Ill Child, pp. 97–98.
2. Physiological integrity
   A. Promote correction of anomaly.
   B. Prevent complications.
3. Psychosocial integrity
   A. See Nursing Care of the Ill Child, pp. 97–98.
   B. Support family.
   C. Prepare family for casting.
   D. Prepare family for surgery.
4. Health promotion and maintenance
   A. Promote optimum health.
   B. Prepare family for home care.
   C. Promote growth and development.

IMPLEMENTATION

1. Implement cast care as in fractures.
2. Explain or reinforce explanation of condition and treatment.
3. Teach family skills needed for home care.

EVALUATION

1. Ensure that cast remains clean and intact and that neurovascular status of toes is intact.
2. Ensure that family demonstrates an understanding of the condition and the ability to provide home care.

Congenital Hip Dysplasia

Description

Congenital hip dysplasia is an imperfect development of the hip that can affect the femoral head, acetabulum, or both.

Pathophysiology

1. Subluxation: incomplete dislocation or dislocatable hip
   A. Femoral head remains in contact with the acetabulum.
   B. Stretched capsule and ligamentum teres cause the head of the femur to be partially displaced.
2. Dislocation
   A. Femoral head loses contact with the acetabulum.
   B. It is displaced posteriorly and superiorly over the rim.
   C. Ligamentum teres is elongated and taut.

Signs and Symptoms

1. Infant
   A. Shortening of limb on affected side (Allis' or Galleazzi sign)
   B. Restricted abduction of hip on affected side
   C. Unequal gluteal folds
   D. Positive Ortolani test (performed by skilled person)
   E. Positive Barlow test (performed by skilled person)
2. Older infant and child
   A. Affected leg shorter than the other
   B. Telescoping or piston mobility of joint

   C. Trendelenburg sign
   D. Prominent greater trochanter
   E. Marked lordosis (bilateral dislocations)
   F. Waddling gait (bilateral dislocations)

Therapeutic Management

Varies with age of child and extent of dysplasia
1. Newborn to 6 months
   A. Application of external device that maintains proximal femur centered in the acetabulum in attitude of flexion: Pavlik harness most common
2. 6–18 months
   A. Traction followed by reduction and plaster cast immobilization
   B. A brace maintaining abduction may be used after cast removed
3. Older child
   A. Surgical reduction

Nursing Care

ASSESSMENT

1. Perform routine physical assessment: apply Barlow's and Ortolani's maneuvers to assess stability of hip.
2. Assess corrective device for proper application and/or maintenance.
3. Assist with diagnostic procedures: ultrasound, CT, MRI.

PLANNING

1. Safe, effective care environment
   A. See Nursing Care of the Ill Child, pp. 97–98.
2. Physiological integrity
   A. Maintain correct position of hip in acetabulum.
   B. Prevent complications related to wearing corrective device.
3. Psychosocial integrity
   A. See Nursing Care of the Ill Child, pp. 97–98.
   B. Support and educate child and family.
   C. Prepare child and family for procedures or surgery.
4. Health promotion and maintenance
   A. Promote optimum health.
   B. Prepare family for home care.
   C. Promote growth and development.

IMPLEMENTATION

1. Explain or reinforce explanation of condition and treatment.
2. Teach family the purpose, function, application, and maintenance of the corrective device (Pavlik harness) or cast.
3. Help family adapt routine nurturing activities and equipment to accommodate corrective device: feeding, sleeping, playing, safety measures (e.g., car seat).

EVALUATION

Ensure that child:
1. Is properly maintained in corrective device.
2. Is able to engage in normal activities.
Ensure that family:
1. Demonstrates an understanding of the condition and its treatment and the ability to provide home care.

Coxa Plana (Legg-Calvé-Perthes Disease)

Description

Coxa plana (Legg-Calvé-Perthes disease) is progressive destruction of the femoral head, producing varying degrees of deformity.

Pathophysiology

Self-limited disease
1. Avascular stage
   A. Aseptic necrosis of femoral capital epiphysis with degenerative changes.
   B. Condition produces flattening of upper surface of femoral head.
2. Revascularization stage: bone absorption and revascularization
3. Reparative stage: new bone formation
4. Regenerative stage: gradual reformation of femoral head; may result in residual deformity

Signs and Symptoms

1. Intermittent appearance of limp on affected side
2. Pain: soreness or aching
   A. Usually in the groin, in lateral hip, or in vicinity of knee
   B. Worse on rising or at end of a long day
   C. Point tenderness felt over hip capsule
3. Joint dysfunction and limited range of motion
4. Stiffness
5. Disuse atrophy of affected thigh
6. Limb length inequality
7. External hip rotation (late sign)

Therapeutic Management

1. Rest, initially, to reduce inflammation and restore motion
2. Traction to stretch tight adductor muscles (sometimes)
3. Containment of femoral head in acetabulum by non-weight-bearing device (abduction brace, leg cast, leather harness)
4. Surgical correction (sometimes)

Nursing Care

ASSESSMENT

1. Perform routine physical assessment.
2. Assess corrective device for proper application, signs of irritation.
3. Assist with diagnostic procedures: radiography.

PLANNING

1. Safe, effective care environment
   A. Alter physical environment as necessary to accommodate corrective device.
2. Physiological integrity
   A. Maintain corrective device.
   B. Prevent complications.
3. Psychosocial integrity
   A. Support and educate child and family.
   B. Prepare child and family for procedures.

4. Health promotion and maintenance
   A. Promote optimum health.
   B. Prepare family for home management.
   C. Promote growth and development.

IMPLEMENTATION

1. Explain or reinforce explanation of condition and treatment.
2. Encourage child to maintain usual activities within limitations imposed by the disorder and its therapy.
3. Teach family purpose, function, application, and maintenance of corrective device.
4. Teach parents skin care measures.

EVALUATION

1. Ensure that child engages in usual activities.
2. Ensure that family demonstrates an understanding of the condition and complies with treatment regimen.

Scoliosis

Description

Lateral curvature of the spine, usually associated with a rotary deformity
   Three types:
1. Congenital: development in utero
2. Neuromuscular: result of muscle imbalance or weakness (e.g., cerebral palsy)
3. Idiopathic: unknown origin

Pathophysiology

Structural scoliosis:
1. Spinal and support structure changes
2. Loss of flexibility
3. Deformity that cannot be corrected

Signs and Symptoms

Undressed subject viewed from posterior aspect:
1. Primary curvature and a compensatory curvature that places head in alignment with gluteal fold.
2. Head and hips not in alignment.
3. Rib hump and flank asymmetry when child bends from waist unsupported by arms (scoliosis with rotary deformity).
4. In girls, hems do not hang straight.

Therapeutic Management

Spinal straightening and realignment
1. Medical
   A. External bracing: Boston and Wilmington braces used for low thoracic, thoracolumbar, and lumbar curves; Milwaukee brace used for high thoracic curves
2. Surgical: internal fixation
   A. Posterior Instrumentation: Harrington, Luque, Wisconsin, Lotrel-Dubosset, Unit rod, Texas Scottish-Rite Hospital
   B. Anterior Instrumentation: Dwyer, Zielke

Nursing Care

ASSESSMENT

1. Perform routine physical assessment.
2. Inspect corrective appliance and skin regularly for possible problems, e.g., skin irritation, correct application and fit.
3. Assist with diagnostic procedures: radiography pulmonary function tests.

PLANNING

1. Safe, effective care environment
   A. Prevent injury.
2. Physiological integrity
   A. Nonsurgical treatment: maintain prescribed appliance
   B. Surgical treatment: provide competent postoperative care.
   C. Prevent complications.
3. Psychosocial integrity
   A. Prepare child and family for long-term therapy.
   B. Support and educate child and family.
   C. Prepare child and family for procedures, surgery.
   D. Help child with adjustment to appliance.
   E. Promote a positive self-image.
4. Health promotion and maintenance
   A. Promote optimum health.
   B. Prepare child and family for home care.
   C. Promote growth and development.

IMPLEMENTATION

1. Explain or reinforce explanation of condition, including:
   A. How appliance corrects defect
   B. Lengthy treatment
   C. Anticipated results of therapy
   D. How they can help achieve desired goals of therapy
   E. Maintenance of therapeutic devices
2. Help child adjust to restricted movement.
3. Maintain skin integrity while child is wearing brace.
4. Refer to Nursing Care of the Hospitalized Child, pp. 97–98, for information on preoperative and postoperative care.
5. Provide guidance regarding selection of appropriate exercises, anticipated problems (e.g., selection of clothing, reactions of peers, etc.).
6. Discuss freedoms and restraints imposed by therapy.
7. Encourage independence and self-care where appropriate.
8. Emphasize positive long-term outcome.
9. Provide feedback and praise for positive behavior and compliance.

EVALUATION

Ensure that child:
1. Engages in activities appropriate to age and capabilities.
2. Displays evidence of positive self-image.
Ensure that child and family:
1. Demonstrate an understanding of the condition and treatment.
2. Comply with therapeutic plan.

Fractures

Description

Fractures are traumatic injuries to bone in which the continuity of bone tissue is broken.

Pathophysiology

1. Complete: Bone fragments are separated.
2. Incomplete: Bone fragments remain attached.
3. Simple, or closed: Fracture does not cause break in skin.
4. Open, or compound: Open wound through which bone protrudes or has protruded.
5. Complicated: Bone fragments cause injury to other organs or tissues.
6. Greenstick: Compressed side of bone bends, and the tension side fails, producing an incomplete fracture similar to the break observed when a green stick is broken.
7. In children, the periosteum remains intact and remarkably stable at fracture site.

Signs and Symptoms

1. Pain or tenderness at site of break.
2. Generalized swelling.
3. Diminished functional use of affected part.
4. Possible bruising, severe muscular rigidity, or crepitus.
5. Child may be able to use affected part because of attached periosteum at fracture site.

Therapeutic Management

1. Reduce fracture: regain alignment of bony fragments.
   A. Closed or open reduction
2. Retain alignment and length of part through immobilization.
3. Restore function to injured parts.

Nursing Care

ASSESSMENT

1. Perform routine physical assessment.
2. Obtain history of trauma.
3. Assist with diagnostic procedures: radiography, MRI scan, tomograms, bone scan.
4. Assess casted extremity regularly for pain, swelling, discoloration (pallor or cyanosis), ability to move part, paresthesia, pulse, odor.
5. Assess extremity in traction for maintenance of desired pull, body alignment, correct functioning of apparatus.
6. Open reduction: assess bleeding over operative site; outline edges of stain to assess increase; monitor for signs of infection.

PLANNING

1. Safe, effective care environment
   A. See Nursing Care of the Ill Child, pp. 97–98.
2. Physiological integrity
   A. Maintain bone immobility.
   B. Promote bone healing.
   C. Prevent complications.
3. Psychosocial integrity
   A. See Nursing Care of the Ill Child, pp. 97–98.
   B. Support and educate child and family.
   C. Prepare child and family for procedures.
4. Health promotion and maintenance
   A. Prepare family for home care.

IMPLEMENTATION

1. Keep casted extremity elevated on pillows or other support for first day, or as directed; apply ice packs as necessary.
2. Apply "petaling" to rough edges of cast.
3. Maintain integrity of cast: keep clean and dry; avoid damage to cast.
4. Prevent child from placing crumbs or small items inside cast.
5. Maintain skin integrity: assess skin for redness and excoriation
6. Maintain physical mobility: encourage use of unaffected extremities (e.g., assistive devices).
7. Promote self-care activities: bathing, hygiene
8. Teach family skills needed for home care: care of cast, signs of complications.
9. Administer pain medication as needed for child with open reduction.
10. Teach crutch walking to child with lower extremity injury.

EVALUATION

Ensure that child:
1. Has a clean and intact cast.
2. Exhibits no evidence of circulatory or neurological impairment.
3. Engages in activities appropriate for age.

Ensure that family:
1. Demonstrates the ability to provide home care.

Cerebral Palsy

Description

Cerebral palsy (CP) is impaired muscular control resulting from a nonprogressive abnormality in the pyramidal motor.

Pathophysiology

The cause of CP has been unclear; however, it is believed the most common cause of CP is existing prenatal brain abnormalities, especially seen in premature deliveries. The pathological picture is noncharacteristic, meaning that some children exhibit gross abnormalities of the brain, and others exhibit vascular occlusion resulting in atrophy and alterations in the structure of the brain. Anoxia has the greatest effect on the pathological state and the area of insult to the brain. Several classifications of CP exist depending on the area of insult to the brain.

CLASSIFICATION

1. Spastic: hypertonicity of voluntary muscles
2. Athetoid: abnormal involuntary movement
3. Ataxic: no muscular control or coordination
4. Mixed type: combination of spasticity and athetosis

Signs and Symptoms

1. Delay in all motor development
2. Impaired fine motor skills
3. Abnormal motor performance
   A. Poor control of posture, balance, and coordinated motion. Neuromuscular scoliosis may develop.
   B. Active attempts at motion increase abnormal postures and movements to other body parts.
   C. Drooling and impaired speech articulation.
   D. Athetosis: slow, wormlike, writhing movements.
   E. Choreoid movements: involuntary, irregular, jerking.
   F. Dystonic movements: disordered muscle tone.
   G. Abnormal and asymmetrical crawl.
   H. Incoordination.
   I. Poor sucking.
   J. Feeding difficulties.
   K. Persistent tongue thrust.
4. Abnormal postures
   A. Scissoring and extension of legs.
   B. Child maintains hips higher than trunk in prone position, with legs and arms flexed or drawn under body.
   C. Persistent infantile resting and sleeping posture.
5. Altered muscle tone
   A. Increased or decreased resistance to passive movements
   B. Opisthotonos
   C. Feels stiff on handling or dressing
   D. Rigid and unbending at hip and knee joints when pulled to sitting position
6. Persistence of primitive reflexes.
7. Seizures (affects 25%).
8. Sensory deficits may occur: hearing difficulties, visual disturbances, and speech problems.
9. Cognitive impairment (mental retardation) may be present.

Therapeutic Management

1. Establish locomotion, communication, and self-help with braces and splints, casting, physical therapy, surgery, mobilizing therapy.
2. Gain optimum appearance and integration of motor functions:
   A. Skeletal muscle relaxants (some older children)
   B. Antianxiety agents for relief of excessive motion
   C. Anticonvulsants for seizures
   D. Dextroamphetamine or Ritalin for hyperactivity
3. Correct any associated defects with surgery: selective posterior rhizotomy, musculoskeletal procedures.
4. Provide educational opportunities adapted to the individual child's needs and capabilities.

Nursing Care

ASSESSMENT

1. Perform routine physical assessment.
2. Obtain history of child's behavior and attainment of developmental milestones.
3. Assist with diagnostic procedures: electroencephalogram, tomography, screening for metabolic defects, serum electrolytes.

PLANNING

1. Safe, effective care environment
   A. Help modify environment to conform to needs of child.
2. Physiological integrity
   A. Promote relaxation.
   B. Establish locomotion and communication.
   C. Prevent complications.

3. Psychosocial integrity
   A. Facilitate acquisition of educational opportunities for child.
   B. Promote a positive self-image in child.
4. Health promotion and maintenance
   A. Promote optimum health.
   B. Support family in its efforts to meet the needs of the child.
   C. Promote growth and development.

IMPLEMENTATION

1. Explain or reinforce explanation of condition and treatment.
2. Provide safe environment with padded furniture, side rails on bed, sturdy furniture that does not slip, no scatter rugs or polished floors.
3. Restrain child when in chair or vehicle.
4. Provide helmet for child who is prone to falls.
5. Apply and correctly use braces and splints.
6. Carry out and teach family to perform physical therapy regimen.
7. Encourage sitting, crawling, and walking at appropriate ages.
8. Incorporate play that encourages desired behavior.
9. Promote use of activities to prevent or minimize effects of disease.
10. Maintain a well-regulated schedule that allows for adequate rest and sleep.
11. Help family devise and modify equipment and activities to meet needs of child.
12. Provide extra calories to meet extra energy demands of increased muscle activity.
13. Encourage child to assist in care.
14. Enlist efforts of speech therapist.
15. Promote verbal and nonverbal communication based on child's competencies.
16. Teach family skills needed for care, including expected results of medications and their possible side effects.
17. See Care of the Child with a Chronic Illness or Disability, pp. 99–100.

EVALUATION

Ensure that child:
1. Is sufficiently rested.
2. Eats a balanced diet with sufficient calories for needs.
3. Is able to communicate his or her needs to caregivers.
4. Achieves maximal potential developmentally based on abilities and competencies.
5. Lives as independently and productively as possible.

Ensure that family:
1. Demonstrates an understanding of the condition and the ability to provide care.
2. Provides a safe environment for the child.

Juvenile Rheumatoid Arthritis

Description

Juvenile rheumatoid arthritis is a chronic inflammatory disease with an unknown inciting agent, a tendency to occur in the prepubertal child, and a slight tendency to occur in families.

Pathophysiology

1. Similar to adult disease.
2. Chronic inflammation of the synovium.

3. Joint effusion.
4. Limited motion caused by muscle spasm and inflammation.
5. Eventual erosion, destruction, and fibrosis of articular cartilage.
6. Adhesions between joint surfaces; ankylosis of joint (longstanding disease).
7. Growth may be retarded during active disease.
8. Disease pursues one of three courses: systemic onset, pauciarticular, polyarticular.

Signs and Symptoms

1. Mode of onset
   A. Systemic: only 20% with joint involvement at diagnosis
      (1) Extra-articular: fever, malaise, myalgia, rash, pleuritis or pericarditis, adenomegaly, splenomegaly, hepatomegaly
   B. Pauciarticular: usually joints of lower extremities (knee, ankle, and eventually sacroiliac; sometimes elbow)
      (1) Extra-articular: acute or chronic iridocyclitis, mucocutaneous lesions, sacroiliitis; eventual ankylosing spondylitis in many (type 2)
   C. Polyarticular: any joints; usually symmetrical involvement of small joints
      (1) Extra-articular: systemic signs minimal (low-grade fever, malaise, weight loss, rheumatoid nodules, and/or vasculitis)
2. Joint characteristics
   A. Stiffness and swelling
   B. Tenderness
   C. May be painful to touch or relatively painless
   D. Warm to touch (seldom red)
   E. Loss of motion
   F. Characteristic morning stiffness or "gelling" on arising in the morning or after inactivity

Therapeutic Management

1. Suppress inflammatory process with:
   A. Nonsteroidal anti-inflammatory drugs
   B. Cytotoxic drugs
   C. Corticosteroids
   D. Slower-acting antirheumatic drugs (e.g., gold, D-penicillamine)
2. Preserve function and/or prevent deformity with physical therapy, occupational therapy, splinting, and positioning.
3. Reduce pain with analgesia, heat application.

Nursing Care

ASSESSMENT

1. Perform routine physical assessment.
2. Observe for joint discomfort and movement.
3. Assist with diagnostic tests: radiography, white blood cell count, rheumatoid factors, erythrocyte sedimentation rate, antinuclear antibodies; latex fixation test used to detect disease in adults is negative in most children.

PLANNING

1. Safe, effective care environment
   A. See Nursing Care of the Ill Child, pp. 97–98.
   B. Modify environment as needed to facilitate child's mobility.

2. Physiological integrity
   A. Relieve discomfort.
   B. Prevent physical deformity and preserve joint function.
3. Psychosocial integrity
   A. See Nursing Care of the Ill Child, pp. 97–98.
4. Health promotion and maintenance
   A. Promote good health practices.
   B. Promote self-care.
   C. Prepare family for home care.
   D. Promote growth and development.

IMPLEMENTATION

1. Explain or reinforce explanation of condition and treatment.
2. Administer and monitor child's response to anti-inflammatory preparations as prescribed.
3. Carry out or assist with physical therapy plan.
4. Provide heat to affected joints via bath, hot compresses, paraffin baths.
5. Carry out range-of-motion activities in appropriate locations (e.g., bath, pool, playroom, etc.).
6. Encourage activity appropriate to capabilities.
7. Apply splints and support equipment (e.g., bolsters, sandbags, pillows) as prescribed.
8. Help modify environment to promote safety and utensils to facilitate self-help.
9. Employ child's natural affinity for play to encourage motion and activity.
10. Teach family skills needed for home care.
    A. Administration of medications and explanation of possible side effects
    B. Purpose and correct application of splints or appliances
    C. Modification of environment, clothing, and utensils to facilitate self-help

EVALUATION

Ensure that child:
1. Demonstrates an understanding of the condition and treatment, as does the family.
2. Is able to move with minimal or no discomfort.
3. Engages in suitable play and self-help activities.

Cognitive and Sensory Disorders

Strabismus

Description

Strabismus is misalignment of the eyes.
1. Esotropia or esophoria: inward deviation of the eye
2. Exotropia or exophoria: outward deviation of the eye

Pathophysiology

1. Image viewed does not fall on corresponding parts of retina in both eyes.
2. Double vision (diplopia) occurs.
3. Child suppresses image in deviating eye to avoid double vision.
4. Disuse causes impaired vision in involved eye (amblyopia).

Signs and Symptoms

1. Deviation apparent on inspection
2. Squinting in attempt to produce clearer vision

Therapeutic Management

1. Patching uninvolved eye to force child to use and strengthen involved eye
2. Corrective lenses to help focus object on retina
3. Surgical correction

Nursing Care

ASSESSMENT

1. Perform routine physical assessment.
2. Assist with diagnostic procedures: ophthalmological examination.

PLANNING

1. Safe, effective care environment
   A. Provide safe environment for child with both eyes patched.
2. Physiological integrity
   A. Provide postoperative care after surgical correction.
   B. Promote compliance in nonsurgical therapies.
   C. Prevent complications.
3. Psychosocial integrity
   A. Support and educate child and family.
   B. Prepare child and family for procedures, surgery.
4. Health promotion and maintenance
   A. Promote optimum health.

IMPLEMENTATION

1. Implement safety precautions as for blind adult (see p. 324).
2. Explain or reinforce explanation of condition and treatment.
3. Teach child and family proper use of patching, eye drops, or glasses.

EVALUATION

Ensure that child:
1. Exhibits desired oculomotor movements and eye alignment.
Ensure that family:
1. Demonstrates an understanding of the condition.
2. Complies with therapy, as does the child.

Mental Retardation

Description

Mental retardation is significantly impaired general intellectual functioning associated with impaired social adaptation and an IQ of 75 or below on an individually administered IQ test.

Pathophysiology

1. Prenatal causes
   A. Inherited diseases (e.g., phenylketonuria, neurofibromatosis)

B. Infection (e.g., rubella)
C. Drugs (e.g., excessive alcohol, chronic lead ingestion)
D. Kernicterus
E. Irradiation
F. Chromosome aberrations (e.g., Down syndrome)
G. Congenital malformations (e.g., microcephaly, hydrocephaly)
2. Perinatal causes
A. Cerebral trauma
B. Anoxia
C. Infections
D. Prematurity
3. Postnatal causes
A. Trauma
B. Seizures
C. Infections
D. Febrile illness
E. Anoxia
F. Chemicals (e.g., lead encephalopathy)
G. Psychological disorders (e.g., autism)
H. Inadequate nutrition
I. Social deprivation (e.g., nonorganic failure to thrive)

Signs and Symptoms

1. Motor delay
2. Cognitive delay: slower than normal rate of acquisition of skills
A. Basic patterns of development maintained
B. Time scale prolonged
3. Delayed vision and hearing development
4. Delayed language
5. Neurobehavioral disturbances

Classification

1. Mild: 50–75 IQ level
2. Moderate: 40–54 IQ level
3. Severe: 25–39 IQ level
4. Profound: below 24 IQ level

Therapeutic Management

1. Infant stimulation
2. Interdisciplinary approach to care: speech and language, special education, physical therapy, occupational therapy, audiologist, nursing, pediatrician, nutritionist, psychologist, social worker, dentist
3. Promotion of inclusionary options in school
4. General health maintenance
5. Correct associated anomalies (e.g., heart defects, facial defects, impaired mobility)

Nursing Care

ASSESSMENT

1. Perform routine physical assessment.
2. Obtain history of possible etiological factors.
3. Obtain developmental history.
4. Perform or assist with diagnostic procedures: developmental screening tests, IQ tests, interdisciplinary assessments, specific diagnostic tests (e.g., chromosome analysis, metabolic studies).

PLANNING

1. Safe, effective care environment
A. Assure protected environment.
2. Physiological integrity
A. Promote development.
3. Psychosocial integrity
A. Support and educate family.
B. Promote acceptance by family.
C. Promote full inclusion for the child.
D. Promote positive self-esteem in child and family.
E. Promote independence, productivity, and inclusion in the community.
4. Health promotion and maintenance
A. Promote optimum health.
B. Help family adjust to future care.
C. Prevent occurrence of secondary problems.

IMPLEMENTATION

1. Explain or reinforce explanation of condition and treatment.
2. Help family to identify both short- and long-term goals.
3. Teach family skills needed for home care.
A. Modify tools for accomplishment of daily living activities.
B. Ensure attainment of developmental milestones and mastery of developmental tasks.
C. Promote self-help and social skills and independence.
D. Provide play materials that stimulate senses and promote self-help.
E. Promote development of interpersonal skills.
4. Help family to investigate and attain special help for the child.
A. Infant stimulation programs
B. Full inclusion in educational settings
C. Supportive living arrangements (adulthood)
5. Help to identify activities that promote independence, productivity and integration.

EVALUATION

Ensure that child:
1. Attains developmental milestones commensurate with cognitive level.
2. Develops optimum self-help within the limits of his or her capabilities.
Ensure that family:
1. Demonstrates an understanding of the condition and accesses community resources and services.

Down Syndrome

Description

Down syndrome is a congenital disorder characterized by varying degrees of mental retardation and multiple defects.

Pathophysiology

1. Syndrome is also called trisomy 21.
2. It is caused by presence of an extra chromosome 21 for a total of 47 chromosomes.

3. In a small number of cases, chromosome 21 is attached to a 14 or 15 chromosome for a total of 46 chromosomes (translocation).
4. Mosaicism: Some cells of developing fetus are normal, and some are trisomy cells.
5. Increased incidence in mothers older than 35 years of age.

Signs and Symptoms

1. Physical characteristics
   A. Small rounded skull with a flat occiput
   B. Inner epicanthal folds and oblique palpebral fissures (eyes slant upward and outward)
   C. Small nose with depressed bridge (saddle nose)
   D. Protruding tongue
   E. Hypoplastic mandible
   F. High-arched palate
   G. Short, thick neck
   H. Hypotonic musculature (floppy infant)
   I. Hyperflexible, lax joints
   J. Broad, short, stubby hands and feet
   K. Simian line (transverse palmar crease)
2. Associated characteristics
   A. Cardiac anomalies most common congenital defects
   B. Atlantoaxial (first and second cervical vertebrae) instability
   C. Highly susceptible to upper respiratory infections
   D. Increased incidence of leukemia

Therapeutic Management

1. See Mental Retardation, pp. 142–143.
2. Correct physical defects.
3. Treat infections.

Nursing Care

ASSESSMENT

1. Perform routine physical assessment.
2. Assist with diagnostic procedures: chromosome analysis, tests to diagnose suspected anomalies.

PLANNING

1. Safe, effective care environment
   A. See Mental Retardation, pp. 142–143.
   B. Prevent infection.
2. Physiological integrity
   A. See Mental Retardation, pp. 142–143.
3. Psychosocial integrity
   A. See Mental Retardation, pp. 142–143.
4. Health promotion and maintenance
   A. See Mental Retardation, pp. 142–143.
   B. Prevent infection.
   C. Prevent additional children with Down's syndrome.

IMPLEMENTATION

1. See Mental Retardation, pp. 142–143.
2. Avoid exposure to persons with upper respiratory infections.
3. Encourage genetic counseling.
4. Prenatal: Encourage prenatal screening for pregnant women older than 35 years of age.

EVALUATION

1. See Mental Retardation, pp. 142–143.
2. Ensure that child remains free of infection.

Skin Disorders

Scabies

Description

Scabies is an endemic infestation produced by the scabies mite, *Sarcoptes scabiei*.

Pathophysiology

1. Impregnated female mite burrows into the stratum corneum of the epidermis and lays eggs.
2. Host is sensitized to mite.
3. Inflammatory response occurs 30–60 days following initial contact.

Signs and Symptoms

1. Pruritus
2. Lesions: papules, vesicles, pustules, and burrows
   A. Eczematous eruption in infants
3. Distribution, in infants: palms, soles, head, neck and face; in older children: primarily interdigital, axillary-cubital, popliteal, and inguinal areas

Therapeutic Management

1. Exterminate mite with scabicide, usually 1% lindane (Kwell).
2. Relieve itching with soothing ointments or lotions.

Nursing Care

ASSESSMENT

1. Perform routine physical assessment.
2. Assist with diagnostic procedures: skin scrapings observed under microscope for evidence of mite.

PLANNING

1. Safe, effective care environment
   A. Prevent spread of mite to others.
2. Physiological integrity
   A. Eliminate scabies mite.
   B. Relieve discomfort.
   C. Prevent or minimize scratching.
3. Psychosocial integrity
   A. Support and educate child and family.
4. Health promotion and maintenance
   A. Promote optimum health.

IMPLEMENTATION

1. Explain or reinforce explanation of condition and treatment.
2. Teach family application of scabicide; instruct them to follow directions accurately.
   A. Apply on cool, dry skin (not after a hot bath).
   B. Leave on for prescribed time.

C. Treat all members of household.
D. Inform family that signs and symptoms may not abate for weeks, although treatment has been effective.
3. Employ methods to prevent scratching.
   A. Keep fingernails short and clean.
   B. Keep child in T-shirt or other soft clothing to cover itching area.
   C. Wrap hands in soft cotton gloves or stockings if needed; pin to shirt.
   D. Apply lotion or ointment to affected areas.
   E. Launder clothing and sheets to prevent reinfection.

EVALUATION

Ensure that child:
1. Keeps skin clean and dry with no evidence of scratching.
2. Rests and plays; has no evidence of discomfort.
3. Exhibits no evidence of infestation.
Ensure that family:
1. Demonstrates an understanding of the condition and therapies.
2. Exhibits no evidence of infestation.

Pediculosis Capitus

Description

Pediculosis capitus is an infestation of the scalp by *Pediculus humanus capitis* (head louse).

Pathophysiology

1. Female louse lays eggs at night on a hair shaft close to junction with skin.
2. Eggs hatch in approximately 7–10 days; located about 4 mm from skin due to hair growth.
3. Lice are blood-sucking organisms that feed approximately 5 times per day.
4. Crawling insect and insect saliva on skin produce itching and irritation.
5. Transmitted by personal contact and contact with shared combs, brushes, clothing, and towels.

Signs and Symptoms

1. Pruritus
2. Nits observable on hair shaft
3. Distribution: hair in occipital area, nape of neck, behind ears

Therapeutic Management

1. Eliminate lice and nits with pediculocidal shampoos (lindane, RID, NIX).
2. Remove nit cases manually by using fine-tooth comb or tweezers.
3. Examine and treat other family members with infestation.

Nursing Care

ASSESSMENT

1. Perform routine physical assessment.
2. Inspect scalp for evidence of nits or nit cases at base of hair shaft.

A. Systematically spread hair with two tongue depressors or popsicle sticks.
B. Observe for:
   (1) Any movement that indicates a louse
   (2) Nits (whitish oval specks adhering to hair shaft)
C. Distinguished from dandruff by adherent nature: dandruff falls off hair readily.

PLANNING

1. Safe, effective care environment
   A. Prevent spread to others.
2. Physiological integrity
   A. Eliminate lice and nits.
3. Psychosocial integrity
   A. Support and educate child and family.
4. Health promotion and maintenance
   A. Promote optimum health.

IMPLEMENTATION

1. Caution children against sharing combs, hats, caps, scarves, coats, and other items used on or near the hair.
2. Explain or reinforce explanation of condition and treatment.
3. Reassure family that anyone can get pediculosis, with no association with age, cleanliness, or socioeconomic level.
4. Teach family application of shampoo.
   A. Follow directions described on label of pediculocide.
      (1) Read directions several times in quiet environment before application.
   B. Make child as comfortable as possible.
   C. Avoid eyes when applying preparation.
      (1) Flush well with tepid water if irritation occurs.
   D. Remove nits with tweezers or fine-tooth comb.
5. Launder washable items of clothing and linens in hot water and dry in dryer.
6. Soak combs, brushes, etc., in pediculocide or lotion and very hot water for 5–10 minutes.
7. Vacuum mattresses and upholstered furniture carefully.
8. Allay child's feelings of shame and embarrassment.
9. Caution family against cutting child's hair or shaving head.

EVALUATION

1. Ensure that child and family exhibit no evidence of infestation.
2. Ensure that family demonstrates an understanding of the condition and treatment.

Dermatophytosis (Ringworm)

Description

Dermatophytosis (ringworm) is a term used for the following infections caused by a group of closely related filamentous fungi:
1. Tinea capitis: ringworm of the scalp
2. Tinea corporis: ringworm of the non-hairy areas of the skin
3. Tinea pedis: "athlete's foot"

Pathophysiology

1. Fungus invades the skin.
2. It produces an enzyme that digests and hydrolyzes keratin of hair, nails, and stratum corneum.
3. Dissolved hair breaks off, producing bald spots.

4. Fungus multiplies at rate equal to the rate of keratin production.

Signs and Symptoms

1. Tinea capitis
   A. Scaly, circumscribed patches
   B. Patchy, scaling areas of alopecia
   C. Pruritus
2. Tinea corpóris
   A. Round or oval erythematous scaling patches that spread peripherally and clear centrally
   B. Pruritus
3. Tinea pedis
   A. Most frequent in adolescents; rare in young children
   B. Maceration, fissuring, and scaling between toes
   C. Patches with pinhead-sized vesicles on plantar surface
   D. Pruritus

Therapeutic Management

Eliminate fungus.
1. Administer oral griseofulvin.
2. Apply topical antifungal preparations.
3. Keep feet dry; avoid wearing occlusive footwear and nylon socks (tinea pedis).

Nursing Care

ASSESSMENT

1. Perform routine physical assessment.
2. Assist with diagnostic procedures: direct microscopic examination of scales from skin scrapings.

PLANNING

1. Safe, effective care environment
   A. Prevent spread to others.
2. Physiological integrity
   A. Help eliminate fungus.
3. Psychosocial integrity
   A. Support and educate child and family.
4. Health promotion and maintenance
   A. Promote optimum health.
   B. Prepare family for home care.

IMPLEMENTATION

1. Explain or reinforce explanation of condition and treatment.
2. Suggest examination of animals in child's environment for evidence of infection (tinea corporis).
3. Teach family how to administer oral medication and apply topical ointments.
4. Teach family desired effects of medications and possible side effects.
5. Teach family strategies to prevent reinfection.

EVALUATION

Ensure that child:
1. Exhibits no evidence of infection.
Ensure that family:
1. Demonstrates an understanding of the condition.
2. Complies with therapy.

Diaper Dermatitis

Description

Diaper dermatitis is an acute inflammatory disorder caused directly or indirectly by the wearing of diapers.

Pathophysiology and Signs and Symptoms

1. Various types and configurations of lesions observed, depending on cause of irritation and inflammation
2. Area of involvement and primary cause:
   A. Convex surfaces, folds spared: contact dermatitis, allergy
   B. Folds: heat, moisture, seborrheic dermatitis
   C. Folds and satellite lesions: candidiasis
   D. Perianal: chemical and/or mechanical irritants
   E. Perianal and satellite lesions: candidiasis
   F. Band at diaper margins: chemical, sweat retention
   G. Small vesicopustules ("heat rash"), miliaria: hot, humid atmosphere under diaper
   H. Bullae or vesicles: bacterial or viral lesions

Therapeutic Management

1. Promote skin healing.
2. Corticosteroids for stubborn inflammations.
3. Topical antifungal or oral preparation (e.g., nystatin [Nilstat, Mycostatin]) for candidiasis.
4. Prevent recurrence.

Nursing Care

ASSESSMENT

1. Perform routine physical assessment.

PLANNING

1. Safe, effective care environment
   A. Promote cleanliness.
2. Physiological integrity
   A. Minimize skin wetness.
   B. Promote normal skin Ph.
   C. Prevent secondary infection.
3. Psychosocial integrity
   A. Support and educate family.
4. Health promotion and maintenance
   A. Promote optimum health.

IMPLEMENTATION

1. Change diaper as soon as wet; change at least once per night.
2. Clean, rinse, and dry area before diapering.
3. Apply occlusive ointment (petrolatum, zinc oxide) over clean, dry, noninflamed skin to prevent moisture reaching skin.
4. Encourage use of diapers that reduce wetness next to skin (e.g., those with absorbent gel).
5. Avoid occlusive diaper covering: plastic pants, some elasticized disposable diapers.
6. Teach diaper care to families.
   A. Encourage use of commercial diaper laundries.
   B. Follow these steps for home care:
      (1) Soak diapers in quaternary ammonium compound.

(2) Wash in hot water with simple laundry soap (Ivory).
(3) Run through rinse cycle twice.
(4) Use dryer to enhance softness.
C. Change plastic diapers frequently.
D. Avoid use of powders, especially those containing cornstarch.
7. Teach families application of any prescribed medication.

EVALUATION

1. Ensure that child is free of dermatitis in the diaper area.
2. Ensure that family demonstrates an understanding of condition, treatment, and prevention.

Atopic Dermatitis (Eczema)

Description

Atopic dermatitis (eczema) is a superficial inflammatory process involving primarily the epidermis.

Pathophysiology

1. Affected individuals have lower threshold for cutaneous itching and tendency to dryness.
2. Characteristic lesions appear following irritation (scratching, rubbing).
3. Appearance and distribution of lesions vary with age of child.
4. Frequently there is a family history of atopy.

Signs and Symptoms

1. Intense itching
2. Unaffected skin dry and rough
3. Infantile form (child 2 months to 3 years)
   A. Generalized distribution: especially cheeks, scalp, trunk, extensor surfaces of extremities
   B. Erythema
   C. Vesicles and papules
   D. Weeping and oozing
   E. Crusting and scaling
4. Childhood form (may follow infantile form; 4–10 years)
   A. Distribution: flexural areas (antecubital and popliteal fossae, neck), wrists, ankles, and feet
   B. Clusters of small erythematous or flesh-colored papules or scaling patches
   C. Dry and possibly hyperpigmented
   D. Lichenification
   E. Gooseflesh appearance to skin (Keratosis pilaris)
   F. Possibly increased number of palmar markings
   G. Possibly extra line along the lower eyelid (atopic pleat)
   H. Generalized pallor
5. Adolescent form (12 to early twenties)
   A. Distribution: face, sides of neck, hands, feet, face, and antecubital and popliteal fossae
   B. Same as childhood
   C. Dry, thick lesions (lichenified plaques) common
   D. Confluent papules
   E. Possibly weeping, crusting, and exudation: usually due to infection

Therapeutic Management

1. Prevent pruritus with antihistamines, mild soaps; and limit bathing: water should be tepid or room temperature.
2. Hydrate the skin with emollients; limit bathing.
3. Reduce inflammation with topical corticosteroids and wet compresses.
4. Prevent or control secondary infection.
5. Diet modification, if indicated.
6. Environmental controls: humidification (winter months), air conditioning (summer months); avoid contact with stuffed and fuzzy animals, cats, and dogs.
7. Avoid wearing harsh clothing (e.g., wool).

Nursing Care

ASSESSMENT

1. Perform routine physical assessment.
2. Assist with elimination diet, if indicated.

PLANNING

1. Safe, effective care environment
   A. Protect from known irritants.
2. Physiological integrity
   A. Prevent or minimize scratching.
   B. Prevent complications.
3. Psychosocial integrity
   A. Support and educate child and family.
4. Health promotion and maintenance
   A. Promote optimum health.

IMPLEMENTATION

1. Explain or reinforce explanation of condition "treatable but not curable" and treatment.
2. Keep fingernails and toenails short and clean.
3. Wrap hands in soft cotton gloves or stockings, and pin to shirt to prevent scratching.
4. Avoid overheating child.
5. Provide soothing and emollient baths or compresses as prescribed.
6. Administer antihistamines, sedatives, topical corticosteroids, and/or antibiotics as prescribed.
7. Teach family diet planning (if food sensitivity is implicated).
8. Teach family skills needed for care, including expected results of medications and their possible side effects, and environmental controls.

EVALUATION

Ensure that child:
1. Has no skin irritation.
2. Exhibits no evidence of secondary infection or trauma.
Ensure that family:
1. Demonstrates an understanding of the condition and the ability to provide care.

Seborrheic Dermatitis

Description

Seborrheic dermatitis is a chronic, recurrent, inflammatory condition of the skin with a predilection to areas well supplied with sebaceous glands.

Pathophysiology

1. Condition occurs most commonly on scalp ("cradle cap"), eyebrows, external ear canal (otitis externa), postauricular region (behind the ears), nasolabial folds, axilla, eyelids (blepharitis), inguinal region (seborrheic diaper dermatitis).
2. It is related to excessive secretion from sebaceous glands.
3. Cause is unknown.

Signs and Symptoms

1. Characterized by thick, adherent, yellowish, scaly, oily patches
2. May or may not be mildly pruritic

Therapeutic Management

1. Symptomatic treatment
2. Corticosteroid ointment for persistent rash
3. Antibiotics for infected rash

Nursing Care

ASSESSMENT

Perform routine physical assessment.

PLANNING

1. Safe, effective care environment
   A. Maintain cleanliness.
2. Physiological integrity
   A. Remove lesions.
   B. Prevent complications.
3. Psychosocial integrity
   A. Support and educate family.
4. Health promotion and maintenance
   A. Promote optimum health.
   B. Prepare family for care.

IMPLEMENTATION

1. Clean scalp (or other affected area).
2. Wash 3–4 times weekly with mild soap or shampoo.
3. Apply oil to lesion prior to shampooing; massage into scalp; allow to penetrate and soften crusts; thoroughly wash out.
4. Remove loosened crusts from hair strands with fine-toothed comb.
5. Apply any prescribed topical preparation.
6. Explain or reinforce explanation of condition and treatment, especially regarding fear of damaging "soft spot."
7. Teach family skills needed for care.

EVALUATION

1. Ensure that child is free of lesions.
2. Ensure that family demonstrates an understanding of the condition and the ability to provide care.

Acne Vulgaris

Description

Acne vulgaris is an inflammatory disease of the pilosebaceous unit.

Pathophysiology, Signs and Symptoms

1. Exact cause unknown; androgens implicated in production of lesions
2. Distribution: face, neck, shoulders, back, and upper chest
3. Noninflamed lesions: comedones
   A. Compact masses of keratin, lipids, fatty acids, and bacteria.
   B. Dilate follicular duct that may be closed (whitehead) or open (blackhead). Open lesions discolored as fatty acids are oxidized by air.
4. Inflamed lesions
   A. Dilated follicular wall ruptures to produce papules, pustules, nodules, and cysts.
   B. Description and possibility of scarring.
5. Secondary infection by *Staphylococcus albus* can complicate lesion.

Therapeutic Management

1. Prevent or reduce formation of new lesions with topical applications of benzoyl peroxide.
2. Reduce lesion formation in older adolescent females with cyclic estrogen-progesterone therapy.
3. Reduce inflammatory process and scarring with antibiotics, intralesional steroids.
4. Prepare selected patients for acne surgery (e.g., comedo extraction, cryosurgery).
5. Improve appearance.

Nursing Care

ASSESSMENT

1. Perform routine physical assessment.

PLANNING

1. Safe, effective care environment
   A. Promote cleanliness.
2. Physiological integrity
   A. Remove comedones.
   B. Reduce number of lesions.
   C. Prevent inflammation and scarring.
   D. Prevent secondary infection.
3. Psychosocial integrity
   A. Support and educate child and family.
   B. Prepare child and family for procedures.
   C. Promote a positive self-image.
4. Health promotion and maintenance
   A. Promote optimum health.
   B. Prepare child and family for care.

IMPLEMENTATION

1. Encourage child to assume responsibility for own care.
2. Teach child how to carry out prescribed regimen.
   A. Skin cleansing and hair shampooing
   B. Application of topical preparations
   C. Expression of comedones
   D. Administration of prescribed medications, including desired effects and possible side effects
3. Teach measures to reduce lesion formation.
   A. Hair styling (off forehead)
   B. Selection and application of makeup (water-based preparations)

C. Avoiding excessive scrubbing or pinching, squeezing, or otherwise manipulating lesions

D. Avoiding contact with oily substances

4. Caution against self-medication with over-the-counter preparations.
5. Emphasize importance of clean skin and hair, hands, and implements coming in contact with lesions.
6. Dispel myths related to cause and treatment of acne.
7. Allow child to express feelings.
8. Provide positive reinforcement for compliance.
9. Emphasize improved appearance, self-limited nature of disorder.
10. Caution family against nagging and/or blaming.

EVALUATION

Ensure that child:
1. Demonstrates an understanding of the condition, as does the family.
2. Complies with treatment plan, as does the family.
3. Assumes responsibility for care.
4. Shows a decrease in the number and severity of acne lesions.
5. Does not develop a secondary infection of the acne lesions.
6. Is supported emotionally by family.

Impetigo Contagiosa

Description

Impetigo contagiosa is a superficial bacterial infection of the skin.

Pathophysiology

1. Infection is caused by staphylococci, streptococci, or both.
2. It begins as discolored spots.
3. These are followed by appearance of vesicles or bullae.
4. Vesicles or bullae rupture, leaving superficial, moist erosion.
5. Germ-laden fluid spreads to surrounding skin.
6. Exudate dries to form heavy, honey-colored, seropurulent crusts and scabs.
7. Infection tends to spread peripherally.

Signs and Symptoms

1. Vesicles, bullae, and weeping crusts as described above.
2. These eruptions are most often observed on face, hands, or perineum.
3. Pruritus is common.

Therapeutic Management

1. Topical application of bactericidal ointment
2. Systemic administration of antibiotics in severe cases

Nursing Care

ASSESSMENT

1. Describe lesion accurately; examine skin for evidence of spread to other areas.
2. Assist with diagnostic procedures: exudate culture.

PLANNING

1. Safe, effective care environment
   A. Prevent spread of infection.
2. Physiological integrity
   A. Help eliminate lesions.
   B. Prevent complications.
3. Psychosocial integrity
   A. Support and educate child and family.
4. Health promotion and maintenance
   A. Promote optimum health.
   B. Prepare family for care.

IMPLEMENTATION

1. Explain or reinforce explanation of condition and treatment.
2. Practice and teach child and family careful hand washing.
3. Caution child against touching lesions to prevent spread; child should not share towels and washcloths.
4. Treat lesions.
   A. Soak crusts with warm-water compresses.
   B. Carefully remove crusts.
   C. Apply antibiotic ointment or bland emollient (e.g., petrolatum) to affected areas.
5. Administer antibiotics, if prescribed.
6. Teach family management of lesions and administration of medications.
7. Depending on geographic region, teach family to observe for signs and symptoms of acute poststreptococcal glomerulonephritis.

EVALUATION

Ensure that:
1. Child's skin is free of lesions.
2. Family demonstrates an understanding of the condition and the ability to provide care.
3. Others remain free of infection.

Thermal Burns

Description

Thermal burns are injuries to tissues caused by application of excessive heat to skin.

Pathophysiology

1. Physiological response directly related to amount of tissue destroyed
2. Extent of injury: expressed as percentage of body surface area involved; varies according to size of child
3. Depth of injury
   A. Superficial (first-degree): involves epidermis, heals without scarring
   B. Partial-thickness (second-degree): involves epidermis and variable portion of corneum (superficial or deep)
      (1) Superficial: heals uneventfully
      (2) Deep: may convert to full-thickness injury
   C. Full-thickness (third-degree): involves all layers of the skin
      (1) Usually combined with extensive partial-thickness damage

      (2) Results in scarring

      (3) May include subcutaneous muscle and bone

4. Severity of injury

  A. Minor burns

      (1) Full-thickness and partial-thickness burns of less than 10% of body surface.

      (2) No other significant injuries.

      (3) Child is 2 years or older.

      (4) Burns do not include hands, feet, face, perineum, or circumferential areas.

  B. Major burns

      (1) Burns complicated by respiratory tract injury

      (2) Burns of face, hands, feet, genitalia, and circumferential areas

      (3) Full-thickness burns of 10% of body surface or greater

      (4) Any child younger than 10 years of age

      (5) Electrical burns that penetrate

      (6) Deep chemical burns

      (7) Burns complicated by fractures or soft tissue injury

      (8) Burns complicated by concurrent illness (e.g., obesity, diabetes, epilepsy, cardiac or renal disorders)

5. Local responses

  A. Edema formation

  B. Fluid electrolyte and protein loss

  C. Circulatory stasis

6. Systemic responses

  A. Circulatory

  B. Anemia from heat-damaged red blood cells (RBCs) at burn site

7. Healing

  A. Superficial burns: Damaged epithelium peels off in small scales or sheets, in 5–10 days, leaving no scarring.

  B. Partial-thickness burns: Crust forms in 3–5 days; healing takes place from underneath.

  C. Deep dermal burns (deep partial-thickness, full-thickness): healing is slow; thin epithelial covering forms in 25–35 days; scarring common.

8. Systemic effects of severe burns

  A. Asphyxia from irritation and edema of lungs and respiratory passages

  B. Shock from fluid and protein loss from denuded skin, edema from increased capillary permeability and vasodilation at burn site, diminished intravascular colloidal osmotic pressure (greatest hazard first 48–72 hours)

  C. Renal shutdown from shock and hemolysis

  D. Potassium excess from tissue breakdown, renal retention

  E. Anemia from direct-heat destruction of RBCs, hemolysis of heat-damaged RBCs, depressed bone marrow

  F. Massive protein loss from burn wound, gluconeogenesis

  G. Accelerated metabolism to maintain body heat and provide for increased energy needs of the body

  H. Neuroendocrine system stimulation

  I. Metabolic acidosis of variable degree

  J. Reduced blood flow to GI tract causing paralytic ileus

Signs and Symptoms

1. Superficial (first-degree) burns

  A. Dry, red surface

  B. Blanches on pressure and refills

  C. Painful

2. Partial-thickness (second-degree) burns

  A. Blistered, moist

  B. Mottled pink or red

  C. Red, blanches on pressure and refills

  D. Very painful

3. Full-thickness (third-degree) burns

  A. Tough, leathery

  B. Dull, dry surface

  C. Brown, tan, red, or black

  D. Does not blanch on pressure

  E. Little pain, but surrounded by painful partial-thickness burns

Therapeutic Management

1. Minor burns

  A. Cleanse and debride wound.

  B. Cover with dry or medicated dressing.

  C. Administer analgesics.

2. Major burns: general care

  A. Hospitalize.

  B. Establish adequate airway and treat pulmonary injuries, complications.

  C. Replace and maintain IV fluids and electrolytes.

      (1) Colloid: albumin, plasma, dextran, etc., and/or

      (2) Crystalloid fluids: Ringer's lactate

  D. Prevent and treat complications.

  E. Provide high-calorie, high-protein diet.

  F. Give the following drugs:

      (1) Morphine sulfate to relieve pain

      (2) Zinc and vitamin A preparations to promote epithelial growth

      (3) Prophylactic antibiotics (controversial)

      (4) Tetanus toxoid (based on immunization history)

3. Wound management

  A. Debride devitalized tissue: hydrotherapy, hosing, surgical, enzymatic.

  B. Apply topical antimicrobial therapy.

  C. Cover: temporary dressing (gauze, homografts, heterografts).

  D. Prepare for skin graft.

      (1) Autografting

      (2) Cultured epithelial autografts

4. Prevent deformity with splinting, compression garments.

Nursing Care

ASSESSMENT

1. Assess respiratory status.

2. Help assess burn injury.

3. Obtain a history of burn injury, especially time of injury, nature of burning agent, duration of contact, whether in enclosed area, any medications given.

4. Obtain pertinent history, especially preburn weight, preexisting illnesses, allergies.

5. Assess pain.

6. Check eyes for evidence of injury or irritation.

7. Observe for signs of respiratory distress.

8. Check nasopharynx for edema or redness.

9. Monitor vital signs frequently.

10. Weight on admission and daily or as prescribed.
11. Measure intake and output.
12. Assess circulation to areas peripheral or distal to burns.
13. Assess level of consciousness.
14. Observe for signs of altered behavior or sensorium.
15. Observe for signs of impending overhydration.
16. Observe wound for evidence of healing, stability of temporary cover or graft, infection.
17. Observe for evidence of complications: pneumonia, wound sepsis (greatest hazard after shock phase), Curling's (stress) stomach ulceration, CNS dysfunction (hallucinations, personality change, delirium, seizures), hypertension.
18. Assess child's level of pain and emotional state.
19. Assess family's coping.
20. Assist with diagnostic tests: CBC, urinalysis, wound cultures, hematocrit.

PLANNING

1. Safe, effective care environment
   A. See Nursing Care of the Ill Child, pp. 97–98.
   B. Prevent heat loss.
   C. Prevent infection and trauma.
2. Physiological integrity
   A. Relieve pain.
   B. Facilitate wound healing.
   C. Preserve graft site.
   D. Provide nutrition.
   E. Prevent complications.
3. Psychosocial integrity
   A. See Nursing Care of the Ill Child, pp. 97–98.
   B. Promote positive self-image.
4. Health promotion and maintenance
   A. Promote good health practices.
   B. Prepare family for home care.

IMPLEMENTATION

1. Monitor respiratory status; provide pulmonary hygiene; assess response to O_2 therapy.
2. Monitor hydration status: hypovolemia, hypervolemia.
3. Monitor intake and output and administration of IV fluids.
4. Place in protective environment according to unit policy.
   A. Prevent contact with infected persons or objects.
   B. Administer good oral hygiene.
5. Maintain environmental temperature to prevent heat loss or place under heat source.
6. Administer analgesics for pain as prescribed.
7. Administer antibiotics as prescribed.
8. Administer tetanus toxoid (or antitoxin), if prescribed.
9. Maintain meticulous medical and surgical asepsis; monitor for signs and symptoms of wound infection, sepsis.
10. Carry out wound care as prescribed.
    A. Avoid injury to crusts and eschar.
    B. Keep child from scratching and picking at wound.
    C. Provide distraction, reasoning (older child).
    D. Restrain infant or younger child as needed.
    E. Position for minimal disturbance of grafted area.
11. Promote appetite by:
    A. Providing highly nutritious meals and snacks
    B. Giving extra calories and protein
    C. Providing attractive meals, preferred foods, companionship during meals
    D. Encouraging self-care

E. Encouraging oral feedings but feeding via other means if necessary: nasogastric tube, hyperalimentation.
F. Administering supplementary vitamins and minerals as prescribed.
12. Administer antacids as prescribed.
13. Carry out active or passive range-of-motion exercises.
14. Encourage mobility of affected area (if it does not disturb graft) and unaffected areas.
15. Have child ambulate as soon as feasible.
16. Encourage and promote self-help activities appropriate to abilities and developmental level.
17. Position in functional attitude for minimum deformity.
18. Apply splints as ordered and designed.
19. Wrap healing tissue with elastic bandage or dress in elastic garments as ordered
20. Convey a positive attitude toward child.
21. Provide reinforcement for positive aspects of appearance and capabilities.
22. Explore child's and family's feeling regarding altered physical appearance.
    A. Discuss aids that camouflage any disfigurement.
    B. Refer to appropriate community supports.
23. Promote positive thinking in child.
24. Encourage continuing schooling.
25. Encourage peer contact.
26. Explain or reinforce explanation of condition and treatment.
27. Teach family skills needed for home care, including wound care, rehabilitation, diet planning, administration of medication (if needed), and diet supplements.
28. Help family set realistic goals for themselves and the child.

EVALUATION

Ensure that child:
1. Exhibits little or no evidence of pain.
2. Has wound healing with minimal disfigurement.
3. Develops no complications.
4. Exhibits a positive attitude toward changed body image.
5. Adheres to rehabilitative efforts, as does the family.

Communicable Diseases

Chickenpox

Description

Chickenpox is a disease characterized by crops of pruritic, vesicular skin eruptions, with few systemic symptoms.

Pathophysiology

1. Highly contagious infection with varicella-zoster virus
2. Source of infection: respiratory tract secretions
3. Mode of transmission: direct contact, droplet spread, and contaminated objects
4. Incubation period: usually 10–21 days
5. Period of communicability 1–2 days before onset of rash to 5 days after crusting of lesions

Signs and Symptoms

1. Slight fever
2. Malaise

3. Anorexia
4. Highly pruritic rash
   A. Lesions: papules, vesicles, and crusts present in varying degrees at any time
   B. Distribution: torso, spreading to face and extremities

Therapeutic Management

1. Symptomatic
2. Aspirin administration: contraindicated because of association with Reye's syndrome

Nursing Care

ASSESSMENT

1. Perform routine physical assessment.
2. Pay particular attention to type and configuration of lesions.

PLANNING

1. Safe, effective care environment
   A. See Nursing Care of the Ill Child, pp. 97–98.
   B. Prevent spread of infection.
2. Physiological integrity
   A. Prevent development of secondary infection of lesions.
3. Psychosocial integrity
   A. See Nursing Care of the Ill Child, pp. 97–98.
4. Health promotion and maintenance
   A. Teach good health practices.

IMPLEMENTATION

1. Isolate infected child and his secretions from others.
2. Implement hospital policy for hospitalized child.
3. Administer soothing lotion (e.g., calamine) to pruritic areas.
4. Prevent scratching.
   A. Keep skin clean.
   B. Keep child's fingernails short.
   C. Apply mittens or elbow restraints, if necessary.
   D. Explain the danger of secondary infection and scarring to older children.
   E. Suggest applying pressure to areas to relieve discomfort.
5. Keep child occupied with diversionary activities.
6. Teach family skills needed for home care, including preventing spread of infection.

EVALUATION

1. Ensure that child makes an uneventful recovery with minimal or no scarring.
2. Ensure that others remain free of infection.

Diphtheria

Description

Diptheria is an infectious disease characterized by the production of a systemic toxin and the formation of a pseudomembrane on the pharyngeal mucosa, often with obstructive laryngotracheitis.

Pathophysiology

1. Infection with the bacterium *Corynebacterium diphtheriae*.
2. Exotoxin can produce toxemia, shock, and life-threatening cardiac and neurological complications.

3. Source of infection: nasopharyngeal secretions, skin, eye, and lesions of affected person.
4. Incubation period: 2–5 days or occasionally longer.
5. Period of communicability: until bacilli are no longer pres-ent, usually 2 weeks; occasionally it can persist for several months if untreated.

Signs and Symptoms

1. Nasal: resembles common cold
2. Pharyngeal
   A. Anorexia
   B. Malaise
   C. Fever
   D. Smooth, adherent white or gray membrane on mucous membrane
   E. Lymphadenitis ("bull's neck")
3. Laryngeal
   A. Fever
   B. Hoarseness
   C. Cough
   D. Possibly signs of airway obstruction

Therapeutic Management

1. Administer antitoxin.
2. Administer antibiotics.
3. Place hospitalized patients in isolation.
4. Provide complete bed rest.
5. Place tracheostomy for airway obstruction.
6. Treat symptomatic treatment of shock.
7. Treat infected contacts and carriers.

Nursing Care

ASSESSMENT

1. Perform routine physical assessment.
2. Observe for evidence of respiratory obstruction.
3. Assist with diagnostic procedures: nose, throat culture, and any lesions and sensitivity testing.

PLANNING

1. Safe, effective care environment
   A. See Nursing Care of the Ill Child, pp. 97–98.
   B. Prevent spread of infection.
2. Physiological integrity
   A. Help eradicate organisms.
   B. Prevent complications.
3. Psychosocial integrity
   A. See Nursing Care of the Ill Child, pp. 97–98.
4. Health promotion and maintenance
   A. Promote good health practices.
   B. Encourage immunization of susceptible persons.

IMPLEMENTATION

1. Maintain strict isolation according to hospital policy.
2. Immunize susceptible individuals.
3. Administer antibiotics and antitoxin as prescribed.
   A. Participate in sensitivity testing; have emergency equipment (tracheostomy set, epinephrine) readily available in the event of a reaction.

4. Provide total care to promote rest and to prevent cardiac complications.
5. Administer humidified O_2, etc., as prescribed.
6. Teach family skills needed for home care, including preventing spread of infection.

EVALUATION

Ensure that child:
1. Exhibits no evidence of complications.
2. Recovers uneventfully.

Ensure that others:
1. Remain free of infection.

Infectious Mononucleosis

Description

Infectious mononucleosis is an acute self-limiting, contagious disease presumed to be of viral origin.

Pathophysiology

1. Mildly contagious disease caused by Epstein-Barr virus
2. Source: oral secretions
3. Mode of transmission: direct intimate contact with oral secretions
4. Incubation period: approximately 30–50 days

Signs and Symptoms

1. Headache
2. Malaise
3. Fatigue
4. Fever
5. Loss of appetite
6. Sore throat
7. Cervical adenopathy
8. Splenomegaly
9. Palatine petechiae
10. Macular eruption (especially on trunk)
11. Exudative pharyngitis
12. Some hepatic involvement
13. CNS involvement; aseptic meningitis, encephalitis, and Guillain-Barré syndrome

Therapeutic Management

1. Supportive treatment
   A. Analgesic (acetaminophen) for headache, fever, malaise
   B. Gargles, hot drinks, analgesic troches for sore throat
2. Steroids for tonsillar swelling and other lymphadenopathy (not for routine cases)
3. Bed rest for fatigue
4. Regulate activities according to tolerance

Nursing Care

ASSESSMENT

1. Perform routine physical assessment.
2. Assist with diagnostic procedures: CBC, heterophil antibody test, enzyme immunoassay test, Monospot.

PLANNING

1. Safe, effective care environment
   A. See Nursing Care of the Ill Child, pp. 97–98.
2. Physiological integrity
   A. Provide comfort.
   B. Prevent secondary infection.
3. Psychosocial integrity
   A. See Nursing Care of the Ill Child, pp. 97–98.
   B. Support and educate child and family.
4. Health promotion and maintenance
   A. Promote optimum health.
   B. Prepare family for home care.

IMPLEMENTATION

1. Provide comfort measures (e.g., analgesics, gargles, etc.).
2. Explain or reinforce explanation of condition and treatment.
3. Help child and family determine appropriate activities according to symptoms and interests.
4. Allow child to express feelings of depression and resentment related to lengthy convalescence, fatigue, and restriction of activities.

EVALUATION

Ensure that child:
1. Complies with therapy, as does the family.
2. Verbalizes feelings and concerns.

Ensure that family:
1. Demonstrates an understanding of the disease.

Measles (Rubeola)

Description

Measles (rubeola) is an acute, highly contagious disease involving the respiratory tract and characterized by a confluent maculopapular rash.

Pathophysiology

1. Highly contagious infection with RNA virus
2. Source of infection: respiratory tract secretions
3. Mode of transmission: direct contact with infectious droplets
4. Incubation period: 14–21 days
5. Period of communicability: from 4 days before to 5 days after appearance of rash
6. Complications: otitis media, bronchopneumonia, encephalitis

Signs and Symptoms

1. Prodromal (catarrhal) stage
   A. Fever and malaise
   B. Coryza, cough, conjunctivitis
   C. Small, irregular red (Koplik's) spots on buccal mucosa opposite molars
2. Rash: appears 3–4 days after onset of prodromal stage
   A. Begins as erythematous maculopapular eruption on face
   B. Gradually spreads downward
3. Photophobia (often)
4. Anorexia
5. Generalized lymphadenopathy

Therapeutic Management

1. Supportive
2. Acetaminophen for fever and discomfort
3. Prophylactic antibiotics

Nursing Care

ASSESSMENT

1. Perform routine physical assessment.

PLANNING

1. Safe, effective care environment
   A. See Nursing Care of the Ill Child, pp. 97–98.
   B. Reduce irritating environmental stimuli.
   C. Prevent spread of infection.
2. Physiological integrity
   A. Promote comfort
   B. Prevent complications
3. Psychosocial integrity
   A. See Nursing Care of the Ill Child, pp. 97–98.
4. Health promotion and maintenance
   A. Promote good health practices.
   B. Prepare family for home care.

IMPLEMENTATION

1. Isolate as appropriate and according to hospital policy.
2. Immunize susceptible individuals.
3. Maintain bed rest and provide quiet activity.
4. Dim light in room if child is photophobic.
5. Administer acetaminophen as prescribed.
6. Avoid chilling.
7. Cleanse eyelids with warm saline to remove secretions and crusts.
8. Encourage fluids and soft, bland foods.
9. Explain or reinforce explanation of condition and treatment.
10. Teach family skills needed for home care, including preventing spread of infection.

EVALUATION

Ensure that child:
1. Exhibits no evidence of discomfort.
2. Recovers without complications.
Ensure that others:
1. Remain free of infection.

Mumps

Description

Mumps is an acute infectious disease characterized by swelling of the salivary glands.

Pathophysiology

1. Highly contagious infection with paramyxovirus
2. Source of infection: saliva of infected persons
3. Mode of transmission: direct contact or droplet spread
4. Incubation period: 16–18 days; but may occur 12–25 days
5. Period of communicability: 7 days prior to swelling to 9 days after onset of gland swelling
6. Unilateral or bilateral involvement of the parotid glands chiefly

7. Complications: orchitis (postpubertal males), arthritis, renal involvement

Signs and Symptoms

1. Prodromal stage: 24 hours
   A. Fever
   B. Headache
   C. Malaise
   D. Anorexia
2. Parotid gland enlarges to maximum size in 1–3 days
3. Accompanied by pain and tenderness
4. May involve submaxillary and sublingual glands

Therapeutic Management

1. Primarily supportive
2. Respiratory isolation advised

Nursing Care

ASSESSMENT

1. Perform routine physical assessment.
2. Assist with diagnostic tests: culture from throat washings, urine, or spinal fluid; viral studies.

PLANNING

1. Safe, effective care environment
   A. See Nursing Care of the Ill Child, pp. 97–98.
   B. Prevent spread of infection.
2. Physiological integrity
   A. Promote comfort.
   B. Prevent complications.
3. Psychosocial integrity
   A. See Nursing Care of the Ill Child, pp. 97–98.
4. Health promotion and maintenance
   A. Promote good health practices.
   B. Prepare family for home care.

IMPLEMENTATION

1. Institute respiratory or other precautions during hospitalization.
2. Avoid contact with susceptible individuals.
3. Offer easily swallowed bland foods; avoid foods that stimulate salivation.
4. Administer analgesics for discomfort.
5. Apply warm or cool compresses to area of neck swelling.
6. Encourage quiet play and nonstrenuous activity, especially for postpubescent males.
7. Explain or reinforce explanation of condition and treatment.
8. Teach family skills needed for home care, including preventing spread of infection.

EVALUATION

1. Ensure that child recovers without complications.
2. Ensure that others remain free of infection.

Pertussis (Whooping Cough)

Description

Pertussis (whooping cough) is an acute, highly contagious respiratory disease characterized by a paroxysmal cough that ends with a loud whooping inspiration.

Pathophysiology

1. Highly contagious infection with the bacillus Bordetella pertussis
2. Source of infection: respiratory tract
3. Transmission: direct contact, droplet spread, freshly contaminated articles
4. Incubation period: 6–20 days, rarely more than 2 weeks
5. Period of communicability: highest during catarrhal stage; risk diminishes rapidly but lasts up to 3 weeks

Signs and Symptoms

1. Catarrhal stage
   A. Coryza
   B. Sneezing
   C. Lacrimation
   D. Cough
   E. Low-grade fever
2. Paroxysmal stage
   A. Frequent attacks
   B. Cough: becomes paroxysmal after 1–2 weeks
      (1) Series of short, rapid bursts during exhalation.
      (2) These are followed by characteristic "whoop": hurried, deep inhalation with a high-pitched crowing sound.
      (3) In infants, whoop can be absent; apnea common.
   C. During attack
      (1) Marked facial redness or cyanosis, vein distention
      (2) Eyes may bulge
      (3) Tongue may protrude
   D. Large amounts of viscous mucus may be expelled during or after paroxysm
   E. Vomiting frequently follows coughing
   F. Stage lasting 4–6 weeks

Therapeutic Management

1. Hospitalization of infants and children with potentially severe disease.
2. Supportive care.
3. Antimicrobials during catarrhal stage may ameliorate symptoms.

Nursing Care

ASSESSMENT

1. Perform routine physical assessment.
2. Observe coughing.
3. Observe for signs of airway obstruction.
4. Assist with diagnostic procedures: throat culture, WBC count, direct immunofluorescence to nasal secretions, enzyme-linked immunosorbent assay.

PLANNING

1. Safe, effective care environment
   A. See Nursing Care of the Ill Child, pp. 97–98.
   B. Reduce or eliminate factors that precipitate coughing.
   C. Prevent spread of infection.
2. Physiological integrity
   A. Reduce coughing.
   B. Ease upper respiratory symptoms.
3. Psychosocial integrity
   A. See Nursing Care of the Ill Child, pp. 97–98.
   B. Reassure child and family during coughing episodes.
4. Health promotion and maintenance
   A. Promote good health practices.
   B. Prepare family for home care.

IMPLEMENTATION

1. Isolate hospitalized child according to hospital policy; intensive-care unit admission may be necessary for severe cases.
2. Avoid contact with nonimmunized children.
3. Immunize susceptible persons.
4. Administer antibiotics as prescribed.
5. Reduce factors that precipitate coughing.
   A. Keep room well ventilated.
   B. Keep environment smoke- and dust-free.
   C. Avoid extremes of temperature or chilling.
   D. Avoid undue excitement or physical activity.
6. Provide comfort measures to prevent distress.
7. Maintain child in mist tent with high humidity.
8. Encourage fluid intake.
9. Refeed if child vomits.
10. Explain or reinforce explanation of condition and treatment.
11. Teach family skills needed for home care, including preventing spread of infection.

EVALUATION

Ensure that child:
1. Exhibits minimal coughing.
2. Recovers without complications.
Ensure that others:
1. Remain free of infection.

Rubella (German Measles)

Description

Rubella (German measles) is a mild contagious disease characterized by maculopapular rash, postauricular and suboccipital lymphadenopathy, and slight fever.

Pathophysiology

1. Contagious infection with RNA virus
2. Source of infection: nasogastric secretions
3. Mode of transmission: direct contact
4. Incubation period: 14–21 days, usually 16–18 days
5. Period of communicability: 10 days before to 15 days after appearance of rash

Signs and Symptoms

1. Postnatal
   A. Low-grade fever, malaise, headache
   B. Lymphadenopathy
   C. Rash
      (1) Pinkish red maculopapular
      (2) Appears on face initially
      (3) Spreads downward to neck, trunk, and extremities
      (4) Disappears in 3 days in same order as it began
   D. Transient polyarthralgia and polyarthritis

2. Congenital rubella syndrome
   A. Ophthalmological defects: cataracts, microphthalmia, glaucoma, chorioretinitis
   B. Cardiac anomalies: patent ductus arteriosus, atrial septal defect, or ventricular septal defect
   C. Sensorineural deafness
   D. Neurological defects: microcephaly, meningoencephalitis, mental retardation
   E. Growth retardation
   F. Hepatosplenomegaly
   G. Jaundice
   H. Thrombocytopenia
   I. Purpuric skin lesions ("blue-muffin" appearance)

Therapeutic Management

1. Supportive care

Nursing Care

ASSESSMENT

1. Perform routine physical assessment.
2. Assist with diagnostic tests: serological tests; throat, blood, urine, or spinal fluid culture; specific IgM antibody titer

PLANNING

1. Safe, effective care environment
   A. See Nursing Care of the Ill Child, pp. 97–98.
   B. Prevent spread of infection.
   C. Prevent prenatal disease.
2. Physiological integrity
   A. Provide comfort measures.
3. Psychosocial integrity
   A. See Nursing Care of the Ill Child, pp. 97–98.
4. Health promotion and maintenance
   A. Promote good health practices.
   B. Prepare family for home care.

IMPLEMENTATION

1. Immunize susceptible persons.
2. Prevent contact of infected child with pregnant women.
3. Administer acetaminophen for discomfort.
4. Teach family skills needed for home care, including preventing spread of infection.

EVALUATION

1. Ensure that child recovers without complications.
2. Ensure that others remain free of infection.

Scarlet Fever

Description

Scarlet fever is an acute infectious disease of childhood characterized by sore throat, fever, and enlarged lymph nodes.

Pathophysiology

1. Contagious infection with group A β-hemolytic streptococci
2. Source of infection: nasopharyngeal secretions
3. Mode of transmission: direct contact or droplet spread, freshly contaminated articles

4. Incubation period: 1–7 days (usually 3 days)
5. Period of communicability: acute stage to 36 hours after antimicrobial therapy
6. Complications: otitis media, peritonsillar abscess, sinusitis, rheumatic fever, glomerulonephritis

Signs and Symptoms

1. Prodromal stage
   A. Abrupt high fever
   B. Pulse increased out of proportion to fever
   C. Chills, malaise, headache
   D. Vomiting, abdominal pain
2. Enanthema
   A. Tonsils: red, enlarged, edematous, and covered with patches of exudate
   B. Tongue: red, swollen, coated with papillae ("white strawberry tongue"); white coat sloughs off, leaving prominent papillae ("red strawberry tongue")
3. Exanthema
   A. Exanthema appears within 12 hours after prodromal signs.
   B. Red, pinhead-sized punctate lesions.
   C. Generalized except for face.
   D. Face flushed.
   E. Desquamation begins at end of first week; usually complete by 3 weeks.

Therapeutic Management

1. Full course of penicillin
2. Supportive measures during febrile phase
3. If hospitalized, isolation for 24 hours until initiation of therapy

Nursing Care

ASSESSMENT

1. Perform routine physical assessment.
2. Assist with diagnostic tests: throat culture.

PLANNING

1. Safe, effective care environment
   A. See Nursing Care of the Ill Child, pp. 97–98.
   B. Prevent spread of infection.
2. Physiological integrity
   A. Promote comfort.
   B. Prevent complications.
3. Psychosocial integrity
   A. See Nursing Care of the Ill Child, pp. 97–98.
4. Health promotion and maintenance
   A. Promote good health practices.
   B. Prepare family for home care.

IMPLEMENTATION

1. Explain or reinforce explanation of condition and treatment.
2. Administer penicillin as prescribed.
3. Promote rest during febrile phase.
4. Administer acetaminophen for sore throat.
5. Teach family skills needed for home care, including preventing spread of infection.
6. Emphasize importance of adherence to penicillin regimen.

EVALUATION

1. Ensure that child recovers without complications.
2. Ensure that others remain free of infection.

Psychosocial Disorders

Failure to Thrive

Description

Failure to thrive (FTT) is deviation from the established growth pattern in a child younger than 3 years of age.
1. Organic FTT: growth failure due to major illness
2. Nonorganic FTT: presence of growth retardation in the absence of organic dysfunction
3. Mixed FTT: combination of organic and nonorganic FTT factors (e.g., child with congenital anomaly who does not feed well living in a high-risk family environment)

Pathophysiology

Causes:
1. Organic FTT: involves principally neurological and GI dysfunction; also includes endocrine, cardiac, or renal dysfunction, inborn errors of metabolism
2. Nonorganic FTT: involves a complexity of constitutional and environmental factors that affect the caregivers, infant, and their relationship (e.g., well-intentioned but uneducated parents, parent psychopathology; poverty [debatable, but principal cause worldwide]; fussy, irritable infant)

Signs and Symptoms

1. Growth failure
   A. A weight that is persistently below the 3rd percentile or 2 standard deviations below the mean on standard growth charts
   B. Developmental delay
   C. Hypotonia, decreased muscle mass
   D. Generalized weakness
   E. Abdominal distention
2. Nonorganic
   A. Apathy
   B. Withdrawal behavior
   C. Feeding or eating dysfunction
   D. No fear of strangers (at age when stranger anxiety is expected)
   E. Avoidance of eye-to-eye contact
   F. Wide-eyed gaze and continual scan of the environment
   G. Stiff and unyielding or flaccid and unresponsive
   H. Minimum smiling
   I. Lack of attachment to parents

Therapeutic Management

1. Organic: determine and treat cause
2. Nonorganic: hospitalize for feeding trial and observation
   A. Home treatment
      (1) Implement feeding program.
      (2) Implement infant stimulation program.
      (3) Provide for stress-relieving services for family.
      (4) Provide for mental health (individual or group counseling).
      (5) Conscientious interdisciplinary follow-up.
   B. Termination of parental rights, if necessary

Nursing Care

ASSESSMENT

1. Perform routine physical assessment.
2. Assess feeding behaviors, temperament, parent-child interaction.
3. Obtain detailed history.
4. Assess family functioning including communication and for marital stress, physical or mental illness, death or illness in a previous child, alcoholism, drug use, financial crisis.
5. Assist with diagnostic procedures.

PLANNING

1. Safe, effective care environment
   A. See Nursing Care of the Ill Child, pp. 97–98.
   B. Provide a nurturing environment for child.
2. Physiological integrity
   A. Plan a feeding program that encourages an adequate caloric intake.
   B. Implement care plan for specific organic disorder (if identified).
3. Psychosocial integrity
   A. See Nursing Care of the Ill Child, pp. 97–98.
   B. Promote a trusting relationship.
   C. Provide appropriate infant stimulation.
   D. Provide nurturing environment for family.
   E. Foster parental self-esteem.
4. Health promotion and maintenance
   A. Promote optimum health.
   B. Achieve and maintain optimum nutrition.
   C. Prepare family for home care.

IMPLEMENTATION

1. Coordinate team plan for care of the child.
2. Provide quiet environment.
3. Maintain structured routine in care.
4. Provide continuity of nursing personnel for care.
5. Monitor stool output.
6. Weigh child daily; monitor fluid intake and output.
7. Implement feeding program.
   A. Provide unlimited feeding of diet for age.
   B. Avoid interruptions of feedings (e.g., laboratory studies, radiological tests, examinations).
   C. Ensure that feeders remain calm, relaxed during feeding.
   D. Follow child's rhythm during feeding.
   E. Persist in the face of protest or other refusal behavior, if exhibited by child.
   F. Maintain accurate record of intake.
8. Provide eye-to-eye contact during care.
9. Praise child for desired behavior.
10. Provide sensory stimulation: tactile, visual, and auditory, appropriate to child's developmental level.
11. Provide nurturing environment for family.
12. Teach family about child's physical care, developmental skills, emotional needs.

13. Serve as role model in child's care.
14. Afford family the opportunity to discuss feelings and concerns.
15. Provide emotional nurturance without encouraging dependency.
16. Build family's self-esteem with praise for positive behaviors and achievements.
17. Prepare for home care.
    A. Continue teaching skills needed for care.
    B. Provide for continued infant stimulation program.
    C. Provide for a consistent contact system.
    D. Refer to services that provide ongoing care and stress-relieving services.
    E. Initiate community referral for financial assistance, mental health, or other needs.
18. Help arrange for alternative placement of child, if indicated.

EVALUATION

Ensure that infant:
1. Attains and maintains desired weight.
2. Exhibits expected developmental accomplishments.

Ensure that family:
1. Demonstrates an understanding of the condition and the ability to provide home care.
2. Exhibits nurturing behaviors toward infant.

Child Maltreatment

Description

Child maltreatment is a term used for intentional physical abuse or neglect, emotional abuse, or sexual abuse of children.
1. Physical abuse (battered child syndrome): deliberate infliction of physical abuse on a child
2. Physical neglect: deprivation of necessities
3. Psychological maltreatment; failure to meet the child's need for affection, attention, and emotional nurturance
4. Sexual abuse: contacts or interactions between child and an adult when the child is being used for the sexual stimulation of that adult or another adult

Pathophysiology

1. Characteristics of child
   A. Usually one child singled out for abuse.
   B. Temperament does not "fit" with caregiver(s).
   C. Child is viewed as difficult or different.
   D. Child reminds caregiver of an unliked person in his or her life.
   E. Often prematurely born child.
   F. Illegitimate or unwanted child.
   G. Child is seriously or chronically ill.
2. Characteristics of parents
   A. Often a history of abuse as a child.
   B. Difficulty in controlling aggressive impulses.
   C. Free expression of violence.
   D. Low self-esteem.
   E. Inadequate understanding of normal growth and development; expectations beyond capabilities of the child.
   F. Role reversal: Parent(s) expect child to be nurturer.
   G. Parents live in social isolation.
   H. Parents do not seek support or assistance from others.

3. Situational characteristics
   A. Environment of chronic stress; unhealthy interpersonal relationships, financial hardship, unemployment, alcoholism, drug addiction, poor housing
   B. No adequate support systems

Signs and Symptoms

1. Physical evidence of abuse and/or neglect
   A. Soft tissue injuries: ecchymoses, hematomas, abrasions, contusions
   B. Traumatic bruises in varying stages of healing, often in shape of a familiar object (belt buckle, utensil, rope burn, or handprint)
   C. Burns: especially symmetrical burns of buttocks, genitalia, legs, or hands; round "dug out" craters (cigarette burns)
   D. Bites, hair loss
   E. Fractures
   F. Drug intoxication
2. Physical neglect
   A. Evidence of noncare; child dirty, ill-fed, and poorly clothed
   B. Evidence of lack of stimulation
   C. Family scapegoat
   D. Unrealistic expectations of child
   E. Suicide attempts
   F. Sleep disorders
3. Sexual abuse
   A. Injuries in genital area
   B. Torn, stained, or bloody underclothing
   C. Evidence of sexually transmitted disease
   D. Pain, discharge from genitals
   E. Withdrawal
   F. Sudden changes in behavior (e.g., anxiety, clinging behavior, loss or gain in weight)
   G. Regressive behaviors
   H. Phobias or fears (e.g., of the dark, men, strangers, particular settings or situations [undue fear of leaving the house for other locations])
   I. Personality changes (e.g., depression, hostility, aggression)
   J. Declining school performance
   K. Suicide attempts
   L. Substance abuse
   M. Inappropriate sexual play, activity
   N. Psychosomatic complaints

Therapeutic Management

1. Protect from further abuse.
2. Treat injuries.
3. Provide nurturing environment.

Nursing Care

ASSESSMENT

1. Perform routine physical assessment.
2. Describe any physical injury.
3. Assess emotional state and evaluate behaviors.
4. Observe parent-child interaction.
5. Identify family strengths and possible support systems.
6. Assist with diagnostic procedures and provide support.

PLANNING

See also Failure to Thrive, pp. 157–158.
1. Safe, effective care environment
   A. Remove child from abusive situation.
2. Physiological integrity
   A. Promote healing of physical injuries.
   B. Prevent complications.
3. Psychosocial integrity
   A. See Nursing Care of the Ill Child, pp. 97–98.
   B. Promote non-threatening, nurturing environment.
   C. Support and educate family.
4. Health promotion and maintenance
   A. Promote optimum health.
   B. Prepare family for home care.
   C. Prevent reoccurrence of abuse.

IMPLEMENTATION

1. Establish protective measures for child as indicated.
2. Report suspected abuse to proper authorities.
3. Keep factual, objective records.
4. See Failure to Thrive, pp. 157–158.
5. Teach family about normal growth and developmental patterns and appropriate expectations for age.
6. Help family accept parenting role.
7. Provide anticipatory guidance.
8. Refer to appropriate community services in an effort to reduce family stresses.
9. Promote family strengths.
10. Help child and new caregivers adjust in situations where family are denied custody.

EVALUATION

Ensure that child:
1. Is free of injury.
2. Exhibits appropriate behavior for developmental level.
3. Exhibits minimal or no evidence of distress.
4. Accepts foster family.
Ensure that family:
1. Demonstrates the ability to provide safe home care.

Anorexia Nervosa

Description

Anorexia nervosa is a disorder characterized by severe weight loss in the absence of obvious physical cause; individuals do not lack hunger but deny its existence.

Pathophysiology

1. A relentless pursuit of thinness and fear of fatness
2. Weight loss usually triggered by a typical adolescent crisis
3. Exaggerated misinterpretation of normal fat deposition of early adolescence
4. In girls, absence of at least three consecutive menstrual cycles

Signs and Symptoms

1. Severe and profound weight loss
2. Signs of altered metabolic activity
   A. Secondary amenorrhea (if menarche attained)
   B. Primary amenorrhea (if menarche not attained)
   C. Bradycardia

D. Lowered body temperature
E. Decreased blood pressure
F. Cold intolerance
G. Dry skin and brittle nails
H. Appearance of lanugo hair
I. Constipation
J. Dependent edema

Therapeutic Management

1. Treat life-threatening malnutrition.
   A. May require IV and tube feeding
2. Promote eating through psychological treatment (e.g., operant conditioning with positive reinforcement).
3. Resolve psychological disorganization.

Nursing Care

ASSESSMENT

1. Perform routine physical and psychosocial assessment.
2. Obtain history of eating behaviors.
3. Assess family interpersonal relationships.
4. Assist with diagnostic procedures.

PLANNING

1. Safe, effective care environment
   A. Provide supportive but firm environment.
2. Physiological integrity
   A. Restore nutritional status.
   B. Reduce energy expenditure.
   C. Alter distorted body image.
3. Psychosocial integrity
   A. Enforce therapeutic plan of care (if implemented).
   B. Support and educate child and family.
   C. Allow patient an appropriate feeling of control.
4. Health promotion and maintenance
   A. Promote optimum health.
   B. Achieve and maintain optimum nutrition.
   C. Prepare family for home care.

IMPLEMENTATION

1. Explain nutritional plan to child and family.
2. Select, with dietitian and child, a balanced diet with incremental increase in calories.
3. Help child prepare a dietary diary.
4. Implement high-calorie diet as prescribed.
5. Monitor intake and output, daily weights.
6. Monitor hydration status.
7. Make certain all members of health team understand the therapeutic plan.
8. Ensure consistent application of plan by team members.
9. Make certain child and family understand the conditions of the plan.
10. Monitor physical activity; supervise selection and performance of selected activities.
11. Maintain open communication with child.
12. Convey an attitude of caring and protection without intrusion.
13. Maintain vigilance to detect signs of sabotaging the therapeutic plan (e.g., self-induced vomiting, hiding or disposing of food, placing weighted material in clothing for weigh-in).

14. Encourage participation in own care.
15. Support psychiatric plan of care.
16. Arrange for follow-up care.

EVALUATION

Ensure that child:
1. Evidences weight gain.
2. Engages in quiet and specified activities.
3. Understands and abides by psychiatric care.
4. Develops insight as to intrapersonal conflicts as manifested by eating disorder.
5. Expresses feelings and concerns.
6. Displays evidence of developing a positive self-image.

Ensure that family:
1. Demonstrates an understanding of the therapeutic plan and the ability to continue at home.

Attention Deficit Hyperactivity Disorder

Description

Attention deficit hyperactivity disorder is a term used for various behavioral problems that in some way impair the child's capacity to profit from new experiences.

Pathophysiology

SUBTYPES:

1. Cause: unknown.
2. Specific learning disabilities: behavioral outcomes of impaired functioning in central processing (e.g., dyslexia, dysphasia, inability to draw or calculate).
3. May develop maladaptive behavior patterns in attempt to cope with cerebral dysfunction.
4. Attention deficit hyperactivity disorder (ADHD) persists in 30% of young adults.

Signs and Symptoms

1. Fidgeting with hands or feet or squirming in seat
2. Difficulty in remaining seated when required to do so
3. Easily distracted by extraneous stimuli
4. Difficulty in awaiting turn in games or group situations
5. Blurting out answers to questions before they have been completed
6. Difficulty in following through on instructions from others (e.g., fails to finish chores)
7. Difficulty in sustaining attention in tasks or play activities
8. Shifting from one uncompleted activity to another
9. Difficulty in playing quietly
10. Talking excessively
11. Interrupting or intruding on others
12. Difficulty in listening to what is being said to him or her
13. Losing things necessary for tasks or activities
14. Engaging in physically dangerous activities without considering possible consequences

Therapeutic Management

1. Family education and counseling.
2. Reduce hyperactivity with medication.
   A. Sympathomimetic amines: methylphenidate (Ritalin) or dextroamphetamine (Dexedrine)

Nursing Care

ASSESSMENT

1. Perform routine physical assessment.
2. Obtain a history of behavior and activity.
3. Observe behaviors.
4. Assist with diagnostic procedures: develop mental tests, IQ tests, psychological tests.

PLANNING

1. Safe, effective care environment
   A. Decrease external stimuli.
2. Physiological integrity
   A. Reduce hyperactivity.
3. Psychosocial integrity
   A. Support and educate child and family.
4. Health promotion and maintenance
   A. Promote optimum health.
   B. Prepare family for care.

IMPLEMENTATION

1. Explain or reinforce explanation of condition and treatment.
2. Teach family administration of medication, expected response, and signs of side effects and untoward reactions.
3. Decrease external stimuli; reduce distractions to a minimum.
4. Provide a stable, predictable environment: regular routines.
5. Control environment whenever possible; reduce number of alternatives.
6. Encourage desired patterns of behavior.
7. Collaborate with schools and other members of health team.

EVALUATION

1. Ensure that child exhibits more relaxed and organized behavior pattern.
2. Ensure that family demonstrates an understanding of the condition and the ability to provide home care.
3. Ensure that school provides appropriate environment and management.

Poisoning

Description

Poisoning is the condition or physical state produced when a substance, in relatively small amounts, is applied to body surfaces, ingested, injected, inhaled, or absorbed and subsequently causes structural damage or disturbance of function.

Pathophysiology

1. Depends on poisonous substance

Signs and Symptoms

1. Sensorium
   A. Anxiety, agitation
   B. Hallucinations
   C. Confusion
   D. Seizures
   E. Coma

2. Neuromuscular
   A. Weakness
   B. Involuntary movements
   C. Teeth gnashing
   D. Ataxia
   E. Dilated pupils
   F. Constricted pupils
   G. CNS depression, lethargy
   H. Headaches
   I. Paralysis
3. GI
   A. Increased salivation
   B. Inability to clear secretions
   C. Dry mouth
   D. Nausea and vomiting
   E. Diarrhea, bloody stools
   F. Constipation
   G. Abdominal pain
   H. Anorexia
4. Cardiovascular
   A. Arrhythmias
   B. Increased blood pressure
   C. Decreased blood pressure
   D. Tachycardia
   E. Bradycardia
   F. Evidence of shock
5. Respiratory
   A. Gagging, choking, coughing
   B. Tachypnea
   C. Bradypnea
   D. Cyanosis
   E. Grunting
6. Renal
   A. Oliguria
7. Metabolic and autonomic
   A. Sweating
   B. Hyperthermia
   C. Hypothermia
   D. Metabolic acidosis
8. Skin
   A. Pallor
   B. Redness
   C. Evidence of burning
   D. Pain
   E. Pruritus
9. Mucous membranes
   A. Evidence of irritation
   B. Red
   C. White
   D. Swollen
   E. Tissue damage (sloughing, erosion)
10. Hematological
    A. Clotting disorders
    B. Leukocytosis

Therapeutic Management

1. Identify toxic substance and antidote.
2. Stabilize cardiovascular and respiratory systems.
3. Terminate or minimize absorption of toxin by removing remaining poison from body.
4. Enhance excretion of toxin.

5. Prevent and/or correct clinical and biochemical effects of absorbed toxin.
6. Prevent complications.

Nursing Care

ASSESSMENT

1. Acquire careful and detailed history regarding what, when, route, and how much of toxic substance has entered the body.
2. Perform physical assessment with particular attention to:
   A. Vital signs
   B. Breath odor
   C. State of consciousness
   D. Skin changes
   E. Neurological signs
   F. Hydration status
3. Assist with diagnostic procedures: blood and urine examination for presence of specific substances.
4. Save all evidence of poison: container, plant, vomitus, urine.
5. Observe for latent symptoms of poisoning.

PLANNING

1. Safe, effective care environment
   A. Protect from injury.
2. Physiological integrity
   A. Ingested poisons
      (1) Dilute poisonous substance
      (2) Remove substance from stomach: syrup of ipecac, gastric lavage.
      (3) Prevent aspiration of vomitus.
      (4) Absorb remaining substance.
   B. Cutaneously absorbed or inhaled poisons
      (1) Reduce absorption.
   C. Prevent complications.
3. Psychosocial integrity
   A. Support and educate child and family.
   B. Prepare child and family for procedures.
4. Health promotion and maintenance
   A. Prevent recurrence.
   B. Prepare family for care.

IMPLEMENTATION

1. Contact local poison control center, emergency facility, or physician for immediate advice regarding treatment.
2. Explain or reinforce explanation of situation.
3. Implement measures to eliminate or reduce effects of poison.
4. Provide the following nursing interventions for ingested poison:
   A. Remove pills, plant parts, or other materials from mouth.
   B. Administer water to dilute substance unless contraindicated.
   C. Administer ipecac to induce vomiting (unless hydrocarbons or corrosives were swallowed, or child is comatose).
   D. Position to prevent aspiration.
   E. Prepare for and assist with gastric lavage, if prescribed.
   F. Administer activated charcoal after vomiting has occurred to absorb remaining poison.

5. Perform the following nursing interventions for inhaled poison:
   A. Remove victim to fresh air.
   B. Provide respiratory support as indicated.
   C. Observe for pulmonary symptoms (later).
6. Perform the following nursing intervention for cutaneous exposure:
   A. Remove contaminated clothing.
   B. Wash skin thoroughly with copious amounts of warm or tepid water.
7. Carry out orders for management of specific poisons (e.g., IV infusion, artificial ventilation, administration of specific antidotes [e.g., chelating agents, antivenom], anticonvulsants).
8. Provide comfort and reassurance to child and family.
9. Teach poison prevention.

EVALUATION

Ensure that child:
1. Eliminates poison.
2. Exhibits no evidence of complications.
3. Does not have recurrent episode of poisoning.

Ensure that family:
1. Demonstrates an understanding of the situation and the ability to provide care.

Lead Poisoning (Plumbism)

Description

Lead poisoning (plumbism) is a toxic condition caused by the ingestion, absorption, or inhalation of lead or lead compounds.

Pathophysiology

1. Lead excreted very slowly by kidneys
2. Retained lead stored chiefly in bone (inert)
3. Chronic ingestion: excess lead deposited in tissues and circulatory system
4. Toxic effects
   A. Hematological
      (1) Lead prevents formation of hemoglobin.
      (2) Anemia.
      (3) Hemoglobin precursors accumulate in blood.
   B. Renal
      (1) Lead damages proximal tubules.
      (2) Abnormal excretion of glucose, protein, phosphate.
   C. CNS: lead encephalopathy
      (1) Increased membrane permeability.
      (2) Fluid shifts to interstitial spaces of brain.
      (3) Increased intracranial pressure.
      (4) Cortical atrophy.

Signs and Symptoms

1. General
   A. Anemia
   B. Acute crampy abdominal pain
   C. Nausea and vomiting
   D. Constipation
   E. Anorexia
   F. Headache
   G. Fever
   H. Decreased height and weight (long-term ingestion)
2. CNS signs
   A. Hyperactivity
   B. Aggression
   C. Impulsiveness
   D. Lethargy
   E. Irritability
   F. Delay or reversal of verbal maturation
   G. Loss of newly acquired motor skills
   H. Clumsiness
   I. Sensory perceptual deficits
   J. Learning difficulties
   K. Short attention span
   L. Distractibility
   M. Seizures
   N. Impaired consciousness
3. Late signs
   A. Mental retardation
   B. Paralysis
   C. Blindness
   D. Convulsions
   E. Coma and death
   F. Behavior problems
   G. Learning difficulties

Therapeutic Management

1. Remove lead from body with chelating agents (e.g., calcium disodium edetate, demercaprol).
2. Correct anemia.
3. Control symptoms: anticonvulsants for seizure activity.
4. Remove source of lead, if possible.

Nursing Care

ASSESSMENT

1. Perform routine physical assessment.
2. Obtain history of possible lead ingestion (pica) or inhalation (gasoline sniffing) and suggestive behavior (aggression, hyperirritability).
3. Observe for evidence of developmental delay, behavior problems.
4. Assist with diagnostic procedures: blood lead concentrations, erythrocyte-protoporphyrin level, hemoglobin, radiography for evidence of "lead line" in bones, urinalysis for hemoglobin precursors.
5. Assess environment for possible sources of lead (e.g., old paint, ceramic dishes with lead-based glaze); question family regarding possibility of lead brought home on clothing from workplace, child playing near area with large amounts of automobile exhaust fumes, etc.

PLANNING

1. Safe, effective care environment
   A. Remove lead from environment.
2. Physiological integrity
   A. Promote removal of lead from body.
   B. Prevent complications.
3. Psychosocial integrity
   A. See Nursing Care of the Ill Child, pp. 97–98.
   B. Prepare child for multiple injections.
   C. Support and educate child and family.

4. Health promotion and maintenance
   A. Promote optimum health.
   B. Evaluate physical surroundings for evidence of lead sources.
   C. Ensure that family demonstrates understanding of condition and ability to provide home care.

IMPLEMENTATION

1. Administer chelating agents as prescribed: plan a rotation schedule for each series of injections IV or deep IM.
2. Administer anticonvulsants, iron preparation, and other medications as prescribed.
3. Maintain and monitor fluid balance.
   A. IV infusion
   B. Intake and output
   C. Related complications (e.g., encephalopathy)

4. Explain or reinforce explanation of condition and treatment.
   A. Explain to child that the "shots" are not a punishment.
   B. Use anxiety-reduction techniques.
   C. Provide needle play after injections.
   D. Provide comfort measures after injections.
5. Explore with family ways of eliminating lead from environment.

EVALUATION

Ensure that child:
1. Submits to therapy with minimal distress.
2. Exhibits no evidence of lead in the body.
Ensure that family:
1. Demonstrates an understanding of the condition and the intent to eliminate lead from the environment.

QUESTIONS

Patricia E. Thompson, EdD, RN

1. A baby was born 2 hours ago by Cesarean section. The newborn has a myelomeningocele with the sac intact and has been placed in an incubator. The nurse, when planning care for the baby, should focus on potential for:

A. Disuse syndrome
B. Infection
C. Fluid volume deficit
D. Decreased cardiac output

2. Appropriate nursing interventions for a newborn's myelomeningocele sac prior to surgery include using sterile technique and:

A. Leaving the sac open to air
B. Applying petrolatum to cover the sac
C. Applying moist saline dressings
D. Applying dry dressings

3. To maintain proper alignment of the hips and lower extremities in a baby with a myelomeningocele, the nurse should position the baby with the:

A. Hips abducted and feet in a neutral position
B. Hips adducted and feet flexed
C. Hips subluxed and feet extended
D. Hips adducted and feet in a natural position

4. Prior to surgery for a myelomeningocele, the nurse would place the baby in which of the following positions?

A. Prone
B. Right side
C. Left side
D. Dorsal

5. A newborn baby is diagnosed with a myelomeningocele. The nurse measures his head circumference daily to assess for the development of what complication?

A. Hydrocele•
B. Hordeolum
C. Hypsarrhythmia
D. Hydrocephalus

6. A 4-month-old infant is admitted to the hospital with acute diarrhea and dehydration. Initial nursing assessment of the infant reveals:

A. Tenting of skin
B. Low hematocrit
C. Bulging fontanelle
D. Weight gain

7. The nurse would place a 4-month-old infant with diarrhea in which of the following types of isolation?

A. Reverse
B. Enteric
C. Strict
D. Wound and skin

8. The nurse should assess a 4-month-old infant who has diarrhea and dehydration for:

A. Metabolic acidosis
B. Metabolic alkalosis
C. Respiratory acidosis
D. Respiratory alkalosis

9. The doctor has ordered that KCl be added to a 4-month-old infant's IV infusion. The nurse should:

A. Give the KCl as soon as ordered to prevent hypocalcemia.
B. Give the KCl within the 1st hour of admission.
C. Wait to give the KCl until an adequate urinary output is documented.
D. Wait to give the KCl until the complete blood count (CBC) results are available and within normal limits.

10. As the nurse monitors the 4 month old's progress, which symptom might indicate she is becoming overhydrated from IV fluids she is receiving?

A. Edema at IV site
B. Vomiting
C. Below normal temperature
D. Bubbling rales

11. As part of the admission history, the nurse asked a mother about a 4-month-old infant's immunization record. Which of the following immunizations is recommended to be given at 4 months?

A. Measles
B. Tetanus
C. Mumps
D. Influenza virus

12. A 13-year-old female client has asthma. The nurse teaches her ways to reduce possible asthma attacks and explains the need to avoid:

A. Mild exercise
B. Turtles as pets
C. Swimming
D. Extremes in temperature

13. The nurse instructs a client that during an asthma attack she may feel more comfortable in which of the following positions?

A. High Fowler
B. Prone
C. Side-lying
D. Dorsal

14. A client is hospitalized with status asthmaticus. The physician has ordered IV theophylline. Which of the following would be a side effect of the drug the nurse should observe for?

A. Seizures
B. Dysrhythmias
C. Drowsiness
D. Headache

15. As the nurse monitors the progress of a 14-year-old client with asthma, she observes for early signs of im-

pending airway obstruction. Which of the following symptoms would cause the nurse concern?

A. Decreased pulse
B. Flaring nares
C. Lethargy
D. Decreased respiratory rate

16. Once a 14-year-old client's post-status-asthmaticus attack has stabilized, which of the following activities would the nurse choose as being the most appropriate for the client while in the hospital?

A. Working a jigsaw puzzle
B. Talking on the phone to friends
C. Watching television
D. Doing arts and crafts

17. A 1-year-old infant is admitted to the hospital with eczema. There is an order for "Diet for age." Which of the following should the nurse avoid in the infant's diet?

A. Milk and wheat cereal
B. Carrots and beef
C. Apple juice and coke
D. Mashed potatoes and tea

18. A 1-year-old infant with eczema is placed in elbow restraints to keep him from scratching. To prevent problems with immobility, the nurse should:

A. Allow him out of restraints when supervised by the nurse or mother
B. Release restraints for meals and bath time
C. Release restraints one at a time every 4 hours
D. Allow him out of restraints when he is asleep at night and during naps

19. The parents of the 1-year-old infant with eczema are concerned about his appearance. He developed a secondary infection that makes him look grotesque. How can the nurse be most supportive of the parents' feelings?

A. Divert the conversation to another topic so they will not focus on the infant's appearance.
B. Encourage them to discuss their fears and concerns.
C. Let them know you do not blame them for being upset.
D. Tell them not to worry, that his condition will improve eventually.

20. The nurse is doing discharge teaching to the mother of the infant with eczema because the infant's pruritus will continue after he goes home. In evaluating the mother's understanding, the nurse would expect her to realize the importance of having the infant:

A. Take cornstarch baths
B. Wear cotton shorts and short-sleeved shirts
C. Wear wool blend long-sleeve jumpsuits
D. Take salt baths 3 times a day

21. A 2-year-old child is admitted to the hospital with Hirschsprung's disease. During the nursing history, the mother describes the child's stool to the nurse as foul-smelling and:

A. Small, hard pebbles
B. Large and frothy

C. Cordlike
D. Ribbonlike

22. The nurse explains to a toddler's parents that the treatment of choice for Hirschsprung's disease (aganglionic colon) would be:

A. Surgical removal of affected colon
B. Modified diet high in fiber
C. Medication to stimulate the colon
D. Permanent colostomy

23. A 7-year-old child is admitted to the hospital with nephrotic syndrome. During the assessment, the nurse is aware that a classic symptom is:

A. Increased urine output
B. Hematuria
C. Elevated blood pressure
D. Proteinuria

24. During the edematous phase of nephrotic syndrome, an important nursing intervention is to:

A. Provide meticulous skin care
B. Encourage fluid intake
C. Encourage moderate activity
D. Weigh the client every other day

25. A 7-year-old boy with nephrotic syndrome is placed on steroid therapy. Which statement by his mother indicates to the nurse an understanding of steroid therapy?

A. "Steroids will improve his acne."
B. "He will have permanent Cushing features."
C. "Steroids will mask infections."
D. "He may get diarrhea."

26. The physician has ordered prednisone for a child who has nephrotic syndrome. The nurse should observe for all side effects, but the one that is most serious is:

A. Cushing features
B. Decreased respirations
C. Metabolic alkalosis
D. Adrenal suppression

27. In evaluating the effectiveness of the prednisone therapy, the nurse realizes that a child with nephrotic syndrome will continue to take the drug until after:

A. Edema has disappeared
B. Urine no longer contains protein
C. Hematuria has resolved
D. His "moon" face has disappeared

28. A 3-year-old child is brought to the emergency room by her parents. She has a broken right leg. The mother tells the admitting nurse that the child had fallen off her tricycle. The father tells the physician that the child had fallen down the stairs. The parents are concerned about their child's condition, and it is obvious she loves them. She is quiet and not talkative. She is the youngest of four children. During the initial assessment, what should clue the nurse to the possibility of child abuse?

A. The child's not being talkative
B. Report of conflicting data

C. The child's being the youngest child

D. Parents' concern about her condition

29. Which of the following data the nurse learns about a mother in conversation support the possibility of child abuse of her 3-year-old daughter?

    A. Has a healthy self-esteem
    B. Has a history of a happy childhood
    C. Viewed the child differently than the other children
    D. Thought the child was developmentally advanced for her age

30. In identifying realistic goals in working with the parents of a 3-year-old abused child, the nurse should understand abusive parents have not mastered the task of:

    A. Developing a trusting relationship
    B. Role gratification
    C. Functioning outside the home
    D. Developing a value system

31. In planning care for a 3-year-old abused child, the nurse realizes that the parents are lacking in knowledge related to:

    A. Appropriate play activities for the child
    B. Normal growth and development
    C. Nutritional needs for the child
    D. Child psychology

32. The nurse has a legal responsibility in child abuse cases to:

    A. Collect additional data before taking further action
    B. Directly report her suspicions to the local child protection agency
    C. Discuss her suspicions with the parents
    D. Notify the physician of her suspicions

33. A 6-year-old child is hospitalized with a urinary tract infection (UTI). The nurse should teach the child that the best way to prevent recurrent UTIs is to:

    A. Void 3 times a day
    B. Wipe from front to back
    C. Drink plenty of milk
    D. Wear nylon underwear

34. A mother brings her 3-month-old son to the emergency room. He is crying with apparent acute abdominal pain. After initial assessment, intussusception is suspected. What type of stool would the nurse expect the mother to report?

    A. Black tarlike
    B. Ribbonlike
    C. Red currant-jellylike
    D. Frothy and foul smelling

35. A 1-month-old infant is at the physician's office for a follow-up visit after surgery for pyloric stenosis. The nurse would identify which of the following as the *best* indicator that the infant is recovering well from his surgery?

    A. Mother reports infant is feeding well every 4 hours.
    B. The infant has demonstrated a satisfactory weight gain.

C. The infant is in the 90th percentile in length on the growth chart.

D. Mother reports infant has a normal stool pattern.

36. A 15-year-old girl is 5 ft 7 inches tall and weighs 98 lb. She perceives herself as overweight. She has been hospitalized with anorexia nervosa. The nurse, when planning care, should focus on prevention of:

    A. Vomiting
    B. Weight loss
    C. Malnutrition
    D. Depression

37. A physician diagnoses a teenager as having anorexia nervosa. The nurse would expect the parents of a patient with anorexia nervosa to describe her as being:

    A. A conformer
    B. Independent
    C. Disruptive
    D. A low achiever

38. With a 15-year-old patient's severe weight loss and disrupted metabolism due to anorexia nervosa, the nurse would expect to observe which of the following symptoms?

    A. Heat intolerance
    B. Decreased temperature
    C. Dysmenorrhea
    D. Tachycardia

39. A baby has died from sudden infant death syndrome (SIDS). SIDS is often initially mistaken for:

    A. Failure to thrive
    B. Viral infection
    C. Meningitis
    D. Child abuse

40. When parents have lost an infant to SIDS, the nurse would plan to insert teaching content about the parents' reactions. The nurse would plan to include content related to:

    A. Anger
    B. Depression
    C. Guilt
    D. Hostility

41. A 5-year-old child is hospitalized with bilateral eye patches in place following surgery. Which of the following is the most important nursing intervention?

    A. Speak to him when entering the room.
    B. Allow his parents to stay with him.
    C. Let him have familiar toys from home.
    D. Keep the side rails up.

42. The nurse is teaching a mother how to administer eye drops to her 5-year-old son. The nurse tells her to place the drops:

    A. Under the upper eyelid
    B. On the sclera as the child looks to the side
    C. In the conjunctival cul-de-sac
    D. Anywhere that makes contact with the eyes, surface

43. During a parenting class for toddlers, the nurse informs parents that the major cause of blindness in children older than 2 years old is:

    A. Glaucoma
    B. Trauma
    C. Hyperopia
    D. Infection

44. The nurse in the newborn nursery is assessing an infant. The nurse observes an opacity of the lens of the eyes, which she knows is a symptom of:

    A. Retinoblastoma
    B. Cataracts
    C. Glaucoma
    D. Blindness

45. During the initial assessment of a child with Reye's syndrome, the mother reports that about a week ago the child had:

    A. Mumps
    B. Meningitis
    C. Influenza
    D. Cellulitis

46. The most important nursing intervention in caring for a child with Reye's syndrome is to:

    A. Prevent skin breakdown
    B. Monitor intake and output
    C. Do range-of-motion exercises
    D. Turn every 2 hours

47. Because of liver involvement associated with Reye's syndrome, the nurse should use which special precaution when caring for children with this condition?

    A. Administering IM injections
    B. Monitoring output from the catheter
    C. Assessing the level of consciousness
    D. Turning the child

48. A 1-year-old infant is admitted to the hospital to rule out cystic fibrosis. During the admission process the infant passes a stool. The nurse, realizing that his stool is symptomatic of cystic fibrosis, charts it as:

    A. Small and constipated
    B. Green and odorous
    C. Large and bulky
    D. Yellow and loose

49. A 15-lb, 1-year-old infant is admitted to rule out cystic fibrosis. He weighed 7 lb at birth. In analyzing data related to the infant's weight, the nurse knows he should currently weigh how many pounds?

    A. 14
    B. 18
    C. 21
    D. 24

50. The nurse would expect the physician to order which of the following tests to diagnose cystic fibrosis?

    A. Sputum culture
    B. Stool culture
    C. Chest x-ray
    D. Sweat test

51. The priority nursing goal for a family whose son is diagnosed with cystic fibrosis is to:

    A. Stabilize his condition
    B. Provide emotional support
    C. Locate financial resources
    D. Develop long-range plans

52. A child is diagnosed with cystic fibrosis. He is receiving pancreatic enzymes. Once the pancreatic enzymes the child is taking are effective, he will:

    A. Have normal bowel movements
    B. Increase 2 lb in weight per week
    C. Have decreased NaCl in his sweat
    D. Have fewer respiratory infections per year

53. A 6-year-old girl is hospitalized with acute lymphocytic leukemia. She is placed on protective isolation, which concerns her parents. The nurse should explain that this will:

    A. Protect her from too many visitors
    B. Protect her from infectious organisms
    C. Provide a quiet, private environment for her
    D. Keep other children away from the child

54. A child who has lymphocytic leukemia is upset about alopecia from her chemotherapy treatments. The nurse should explain to her that:

    A. She can wear a wig
    B. This is an unavoidable side effect
    C. Her hair will grow back in a few months
    D. She can stay home until she adjusts to her hair loss

55. The nurse discusses mouth care with a 6-year-old girl who has acute lymphocytic leukemia and her mother. The nurse explains that when toothbrushing is contraindicated, the most effective way to clean teeth is:

    A. Rinsing with water
    B. Chewing gum after eating
    C. Rinsing with hydrogen peroxide
    D. Use of a Water Pik

56. A 12-year-old girl is hospitalized with a diagnosis of rheumatic fever. To minimize her joint pain during acute episodes, the nurse should teach the parents to:

    A. Immobilize the joints in a functional position
    B. Do full range of motion on all joints daily
    C. Apply heat to the involved joints
    D. Massage joints briskly with lotion after her bath

57. Discharge planning of a child with rheumatic fever should include teaching the child and parents to recognize which of the following toxic symptoms of sodium salicylate?

    A. Blurred vision and itching
    B. Chills and fever
    C. Acetone breath odor
    D. Tinnitus and nausea

58. A neonate in the newborn nursery is suspected of having a tracheoesophageal fistula. A major symptom the nurse observed was:

    A. Hypersensitive gag reflex
    B. Dry mouth with no drooling
    C. Cyanosis
    D. Lethargy

59. A 3-year-old child is diagnosed with Kawasaki's disease. The nurse observes which of the following symptoms?

    A. Below-normal temperature
    B. Strawberry tongue
    C. Edema of the face
    D. Swelling in the groin

60. The therapeutic management for a child who has been diagnosed with Kawasaki's disease will include administering which of the following medications?

    A. Acetaminophen (Tylenol)
    B. γ-Globulin
    C. Antibiotics
    D. Steroids

61. A 14-year-old child has come to the clinic to receive a measles, mumps, rubella (MMR) immunization. What is the major concern when administering the MMR vaccine to children 12–18 years of age?

    A. It cannot be given with oral polio virus vaccine (OPV).
    B. Allergy to horse serum makes it contraindicated.
    C. The children should not have an upper respiratory infection.
    D. Girls should not be pregnant or plan on being pregnant within 3 months

62. A mother is being instructed on the best method of administering syrup of ipecac in the initial home management of an accidental ingestion. The nurse should inform her that syrup of ipecac should be administered with:

    A. Milk
    B. Activated charcoal
    C. One to two glasses of tepid water
    D. Large amounts of cold water

63. A 4-year-old child will begin taking medication for the treatment of attention deficit hyperactivity disorder (ADHD) to help control his hyperactivity. Which of the following is the drug of choice for this problem?

    A. Phenobarbital
    B. Prednisone
    C. Phenytoin (Dilantin)
    D. Methylphenidate (Ritalin)

64. A 7-year-old child has been taking phenytoin and phenobarbital for control of chronic recurrent seizures. In the physical exam, the nurse notes that the child has hyperplasia of the gums. The nurse should recognize that hyperplasia of the gums is:

    A. A common occurrence with chronic recurrent seizures
    B. A common side effect of phenytoin

C. Not related to the drugs or the disease
D. An unusual side effect of phenobarbital

65. A 7-month-old infant has been on antibiotic therapy. The nurse notes that the child has white patches in his mouth that will not rub off. The physician orders nystatin (Mycostatin) 1 mL, po, qid. The nurse should realize that the appropriate technique in administering this medication is to:

    A. Give 0.5 mL in each side of the mouth
    B. Give with milk or food
    C. Give through a nipple
    D. Follow with water

66. A primary objective for planning nursing care of an edematous child with nephrotic syndrome would be to encourage:

    A. Ambulation
    B. A low-carbohydrate diet
    C. A high-protein diet
    D. A low-protein diet

67. Which would be the most appropriate toy for the nurse to choose for enhancing imagination in a preschool child?

    A. Books
    B. Costumes
    C. Coloring books
    D. Wagon

68. When trouble shooting for error in a continuous pulse oximetry measurement, the nurse would check the child for which of the following?

    A. Hypothermia
    B. Hypertension
    C. Increased hemoglobin level
    D. Skin intact at site of sensor

69. The nurse is preparing to suction a tracheostomy in a 9 month old. What would be the most appropriate setting for the suction machine?

    A. 20–40 mm Hg
    B. 60–80 mm Hg
    C. 80–100 mm Hg
    D. 100–120 mm Hg

70. The nurse is teaching anticipatory guidance to a mother of a 3 year old. Which is appropriate for the nurse to recommend for play?

    A. Board games
    B. Cradle gym
    C. Soap bubbles
    D. Costumes for dress-up

71. An infant has returned to the unit after revision of a malfunctioning VP shunt. Which of the following would indicate to the nurse that a problem could be developing with the shunt?

    A. Irritability
    B. Bradycardia
    C. Sunken fontanel
    D. Increased urine output

72. The emergency department nurse notifies the charge nurse on the pediatric unit that a child with tuberculosis is being admitted. The charge nurse surveys the rooms and realizes there are no private rooms available and no other patients with tuberculosis. What action by the charge nurse would be most appropriate at this time?

    A. Notify the infection control nurse.
    B. Place the child in a room with another uninfected child, but space them at least 6 feet apart.
    C. Place the child in a room with another child infected with bacteria and space them 6 feet apart.
    D. Refuse the admittance of the child to the pediatric unit.

73. The nurse observes a mother suctioning her infant with a bulb syringe. Which behavior by the mother lets the nurse know the mother needs further instructions on how to use the bulb syringe?

    A. Compressing the bulb of the syringe once inside the nostrils
    B. Holding the infant's head upright during suctioning
    C. Placing the infant on the side after suctioning
    D. Suctioning the nares before the mouth

74. Which food would the nurse teach a mother of a child with celiac disease to avoid in the diet?

    A. Oatmeal or oat products
    B. Fresh fruits or vegetables
    C. Chicken or poultry products
    D. Cow's milk and products containing milk

75. The nurse is taking care of a newborn in transition, and the newborn is requiring more suctioning and seems to be choking on secretions. Which of the following behaviors by the nurse would promote the safest environment for the newborn?

    A. Assessing for cyanosis
    B. Obtaining a culture on the secretions
    C. Measuring the abdomen
    D. Positioning on the back with the head elevated.

76. The nurse is performing an assessment on a 2-year-old child who is 1 day post-op after having a gastrostomy tube inserted. Which assessment finding would the nurse report to the surgeon?

    A. A specific gravity of 1.032
    B. A reduction in gastric drainage
    C. A potassium of 3.8
    D. A bulging fontanel

77. A mother brings her 4 month old to the clinic for immunizations. The record indicates the infant is on schedule with immunizations. Which immunizations would the clinic nurse administer to the infant at this visit?

    A. DTP & HIB
    B. DTP, Polio, and Hepatitis B
    C. DTP, HIB, and Polio
    D. DTP, HIB, and Hepatitis B

78. A 4-month-old male is admitted for pyloric stenosis repair. When planning care, the nurse would emphasize:

    A. Fluid volume deficit related to improper intake

    B. Fluid volume deficit related to diarrhea
    C. Malnutrition due to improper diet
    D. Malnutrition due to gastrointestinal alteration

79. A 9-year-old male is brought to the emergency room by his mother for complaints of fatigue. History reveals the child has a congenital heart defect and has been on digoxin for a long time. Which of the following behaviors would cause the nurse to suspect digoxin toxicity?

    A. Bradycardia
    B. Confusion
    C. Dyspnea
    D. Weight loss

80. A 4-year-old female is receiving her first dose of intravenous γ-globulin infusion. The nurse would suspect a reaction to the infusion if the child exhibited:

    A. Chest tightness
    B. Increased blood pressure
    C. Poor appetite
    D. Redness at the IV site

81. The charge nurse receives a call that an 18 month old with pneumonia is being admitted. Which would be the most appropriate room assignment by the nurse?

    A. Private room
    B. Rooming with a 12 month old diagnosed with pneumonia who has been taking antibiotics for 3 days.
    C. Rooming with an 18 month old admitted with FTT
    D. Rooming with a 14 month old with viral pneumonia

82. A 6 month old presents to the emergency department with a history of low-grade fever for 2 days. The mother reports increasing nasal congestion and irritability today with poor oral intake. The physician admits the infant to the hospital and orders a viral panel and IV fluids. What room assignment by the charge nurse would be appropriate?

    A. Private room only
    B. Rooming with a 2 year old admitted 2 days ago with RSV
    C. Rooming with a 12 month old diagnosed with viral pneumonia
    D. Rooming with a 6 month old diagnosed with otitis media

83. A 5-year-old female is being admitted with a UTI. An appropriate room assignment by the charge nurse would be:

    A. Rooming with another 5-year-old female diagnosed with pneumonia
    B. Rooming with a 5-year-old male with a UTI
    C. Rooming with a 4-year-old female with celiac disease
    D. Rooming with a 10-year-old female with dehydration

84. An LPN was pulled to the pediatric unit. Which of the following patients would be most appropriate for the charge nurse to include in this nurse's assignment?

    A. A child with developmental delays admitted for diagnostic tests

B. A second-day post-op child who underwent a urinary diversion surgery

C. A first day post-op child who underwent hypospadius repair

D. A 2 year old diagnosed with bronchial pneumonia being transferred from PICU

85. Which of the following would be inappropriate for the charge nurse to assign to a nurse that is pregnant?

A. A child with a UTI

B. A 4 month old receiving riboviran

C. A child requiring numerous diagnostic x-rays

D. A ventilator-assisted child with bronchial pneumonia

86. What should be the initial action by the charge nurse when there has been a chemotherapy spill in the medication room?

A. Notify the nursing supervisor.

B. Notify the housekeeping department.

C. Implement clean-up by using the chemotherapy spill kit.

D. Instruct visitors to stay in the patient's room until fumes disappear.

87. What isolation precaution is appropriate for the nurse to assign to a patient with giardia?

A. Airborne precautions

B. Contact precautions

C. Droplet precautions

D. Standard precautions

88. A nurse taking care of a child with RSV knows the virus is viable on a nonporous surface for:

A. Less than 30 minutes

B. Up to 1 hour

C. 6 hours

D. A 12-hour period

89. The nurse would choose which of the following for visual stimulation in the neonate?

A. Red mobile

B. Pastel color mobile

C. Primary color mobile

D. Black and white mobile

90. A 4-year-old child had a glucose level of 60 at the 4:00 PM glucose check. What snack would the nurse choose to give 15 g of carbohydrate?

A. Six Life Savers

B. One half cup of milk

C. One cup of orange juice

D. One half cup of orange juice with two packs of sugar

91. A child took an injection of NPH and regular insulin at 8:00 AM. The nurse would expect the combination peak time of these two insulins to occur at:

A. 9:00 AM

B. 10:00 AM

C. 12 noon

D. 2:00 PM

ANSWERS

1. **(B)** Client need: physiological integrity; subcategory: reduction of risk potential; content area: pediatrics

   RATIONALE

   (A) Varying degrees of neurological involvement affecting the lower musculoskeletal system occur; however, this is not a life-threatening problem. (B) There is potential for infection spreading into the CNS through the meningeal sac, which could be life threatening. (C) Electrolyte imbalance is not a problem. (D) Renal complications often occur, but cardiac complications would not occur from myelomeningocele.

2. **(C)** Client need: physiological integrity; subcategory: reduction of risk potential; content area: pediatrics

   RATIONALE

   (A) The sac should be kept moist. Leaving the sac open to air, especially in an incubator, has a drying effect. (B) Prolonged use of ointments can cause breakdown of the tissue. (C) The sac should be kept moist to maintain the integrity of the sac prior to surgery. (D) A dry dressing may be irritating to the sac.

3. **(A)** Client need: physiological integrity; subcategory: reduction of risk potential; content area: pediatrics

   RATIONALE

   (A) This position maintains proper alignment of the hips and lower extremities. (B, C, D) This position will pull the hips out of alignment.

4. **(A)** Client need: physiological integrity; subcategory: reduction of risk potential; content area: pediatrics

   RATIONALE

   (A) This position minimizes the tension on the sac and reduces the potential for trauma to the area. (B, C) A side-lying position puts pressure on the sac with potential for leaks or breaks. (D) This would cause trauma to the sac and cause it to leak or break.

5. **(D)** Client need: physiological integrity; subcategory: physiological adaptation; content area: pediatrics

   RATIONALE

   (A) This is fluid in the tunica vaginalis testes and is not associated with myelomeningocele. (B) This is a stye and not a complication of myelomeningocele. (C) This occurs in infantile spasms and is not a complication of myelomeningocele. (D) There is greater production than absorption of cerebrospinal fluid in the ventricular system, which is a complication associated with myelomeningocele.

6. **(A)** Client need: physiological integrity; subcategory: physiological adaptation; content area: pediatrics

   RATIONALE

   (A) Skin turgor, fever, lethargy, and a whining cry would be initial symptoms. (B) The hematocrit would be elevated owing to fluid volume loss. (C) The fontanelle is depressed with dehydration. (D) Weight loss from fluid occurs with diarrhea and dehydration.

7. **(B)** Client need: safe, effective care environment; subcategory: safety and infection control; content area: pediatrics

   RATIONALE

   (A) Reverse isolation protects the infant from other people's germs. (B) The infant needs to be on stool precautions until culture results are known. (C) This is for diseases transmitted through the respiratory route. (D) The infant has no wound, so this type of isolation is not appropriate.

8. **(A)** Client need: physiological integrity; subcategory: physiological adaptation; content area: pediatrics

   RATIONALE

   (A) With diarrhea, the loss of bicarbonate, sodium, and potassium results in metabolic acidosis. (B) Loss of bicarbonate with diarrhea results in acidosis. (C, D) Diarrhea and dehydration are metabolic, not respiratory, disorders.

9. **(C)** Client need: safe, effective care environment; subcategory: safety and infection control; content area: pediatrics

   RATIONALE

   (A, B) IV KCl should never be given until kidney function is established, or hypercalcemia and death may occur. (C) Kidney function must be established prior to administering IV KCl, or hypercalcemia and death may occur. (D) CBC results are not related to the administration of IV KCl.

10. **(D)** Client need: safe, effective care environment; subcategory: safety and infection control; content area: pediatrics

    RATIONALE

    (A) This would indicate infiltration of the IV. (B, C) This is not a symptom of overhydration. (D) Rales are a symptom of fluid overload produced from left-sided heart failure.

11. **(B)** Client need: health promotion and maintenance; subcategory: prevention and early detection of disease; content area: pediatrics

    RATIONALE

    (A, C) Recommended at 12 or 15 months. (B) Recommended at 2, 4, 6 months and 15 years. (D) Recommended at 2, 4, 6 months, and a booster at 12–15 months.

12. **(D)** Client need: health promotion and maintenance; subcategory: prevention and early detection of disease; content area: pediatrics

    RATIONALE

    (A) Mild exercise is usually not a problem; however, extremes in exercise can be. (B) Animal dander from dogs, cats, and birds can cause asthma attacks. Turtles are acceptable pets. (C) Swimming is a recommended exercise for asthmatic clients. (D) Extremely cool or warm temperatures can cause an asthma attack.

13. **(A)** Client need: safe, effective care environment; subcategory: prevention and early detection of disease; content area: pediatrics

    RATIONALE

    (A) The sitting position facilitates the breathing process for children during an attack. (B, C, D) Children do not find this position comfortable during an asthma attack.

14. **(D)** Client need: physiological integrity; subcategory: pharmacological and parenteral therapies; content area: pediatrics

    RATIONALE

    (A) This is a symptom of toxicity, not a side effect. (B) This is a symptom of toxicity, not a side effect. (C) Insomnia is not a side effect. (D) Headache is a side effect.

15. **(B)** Client need: physiological integrity; subcategory: physiological adaptation; content area: pediatrics

    RATIONALE

    (A) The pulse rate increases. (B) The nares flare prior to airway obstruction as the body attempts to exchange more air. (C) There is increased restlessness. (D) Respirations increase.

16. **(B)** Client need: psychosocial integrity; subcategory: coping and adaptation; content area: pediatrics

    RATIONALE

    (A, C, D) This would not provide an opportunity to interact with peers, which is important for adolescents. (B) She can talk to peers and have an outlet to express concerns she may have about her disease.

17. **(A)** Client need: physiological integrity; subcategory: reduction of risk potential; content area: pediatrics

    RATIONALE

    (A) These foods commonly cause sensitivity and can trigger eczema. (B, C, D) These foods are allowed on a hypoallergenic diet.

18. **(C)** Client need: safe, effective care environment; subcategory: safety and infection control; content area: pediatrics

    RATIONALE

    (A) Both restraints should never be released at the same time, even with the child supervised. Children are very quick and can scratch before anyone realizes it. (B) Both restraints should never be released at the same time. (C) Restraints should be released one at a time several times a day to do range-of-motion exercise. (D) He can still scratch while he is asleep.

19. **(B)** Client need: psychosocial integrity; subcategory: coping and adaptation; content area: pediatrics

    RATIONALE

    (A) The nurse is avoiding the parents' current feelings and not dealing with them. (B) Once the fears and concerns are verbalized, the nurse can help the parents deal with them. (C) The word "blame" is negative. This is not a supportive statement. (D) It is inappropriate to tell them not to worry. Their feelings need to be dealt with now.

20. **(A)** Client need: health promotion and maintenance; subcategory: prevention and early detection of disease; content area: pediatrics

    RATIONALE

    (A) Cornstarch relieves itching for short periods of time. (B) Large areas of skin should not be exposed because the child will scratch. (C) Wool is irritating and could increase itching. (D) Salt may sting if there are open lesions.

21. **(D)** Client need: physiological integrity; subcategory: reduction of risk potential; content area: pediatrics

    RATIONALE

    (A, C) This stool pattern is not characteristic of Hirschsprung's disease. (B) This stool pattern is characteristic of cystic fibrosis. (D) This stool pattern is characteristic of an aganglionic colon.

22. **(A)** Client need: physiological integrity; subcategory: reduction of risk potential; content area: pediatrics

    RATIONALE

    (A) The aganglionic section of the colon is removed so the remaining intestines can function. (B) Diet changes will not make a difference owing to the lack of peristalsis. (C) There is no medication that will make an aganglionic colon function. (D) A permanent colostomy is not necessary. A temporary colostomy is performed using a two- or three-stage procedure to correct the problem.

23. **(D)** Client need: physiological integrity; subcategory: reduction of risk potential; content area: pediatrics

    RATIONALE

    (A) There is decreased urine output. (B) This is a symptom of glomerulonephritis. (C) The blood pressure is normal or slightly below normal. (D) There is massive proteinuria.

24. **(A)** Client need: physiological integrity; subcategory: reduction of risk potential; content area: pediatrics

    RATIONALE

    (A) Edema increases the potential for skin breakdown, so skin care is extremely important. (B) Fluid intake is monitored carefully and often limited. (C) Activity is limited to decrease the workload on the circulatory system with the excess fluid. (D) The child should be weighed at least daily and often twice a day.

25. **(C)** Client need: safe, effective care environment; subcategory: safety and infection control; content area: pediatrics

    RATIONALE

    (A) Steroid therapy aggravates acne. (B) Cushing features are temporary. (C) Infections are "masked," and this could lead to a life-threatening situation. (D) This is not associated with steroid therapy.

26. **(D)** Client need: physiological integrity; subcategory: pharmacological and parenteral therapies; content area: pediatrics

    RATIONALE

    (A) This is a side effect of the drug but is not life threatening. (B, C) This is not a side effect of prednisone. (D) This is a serious and potentially life-threatening side effect.

27. **(B)** Client need: physiological integrity; subcategory: pharmacological and parenteral therapies; content area: pediatrics

    RATIONALE

    (A) Some edema may continue even after the drug has been stopped. (B) Prednisone is continued as long as there is protein in the urine. (C) Hematuria is a symptom of glomerulonephritis and not nephrosis. (D) His "moon" face is a side effect of the drug and will continue as long as prednisone is taken.

28. **(B)** Client need: psychosocial integrity; subcategory: psychosocial adaptation; content area: pediatrics

    RATIONALE

    (A) It is not unusual for a 3-year-old child who is hurt and in a strange environment to not be talkative. (B) There is conflicting data between what each parent reported happened and her physical injuries. (C, D) This does not necessarily indicate child abuse.

29. **(C)** Client need: psychosocial integrity; subcategory: psychosocial adaptation; content area: pediatrics

    RATIONALE

    (A) Abusive parents have a low self-esteem. (B) Most abusive parents were abused as children and did not experience a happy childhood. (C) Abusive parents usually select one child to abuse that they see as being different. (D) Abused children are usually perceived by the abusive parent as developmentally delayed.

30. **(A)** Client need: health promotion and maintenance; subcategory: growth and development through the life span; content area: pediatrics

    RATIONALE

    (A) Parents that are abusive have not mastered the developmental task of trust. (B) Through role reversal with their children, abusive parents do receive some role gratification. (C) These parents are able to function outside the home; they just do not develop friendships easily. (D) Everyone has a value system.

31. **(B)** Client need: health promotion and maintenance; subcategory: growth and development through the life span; content area: pediatrics

    RATIONALE

    (A, C, D) This is not a major area of knowledge deficit that results in child abuse. (B) Abusive parents are not realistic in their expectations related to growth and developmental tasks for their children owing to a lack of knowledge.

32. **(B)** Client need: psychosocial integrity; subcategory: psychosocial adaptation; content area: pediatrics

    RATIONALE

    (A) If there are adequate data to suspect child abuse, no additional data are necessary to take action. (B) The nurse has a legal responsibility to report any suspected cases of child abuse. (C) This could result in the parents' taking the child and leaving the hospital. (D) Discussing the situation with the physician does not guarantee that the authorities will be notified.

33. **(B)** Client need: health promotion and maintenance; subcategory: prevention and early detection of disease; content area: pediatrics

    RATIONALE

    (A) Frequent voiding is important, but there is no specific number of times a day a child should void. (B) This prevents contamination of bacteria from the anal area. (C) Increased fluid intake, especially with acid juices, aids in acidifying the urine. (D) The child should wear cotton underwear.

34. **(C)** Client need: physiological integrity; subcategory: physiological adaptation; content area: pediatrics

    RATIONALE

    (A) This would indicate old blood in the stool. (B) This stool pattern is characteristic of Hirschsprung's disease. (C) This stool pattern is characteristic of intussusception and indicates fresh blood. (D) This stool pattern is characteristic of cystic fibrosis.

35. **(B)** Client need: health promotion and maintenance; subcategory: prevention and early detection of disease; content area: pediatrics

    RATIONALE

    (A) This is subjective information and therefore not the best answer. (B) This is objective information that indicates the infant is maintaining and absorbing his feedings. (C) This is not directly related to food absorption. (D) This is subjective information and not the best indicator of food intake and absorption.

36. **(C)** Client need: physiological integrity; subcategory: reduction of risk potential; content area: pediatrics

    RATIONALE

    (A) This by itself is not a life-threatening problem. (B) This is important, but by itself is not life threatening. (C) Malnutrition alters metabolic functioning and eventually results in starvation and death. (D) Behavior changes and mood swings are usually present and not depression.

37. **(A)** Client need: psychosocial integrity; subcategory: psychosocial adaptation; content area: pediatrics

    RATIONALE

    (A) Adolescents with anorexia nervosa try very hard to do what is expected of them at home and school and with their peers. (B) Anorexic clients are very dependent. (C) Anorexic clients tend to follow the rules and are described as "good kids." (D) Anorexic clients are high achievers.

38. **(B)** Client need: physiological integrity; subcategory: physiological adaptation; content area: pediatrics

    RATIONALE

    (A) There would be cold intolerance. (B) With little or no body fat for insulation, the body temperature is decreased. (C) There would be amenorrhea. (D) There would be bradycardia.

39. **(D)** Client need: safe, effective care environment; subcategory: management of care; content area: pediatrics

RATIONALE

(A, B, C) This condition has no symptoms that could be mistaken for SIDS. (D) Bruising occurs due to the pooling and settling of blood once the infant has died. This gives the appearance that the child has been beaten.

40. **(C)** Client need: psychosocial integrity; subcategory: coping and adaptation; content area: pediatrics

    RATIONALE

    (A) Anger is felt, but it is not the main feeling consistently expressed by parents. (B) Depression may occur, but it is not the main feeling expressed by parents. (C) Parents consistently experience guilt. They always question whether they could have done something differently (i.e., checked on the infant more often) to have prevented their baby's death. (D) Hostility is felt, but it is not the main feeling expressed by parents.

41. **(D)** Client need: safe, effective care environment; subcategory: safety and infection control; content area: pediatrics

    RATIONALE

    (A, B, C) These are appropriate interventions, but not as important as the child's safety. (D) This intervention prevents the child from sustaining further injury from falling out of the bed.

42. **(C)** Client need: physiological integrity; subcategory: pharmacological and parenteral therapies; content area: pediatrics

    RATIONALE

    (A, B, D) Even distribution of the medication will not occur with this placement. (C) This is the correct placement for eye drops.

43. **(B)** Client need: health promotion and maintenance; subcategory: prevention and early detection of disease; content area: pediatrics

    RATIONALE

    (A) This is not usually found in children older than 2 years of age. (B) Injuries to the eyes, especially related to accidents, are the major cause. (C) Farsightedness does not result in blindness. (D) This does not usually cause blindness.

44. **(B)** Client need: physiological integrity; subcategory: physiological adaptation; content area: pediatrics

    RATIONALE

    (A, C, D) Opacity is not a symptom of this condition. (B) Cloudiness of the lens is a symptom of congenital cataracts.

45. **(C)** Client need: physiological integrity; subcategory: physiological adaptation; content area: pediatrics

    RATIONALE

    (A, B, D) This condition is not associated with Reye's syndrome. (C) Influenza usually precedes Reye's syndrome.

46. **(B)** Client need: physiological integrity; subcategory: physiological adaptation; content area: pediatrics

    RATIONALE

    (A) This is not a life-threatening problem. (B) Careful monitoring of intake and output aids in preventing cerebral edema or dehydration. (C) This intervention is not associated with a life-threatening problem. (D) This intervention is not as important as preventing cerebral edema or dehydration.

47. **(A)** Client need: safe, effective care environment; subcategory: safety and infection control; content area: pediatrics

    RATIONALE

    (A) Prolonged bleeding may occur owing to impaired coagulation. Pressure should be applied to the injection site for a longer period of time. (B, C, D) This intervention is not related to liver function.

48. **(C)** Client need: physiological integrity; subcategory: physiological adaptation; content area: pediatrics

RATIONALE
(A, D) This type of stool is not symptomatic of cystic fibrosis. (B) Stools are not green but are foul smelling. (C) Undigested food, owing to malabsorption, is excreted, causing an increase in amount and bulk of stools.

49. **(C)** Client need: physiological integrity; subcategory: physiological adaptation; content area: pediatrics
    RATIONALE
    (A) This is incorrect because the birth weight is usually doubled by 6 months. (B) This is incorrect because it is approximately 2.5 times his birth weight. (C) An infant should triple his birth weight by 1 year of age. (D) This is incorrect because it is approximately 3.5 times his birth weight.

50. **(D)** Client need: safe, effective care environment; subcategory: management of care; content area: pediatrics
    RATIONALE
    (A, C) This is not a diagnostic test for cystic fibrosis. (B) Stool specimens are checked for pancreatic enzymes to diagnose cystic fibrosis. Stool cultures are not diagnostic for this disease. (D) Children with cystic fibrosis have above-normal levels of sodium and chloride in their sweat.

51. **(B)** Client need: psychosocial integrity; subcategory: coping and adaptation; content area: pediatrics
    RATIONALE
    (A) His condition is stable. (B) The parents need emotional support to adjust to this chronic condition, the genetic implications, the treatment and prognosis. (C, D) This is not an immediate goal but may be a long-term goal.

52. **(A)** Client need: physiological integrity; subcategory: pharmacological and parenteral therapies; content area: pediatrics
    RATIONALE
    (A) Pancreatic enzymes aid in absorption of nutrients from the intestines so the stools become normal. (B) This is not a realistic weight gain. (C) Pancreatic enzymes are not related to the respiratory system. (D) Pancreatic enzymes are not related to the NaCl level in the sweat.

53. **(B)** Client need: safe, effective care environment; subcategory: safety and infection control; content area: pediatrics
    RATIONALE
    (A) The purpose of protective isolation is to protect the child from exposure to organisms from other people. (B) With leukemia, changes in the blood cell number and composition make the child susceptible to infection. (C) The purpose of protective isolation is to protect the child from exposure to organisms from other people. (D) This is not the purpose of protective isolation. Preventing infection through direct contact with anyone is the purpose.

54. **(C)** Client need: psychosocial integrity; subcategory: coping and adaptation; content area: pediatrics
    RATIONALE
    (A) This explanation does not deal with her immediate feelings of loss. (B) Knowing that this is a side effect does not make her feel better. (C) Understanding that the condition is temporary and her hair will grow back is comforting. (D) This explanation is not realistic and does not deal with the feelings of loss.

55. **(D)** Client need: health promotion and maintenance; subcategory: prevention and early detection of disease; content area: pediatrics
    RATIONALE
    (A) This is not very effective and does not stimulate the gums. (B) This is not very effective and does not stimulate the gums. (C) This does not stimulate the gums and prevent gingivitis. (D) This will effectively rinse the mouth and stimulate the gums.

56. **(A)** Client need: physiological integrity; subcategory: physiological adaptation; content area: pediatrics
    RATIONALE
    (A) Immobilization allows rest and healing. The pain can be so intense that even the weight of a blanket can hurt. (B, D) Movement of the joints causes pain. (C) The pressure of the heating pad or hot water bottle can cause pain.

57. **(D)** Client need: physiological integrity; subcategory: physiological adaptation; content area: pediatrics
    RATIONALE
    (A, B, C) These are not toxic symptoms. (D) These are common toxic symptoms of salicylates.

58. **(C)** Client need: physiological integrity; subcategory: physiological adaptation; content area: pediatrics
    RATIONALE
    (A, D) This is not a symptom of this condition. (B) Symptoms are excessive salivation and drooling. (C) Cyanosis is due to the fistula from the trachea and the esophagus.

59. **(B)** Client need: physiological integrity; subcategory: physiological adaptation; content area: pediatrics
    RATIONALE
    (A) With this disease there is a fever for more than 5 days. (B) This is a symptom of the disease. There is also reddening of the rest of the oropharynx. (C) There is edema of the hands and feet, as well as redness. (D) Swelling occurs in the cervical lymph nodes with this disease.

60. **(B)** Client need: physiological integrity; subcategory: physiological adaptation; content area: pediatrics
    RATIONALE
    (A) Aspirin is usually given to reduce inflammation. (B) γ-Globulin is given to minimize possible cardiac complications. (C, D) This is not a drug usually given for this condition.

61. **(D)** Client need: health promotion and maintenance; subcategory: prevention and early detection of disease; content area: pediatrics
    RATIONALE
    (A) MMR can be given with OPV. (B) Allergies to horse serum are a significant consideration with tetanus antitoxin. (C) There is concern with children who have an upper respiratory infection, but it is not the major concern specific to MMR vaccine. (D) MMR vaccine is dangerous to the fetus in pregnant women. Pregnancy should be avoided for at least 3 months after the MMR vaccination.

62. **(C)** Client need: health promotion and maintenance; subcategory: prevention and early detection of disease; content area: pediatrics
    RATIONALE
    (A) Milk or carbonated drinks should be avoided with administration of syrup of ipecac because they may delay emesis. (B) The purpose of administering activated charcoal is to bind with the poison so that body absorption of the poison will be decreased. Because the purpose of syrup of ipecac is to induce vomiting, these drugs would decrease the effectiveness of each other. (C) The therapeutic action of syrup of ipecac is facilitated by following the dose with 100–200 mL of tepid water or other clear liquid in children (200–300 mL in adults). (D) There could be a problem with water intoxication and decreased effectiveness of syrup of ipecac with the administration of large amounts of cold water.

63. **(D)** Client need: physiological integrity; subcategory: pharmacological and parenteral therapies; content area: pediatrics

RATIONALE

(A) Sedative-type drugs usually have a paradoxical effect and cause increased activity. Consequently, they would not be used unless indicated in the treatment of some other problem exhibited by the child. (B) Prednisone would not be indicated in the treatment of hyperactivity. (C) Dilantin is an anticonvulsant and is inappropriate. (D) Ritalin is the drug of choice in the management of hyperactive behavior in children with ADHD.

64. **(B)** Client need: physiological integrity; subcategory: pharmacological and parenteral therapies; content area: pediatrics

RATIONALE

(A) Many children who have seizures do have this side effect. However, it has nothing specifically to do with the seizure. (B) Hyperplasia of the gums is a side effect of phenytoin. Phenytoin administration is seen most commonly in children and adolescents. It never occurs in edentulous clients. (C) Hyperplasia of the gums is an effect of phenytoin. Phenytoin administration is seen most commonly in children and adolescents. It never occurs in edentulous clients. (D) Hyperplasia of the gums is not a side effect of phenobarbital.

65. **(A)** Client need: physiological integrity; subcategory: pharmacological and parenteral therapies; content area: pediatrics

RATIONALE

(A) Nystatin is a local antibiotic and must come into contact with the infected area to be effective. Giving half of the dose on each side of the mouth will increase the area of contact and consequently increase the effectiveness of the drug. (B, C, D) Giving with milk or food, through a nipple, or following medication with water would decrease effectiveness by decreasing direct contact of the medication with the infected area.

66. **(C)** Client need: physiological integrity; subcategory: physiological adaptation; content area: pediatrics

RATIONALE

(A) The child with nephrosis should be on bed rest in the edematous state. (B) High-carbohydrate diet is needed for energy and the caloric intake. (C) Protein replacement is critical because of the massive proteinuria and hypoalbuminemia with nephrosis. (D) High-protein diet is needed for protein replacement.

67. **(B)** Client need: health promotion and maintenance; subcategory: growth and development through the life span; content area: pediatrics

RATIONALE

(A) Books are appropriate for this age and do enhance a child's mental development. (B) Costumes would allow the child an increase in self-expression. The most characteristic play of this age group is imaginative, dramatic, and imitative play. (C) Coloring books are appropriate play and will enhance creativity and mental development. (D) A wagon will enhance physical development.

68. **(A)** Client need: physiological integrity; subcategory: reduction of risk potential; content area: pediatrics

RATIONALE

(A) Pulse oximetry measures the oxygen saturation and perfusion. Hypothermia can give an inaccurate reading. (B) Hypotension will alter the pulse oximetry measurement, not hypertension. (C) A low hemoglobin level will alter the reading. (D) Good skin integrity will promote an accurate measurement.

69. **(C)** Client need: physiological integrity; subcategory: reduction of risk potential; content area: pediatrics

RATIONALE

(A) This is too low a setting to suction a tracheostomy. (B) This is the appropriate setting for a neonate. (C) This is the appropriate setting for an infant. (D) This is the appropriate setting for a larger child.

70. **(C)** Client need: health promotion and maintenance; subcategory: growth and development through the life span; content area: pediatrics

RATIONALE

(A) Board games are appropriate for a school-age child. (B) Cradle gym is appropriate for an infant. (C) Soap bubbles are appropriate for a 3-year-old child. (D) Costumes for dress-up are appropriate for preschool age.

71. **(A)** Client need: physiological integrity; subcategory: physiological adaptation; content area: pediatrics

RATIONALE

(A) Irritability is an early sign of increased intracranial pressure in an infant. (B) Bradycardia would not be an initial sign of increased intracranial pressure. It is a late sign after tachycardia. (C) The fontanel would be bulging. (D) Increased urine output does not apply to this situation.

72. **(A)** Client need: safe, effective care environment; subcategory: safety and infection control; content area: pediatrics

RATIONALE

(A) This is the appropriate response. Consulting the infection control nurse for alteratives for patient placement is best. (B) The uninfected child could become infected because this disease can be transmitted through airborne droplets. (C) The child can become infected with TB through airborne droplets. (D) The best choice would be to consult someone for placement before refusing to accept a child for admission.

73. **(D)** Client need: health promotion and maintenance; subcategory: prevention and early detection of disease; content area: pediatrics

RATIONALE

(A) This is the correct procedure to compress once inside the nostrils. (B) This is an acceptable position and will help prevent aspiration. (C) Placing on the side will facilitate drainage and help prevent aspiration. (D) The mouth should be suctioned before nares when suctioning both.

74. **(A)** Client need: physiological integrity; subcategory: physiological adaptation; content area: pediatrics.

RATIONALE

(A) Oats, rye, barley, and wheat all have the protein gluten. People with celiac disease are unable to digest the by-product of gluten, gliadin, resulting in GI problems. (B) Fresh fruits and vegetables are acceptable in the diet. (C) Chicken and poultry products are acceptable and do not cause a toxic buildup in the intestines. (D) Milk products are acceptable.

75. **(D)** Client need: physiological integrity; subcategory: physiological adaptation; content area: pediatrics

RATIONALE

(A) The nurse would assess for cyanosis, but this does not change the environment the newborn is in. (B) The newborn is exhibiting s/sx of a tracheal atresia; therefore, the culture is not warranted. (C) Measuring the abdomen would be appropriate assessment just as checking for cyanosis, but will not alter the environment. (D) Positioning on the back and elevating the head will help prevent aspiration and place the newborn in the safest environment.

76. **(A)** Client need: physiological integrity; subcategory: physiological adaptation; content area: pediatrics

RATIONALE

(A) A high specific gravity can indicate dehydration, which could be a complication this child could develop. (B) A reduction in gastric drainage is expected and indicates the GI tract is recovering from surgery. (C) This is a normal potassium level. (D) Fontanels are closed in children that are 2 years old.

77. **(C)** Client need: health promotion and maintenance; subcategory: prevention and early detection of disease; content area: pediatrics

RATIONALE

(A) These should be administered along with the polio vaccine. (B) The Hepatitis B could be administered, but since the record indicates the infant is on schedule this was probably given at the 2-month clinic visit. (C) These are the immunizations needed at this visit. (D) The polio vaccine should be given in addition. The Hepatitis B should only be given if not given at the 2-month visit.

78. **(A)** Client need: physiological integrity; subcategory: physiological adaptation; content area: pediatrics

RATIONALE

(A) Infants with pyloric stenosis have a tendency toward dehydration since they cannot keep their formula down. (B) Diarrhea is not an issue with this illness. (C) This illness is usually corrected before malnourishment occurs. However, the malnourishment would not be due to improper diet, but due to inability to keep formula down. (D) This could occur, but the stenotic pylorus is usually corrected before malnourishment.

79. **(A)** Client need: physiological integrity; subcategory: reduction of risk potential; content area: pediatrics

RATIONALE

(A) This is a classic symptom of digoxin toxicity. (B) Confusion is not usually a symptom, but lethargy can be. (C) Dyspnea is usually not associated with digoxin toxicity. (D) Anorexia is a symptom of digoxin toxicity. Typically, these children have poor weight gain due to underlying heart condition.

80. **(A)** Client need: physiological integrity; subcategory: reduction of risk potential; content area: pediatrics

RATIONALE

(A) Chest tightness should alert the nurse to a reaction. (B) In allergic reactions the BP usually decreases. (C) This is usually not associated with this type of infusion. (D) The nurse should watch redness at the site for further problems.

81. **(A)** Client need: safe, effective care environment; subcategory: safety and infection control; content area: pediatrics

RATIONALE

(A) Private room is recommended for at least 24 hours post antibiotics to prevent the spread of infection. (B) The pneumonia could be from a different type of bacteria or virus, and cross contamination could result. (C) The child with FTT is at high risk and more susceptible to illness. (D) Cross contamination could result if these two patients roomed together.

82. **(A)** Client need: safe, effective care environment; subcategory: safety and infection control; content area: pediatrics

RATIONALE

(A) Private room is recommended because the cause of illness is undetermined and respiratory viruses are contagious. (B) The child being admitted may not have RSV, and cross-contamination can occur. (C) A virus other than RSV could have caused this child's pneumonia. (D) The child with otitis media could be contaminated with a viral illness.

83. **(C)** Client need: safe, effective care environment; subcategory: management of care; content area: pediatrics

RATIONALE

(A) The child being admitted could contract respiratory illness due to exposure to the child with pneumonia. (B) At this age, males and females are usually not assigned to the same room. (C) This would be an acceptable assignment because the patient is a female and has a noncontagious disease. (D) This is not preferred due to the age difference.

84. **(A)** Client need: safe, effective care environment; subcategory: management of care; content area: pediatrics

RATIONALE

(A) This child is in for diagnostic work-up for a chronic problem. Assessment needs for this child are not as critical as the other acutely ill children. (B) These children need much attention after surgery and require higher skill level. The pulled nurse may not be familiar with this surgery. (C) The first 24 hours after surgery will require increased assessment for complications and pain management. (D) This child will need close observation to assess for signs of respiratory difficulty/distress.

85. **(B)** Client need: safe, effective care environment; subcategory: management of care; content area: pediatrics

RATIONALE

(A) This is an acceptable assignment. Proper handwashing precautions and contact precautions will prevent spread of any bacteria. (B) Ribavirin has been reported to cause problems with pregnancy; therefore it would be best not to assign this nurse to take care of this infant. (C) This is an acceptable assignment; the nurse does not have to expose herself to the x-rays. (D) This assignment would be acceptable; the nurse should take proper isolation precautions.

86. **(C)** Client need: safe, effective care environment; subcategory: safety and infection control; content area: pediatrics

RATIONALE

(A) This can be done but should not be the initial response. (B) Housekeeping should be notified, especially if it was a large spill. (C) The initial action should be to cover the chemotherapy agent and implement cleanup. (D) Personnel should be asked to stay away from the area until the spill is cleaned up. Visitors should not be in the area of the medication room even when there is not a spill.

87. **(B)** Client need: safe, effective care environment; subcategory: safety and infection control; content area: pediatrics

RATIONALE

(A) This is not an airborne illness. (B) This illness is spread through direct contact. Therefore, contact and standard precautions should be taken when caring for this patient. (C) This illness is not spread by droplets. (D) Standard precautions should be taken along with contact precautions.

88. **(C)** Client need: safe, effective care environment; subcategory: safety and infection control; content area: pediatrics

RATIONALE

(A) The virus is viable for a longer period of time. (B) The virus is viable for a longer period of time. (C) The virus can live on a nonporous surface for 6 hours. (D) The virus is viable for 6 hours.

89. **(D)** Client need: health promotion and maintenance; subcategory: growth and development through the life span; content area: pediatrics

RATIONALE

(A) Red mobile would be good for an infant 2–3 months old. (B) An infant does not recognize pastel colors until around 3 months. (C) Primary colors cannot be distinguished by a neonate; these colors would be best for an older infant. (D) Black and white is the best choice to help the neonate focus.

90. **(A)** Client need: physiological integrity; subcategory: reduction of risk potential; content area: pediatrics

    RATIONALE

    (A) Six Lifesavers equals 15 g of carbohydrates. (B) One cup of milk equals 15 g of carbohydrates. (C) One half cup of orange juice equals 15 g of carbohydrates. (D) This exceeds 15 g of carbohydrates.

91. **(C)** Client need: physiological integrity; subcategory: reduction of risk potential; content area: pediatrics

    RATIONALE

    (A) The onset of regular insulin is one half to 1 hour with the onset of NPH being 1–2 hours; therefore, the insulins are just beginning to take effect. (B) The regular insulin is peaking, but the NPH insulin is just beginning to peak. (C) Twelve noon is the expected combination peak time. The peak of the regular insulin is tapering off and the NPH insulin is reaching its peak. (D) The regular insulin peak occurs within 4 hours, which has already occurred at 2:00 PM, and the NPH is still at its peak at 2:00 PM, but the child is not getting the peak effect of both insulins at this time.

CHAPTER **5**

Medical-Surgical Nursing: Content Review and Test

Patricia G. Beare, RN, PhD
Helen Ptak, PhD, RN
Louise Plaisance, RN, C, DNS

Respiratory System

Assessment

SUBJECTIVE

1. Signs and symptoms
   A. Cough
   B. Difficulty in breathing
   C. Pain
   D. Weakness, tiredness
   E. Sputum color and consistency
2. History
   A. Respiratory illness or difficulty
   B. Injuries
   C. Use of extra pillows when sleeping
   D. Smoking
   E. Occupation
   F. Use of medications

OBJECTIVE

1. Respirations
   A. Rate, depth, rhythm, and type
   B. Difficulty in breathing
2. Symptoms of lack of O_2
   A. Yawning
   B. Restlessness
   C. Drowsiness
   D. Anxiety
   E. Confusion
   F. Disorientation
3. Skin
   A. Color
      (1) Pale or ruddy (reddened)
      (2) Cyanotic—color of lips, nails, inside of mouth

   B. Temperature
   C. Excessive sweating
4. Cough
   A. Frequency—continuous, sporadic
   B. Type—productive, moist, hacking, dry, nonproductive
5. Sputum
   A. Presence or absence
   B. Type—thick, frothy, watery
   C. Color—white, yellow, rusty, blood tinged, purulent, green
   D. Amount—scant, moderate, abundant
   E. Odor
6. Vital signs
   A. Pulse—rate, quality, type
   B. Blood pressure
   C. Temperature—rectal, unless ordered otherwise

DIAGNOSTIC TESTS AND METHODS

1. Complete blood count (CBC)
2. White blood cell (WBC) count
3. Arterial blood gases (ABGs)
4. Culture and sensitivity tests
5. Specimen of throat or nasopharyngeal secretions
6. Sputum culture
7. Sputum for acid-fast bacillus—check for tuberculosis (TB) infection
8. Chest x-ray
9. Bronchoscopy
10. Biopsy examination of tissue for diagnosis
11. Thoracentesis
12. Pulmonary function tests
    A. Vital capacity
    B. Tidal volume
    C. Total lung capacity
13. Lung scan

Implementation

1. Mouth breathing
   A. Give mouth care every 2 hours.
   B. Increase fluid intake (if allowed).
   C. Lubricate lips.
2. Dyspnea
   A. Give O_2 as ordered.
   B. Position in semi-to-high Fowler position; use extra pillows.
   C. Plan rest periods.
   D. Organize care in order to save client's energy.
   E. Use rectal thermometer to take temperature.
   F. Give small, frequent feedings of soft diet.
   G. Prevent constipation and straining.
3. Cough, sputum
   A. Accurately record and report observations about cough and sputum.
   B. Provide tissues and receptacle for disposal.
   C. Provide sputum cup.
   D. Encourage deep breathing.
   E. Turn client every 2 hours.
   F. Force fluid unless contraindicated.
   G. Give mouth care every 2 hours.
   H. Obtain sputum specimen as ordered.
   I. Give expectorants, if ordered.
   J. Use postural drainage, if ordered.
4. Weakness, dizziness (client tires easily if demand for O_2 by cells not met; dizziness caused by decreased O_2 supply to brain cells)
   A. Provide care—assist client to decrease exertion.
   B. Give humidified O_2 as ordered.
   C. Limit conversation.
   D. Use side rails.
   E. Make frequent neurological assessments.
   F. Minimize loss of appetite and its effects—odor from sputum, bad taste, dry mouth from mouth breathing affects appetite.
      (1) Give mouth care before each meal.
      (2) Serve small, frequent, and attractive meals.
5. Orthopnea (difficulty in breathing when lying flat)
   A. Place bed in semi-to-high Fowler position.
   B. Use overbed table with pillow for headrest in extreme cases.
   C. Place footboard at end of bed to prevent client from slipping down.

Evaluation

1. Reports increased comfort, decreased anxiety
2. Shows no evidence of laryngitis
3. Reports relief of pain
4. Maintains stable vital signs
5. Is able to communicate vocally without frustration
6. Demonstrates understanding of disease process, treatment, home care, and need for follow-up

Carcinoma of the Larynx

Description

1. The most common form of carcinoma of the larynx is squamous cell carcinoma (95%).
2. Rare forms include adenocarcinoma, sarcoma, and others.
3. Intrinsic tumors are found on the true vocal cord and do not tend to spread because nearby tissue lacks lymph nodes.
4. Extrinsic tumors are found on the larynx outside of the true vocal cord and tend to spread early, involving the epiglottis, false vocal cords, and piriform sinuses, which are rich in lymph nodes.
5. Cancer of the larynx is more common in men than in women; most are between the ages of 55 and 70.
6. Early diagnosis and treatment can lead to an 80%–90% cure rate for small lesions of the vocal cords.
7. Cause—unknown
8. Predisposing factors
   A. Smoking—especially in heavy smokers
   B. Alcoholism
   C. Combined use of tobacco and alcohol—causes a synergistic effect
   D. Chronic inhalation of noxious fumes
   E. Familial tendency
   F. History of frequent laryngitis and vocal straining
   G. Prior exposure to radiation
   H. Certain diets in different cultures
9. Classification by location
   A. Supraglottic—posterior surface of epiglottis, false vocal cords
   B. Glottis—true vocal cords
   C. Subglottic—downward from vocal cords (rare)

Assessment

SUBJECTIVE

1. Hoarseness longer than 3 weeks
2. Voice change
3. Cough
4. Pain or burning in throat after drinking citrus juice or hot liquid
5. Dysphagia
6. Pain around thyroid or Adam's apple radiating to ear on affected side
7. Anxiety

OBJECTIVE

1. Hoarseness
2. Mass in throat
3. Dysphagia (difficulty in swallowing)
4. Cough
5. Hemoptysis
6. Enlarged cervical lymph nodes
7. Weight loss
8. Erosion into major blood vessels with hemorrhage if left untreated

DIAGNOSTIC TESTS AND METHODS

1. Detailed history
2. Detailed physical examination
3. Visual examination—indirect laryngoscopy
4. Direct laryngoscopy with biopsy of tissue
5. Needle biopsy of enlarged lymph nodes
6. Laryngeal tomography
7. Chest x-ray—to detect metastases
8. Staging—to determine:
   A. Tumor size and location of laryngeal cancerous growth

B. Number of nodes found
C. Presence or absence of metastases

Planning

1. Safe, effective care environment
   A. Prevent avoidable injury and/or infection.
   B. Increase client's knowledge of disease process, diagnostic procedures, and treatment.
2. Physiological integrity
   A. Increase comfort.
   B. Maintain effective airway clearance.
   C. Maintain oral hygiene.
3. Psychosocial integrity
   A. Maintain effective communication.
   B. Reduce anxiety.
   C. Counsel on alterations of body image and self-concept.
4. Health promotion and maintenance
   A. Increase client's knowledge of home care and follow-up.

Implementation

1. Assess, record, and report signs and symptoms and reactions to treatment.
2. Give emotional support.
3. Prepare client for surgical intervention—assess emotional and knowledge needs.
4. Encourage client to practice deep breathing and coughing to be used postoperatively.
5. Clarify and reinforce physician's directions.
6. Arrange for visit by hospital chaplain, psychiatric nurse, or private clergy to counsel client, if needed.
7. Arrange for visit by laryngectomy volunteer.
8. Provide general preoperative and postoperative care as required for:
   A. Excisional biopsy—for small, localized cancers, client may be discharged the same day.
   B. Laryngectomy (partial or complete).
   C. Radical neck dissection—excision includes lymph nodes, epiglottis, muscle tissue, thyroid cartilage, sternocleidomastoid muscle, internal jugular vein, and spinal accessory nerve.
   D. Permanent tracheostomy.
   E. Radiotherapy.
   F. Radiotherapy in conjunction with surgery and/or chemotherapy.
9. Provide the following additional care after radical neck dissection:
   A. Monitor the drain or drainage collection device frequently for proper function.
   B. Empty, measure, and record amount of drainage—approximately 70–120 mL of serosanguineous drainage is expected during the first postoperative day.
   C. Provide specific care as ordered for skin flap and donor site.
   D. Monitor for adequate ventilation to graft area.
   E. Monitor for friction or pressure on graft area.
   F. Monitor for presence of hematoma formation.
      (1) Excessive swelling
      (2) Changes in skin coloration
      (3) Blanching of skin
      (4) Changes in rate or type of drainage
      (5) Airway compression
      (6) Changes in hemoglobin and hematocrit levels
   G. Monitor and report signs of infection of suture line immediately.
      (1) Danger of carotid artery rupture if suture line is disrupted.
      (2) Emergency equipment should be available.
   H. Monitor and report presence of salivary fistulas.
      (1) Saliva abrades the suture line.
      (2) It causes a channel to the skin.
      (3) It delays healing of suture sites.
   I. Provide the following care for these effects of external carotid removal during radical neck dissection:
      (1) Results in decreased O_2 to area
         (a) Monitor client's skin color until collateral blood vessels are established.
      (2) May have decreased oxygenation to brain
         (a) Monitor for vertigo.
         (b) Monitor for spatial disorientation.
         (c) Check for gait alterations.
         (d) Instruct client to change position slowly.
         (e) Assist with self-care and ambulation.
         (f) Keep side rails up for several days following operation.
      (3) May produce emboli due to manipulation of major blood vessels during surgery.
         (a) Monitor and report changes in mental status immediately.
         (b) Check for signs of cerebrovascular accident (CVA).
10. Instruct client regarding disease process, diagnostic procedures, treatment, home care, and follow-up.

Evaluation

1. Maintains normal rate and depth of breathing
2. Maintains patent airway without mucous plugging
3. Maintains ABGs within normal range
4. Reports relief of pain
5. Is able to communicate effectively
6. Remains free of infection at operative site
7. Maintains adequate nutritional intake
8. Regains usual body weight
9. Reports increased comfort, decreased anxiety
10. Uses effective coping strategies
11. Accepts new appearance as shown by self-care and social interaction
12. Demonstrates proper care of tracheostomy tube and suctioning
13. Verbalizes feelings about disfigurement
14. Demonstrates understanding of disease process, diagnostic procedures, treatment, home care, and need for follow-up

Pneumonia

Description

1. Pneumonia is acute inflammation of lung parenchyma associated with the production of exudate.
2. Secretions fill the alveolar sacs, which allows bacterial or viral growth.

3. Inflammation spreads to neighboring sacs, bronchioles, and bronchi, resulting in consolidation accompanied by a thick exudate in the spaces of the lung.
4. This process prevents ventilation of the affected lung structures, resulting in arteriovenous shunting, which in turn causes:
   A. Hypoxemia.
      (1) Severity is correlated with the size of the shunt.
      (2) Extent of hypoxic vasoconstriction compensation in affected area depends on severity of the hypoxemia produced.
   B. Characteristic rusty color of sputum
   C. Breathing becomes difficult.
5. Classification by cause
   A. Types of bacterial causative organisms
      (1) Pneumococci
      (2) *Staphylococcus aureus, Streptococcus pneumoniae,* and *Streptococcus pyogenes*
         (a) Most cases occur in winter or early spring.
         (b) Pneumonia often follows upper respiratory tract infection.
         (c) Exact mode of transmission is unknown.
      (3) *Haemophilus influenzae*
         (a) Gram-negative bacillus often invades airways of patients with chronic obstructive pulmonary disorder (COPD).
         (b) Infection is believed to be spread through aerosolized respiratory droplets.
         (c) Older clients with COPD, diabetes mellitus, or chronic alcoholism are at risk.
         (d) Death rates, especially in the elderly, are about 30%.
      (4) *Mycoplasma pneumoniae*
         (a) Nonmotile bacteria with no cell walls.
         (b) Bacteria produce mild pneumonia in healthy individuals.
         (c) Infection is transmitted from one person to another by water droplets suspended in the air.
         (d) It often spreads rapidly to family members.
   B. Viral infections
   C. Irritating chemicals
      (1) Aspiration of chemicals in stomach contents
      (2) Inhalation of chemicals (e.g., chlorine)
   D. Fungal infection
      (1) Histoplasmosis caused by *Histoplasma capsulatum*
         (a) Infection is transmitted by spores living in soil.
         (b) It is endemic in certain areas of the United States.
         (c) It thrives in soil high in nitrogen—soil high in compost heaps, bird droppings.
         (d) It invades lungs and spreads through body via the circulatory system.
         (e) It is characterized by a brief infection of lower respiratory tract.
         (f) Clients may be asymptomatic.
         (g) It requires no special treatment unless severe.
         (h) Severe pneumonia is treated with amphotericin B (Fungizone).
      (2) Coccidioidomycosis caused by *Coccidioides immitis*
         (a) Infection is endemic in southwestern United States and northern Mexico.
         (b) It is transmitted by inhalation of spores that live in the soil.
         (c) Following inhalation into the alveoli, the spores cause a granulomatous and suppurative response.
         (d) Clients are usually asymptomatic.
         (e) Infection may produce a mild respiratory illness.
         (f) It occasionally causes a severe pneumonia.
         (g) Amphotericin B is used when treatment is required.
   E. Mycobacteria
6. Classification as community acquired
   A. Pneumonia acquired in the community.
   B. It usually begins as common respiratory illness and evolves into fulminant pulmonary infections.
   C. *S. pneumoniae* is the most common cause.
   D. Infection is commonly due to the following anaerobic bacteria, which are prevalent in the upper respiratory tract:
      (1) *Fusobacterium nucleatum*
      (2) Pigmented bacteroides
      (3) *Peptostreptococcus*
      (4) Microaerophilic streptococcus
   E. Community-acquired pneumonia occurs in the very young and the elderly.
7. Classification as hospital acquired
   A. Pneumonia acquired in the hospital (nosocomial pneumonia).
   B. It is commonly caused by bacteria.
      (1) *Klebsiella pneumoniae*
      (2) *S. aureus*
      (3) *Pseudomonas aeruginosa*
   C. Infection may be transmitted directly by the hands of hospital personnel.
   D. It accounts for 16% of infections and associated death rates.
      (1) Related to the causative agent
      (2) Related to the clinical status of the patient
   E. Mortality ranges from 30%–50%.
   F. Most deaths occur in intensive care unit (ICU), usually due to client's critical condition.
8. Classification by anatomical location
   A. Bronchopneumonia
      (1) Patchy consolidations of the lung.
      (2) Infection usually involves both lungs and more than one lobe.
      (3) It may be limited to one lobe.
   B. Lobar pneumonia
      (1) Infection involves the entire lung.
      (2) It may involve a major portion of the lung.
9. Classification as other pneumonia
   A. Protozoa and helminths
      (1) Rare causes of pneumonia.
      (2) The unicellular protozoan *Pneumocystis carinii* is the cause of pneumonia in clients with immunosuppression.
         (a) Infection is believed to be transmitted by airborne droplets.
         (b) It may be due to reactivation of a latent infection.
         (c) Death rates are high.
         (d) Client has depressed immune system, predisposing to opportunistic infection.

10. Once the specific causative organism is identified, it is used to classify the pneumonia.
11. The onset of pneumonia depends on:
    A. Condition of the respiratory defenses
    B. Number of the causative organisms
    C. Virulence of the causative organisms
12. Mode of transmission
    A. Aspiration
        (1) Causative organisms are transmitted from the oropharynx and gastrointestinal (GI) system to the lungs by direct contact.
        (2) Many bacteria are found in the oropharyngeal secretions.
        (3) Clients who are at risk include those with:
            (a) Decreased gag and cough reflexes
            (b) Esophageal disorders
            (c) Endotracheal tubes
            (d) Nasogastric (NG) tubes
    B. Inhalation
        (1) Causative organisms are suspended in water droplets.
        (2) Organisms enter air when infected individual coughs, sneezes, or talks.
        (3) Minute water drops remain suspended in the air, allowing water to evaporate.
        (4) A droplet nucleus with the causative organism can then be inhaled deeply into the lungs of individuals.
        (5) Lung defenses may be overcome when a sufficient number of the causative organisms are inhaled.
        (6) Lungs become infected.
        (7) The more virulent the organism is, the smaller the number required to infect the lungs.
    C. Circulation
        (1) Causative organisms transmitted to lungs via the circulatory system from infections in other parts of the body.
        (2) Examples include clients with:
            (a) Septicemia
            (b) Endocarditis
            (c) Other lung disease
            (d) Immunosuppression
13. Pneumonia in the elderly
    A. Pneumonia is listed as the fourth leading cause of death among individuals older than 65 years of age, usually secondary to other chronic conditions.
    B. Condition does not fit the typical clinical picture of fever and pulmonary symptoms.
        (1) Symptoms include:
            (a) Lethargy
            (b) Confusion
            (c) Tachypnea
            (d) Dehydration
    C. Elderly persons in nursing homes are at highest risk.
        (1) Predisposing factors
            (a) Changes in immune function
            (b) Decrease in mobility
            (c) Decreased cough reflex
            (d) Decreased gag reflex
            (e) Decrease in functional reserve
            (f) Bedridden client at risk for aspiration pneumonia
            (g) Presence of underlying chronic disease

14. Other individuals at risk include those with:
    A. Bronchiectasis
    B. COPD
    C. Cystic fibrosis
    D. Diabetes mellitus
    E. Renal failure
    F. Hepatic failure
    G. Chronic congestive heart failure (CHF)
    H. Pulmonary valvular heart disease
    I. Triscupid valvular heart disease
    J. Severe nutritional problems
    K. Alcohol and drug abusers
    L. Neurological problems with concomitant decreased gag and swallowing reflexes

Assessment

SUBJECTIVE

1. Chills
2. Pain on inspiration
3. Weakness
4. Chest pain—pleuritic type
5. Anorexia

OBJECTIVE

1. Painful, dry cough, changing to a productive cough with green, yellow, or rusty sputum depending on organism
2. Marked elevation in temperature
3. Elevated WBC count with increased immature polymorphonuclear leukocytes
4. Positive diagnosis by chest x-ray
    A. Patchy infiltrates or consolidation over affected area.
    B. X-ray may show small pleural effusion.
5. Positive sputum culture
6. Presence of rales
7. ABGs indicative of hypoxemia
    A. Initial increase in heart rate and blood pressure accompanying severe hypoxemia.
    B. Decreased O_2 saturation accompanied by changes in level of consciousness.
    C. These changes may be accompanied by dyspnea and rapid, shallow breathing.
8. Lethargy
9. Confusion
10. Evidence of lung consolidation on physical examination
11. Dullness to percussion over affected areas
12. Increased fremitus
13. Bronchophony
14. Egophony
15. Bronchial breath sounds
16. Crackles

NOTE: Temperature is not a reliable sign in the elderly.

SUBJECTIVE—ATYPICAL PNEUMONIA (GRADUAL INSIDIOUS ONSET)

1. Headache
2. Sore throat
3. Muscle soreness
4. Fatigue

OBJECTIVE

1. Dry cough
2. Presence of mucoid sputum
3. Scattered wheezes and crackles
4. Minimal or no consolidation over area
5. Findings on chest x-ray
   A. Ranges from minimal infiltrates to substantial bilateral infiltrates
   B. WBC count slightly elevated—usually less than 10,000/mL.

   NOTE: Viral infections and mycoplasma pneumonia are the most common causes of atypical pneumonia.

DIAGNOSTIC TESTS AND METHODS

1. History
   A. Elderly client
2. Physical assessment with auscultation of chest
3. Chest x-ray and examination
4. CBC
5. Sputum culture and sensitivity test
6. ABGs—to detect presence of hypoxemia
7. O_2 saturation measured by pulse oximetry, heart rate, blood pressure, respiratory rate, and level of consciousness

Planning

1. Safe, effective care environment
   A. Prevent avoidable injury and/or infection.
   B. Increase client's and family's knowledge of disease process, diagnostic procedures, and treatment.
2. Physiological integrity
   A. Maintain effective airway clearance and breathing.
   B. Increase comfort.
   C. Maintain adequate nutritional and fluid intake.
3. Psychosocial integrity
   A. Reduce anxiety.
4. Health promotion and maintenance
   A. Increase client's and family's knowledge of prevention, home care, and follow-up.

Implementation

1. Assess, record, and report signs and symptoms and reactions to treatment.
2. Assess adequacy of airway clearance—auscultation of chest.
3. Keep personal items and call bell within easy reach.
4. Help client conserve energy—schedule rest periods.
5. Monitor nutritional intake and weight changes.
   A. Consult with client, family, and dietitian.
   B. Ensure sufficient nutritional intake to:
      (1) Meet energy needs
      (2) Prevent loss of muscle mass
   C. Encourage eating small, frequent meals and increasing fluid intake.
6. Monitor fluid intake and output.
7. Position in semi-to-high Fowler position.
8. Give humidified O_2 as prescribed.
9. Check vital signs every 4 hours; use rectal thermometer.
10. Check breathing effort.
11. Check sputum color, thickness.
12. Collect sputum specimens.
13. Encourage good hand-washing technique.
14. Isolate as indicated; provide for proper disposal of oral and nasal secretions.
15. Provide mouth care.
16. Assist with loosening secretions.
17. Have client turn, cough, and deep breathe every 2 hours or as prescribed.
18. Maintain IV fluids and medication schedule as ordered.
19. Give prescribed antibiotics, antipyretics, analgesics, expectorants, bronchodilators as ordered.
20. Give inhalation therapy as ordered.
21. Avoid cough suppressants if client is producing sputum.
22. Perform chest physiotherapy.
   A. Perform percussion and postural drainage as tolerated.
   B. Suction airway if client is unable to mobilize secretions using nasopharyngeal or oropharyngeal airway.
23. Gradually increase activity levels as condition improves.
   A. Monitor O_2 saturation with a pulse oximeter.
   B. Accompany client during initial ambulation efforts.
      (1) Reduces client's anxiety
      (2) Builds confidence
24. Assess older clients for confusion.
   A. Assess and maintain safety requirement.
   B. Involve family members.
25. Instruct client and family regarding disease process, diagnostic procedures, treatment, prevention, home care, and follow-up.
   A. Percussion and postural drainage if client has excessive secretions at time of discharge
   B. Risk factors, including age, chronic pulmonary disease, immunosuppression
   C. Appropriate behaviors to prevent reinfection
   D. Importance of influenza and pneumococcus vaccination for high-risk groups
   E. Ways to promote good nutrition

Evaluation

1. Reports increased comfort, decreased anxiety
2. Keeps airway free of secretions
3. Maintains clear breath sounds throughout lung fields
4. Maintains $PaO_2 > 70$ mm Hg
5. Resumes usual breathing pattern
6. Resumes or maintains normal mental status
7. Performs activities without undue fatigue
8. Resumes normal sleep pattern
9. Has no complications from infection
10. Maintains adequate fluid and nutritional intake
11. Demonstrates understanding of disease process, diagnostic procedures, treatment, prevention, home care (especially taking medications as ordered), and need for follow-up; similar understanding demonstrated by family

Empyema, Suppurative Pleurisy, and Pleural Effusion

Description

1. **Empyema** is a collection of pus and necrotic (dead) tissue within the pleural space.
   A. Normally this space contains a small amount of extracellular fluid that lubricates the surfaces of the pleura.

B. Causes
    (1) Pneumonia
    (2) Lung abscess
    (3) Chest trauma or surgery
    (4) Liver disease with ascites
    (5) Peritoneal dialysis
    (6) Fungus infections

2. **Suppurative pleurisy** is purulent inflammation of the pleura, causing pain and a pleural rub.
  A. Causes
    (1) Pneumonia
    (2) Lung abscess
    (3) Pancreatitis
    (4) Pulmonary infarction
    (5) Chest trauma or surgery
    (6) Pulmonary TB

3. **Pleural effusion** is accumulation of fluid within the pleural space.
  A. Causes
    (1) Pulmonary TB
    (2) Lung cancer
    (3) Other infections of lung—pneumonia, lung abscess
    (4) CHF
    (5) Liver disease with ascites
    (6) Peritoneal dialysis
    (7) Chest trauma

Assessment

SUBJECTIVE

1. Chest pain
2. Empyema
3. Unilateral
4. Sharp pain on inspiration—referred to shoulder, abdomen, or affected side
5. Malaise
6. Difficulty in breathing
7. Cough
8. Complaints of shortness of breath

OBJECTIVE

1. Elevated temperature
2. Cough
3. Decreased breath sounds
4. Chest expansion not symmetrical
5. Increase in WBC count
6. Presence of pleural rub (suppurative pleurisy)
7. Findings from chest x-ray
8. Anxiety

DIAGNOSTIC TESTS AND METHODS

1. History
2. Chest x-ray
3. Physical examination—including listening to lung sounds
4. Laboratory study of pleural fluid specimen obtained via thoracentesis

Planning

1. Safe, effective care environment
  A. Prevent avoidable injury and/or infection.
  B. Increase client's and family's knowledge of disease process, diagnostic procedures, and treatment.

2. Physiological integrity
  A. Increase comfort.
  B. Maintain effective breathing pattern.
3. Psychosocial integrity
  A. Promote effective coping.
4. Health promotion and maintenance
  A. Increase client's and family's knowledge of home care and follow-up.

Implementation

1. Assess, record, and report signs and symptoms and reactions to treatment.
2. Monitor respirations, breath sounds, and vital signs.
3. Administer antibiotics, anti-inflammatory, and analgesic medications as ordered.
4. Position in semi-to-high Fowler position to assist in breathing.
5. Plan care to allow client adequate rest.
6. Demonstrate splinting chest for coughing.
7. Encourage coughing and deep breathing.
8. Encourage good hand-washing technique.
9. Encourage fluid intake.
10. Encourage good oral hygiene.
11. Prepare client and assist with thoracentesis and/or chest tube insertion as ordered for pleural effusion and empyema.
12. Instruct client and family regarding disease process, diagnostic procedures, home care, and follow-up.

Evaluation

1. Reports increased comfort, decreased anxiety
2. Maintains effective breathing pattern
3. Demonstrates that chest tube system is working correctly
4. Has no complications from infection
5. Demonstrates understanding of disease process, diagnostic procedures, treatment, home care, and need for follow-up; family demonstrates similar understanding

Chronic Obstructive Pulmonary Disease

Description

1. Chronic obstructive pulmonary disease (COPD) includes a group of lung conditions (e.g., asthma, emphysema, and bronchitis) that are frequently progressive and obstruct pulmonary airflow.
2. COPD affects expiratory airflow.
3. Difficulty in emptying lungs when asked to exhale rapidly and forcefully.
4. COPD is a chronic, progressive condition characterized by periodic exacerbations.
5. During periods of exacerbation:
  A. Symptoms are exaggerated.
  B. Clients are acutely ill.
6. Between exacerbation periods:
  A. Symptoms remain, but to a lesser extent.
  B. Clinically, the client remains generally stable.
7. COPD is the most common chronic lung disease, affecting over 17 million Americans.
  A. Incidence is rising.

B. Males are affected more often than females.

C. Condition tends to worsen with time.

8. Predisposing factors

A. Cigarette smoking

(1) Smoking impairs ciliary action.

(2) It impairs macrophage function.

(3) Smoking causes:

(a) Inflammation in airways

(b) Increased mucus production

(c) Destruction of alveolar septic

(d) Peribronchiolar fibrosis

(4) Cessation of smoking before lung destruction becomes extensive may reverse inflammatory changes.

B. Recurrent or chronic respiratory infections

C. Allergies

D. Air pollutants

E. Familial and hereditary factors (e.g., deficiency of α_1 antitrypsin)

9. Complications of COPD

A. Acute respiratory failure (ARF)

(1) ARF usually occurs during exacerbation of COPD.

(2) Both ventilation and oxygenation are inadequate to meet resting requirements of the body.

(3) COPD is characterized by a significant decrease in PaO_2 and/or a combined increase in $PaCO_2$ and decrease in pH.

B. Cor pulmonale

C. Pneumothorax

D. Giant bullae

10. Three major conditions are associated with COPD—asthma, emphysema, and chronic bronchitis.

A. Usually more than one of these underlying conditions coexist.

B. Most often, bronchitis and emphysema occur together.

Asthma

Description

1. Asthma produces sudden narrowing of the trachea and bronchi, obstructing airflow and causing hyperinflation resulting in spasms of the muscle of the bronchi, edema, and swelling of mucous membrane. These changes produce thick tenacious mucus that tends to plug peripheral airways.

2. Condition is characterized by:

A. Reversible airway obstruction

B. Airway inflammation

C. Airway hyperresponsiveness

3. Air enters and is trapped.

A. Characteristic wheeze when client tries to exhale through narrowed bronchi; difficulty in breathing.

B. Inability to expectorate in sufficient amounts by coughing.

C. Attacks last 30–60 minutes with normal breathing between attacks.

D. Status asthmaticus may occur, which is difficult to control.

4. Changes in airways eventually interfere with gas exchange and ventilation through:

A. A mismatch of ventilation-perfusion

(1) Imbalance occurs due to varying degrees of obstruction to airflow throughout lungs.

(2) A portion of the pulmonary circulation is distributed to sections of the lungs that are underventilated.

B. Impaired diffusion due to excessive secretions in airways

C. Shunting in areas of atelectasis

D. Hypoventilation

(1) In early stages, there is a tendency to hyperventilate.

(2) When work of breathing exceeds ability of respiratory muscles to ventilate lungs, hypoventilation occurs.

5. Paroxysmal airway obstruction.

A. May be associated with nasal polyps

B. May be due to aspirin or indomethacin ingestion

6. Magnitude and extent of physiological alterations correlate with the severity of the asthmatic episode, which can range from mild increases in airflow obstruction to respiratory failure and death.

7. Causes include:

A. Inhalation of irritating chemicals. Hyperresponsiveness is more generalized, caused by inflammation of airways.

(1) Common irritants include:

(a) Cigarette smoke

(b) Perfume

(c) Automobile emissions

(d) Vapors from cleaning solvents

(e) Industrial pollutants

(f) Paint

(g) Paint thinners

(h) Sprays—hair spray, furniture polish, household cleaning products, cold air

B. Recurrent respiratory infections.

(1) Generalized hyperresponsiveness due to inflamed airways.

(2) β-agonist bronchodilator action is interfered with by β-adrenergic blockers, resulting in bronchoconstriction.

C. Exercise probably correlated with effects of cold air on airways.

(1) Allergic-induced reaction.

(a) Hyperresponsiveness is an IgE-mediated inflammatory response.

(b) Common allergens include dust, pollens, animal dander, specific foods, and additives.

D. Physical or emotional stress.

E. Familial tendency.

F. Seasonal occurrence.

G. Possible occurrence without any apparent precipitating event.

Assessment

SUBJECTIVE

1. Shortness of breath

2. Wheezing

3. Thick, tenacious sputum (following an acute attack)

4. Chest tightness

5. Anxiety—feeling of suffocation

6. Feelings of severe panic—scared, afraid of dying

7. Irritable, short tempered, and edgy

8. Vertigo

9. Tingling sensations
10. Headaches
11. Nausea
12. Feeling of chest tightening
13. Choking
14. Lack of energy, worn out, fatigued

NOTE: All symptoms are not experienced with each attack.

OBJECTIVE

1. Dyspnea
2. Wheezing on expiration
3. Thick, tenacious sputum
4. Flaring nostrils
5. Use of accessory muscles of respiration
6. Tachypnea
7. Tachycardia
8. Diaphoresis
9. Flushing
10. Evidence of airway obstruction
11. Nature of breathing patterns
12. Changes in level of consciousness
13. During severe attack:
    A. Diaphoretic
    B. Extremely anxious
    C. Inability to talk due to severe dyspnea
    D. Evidence of severe airflow obstruction
    E. Presence of hypoxemia
    F. Use of accessory muscles to breathe
    G. Presence of paradoxical pulse due to:
       (1) Large deviations in intrathoracic pressure during expiration and inspiration.
       (2) Respiratory muscles generate large pressures to ventilate lungs when bronchoconstriction is severe.
       (3) These pressures effect the return of venous blood to right side of heart.
       (4) During inspiration, negative intrathoracic pressures increase venous return.
       (5) During expiration, positive intrathoracic pressures decrease venous return.
       (6) This results in fluctuations in the systolic blood pressure of <10 mm Hg.
    H. Decrease in level of consciousness
    I. Presence of lethargy and drowsiness an indication of exhaustion, which commonly accompanies onset of respiratory failure

NOTE: Dyspnea tends to be more pronounced in younger individuals than in older individuals. Individuals having frequent attacks report lower levels of dyspnea than do individuals having few attacks.

DIAGNOSTIC TESTS AND METHODS

1. History
   A. Intermittent attacks of dyspnea and wheezing
2. Physical examination
   A. Usually normal between attacks
   B. Auscultation shows rhonchi and wheezing throughout lung fields on:
      (1) Expiration
      (2) Inspiration (at times)
   C. Absent or decreased breath sounds during severe obstruction

D. Loud bilateral wheezing—may be audible without stethoscope
   E. Hyperinflated chest
3. Chest x-ray
   A. Hyperinflated lungs with air trapping during asthmatic attack
   B. Normal during remission
4. Sputum analysis shows presence of:
   A. Curschmann's spirals (spirals of mucus)
   B. Charcot-Leyden crystals
   C. Eosinophils
5. ABGs
   A. Decreased PO_2
   B. Decreased or normal PCO_2 (in severe attack)
6. Pulmonary function tests
   A. During attacks—decreased forced expiratory volumes that improve following inhalation of bronchodilator
7. Pulse oximetry
8. Electrocardiogram (ECG)
   A. Sinus tachycardia during asthma attack
   B. Signs of cor pulmonale during severe attack that resolve after attack
      (1) Right-axis deviation
      (2) Peaked P wave
9. Skin tests for allergies

PLANNING

1. Safe, effective care environment
   A. Prevent avoidable injury and/or infection.
   B. Increase client's and family's knowledge of disease process, diagnostic procedures, and treatment (especially medication).
2. Physiological integrity
   A. Maintain effective airway clearance and gas exchange.
   B. Maintain effective breathing pattern.
   C. Maintain fluid balance.
   D. Promote undisturbed sleep perfusion.
   E. Maintain adequate tissue perfusion.
   F. Maintain adequate nutritional intake.
   G. Increase comfort.
3. Psychosocial integrity
   A. Reduce anxiety.
4. Health promotion and maintenance
   A. Increase client's and family's knowledge of prevention, home care, and follow-up.

Implementation

1. Assess, record, and report signs and symptoms and reactions to treatment.
2. Decrease anxiety—provide time to listen; do not leave client alone during attack.
3. Keep environment free from dust and allergens.
4. Place client in semi-to-high Fowler position with arms supported by overbed table.
5. Prevent infection—discourage visits by persons with upper respiratory infections.
6. Discourage smoking.
7. Monitor vital signs, particularly respirations; and check skin color frequently.
   A. Check use of accessory muscles of respiration.
   B. Auscultate breath sounds and pulse rate.
8. Monitor ABGs frequently.
   A. Check indwelling arterial catheter, if used.

9. Assess intensity of dyspnea frequently.
10. Explain and assist with respiratory therapy treatments.
11. Administer prescribed antibiotics and bronchodilators as ordered.
12. Administer prescribed medications such as β-agonists, methylxanthines, and corticosteroids as ordered.
13. Give O_2 therapy as ordered.
14. Note sputum characteristics.
15. Provide adequate fluid intake.
16. Monitor fluid intake and output.
17. Encourage adequate nutritional intake—small, frequent, high-protein, high-caloric meals.
18. Teach breathing exercises.
19. Explain dietary and fluid requirements.
20. Have client and family assist in planning care.
21. Instruct client and family regarding disease process, diagnostic procedures, treatment (especially medications), prevention, home care, and follow-up (especially signs and symptoms indicating need for immediate medical attention).
    A. General guidelines for bronchodilator use
       (1) Instruct client to use β-agonist inhaler at first evidence of an attack.
       (2) Instruct client to seek medical assistance if bronchodilator does not stop the attack within a reasonable period of time.
    B. Drug protocol for clients with mild asthma
       (1) Maintenance therapy—inhaled β-agonists on as-needed basis
    C. Drug protocol for clients with moderate to severe asthma
       (1) A routine regimen of drugs prescribed to reduce frequency of attacks.
       (2) Inhaled corticosteroids are taken on a routine basis to decrease inflammation.
          (a) Localized side effects may include oropharyngeal candidiasis and coughing.
          (b) Seldom produce systemic side effects like those seen with oral corticosteroids.
       (3) Inhaled cromolyn sodium (nonsteroid anti-inflammatory effect) produces fewer side effects.
       (4) Inhaled β-agonists and theophylline are used as maintenance therapy for their bronchodilator effects.
       (5) Use of β-agonists may produce side effects related to cardiac stimulation in persons with cardiac disease and in the elderly.
       (6) Theophylline needs to be administered with caution because there is a fine line between therapeutic and toxic levels.
          (a) Optimal levels are between 10 and 20 mL.
          (b) Signs and symptoms of toxicity include GI disturbances, seizures, arrhythmias, and tachycardia.
       (7) Oral corticosteroids are prescribed only when absolutely necessary because severe side effects can occur from long-term use.
    D. Home monitoring of airway obstruction
       (1) Patient and family are taught to monitor peak expiratory flow rate (PEFR) on a regular basis.
       (2) PEFR is an indicator of airflow obstruction.
       (3) PEFR can be measured by clients with a small affordable peak flowmeter.
       (4) Routine monitoring helps clients to manage their asthma.
       (5) Early changes in airflow obstruction call for early treatment and prevent severe asthma attacks.
       (6) Home monitoring allows for adjustment of medications to meet clients' needs.
    E. Emergency room procedures
       (1) Administer O_2 therapy.
       (2) Give drugs in the following order until client responds:
          (a) Inhaled β-agonists or subcutaneous β-agonists for three doses
          (b) Systemic corticosteroids
       (3) Administer inhaled medications via a nebulizer during an acute attack.
       (4) Monitor for deteriorating respiratory status.
          (a) Note characteristics of sputum.
          (b) Provide adequate fluid intake and O_2 as ordered.
    F. Preventive measures
       (1) Instruct client to avoid possible allergens.
       (2) Use antihistamines, decongestants, inhalation of cromolyn powder, and oral or aerosol bronchodilators as ordered.
       (3) Explain the influence of stress and anxiety and association with exercise (especially running) and cold air.

Evaluation

1. Reports increased comfort, decreased anxiety
2. Has no complications from infection
3. Maintains effective breathing pattern
4. Maintains open airway and adequate gas exchange
5. Verbalizes feelings regarding condition
6. Discusses intention to stop smoking and to check home and work environment for potential irritants.
7. Maintains fluid balance
8. Maintains effective sleep pattern
9. Maintains adequate nutritional intake
10. Reports no shortness of breath at rest and minimal shortness of breath with activities
11. Expresses realistic expectations regarding current health status
12. Maintains $PaCO_2$ at normal baseline—about 40 mm Hg
13. Maintains PaO_2 at normal baseline—approximately 80–100 mm Hg
14. Demonstrates evidence of clear breath sounds on auscultation, with little or no evidence of wheezing
15. Demonstrates understanding of disease process, diagnostic procedures, treatment, prevention, home care, and need for follow-up; similar understanding demonstrated by family

Emphysema

Description

1. Emphysema is a chronic, progressive condition in which the alveolar sacs distend, rupture, and destroy the capillaries.
2. The alveoli lose elasticity, resulting in trapping of inspired air.
3. Inspiration becomes difficult.
4. Expiration is prolonged.
5. Lung tissue becomes fibrotic.

6. Exchange of O_2 and CO_2 decreases due to destruction of alveolar walls, which decreases surface area for gas exchange.
7. The mechanism of destruction is believed to be an imbalance between:
   A. Proteolytic enzymes, which destroy the lung parenchyma, and protease inhibitors, which inactivate proteolytic enzymes.
   B. This mechanism is referred to as the *proteaseantiprotease imbalance hypothesis.*
   C. Increased levels of proteases are released from neutrophils or macrophages in the lung to destroy lung tissue.
8. Loss of lung supporting structures results in:
   A. Decreased elastic recoil
   B. Airway collapse on expiration
9. Causes
   A. Asthma
   B. Recurrent inflammation (pneumonia, air pollution)
   C. Deficiency of α_1-antitrypsin
   D. Cigarette smoking
   E. Pulmonary fibrosis
   F. Familial tendency

Assessment

SUBJECTIVE

1. Insidious onset with dyspnea as the predominant symptom
2. Chronic cough
3. Difficulty in breathing
4. Anorexia (loss of appetite)
5. Malaise

OBJECTIVE

1. Chronic cough—productive, purulent sputum
2. Barrel chest
3. Use of accessory muscles of respiration
4. Prolonged expiratory period—grunting, pursed-lip breathing, abnormal rapidity of breathing
5. Weight loss
6. Peripheral cyanosis
7. Clubbing of fingers
8. Dyspnea on exertion
9. Orthopnea
10. Difficulty in talking—short, jerky sentences
11. Drowsiness, confusion, possible unconsciousness—lack of O_2 to brain

DIAGNOSTIC TESTS AND METHODS

1. History
2. Physical examination
   A. Hyperresonance on percussion
   B. Decreased breath sounds
   C. Expiratory prolongation
   D. Quiet heart sounds
3. Chest x-ray—advanced stages
   A. Flattened diaphragm
   B. Reduced vascular markings at lung periphery
   C. Overaeration of lungs
   D. Vertical heart
   E. Enlarged anteroposterior chest diameter
   F. Large retrosternal air space

4. Pulmonary function tests
   A. Increased residual volume
   B. Total lung capacity and compliance
      (1) Decreased vital capacity
      (2) Decreased diffusing capacity
      (3) Decreased expiratory volumes
5. ABGs
   A. Reduced PO_2
   B. Normal PCO_2 until late in disease
6. Sputum analysis
7. ECG
   A. Tall, symmetrical P waves in leads II, III, and aVF
   B. Vertical QRS axis
   C. Signs of right ventricular hypertrophy late in disease
8. Red blood cells (RBCs)—increased hemoglobin late in disease in presence of persistent severe hypoxia

Planning

1. Safe, effective care environment
   A. Prevent avoidable injury and/or infection.
   B. Increase client's knowledge of disease process, diagnostic procedures, and treatment (especially medications).
2. Physiological integrity
   A. Maintain effective airway clearance and gas exchange.
   B. Maintain effective breathing pattern.
   C. Maintain fluid balance.
   D. Promote undisturbed sleep pattern.
   E. Maintain adequate tissue perfusion.
   F. Maintain adequate nutritional intake.
   G. Increase comfort.
3. Psychosocial integrity
   A. Reduce anxiety.
4. Health promotion and maintenance
   A. Increase client's knowledge of prevention, home care, and follow-up

Implementation

1. Assess, record, and report signs and symptoms and reactions to treatment.
2. Loosen, liquefy, and remove secretions (clapping, chest physiotherapy, postural drainage) as ordered.
3. Promote breathing exercises and coughing to increase respiratory function.
4. Prevent and control infections.
5. Encourage cessation of smoking.
6. Prevent exposure to air pollution.
7. Give antibiotics to treat respiratory infection on time as ordered.
8. Give flu vaccine to prevent flu, if ordered.
9. Give pneumovax to prevent pneumococcal pneumonia, if ordered.
10. Discourage visits by persons with upper respiratory infections.
11. Give O_2 in low concentrations (1–2 liters) to treat hypoxia.
    A. Higher levels of O_2 are dangerous when CO_2 level is high.
    B. Respiratory center of brain becomes used to low blood O_2 level.
    C. Increase in O_2 level causes respiratory rate to decrease—may lead to unconsciousness and death.

12. Encourage adequate fluid intake.
13. Provide humidity.
14. Use nebulizers and intermittent positive pressure breathing as ordered.
15. Give expectorants as ordered.
16. Ensure adequate rest.
17. Organize care.
18. Limit exertion.
19. Assist client with turning and getting in and out of bed.
20. Instruct client regarding disease process, diagnostic procedures, treatment, prevention, home care, and follow-up.

Evaluation

1. Reports increased comfort, decreased anxiety
2. Shows no signs of avoidable injury and/or infection
3. Maintains effective airway clearance and gas exchange
4. Maintains adequate tissue perfusion
5. Maintains adequate nutritional status
6. Develops undisturbed sleep pattern
7. Uses effective coping strategies
8. Verbalizes feelings about condition
9. Discusses intention to stop smoking
10. Demonstrates understanding of disease process, diagnostic procedures, treatment, prevention, home care, and need for follow-up

Chronic Bronchitis

Description

1. Chronic bronchitis is a chronic, progressive condition accompanied by excessive secretions from overactive mucous glands.
2. Diagnostic criteria include:
   A. Production of excessive tracheobronchial secretions on a daily basis for at least 3 months of the year for a period of 2 consecutive years.
   B. No other cause for chronic cough, such as lung cancer, CHF, or TB.
3. Edema and infection within bronchi obstructing airflow and gas exchange.
4. Extension and destruction of alveolar sacs and capillaries may occur if acute attacks are not prevented or treated.
5. Associated with:
   A. Enlargement, or hyperplasia, of the bronchial mucous glands.
   B. Increased goblet cells.
   C. Damage to cilia.
   D. Squamous metaplasia of columnar epithelium.
   E. Chronic WBC and lymphocytic infiltration of bronchial walls.
   F. Narrowing of airways.
   G. Mucus in airways produces resistance in small airways, causing severe ventilation-perfusion imbalance.
6. It is believed that airflow obstruction may be due to infringement of the bronchial mucous glands on the bronchial lumen.
7. Causes
   A. Asthma
   B. Inhalation of irritating chemicals such as cigarette smoke
   C. Recurrent respiratory infections
   D. Air pollution
   E. Familial tendency

Assessment

SUBJECTIVE

1. Insidious onset, with productive cough and exertional dyspnea as predominant symptoms
2. Dyspnea on exertion
3. Swelling of legs
4. Tachypnea (abnormal rapid breathing)
5. Wheezing
6. Anxiety

OBJECTIVE

1. Productive cough with tenacious gray, white, or blood-tinged sputum
2. Tachypnea
3. Use of accessory respiratory muscles
4. Edema
5. Dyspnea on exertion
6. Wheezing
7. Neck vein distention
8. Weight loss
9. Cyanosis
10. Prolonged expiratory time

DIAGNOSTIC TESTS AND METHODS

1. History
2. Physical examination
   A. Presence of rhonchi and wheezes on auscultation
   B. Expiratory elongation
   C. Neck vein distention
   D. Pedal edema
3. Chest x-ray
   A. Hyperinflation
   B. Increased bronchovascular markings
4. Pulmonary function tests
   A. Increased residual volume
   B. Decreased vital capacity
   C. Forced expiratory volumes
   D. Normal static compliance and diffusing capacity
5. ABGs
   A. Decreased PO_2
   B. Normal or increased PCO_2
6. Sputum analysis
   A. Many organisms
   B. Increased number of neutrophils
7. ECG
   A. Atrial arrhythmias
   B. Peaked P waves in leads II, III, and aVF
   C. Occasionally right ventricular hypertrophy

Planning

1. Safe, effective care environment
   A. Prevent avoidable injury and/or infection.
   B. Increase client's and family's knowledge of disease process, diagnostic procedures, and treatment (especially medications).
2. Physiological integrity
   A. Maintain effective airway clearance and gas exchange.

B. Maintain effective breathing pattern.
C. Maintain fluid balance.
D. Promote undisturbed sleep perfusion.
E. Maintain adequate tissue perfusion.
F. Maintain adequate nutritional intake.
G. Increase comfort.
3. Psychosocial integrity
   A. Reduce anxiety.
4. Health promotion and maintenance
   A. Increase client's and family's knowledge of prevention, home care, and follow-up.

Implementation

1. Assess, record, and report signs and symptoms and reactions to treatment.
2. Loosen, liquefy, and remove secretions.
3. Provide postural drainage, clapping, chest physiotherapy as ordered.
4. Force fluids as ordered.
5. Monitor fluid intake and output.
6. Ensure adequate rest.
7. Provide high-protein diet.
8. Discourage visits from persons with upper respiratory infections.
9. Administer bronchodilators, expectorants, antibiotics, corticosteroids as ordered.
10. Administer ultrasonic or mechanical nebulizer treatments to loosen secretions and to aid in mobilization.
11. Administer diuretics for edema as ordered.
12. Administer O_2 as ordered for relief of hypoxia.
13. Discourage smoking.
14. Include client and family in planning care.
15. Instruct client and family regarding disease process, diagnostic procedures, treatment (especially medications), prevention, home care, and follow-up.

Evaluation

1. Reports increased comfort, decreased anxiety
2. Maintains open airway for increased gas exchange
3. Has no complications from infection
4. Reports improved sleeping pattern
5. Maintains adequate nutritional intake
6. Maintains adequate fluid intake
7. Discusses intention to stop smoking
8. Demonstrates understanding of disease process, diagnostic procedures, treatment, prevention, home care, and need for follow-up; similar understanding demonstrated by family

Acute Respiratory Failure in COPD

Description

1. Acute respiratory failure (ARF) occurs when acute ventilatory and oxygenation failure has not been corrected by conservative measures.
2. Management of COPD patients at this stage differs from the management of ARDS patients.
3. During this stage, mechanical ventilation is required.
4. Patients with ARF usually have consistently high PCO_2 and low PO_2 values.
5. In patients with COPD, only acute deterioration in blood gas values, with associated clinical deterioration, indicates adult respiratory distress syndrome (ARDS).
6. Causes
   A. Any condition of a patient with COPD that increases the work of breathing and decreases respiratory drive
      (1) Respiratory tract infections (bronchitis or pneumonia)
      (2) Bronchospasms (common precipitating factor)
      (3) Accumulation of secretions secondary to cough suppression
   B. Central nervous system (CNS) depression due to injudicious use of:
      (1) Tranquilizers
      (2) Sedatives
      (3) Narcotics
      (4) O_2
   C. CNS depression due to head injury
   D. Airway irritants
      (1) Smoke
      (2) Fumes
      (3) Air pollution
   E. Cardiovascular disorders
      (1) CHF
      (2) Myocardial infarction (MI)
      (3) Pulmonary emboli
   F. Thoracic disorders
      (1) Chest trauma
      (2) Thoracic surgery
      (3) Abdominal surgery
      (4) Pneumothorax
   G. Endocrine and metabolic disorders
      (1) Metabolic alkalosis
      (2) Myxedema

Assessment

1. Signs and symptoms
   A. Hypoxemia
   B. Hypercapnia
      (1) Headache
      (2) Lethargy
      (3) Increased cranial pressure
      (4) Flushed, dry skin
      (5) Papilledema
      (6) Vasodilation
   C. Acidosis
   D. Potential respiratory problems
      (1) Respiratory rate may increase or remain normal depending on cause.
      (2) Respirations may be shallow or deep, or alternate between these two types.
      (3) Air hunger may occur.
      (4) Presence of cyanosis depends on hemoglobin level and arterial oxygenation.
      (5) Presence of rales (crackles), wheezes, rhonchi, or decreased breath sounds on auscultation.
      (6) Bronchospasms.
   E. Potential cardiovascular problems
      (1) Tachycardia
         (a) Increased cardiac output
         (b) Mildly elevated blood pressure as a result of adrenal release of catecholamine due to early response to low PO_2

  (2) Possible arrhythmias due to myocardial hypoxia
  (3) Pulmonary hypertension
F. Potential CNS problems
  (1) Restlessness
  (2) Loss of concentration
  (3) Confusion
  (4) Tremors
  (5) Irritability
  (6) Diminished tendon reflexes
  (7) Papilledema
  (8) Coma
G. Drug toxicity
  (1) Aminophylline toxicity
    (a) CNS stimulation
    (b) Nausea
    (c) Diarrhea
    (d) Seizures
    (e) Cardiac dysrhythmias
    (f) Insomnia
H. Fluid volume excess due to hormonal imbalances
  (1) Hyponatremia
    (a) Edema

DIAGNOSTIC TESTS AND METHODS

1. History
2. Physical examination
3. Laboratory findings
   A. Progressive deterioration in blood gas values and pH
   B. Increased levels of bicarbonate (HCO_3)
      (1) May be indicative of metabolic alkalosis or
      (2) Reflect metabolic compensation for chronic respiratory acidosis
   C. Abnormally low levels of hematocrit and hemoglobin
      (1) May be due to blood loss
      (2) Indicate decrease in oxygen-carrying capacity
   D. Possible elevated WBC count if ARF is due to bacterial infection
   E. Serum electrolytes
      (1) Hyperkalemia due to compensatory hyperventilation
      (2) Hypochloremia due to metabolic alkalosis
4. Chest x-ray
   A. Pulmonary pathology—findings may include:
      (1) Emphysema
      (2) Atelectasis
      (3) Infiltrates
      (4) Lesions
      (5) Pneumothorax
      (6) Effusions
5. ECG
   A. Arrhythmias characteristic of myocardial hypoxia and cor pulmonale

Planning

1. Safe, effective care environment
   A. Prevent avoidable injury.
   B. Increase client's and family's knowledge of disease process, diagnostic procedures, and treatment.
2. Physiological integrity
   A. Maintain effective gas exchange and breathing pattern.
   B. Maintain effective airway clearance.
   C. Maintain adequate tissue perfusion.

D. Maintain adequate nutritional status.
3. Psychosocial integrity
   A. Reduce anxiety.
   B. Maintain effective communication.
4. Health promotion and maintenance
   A. Increase client's and family's knowledge of home care and follow-up.

Implementation

NOTE: Most ARF clients are treated in the ICU.

1. Assess, record, and report signs and symptoms and reactions to treatment.
2. Reduce or minimize anxiety by:
   A. Orienting clients to ICU environment
   B. Explaining procedures
   C. Explaining routines
3. Give appropriate concentrations of O_2 to raise client's PO_2 levels, if ordered.
   A. Use nasal prongs or Venturi mask.
   B. Maintain PO_2 at a minimum of 40–60 mm Hg.
4. Monitor for a positive response to O_2 therapy.
   A. Improved breathing
   B. Improved skin color
   C. Improvement in ABG results
5. Maintain a patent airway.
6. Encourage coughing and deep breathing with "pursed lips" to remove excess CO_2.
   A. Turn client while awake.
   B. Give postural drainage and chest physiotherapy, if tolerated, to facilitate expectoration of secretions.
7. Carry out drug therapy measures as ordered to increase bronchodilation.
   A. Administer IV aminophylline to maintain a therapeutic drug level.
      (1) Maintenance dosage varies.
      (2) Drug levels need to be monitored closely for evidence of toxicity.
   B. Administer inhaled β-agonists via ventilator circuits as ordered.
      (1) Dosage depends on medication ordered.
      (2) Metaproterenol, isoproterenol, isoetharine, and albuterol are usually administered q3–4h.
   C. Administer corticosteroids IV, if ordered—usually q6h.
      (1) These drugs may speed recovery and decrease length of time that client remains on mechanical ventilation.
      (2) They are advocated by some for their anti-inflammatory effect, depression of lung fibroblasts, and depression of platelets.
      (3) Results of some studies indicate increase in lung injury with resultant death due to secondary infection.
      (4) Corticosteroids may be used early in course of disease and then rapidly tapered off.
   D. Monitor for signs and symptoms of infection during steroid administration.
   E. Administer antibiotics for infection as ordered following culture and sensitivity test results.
   F. Administer digoxin as ordered for left-sided heart failure.
   G. Administer antidysrhythmic agents, if ordered.
   H. Administer low-dose subcutaneous heparin, if ordered, to prevent pulmonary embolism.

8. Provide the following nursing interventions for intubated clients:
   A. Suction tracheal hourly after hyperoxygenation.
   B. Provide humidification to liquefy secretions.
   C. Check sputum for change in quantity, consistency, and color.
9. Observe client for signs of respiratory arrest.
   A. Auscultate chest for breath sounds.
   B. Monitor and record ABGs.
   C. Report ABG changes immediately.
10. Monitor and record serum electrolytes.
    A. Report changes immediately.
11. Monitor fluid balance.
    A. Intake and output
    B. Daily weights
12. Check cardiac monitor frequently for arrhythmias.

NOTE: Mechanical ventilation of COPD clients is avoided if at all possible because the use of an endotracheal tube causes increased airway resistance and makes it harder to breathe. Mechanical ventilation is usually ordered if: (1) significant respiratory acidosis persists following correction of severe hypoxemia; (2) client is unable to cooperate with conservative therapy owing to altered mental state; (3) client is exhausted; or (4) secretions cannot be expectorated, resulting in progressive clinical deterioration.

13. Provide the following nursing interventions for clients on mechanical ventilation through endotracheal or tracheostomy tube:
    A. Check ventilator settings frequently.
       (1) Ventilation mode
       (2) FIO_2
       (3) Respiratory rate
       (4) Tidal volume
       (5) Peak inspiratory pressure
       (6) Level of positive end-expiratory pressure (PEEP)
       (7) Status of alarm settings
       (8) Breathing patterns for evidence that patient is "fighting the ventilator"
          (a) Signs of asynchronous breathing
          (b) Signs of triggering the high-pressure alarm (attempting to exhale when ventilator is delivering a breath)
    B. Check ABGs frequently.
       (1) FIO_2 setting depends on results of ABGs.
       (2) ABG specimens should be drawn 20–30 minutes after every FIO_2 change.
    C. Prevent infection by:
       (1) Using sterile technique when suctioning
       (2) Changing ventilator circuits every 24 hours
    D. Monitor for signs and symptoms of stress ulcers (common in intubated clients).
       (1) Check gastric secretions for signs of bleeding if client complains of:
          (a) Epigastric tenderness
          (b) Nausea
          (c) Vomiting
       (2) Monitor all stools for presence of occult blood.
          (a) Report abnormal findings immediately.
          (b) Administer antacids or Tagamet (cimetidine) as ordered.
       (3) Monitor hemoglobin and hematocrit levels—report changes immediately.

E. Keep head of bed elevated to optimize pattern of breathing.
F. Prevent tracheal erosion owing to artificial airway cuff overinflation due to:
   (1) Compression of blood vessels in tracheal wall when minimal-leak technique is used with:
      (a) Low-pressure cuffed tube *or*
      (b) Foam cuff *or*
      (c) Pressure-regulating valve on cuff
G. Prevent nasal necrosis by:
   (1) Keeping nasotracheal tube midline within nostrils
   (2) Providing good oral hygiene
   (3) Loosening tape periodically to prevent skin breakdown
   (4) Avoiding excessive movement of tubes
   (5) Ensuring that ventilator tubing interface is adequately supported
H. Monitor fluid balance to avoid overhydration or underhydration.
   (1) Overhydration increases extravascular lung fluid.
   (2) Dehydration results in enhanced cardiovascular depression related to PEEP therapy.
   (3) Monitor fluid balance hourly.
      (a) Signs of decreased urine output are indicative of poor renal perfusion due to low cardiac output.
      (b) Humidity in the ventilator circuit should be calculated as insensible fluid intake (300–500 mL/day).
      (c) Increased levels of antidiuretic hormone (ADH) occur with mechanical ventilation, which increases fluid retention.
I. Monitor amount of calories and protein based on patient's hypermetabolic state.
   (1) Client may be fed via the enteral route.
      (a) Monitor for gastric distention, which can increase respiratory insufficiency.
      (b) Gastric distention is caused by poor GI perfusion and motility, which interferes with absorption of nutrients.
   (2) Client may be fed via hyperalimentation.
   (3) Fluid balance and electrolytes (sodium, potassium, chloride, phosphate magnesium, and calcium) must be monitored carefully.
J. Monitor for signs of barotrauma owing to use of high-peak airway pressures and high levels of PEEP to prevent decreased lung compliance.
   (1) Agitation
   (2) Hypotension and tachycardia
   (3) Progressive hypoxemia
   (4) Cardiovascular collapse
   (5) Increased central venous pressure (CVP)
   (6) Crepitation in neck, face, axillae, chest, or abdomen
   (7) Mediastinal crunch
   (8) Pulmonary interstitial emphysema on chest x-ray
   (9) Absence of breath sound accompanied by distended neck veins and distant heart sounds
   (10) Rising peak airway pressure
K. Provide reassurance to client and family.
   (1) Explain procedures.
   (2) Provide opportunity for client to participate in some decision making.

(3) Support clients during periods of anxiety and frustration.

(4) Use speech and touch.

14. Assist with weaning client from mechanical ventilation.
    A. Begin when client is stabilized.
       (1) Heart failure corrected
       (2) Nutritional status improved
       (3) Infection cleared
       (4) Bronchospasms relieved
    B. Assist client into chair as soon as client is clinically stable.
       (1) Gradually increase time in chair.
       (2) Coach client to adopt a breathing pattern using:
          (a) Deep inspirations
          (b) Slow, controlled exhalation
    C. Monitor nutritional status—nutritional support should begin as soon as client is stabilized.
       (1) Encourage client to eat to prevent:
          (a) Wasting of inspiratory muscles
          (b) Additional cachexia
       (2) Avoid use of high-glucose loads to prevent impairment of oxygenation.
          (a) Use may increase CO_2 production.
          (b) Use may increase hypophosphatemia.
       (3) Use a higher proportion of lipids than glucose in diet.
15. Provide the following nursing interventions for clients requiring long-term ventilator support:
    A. Encourage nutritional intake.
    B. Maintain skin integrity.
    C. Establish communications and psychological support.
    D. Encourage family to support client.
    E. Continue efforts to improve lung function.
    F. Continue efforts to wean client off the ventilator.
16. Instruct client and family regarding disease process, diagnostic procedures, treatment, home care, and follow-up.

Evaluation

Ensure that client remaining on the ventilator:
1. Maintains patent airway
2. Breathes in synchrony with the ventilator
    A. Rate is adjusted to maintain a normal level of ventilation—$PaCO_2$ 35–45 mm Hg
3. Maintains PaO_2 above 60 mm Hg on 40% FIO_2 with a shunt fraction of <20%
4. Keeps peak airway pressure below 40–50 mm Hg
5. Maintains stable cardiac output, heart rate, and blood pressure
6. Maintains balanced intake and output of fluid
7. Keeps weight stable
8. Is able to communicate needs using nonverbal measures
9. Maintains skin integrity
10. Keeps oral mucous membranes intact and moist
11. Demonstrates understanding of disease process, diagnostic procedures, treatment, home care, and need for follow-up; similar understanding demonstrated by family

Ensure that client weaned from the ventilator:
1. Maintains stable clinical condition
2. Maintains patent airway
3. Keeps body weight stable
4. Maintains balanced fluid intake and output
5. Demonstrates return of breathing pattern to prefailure levels
6. Demonstrates return of ABGs to prefailure levels
7. Has clear lungs on auscultation
8. Demonstrates understanding of disease process, diagnostic procedures, treatment, home care, and need for follow-up; similar understanding demonstrated by family

NOTE: If client cannot be successfully weaned from the ventilator, evaluation of condition is required to determine nursing home or home-care placement with long-term ventilator support.

Pneumothorax and Hemothorax

Description

1. Pneumothorax is an accumulation of air or gas in pleural space, causing collapse of the lung.
2. The amount of air or gas trapped in the pleural space determines the degree of lung collapse, which may be partial or complete.
3. In tension pneumothorax, air in pleural space is under higher pressure than air in opposite lung and vascular structures.
4. In open pneumothorax (usually result of trauma), air flows between pleural space and outside of body.
5. In closed pneumothorax, air reaches pleural space directly from the lung.
6. Prompt treatment is required for tension or large pneumothorax.
7. Without prompt treatment, fatal pulmonary and circulatory impairment will result.
8. Hemothorax is an accumulation of blood in pleural space.
9. Blood from intercostal, pleural, mediastinal, and sometimes blood vessels in lung enter the pleural cavity.
10. Amount of lung collapse and mediastinal shift depends on amount of bleeding and underlying cause.
11. Pneumothorax often accompanies hemothorax.
12. Causes
    A. Possibly spontaneous—air leakage from congenital blebs next to pleural surface, rupture of emphysematous bulla (large vesicle) following exercise or coughing, tubercular lesions or cancerous lesions that erode into pleural space
    B. Trauma—knife wound, fractured ribs, venous pressure line insertion, gunshot wound, following thoracentesis
    C. Postoperative procedure where chest cavity has been entered
    D. Diagnostic, treatment procedures
    E. Thoracentesis
    F. Insertion of CVP line
    G. Closed pleural biopsy

Assessment

SUBJECTIVE

1. Spontaneous—sudden sharp pleuritic pain increased by breathing and coughing
2. Anxiety
3. Dizziness

OBJECTIVE

1. Profuse sweating
2. Shortness of breath

3. Rapid pulse
4. Dizziness
5. Weak, rapid pulse
6. Pallor
7. Neck vein distention
8. Asymmetrical (uneven) chest movements
9. Crackling under skin (crepitus)
10. Hypotension
11. Tachycardia
12. Decreased vocal fremitus
13. Decreased or absent breath sounds over collapsed lung
14. ABG findings—pH < 7.35, PO_2 < 80 mm Hg, PCO_2 > 45 mm Hg
15. Respiratory distress
16. Spontaneous pneumothorax with only a small amount of air moved into pleural space—may cause no or few symptoms

DIAGNOSTIC TESTS AND METHODS

1. History
2. Physical examination
3. Chest x-ray

Planning

1. Safe, effective care environment
   A. Prevent avoidable injury.
   B. Increase client's knowledge of disease process, diagnostic procedures, and treatment.
2. Physiological integrity
   A. Maintain effective airway clearance.
   B. Maintain adequate cardiopulmonary tissue perfusion.
   C. Increase comfort.
3. Psychosocial integrity
   A. Prevent social isolation.
4. Health promotion and maintenance
   A. Increase client's knowledge of home care and follow-up.

Implementation

1. Assess, record, and report signs and symptoms and reactions to treatment.
2. Provide the following nursing interventions for spontaneous pneumothorax with no signs of increased pleural pressure, lung collapse of <30%, and no signs of dyspnea or other indications of compromise or complications:
   A. Provide bed rest.
   B. Monitor vital signs every hour for indications of shock.
   C. Administer O_2 as prescribed.
   D. Assist in needle aspiration of air, if required.
3. For lung collapse >30%
   A. Prepare client for thoracotomy and chest tubes.
   B. Prepare client for possible surgical repair.
   C. Give mouth care.
   D. Check nutritional status.
   E. Watch for pallor, gasping respirations, and sudden chest pain.
   F. Check for increased respiratory distress or mediastinal shift.
   G. Listen for breath sound over both lungs.
   H. Encourage client to control coughing and gasping during thoracentesis or thoracotomy procedure.
   I. Encourage coughing and deep breathing once chest tubes are in place to facilitate lung expansion.
4. Provide the following nursing interventions for clients undergoing chest tube drainage:
   A. Watch for air leakage (bubbling)—indicates lung defect has not closed.
   B. Check around neck or at tube insertion site for crackling beneath the skin—sign of subcutaneous emphysema.
5. Provide the following nursing interventions for clients on ventilators:
   A. Check for difficulty in breathing in time with ventilator.
   B. Check pressure changes on ventilator gauges.
   C. Check, record, and report amount and color of drainage.
   D. Assist in changing dressings around chest tube insertion site as necessary.
   E. Do not dislodge or reposition tube.
   F. If tube dislodges, place petrolatum gauze dressing over opening immediately to prevent rapid lung collapse and call for help.
   G. Reassure client and family.
6. Instruct client regarding disease process, diagnostic procedures, treatment, home care, and follow-up.

Evaluation

1. Reports increased comfort, decreased anxiety
2. Maintains stable vital signs.
3. Demonstrates lung re-expansion
4. Reports relief of pain
5. Shows no evidence of respiratory problems
6. Maintains effective breathing pattern
7. Maintains effective gas exchange—normal ABGs
8. Maintains adequate nutritional status
9. Demonstrates understanding of disease process, diagnostic procedures, treatment, home care, and need for follow-up

Pulmonary Tuberculosis

Description

1. Pulmonary tuberculosis is an acute or chronic infection caused by the tubercle bacillus organism that leads to inflammation and formation of a permanent nodule containing the tubercle bacillus.
2. The person who has been infected harbors the bacillus for life. It is dormant unless it becomes active during physical or emotional stress.
3. The nodules become fibrosed, and the area becomes calcified and can be identified by x-ray.
4. The incidence of TB is currently increasing, and a drug-resistant strain is becoming a problem.
5. High incidence in individuals with AIDS; the homeless; and others living in crowded, poorly ventilated conditions.
6. Transmission of the organism is by airborne droplets.
7. Causes:
   A. Exposure to airborne droplets containing the tubercle bacillus from infected person
   B. Inhalation of airborne droplets containing tubercle bacilli

8. Factors contributing to activation of infection
   A. Uncontrolled diabetes mellitus
   B. Hodgkin's disease
   C. Leukemia
   D. Treatment with corticosteroids
   E. Immunosuppressive conditions such as AIDS
   F. Silicosis

Assessment

SUBJECTIVE

1. Early phase may be asymptomatic
2. Fatigue
3. Weakness
4. Weight loss
5. Anorexia
6. Night sweats
7. Low-grade fever
8. Cough with micropurulent sputum
9. Occasional hemoptysis (coughing up of blood from the lungs)
10. Chest pains
11. Anxiety, fear of public rejection

OBJECTIVE

1. Productive cough with micropurulent sputum
2. Elevated afternoon temperature
3. Positive chest x-ray
4. Positive sputum for acid-fast bacilli
5. Presence of hemoptysis
6. Positive tuberculin test

DIAGNOSTIC TESTS AND METHODS

1. History of tuberculin exposure
2. Physical examination
3. Chest x-ray
4. Tuberculin test
5. Sputum smears and cultures
6. Auscultation of chest
7. Chest percussion

Planning

1. Safe, effective care environment
   A. Prevent avoidable injury and/or infection.
   B. Assess appetite and maintain adequate nutritional status.
   C. Increase client's and family's knowledge of disease process, diagnostic procedures, and treatment.
2. Psychological integrity
   A. Maintain effective airway clearance and gas exchange.
   B. Increase comfort.
3. Psychosocial integrity
   A. Reduce anxiety.
4. Health promotion and maintenance
   A. Increase client's and family's knowledge of prevention, home care, and follow-up.

Implementation

1. Assess, record, and report signs and symptoms and reactions to treatment.

2. Isolate client in quiet, well-ventilated room during infective period.
3. Assist with comfort measures.
4. Assess respirations, breath sounds, and vital signs.
5. Instruct client to cough, sneeze, or laugh into tissue.
6. Instruct client to dispose of tissues in receptacle provided for this purpose.
7. Instruct client to wear mask when outside of room.
8. Instruct staff and visitors to wear masks (recommended by Occupational Health and Safety Administration).
9. Encourage rest.
10. Encourage client to eat well-balanced meals.
11. If anorexic, encourage client to eat small meals more frequently.
12. Record weight weekly.
13. Observe, report, and record hemoptysis.
14. Administer antituberculosis drugs as ordered.
15. Explain need for taking medications (combinations of 2 or 3) as ordered to prevent resistant strains.
16. Watch for drug side effects—isoniazid sometimes leads to hepatitis or peripheral neuritis.
17. Monitor aspartate transaminase (AST) and alanine transaminase (ALT) levels.
18. Give pyridoxine (vitamin B_6) as ordered for peripheral neuritis.
19. Use of ethambutol may cause optic neuritis (drug will probably be discontinued).
20. Use of rifampin may cause hepatitis and purpura.
21. Instruct client and family regarding disease process, diagnostic procedures, treatment, prevention, home care, and follow-up. Include teaching on:
    A. Reporting side effects of medications immediately
    B. Importance of regular follow-up examinations
    C. Reporting signs and symptoms of recurring TB
    D. Need for long-term treatment
    E. Persons exposed to infected clients receiving tuberculin tests and, if ordered, chest x-rays and prophylactic isoniazid

Evaluation

1. Reports increased comfort, decreased anxiety
2. Shows no evidence of hemoptysis
3. Maintains adequate nutrition
4. Reports absence of cough and sputum
5. Maintains effective airway clearance
6. Negative sputum culture
7. Demonstrates understanding of disease process, mode of transmission, diagnostic procedures, treatment (long term), home care, and need for follow-up

Adult Respiratory Distress Syndrome, or Shock Lung

Description

1. Adult respiratory distress syndrome (ARDS) is a form of pulmonary edema that causes ARF in previously healthy persons.
2. It results from increased permeability of the alveolar capillary membrane.
3. Fluid accumulates in the tissues of the lung, alveolar spaces, and small airways, causing the lungs to stiffen.

4. Impairment of ventilation occurs, which prohibits adequate oxygenation of pulmonary capillary blood.
5. ARDS is characterized by hypoxia, dyspnea, pulmonary edema, destruction of alveoli, and inflammation, resulting in decreased O_2 and CO_2 exchange.
6. Severe ARDS can cause irreversible and fatal hypoxia; however, clients who recover usually have little or no permanent damage.
7. Predisposing factors:
   A. Shock
   B. Sepsis—primarily gram-negative bacteria
   C. Drug overdose—barbiturates, glutethimide, narcotics
   D. Blood transfusion reaction
   E. Smoke or chemical inhalation—chlorine, ammonia
   F. Pancreatitis, uremia
   G. Near-drowning
   H. Viral, bacterial, or fungal pneumonia
   I. Trauma—lung contusion, head injury, long bone fracture with fat emboli
   J. Disseminated intravascular coagulation (DIC)
   K. O_2 toxicity
   L. Aspiration of gastric contents
   M. Infection

Assessment

SUBJECTIVE

1. Rapid breathing
2. Dyspnea
3. Confusion, anxiety
4. Restlessness, apprehension
5. Mental sluggishness
6. Increased heart rate
7. Decreased urinary output

OBJECTIVE

1. Dyspnea
2. Cough
3. Tachypnea
4. Cyanosis
5. Elevated temperature
6. Rapid, shallow breathing
7. Intercostal and suprasternal retractions
8. Presence of rales and rhonchi
9. Restlessness, confusion, apprehension due to hypoxia
10. Motor dysfunction due to hypoxia
11. Decreased urinary output
12. Evidence of initial respiratory alkalosis (decreased PCO_2) and a decrease in PO_2
13. Evidence of more severe ARDS
14. Increased PCO_2—presence of respiratory acidosis
15. Decreasing HCO_3—presence of metabolic acidosis
16. Continued decrease in PO_2 despite O_2 therapy
17. Severe ARDS—severe hypoxemia (very low blood O_2 levels)
18. Hypotension due to severe hypoxemia
19. Ventricular fibrillation (in late stages of ARDS)

DIAGNOSTIC TESTS AND METHODS

1. ABGs
2. Pulmonary artery catheterization—to identify cause of pulmonary edema
3. Serial chest x-rays
4. Laboratory tests
5. Sputum Gram's stain, culture, and sensitivity
6. Blood cultures—to detect infections
7. Toxicology screen—to detect drug ingestion
8. Serum amylase determination if pancreatitis is suspected

Planning

1. Safe, effective care environment
   A. Prevent avoidable injury and/or infection.
   B. Increase client's and family's knowledge of disease process, diagnostic procedures, and treatment.
2. Physiological integrity
   A. Increase comfort.
   B. Maintain effective breathing pattern.
3. Psychosocial integrity
   A. Promote effective coping.
4. Health promotion and maintenance
   A. Increase client's and family's knowledge of prevention, home care, and follow-up.

Implementation

1. Assess, record, and report signs and symptoms and reactions to treatment.
2. Maintain bed rest in high Fowler position.
3. Administer humidified O_2 via a tight-fitting mask—allows for use of continuous positive airway pressure as ordered.
4. Administer ventilator support using PEEP, if ordered.
5. Administer sedatives, narcotics, and neuromuscular blocking agents as ordered to minimize restlessness, O_2 consumption, and CO_2 production and to facilitate ventilation.
6. Monitor ventilator, ABGs, and vital signs hourly.
7. Administer prescribed IV fluids, bronchodilators, vasodilators to facilitate ventilation.
8. Maintain open airway; suction as necessary.
9. Check extremities for color, temperature, and capillary refill hourly
10. Restrict fluids as ordered.
11. Administer diuretics to reduce edema as ordered.
12. Monitor intake and output hourly.
13. Administer a short course of high-dose steroids as ordered in cases where fat emboli or chemical injuries are the cause of ARDS.
14. Administer IV fluids and vasopressors as ordered to maintain blood pressure if hypotension occurs.
15. Administer antimicrobial drugs as ordered for nonviral infections.
16. Monitor respiratory status at least every 2 hours. Watch for retractions on inspiration.
    A. Note rate, rhythm, and depth of respirations.
    B. Watch for use of accessory muscles of respiration.
    C. Listen for abnormal breath sounds with stethoscope.
17. Check characteristics of sputum—clear, frothy sputum is indicative of pulmonary edema.
18. Monitor for signs of confusion due to hypoxia.
19. Prepare client and assist with insertion of Swan-Ganz catheter; monitor placement and dressing of Swan-Ganz catheter.
20. Give emotional support to client and family.
21. Communicate frequently with client using appropriate communication aids.
22. Instruct client and family regarding disease process, diag-

nostic procedures, treatment, prevention, home care, and follow-up.

Evaluation

1. Reports increased comfort, decreased anxiety
2. Maintains effective gas exchange (O_2 and CO_2)
3. Maintains effective breathing pattern
4. Maintains adequate nutritional status
5. Shows no evidence of edema
6. Maintains PaO_2 between 50 mm Hg and 60 mm Hg during acute phase
7. Maintains normal ABGs as condition improves
8. Verbalizes feelings about condition
9. Communicates needs
10. Demonstrates understanding of disease process, diagnostic procedures, treatment, prevention, home care, and need for follow-up; similar understanding demonstrated by family

Respiratory Failure

Description

1. In patients with normal lung tissue, acute respiratory failure (ARF) usually means $PCO_2 > 50$ mm Hg and $PO_2 < 50$ mm Hg as a result of inadequate ventilation.

   NOTE: These limits do not apply to patients with exacerbation of chronic obstructive lung disease, who often have consistently high PCO_2 and low PO_2 values.

2. Predisposing factors
   A. Pulmonary edema
   B. Chest trauma
   C. Infections—pneumonia, bronchitis
   D. Bronchospasms or accumulating secretions secondary to cough suppression
   E. ARDS
   F. Cancer
   G. Pulmonary emboli
   H. CHF
   I. Neuromuscular problems
   J. Extended mechanical ventilation
   K. Head injury
   L. Drug overdose leading to CNS depression
   M. Anesthesia
   N. AIDS

Assessment

SUBJECTIVE

1. Headache
2. Confusion
3. History of contributing factors
4. Difficulty in breathing
5. Increased heart rate
6. Restlessness

OBJECTIVE

1. ABGs—$PaO_2 < 50$–60 mm Hg, $PaCO_2 > 50$ mm Hg, and pH < 7.35
2. Dyspnea
3. Cyanosis

4. Hypertension and tachycardia or hypotension and bradycardia
5. Tachypnea
6. Dysrhythmias
7. Restlessness
8. Confusion or irritability
9. Diaphoresis
10. Decreased level of consciousness
11. Alterations in respirations and breath sounds

DIAGNOSTIC TESTS AND METHODS

1. ABGs
2. Serial chest x-ray
3. pH blood levels
4. Tidal volume measurements
5. Hematocrit and hemoglobin—to detect blood loss indicative of decreased oxygen-carrying capacity
6. Serum electrolyte measurements

Planning

1. Safe, effective care environment
   A. Prevent avoidable injury.
   B. Assess appetite and maintain adequate nutritional status.
   C. Increase client's and family's knowledge of disease process, diagnostic procedures, and treatment.
2. Physiological integrity
   A. Maintain effective airway clearance and gas exchange.
   B. Increase comfort.
3. Psychosocial integrity
   A. Reduce anxiety.
4. Health promotion and maintenance
   A. Increase client's and family's knowledge of home care and follow-up.

Implementation

1. Assess, record, and report signs and symptoms and reactions to treatment.
2. Maintain bed rest with high Fowler position; turn every 2 hours.
3. Monitor vital signs, breath sounds.
4. Monitor ABGs, pH.
5. Give O_2 as prescribed.
6. Monitor for signs of hypoxia.
7. Suction only when secretions are present (preoxygenate before suctioning).
8. Administer prescribed bronchodilators.
9. Prepare client and assist with endotracheal and mechanical ventilation, if necessary.
10. Administer sedatives, narcotics, and neuromuscular blocking agents as ordered to minimize restlessness, O_2 consumption, and CO_2 production and to facilitate ventilation.
11. Give sedatives to promote relaxation while client is on mechanical ventilator.
12. Have resuscitation bag with mask available—clients may be temporarily pharmacologically paralyzed.
13. Make sure ventilator alarms are turned on.
14. Stabilize artificial airway securely.
15. Assess client for retained secretions. While client is temporarily paralyzed, cough reflex is lost.

16. Keep eyes lubricated to avoid corneal abrasions (temporary loss of corneal reflex).
17. Check ECG monitor, indwelling arterial catheter, and pulmonary artery catheter continually for changes in cardiovascular status.
18. Monitor CNS—level of consciousness, movement, and sensation.
19. Monitor renal status—hourly urine output, blood urea nitrogen (BUN), and serum creatinine.
20. Check nutritional status—administer total parenteral nutrition (TPN) or tube feedings as ordered.
21. Regulate amount of protein and calories based on client's metabolic state.
22. Ensure adequate GI perfusion and motility—poor perfusion and motility interfere with absorption of nutrients.
23. Prevent gastric distention—may lead to respiratory insufficiency owing to upward pressure against diaphragm.
24. Check fluid balance and electrolytes—sodium, potassium, chloride, calcium, phosphate, and magnesium blood levels.
25. Give emotional support to client and family.
26. Instruct client and family regarding disease process (including predisposing factors), diagnostic procedures, treatment, home care, and follow-up.

Evaluation

1. Reports increased comfort, decreased anxiety
2. Maintains effective airway clearance
3. Maintains adequate exchange of O_2 and CO_2
4. Maintains effective breathing patterns
5. Maintains improved ABGs and pH
6. Maintains adequate nutritional status
7. Maintains adequate cardiac output
8. Maintains adequate CNS response
9. Maintains adequate renal status
10. Demonstrates understanding of disease process, diagnostic procedures, treatment, home care, and need for follow-up; similar understanding demonstrated by family

Carcinoma of the Lung

Description

1. Carcinoma of the lung is a primary or secondary (metastatic from a primary site) malignant tumor in the lung or bronchi.
2. Bronchiogenic carcinoma usually develops within wall or epithelium of the bronchial tree and is the most common primary tumor.
3. It is usually without symptoms until late stages when metastasis has spread to brain, spinal cord, or esophagus.
4. Treatment in late stages is usually symptomatic.
5. Prognosis is poor unless detected early and treated early.
6. Types
   A. Epidermoid (squamous cell) carcinoma
   B. Small cell (oat cell) carcinoma
   C. Adenocarcinoma
   D. Large cell (anaplastic) carcinoma
7. Precipitating factors for susceptible host
   A. Cigarette smoking
   B. Exposure to asbestos
   C. Exposure to other carcinogens (uranium, arsenic, nickel, iron oxides, chromium, radioactive dust, and coal dust)
   D. Familial susceptibility
8. Primary prevention begins with cessation or avoidance of cigarette smoking and avoidance of particular industrial and air pollutants.

Assessment

SUBJECTIVE

1. Asymptomatic in early stages
2. Later symptoms—depend on location of lesion
   A. Squamous cell and small cell carcinomas
      (1) Cough
      (2) Wheezing
      (3) Dyspnea
      (4) Hemoptysis
      (5) Chest pain
   B. Adenocarcinoma and large cell carcinomas
      (1) Fever
      (2) Weakness
      (3) Weight loss
      (4) Anorexia
   C. Lesions that penetrate into pleural space
      (1) Pleural friction rub
      (2) Pleural effusion
      (3) Clubbing of fingers
   D. Hormonal paraneoplastic syndromes (alteration of hormones that regulate body function or homeostasis)
      (1) Gynecomastia from large cell carcinoma
      (2) Hypertrophic pulmonary osteoarthropathy (bone and joint pain from erosion of cartilage due to abnormal production of growth hormone)
      (3) Cushing's and carcinoid syndromes from small cell carcinomas
      (4) Hypercalcemia (increased blood calcium levels) from squamous cell carcinomas
   E. Metastatic symptoms involving intrathoracic structures
      (1) Bronchial obstruction—hemoptysis (expectoration of blood), atelectasis, pneumonia, dyspnea
      (2) Thoracic wall invasion—increased dyspnea, severe shoulder pain radiating down arm, severe chest pain.
      (3) Spread to local lymph nodes—cough, hemoptysis, pleural effusion, stridor
      (4) Recurrent nerve invasion—hoarseness, paralysis of vocal cord
      (5) Phrenic nerve involvement—shoulder pain, dyspnea, one-sided paralysis of diaphragm
      (6) Pericardial involvement—pericardial effusion, arrhythmias
      (7) Esophageal compression—difficulty in swallowing
      (8) Vena cava obstruction—edema of face, neck, chest, and back; venous distention of neck
   F. Metastasis to distant structures—may involve any part of body—CNS, abdomen, bone, connective and vascular tissues

DIAGNOSTIC TESTS AND METHODS

1. Chest x-ray
2. Examination of sputum for cells—requires sputum coughed up from lungs and tracheobronchial tree

3. Bronchoscopy
4. Needle biopsy
5. Tissue biopsy
6. Thoracentesis
7. Chest tomography
8. Esophagography
9. Bronchography
10. Angiocardiography—contrast studies of bronchial tree, esophagus, and cardiovascular tissue
11. Tests for detection of metastasis
    A. Bone scan
    B. Bone marrow biopsy
    C. Computed tomography (CT) scan of brain
    D. Liver function tests
    E. Gallium scan (noninvasive nuclear scan) of liver, bone, and spleen
    F. Staging—determines extent of disease and aids in planning treatment

Planning

1. Safe, effective care environment
   A. Prevent avoidable injury and/or infection.
   B. Assess appetite and maintain adequate nutritional status.
   C. Increase client's and family's knowledge of disease process, diagnostic procedures, and treatment.
2. Physiological integrity
   A. Maintain effective airway clearance and gas exchange.
   B. Increase comfort.
3. Psychosocial integrity
   A. Reduce anxiety.
   B. Assist client and family in coping with fear.
4. Health promotion and maintenance
   A. Increase client's and family's knowledge of home care and follow-up.

Implementation

1. Assess, record, and report signs and symptoms and reactions to treatment.
2. Prevent avoidable complications.
3. Maintain adequate nutritional status.
4. Reduce anxiety.
5. Assist client and family in coping with fear.
6. Provide preoperative care.
   A. Monitor vital signs, breath sounds, skin color.
   B. Monitor cough and sputum.
   C. Supplement and reinforce physician's information about disease and surgical procedure.
   D. Explain postoperative procedures.
      (1) Foley catheter insertion
      (2) Endotracheal tube
      (3) IV therapy
      (4) Dressing changes
      (5) Coughing, deep diaphragmatic breathing
      (6) Range-of-motion (ROM) exercises
7. Provide postoperative care.
   A. Maintain open airway for adequate gas exchange.
   B. Monitor chest tubes.
   C. Prevent postoperative and pulmonary complications.
   D. Check vital signs every 15 minutes for 1st hour, every 30 minutes for next 4 hours, then every 4 hours.
   E. Observe and report abnormal respirations and other changes immediately.
   F. Suction as necessary—encourage deep breathing and coughing.
   G. Check secretions—initial sputum will be thick and contain dark blood, changing to thin and grayish yellow within 24 hours.
   H. Monitor and record closed chest drainage—watch for air leaks; report immediately.
   I. Position patient on surgical side to promote drainage and re-expansion of lung.
   J. Monitor intake and output—maintain adequate hydration.
   K. Check for potential infection, shock, hemorrhage, dyspnea, mediastinal shift, atelectasis, and pulmonary embolus.
   L. Use antiembolism stockings, and encourage ROM exercises to prevent pulmonary embolus.
   M. Check and report foul-smelling discharge or excessive drainage on dressing.
8. Provide the following nursing interventions for clients receiving chemotherapy and radiation:
   A. Encourage client to eat soft, nonirritating foods high in protein.
   B. Explain and watch for possible side effects of chemotherapy and radiation.
   C. Administer antiemetics and antidiarrheals as needed.
   D. Give good skin care to decrease skin breakdown.
   E. Use good handwashing and scrupulous standard precautions if bone marrow suppression occurs.
9. Instruct client and family regarding disease process, diagnostic procedures, treatment, home care, and follow-up. Include teaching on:
   A. Avoidance of sunburn and tight-fitting clothing by clients receiving radiotherapy as outpatients
   B. Exercises for prevention of shoulder stiffness
   C. Cessation of smoking

Evaluation

NOTE: Depends on prognosis

1. Reports increased comfort, decreased anxiety
2. Maintains effective airway for gas exchange
3. Uses effective coping strategies
4. Verbalizes feelings on condition
5. Maintains normal ABGs
6. Has no complications
7. Maintains adequate nutritional status
8. Demonstrates understanding of disease process, diagnostic procedures, treatment, home care, and need for follow-up.

Chest Injury

Description

1. Chest injury includes trauma to rib cage, the diaphragm, mediastinum, or pleura caused by blunt or penetrating injuries.
2. Blunt chest injuries
   A. Damage to internal structures without chest wall penetration.
   B. Common cause is vehicular accidents.

C. Types include myocardial contusions, pulmonary contusions, rib and sternal fractures, and flail chest, which may be simple, multiple, jagged, and/or displaced.
   (1) Myocardial contusion—bruising of heart muscle.
   (2) Pulmonary contusion—bruising of lung tissue or pleura.
   (3) Rib and sternal fractures—displacement of ribs and sternum due to fractures caused by a powerful impact.
   (4) Flail chest—asymmetrical (uneven) chest movement during respiration due to multiple rib or sternal fractures. Such fractures may cause fatal complications such as hemorrhagic shock, diaphragmatic rupture, pneumothorax, and hemothorax if not treated correctly.
3. Penetrating chest injuries
   A. Blunt or sharp object pierces chest wall, causing injury and changes in pressures within chest cavity.
   B. Depending on size of injury, it may cause varying degrees of damage to soft tissue, bones, nerves, and blood vessels.
   C. Common cause is knife stabs or gunshot wounds.
   D. Gunshot wounds are usually more severe than stab wounds because of more severe lacerations and rapid blood loss. Also, bullet ricochet often damages large areas and multiple organs.
   E. Such injury may cause hemothorax and pneumothorax, including tension pneumothorax, mediastinal shift, arrhythmias, subcutaneous emphysema, esophageal perforation, and broncho-pleural fistula.

Assessment

1. Blunt injury
   A. Rib fractures
   B. Pain at site of injury, increases with deep breathing and movement
   C. Shallow, splinted respirations possibly leading to hypoventilation
   D. Evidence of fracture noted on x-ray
   E. Sternal fractures
   F. Persistent chest pains even at rest
   G. Shallow, splinted respirations
   H. Evidence of fracture noted on x-ray
   I. Flail chest
      (1) Poor lung expansion due to loss of chest wall integrity
      (2) Bruised skin
      (3) Extreme pain
      (4) Asymmetrical chest movement
      (5) Dyspnea
      (6) Shallow respirations
      (7) Tachypnea
      (8) Tachycardia
      (9) Hypotension
      (10) Respiratory acidosis
      (11) Cyanosis
      (12) Use of accessory muscles during respiration
      (13) Decreased breath sounds
   J. Pulmonary contusion
      (1) Hemoptysis
      (2) Restlessness

      (3) Difficulty in breathing
      (4) Abnormal breath sounds
      (5) Increased respiratory rate and rhythm
2. Penetrating injuries
   A. Symptoms as in blunt injuries
   B. Pneumothorax
   C. Dyspnea
   D. Tachycardia
   E. Absent breath sounds on affected side
   F. Sucking sound with open wound
   G. Cyanosis
   H. Hypotension
   I. Mediastinal shift with tension pneumothorax
   J. Varying levels of consciousness
   K. Weak, thready pulse
   L. Tachycardia
   M. Possibly hemothorax

DIAGNOSTIC TESTS AND METHODS

1. History
2. Chest x-ray
3. Auscultation of chest
4. ECG
5. Serial AST, ALT, lactic dehydrogenase (LDH), creatine phosphokinase (CPK)
6. Retrograde aortography—to check aortic laceration or rupture
7. Contrast studies and liver and spleen scans—to help detect rupture of diaphragm
8. ABGs
9. CBC including hemoglobin, hematocrit, and differential
10. Palpation and auscultation of abdomen—to evaluate damage to nearby organs and structures

Planning

1. Safe, effective care environment
   A. Prevent avoidable injury.
   B. Increase client's knowledge of condition, diagnostic procedures, and treatment.
2. Physiological integrity
   A. Maintain effective airway clearance.
   B. Maintain adequate cardiopulmonary tissue perfusion.
   C. Increase comfort.
3. Psychosocial integrity
   A. Prevent social isolation.
4. Health promotion and maintenance
   A. Increase client's knowledge of home care and follow-up.

Implementation

1. Assess, record, and report signs and symptoms and reactions to treatment.
2. Assess airway, breathing, and circulation.
3. Place an occlusive dressing over sucking wound.
4. Check level of consciousness.
5. Evaluate color and temperature of skin.
6. Look for distended jugular veins.
7. Check for subcutaneous emphysema.
8. Have blood typed and cross-matched.
9. Check breath sounds and vital signs.

10. Assist in establishing an open airway and support ventilation as needed.
11. Monitor for signs of tension pneumothorax.
12. Stabilize injury.
13. Assist with insertion of chest tubes or aspiration in pneumothorax.
14. Support flail chest.
15. Splint fractured ribs.
16. Control blood loss—remember to look under client to estimate loss.
17. Monitor for shock.
18. Provide O_2 as ordered.
19. Place client in Fowler position unless client requires shock position.
20. Administer analgesics, antibiotics, and supportive medications as ordered.
21. Provide emotional support.
22. Prepare client for necessary surgical intervention.
23. Provide postoperative care.
24. Instruct client regarding condition, diagnostic procedures, treatment, home care, and follow-up.

Evaluation

1. Maintains effective, open airway for adequate gas exchange and clearance
2. Maintains effective breathing patterns
3. Reports increased comfort, decreased anxiety
4. Resumes prior lung capacity
5. Maintains adequate nutritional status
6. Demonstrates understanding of condition, treatment, home care, and need for follow-up

Cardiovascular System

Basic Information

The heart, arteries, veins, and lymphatics form the cardiovascular system, which serves as the body's transport system. It brings life-supporting O_2 and nutrients to cells, removes metabolic waste products, and carries hormones from one part of the body to another. It is divided into two branches: pulmonary circulation and systemic circulation. Circulation requires normal function of the heart, which pushes blood through the system by continuous rhythmic contractions.

Diseases related to the cardiovascular system are the leading cause of death in the United States. Conditions affecting this system occur across the age continuum. Three major strategies to reduce death and disability due to disorders of the cardiovascular system include: early detection, appropriate treatment to control the progress of the disease, and a reduction of risk factors that predispose individuals to the disease.

Assessment

SUBJECTIVE

1. History
2. Chest pain during periods of physical and emotional stress
3. Dyspnea on exertion
4. Dizziness, fainting
5. Hemoptysis
6. Easily fatigued
7. Family history of heart disease and hypertension

OBJECTIVE

1. Signs and symptoms
   A. Irregular pulse, abnormal rhythm
   B. Abnormal respirations
   C. Skin temperature, color—pallor, cyanosis
   D. Distended neck veins
   E. Abnormal heart sounds
   F. Clubbing of fingers and toes
   G. Presence of edema
   H. Abnormal peripheral pulses
   I. Bruits, thrills over carotid arteries
   J. Pulsations in jugular vein
   K. Pericardial friction rub
2. Physical assessment

DIAGNOSTIC TEST AND METHODS

1. ECG
   A. Primary tool used to evaluate cardiac status
2. Chest x-ray
   A. Diagnostic tool used to determine heart size and shape
3. Stress test
   A. Test used to detect cardiac ischemia developing during exercise or exertion
4. Blood tests
   A. Hemoglobin and hematocrit to detect anemia
   B. WBC count to detect inflammation and infection
   C. BUN and creatinine to detect effect of heart disease on kidneys
   D. Erythrocyte sedimentation rate (ESR) to detect inflammation
   E. Serum enzymes and isoenzymes (AST, CPK, and LDH) to detect myocardial infarction or severe cardiac trauma
   F. Serum lipids to detect presence of heart disease
   G. Blood cultures to detect presence of bacterial endocarditis
5. Urinalysis to detect effects of heart disease on kidneys
6. Cardiac catheterization to detect defects: evaluates chest pain, need for coronary artery surgery, congenital heart defects, and valvular heart disease; determines extent of heart failure
7. Ventriculography (conducted during left heart catheterization—injection of radiopaque dye into left ventricle) to measure ejection fraction (portion of ventricular volume ejected per beat) and to detect abnormal heart wall motion or mitral valve incompetence
8. Coronary arteriography (radiopaque dye injected into coronary arteries) to allow visualization of internal architecture of coronary arteries
9. Echocardiography (use of echos from high-frequency sound waves [ultrasound]) to evaluate heart structures
10. Holter monitor (external ambulatory monitoring device) to detect arrhythmias, congestive heart failure, pacemaker failure, or response to new drug therapy.
11. Nuclear cardiology (Small amounts of radioactive material are injected intravenously) to evaluate left ventricular function, detect and locate myocardial infarctions, and determine development of collateral circulation or patency of grafts.

12. Magnetic Resonance Imaging (MRI) to diagnose thoracic aortic aneurysm, evaluate coronary heart disease and cardia masses.

Implementation

1. Chest pain
   A. Assess and record onset, duration, and intensity.
   B. Monitor and record vital signs.
   C. Check for presence of nausea, vomiting, dyspnea.
   D. Administer vasodilators as ordered; monitor response and report side effects.
   E. Notify physician if chest pain persists more than 15 minutes after administration of nitroglycerine.
   F. Record reactions to treatment and nursing care.
   G. Instruct client regarding diet, medications, and other treatments.
2. Fatigue, weakness
   A. Monitor for signs of fatigue.
   B. Provide adequate rest periods.
   C. Provide prescribed diet, medications.
   D. Encourage progressive ambulation.
   E. Encourage progressive return to activities of daily living (ADL).
   F. Perform ROM exercises.
   G. Record and report response to activity.
   H. Instruct client in planned exercise regimen.
3. Dyspnea
   A. Monitor and record respiratory rate and rhythm.
   B. Monitor and record vital signs.
   C. Place in semi-to-high Fowler position if necessary.
   D. Listen for abnormal lung and heart sounds.
   E. Record intake and output.
   F. Administer diuretics, bronchodilators, and cardiotonic drugs as prescribed; monitor response and report side effects.
   G. Administer and monitor O_2 as ordered.
   H. Observe and record sputum characteristics.
4. Arrhythmias
   A. Monitor and record vital signs—check for changes.
   B. Auscultate chest; report any abnormal heart sounds.
   C. Administer antiarrhythmic medications as ordered—monitor response and report side effects.
5. Hypotension
   A. Monitor vital signs; record and report findings.
   B. Check for postural hypotension.
   C. Instruct client to get out of bed slowly.
   D. Check pulse before and after client stands.
   E. Have client sit on side of bed before standing.
6. Hypertension
   A. Monitor vital signs; record and report findings.
   B. Administer diuretics and antihypertensive medications as prescribed; monitor response and report side effects.
   C. Provide special diet as prescribed (sodium restricted).
   D. Provide low-cholesterol diet, if ordered.
   E. Instruct client in regard to diet, weight control, monitoring of blood pressure, medications, and removal of stressful situations.
7. Edema
   A. Note location and degree.
   B. Change position.
   C. Elevate legs.
   D. Check skin for breakdown.
   E. Check degree of pitting.
   F. Administer prescribed diuretics and cardiotonic drugs; monitor response and report side effects.
   G. Check for ascites.
   H. Check daily weights.
   I. Record intake and output.
   J. Restrict fluids as ordered.
   K. Instruct client in regard to reducing dependent edema.
8. Fluid and electrolyte imbalance
   A. Monitor serum electrolytes.
   B. Record intake and output.
   C. Check daily weight.
   D. Restrict fluids as ordered.
   E. Administer diuretics, if ordered.
   F. Instruct client in regard to diet, medications, and weight.

Angina Pectoris

Description

Angina pectoris involves episodes of acute chest pain as a result of an inadequate O_2 supply to the myocardium due to a decrease in blood flow from the coronary arteries

1. Pain either has a gradual or a sudden onset; pain usually lasts <15 minutes and not >30 minutes (average duration: 3 minutes).
2. Chest pain located behind or under sternum, often radiating to back, neck, left arm, jaws, even upper abdomen or fingers.
3. Mild to moderate pressure, deep sensation; varied pattern of attacks: "tightness," "squeezing," "crushing" sensations.
4. Causes
   A. Major cause—atherosclerotic plaque within coronary arteries
   B. Thrombus formation within vessel
   C. Vasospasms
   D. Low blood volume
   E. Cardiac arrhythmias
   F. Sustained hypertension
   G. Cardiomyopathy
   H. Mitral valve disease
5. Predisposing factors
   A. Exercise
   B. Cigarette smoking
   C. Eating a heavy meal
   D. Environmental temperature extremes—cold, hot, or humid weather
   E. Alcohol use
   F. Drugs
   G. Anemia, thyrotoxicosis, fever

Assessment

SUBJECTIVE

1. Substernal chest pain lasting an average of 3–5 minutes
2. Report of exertion prior to episode
3. Radiation of pain to neck, jaw, left arm
4. Sensation of heaviness, tightness, suffocation

5. Indigestion
6. Pain alleviated by Nitrostat (nitroglycerin) or rest
7. Verbalization of feelings of fear, impending doom, apprehension

OBJECTIVE

1. Presence of nausea or vomiting
2. Dyspnea
3. Potential increase in heart rate
4. Potential increase in blood pressure
5. Skin condition—warm and dry or cool and clammy

DIAGNOSTIC TESTS AND METHODS

1. History
2. Physical examination
3. ECG
4. Holter monitoring
5. Coronary angiography
6. Treadmill exercise testing
7. Serum lipid and enzyme values

Planning

1. Safe, effective care environment
   A. Provide a restful environment.
   B. Increase client's and family's knowledge of disease process, diagnostic procedures, and treatment.
2. Physiological integrity
   A. Control or relieve pain.
   B. Maintain adequate tissue perfusion.
3. Psychosocial integrity
   A. Promote effective coping mechanisms.
4. Health promotion and maintenance
   A. Increase client's and family's knowledge of prevention (including lifestyle changes to reduce risk factors), home care, and follow-up.

Implementation

1. Assess, record, and report signs and symptoms and reactions to treatment.
2. Monitor vital signs, especially during attack.
3. Monitor ECG; record and report any changes.
4. Provide restful environment—remove stressors such as noise, bright lights, interruptions.
5. Administer O_2 as ordered.
6. Decrease activity level.
7. Monitor weight.
8. Provide fat- and cholesterol-restricted diet as prescribed.
9. Monitor angina attacks.
   A. Instruct client to notify staff at the onset of an angina attack.
   B. Record and report onset, duration, location, symptoms, quality, and intensity.
   C. Administer vasodilating medication as prescribed; monitor response and report side effects.
10. Provide emotional support to client and family.
11. Instruct client and family regarding disease process, diagnostic procedures, treatment, prevention, home care, and follow-up. Include teaching on:
    A. Predisposing factors
    B. Medication

C. Diet
D. Lifestyle changes to reduce risk factors

Evaluation

1. Reports increased comfort, relief of pain
2. Maintains stable vital signs
3. Has normal ECG
4. Uses effective coping strategies
5. Demonstrates understanding of disease process, diagnostic procedures, treatment, prevention, home care, and need for follow-up

Hypertension

Description

1. Hypertension is an intermittent or sustained elevation in diastolic or systolic blood pressure; systolic pressure > 140 mm Hg and diastolic pressure > 90 mm Hg.
2. Arterioles are primarily affected, resulting in an increase in peripheral resistance with rise in blood pressure that may be due to responses of the sympathetic nervous system, which in turn stimulates the renin-angiotensin mechanism.
3. Damage occurs to organ supplied by these blood vessels over time.
4. Classification by stage.
5. Types
   A. Genetic (nonmodifiable) factors
   B. Environmental (modifiable) factors
6. Predisposing factors for secondary hypertension
   A. Smoking
   B. Obesity
   C. Diet
   D. Occupation
   E. Stress
   F. Familial history
   G. Sex—primarily among men over 35 years and women over 45 years of age
   H. Race—primarily among blacks; twice the incidence of whites
   I. Birth control pills, estrogen use
7. Associations with other diseases
   A. Renal disease
   B. Pheochromocytoma
   C. Atherosclerosis
   D. Cushing's syndrome
   E. Thyroid, parathyroid, or pituitary dysfunction
   F. Primary aldosteronism
8. Malignant hypertension is a severe form of hypertension common to primary and secondary types of hypertension.
9. Hypertensive crisis (profoundly elevated blood pressure) may be fatal.
10. Isolated systolic hypertension (above 160 mm Hg) is common in elderly persons.

Assessment

SUBJECTIVE

1. Asymptomatic or vague symptoms; may have condition and not know it

2. Complaints of
   A. Chest pain
   B. Fatigue
   C. Blurred vision
   D. Morning headache
   E. Irritability
   F. Dizziness
   G. Ringing in ears
   H. Tachycardia and palpitations
   I. Nausea or vomiting
   J. Shortness of breath
   K. Nosebleeds
   L. Anxiety

OBJECTIVE

1. BP > 140/90
2. Epistaxis
3. Changes in retina
4. Evidence of other associated diseases
5. Hematuria
6. Proteinuria
7. Restlessness

DIAGNOSTIC TESTS AND METHODS

1. History
2. Physical examination
3. Series of resting blood pressure readings
4. Tests and examinations to check for other organ involvement
   A. Chest x-ray examination—to check for increased heart size
   B. ECG—to check for left ventricular hypertrophy or ischemia
   C. Routine urinalysis, BUN, and serum creatinine—to check for renal involvement
   D. Serum potassium levels—to check for adrenal dysfunction
   E. Intravenous pyelogram (IVP)—to check for renal disease
   F. Eye examination—to check for A-V nicking and papilledema
   G. Serum electrolytes—to check for adrenal involvement
   H. Blood glucose levels—to check for endocrine involvement

Planning

1. Safe, effective care environment
   A. Prevent avoidable injury and/or complications.
   B. Increase client's knowledge of disease process, diagnostic procedures, and treatment.
2. Physiological integrity
   A. Ensure that blood pressure remains normal.
   B. Stabilize hemodynamic status.
   C. Prevent dysrhythmias and other complications.
3. Psychosocial integrity
   A. Prevent anxiety and sensory overload from environment.
4. Health promotion and maintenance
   A. Increase client's knowledge of home care (including lifestyle changes such as diet, activity, medication, and stress reduction) and follow-up.

Implementation

1. Assess, record, and report signs and symptoms and reactions to treatment.
2. Provide a quiet, calm environment; rest periods.
3. Provide emotional support to decrease anxiety.
4. Administer prescribed medications; monitor and report side effects.
   A. Diuretics: thiazide loop and potassium sparing
   B. Adrenergic inhibitors: central agonists, α- and β-blockers
   C. Vasodilators: direct vasodilators, calcium channel blockers, angiotensin-converting enzyme (ACE) inhibitors
5. Monitor weight daily to assess response to diuretic therapy.
6. Monitor intake and output to evaluate response to diuretic therapy.
7. Monitor vital signs including blood pressure at the same time every day.
8. Provide adequate nutrition.
   A. Calorie controlled
   B. Sodium restricted
   C. Cholesterol controlled
   D. Increased intake of calcium, potassium, and vitamins A and C and omega-3 fatty acids as ordered.

   NOTE: Controversies remain in regard to the role of calcium and sodium in hypertension.

9. Discourage smoking.
10. Instruct client regarding disease process, diagnostic procedures, treatment, prevention, home care, and follow-up. Include teaching on:
    A. Risk factors
    B. Blood pressure monitoring
    C. Medications
    D. Weight
    E. Dietary restrictions
    F. Planned exercise
    G. Stress management

Evaluation

1. Reports increased comfort, decreased anxiety
2. Decreases blood pressure to acceptable level
3. Reduces risk factors when possible
4. Expresses willingness to comply with medications and dietary restrictions
5. States plan for taking blood pressure measurements
6. Practices methods to control stress
7. Engages in regular exercise
8. Limits alcoholic intake
9. Expresses willingness to lose weight (if overweight)
10. Demonstrates understanding of disease process, diagnostic procedures, treatment, prevention, home care, and need for follow-up

Myocardial Infarction

Description

1. Myocardial infarction (MI) is necrosis of an area of the myocardium as a result of obstruction to blood flow through the coronary artery or one of its branches.

2. The myocardium tissue dies as a result of O_2 deprivation, which causes cell ischemia.
3. The location and size of the necrosed area affects the heart's ability to regain or maintain its function.
4. The leading cause of death in cardiovascular disease; death usually results from cardiac damage or complications of MI.
5. Mortality is high when treatment is delayed.
6. Approximately one half of sudden deaths due to MI occur within 1 hour of onset of symptoms and prior to hospitalization.
7. Prognosis improves if vigorous treatment is started immediately unless location and size of infarct are profound.
8. Complications
   A. Cardiogenic shock
   B. Dysrhythmias
   C. CHF
   D. Ventricular aneurysm
   E. Ventricular rupture
   F. Pericarditis
   G. Pulmonary embolism
   H. Postmyocardial infarction
9. Risk factors
   A. Smoking
   B. Positive family history
   C. Hypertension
   D. Elevated serum triglycerides and cholesterol levels
   E. Obesity or excessive intake of saturated fats
   F. Sedentary lifestyle
   G. Aging
   H. Stress
   I. Sex—males more susceptible, although incidence in females is increasing
   J. Diabetes mellitus
10. Causes
   A. Atherosclerosis—approximately 90% of cases
   B. Constriction or spasm of the coronary artery
   C. Coronary artery embolus
   D. Coronary artery thrombus

Assessment

SUBJECTIVE

1. Chest pain
   A. Tightness, heaviness, squeezing, crushing sensations in substernal area—may radiate to other areas such as neck, jaw, left arm, shoulder.
   B. Pain is not relieved by rest or drugs (nitroglycerin) and can last 30 minutes or more.
   C. In elderly and those with diabetes, pain may not occur or may be mild and confused with indigestion.
2. Precipitating factors
   A. Exertion
   B. Stress
   C. Exercise
3. Predisposing factors
   A. Respiratory tract infection
   B. Pulmonary emboli
   C. Hypoxemia
   D. Blood loss
4. Anxiety, fear, apprehension, feeling of doom, denial, depression

OBJECTIVE

1. Dyspnea
2. Nausea and vomiting
3. Profuse diaphoresis and pallor
4. Presence of rale
5. Tachycardia, decreased blood pressure
6. Temperature rises after 24–48 hours
7. Elevation of cardiac enzymes
   A. CPK peaks 12–18 hours after onset.
   B. CPK-MB elevated 2–4 hours after onset.
   C. AST peaks 24–36 hours after onset.
   D. LDH peaks 48–72 hours after onset.
   E. LDH_1 and LDH_2 may show a flipped pattern in which LDH_1 is greater than LDH_2; present in 48 hours in most infarctions.

DIAGNOSTIC TESTS AND METHODS

1. Detailed history
2. Physical examination
3. Serial 12-lead ECG—abnormalities may be absent or inconclusive during the first few hours
   A. Characteristics include serial ST-T changes in subendocardial MI and Q waves indicative of transmural MI
4. Cardiac enzyme studies (AST, LDH, CPK-MB)
5. Serial chest x-rays
   A. Normal in MI, but if CHF develops, shows cardiomegaly, pulmonary vascular congestion, or bilateral pleural effusion
6. ESR and WBC count
7. Blood lipids study
8. Test for myoglobin
9. CT
10. Nuclear cardiology—scans using prescribed radioactive substance to identify damaged muscle by showing hot spots
11. Radionuclide angiography
12. Myocardial perfusion scan (thallium imaging)
13. Technetium 99mm pyrophosphate imaging
14. Cardiac positron emission tomography scan
15. Magnetic resonance imaging (MRI)
16. Cardiac catheterization
17. Cardiac biopsy

Planning

1. Safe, effective care environment
   A. Allow client to rest.
   B. Increase client's and family's knowledge of disease process, diagnostic procedures, and treatment.
2. Physiological integrity
   A. Maintain adequate oxygenation.
   B. Maintain adequate cardiac output.
3. Psychosocial integrity
   A. Reduce anxiety.
4. Health promotion and maintenance
   A. Increase client's and family's knowledge of home care (including medication, nutrition, and activity) and follow-up.

Implementation

1. Assess, record, and report signs and symptoms and reactions to treatment.

2. Provide quiet, calm environment.
3. Keep client on bed rest for first 24–48 hours, then progressive activity as prescribed.
   A. Turn every 2 hours with assistance.
   B. Use antiembolism stockings to prevent venostasis and thrombophlebitis.
   C. Allow client out of bed to use commode—less strain placed on cardiovascular system.
   D. Avoid activities that may strain the cardiovascular system (e.g., Valsalva's maneuver).
4. Administer stool softeners as prescribed; instruct client not to strain during bowel movement.
5. Monitor pulse during periods of activity.
6. Administer sedatives as prescribed to decrease anxiety and apprehension.
7. Administer vasopressor drugs as prescribed to prevent circulatory collapse (cardiogenic shock).
8. Monitor laboratory data for presence of abnormalities—cardiac enzymes, electrolytes, blood gases, blood counts, blood studies, chemistries, lipids, and drug levels.
9. Assess parameters, waveforms, and signs of complications for clients who have undergone invasive hemodynamic monitoring including arterial and pulmonary arterial lines.
10. Monitor mental state—sensitive indicator of decreased cerebral perfusion due to decrease in cardiac output.
11. Assess peripheral pulses, temperature, and for presence of edema.
12. Monitor for signs of bleeding in patients receiving thrombolytic drugs or anticoagulants.
13. Observe condition of skin—pallor and diaphoresis may indicate a decreasing cardiac output.
14. Perform internal monitoring of blood pressure and pulmonary artery pressure (PAP) (hemodynamic monitoring).
15. Keep IV line open as ordered to provide means for IV drug administration.
16. Relieve chest pain with prescribed medications.
17. Monitor heart rhythm to detect arrhythmias.
18. Administer and monitor O_2 as prescribed to relieve respiratory distress.
19. Administer anticoagulant medications as prescribed.
20. Record vital signs every hour during acute episode.
21. Monitor pulmonary-artery catheter readings for cardiac function.
22. Assist with progressive activity when condition stabilizes.
23. Continue assessment and documentation of signs and symptoms and reactions to treatment.
24. Monitor for signs of complications.
   A. Pulmonary edema—left ventricle failure resulting in decrease in blood pumped out by the diseased heart per minute
   B. CHF
   C. Cardiogenic shock caused by a decrease in cardiac output
25. Assist with cardiopulmonary resuscitation in event of cardiac arrest.
26. Instruct client and family regarding disease process, diagnostic procedures, treatment, home care, and follow-up. Include teaching on:
   A. Reporting any chest pain to the physician immediately.
   B. Lifestyle modifications—activity, diet, stress management, cessation of smoking
   C. Counseling in regard to resuming sexual activity

Evaluation

1. Reports increased comfort, decreased anxiety
2. Reports decrease or relief of chest pain
3. Maintains hemodynamic status
4. Progresses with activity with decreased fatigue
5. Demonstrates adequate cardiac output as evidenced by:
   A. Absence of hypotension
   B. Absence of dysrhythmias
   C. Absence of dyspnea
   D. Clear breath sounds—no rales present
   E. Urinary output >30 mL/hr
   F. Good peripheral pulses
   G. Absence of peripheral edema
   H. Normal mentation
   I. Warm and dry skin
6. Demonstrates ability to do ADL without pain or fatigue
7. Demonstrates understanding of disease process, diagnostic procedures, treatments, home care (including drug compliance and lifestyle modifications), and need for follow-up; similar understanding demonstrated by family

Congestive Heart Failure

Description

1. Congestive heart failure (CHF) is a condition in which the pumping mechanism of the heart is impaired, resulting in an insufficient blood supply to meet the metabolic needs of the body.
2. A build-up of pressure occurs in the vascular beds of the affected side of the heart.
3. Congestion of systemic venous circulation results in peripheral edema or enlarged liver.
4. Congestion of pulmonary circulation may result in pulmonary edema.
5. CHF usually occurs in the left ventricle (left heart failure) but can occur in the right ventricle (right heart failure) primarily or secondary to left heart failure.
6. Sometimes left and right heart failure occur at the same time.
7. CHF is generally considered a chronic disorder with retention of sodium and water by the kidneys.
8. It may be acute as a direct result of MI.
9. Prognosis depends on underlying cause and response to treatment.
10. Causes
   A. MI
   B. Ischemic heart disease
   C. Cardiomyopathy
   D. Myocarditis
   E. Valvular heart disease
   F. Ventricular aneurysm
   G. Aortic or mitral regurgitation, stenosis
   H. Cardiac tamponade
   I. Dysrhythmias
   J. Hypertension
   K. Ventricular or atrial septal defects
   L. Therapeutic interventions such as drug therapy and fluid replacement therapy
11. CHF may become progressively worse from:
   A. Respiratory tract infections
   B. Pulmonary embolism
   C. Added emotional stress

D. Increased sodium or water intake

E. Failure to comply with prescribed therapy

Assessment

SUBJECTIVE

1. Anxiety or restlessness
2. Fatigue
3. Dyspnea
4. Confusion

OBJECTIVE

1. Left-sided heart failure
   A. Dyspnea
   B. Orthopnea
   C. Nonproductive cough—worsens at night
   D. Later, productive cough with frothy, blood-tinged sputum
   E. S-3 heart tone
   F. Cardiomegaly
2. Right-sided heart failure
   A. Weight gain due to fluid accumulation in tissues
   B. Pitting, dependent edema (ankle edema and leg edema, sacral edema)
   C. Ascites from portal hypertension—resulting in accumulation of fluid in abdominal cavity; may interfere with respirations owing to pressure against diaphragm
   D. Decreased urine output
   E. Distended neck veins (jugular venous distention [JVD])
   F. Nausea, vomiting, and anorexia

DIAGNOSTIC TESTS AND METHODS

1. Detailed history
2. Physical examination
3. Chest x-ray examination
4. ECG
5. Pulmonary artery monitoring
6. ABGs
7. Renal function tests
8. Liver function tests

Planning

1. Safe, effective care environment
   A. Maintain restful environment.
   B. Prevent infection and other complications.
   C. Increase client's and family's knowledge of disease process, diagnostic procedures, and treatment.
2. Physiological integrity
   A. Maintain adequate cardiac output.
3. Psychosocial integrity
   A. Reduce anxiety; promote self-esteem.
4. Health promotion and maintenance
   A. Increase client's and family's knowledge of home care (especially antibiotic prior to dental work, surgery, or other invasive procedures) and follow-up.

Implementation

1. Assess, record, and report signs and symptoms and reactions to treatment.
2. Administer and monitor O_2 therapy as ordered.
3. Place client in high Fowler position; elevate extremities.
4. Record vital signs every 15 minutes to 2 hours during acute phase.
5. Restrict fluids as ordered.
6. Provide adequate nutrition.
   A. Restrict salt intake.
7. Record intake and output every hour during acute phase.
8. Monitor for progression of failure.
   A. Evaluate blood pressure and pulse.
   B. Check for presence of JVD and peripheral edema.
9. Assist with use of rotating tourniquets as ordered.
   A. Check radial and pedal pulses often to ensure tourniquets are not too tight.
   B. Remove one tourniquet at a time in a clockwise pattern to prevent sudden upsurge in circulating volume.
10. Assess invasive hemodynamic monitoring data.
11. Monitor CVP in clients with right ventricular failure and monitor pulmonary capillary wedge pressure (PCWP) for left ventricular failure.
12. Ausculate lung fields for presence of abnormal sounds such as crackles and wheezes.
13. Weigh patient daily—check for weight gain or loss in response to fluid retention or therapeutic intervention.
14. Measure abdominal girth to detect presence or absence of hepatomegaly or ascites.
15. Provide quiet, calm environment.
16. Plan care to provide adequate rest—conserves energy, prevents fatigue.
17. Monitor and record daily weights; report any changes.
18. Monitor mental status.
19. Monitor IV intake as prescribed.
20. Monitor BUN, creatinine and serum potassium, sodium, chloride, and magnesium levels.
21. Assess amount of activity that results in the least discomfort to client.
22. Monitor for signs of embolic complications due to forced inactivity or dysrhythmias.
23. Assist with ROM exercises to prevent deep vein thrombosis due to vascular congestion.
24. Apply antiembolism stockings—watch for calf pain and tenderness.
25. Assist with ADL until client is able to show gradual progress.
26. Administer medications such as digitalis, diuretics, vasodilators as prescribed.
   A. Check apical-radial pulse when giving digitalis.
   B. Monitor, record, and report responses to medications, including any side effects.
27. Monitor digitalis toxicity tests.
28. Assist client to turn, cough, deep breathe.
29. Instruct client and family regarding disease process, diagnostic procedures, treatment, home care, and follow-up. Include teaching on:
   A. Avoiding foods high in sodium, such as canned or processed foods and dairy products, to reduce fluid overload
   B. Loss of potassium through use of diuretics and replacement with prescribed potassium supplement and eating high-potassium foods (unless taking potassium-sparing diuretics)
   C. Need for regular checkups
   D. Importance of taking digitalis exactly as prescribed

E. Watching for signs of digitalis toxicity—anorexia, nausea, vomiting, yellow vision, cardiac arrhythmias
F. Importance of notifying physician immediately of irregular pulse or pulse <60 bpm, persistent dry cough, palpitations, increased fatigue, paroxysmal nocturnal dyspnea, swollen ankles, decreased urinary output, or weight gain of 3–5 lb in a week

Evaluation

1. Reports increased comfort, decreased anxiety
2. Displays decreased confusion
3. Experiences decreased respiratory difficulties.
4. Tolerates progressive activity
5. Experiences decreased edema
6. Demonstrates increase in cardiac output
    A. Skin color is improved.
    B. Skin is warm.
    C. Absence of orthostasis.
    D. Blood pressure levels are within normal limits.
    E. Absence of tachycardia.
    F. Decreased dysrhythmias.
7. Demonstrates improvement in gas exchange
    A. Respirations within normal range.
    B. Good skin color, pink nail beds.
    C. Lungs are clear to auscultation.
    D. Improved breathing.
    E. Improved activity tolerance.
8. Is able to sleep without dyspnea.
9. Demonstrates reduction in excess fluid volume
    A. Loss of water weight.
    B. Reduction in abdominal girth.
    C. Intake is less than or equal to output.
    D. Reduction of edema in dependent areas.
10. Shows signs of improved mental acuity
    A. Aware of current events, surroundings
    B. Intact memory
    C. Logical and clear communication
    D. Ability to follow directions
11. Demonstrates improved renal flow
    A. Intake and output are balanced.
    B. BUN and electrolytes are within normal range.
12. Demonstrates restoration and maintenance of activity level.
    A. Decreased fatigue
    B. Regular exercise
    C. Need to avoid certain activities that induce symptoms
13. Demonstrates improvement of sleeping habits.
    A. Adequate rest periods at night without dyspnea
    B. Increased solid sleep time
    C. Respiratory status does not interfere with sleep.
14. Reports improved sexual function
15. Demonstrates understanding of disease process, diagnostic procedures, treatment, home care (including drug compliance and daily weights), and need for follow-up; similar understanding demonstrated by family

Shock

Description

1. Shock indicates insufficient cardiac output or tissue perfusion. The types of shock are described as follows.
2. Cardiogenic shock.

A. Cardiogenic shock is a condition of decreased cardiac output due to pump failure.
B. Condition reflects severe left ventricular failure.
C. It occurs as a serious complication in approximately 15% of clients hospitalized with acute MI.
3. Coronary cardiogenic shock
    A. Condition is associated with atherosclerotic artery disease.
    B. Cells become ischemic and MI occurs.
    C. Heart's ability to contract normally is compromised.
    D. It typically affects clients who have infarcts exceeding 40% of myocardial mass.
    E. It often involves anterior wall of left ventricle.
    F. Damage may be cumulative, resulting from previous MIs.
    G. Fatality rate may exceed 85% in these clients.
    H. Most clients expire within 24 hours of onset.
    I. Prognosis is extremely poor for those who survive.
4. Noncoronary cardiogenic shock
    A. Condition can develop in absence of coronary artery diseases and is related to a variety of causes:
        (1) MI
        (2) CHF
        (3) Cardiac tamponade
        (4) Severe valvular heart disease
        (5) Restrictive pericarditis
        (6) Papillary muscle dysfunction
        (7) End-stage cardiomyopathy
        (8) Massive left ventricular aneurysm
5. Hypovolemic shock
    A. Condition occurs due to reduction in intravascular blood volume, resulting in insufficient perfusion of the tissues (loss of fluid within vascular space).
    B. It may lead to irreversible cerebral and renal damage, cardiac arrest, and finally death.
    C. Condition requires immediate recognition of signs and symptoms and prompt, aggressive treatment to improve prognosis.
    D. Causes
        (1) Acute blood loss due to GI bleeding, internal hemorrhage, or external hemorrhage
        (2) Acute loss of fluids other than blood due to dehydration from excessive perspiration, severe diarrhea, protracted vomiting; diabetes insipidus; diuresis
        (3) Fluid shift from vascular space into another space (third spacing) due to intestinal obstruction, peritonitis, ascites
6. Vasogenic (or neurogenic) shock
    A. Vasogenic shock is a disruptive type of shock characterized by massive vasodilation due to loss of sympathetic tone.
    B. Condition occurs from acute vasodilation of vascular beds with pooling of blood within peripheral blood vessels, resulting in inadequate perfusion of tissues.
    C. Condition is rare and often transitory.
    D. Loss of sympathetic tone may develop owing to injury and disease of the spinal cord above the midthoracic region.
    E. High levels of spinal anesthesia can impair nerve impulse transmission and decrease sympathetic tone.
    F. Sympathetic outflow from vasomotor center in brain

can be blocked or temporarily decreased by emotional stress, drug overdose, or severe pain.
  G. Manifestation of low blood pressure and a normal or slow heart rate because the absence of sympathetic outflow prevents an increase in heart rate.
7. Anaphylactic shock
  A. Condition is characterized by massive vasodilation and increase in capillary permeability.
  B. A severe form of hypersensitivity (allergic reaction).
  C. It presents a dramatic picture that is potentially life threatening.
  D. Causes
    (1) Severe allergic reaction to antigen ingestion or injection to which previously sensitized
    (2) Antibiotics such as penicillin, tetracycline, and sulfonamides; narcotics and barbiturates
    (3) Contrast media such as those used for diagnostic studies
    (4) Transfused blood and blood products
    (5) Insect bites, stings, (honeybees, bumblebees, hornets, yellow jackets, wasps, and fire ants)
8. Septic shock
  A. Condition is associated with severe, overwhelming infection.
  B. It develops secondary to the invasion of the body by foreign microorganisms and subsequent failure of body's defense system.
  C. Approximately 1 in every 100 hospitalized patients develops sepsis, and 40% of these develop septic shock.
  D. Mortality ranges from 40%–90%.
  E. Client-related risk factors
    (1) Malnutrition
    (2) General debilitation
    (3) Chronic illness
    (4) CHF
    (5) Chronic obstructive lung disease
    (6) Cancer
    (7) Cirrhosis
    (8) Pregnancy
    (9) Extremes of age
  F. Treatment-related risk factors
    (1) Insertion of invasive lines and catheters
    (2) Surgical procedures, wounds, and drains
    (3) Traumatic wounds, thermal injuries
    (4) Invasive diagnostic procedures
    (5) Drugs
      (a) Antibiotics
      (b) Cytotoxic drugs
      (c) Immunosuppressive drugs
  G. Causative microorganisms
    (1) Gram-negative bacteria such as *Escherichia coli, Klebsiella-Enterobacter-Serratia,* and *Pseudomonas aeruginosa.*
    (2) Gram-positive bacteria such as *S. pneumoniae* and *S. aureus.*
    (3) Viruses, fungi, and rickettsiae.
9. Progression
  A. Initial: Inadequate O_2 delivery causes cellular changes—increase in serum lactic acid.
  B. Compensatory: Decrease in cardiac output triggers neural, hormonal, and chemical mechanisms that restore tissue perfusion to vital organs.

  C. Progressive: Compensatory mechanisms start to fail, resulting in inadequate perfusion to vital organs.
  D. Refractory: Severe prolonged shock state results in death from multiple organ system failure.
10. Complications
  A. ARDS
  B. Renal failure
  C. DIC
  D. Cerebral infarction
  E. Liver dysfunction
  F. GI ulcerations
  G. Pancreatic failure
  H. Ischemic changes in brain

Assessment

SUBJECTIVE

1. Confusion, lethargy, restlessness

OBJECTIVE

1. Blood pressure—initially normal, then drops
2. Rapid, weak pulse
3. Cold, clammy skin
4. Low urine output
5. Diaphoresis, pallor
6. Increased respiratory rate, dyspnea, cough
7. Decrease in CVP readings in hypovolemic and vasogenic shock
8. Increase in CVP readings in cardiogenic shock
9. Increased P_{CO_2} and decreased Pa_{O_2}
10. Decreased level of consciousness
11. Abnormal clotting with DIC
12. Decreased or absent bowel sounds (paralytic ileus)

DIAGNOSTIC TESTS AND METHODS

1. History
2. Physical examination
3. Cardiogenic shock
  A. PAP monitoring
  B. Invasive arterial pressure monitoring
  C. ABGs
  D. ECG
  E. Serum enzyme levels
  F. X-rays—to identify internal bleeding sites
4. Hypovolemic shock
  A. Laboratory tests
  B. Serum potassium, lactate, and BUN levels
  C. Urine specific gravity
  D. Blood pH, P_{O_2}, and P_{CO_2}
5. Septic shock
  A. Urine cultures
  B. Blood cultures
  C. Sputum cultures
  D. Chest x-ray
6. Gastroscopy
7. Aspiration of gastric contents
8. Coagulation studies

Planning

1. Safe, effective care environment
  A. Prevent complications.

B. Increase client's knowledge of disease process, diagnostic procedures, and treatment (including surgery, if needed).
2. Physiological integrity
   A. Increase comfort and rest.
   B. Maintain adequate cardiac function.
3. Psychosocial integrity
   A. Assist with effective coping.
4. Health promotion and maintenance
   A. Increase client's knowledge of home care and follow-up.

Implementation

1. Assess, record, and report signs and symptoms and reactions to treatment.
2. Establish and maintain an open airway.
3. Remove secretions from trachea and tracheobronchial tree via bronchial hygiene such as suctioning, postural drainage, and chest physiotherapy through trachea.
4. Provide adequate systemic hydration and frequent turning to mobilize secretions.
5. Provide O_2 to promote adequate oxygenation of tissues.
6. Encourage deep breathing and coughing.
7. Have ventilator on hand if respiratory function deteriorates.
8. Assist with ventilator support.
9. Monitor blood pressure and heart rate immediately.
10. Keep IV line open as means for IV drug administration.
11. Monitor vital signs (watch for drop in systolic blood pressure to <80 mm Hg—usually results in insufficient coronary artery blood flow).
    A. May produce cardiac arrhythmias or cardiac ischemia.
    B. Report hypotension immediately.
12. Monitor ABGs.
13. Monitor CBC and serum electrolyte levels.
14. Administer prescribed vasoactive drugs and antibiotics.
15. Monitor CVP and/or PAPs.
16. Monitor urinary output (use Foley catheter)—notify registered nurse if output drops below 30 mL/hr.
17. Administer osmotic diuretic if prescribed to prevent renal tubular necrosis.
18. Turn client every 2 hours to prevent skin breakdown.
19. Monitor for signs of infection.
20. Provide safe environment for client who is confused, restless.
21. Provide environment for client to rest; assist in comfort measures.
22. Instruct client regarding disease process, diagnostic procedures, treatment, home care, and follow-up.

Evaluation

1. Demonstrates normal sensorium—able to follow directions, and responds to verbal stimuli
2. Maintains adequate hemodynamic status
3. Maintains adequate gas exchange
4. Maintains vital signs within normal limits
5. Maintains urine output of >30 mL/hr (in adults)
6. Displays reduction in anxiety, confusion, restlessness
7. Maintains serum electrolyte levels within normal range

8. Maintains BUN, creatinine levels within normal range
9. Maintains good skin hygiene
10. Maintains laboratory test levels within normal range
11. Decreases metabolic demands
12. Maintains normal arterial blood pressure
13. Maintains a heart rate >50–60 bpm but <110–120 bpm
14. Demonstrates full, strong, and regular bilateral peripheral pulses
15. Maintains pulmonary artery and cardiac output at a normal level
16. Maintains venous O_2 saturation at least between 70% and 90%
17. Maintains normal respiratory rate
18. Maintains regular and unlabored respiratory levels
19. Shows no evidence of moist crackles in lung field
20. Shows no evidence of cyanosis
21. Maintains PaO_2 at >80 mm Hg on 50% O_2
22. Maintains $PaCO_2$ between 35 mm Hg and 45 mm Hg
23. Demonstrates understanding of disease process, diagnostic procedures, treatment, home care, and need for follow-up

Acquired Inflammatory Disorders of the Heart

Description

Acquired inflammatory disorders of the heart are diseases that occur due to an acute or chronic inflammation of the heart lining and valves caused by bacteria, viruses, trauma, or other factors. There are three types of rheumatic heart disease—pericarditis, myocarditis, and endocarditis. Rheumatic heart disease can cause valvular heart disease, which in turn can cause acute pulmonary edema.

Pericarditis

Description

1. Pericarditis is an inflammation of the pericardium, the fibroserous sac that envelops and protects the heart. It can be acute or chronic.
2. Acute pericarditis can be either fibrinous or effusive with purulent serous or hemorrhagic exudate.
3. The chronic type is characterized by thickening of the pericardial wall. The result is either loss of elasticity or accumulation of fluid within the pericardial sac.
4. Complications include heart failure and cardiac tamponade. Prognosis depends on underlying cause.
5. *Coccus faecalis* (enterococcus) usually found in perineal and GI flora.
6. Causes
   A. Bacterial, fungal, or viral infections
   B. Neoplasms (primary) or secondary from lungs, breasts, and other organs
   C. High-dose radiation to chest
   D. Hypersensitivity or autoimmune disease such as rheumatic fever, systemic lupus erythematosus, and rheumatoid arthritis
   E. Postcardiac injury
   F. Drugs such as procainamide
   G. Idiopathic factors
   H. Aortic aneurysm with pericardial leakage
   I. Myxedema

Assessment

SUBJECTIVE

1. Sharp pain over sternum radiating to neck, shoulders, back, and arms.
2. Pain increases with deep inspiration, decreases when sitting up or leaning forward (pulls heart away from diaphragmatic pleurae of the lungs).
3. Difficulty in breathing.
4. Tachycardia.
5. Feeling of fullness in chest.

OBJECTIVE

1. Dyspnea, orthopnea
2. Tachycardia
3. Substernal chest pain
4. Pallor; cold, clammy skin
5. Neck vein distention
6. Hypotension
   A. Signs of constrictive pericarditis
      (1) Increase in systemic venous pressure
      (2) Pericardial friction rub
7. Symptoms similar to right heart failure—fluid retention, hepatomegaly, ascites

DIAGNOSTIC TESTS AND METHODS

1. History
2. Physical examination
3. WBC count, ESR
4. Serum cardiac enzymes
5. Cardiocentesis
6. ECG
7. Pericardial fluid culture
8. Echocardiography—to assess valvular disease

Planning

1. Safe, effective care environment
   A. Increase client's and family's knowledge of disease process, diagnostic procedures (such as pericardiocentesis, pericardial window, or pericardiotomy), and treatment.
2. Physiological integrity
   A. Control or alleviate chest pain.
   B. Prevent cardiac tamponade or CHF.
   C. Maintain adequate comfort.
3. Psychosocial integrity
   A. Reduce anxiety.
4. Health promotion and maintenance
   A. Increase client's and family's knowledge of home care and follow-up.

Implementation

1. Assess, record, and report signs and symptoms and reactions to treatment.
2. Assess pain in relation to respiration and body position.
3. Place client in upright position to relieve dyspnea and pain.
4. Provide bed rest.
5. Administer salicylates, antibiotics, and other prescribed medications.
6. Administer O_2 as prescribed.

7. Assist with procedures as necessary.
8. Monitor for signs of infection.
9. Monitor blood pressure and venous pressure; decreased blood pressure and increased venous pressure indicate pericardial effusion.
10. Prepare client and family for surgical intervention, if required by client.
11. Provide postoperative care.
12. Instruct client and family regarding disease process, diagnostic procedures, treatment, home care, and follow-up.

Evaluation

1. Shows no signs of pericardial friction rub, pericardial effusion, or infection
2. Reports increased comfort, relief of pain
3. Maintains stable vital signs
4. Has normal laboratory values
5. Demonstrates understanding of disease process, diagnostic procedures, treatment, home care, and need for follow-up; similar understanding demonstrated by family

Myocarditis

Description

1. Myocarditis is an inflammation of the cardiac muscle. It may be acute or chronic and occurs at any age.
2. The result is impairment of contractility. Often, this condition does not produce specific symptoms or ECG abnormalities.
3. Complications associated with myocarditis include CHF, myocardial ischemia, necrosis, and, rarely, cardiomyopathy.
4. Causes
   A. Viral infections—influenza, measles, German measles, echoviruses
   B. Bacterial infections—diphtheria; TB; typhoid fever; tetanus; staphylococcal, pneumonococcal, and gonococcal variety
   C. Hypersensitive immune reactions—acute rheumatic fever
   D. Radiation therapy—large doses to chest for treatment of lung or breast cancer
   E. Chemical poisons—chronic alcoholism
   F. Parasitic infections, viral infections—influenza, measles, German measles, echoviruses

Assessment

SUBJECTIVE

1. Fatigue
2. Difficulty in breathing
3. Feeling of soreness in chest

OBJECTIVE

1. Dyspnea
2. Neck vein distention, tachycardia, fever, arrhythmias (in severe cases)

DIAGNOSTIC TESTS AND METHODS

1. History
2. Physical examination

3. Serum cardiac enzymes, WBC count, and ESR
4. ECG
5. Throat culture
6. Stool culture

Planning

1. Safe, effective care environment
   A. Increase client's and family's knowledge of disease process and diagnostic procedures.
2. Physiological integrity
   A. Prevent CHF.
   B. Promote rest.
   C. Maintain cardiovascular status.
3. Health promotion and maintenance
   A. Increase client's knowledge of prevention and reporting of signs and symptoms of infection.

Implementation

1. Assess, record, and report signs and symptoms and reactions to treatment.
2. Monitor cardiovascular status frequently.
   A. Listen for rales.
   B. Take vital signs.
   C. Weigh daily.
   D. Record intake and output.
3. Monitor cardiac rhythm and conduction.
   A. Observe for signs of digitalis toxicity.
4. Check serum electrolyte levels.
5. Stress importance of bed rest.
6. Assist with activities; provide rest periods.
7. Provide bedside commode.
8. Instruct client to resume normal activities slowly.
9. Instruct client and family regarding disease process, diagnostic procedures, treatment, home care, and follow-up.

Evaluation

1. Reports increased comfort, decreased anxiety
2. Maintains normal cardiovascular status
3. Shows no signs of infection
4. Demonstrates understanding of disease process, diagnostic procedures, treatment, home care, and need for follow-up; similar understanding demonstrated by family

Endocarditis

Description

1. Endocarditis is an inflammation of the endocardium, heart valves, or cardiac prosthesis due to infectious organisms.
2. Organisms such as staphylococci and *Streptococcus viridans* and *faecalis* produce vegetative growths on the heart valves, endocardial lining of the heart chambers, or endothelium of blood vessels that may break off and embolize to the CNS, spleen, kidneys, and lungs.
3. Condition is usually fatal if untreated, but with treatment, approximately 70% recover.
4. Prognosis is worse when severe vascular damage occurs, resulting in insufficiency of blood flow and CHF, or when a prosthetic valve is involved.

5. Causes
   A. In acute form, bacteremia following septic thrombophlebitis; open heart surgery involving prosthetic valves; or skin, bone, and pulmonary infections.
   B. Most common organisms are group A nonhemolytic streptococcus (rheumatic endocarditis), pneumococcus, staphylococcus.
   C. Occurs in IV drug users due to *S. aureus, Pseudomonas,* or *Candida.*
   D. In subacute infections, associated with acquired valvular or congenital cardiac disorders.
   E. Condition is also associated with dental, genitourinary (GU), GI, and gynecological procedures.

Assessment

SUBJECTIVE

1. Anorexia, weight loss
2. Malaise, weakness
3. Chest pain
4. Chills
5. Night sweats

OBJECTIVE

1. Low-grade fever (99°–102°F)—subacute endocarditis
2. High-grade fever (103°–104°F)—acute infective endocarditis
3. Positive blood cultures
4. Murmurs over valves
5. Clubbing of fingers
6. Petechiae (in 49% of cases)
7. Typical symptoms of complications due to emboli reaching other organs, including spleen, kidney, lungs, peripheral vascular beds. Symptoms include hematuria, pleuritic chest pain, upper left quadrant pain.

DIAGNOSTIC TESTS AND METHODS

1. Blood culture studies
2. WBC count, ESR
3. Histocyte studies
4. Rheumatoid factor (RF)
5. Echocardiography—to identify valvular damage
6. ECG—may show arterial fibrillation and other arrhythmias

Planning

1. Safe, effective care environment
   A. Increase client's and family's knowledge of disease process and therapeutic management.
2. Physiological integrity
   A. Reduce anxiety.
3. Health promotion and maintenance
   A. Teach prophylactic care.

Implementation

1. Assess, record, and report signs and symptoms and reactions to treatment.
2. Obtain history of allergies, sore throats, dental surgery, rheumatic fever.
3. Administer antibiotics on time to maintain consistent antibiotic blood levels.
4. Monitor for signs of heart failure, embolization.

5. Provide mouth care.
6. Avoid invasive procedures.
7. Monitor renal status—BUN creatinine, urinary output to check for signs of renal emboli or drug toxicity.
8. Provide reassurance to client and family.
9. Instruct client regarding disease process, diagnostic procedures, treatment, home care, and follow-up. Include teaching on:
   A. Need for prophylactic antibiotics before, during, and after dental work; childbirth; GU and GI procedures
   B. Need to notify physician immediately if these symptoms reappear

Evaluation

1. Shows no signs of infection (e.g., fever) or other avoidable complications
2. Maintains adequate cardiac function
3. Demonstrates understanding of disease process, diagnostic procedures, treatment, home care (including drug precautions for invasive procedures), and need for follow-up

Valvular Heart Disease

Description

1. Valvular heart disease results in either stenosis or insufficiency (regurgitation) of heart valves.
2. In valvular stenosis, the valve cusps become fibrotic and thicken; may fuse together, hindering blood flow
3. In valvular insufficiency, valve cusps become inflamed and scarred; no longer close completely.
4. Alteration of blood flow through the heart occurs, resulting in a decrease in cardiac output, systemic and pulmonary congestion, and dilation of heart chambers.
5. Types
   A. Mitral stenosis: Mitral valve becomes calcified and stiff. It leads to left atrial hypertrophy with an increase in left atrial and pulmonary pressures. Right-sided heart failure results.
      (1) Causes
         (a) Rheumatic fever
      (2) Complications
         (a) Atrial fibrillation
         (b) Thrombus formation
         (c) CHF
   B. Mitral regurgitation: Insufficient valves allow blood to backflow from ventricle to atria during systole. Atrial and left ventricular hypertrophy result.
      (1) Causes
         (a) Rheumatic fever
         (b) Myocardial infarction
         (c) Ventricular aneurysm
         (d) Papillary muscle rupture
         (e) Endocarditis
      (2) Complications
         (a) Atrial fibrillation
         (b) Elevated left-sided heart pressures
         (c) CHF
         (d) Systemic embolization
   C. Aortic stenosis: Aortic valve becomes stiffened and fibrotic, impeding blood flow during left ventricular emptying. It results in left ventricular hypertrophy, increased O_2 demands, and pulmonary congestion.
      (1) Causes
         (a) Rheumatic fever
         (b) Congenital valve defects
         (c) Atherosclerosis
      (2) Complications
         (a) Right-sided heart failure
         (b) Pulmonary edema
         (c) Atrial fibrillation
   D. Aortic regurgitation: Aortic valve becomes insufficient owing to deformed or contracted valve cusps. Valves cannot close completely, resulting in backflow of blood into left ventricle. Left ventricular hypertrophy occurs.
      (1) Causes
         (a) Rheumatic fever
         (b) Congenital defects
         (c) Endocarditis
      (2) Complications
         (a) Left-sided heart failure
         (b) Dysrhythmias
   E. Tricuspid stenosis: Chordae tendinae become fused and shortened, resulting in a narrowing of the valvular opening. Blood flow is obstructed to the right atrium, causing right-sided heart failure and decreased cardiac output.
      (1) Causes
         (a) Rheumatic fever
         (b) Right atrial myxomas
   F. Tricuspid regurgitation: The valve becomes insufficient as a result of papillary muscle dysfunction or dilation of the valvular ring. Blood flows back into the right atrium with resultant venous overload and decreased cardiac output.
      (1) Causes
         (a) Rheumatic fever
         (b) Congenital defect
         (c) Dilation of right ventricle
         (d) Endocarditis

Assessment

SUBJECTIVE

1. Fatigue, weakness
2. General malaise
3. Dyspnea on exertion
4. Dizziness
5. Chest pain, discomfort
6. Weight gain
7. Prior history of rheumatic fever

OBJECTIVE

1. Orthopnea
2. Dyspnea, rales
3. Pink-tinged sputum (mitral stenosis)
4. Heart murmurs
5. Palpitations
6. Cyanosis, capillary refill
7. Edema
8. Dysrhythmias
9. Restlessness
10. Left-sided or right-sided elevated pressures

DIAGNOSTIC TESTS AND METHODS

1. History
2. Physical examination
3. ECG
4. Chest x-ray—to determine size of heart
5. Cardiac catheterization—to identify pressure changes
6. Echocardiogram—to obtain information regarding structure and function of valves

Planning

1. Safe, effective care environment
   A. Prevent avoidable injury and/or infection.
   B. Increase client's and family's knowledge of disease process, diagnostic procedures, and treatment.
2. Physiological integrity
   A. Increase comfort (for pain, rest, and sleep).
   B. Maintain adequate cardiac output.
   C. Maintain effective breathing pattern.
3. Psychosocial integrity
   A. Reduce anxiety
4. Health promotion and maintenance
   A. Increase client's and family's knowledge of home care including medication, diet, activity, and follow-up.

Implementation

1. Assess, record, and report signs and symptoms and reactions to treatment.
2. Elevate head of bed.
3. Provide O_2 therapy as prescribed.
4. Provide emotional support to client and family.
5. Administer prescribed medication—antibiotics, digitalis, diuretics, and anticoagulants; monitor response and report side effects.
6. Check digitalis toxicity reports.
7. Provide a calm, quiet environment to conserve client's energy.
8. Monitor and record vital signs.
9. Monitor intake and output.
10. Check for edema, capillary refill.
11. Weigh daily.
12. Provide sodium-restricted diet as prescribed.
13. Provide progressive activity based on client's limitations.
14. Instruct client and family regarding disease process, diagnostic procedures, treatment, home care, and follow-up. Include teaching on:
    A. Diet
    B. Medications
    C. Activity
    D. Need for treatment compliance

Evaluation

1. Maintains effective cardiac output
2. Maintains effective breathing pattern
3. Reports reduction in edema
4. Reports increased comfort, decreased anxiety
5. Demonstrates understanding of disease process, diagnostic procedures, treatment (including need for compliance and precautions for invasive procedures), home care, and need for follow-up; similar understanding demonstrated by family

Acute Pulmonary Edema

Description

1. In cardiogenic pulmonary edema, fluid accumulation in alveoli, bronchioles, and bronchi is a result of elevations in pulmonary venous and capillary pressures. Gas exchange is decreased.
2. Pulmonary edema is a common complication of cardiac disorders; it can occur as a chronic condition or develop quickly with rapid fatal consequences.
   A. Causes
      (1) CHF
      (2) Valvular heart disease
      (3) Fluid overload
      (4) Inhalation of irritating chemicals
      (5) Nephrosis, extensive burns, liver disease, nutritional deficiency—due to decreased serum colloid osmotic pressure
      (6) Hodgkin's disease—due to impaired lung lymphatic drainage

Assessment

SUBJECTIVE

1. Difficulty in breathing
2. Anxiety, apprehension
3. Weakness
4. Cough

OBJECTIVE

1. Dyspnea
2. Restlessness, confusion
3. Productive cough with frothy pink sputum
4. Weak, rapid pulse
5. Wheezing
6. Cyanosis
7. Increased CVP readings
8. Tachycardia
9. Orthopnea
10. Arrhythmias
11. Cold and clammy skin
12. Decreased blood pressure

DIAGNOSTIC TESTS AND METHODS

1. History
2. Physical examination
3. ABGs
4. Chest x-ray
5. Pulmonary artery catheterization

Planning

1. Safe, effective care environment
   A. Increase client's and family's knowledge of disease process (dysrhythmia), diagnostic procedures (monitor, catheterization, etc.), and treatment (pacemaker).
2. Physiological integrity
   A. Maintain adequate cardiac output.
   B. Maintain adequate gas exchange.
3. Psychosocial integrity
   A. Reduce anxiety and fear.
4. Health promotion and maintenance
   A. Increase client's and family's knowledge of home care

(lifestyle changes such as diet, pacemaker, medication, activity, etc.) and follow-up.

Implementation

1. Assess, record, and report signs and symptoms and reactions to treatment.
2. Provide complete bed rest.
3. Place client in high Fowler position.
4. Monitor vital signs.
5. Monitor breath sounds.
6. Check for peripheral edema.
7. Administer O_2 as ordered.
8. Administer prescribed medications such as morphine, diuretics, digitalis, and vasodilators.
9. Observe effects of medications including side effects.
10. Assess client's condition frequently.
11. Monitor ABGs.
12. Check cardiac monitor frequently; report any changes.
13. Assist with rotating tourniquets, if prescribed; record sequence and timing.
14. Reassure client and family.
15. Instruct client and family regarding disease process, diagnostic procedures, prevention, treatment, home care, and follow-up.

Evaluation

1. Demonstrates decreased venous return
2. Maintains effective gas exchange
3. Maintains effective cardiovascular function
4. Reports increased comfort, decreased anxiety, apprehension
5. Demonstrates understanding of disease process, diagnostic procedures, treatment, home care, and need for follow-up; similar understanding demonstrated by family

Peripheral Vascular System

Basic Information

1. The peripheral vascular system includes the branching network of vessels that carry blood from the left side of the heart to tissues and then back to the right side of the heart.
2. Alterations of the vascular system usually occur in adulthood.
3. Peripheral vascular disease refers to vascular disorders other than those specifically affecting the heart.
4. Exercise, diet, and other health promotion practices affect the integrity of the peripheral vascular system.
5. Risk factors for peripheral vascular disease include high fat intake, sedentary lifestyle, smoking, and obesity.
6. Females are prone to peripheral vascular disease, particularly in terms of obstruction to the circulation in the lower extremities during pregnancy.
7. Certain disease processes, such as diabetes mellitus, are associated with the development of peripheral vascular impairment.
8. Blood flow is decreased owing to narrowing or obstructed blood vessels. The underlying factor is the arteriosclerotic process. The decreased blood flow causes changes in the tissues.

Assessment

SUBJECTIVE

1. Aching calves
2. Numbness in legs
3. Leg cramps
4. Loss of sensation in legs
5. Pain in legs during exercise (intermittent claudication)
6. History of diabetes mellitus, thrombophlebitis, hypertension, alcoholism

OBJECTIVE

1. Arterial Insufficiency
   A. Pain in region of the affected vessel
   B. Numbness in affected limb
   C. Pallor or mottling in the affected limb
   D. Muscle spasms
   E. Pulselessness in distal limb (due to blockage)
   F. Possible paralysis
2. Venous Insufficiency
   A. Lower leg edema
   B. Discolored skin in affected lower limb
   C. Affected subcutaneous tissue feels hard
   D. Stasis ulcers over the ankle
   E. Redness of leg in dependent position
3. Other
   A. Sparse hair distribution
   B. Varicose veins
   C. Delay in capillary filling
   D. Bruits heard in major arteries
   E. Difference in circumference of legs

DIAGNOSTIC TESTS AND METHODS

1. Oscillometry—an instrument to measure pulsations over an artery
2. Chest x-ray
3. Doppler ultrasonography—an instrument to measure blood flow through a vessel
4. Venography—an invasive procedure to determine vessel distention, development of collateral circulation, and location and size of blood clot
5. Trendelenburg test—a tool to determine valvular competency in legs
6. ABG analysis—a tool to determine adequacy of ventilation
7. X-ray of abdomen—a tool to determine presence or absence of aneurysm
8. Lung scan—a tool to determine presence or absence of pulmonary embolism and lung damage
9. Oculoplethysmography—a noninvasive procedure used to assess the blood flow to the carotid artery by an indirect measurement of blood flow in the ophthalmic artery, a major branch of the carotid artery
10. Carotid phonangiography—a noninvasive procedure to determine the location and severity of the stenosis of the carotid artery
11. Impedance plethysmography—a noninvasive procedure useful in diagnosing deep vein thrombosis, especially in the popliteal and ileofemoral veins
12. Ultrasound arteriography—a noninvasive procedure to determine high-grade narrowing and occlusion of the internal carotid artery in clients with complaints of claudication, transient ischemic attacks, or asymptomatic bruits

13. Contrast arteriography—an invasive procedure used to assess the presence of arterial emboli or thrombosis, arterial trauma, and aneurysms
14. Digital vascular imaging—an invasive radiographic procedure used to visualize arterial vessels
15. Laboratory tests—a CBC to perform routine evaluation, coagulation studies to determine presence or absence of blood disorders, an ESR to determine presence or absence of inflammatory process

Raynaud's Disease

Description

1. Raynaud's disease is characterized by episodic vasospasm in small peripheral arteries and arterioles, resulting in interruption of blood flow to distal parts of affected extremities.
2. It occurs bilaterally, usually affects hands; feet are less often affected.
3. It is characterized by triphasic color change from white to blue to red of involved body parts.
4. It is most prevalent in females, especially between puberty and age 40.
5. Over time, disease may progress to occlusion of the arteries, resulting in digital gangrene; eventually amputation may be required.
6. Cause—unknown
7. Precipitating factors
   A. Cold, stress, smoking
   B. Associated with collagen diseases in women
8. Predisposing factors
   A. Pressure to fingertips—affects typists, pianists, users of hand-held vibrating equipment
9. Raynaud's phenomenon may occur with no underlying or concomitant disease and is associated with connective tissue disease, which is considered to be an early indicator of these conditions when it occurs in well individuals.

Assessment

SUBJECTIVE

1. Numbness, coldness of hands or feet
2. Pain in hands or feet

OBJECTIVE

1. Hands or feet feel cold to touch
2. Color changes—pallor, cyanosis, rubor
3. Numbness and tingling
4. Dryness and atrophy of nails
5. Ulcerations or gangrene, especially on fingertips

DIAGNOSTIC TESTS AND METHODS

1. Detailed history
2. Physical examination
3. Arteriography
4. ECG
5. Doppler ultrasonography
6. Chest x-ray

Planning

1. Safe, effective care environment
   A. Prevent injury to tissues and extremities.

B. Increase client's and family's knowledge of disease process, diagnostic procedures, and treatment.
2. Physiological integrity
   A. Increase comfort; decrease pain in extremities.
   B. Promote adequate tissue perfusion.
3. Psychosocial integrity
   A. Promote effective coping.
4. Health promotion and maintenance
   A. Increase client's and family's knowledge of prevention, home care (including medication), and follow-up.

Implementation

1. Assess, record, and report signs and symptoms and reactions to treatment.
2. Ask client about situations that stimulate pain and skin-color change.
3. Record location and characteristics of pain.
4. Monitor peripheral extremities for changes in skin color and temperature.
5. Monitor peripheral pulses—may be diminished or absent during acute episodes.
6. Check capillary refill time.
7. Administer prescribed vasodilators and analgesics; record response and side effects.
8. Observe affected areas every day for color, sensation, diminished pulse.
9. Keep extremities warm and protected.
10. Provide safe environment to prevent injury.
11. Provide emotional support.
12. Instruct client and family regarding disease process, diagnostic procedures, treatment, prevention, home care, and follow-up. Include teaching on:
    A. Avoiding exposure of hands and feet to cold—using gloves, warm socks
    B. Dressing in warm, nonconstrictive clothing
    C. Maintaining adequate caloric intake
    D. Rest following exercise
    E. Cessation of smoking
    F. Practicing stress-reduction techniques
    G. Avoiding use of hot water bottles and heating pads
    H. Protection from trauma

Evaluation

1. Reports relief of pain
2. Demonstrates techniques to control acute episodes; shows evidence of decreased episodes of arterial spasms
3. Maintains effective tissue perfusion and good skin hygiene
   A. Demonstrates capillary refill time of <3 seconds
   B. Shows evidence of full peripheral pulses
   C. Has warm skin with no color changes
4. Demonstrates understanding of disease process, diagnostic procedures, treatment, prevention, home care, and need for follow-up; similar understanding demonstrated by family

Buerger's Disease (Thromboangiitis Obliterans)

Description

1. Buerger's disease is an inflammatory occlusive condition involving the small and medium arteries (sometimes

veins), resulting in decrease in blood flow to feet and legs.

2. Pain is the result of ischemia, which occurs with inflammation of vessel layers.
3. Condition causes segmental lesions and eventual thrombus formation.
4. It may produce ulcerations and eventually gangrene.
5. Incidence is highest among males of Jewish ancestry aged 20–40.
6. Causes—unknown
7. Predisposing factor—associated with smoking (hypersensitivity to nicotine)

Assessment

SUBJECTIVE

1. History of cigarette smoking, exposure to cold, stress
2. Pain in fingers and feet at rest (aggravated by arm elevation and hyperextension)
3. Pain in neck, shoulder, and hand due to compression of brachial plexus
4. Instep claudication (pain) with exercise
5. Numbness or tingling
6. Cold extremities

OBJECTIVE

1. Diminished or absent pulses
2. Skin ulceration
3. Changes in appearance of extremities
4. Skin color—white (pallor at first) changes to cyanotic, then red
5. Redness and hardness along vessels—indication of recurring superficial phlebitis
6. Muscle atrophy
7. Slow-healing cuts
8. Presence of ischemic ulcers or blisters on toes
9. Gangrene

DIAGNOSTIC TESTS AND METHODS

1. History
2. Physical examination
3. Doppler ultrasonography
4. ECG
5. Arteriography
6. Chest x-ray
7. Cervical spine x-ray—to rule out cervical fracture or fractured clavicle
8. Nerve conduction tests—to determine level of nerve compression

Planning

1. Safe, effective care environment
   A. Prevent injury to skin.
   B. Increase client's and family's knowledge of disease process, diagnostic procedures, and treatment.
2. Physiological integrity
   A. Increase comfort; decrease pain in extremities.
   B. Promote adequate tissue perfusion.
3. Psychosocial integrity
   A. Promote effective coping.

4. Health promotion and maintenance
   A. Increase client's and family's knowledge of prevention, home care (including medication), and follow-up.

Implementation

1. Assess, record, and report signs and symptoms and reactions to treatment.
2. Document location and character of pain.
3. Monitor extremities for changes in color.
4. Provide safe environment to prevent injury.
5. Monitor bilateral pulses.
6. Keep extremities warm and protected in slightly dependent position—elevating legs interferes with arterial blood flow.
7. Administer prescribed medications—vasodilators, analgesics.
8. Prepare client and family for surgical intervention, if client requires sympathectomy.
9. Provide preoperative and postoperative care.
10. Instruct client and family regarding disease process, diagnostic procedures, treatment, prevention, home care, and follow-up. Include teaching on:
    A. Avoidance of exposure to cold
    B. Cessation of smoking—surgical wounds may stop healing
    C. Dressing in warm, nonconstrictive clothing
    D. Using tepid bath water
    E. Rest following exercise
    F. Maintaining effective caloric intake
    G. Medications

Evaluation

1. Reports relief of pain or tolerable pain
2. Maintains adequate tissue perfusion and skin integrity
3. Demonstrates understanding of disease process (including risk factors), diagnostic procedures, treatment (including surgery), prevention, home care (including medications), and need for follow-up; similar understanding demonstrated by family

Thrombophlebitis (Venous Thromboembolic Disease)

Description

1. Thrombophlebitis is characterized by inflammation and thrombus formation. It may occur in deep or superficial veins.
2. Phlebothrombosis is a clot in the vein without accompanying inflammation.
3. Superficial thrombophlebitis begins with localized inflammation alone (phlebitis); thrombus formation is frequently provoked by the inflammatory process. Platelets, RBC, and fibrin form a clot within the vein, which potentially can break loose and lead to emboli.
   A. Causes
      (1) Trauma or irritation of a vein from an IV catheter or administration of an irritating solution
      (2) IV administration of potassium chloride and antibiotics
      (3) IV drug abuse

4. Deep vein thrombophlebitis
   A. Presence of unilateral edema in affected limb.
   B. Edema may be mild or severe.
   C. Pain on dorsiflexion of foot (Homans' sign) when leg is affected. This sign is accurate less than 1/3 of the time.
   D. Condition may frequently lead to pulmonary embolism.
   E. Causes
      (1) Damage to vessel lining
      (2) Venous pooling and stasis
      (3) Increased clotting ability of blood
   F. Predisposing factors
      (1) Immobilization such as paralysis, being bedridden or chairfast, long plane or car rides
      (2) Disease processes such as sepsis, hematological disorders, malignancy, CHF, MI
      (3) Increased abdominal pressure due to obesity, pregnancy, or tumor
      (4) Trauma such as fractures, venipuncture
      (5) Clotting deficiencies such as antithrombin III deficiency, disorders of plasminogen activators, and abrupt heparin withdrawal
      (6) Surgical procedures such as hip pinning, craniotomy, transurethral resection, hysterectomy
   G. Other factors
      (1) Dehydration
      (2) Advancing age
      (3) Prior thrombosis or thromboembolic event
      (4) Use of oral contraceptives

Assessment

SUBJECTIVE

1. Pain in affected extremity
2. History of causes and contributing factors

OBJECTIVE

1. Warmth and redness of extremity—superficial thrombophlebitis
2. Elevation of temperature
3. Swelling
4. Pain elicited by palpation of calf muscle for deep vein thrombosis
5. Area sensitive to touch
6. Quality of pulse in affected extremity

DIAGNOSTIC TESTS AND METHODS

1. History
2. Physical examination
3. Homans' sign
4. Palpation of calf muscles
5. Doppler ultrasonography
6. Venography
7. Impedance plethysmography
8. Noninvasive venous ultrasound—to assess deep vein thrombosis
9. Laboratory tests—CBC, ESR, coagulation studies
10. Lung scan—to rule out pulmonary embolism

Planning

1. Safe, effective care environment
   A. Prevent avoidable injury.

   B. Increase client's and family's knowledge of disease process, diagnostic procedures, and treatment.
2. Physiological integrity
   A. Increase comfort.
   B. Maintain adequate tissue perfusion.
   C. Reduce swelling.
3. Psychosocial integrity
   A. Promote effective coping.
4. Health promotion and maintenance
   A. Increase client's and family's knowledge of prevention (to avoid recurrence), home care, and follow-up.

Implementation

1. Assess, record, and report signs and symptoms and reactions to treatment.
2. Provide bed rest.
3. Use moist heat as prescribed to reduce comfort.
4. Elevate affected limb to decrease swelling and to prevent blood stasis.
5. Administer analgesics as ordered; monitor for side effects.
6. Take thigh and calf measurements daily.
7. Monitor vital signs every 4 hours.
8. Avoid massaging affected leg.
9. Use compression stockings.
10. Administer anticoagulants, vasodilators, and thrombolytic medications as prescribed; monitor response.
11. Assist with ROM exercises to unaffected extremity.
12. Monitor for bleeding tendencies.
    A. Check gums.
    B. Check skin for bruises, petechiae.
    C. Watch for nosebleeds.
    D. Monitor hemoglobin and hematocrit levels.
13. Monitor for signs and symptoms of complications, such as embolism.
14. Inform client and family in regard to thrombectomy procedure.
15. Provide preoperative and postoperative care.
16. Watch for complications of postoperative rethrombosis of vessel.
17. Instruct client and family regarding disease process, diagnostic procedures, treatment, prevention, home care, and follow-up. Include teaching on:
    A. Avoidance of long periods of sitting or standing
    B. Routine exercise plan
    C. Avoidance of tight, constrictive clothing
    D. Use of elastic or support hose for extended periods of sitting or standing
    E. Early ambulation of postoperative client as a preventive measure

Evaluation

1. Reports increased comfort, decreased anxiety
2. Reports decrease or absence of swelling
3. Has no redness along affected superficial vein
4. Reports relief of pain
5. Maintains effective tissue perfusion
   A. Skin color returns to normal.
   B. Peripheral pulses are palpable.
6. Has no signs of pulmonary emboli
7. Reports that bleeding is easily controlled

8. Demonstrates understanding of disease process, diagnostic procedures, treatment, prevention, home care, and need for follow-up; similar understanding demonstrated by family

Varicose Veins

Description

1. Varicose veins are dilated, tortuous leg veins due to backflow of blood caused by incompetent venous valve closure. Results in venous congestion and further enlargement of veins.
2. Condition usually affects subcutaneous leg veins (saphenous veins and branches).
3. Classification
   A. Primary varicosities
      (1) Venous valve insufficiency.
      (2) Incompetence of superficial veins resulting in reflux of blood from deep to superficial veins.
      (3) Increased hydrostatic pressure from long column of blood extending from inferior vena cava to the saphenous vein.
      (4) Veins become dilated and tortuous with characteristic bulging appearance of varicose veins.
      (5) Varicosities usually found in greater saphenous vein along thigh, but may extend laterally.
   B. Secondary varicosities
      (1) Deep venous disease
      (2) May produce postphlebitic syndrome—chronic problem that cannot be cured by the removal of the superficial veins
4. Causes—unknown
5. Predisposing factors
   A. Congenital weakness of venous valves or venous wall
   B. Diseases of venous system such as thrombophlebitis
   C. Conditions that produce venostasis—pregnancy, prolonged standing, obesity
   D. Familial tendency

Assessment

SUBJECTIVE

1. Aching
2. Cramping and pain
3. Heavy feeling in legs

OBJECTIVE

1. Palpable nodules—primary varicose veins
2. Foot and ankle edema exacerbated by prolonged standing or immobility
3. Edema relieved by bed rest and elevation of legs
4. Dilated veins—primary varicose veins
5. Status pigmentation of calves and ankles

DIAGNOSTIC TESTS/METHODS

1. Client and family history
2. Physical examination
3. Venography
4. Trendelenburg test

Planning

1. Safe, effective care environment
   A. Prevent avoidable injury.

   B. Increase client's knowledge of disease process, diagnostic procedures, and treatment.
2. Physiological integrity
   A. Increase comfort.
   B. Maintain adequate tissue perfusion.
   C. Reduce swelling.
3. Psychosocial integrity
   A. Promote effective coping.
4. Health promotion and maintenance
   A. Increase client's knowledge of prevention (to avoid recurrence), home care, and follow-up.

Implementation

1. Assess, record, and report signs and symptoms and reactions to treatment.
2. Provide rest with legs elevated.
3. Apply support stockings.
4. Discourage prolonged standing, sitting, and crossing legs.
5. Encourage weight management.
6. Encourage walking and swimming.
7. Instruct client to avoid constrictive clothing and hosiery.
8. Prepare client with primary varicosities for surgical intervention—surgical vein stripping, ligation, vein sclerosing.
9. Provide postoperative care:
   A. Administer analgesics as prescribed to alleviate pain.
   B. Elevate affected leg.
   C. Check circulation in toes frequently (color and temperature).
   D. Observe elastic bandages for bleeding.
   E. Rewrap bandage, if ordered, once per shift (wrap from toe to thigh with leg elevated).
   F. Watch for signs of complications.
      (1) Sensory loss in leg (indicative of saphenous nerve damage)
      (2) Calf pain (indicative of thrombophlebitis)
      (3) Fever (indicative of infection)
10. Instruct client regarding disease process, diagnostic procedures, treatment, prevention, home care, and follow-up.

Evaluation

1. Reports relief of pain
2. Reports increased comfort, decreased anxiety
3. Demonstrates measures to increase venous return
4. Verbalizes positive attitude toward physical appearance
5. Maintains adequate tissue perfusion
6. Shows no signs of complications
7. Demonstrates understanding of disease process, diagnostic procedures, treatment, prevention, home care, and need for follow-up

Aneurysms

Description

1. An aneurysm is the enlargement or ballooning of an artery. The aneurysm may be dissecting, saccular, or fusiform.
2. Damage to the tunica media leads to enlargement of the area.
3. Some aneurysms progress to serious and eventually fatal complications, such as rupture.

4. Types
   A. Dissecting aneurysm—a hemorrhagic separation of the inner layer of the arterial wall
   B. Saccular aneurysm—an outpouching of one side of the arterial wall with a narrow neck
   C. Fusiform aneurysm—a spindle-shaped enlargement including the entire circumference of the artery
5. Causes
   A. Connective tissue disease
   B. Infections
   C. Familial tendency
   D. Trauma
   E. Syphilis
   F. Hypertension.
   G. Arteritis
   H. Atherosclerosis

Assessment

Thoracic aneurysms involve the transverse or descending portion of the aorta. They are most common in males between 50 and 70 years of age. Dissecting aneurysms are most common in African Americans. Abdominal aortic aneurysms may be nonthreatening, but they usually expand and rupture.

SUBJECTIVE—DISSECTING ANEURYSM

1. Possibly asymptomatic
2. Dyspnea
3. Severe chest pain
4. Dysphagia (difficulty in swallowing)
5. Dizziness

OBJECTIVE—DISSECTING ANEURYSM

1. Diaphoresis.
2. Increased pulse rate.
3. Cyanosis.
4. Neck vein distention.
5. Leg weakness or transient paralysis.
6. Diastolic murmur—due to aortic regurgitation.
7. Abrupt loss of femoral and radial pulses or wide variations in pulses of arms and legs.
8. Shock appearance, but systolic blood pressure often normal or significantly increased.
9. Symptoms vary according to size and location of defect, and the effects of compression or erosion of surrounding structures. Abdominal aortic aneurysm generally occurs between the renal arteries and iliac branches, the most common site for aneurysm development. It is approximately four times more common in white men between the ages of 50 and 80.

SUBJECTIVE—ABDOMINAL AORTIC ANEURYSM

1. Tenderness or pain in abdomen or back
2. Chest pain in dissecting aneurysms

OBJECTIVE—ABDOMINAL AORTIC ANEURYSM

1. Pulsating mass in periumbilical area of abdomen
2. Systolic bruit over aorta
3. Elevated blood pressure
4. Pulse changes in lower extremities
5. Large aneurysm may mimic renal calculi, lumbar disk disease, and duodenal compression

DIAGNOSTIC TESTS AND METHODS

1. History
2. Physical examination
3. Angiography to determine location of aneurysm
4. X-rays to visualize thoracic aortic aneurysm
5. Abdominal ultrasonography
6. Aortography
7. CT with contrast or MRI
8. Routine ECG
9. Laboratory studies—hemoglobin, hematocrit

Planning

1. Safe, effective care environment
   A. Prevent avoidable injury.
   B. Increase client's knowledge of disease process, diagnostic procedures, and treatment.
2. Physiological integrity
   A. Maintain adequate hemodynamic perfusion.
   B. Maintain fluid balance.
3. Psychosocial integrity
   A. Reduce anxiety.
4. Health promotion and maintenance
   A. Increase client's knowledge of home care, postoperative care, and follow-up.

Implementation

1. Assess, record, and report signs and symptoms and reactions to treatment.
2. Monitor vital signs and peripheral pulses every 15 minutes until stable.
3. Monitor for signs of decreased tissue perfusion—low blood pressure; bleeding; rapid, weak pulse.
4. Assess pain; respirations; and carotid, radial, and femoral pulse.
5. Administer prescribed medications to decrease pain.
6. Administer prescribed prophylactic antibiotics.
7. Listen to lung and bowel sounds at least every 4 hours.
8. Monitor for arrhythmias.
9. Apply antiembolism stockings; do not massage lower extremities. Monitor for signs of arterial thrombosis or embolism: absent peripheral pulses, pale or cyanotic extremities, cool extremities, diffuse abdominal pain, or increased pain in the groin, lumbar areas, or lower extremities
10. Compare extremities for warmth and color.
11. Administer IV fluids as ordered.
12. Monitor O_2 therapy.
13. Monitor CVP, PAP, pulmonary capillary wedge pressure (PCWP) for elevated pressures.
14. Check for blood type and cross-matching; have blood available.
15. Monitor intake and output for fluid balance.
16. Provide emotional support to client and family.
17. Encourage deep breathing and coughing exercises.
18. Maintain bed rest preoperatively.
19. Encourage prescribed leg exercises to prevent venous stasis.
20. Instruct client regarding disease process, diagnostic procedures, treatment, home care, postoperative care (including activity and care of incision), and follow-up.

Evaluation

1. Reports increased comfort, decreased anxiety
2. Maintains stable vital signs
3. Maintains stable fluid balance
4. Reports relief of pain
5. Has no avoidable complications
6. Goes to emergency room immediately if signs of bleeding occur
7. Demonstrates understanding of disease process, diagnostic procedures, treatment (including surgery), postoperative care, home care, and need for follow-up

Hematological System

Basic Information

Blood is a major body fluid tissue that continuously circulates through the heart and blood vessels, carrying vital elements to all parts of the body. RBCs (erythrocytes) carry O_2 to the tissues and remove carbon dioxide from them. WBCs (leukocytes) assist in inflammatory and immune responses. Plasma carries antibodies and nutrients to tissues and wastes from tissues. Coagulation factors found in plasma along with platelets (thrombocytes) control blood clotting. The average individual has 5–6 liters of circulating blood, which makes up 5%–7% of body weight. The pH of blood ranges between 7.35 and 7.45 and the color is either dark red (venous blood) or bright red (arterial blood) depending on the level of hemoglobin and the degree of O_2 saturation.

Assessment

SUBJECTIVE

1. Weakness, fatigue, and palpitations
2. Nausea, dyspnea
3. Pain, numbness, prickling or tingling sensations; bone and joint pain a predominant symptom
4. Irritability, bleeding from nose and mouth, bruising
5. Ashen, pale, cyanotic, or jaundiced sclera (reflect nutritional and circulatory dysfunction); headache
6. Reports of skin breakdown and delayed healing
7. Numbness, burning of feet
8. Complaints of persistent or sporadic fever

OBJECTIVE

1. Tachycardia
2. Pallor and jaundice, the latter possibly indicating destruction of red blood cells or specific liver, gallbladder, or splenic alterations
3. Pruritus
4. Petechiae, ecchymosis, and purpura
5. Skin lesions
6. Excess joint edema
7. Mouth ulcerations; red, beefy, or smooth tongue
8. Hypotension
9. Painful lymph nodes
10. Macular rash
11. Blood in stools
12. Hemoptysis
13. Hematuria

DIAGNOSTIC TESTS AND METHODS

1. Detailed history
2. Past history of:
   A. Malignancy
   B. Excessive bleeding from injury or surgical procedures
   C. Blood or blood product transfusions and reasons for use
   D. Record of client's blood ABO group and Rh type
   E. Record of medications and treatments
   F. Record of chest x-rays
3. Physical examination
4. RBC count
5. Hemoglobin and hematocrit levels
6. Reticulocyte count
   A. Provides information regarding the cause of the anemia
   B. Distinguishes between decreased production or excessive loss or destruction of RBCs
7. Erythrocyte indices
   A. Aids in describing anemias
   B. Provides information regarding relationship between size, number, and hemoglobin content of RBCs
8. Serum iron and total iron-binding capacity
   A. Aids in classification of anemia
   B. Aids in differentiating between acute and chronic anemias
9. Platelet count
   A. Check of platelet level (low platelet level—potential for spontaneous hemorrhage)
10. Serum bilirubin
    A. Aids in evaluating degree of hemolysis of red blood cells.
    B. Increased levels may indicate destruction of RBCs.
11. Vitamin B_{12} level
    A. Determines adequacy of B_{12} levels
12. Serum folate level
    A. Aids in classification of anemia
13. Sickle cell preparation
    A. Analysis of reaction to hypoxia.
    B. Sickling of cells suggests sickle cell anemia or sickle cell trait.
14. Hemoglobin electrophoresis
    A. Separation into various hemoglobin types through the utilization of an electric field.
    B. Presence of hemoglobin A or S indicates presence of sickle cell anemia or sickle cell trait.
    C. Presence of hemoglobin F indicates presence of thalassemia.
15. WBC count and differential
    A. Determines total number of leukocytes
    B. Evaluates each type and proportion of WBCs
    C. Aids in diagnosis of infection and blood disorders such as leukemia
16. Gastric analysis
    A. Absence of hydrochloric acid in gastric contents indicates pernicious anemia.
17. Schilling test
    A. Used in classifying anemias, especially vitamin B_{12} disorders
    B. Aids in differentiating between intrinsic factor deficiency and an intestinal malabsorption disorder
18. Bone marrow biopsy
    A. Provides information about blood cell production

B. Used in suspected cases of leukemia, aplastic anemia, and other blood disorders
19. Human immunodeficiency virus (HIV) serum study
    A. Provides information in regard to presence or absence of the AIDS virus

Implementation

1. Weakness, fatigue
   A. Monitor for signs and symptoms.
   B. Provide rest periods.
   C. Assist with ADL.
2. Dyspnea
   A. Check activities that cause dyspnea.
   B. Assist in planning activities to decrease occurrence of dyspnea.
   C. Monitor rate, character of respirations during dyspneic episodes.
3. Mouth and tongue ulcerations
   A. Check oral cavity daily.
   B. Provide oral hygiene as prescribed, including mouthwash every 2 hours.
   C. Instruct client to avoid food or liquids that irritate ulcers.
4. Hemorrhage
   A. Signs of bleeding
   B. Bleeding gums
   C. Bruising
   D. Epistaxis
   E. Hematuria
   F. Tarry, black stools
5. Monitor vital signs every 4 hours.
6. Monitor lab studies—hemoglobin, hematocrit.
7. Avoid parenteral injections.
8. Protect against injury.
9. Encourage fluid intake and prescribed diet.
10. Infection
    A. Check for signs and symptoms of infection.
    B. Administer medications as prescribed; check for side effects.
    C. Place in protective isolation, if required.

Anemias Due to Decreased RBC Production

Description

1. Anemias involving a deficiency of RBCs are caused by conditions affecting production of red blood cells.
2. Types
   A. Pernicious anemia
      (1) Condition is due to lack of intrinsic factor in GI system, which is required for the absorption of vitamin B_{12}
      (2) Deficiency of mucosal surface of GI tract, which secretes intrinsic factor.
      (3) Clients at risk include those who have had gastrectomies and small bowel resections.
   B. Folic acid deficiency
      (1) Folic acid is necessary for the synthesis of DNA; DNA is required for the production of RBCs.
      (2) Causes include poor nutrition (lack of citrus fruits, liver, grains, leafy green vegetables); drugs; malabsorption disorders, which interfere with absorption of folic acid.

C. Iron-deficiency anemia
   (1) Is due to insufficient intake of dietary iron—necessary for production of hemoglobin and RBCs
   (2) May be due to malabsorption, hemolysis of RBCs, and blood loss

Assessment

SUBJECTIVE

1. Pallor
2. Fatigue
3. Dyspnea
4. Anginal pain
5. Blurred vision
6. Vertigo
7. Irritability
8. Depression
9. Nausea
10. Anorexia
11. Weight loss
12. Bone pain
13. Numbness, tingling of feet

OBJECTIVE

1. CHF
2. Positive bone marrow findings
3. Lack of coordination
4. Confusion
5. Vomiting
6. Splenomegaly
7. Hepatomegaly
8. Signs of bleeding, bruising

DIAGNOSTIC TESTS AND METHODS

1. History
2. Physical examination
3. Routine chest x-ray, ECG
4. CBC
5. Schilling test
6. Bone marrow aspiration

Planning

1. Safe, effective care environment
   A. Prevent avoidable injury.
   B. Promote rest.
   C. Increase client's and family's knowledge of disease process, diagnostic procedures, and treatment.
2. Physiological integrity
   A. Increase comfort.
   B. Maintain adequate cardiac output.
   C. Promote hygiene care.
   D. Maintain effective gas exchange.
   E. Maintain tissue perfusion.
   F. Maintain adequate nutritional intake.
3. Psychosocial integrity
   A. Reduce anxiety.
   B. Promote effective coping.
   C. Discuss alterations in self-concept or self-esteem.
4. Health promotion and maintenance
   A. Increase client's and family's knowledge of prevention, home care, and follow-up.
   B. Counsel on stress reduction.

Implementation

1. Assess, report, and record signs and symptoms and reactions to treatment.
2. Monitor vital signs, intake and output, skin color.
3. Provide planned activity and rest periods.
4. Administer prescribed supplemental O_2.
5. Administer prescribed medications such as iron supplements, Vitamin B_{12}, oral folic acid.
6. Assist with comfort and hygienic needs.
7. Monitor blood transfusions; check for reactions.
8. Provide oral hygiene.
9. Provide prescribed diet and fluid intake.
10. Provide emotional support to allay anxiety.
11. Instruct client and family regarding disease process, diagnostic procedures, treatment, home care, and follow-up.

Evaluation

1. Reports increased comfort, decreased anxiety
2. Maintains adequate cardiac output and tissue perfusion
3. Maintains normal laboratory values
4. Demonstrates understanding of disease process, diagnostic procedures, treatment, prevention, home care, and need for follow-up; similar understanding demonstrated by family

Anemia Due to RBC Destruction

Description

1. Some types of anemia are due to destruction of RBCs at a faster pace than their production
2. Causes
   A. Infections
   B. Drugs, chemicals
   C. Antigen-antibody reactions
   D. Disorders of the spleen
   E. Organic compounds
   F. Congenital disorders
3. Types
   A. Thalassemia
      (1) Genetic disorder causing abnormal hemoglobin synthesis. Individuals at risk are of Mediterranean ancestry, especially Italian and Greek, but blacks and persons from southern China, Southeast Asia, and India are also at risk.
      (2) Thalassemia minor, a mild form of the disease, may be asymptomatic.
      (3) Thalassemia major, a severe form of the disease, may have hepatomegaly, jaundice, splenomegaly, and hypertrophy of the bone marrow. Individuals with this type seldom survive to adulthood.
   B. Glucose-6-phosphate dehydrogenase deficiency
      (1) Genetic disorder in which hemolytic anemia occurs owing to stressors such as infection, specific types of drugs, acidosis, and toxic substances

Assessment

SUBJECTIVE

1. Weakness, fatigue
2. Pallor
3. Weight loss
4. Painful episodes, history of stress—sickle cell anemia

OBJECTIVE

1. Positive Coombs' test—acquired anemia due to drugs or autoimmune disorder
2. Elevated serum bilirubin level
3. Elevated reticulocyte count
4. Enlarged spleen
5. Low-grade fever
6. Renal insufficiency
7. Jaundice
8. Low mean corpuscular volume, mean corpuscular hemoglobin concentration, positive hemoglobin electrophoresis in thalassemia

DIAGNOSTIC TESTS AND METHODS

1. History
2. Physical examination
3. Laboratory studies—serum bilirubin, CBC, Coombs' test
4. Renal studies—to check renal function
5. Routine chest x-ray
6. Routine ECG
7. Bone marrow biopsy

Planning

1. Safe, effective care environment
   A. Prevent avoidable injury and/or infection.
   B. Promote rest.
   C. Increase client's and family's knowledge of disease process, diagnostic procedures, and treatment.
2. Physiological integrity
   A. Increase comfort.
   B. Maintain adequate cardiac output.
   C. Promote hygiene care.
   D. Maintain effective gas exchange.
   E. Maintain tissue perfusion.
   F. Maintain adequate nutritional intake.
3. Psychosocial integrity
   A. Reduce anxiety.
   B. Promote effective coping.
   C. Discuss alterations in self-concept or self-esteem.
4. Health promotion and maintenance
   A. Increase client's and family's knowledge of prevention, home care, and follow-up.
   B. Counsel on stress reduction.

Implementation

1. Assess, report, and record signs and symptoms and reactions to treatment.
2. Provide rest periods to avoid fatigue.
3. Protect client from exposure to infection sources.
4. Monitor for bleeding, bruising.
5. Assist in administration of blood transfusions; check reaction to transfusion.
6. Administer prescribed medications; check for side effects.
7. Administer prescribed O_2.
8. Monitor fluid intake and output.
9. Monitor laboratory studies.
10. Provide for genetic counseling.
11. Instruct client and family regarding disease process, diagnostic procedures, treatment, prevention, home care, and follow-up.

Evaluation

1. Reports increased comfort, decreased anxiety
2. Maintains adequate gas exchange
3. Maintains adequate cardiac output and tissue perfusion
4. Verbalizes feelings about condition
5. Demonstrates understanding of disease process, diagnostic procedures, treatment, prevention, home care (including medication), and need for follow-up; similar understanding demonstrated by family

Leukemia

Description

Leukemia is a disorder of the hematological system characterized by an overproduction of immature WBCs. Fewer normal WBCs are produced as the disease progresses. Abnormal WBCs increase, infiltrate, and damage bone marrow, lymph nodes, spleen, and other organs. RBC production is disrupted, leading to anemia, immature cells, thrombocytopenia, and decline in immunity. Cause is unknown, considered to be a neoplastic process.

1. Predisposing factors
   A. Viral origin
   B. Exposure to radiation
   C. Exposure to chemicals
   D. Familial tendency
2. Classification as acute or chronic and according to cell type
   A. Acute lymphocytic leukemia (ALL)
      (1) Lymphoblasts mostly present in bone marrow.
      (2) Incidence peaks at 2–4 years of age.
      (3) Treatment induces remissions in 90% of children.
      (4) Average survival time is 5 years.
      (5) Treatment induces remissions in 40%–65% of adults.
   B. Acute myelogenous leukemia (AML)
      (1) Myeloblasts mostly present in bone marrow.
      (2) Incidence peaks at 12–20 years and after 55 years of age.
      (3) Average survival rate is 1 year after diagnosis, even with aggressive therapy.
   C. Chronic myelogenous leukemia (CML)
      (1) Granulocytes mostly present in bone marrow.
      (2) Incidence peaks at 30–50 years of age.
   D. Chronic lymphocytic leukemia (CLL)
      (1) Lymphocytes mostly present in bone marrow.
      (2) Incidence peaks at 50–70 years of age.

Assessment

SUBJECTIVE—ALL AND AML

1. Sudden onset of high fever
2. Abnormal bleeding such as nosebleeds, easy bruising, prolonged menses
3. Fatigue
4. Chills
5. Recurrent infections
6. Dyspnea
7. Abdominal or bone pain
8. Confusion, lethargy, headache when leukemic cells cross blood-brain barrier

SUBJECTIVE—CLL AND CML

1. Fatigue
2. Weakness
3. Anorexia
4. Weight loss
5. Lymph node enlargement
6. Recurrent infections
7. Bone tenderness

OBJECTIVE—ALL AND AML

1. Anemia
2. Elevated temperature
3. Abnormal bleeding
4. Lymphadenopathy
5. Ecchymoses
6. Tachycardia
7. Palpitations
8. Systolic ejection murmur
9. Positive bone marrow biopsy
10. Normal, elevated, or decreased WBC count

OBJECTIVE—CLL AND CML

1. Skin lesions
2. Elevated WBC count
3. Anorexia
4. Enlarged spleen and liver
5. Positive bone marrow biopsy
6. Recurrent opportunistic fungal, viral, and bacterial infections

DIAGNOSTIC TESTS AND METHODS

1. History
2. Physical examination
3. Laboratory studies—CBC, hemoglobin, hematocrit, platelet count, differential WBC count for determination of cell type
4. Bone marrow biopsy
5. Routine chest x-ray
6. Routine ECG
7. Lumbar puncture for detection of meningeal involvement

Planning

1. Safe, effective care environment
   A. Prevent avoidable injury and/or infections.
   B. Increase client's and family's knowledge of disease process, diagnostic procedures, and treatment (including medication).
2. Physiological integrity
   A. Maintain adequate hemodynamic status, tissue perfusion, and gas exchange.
   B. Support immunological defense.
   C. Increase comfort.
3. Psychosocial integrity
   A. Promote effective coping and provide support.
4. Health promotion and maintenance
   A. Increase client's and family's knowledge of home care (including medication) and follow-up.

Implementation

1. Assess, report, and record signs and symptoms and reactions to treatment.

2. Provide comfort.
3. Monitor laboratory data.
4. Check for signs of bleeding or infection.
5. Monitor vital signs.
6. Assist in administration of prescribed medications such as chemotherapeutic drugs, antiemetics, antihistamines, anxiolytics analgesics, IV fluids, and blood or blood-product transfusions.
7. Monitor for side effects of medications, transfusions
8. Minimize side effects of chemotherapy.
9. Monitor fluid intake and output.
10. Prevent exposure to infection.
11. Assist client with activities; provide rest periods.
12. Provide emotional support.
13. Allay anxiety, fears.
14. Monitor supplemental O_2, if ordered.
15. Provide, encourage adherence to prescribed diet.
16. Provide oral hygiene.
17. Provide skin care; use protective devices.
18. Allow client to verbalize feelings about condition.
19. Instruct client and family regarding disease process, diagnostic procedures, treatment, home care, and follow-up. Include teaching on:
   A. Drug therapy
   B. Diet
   C. Activity
   D. Avoidance of injury and infection
   E. Checking for abnormal bleeding
   F. Available community resources and support groups

Evaluation

1. Reports increased comfort, decreased anxiety
2. Maintains adequate tissue perfusion and gas exchange
3. Shows no signs of avoidable injury and/or infection
4. Demonstrates understanding of disease process, diagnostic procedures, treatment (including medications and their side effects), home care, and need for follow-up; similar understanding demonstrated by family

Multiple Myeloma

Description

1. Multiple myeloma is a disseminated neoplasm of immature plasma cells that infiltrates bone to produce tumors throughout the skeleton—vertebrae, skull, pelvis, flat bones, ribs.
2. During the late stages, it infiltrates body organs—lungs, liver, spleen, adrenals, lymph nodes, GI tract, kidneys, skin.
3. Death usually occurs following complications such as infection, fractures, hypercalcemia, hyperuricemia, or renal failure.
4. Cause—unknown.

Assessment

SUBJECTIVE

1. Bone pain
2. Fatigue
3. Achiness
4. Joint swelling

5. Tenderness
6. Fever
7. Weight loss
8. Decreased body height

OBJECTIVE

1. Anemia
2. Renal complications—renal insufficiency due to tubular damage
3. Elevated serum calcium and uric acid levels
4. Severe recurrent infections such as pneumonia due to damaged nerves associated with respiratory function
5. Pathological fractures, symptoms of vertebral compression
6. Decreased platelet count
7. Elevated ESR
8. Possible hypercalciuria
9. Presence of Bence Jones protein in urine
10. Positive bone marrow aspiration for myeloma cells
11. Elevated globulin

DIAGNOSTIC TESTS AND METHODS

1. History
2. Physical examination
3. CBC—to determine presence of anemia
4. ESR
5. Urine studies
6. Bone marrow biopsy
7. Serum electrophoresis for abnormal globulin
8. X-rays of skeleton
9. Intravenous pyelography (IVP)

Planning

1. Safe, effective care environment
   A. Prevent avoidable injury and/or infections.
   B. Provide skeletal support during activity.
   C. Increase client's and family's knowledge of disease process, diagnostic procedures, and treatment.
2. Physiological integrity
   A. Maintain balanced intake and output.
   B. Increase comfort.
3. Psychosocial integrity
   A. Promote support network.
   B. Reduce anxiety.
4. Health promotion and maintenance
   A. Increase client's and family's knowledge of prevention (of infection), home care, and follow-up.

Implementation

1. Assess, report, and record signs and symptoms and reactions to treatment.
2. Monitor vital signs, intake and output, and laboratory studies.
3. Check for bleeding, infection, or presence of fractures.
4. Encourage fluid intake.
5. Monitor intake and output—immediately report daily output of <1500 mL.
6. Encourage client to ambulate—decreases potential for bone demineralization and pneumonia.
7. Assist client in walking with use of walker or other supportive devices to prevent falls.

8. Protect client from others with infections.
9. Administer prescribed medications such as antineoplastic drugs, corticosteroids, antibiotics, and analgesics.
10. Assist with good hygienic measures to prevent infection.
11. Provide emotional support to client and family.
12. Prevent complications—watch for presence of fever or malaise.
13. Turn client every 2 hours if on complete bed rest.
14. Give passive ROM and deep breathing exercises.
15. Assure that blood is drawn for platelet and WBC counts prior to administration of chemotherapy.
16. Prepare client and family for laminectomy if required by client owing to spinal cord compression.
17. Prepare client and family for dialysis if required by client owing to renal complications.
18. Provide comfort measures.
19. Instruct client and family regarding disease process, diagnostic procedures, treatment, prevention, home care, and follow-up. Include teaching on:
    A. Drug therapy
    B. Available community resources and support groups

Evaluation

1. Shows no signs of avoidable injury and/or infection
2. Reports increased comfort, decreased anxiety
3. Maintains adequate intake and output
4. Has access to community resources for support
5. Maintains adequate urine output
6. Demonstrates understanding of disease process, diagnostic procedures, treatment (including medication), prevention, home care, and need for follow-up; similar understanding demonstrated by family

Hodgkin's Disease

Description

1. Hodgkin's disease is a neoplastic disease with painless, progressive enlargement of lymph nodes, spleen, and other lymphoid tissue.
2. Results from proliferation of Reed-Sternberg giant cells, lymphocytes, eosinophils, and histiocytes.
3. Condition is potentially curable owing to recent advances in therapeutic measures.
4. Prognosis depends on stage of the disease.
5. Four stages are defined by the Ann Arbor clinical staging classification of Hodgkin's. Treatment yields a 15-year survival rate of approximately 54% of clients. Disease occurs most often in young adults, with a higher incidence in males than in females. It occurs in all races; slightly more common in whites. Incidence peaks in two age groups (15–38 and after 50).

Assessment

SUBJECTIVE

1. Fatigue
2. Loss of appetite
3. Weakness
4. History of recent upper respiratory infection
5. Persistent fever
6. Night sweats
7. Weight loss
8. Malaise
9. Pruritus

OBJECTIVE

1. Enlarged lymph nodes, spleen, and liver
2. Positive biopsy of lymph nodes (cervical nodes most often affected)
3. Anemia
4. Positive CT scan of liver and spleen
5. Elevated temperature
6. Thrombocytopenia
7. Elevated serum alkaline phosphatase (indicating liver or bone involvement)
8. Evaluation of stage by results of lymphangiography and laparotomy
9. Positive bone marrow biopsy (if affected)

DIAGNOSTIC TESTS AND METHODS

1. History
2. Physical examination
3. Lymph node biopsy—to check for presence of the Reed-Sternberg cell, nodular fibrosis, and necrosis
4. Bone marrow, liver, and spleen biopsies
5. CT scan of lung, bone, liver, spleen
6. Lymphangiography—to detect involved lymph nodes or organ involvement
7. Hematological tests (CBC, blood chemistries)—to check serum alkaline phosphatase levels
8. Staging laparotomy for patients under age 55 or with no obvious stage III or IV disease, or medical contraindications.
9. Measures to rule out other disorders characterized by enlarged lymph nodes.

Planning

1. Safe, effective care environment
    A. Increase client's and family's knowledge of disease process, diagnostic procedures, and treatment (such as surgery, radiation, or chemotherapy).
    B. Prevent avoidable injury and/or infection.
2. Physiological integrity
    A. Increase comfort.
    B. Maintain skin integrity (compromised by invasive procedures, pruritus, radiation).
3. Psychosocial integrity
    A. Promote effective coping.
    B. Reduce anxiety.
4. Health promotion and maintenance
    A. Increase client's and family's knowledge of prevention (of infection), home care, and follow-up.

Implementation

1. Assess, report, and record signs and symptoms and reactions to treatment.
2. Assist with comfort measures for night sweats, itching, and fever.
3. Prepare and explain to client and family treatments such as radiation, chemotherapy, and surgical procedures, if needed.
4. Protect patient from contact with others who have infections.

5. Provide safe environment.
6. Provide emotional support to client and family.
7. Monitor for signs of infection and changes in skin integrity.
8. Monitor for radiation and chemotherapeutic side effects—anorexia, nausea, vomiting, diarrhea, hair loss.
9. Administer good oral hygiene using a soft toothbrush, cotton swab, or anesthetic mouthwash (if prescribed) to control pain and bleeding from stomatitis.
10. Instruct client and family regarding disease process, diagnostic procedures, treatment (including medications), prevention, home care, and follow-up.

Evaluation

1. Shows no signs of avoidable injury and/or infection
2. Reports increased comfort, decreased anxiety
3. Maintains good hygienic measures, skin integrity
4. Uses effective coping strategies
5. Demonstrates understanding of disease process, diagnostic procedures, treatment, prevention, home care, and need for follow-up; similar understanding demonstrated by family

Thrombocytopenia

Description

1. Thrombocytopenia is the most common cause of hemorrhagic disorders. It is characterized by a decreased number of circulating platelets and an abnormally low platelet count (normal range is 150,000–400,000/mm^3).
2. Prognosis is good if thrombocytopenia is drug induced, by withdrawing drug. Prognosis for thrombocytopenia in other cases depends on response to treatment of underlying cause.
3. Causes
   A. Congenital or acquired
4. Condition usually results from:
   A. Decreased production of platelets in marrow—leukemia, aplastic anemia, or toxicity of certain drugs.
   B. Increased destruction of platelets outside the marrow—cirrhosis of liver, DIC, severe infections.
   C. Reduction in platelet survival time.
   D. Collection of blood (sequestration) in spleen.
   E. Acquired thrombocytopenia may be due to certain drugs such as quinine, quinidine, chlorothiazide, Gantrisin (sulfisoxazole), phenylbutazone, rifampin, heparin, and cyclophosphamide.

Assessment

SUBJECTIVE

1. History of current medication intake
2. Bleeding from oral cavity, nose
3. Easy bruising
4. Malaise
5. Fatigue
6. General weakness

OBJECTIVE

1. Petechiae
2. Ecchymoses
3. Epistaxis or gingival bleeding
4. Low platelet count
5. Presence of megakaryocytes (platelet precursors) in bone marrow aspirations
6. Hematuria
7. Tachycardia, dyspnea, loss of consciousness, and death due to hemorrhage

DIAGNOSTIC TESTS AND METHODS

1. History
2. Physical examination
3. Laboratory tests—coagulation tests, platelet count, hemoglobin, hematocrit
4. Bone marrow biopsy

Planning

1. Safe, effective care environment
   A. Prevent avoidable injury.
   B. Increase client's knowledge of disease process, diagnostic procedures, and treatment (including medication).
2. Physiological integrity
   A. Maintain skin integrity.
   B. Maintain adequate tissue perfusion.
3. Psychosocial integrity
   A. Reduce anxiety.
4. Health promotion and maintenance
   A. Increase client's knowledge of prevention, home care, and follow-up.

Implementation

1. Assess, report, and record signs and symptoms and reactions to treatment.
2. Monitor for signs of bleeding.
3. Protect from injury or trauma.
4. Avoid invasive procedures such as venipuncture, intramuscular injections, urinary catheterization, rectal temperature, if possible.
5. Exert pressure on puncture site for at least 20 minutes or until bleeding stops if venipuncture used.
6. Assist in administration of prescribed platelet transfusions.
7. Monitor platelet count, blood count, and bleeding times.
8. Test stool for presence of blood; perform dipstick urine and emesis testing for blood.
9. Instruct client to avoid aspirin and other drugs that prolong clotting time.
10. Instruct client to avoid straining to pass stool or coughing—increases intercranial pressure with potential for causing cerebral hemorrhage. Provide stool softener, if necessary.
11. Enforce bed rest if bleeding occurs.
12. Instruct client regarding disease process, diagnostic procedures, treatment, prevention, home care, and follow-up.

Evaluation

1. Reports increased comfort
2. Reports decreased anxiety
3. Shows no avoidable injury

4. Maintains skin integrity
5. Has no bleeding
6. Demonstrates understanding of disease process, diagnostic procedures, treatment, prevention, home care, and need for follow-up

Immune System

Acquired Immunodeficiency Syndrome

Description

1. Acquired immunodeficiency syndrome (AIDS) is a viral disorder caused by the human immunodeficiency virus (HIV-1). The virus infects helper T4/CD4 lymphocytes, B lymphocytes, macrophages, promyelocytes and fibroblasts. It causes an immune deficiency that results in inability of the body to defend itself against infection.
2. Disease is progressive and usually fatal; death occurs due to opportunistic complications. The incubation period varies from 1 to 10 or more years.
3. Transmission
   A. Intimate sexual contact (vaginal or anal)
   B. Parenterally
      (1) Sharing of infected needles
      (2) Contaminated blood or blood product transfusions
      (3) Occupational exposure
   C. Perinatally
      (1) Across the placenta, by the infected woman to the fetus through exposure in utero
      (2) During the birth process
      (3) Via breast-feeding.
4. HIV disease consists of 4 stages, which the client may not progress through systematically:
   A. Primary or acute HIV infection—resembles a flu-like syndrome with fever, chills, sore throat, myalgia, arthralgia, malaise, and rash.
   B. Asymptomatic infection—infected clients generally appear well, however, their T4/CD4 cell counts may be declining
   C. Mild symptomatic infection—Symptoms such as fever, weight loss, diarrhea, night sweats, and fatigue along with other manifestations such as thrush, seborrhea, and generalized lymphadenopathy may be exhibited.
   D. Advanced HIV disease—characterized by severe immunosuppression and life-threatening opportunistic infections, malignancies, and HIV-related encephalopathy.

Assessment

SUBJECTIVE

1. Recurrent fever, night sweats
2. Weight loss
3. Anorexia
4. Chronic diarrhea
5. Fatigue, weakness
6. Chronic vaginal infection

OBJECTIVE

1. Swollen lymph glands
2. White spots or lesions in oral cavity
3. Dry cough
4. Shortness of breath

5. Presence of opportunistic infections:
   A. Viral, such as herpes simplex, varicella zoster, cytomegalovirus (CMV), and others
   B. Protozoal, such as *Pneumocystis carinii* pneumonia (PCP), and others
   C. Fungal, such as *Candida, Cryptococcus*, histoplasmosis, and others
   D. Bacterial, such as *Mycobacterium avium-intracellulare* complex (MAC), *Mycobacterium tuberculosis* (TB), and others
   E. Malignancies, such as Kaposi's sarcoma and others
6. Presence of AIDS dementia complex or HIV encephalopathy; includes cognitive, motor and behavioral changes

DIAGNOSTIC TESTS AND METHODS

1. History
2. Physical examination
3. Serum using the enzyme-linked immunosorbent assay (ELISA), confirmed by the Western blot test
4. Presence of opportunistic infections
5. Lumbar puncture
6. CT scan
7. Bronchial biopsy
8. Home HIV testing kits; Accuracy depends on adherence to testing instructions
9. Viral load monitoring—Serial comparisons of the serum viral load are used to predict progression of the disease and the effectiveness of medication therapy. The Centers for Disease Control (CDC) case definition for AIDS includes a CD4 lymphocyte count of below 200/mm^3 or below 14%.

Planning

1. Safe, effective care environment
   A. Prevent avoidable injury and/or infection.
   B. Increase client's and family's knowledge of disease process, diagnostic procedures, and treatment.
2. Physiological integrity
   A. Promote nutritional support.
   B. Maintain skin integrity.
   C. Monitor for opportunistic infections.
3. Psychosocial integrity
   A. Provide support for coping with chronic/fatal disease.
4. Health promotion and maintenance
   A. Increase client's and family's knowledge of prevention, home care, and follow-up.

Implementation

1. Assess, report, and record signs and symptoms and reactions to treatment.
2. Protect client from opportunistic infections. Reinforce good personal hygiene to decrease infections.
3. Administer antiretroviral (protease inhibitors and reverse transcriptase inhibitors) and other prescribed medications at precisely prescribed times. Some medications must be given with food; others must be given between meals. Monitor for side effects.
4. Provide nutritional support.
5. Label specimens carefully.
6. Dispose of contaminated articles appropriately.

7. Encourage physical independence.
8. Monitor O_2 therapy.
9. Administer analgesics for pain.
10. Provide rest periods.
11. Provide emotional support to client and family.
12. Provide information for support network, including available community resources.
13. Instruct client and family regarding disease process (including modes of transmission), diagnostic procedures, treatment, prevention, home care, and follow-up.

Evaluation

1. Reports increased comfort
2. Shows no evidence of avoidable injury and/or infection
3. Demonstrates understanding of disease process (including modes of transmission), diagnostic procedures, treatment, prevention, home care, need for follow-up, and available community resources; similar understanding demonstrated by family

GI System

Basic Information

The GI system breaks down food—carbohydrates, fats, and proteins into molecules small enough to pass through cell membranes.

1. It provides cells with necessary energy to function properly; prepares food for cellular absorption by altering its physical and chemical composition.
2. Other systems influence the GI system. The endocrine, central nervous, and autonomic nervous systems serve as regulators to the GI system.
3. Malfunction of the GI tract has far-reaching metabolic effects on the body.
4. It excretes insoluble and unabsorbed food materials.

Nursing Assessment

SUBJECTIVE

1. Nausea and vomiting
2. Difficulty in swallowing
3. Difficulty in chewing
4. Weight changes
5. Pain and location
6. Burning sensation beneath sternum
7. Indigestion
8. Appetite change
9. Flatus
10. Changes in bowel habits
11. Intolerance to certain foods
12. Personal and family history of GI-related problems

OBJECTIVE

1. Stomatitis
2. Hematemesis, hemachezia
3. Difficulty in swallowing
4. Poor dentition
5. Bleeding gums
6. Abdominal distention
7. Jaundice
8. Constipation or diarrhea
9. Edema
10. Hemorrhoids
11. Stool changes—clay colored, black, frothy
12. Dark urine

DIAGNOSTIC TESTS AND METHODS

1. History
2. Physical examination
3. Esophageal function tests
4. Stool examination
5. Upper GI series—barium enema
6. Esophagogastroduodenoscopy for direct visualization of the lining of the esophagus, stomach, and duodenum
7. Lower GI series—barium enema
8. Upper GI endoscopy
9. Sigmoidoscopy
10. Proctosigmoidoscopy
11. Colonoscopy
12. Gallbladder series
13. Oral cholecystography
14. Intravenous cholangiography
15. Percutaneous transhepatic cholangiogram (PTC)
16. Ultrasonography
17. Scans (liver and pancreas)
18. Liver biopsy
19. Gastric analysis
20. A CT of the abdomen—used in diagnosis of acute and chronic pancreatitis, pancreatic cysts, cirrhosis of the liver, ascites, aneurysms, and pancreatic cancer
21. Ultrasonography—used in evaluating organ shape, size, and structure; also aids in diagnosis of gallstones, differentiation of obstructive and nonobstructive jaundice, detection of pancreatic cysts and enlargement, screening for hepatocellular disease
22. Endoscopic retrograde cholangiopancreatography—used for diagnosis of diseases of the pancreas
23. Laboratory studies
    A. Serum amylase
    B. Serum lipase
    C. Urine amylase
    D. Liver enzyme studies (AST and LDH)
    E. Coagulation studies
    F. Hepatitis B surface antigen (HB_sM_g) study
    G. Stool: for cultures, fecal fat, urobilinogen or occult blood

Assessment

1. Problems
   A. Stomatitis
      (1) Provide cool, soft, bland foods.
      (2) Encourage mouth care with soothing mouth rinses.
      (3) Administer prescribed topical medication.
      (4) Encourage fluid intake.
         (a) Nausea and vomiting
      (5) Observe amount and character of emesis.
      (6) Observe other symptoms.
      (7) Observe for contributing factors.
      (8) Offer ice chips.

(9) Administer antiemetics as prescribed.
(10) Offer sips of clear liquids.
(11) Provide an environment free of unpleasant odors.
(12) Limit food servings; serve favorite foods.
(13) Encourage rest and deep breathing.
(14) Provide mouth care after each episode of emesis.
(15) Daily weight.
B. Anorexia
   (1) Evaluate status of anorexia.
   (2) Monitor intake of fluids and food.
   (3) Obtain information of food likes and dislikes.
   (4) Provide an environment free of unpleasant stimuli.
   (5) Prepare client for meals.
      (a) Give mouth care before eating.
      (b) Place client in a comfortable position for eating.
      (c) Provide privacy.
   (6) Daily weight
C. Dysphagia
   (1) Provide mouth care.
   (2) Provide small, frequent feedings of soft, bland foods that can be easily chewed.
   (3) Arrange tray attractively with client's favorite foods.
   (4) Monitor intake of fluids and foods.
   (5) Administer prescribed topical medications.
D. Diarrhea
   (1) Evaluate associated symptoms.
   (2) Record character, consistency.

Esophagitis (Gastroesophageal Reflux)

Description

1. Esophagitis is an inflammation of the esophagus, more common in middle age.
2. It often occurs with a sliding hiatal hernia, but may occur in the absence of hiatal hernia.
3. Reflux esophagitis—incompetent esophageal sphincter that allows a backward flow of gastric contents into the esophagus.
   A. Corrosive esophagitis—following ingestion of harmful chemicals, such as lye or other strong alkalies or acids
      (1) May be temporary or may lead to a permanent stricture (narrowing) of the esophagus that needs correction by surgical means
      (2) Is similar to a burn—severe burns may result in esophageal perforation; inflammation of the mediastinum; and death due to infection, shock, and hemorrhage
   B. Cause—unknown
   C. Contributing factors include:
      (1) Irritants such as food, tobacco, bacteria; or trauma
      (2) Malignancy
      (3) Repeated bouts of vomiting
      (4) Prolonged use of NG intubation

Assessment

SUBJECTIVE

1. Heartburn
2. Dysphagia (difficulty in swallowing)
3. Pain with eructation (belching) or regurgitation
4. Pain in anterior chest
5. Burning sensation retrosternally shortly after eating, bending over, or while lying down
6. Pain on ingestion of hot or cold fluids
7. Anxiety

OBJECTIVE

1. Repeated vomiting
2. Tachypnea
3. Bloody vomitus with pieces of tissue—indication of severe damage
4. Sign of esophageal perforation and inflamed mediastinum
   A. Crepitation (crackling sound)
5. Inability to speak—indication of damage to larynx

DIAGNOSTIC TESTS AND METHODS

1. History
2. Physical assessment
3. Chest x-ray
4. Manometry—assesses pressures in esophagus
5. Barium swallow
6. Endoscopy—determines extent of damage
7. Esophagoscopy, biopsy

Planning

1. Health promotion and maintenance
   A. Increase client's knowledge of ways to prevent or diminish symptoms.
2. Physiological integrity
   A. Reduce or eliminate contributing factors

Implementation

1. Assess, report, and record signs and symptoms and reactions to treatment.
2. Explain procedures to client to decrease anxiety and to obtain cooperation.
3. Provide small, frequent bland, low-roughage feedings.
4. Administer medications such as antacids, analgesics, and sedatives as prescribed; monitor for side effects.
5. Discourage food intake at bedtime.
6. Place client in semi-Fowler position.
7. Provide the following nursing interventions for corrosive esophagitis:
   A. Do not induce vomiting—burns the esophagus.
   B. Do not use gastric lavage—chemical may cause further damage to mucous membrane and lining of the GI tract.
   C. Assist in administration of O_2, mechanical ventilation, IV fluids, and treatment of shock as needed.
   D. Administer corticosteroids, cholinergics and antibiotics as prescribed.
   E. Prepare client for surgery if required.
   F. Assist client and family to seek psychological counseling if ingestion is due to suicidal attempt.
   G. Provide emotional support to parents or guardians if client is a child.
   H. Teach appropriate preventive measures.
      (1) Locking cabinets where corrosive chemicals are kept
      (2) Keeping chemicals out of child's reach

8. Instruct client regarding disease process, diagnostic procedures, treatment prevention, home care, and follow-up.

Evaluation

1. Reports increased comfort, decreased anxiety
2. Reports absence of dysphagia
3. Reports absence of pain
4. Demonstrates healing of mucous membrane and esophageal tissues
5. Maintains stable vital signs
6. Demonstrates understanding of disease process, diagnostic procedures, treatment, prevention, home care, and need for follow-up

Esophageal Varices

Description

1. Esophageal varices represent a dilation of blood vessels (varicose veins) at the lower end of esophagus.
2. Causes
   A. Elevated pressure in portal vein (vessel bringing blood into liver) due to
      (1) Cirrhosis of the liver
      (2) Mechanical obstruction of portal vein by blood clot or tumor or obstruction of the hepatic veins
3. Varices may rupture causing hemorrhage and shock.
4. Death due to hemorrhage is approximately 67%.

Assessment

SUBJECTIVE

1. Anxiety
2. History of cirrhosis, portal hypertension
3. Weakness, vertigo

OBJECTIVE

1. Blood in emesis
2. Melena (black, tarry stools due to bleeding)
3. Low hemoglobin and hematocrit values
4. Elevated AST, ALT, amylase, bilirubin; low albumin
5. Hypotension
6. Tachycardia
7. Decreased level of consciousness
8. Signs of shock
9. Ascites

DIAGNOSTIC TESTS/METHODS

1. History
2. Physical examination
3. Endoscopy (identifies bleeding site)
4. Laboratory studies—hematocrit, hemoglobin, liver function
5. Tests
6. Angiography

Planning

1. Safe, effective care environment
   A. Prevent avoidable injury.
   B. Increase client's knowledge of disease process, diagnostic procedures, and treatment.

2. Physiological integrity
   A. Maintain adequate cardiac output.
   B. Maintain adequate tissue perfusion.
   C. Maintain adequate fluid and electrolyte balance.
   D. Maintain effective breathing pattern.
   E. Increase comfort.
3. Psychosocial integrity
   A. Reduce anxiety.
4. Health promotion and maintenance
   A. Increase client's knowledge of home care and follow-up.

Implementation

1. Assess, record, and report signs and symptoms and reactions to treatment.
2. Monitor for hemorrhage, hypotension.
3. Monitor emesis and stool for presence of blood.
4. Monitor laboratory test results; report abnormal findings.
5. Administer O_2 therapy, if prescribed.
6. Monitor vital signs at least every 4 hours (every ½ hour if bleeding occurs).
7. Monitor fluid intake, urinary output, and CVP for volume determination.
8. Evaluate level of consciousness.
9. Provide emotional support and reassurance to client and family.
10. Administer mouth care.
11. Give prescribed medications; monitor for side effects.
12. Administer and monitor IVs and blood transfusions as prescribed.
13. Keep client quiet and comfortable. (**NOTE:** Tolerance for sedatives and tranquilizers may be decreased owing to liver disease.)
14. Control bleeding by use of:
    A. Ice water lavages
    B. Sengstaken-Blakemoor tube, if ordered (keep scissors taped to head of bed in case of emergency)
15. Administer vitamin K as prescribed.
16. Monitor vasopressin (Pitressin) effects (used to constrict splanchnic vessels).
17. Monitor patient with Sengstaken-Blakemoor tube for:
    A. Bleeding in gastric drainage
    B. Signs of asphyxiation
    C. Tube displacement—correct traction to keep tube in correct placement
    D. Proper inflation of balloons
18. Assist with injection of sclerosing agent to control bleeding.
19. Monitor for signs of hepatic encephalopathy.
20. Prepare client for surgery if required to control bleeding
21. Provide postoperative care.
22. Instruct client regarding disease process, diagnostic procedures, treatment, home care, and follow-up.

Evaluation

1. Reports decreased anxiety, increased comfort
2. Has decreased or no hematemesis
3. Has decreased or no melena
4. Maintains stable vital signs
5. Maintains adequate fluid intake and output

6. Maintains adequate nutritional intake
7. Shows evidence of laboratory values returning to normal
8. Demonstrates understanding of disease process, diagnostic procedures, treatment, prevention, home care, and follow-up

Gastritis

Description

1. Gastritis is inflammation of the gastric mucosa, acute or chronic.
2. Acute type—produces reddening of mucosa, edema, hemorrhage, and erosion.
3. Common in clients with pernicious anemia (chronic atrophic gastritis).
4. It can occur at any age, but more common in elderly.
5. Back diffusion of acid and pepsin occur once mucosal injury is present.
6. Causes
   A. Drugs such as aspirin and nonsteroidal anti-inflammatory drugs (NSAIDs)
   B. Poisons such as DDT, ammonia, mercury, and carbon tetrachloride
   C. Bacterial infections of stomach wall—usually streptococci
   D. Irritating foods such as hot peppers—may be allergic reaction to certain foods
   E. GI injury such as ingestion of hot fluids, swallowing a foreign object
   F. overuse of alcoholic beverages
7. Associated factors
   A. Liver disorders
   B. GI disorders
   C. Infectious diseases—viruses, influenza, typhoid fever
   D. Curling's ulcer (following a severe burn)

Assessment

SUBJECTIVE

1. Nausea, vomiting
2. Anorexia
3. Feeling of fullness
4. Cramping
5. Upper abdominal pain
6. Belching
7. Malaise
8. Anxiety

OBJECTIVE

1. Presence of vomiting, diarrhea
2. Epigastric tenderness
3. Melena
4. Increased temperature

DIAGNOSTIC TESTS AND METHODS

1. History
2. Physical examination
3. Stool culture
4. Stool examination for occult blood
5. Laboratory tests—hemoglobin, hematocrit, electrolytes, CBC

6. Gastric analysis—to determine presence of *Helicobacter pylori*
7. Endoscopy with biopsy—to rule out cancer
8. **NOTE:** Gastroscopy is contraindicated after ingestion of corrosive agent
9. X-ray

Planning

1. Safe, effective care environment
   A. Prevent avoidable injury.
   B. Increase client's and family's knowledge of disease process, diagnostic procedures, and treatment.
2. Physiological integrity
   A. Maintain adequate cardiac output.
   B. Maintain adequate tissue perfusion.
   C. Maintain adequate fluid and electrolyte balance.
   D. Maintain effective breathing pattern.
   E. Increase comfort.
3. Psychosocial integrity
   A. Reduce anxiety.
4. Health promotion and maintenance
   A. Increase client's and family's knowledge of home care and follow-up.

Implementation

1. Assess, record, and report signs and symptoms and reactions to treatment.
2. Administer antacids, anticholinergics, and antibiotics as prescribed; monitor for side effects.
3. Monitor fluid intake and output.
4. Monitor electrolytes; report abnormal values.
5. Assist with insertion of NG tube, if ordered.
6. Monitor for signs of GI bleeding—bloody NG drainage, melena.
7. Monitor for signs of hemorrhagic shock—hypotension, tachycardia.
8. Administer iced saline lavage, vasopressin or epinephrine to control bleeding as prescribed.
9. Watch for nausea, vomiting, diarrhea, abdominal pain, or fever, in cirrosive gastritis which are indicative of:
   A. Signs of obstruction
   B. Perforation
   C. Peritonitis
10. Prepare client for endoscopic laser photocoagulation to control bleeding.
11. Instruct client and family regarding disease process, diagnostic procedures, treatment, home care, and follow-up. Include teaching on:
    A. Drug therapy
    B. Diet
    C. Activity
    D. Restrictions

Evaluation

1. Reports increased comfort, decreased anxiety
2. Has no nausea, vomiting, bleeding
3. Maintains stable vital signs
4. Shows evidence of laboratory test results returning to normal values

5. Demonstrates understanding of disease process, treatment, prevention, home care, and need for follow-up; similar understanding demonstrated by family

Hiatal Hernia

Description

1. Hiatal hernia is a condition in which part of the stomach and other abdominal viscera protrudes through a weakened area of the diaphragm into the thoracic cavity.
2. Gastric reflux (regurgitation) occurs when the lower esophageal sphincter (muscle) pressure is less than that of the pressure in the stomach.
3. Gastric reflux may enter esophagus resulting in inflammation and ulceration.
4. Two types
   A. Type I—sliding hiatal hernia
      (1) Portion of stomach herniates slightly upward into the enlarged diaphragmatic hiatus.
      (2) Most individuals are asymptomatic.
      (3) Approximately 5% of population diagnosed with type I also have symptoms of gastroesophageal reflux.
   B. Type II—rolling hiatal hernia
      (1) Portion of stomach herniates alongside esophagus.
      (2) Herniated stomach extends above the gastroesophageal junction.
      (3) Gastroesophageal reflux is not usually associated with type II disorder.
      (4) Type II is larger and less common than type I.
5. Cause—unknown
6. Contributing factors include:
   A. Congenital weakness of diaphragm
   B. Trauma
7. Related factors
   A. Increased abdominal pressure
   B. Relaxed esophageal sphincter
   C. Pregnancy
   D. Obesity
   E. Smoking, alcohol, caffeine ingestion

Assessment

SUBJECTIVE

1. Heartburn
2. Regurgitation
3. Dysphagia (difficulty in swallowing)
4. Feeling of fullness
5. History of trauma, obesity, pregnancy
6. Anxiety

OBJECTIVE

1. Dyspnea (difficulty in breathing)
2. Discovered via diagnostic methods

DIAGNOSTIC TESTS AND METHODS

1. History
2. Physical examination
3. Chest x-ray
4. Upper GI series (barium swallow)
5. Esophagoscopy

Planning

1. Safe, effective care environment
   A. Increase client's and family's knowledge of disease process, diagnostic procedures, treatment (including medication and surgery).
2. Physiological integrity
   A. Increase comfort.
   B. Maintain adequate nutritional intake.
3. Psychosocial integrity
   A. Reduce anxiety.
4. Health promotion and maintenance
   A. Increase client's and family's knowledge of home care and follow-up.

Implementation

1. Assess, record, and report signs and symptoms.
2. If patient is asymptomatic, no treatment is required.
3. Provide small, frequent meals—bland diet (high protein, low fat).
4. Keep head of bed elevated when eating and up to 3 hours following meal.
5. Administer medications such as urecholine, cimetidine, antacids as prescribed.
6. Instruct client not to perform activities that will increase abdominal pressure, such as lifting heavy objects, bending over; not to wear tight clothing around waist.
7. Instruct obese clients regarding weight management.
8. Keep head of bed slightly elevated during sleep periods.
9. Instruct client to avoid alcohol and caffeine.
10. Prepare client and family for surgical intervention if conservative measures fail.
11. Provide postoperative care.
12. Administer, monitor IV therapy, blood transfusion.
13. Assist in insertion of NG tube; monitor effects.
14. Administer analgesics and antiemetics as prescribed.
15. Monitor medications for side effects.
16. Monitor fluid intake and output.
17. Monitor vital signs.
18. Report incidence of gastric reflux immediately.
19. Instruct client and family regarding disease process, diagnostic procedures, treatment (including need for compliance), home care, and follow-up.

Evaluation

1. Reports increased comfort, decreased anxiety
2. Maintains adequate nutritional intake
3. Has no symptoms
4. Demonstrates understanding of disease process, diagnostic procedures, treatment (including need for compliance), home care, and follow-up; similar understanding demonstrated by family

Peptic Ulcers

Description

1. Peptic ulcers are ulcerations that penetrate the mucous membrane or deeper structures of the GI tract.
2. All peptic ulcers require the presence of gastric acid.

3. The development of an ulcer reflects an imbalance of acid and pepsin and the natural ability of the GI mucosa to protect itself from acid and pepsin.

Duodenal Ulcers

Description

1. Usually duodenal ulcers are caused by hypersecretion of gastric acids, whereas gastric ulcers represent a breakdown in the body's protective mechanisms.
2. They can develop in lower esophagus, stomach, pylorus, duodenum, or jejunum.
3. Approximately 80% occur in proximal part of small intestine.
4. Duodenal ulcers occur most often in males between 20 and 50 years of age.
5. They often become chronic with remissions and exacerbations.
6. Hypersecretion of acid may be caused by:
   A. Excessive parietal cell mass
   B. Increased gastrin release after a meal
   C. Increased sensitivity to gastrin
   D. An uncontrolled source of gastrin release (Zollinger-Ellison syndrome)
7. Complications may occur requiring surgical intervention.

Gastric Ulcers (Stomach)

Description

1. Gastric ulcers occur most often in middle-aged and elderly men.
2. They are especially common among poor and undernourished individuals.
3. Benign gastric ulcers tend to recur.
4. Most common site is the distal half of the stomach.
5. Majority of affected individuals have a lower acid secretion than those with duodenal ulcers.
6. Disruption of the gastric mucosal barrier occurs, causing hydrogen ions to diffuse into cells and cells to release histamine.
7. Histamine stimulates acid secretion and capillary leakage of serum and blood.
8. The back diffusion of hydrogen ions is correlated with a decrease in acid and an increase in sodium levels.
9. Mucosal cells die owing to absence of blood and O_2 supply, leading to erosions and ulcers.
10. Both types of ulcers may be asymptomatic.
11. Complications of ulcers
    A. Penetration to pancreas causing severe back pain
    B. Perforation of area involved
    C. Hemorrhage
    D. Pyloric obstruction
12. Possible causes
    A. Decreased mucous resistance or defense mechanism
    B. Imbalance of acid and pepsin
    C. Defective mucus
    D. Acid hypersecretion due to possible overactive vagus nerve may contribute to duodenal ulcer formation.
13. **NOTE:** Exact cause not determined.
14. Related factors
    A. Chronic use of salicylates, alcohol and NSAIDs
    B. Cigarette smoking

C. Heredity
D. Emotional stress
E. Drugs such as ibuprofen, corticosteroids
F. Infection by *Helicobacter pyloris*

Assessment

SUBJECTIVE

1. Gastric ulcer
   A. Heartburn
   B. Indigestion and belching
   C. Feeling of fullness and distention following a large meal
2. Duodenal ulcer
   A. Heartburn and belching
   B. Pain (gnawing, burning) in middle upper abdomen relieved by food ingestion.
   C. Attacks follow in approximately 2 hours after meals or when stomach is empty.
   D. Pain follows ingestion of citric juices, coffee, aspirin, or alcohol.

OBJECTIVE

1. Gastric ulcer
   A. Loss of appetite
   B. Possibly repeated episodes of GI bleeding
   C. Weight loss
   D. Anemia
   E. GI bleeding
   F. Melena
   G. Vomiting (coffee-ground appearance with bleeding)
2. Duodenal ulcer
   A. Weight gain from eating to relieve discomfort.
   B. Vomiting and other digestive symptoms are rare.
   C. If complications occur, watch for GI bleeding, melena.

DIAGNOSTIC TESTS AND METHODS

1. History
2. Physical examination
3. Upper GI series
4. Gastric analysis
5. Gastroscopy
6. Fiber-optic endoscopy—to diagnose both gastric and duodenal ulcer
7. Radiological examination of upper GI tract—standard and double air contrast studies
8. Laboratory studies—hematocrit, hemoglobin, electrolytes, CBC
9. Biopsy of tissue—to rule out malignancy

Planning

1. Safe, effective care environment
   A. Prevent avoidable injury.
   B. Increase client's and family's knowledge regarding disease process, diagnostic procedures, and treatments.
2. Physiological integrity
   A. Increase comfort; reduce pain.
   B. Promote adequate nutrition.
3. Psychosocial integrity
   A. Assist with stress management.
4. Health promotion and maintenance
   A. Increase client's and family's knowledge regarding

home care (including medication, diet, smoking, stress management, and self-care), and follow-up.

Implementation

1. Assess, record, and report signs and symptoms and reaction to treatment.
2. Provide a quiet environment, assist with comfort measures.
3. Administer prescribed medications such as analgesics, sedatives, antacids, anticholinergics, histamine receptor antagonists (Zantac, ranitidine, or cimetidine) to neutralize or inhibit gastric secretions, sedatives.
4. Monitor and report medication side effects such as dizziness, rash, mild diarrhea, muscle pain, leukopenia, gynecomastia, dry mouth, blurred vision, headache, constipation, and urinary retention.
5. Monitor vital signs.
6. Monitor laboratory test results—hematocrit, hemoglobin, CBC, electrolytes.
7. Watch for signs of bleeding; changes in vital signs, vomiting (coffee-ground appearance); anemia; black, tarry stools or bloody stools.
8. Provide prescribed diet—avoid irritating foods such as coffee, spices.
9. Discourage cigarette smoking.
10. Prepare client and family for surgical intervention if required for recurrent ulcers, perforation, or hemorrhage.
    A. Closure if perforation has occurred.
    B. Total or partial resection of stomach or duodenum to remove ulcerated area(s).
    C. Pyloroplasty and vagotomy if gastric outlet is obstructed.
11. Provide preoperative care
    A. Correct nutritional deficiencies.
    B. Assist in administration of blood replacement.
    C. Assist with insertion of NG tube for gastric decompression.
    D. Provide reassurance to client and family.
12. Provide postoperative care
    A. Monitor vital signs—report abnormalities immediately.
    B. Administer narcotics and analgesics as prescribed for pain.
    C. Monitor fluid intake and output.
    D. Assess for signs of dehydration, sodium deficiency, and metabolic alkalosis—may occur secondary to gastric suction.
    E. Assist in administration of blood transfusions, IVs, monitor for side effects.
    F. Monitor patency of NG tube; check, record, and report characteristics of drainage.
    G. Monitor and report signs of bleeding.
    H. Encourage coughing and deep breathing.
    I. Monitor elimination—check bowel sounds—NPO until peristalsis resumes and NG tube is removed or clamped.
    J. Watch for complications:
       (1) Hemorrhage, shock
       (2) Iron, folate, or vitamin B_{12} deficiency anemia (from continued blood loss or malabsorption)
       (3) Dumping syndrome (weakness, nausea, diarrhea, gas pains, distention, and palpations within 30 minutes after a meal)

K. Perform the following nursing interventions if complications such as hemorrhage occur.
   (1) Monitor vital signs every half hour, report abnormalities immediately.
   (2) Monitor fluid intake and output.
   (3) Check palms of hands—pale palmar creases indicate a hemoglobin level of <10 g/dL.
   (4) Check for presence of red-maroon stool on digital rectal examination.
   (5) Check for bloody aspirate from NG tube.
   (6) Monitor for signs of:
       (a) Hypovolemia—related to hemorrhage and dehydration—due to excessive fluid loss and inadequate fluid replacement
       (b) Altered electrolyte balance—presence of hypernatremia, hypokalemia as a result of body's attempt to compensate for lost fluid
       (c) Altered tissue perfusion—due to vasoconstriction as a result of blood loss
       (d) Altered clotting factors associated with body's attempt to restore hemostasis through clotting mechanisms
       (e) Altered thought processes such as confusion due to cerebral hypoxia associated with decreased O_2 supply, anemia, and elevated ammonia levels
   (7) Provide complete bed rest, NPO.
   (8) Provide quiet environment, allay anxiety.
   (9) Monitor NG drainage, presence of vomitus, bloody stools; report changes immediately.
   (10) Assist in administration of blood, IV fluids, and medications as prescribed.
L. Monitor for symptoms of complications such as peritonitis, infection due to anastomotic leak, intestinal obstruction, and impaired healing.
M. Monitor for signs of paralytic ileus due to decreased neuromuscular activity as a result of gut manipulation during surgery and electrolyte imbalance.
N. Monitor for signs of fluid and electrolyte imbalance as a result of NG decompression, NG irrigation, surgical drains, and fistulas.
O. Monitor nutritional status—altered nutritional status may be related to dumping syndrome.
P. Instruct client in prevention of dumping syndrome.
   (1) Eating four to six small, high-protein, low-carbohydrate meals during the day.
   (2) Resting after meals.
   (3) Drink fluids between meals rather than with meals.
Q. Instruct client that magnesium-containing antacids may cause diarrhea, and aluminum-containing antacids may cause constipation.
R. Instruct client to avoid drugs containing aspirin—they cause irritation of gastric mucosa.
S. Advise client to avoid excessive use of coffee, alcohol, and stressful situations.
T. Advise client to stop smoking—smoking stimulates gastric secretions.
U. Instruct client and family regarding disease process, diagnostic procedures, treatment, home care (including medication, diet, smoking, stress management, and self-care) and follow-up.

Evaluation

1. Reports increase in comfort, decreased anxiety
2. Maintains a normal fluid balance as evidenced by:
   A. Stable weight
   B. Blood pressure and pulse rate within normal limits
   C. Absence of edema or distended neck veins
   D. Normal serum osmolality
   E. Balanced intake and output
   F. Specific gravity within normal limits
   G. Respirations within normal limits
3. Maintains adequate nutrition
4. Has no symptoms of infection
5. Maintains normal temperature
6. Shows no signs of redness or drainage at incision site
7. Demonstrates adequate wound healing
8. Shows no signs of paralytic ileus
9. Has normal bowel sounds
10. Shows no signs of abdominal distention
11. Shows evidence of ulcer healing as revealed by endoscopic examination
12. Has normal laboratory values
13. Demonstrates understanding of disease process, diagnostic procedures, treatment, home care (including need for compliance to prescribed therapy and lifestyle changes), and follow-up; similar understanding demonstrated by family

Crohn's Disease (Regional Enteritis)

Description

1. Crohn's disease is inflammation of any part of the GI tract (usually the terminal ileum).
2. Lacteal blockage in intestinal wall leads to edema.
3. Blockage eventually leads to inflammation, ulceration, stenosis, abscess, and fistula formation.
4. Process extends through all layers of the intestinal wall.
5. Cobblestone ulcerations occur in intestinal lining, and scar tissue forms.
6. Bowel becomes thick and narrow.
7. Condition may also involve regional lymph nodes and the mesentery.
8. Ulcerations may perforate resulting in fistulas (common), which in turn lead to colon, bladder, or vaginal, perianal, and perirectal abscesses and perforations.
9. Normal absorption of nutrients is decreased due to scar tissue formation.
10. Strictures may develop with potential for intestinal obstruction.
11. Condition is most prevalent in adults aged 20 to 40.
12. It is 2–3 times more common in Jews and least common in blacks.
13. Up to 5% of affected patients have one or more affected relatives with condition (inheritance pattern is not clear).
14. Possible causes
    A. Allergies, other immune disorders
    B. Lymphatic obstruction
    C. Infection
    D. Environmental or genetic factors
    E. Emotional stress
    F. Heredity (genetic cause)

Assessment

SUBJECTIVE

1. Abdominal pain and cramping
   A. Mimics appendicitis symptoms
2. Tenderness
3. Gas pains
4. Nausea
5. Loss of appetite
6. Malaise, weakness, fatigue
7. Anxiety
8. Inability to cope with everyday stress

OBJECTIVE

1. Elevated temperature
2. Diarrhea containing pus, mucus, or blood (four to six stools a day)
3. Marked weight loss
4. Anemia
5. Laboratory test results
   A. Elevated WBC and ESR counts
   B. Hypokalemia
   C. Hypocalcemia
   D. Hypomagnesemia
   E. Depressed hemoglobin
   F. Stool specimen studies
6. Signs of dehydration—poor skin turgor, dry mucous membranes
7. Lower right quadrant tenderness

DIAGNOSTIC TESTS AND METHODS

1. History
2. Physical examination
3. Stool specimen examination for occult blood
4. Laboratory studies—CBC, ESR, electrolytes, hemoglobin, hematocrit
5. Barium enema—shows string sign (segments of stricture separated by normal bowel)
6. Endoscopy
7. Sigmoidoscopy, colonoscopy—may show patchy areas of inflammation (helps to rule out ulcerative colitis)
8. Biopsy—provides definitive diagnosis
9. Colonoscopy

Planning

1. Safe, effective care environment
   A. Prevent avoidable injury and/or infection.
   B. Increase client's and family's knowledge of disease process, diagnostic procedures, and treatment.
2. Physiological integrity
   A. Increase comfort and rest.
   B. Maintain fluid and electrolyte balance.
   C. Maintain adequate nutritional intake.
   D. Resume progressive activity.
3. Psychosocial integrity
   A. Reduce anxiety.
   B. Discuss sexuality disturbances.
   C. Promote effective coping of client and family.
4. Health promotion and maintenance
   A. Increase client's and family's knowledge regarding home care (including self-care) and follow-up.

Implementation

1. Assess, record, and report signs and symptoms and reactions to treatment.
2. Provide emotional support, rest.
3. Record intake and output—include amount of stool.
4. Weigh client daily.
5. Watch for dehydration—decrease in urinary output, poor skin turgor.
6. Monitor fluid and electrolyte balance.
7. Monitor vital signs every 4 hours.
8. Watch for signs of intestinal bleeding—check stools daily for occult blood.
9. Provide prescribed diet.
   A. Restricted fiber diet with no fruit or vegetables for intestinal stenosis
   B. Low-fat diet for steatorrhea
   C. Elimination of dairy products for lactose deficiency
10. Administer prescribed medications and monitor for side effects.
    A. Sulfasalazine—to reduce inflammation
    B. Steroids—to reduce inflammation (watch for GI bleeding—steroids mask signs of infection)
    C. Antibiotics—to reduce risk of infection from peritoneal irritation, abscess, or fistulas.
    D. Sedatives
    E. Analgesics
       (1) Anticholinergics
    F. Bulk hydrophilic drugs—to treat diarrhea
11. Check hemoglobin and hematocrit daily.
12. Administer iron supplements and blood transfusions as prescribed.
13. Provide mouth care.
14. Provide good skin care following each bowel movement.
    A. Keep clean, covered bedpan within client's reach.
15. Ventilate room to eliminate odors.
16. Monitor client for fever or pain on urination (may be a sign of a bladder fistula).
17. Monitor client for abdominal pain; fever; and hard, distended abdomen—may indicate intestinal obstruction.
18. Provide information regarding surgical intervention and postoperative course, if required. (Colectomy with ileostomy often required in clients with extensive disease of large intestine and rectum.)
    A. Request that an enterostomal therapist visit client before ileostomy.
    B. Provide care during postoperative period.
    C. Monitor IV and NG tube for proper functioning.
    D. Monitor fluid intake and output.
    E. Monitor vital signs.
    F. Watch for signs of wound infection.
19. Provide meticulous stoma care.
20. Instruct client and family regarding disease process, diagnostic procedures, treatment, home care, and follow-up. Include teaching on:
    A. Stoma care—offer reassurance and emotional support (ileostomy changes client's body image).
    B. Importance of diet, bed rest, medications, and sexuality.
    C. Stress reduction—may need to refer for counseling.

Evaluation

1. Reports increased comfort, decreased anxiety
2. Maintains adequate nutrition and hydration
3. Tolerates progressive activity
4. Verbalizes concerns
5. Uses effective coping strategies
6. Demonstrates understanding of disease process, diagnostic procedures, treatment, prevention, home care, and need for follow-up; similar understanding demonstrated by family

Ulcerative Colitis

Description

1. Ulcerative colitis is an inflammatory, often chronic, disorder of the large bowel. The rectal and sigmoid colon mucosae and submucosae become edematous and develop small bleeding lesions that result in ulcerations.
2. Ulcerations often extend upward into entire colon; they rarely affect small intestine, except for the terminal ileum.
3. Congestion, edema results in mucosal friability.
4. Ulcerations develop into abscesses.
5. The colon eventually loses elasticity with a reduction in nutrient absorptive capability.
6. Severity ranges from a mild, localized condition to a severe disease, which may result in a perforated colon, progressing to potentially fatal peritonitis and toxemia.
7. Condition may lead to complications affecting various body systems.
   A. Vascular system—anemia from iron deficiency, clotting defects due to vitamin K deficiency
   B. Liver—pericholangitis, cirrhosis, sclerosing cholangitis
   C. GI—strictures, pseudopolyps, anal fissures, abscesses, perforated colon, resulting in peritonitis and toxemia
      (1) Toxic megacolon is a life-threatening complication
   D. Musculoskeletal—arthritis, loss of muscle mass
8. Those with condition are at risk for development of colorectal cancer.
9. It occurs primarily in young adults, especially females.
10. It is more prevalent in Jews and upper socioeconomic groups.
11. Overall, incidence rates are increasing.
12. Cause is unknown.
13. Predisposing factors
    A. Family history of disease
    B. Bacterial infection
    C. Allergic reaction to food, milk, or substances that release inflammatory histamine in the bowel
    D. Overproduction of enzymes that break down mucous membrane
    E. Autoimmune reactions such as arthritis, hemolytic anemia
    F. Environmental factors
    G. Emotional stress

Assessment

SUBJECTIVE

1. Abdominal cramping, pain, distention
2. Nausea
3. Loss of appetite
4. Irritability

5. Anxiety
6. Weakness
7. Loss of appetite

OBJECTIVE

1. Bloody diarrhea containing pus and mucus
2. Spastic rectum and anus
3. Weight loss
4. Vomiting
5. Temperature as high as 104°F

DIAGNOSTIC TESTS AND METHODS

1. History
2. Physical examination
3. Stool examination
4. Sigmoidoscopy—shows increased mucosal friability, thick inflammatory exudate
5. Colonoscopy with biopsy—to determine extent of disease and to evaluate strictures and pseudopolyps
6. Barium enema—to assess extent of disease and to detect complications
7. Laboratory tests—electrolytes, CBC, hemoglobin, hematocrit, ESR

Planning

1. Safe, effective care environment
   A. Prevent avoidable injury.
   B. Increase client's and family's knowledge regarding disease process, diagnostic procedures, and treatment.
2. Physiological integrity
   A. Increase comfort and rest.
   B. Maintain fluid and electrolyte balance.
   C. Maintain adequate nutritional intake.
   D. Resume progressive activity.
3. Psychosocial integrity
   A. Reduce anxiety.
   B. Discuss sexuality disturbances.
   C. Promote effective coping of client and family.
4. Health promotion and maintenance
   A. Increase client's and family's knowledge regarding home care (including self-care) and follow-up.

Implementation

1. Assess, record, and report signs and symptoms and reactions to treatment.
2. Provide emotional support and rest.
3. Provide good skin care to prevent anal excoriation.
4. Monitor the number, amount, time, and characteristics of stools.
5. Provide client with air mattress or sheepskin to prevent breakdown.
6. Monitor bowel sounds every 4 hours.
7. Administer prescribed medications; monitor for side effects.
   A. Corticosteroids—prolonged therapy causes moon face, hirsutism, edema, gastric irritation
8. Monitor vital signs.
9. Monitor intake and output.
10. Watch for signs of dehydration—dry skin and mucous membranes, sunken eyes, fever, decreased urine output and weight loss.
11. Monitor hemoglobin, hematocrit, and electrolyte levels.
12. Assist with blood transfusions and IV therapy as prescribed.
13. Provide mouth care for those on NPO.
14. Weigh patient daily.
15. Provide prescribed diet.
16. Assist with ADL.
17. Monitor for signs of complications such as perforated colon or peritonitis.
    A. Fever
    B. Severe abdominal pain
    C. Rigid and tender abdomen
    D. Cool, clammy skin
    E. Abdominal distention, decreased or absent bowel sounds.
18. Prepare client for surgery if complications occur.
    A. Arrange for visit by an enterostomal therapist.
19. Provide postoperative care
    A. Give meticulous stoma care, and teach correct stoma care to client and family.
    B. Monitor NG tube for patency.
    C. Following nasogastric tube removal, provide a clear-liquid diet; advance to low-residue diet.
    D. Prepare client for discharge—encourage regular physical examinations.
20. Instruct client and family regarding disease process, diagnostic procedures, treatment, prevention, home care (including self-care and compliance with prescribed therapy), and follow-up.

Evaluation

1. Reports increased comfort, decreased anxiety
2. Maintains adequate hydration, nutritional status
3. Continues progressive activity
4. Verbalizes concerns
5. Identifies stressors and measures to reduce them
6. Demonstrates understanding of disease process, diagnostic procedures, treatment, prevention, home care (including self-care, need for follow-up, and compliance with prescribed therapy); similar understanding demonstrated by family

Diverticulosis and Diverticulitis

Description

1. Diverticula are bulging pouches found in the GI wall.
2. Diverticula push mucosal lining through surrounding muscle.
3. Most common site is in sigmoid colon, although pouches may develop from proximal end of pharynx to anus.
4. Diverticular disease of ileum (Meckel's diverticulum) is the most common congenital anomaly of GI tract.
5. Diverticular disease has two clinical forms:
   A. Diverticulosis
      (1) Diverticula are present but do not cause symptoms.
      (2) Client may be asymptomatic—usual occurrence before age 35.
      (3) Treatment is primarily medical.

B. Diverticulitis
   (1) Diverticula are inflamed and may cause severe obstruction, infection, or hemorrhage.
      (a) Retained, undigested food mixes with bacteria in diverticular sac, resulting in a hard mass.
      (b) Blood supply is cut off to thin walls of the diverticular sac, which become susceptible to bacteria found in the colon.
      (c) Inflammation results.
   (2) Condition usually occurs in adults between 50 and 70 years of age.
   (3) It may result in spasms, obstruction, perforation, or bleeding.
   (4) Inflamed colon segment may result in a fistula leading to the bladder or other organs.
6. Causes
   A. Result of high pressure within lumen of GI tract on weakened areas of GI wall where blood vessels enter
   B. Low-fiber diet resulting in lack of roughage
      (1) It reduces fecal residue.
      (2) It narrows bowel lumen.

Assessment

SUBJECTIVE

1. Diverticulosis (usually asymptomatic)
   A. Rare complication in elderly is hemorrhage from diverticula located in rectum (usually mild).
   B. Condition may cause recurrent pain in left lower quadrant.
2. Diverticulitis
   A. Recurrent pain in lower left quadrant radiating to the back, often relieved by bowel movement or passage of gas
   B. Increased flatus
   C. Rectal bleeding
   D. Symptoms of partial obstruction
   E. Mild nausea
   F. Vomiting when obstruction is present

OBJECTIVE

1. Alternating constipation and diarrhea
2. Irregular bowel movements
3. Low-grade fever
4. Increased WBC count
5. Occult bleeding
6. If rupture occurs—abdominal rigidity, severe lower left-quadrant pain, signs of sepsis and shock (high fever, chills, hypotension)
7. If rupture near blood vessel—mild to severe hemorrhage based on size of affected blood vessel
8. Constipation, ribbonlike stools, intermittent diarrhea, abdominal distention (signs of incomplete bowel obstruction usually a result of chronic condition)
9. Abdominal rigidity, decreased or absent bowel sound, nausea, vomiting, abdominal pain (signs of increasing bowel obstruction).

DIAGNOSTIC TESTS AND METHODS

1. History.
2. Physical examination.
3. Laboratory values—CBC, ESR, hemoglobin, hematocrit, RBC count.
4. Stool for occult blood.
5. X-ray series—may reveal spasms of the colon.
6. Upper GI series—assess for diverticulosis of esophagus and upper bowel.
7. Barium enema—assess for diverticulosis of lower bowel. In acute diverticulitis, enema may rupture bowel.
8. Sigmoidoscopy.
9. Colonoscopy.

Planning

1. Safe, effective care environment
   A. Prevent avoidable injury.
   B. Increase client's knowledge of disease process, diagnostic procedures, and treatment.
2. Physiological integrity
   A. Increase comfort and rest.
   B. Maintain fluid balance.
   C. Support adequate nutrition.
3. Psychosocial integrity
   A. Reduce anxiety.
4. Health promotion and maintenance
   A. Increase client's knowledge regarding prevention, home care, and follow-up.

Implementation

1. Assess, record, and report signs and symptoms and reactions to treatment.
2. Provide emotional support.
3. Provide the following nursing interventions for diverticulosis with pain, constipation, mild GI distress, or difficulty with bowel movements:
   A. Provide prescribed diet—liquid or soft diet during acute phase. (It helps to relieve symptoms, decrease irritation, and decrease progression to diverticulitis.)
   B. Administer stool softeners, other medications as prescribed.
   C. Monitor stools, check frequency, color, and consistency.
   D. Monitor vital signs—changes may indicate progression of condition.
   E. Encourage fluid intake.
   F. Provide high-roughage diet and bulk-forming agents once pain subsides.
4. Provide the following nursing interventions for mild diverticulosis without complications.
   A. Provide quiet environment, bed rest.
   B. Provide a liquid diet.
   C. Administer prescribed medications such as stool softeners, broad-spectrum antibiotics, analgesics for pain, smooth muscle relaxants, antispasmodics.
   D. Observe stools; record, report abnormalities.
   E. Monitor vital signs for changes.
   F. Monitor fluid intake and output.
5. Provide the following nursing interventions for hemorrhage:
   A. Administer blood transfusions, IV therapy as prescribed.
   B. Monitor fluid and electrolyte balance.
   C. Monitor catheter patency and placement if angiography required for catheter placement to infuse vasopressin into bleeding vessel.

6. Monitor for vasopressin-induced fluid retention.
   A. Apprehension
   B. Decreased or absence of urinary output
   C. Abdominal cramps
   D. Severe decrease in serum sodium (hypotension, cold, clammy skin, rapid, thready pulse, and cyanosis)
7. Prepare client for surgical treatment of diverticulitis if client does not respond to conservative therapy.
   A. Colon resection
   B. Temporary colostomy in cases of perforation, peritonitis, obstruction, fistula formation—to drain abscesses, rest colon prior to anastomosis
8. Provide postoperative care.
   A. Provide meticulous wound care.
   B. Watch for signs of infection.
   C. Check drain sites frequently—observe for pus, foul odor, or fecal drainage.
   D. Change dressings as necessary.
   E. Monitor fluid intake and output.
   F. Observe for postoperative bleeding—decreased hemoglobin and hematocrit.
   G. Monitor other laboratory values—electrolytes, WBC, and RBC counts.
   H. Instruct patient to cough and deep breathe—to prevent atelectasis.
   I. Monitor IVs.
   J. Monitor patency and placement of NG tube.
9. Instruct client regarding disease process, diagnostic procedures, treatment, prevention, home care, and follow-up. Include teaching on:
   A. Colostomy care, if needed—arrange for visit by enterostomal therapist. Temporary colostomy may be closed 6–12 weeks after initial surgery.
   B. Avoidance of any activity that increases abdominal pressure, such as bending, wearing tight clothing around waist, and straining during bowel movement.
   C. Diet, stress management.

Evaluation

1. Reports increased comfort, decreased anxiety
2. Maintains adequate hydration and nutritional intake
3. Has no signs and symptoms
4. Demonstrates understanding of diagnostic procedures, treatment, prevention, home care (particularly colostomy care, if needed), and need for follow-up

Intestinal Obstruction

Description

1. Intestinal obstruction is partial or complete blockage of the lumen in the small or large intestine.
2. Decreased or absent peristaltic movement of intestinal contents due to mechanical or neurological disorders.
3. Mechanical disorders include such conditions as scar tissue, strangulated hernias, and tumors.
4. Neurological disorders include such conditions as paralytic ileus, which interferes with innervation, preventing normal peristaltic activity.
5. Pressure increased as peristaltic activity attempts to move intestinal contents within intestine resulting in:
   A. Dilation, atonicity of smooth muscle

B. Inhibition of flatus due to edema and decreased blood supply for elevated pressures
6. Collection of gas occurs in distended intestine.
   A. Bowel begins to secrete water, sodium, and potassium into fluid pooled in intestine.
   B. Loss of fluid and electrolytes cause electrolyte imbalance, dehydration, and hypovolemia.
7. Upper intestinal obstruction results in metabolic alkalosis from dehydration and loss of gastric hydrochloric acid.
8. Lower intestinal obstruction results in slower dehydration and loss of alkaline fluids leading to metabolic acidosis.
9. Small bowel obstruction is more common (90% of patients) and usually more serious.
10. Complete obstruction, if untreated, can cause death within hours from ischemia, necrosis, shock, and vascular collapse.
11. Intestinal obstruction more likely to occur after abdominal surgery or in persons with congenital defects of the bowel.
12. Causes
    A. Small-bowel obstruction
       (1) Adhesions, strangulated hernias
    B. Large-bowel obstruction
       (1) Carcinomas, tumors
    C. Obstruction due to mechanical disorders
       (1) Presence of foreign bodies such as fruit pits, gallstones, worms
       (2) Compression of intestinal wall due to:
          (a) Stenosis
          (b) Intussusception (telescoping of bowel)
          (c) Volvulus (twisting) of sigmoid or cecum
          (d) Tumors
          (e) Atresia
       (3) Obstruction due to physiological disturbances
          (a) Electrolyte imbalances
          (b) Toxicity (uremia, generalized infections)
          (c) Paralytic ileus
          (d) Spinal cord lesions
          (e) Thrombosis or embolism of mesenteric blood vessels
13. Three forms of intestinal obstruction
    A. Simple—intestinal contents blocked from passing, no other complications
    B. Strangulated—blockage of intestinal lumen causing lack of blood supply to part or all of obstructed section
    C. Close-looped—occlusion of both ends of the bowel section, isolated from rest of intestine

Assessment

SUBJECTIVE—SMALL-BOWEL OBSTRUCTION

1. Nausea
2. Colicky pain
3. Drowsiness
4. Thirst
5. Malaise, fatigue
6. Aching
7. Dry mucous membranes
8. Intestinal spasms
9. Persistent epigastric pain

SUBJECTIVE—LARGE-BOWEL OBSTRUCTION

1. Constipation
2. Colicky abdominal pain with spasms
3. Continuous hypogastric pain
4. Nausea

OBJECTIVE—SMALL-BOWEL OBSTRUCTION

1. Vomiting
2. Constipation
3. Abdominal distention
4. Presence of bowel sounds, borborygmi (rumbling in bowels)

OBJECTIVE—LARGE-BOWEL OBSTRUCTION

1. Constipation
2. Leakage of liquid stool around obstruction common in partial obstruction
3. Intestinal spasms
4. Fecal vomiting (usually absent at first)
5. Severe abdominal distention

DIAGNOSTIC TESTS AND METHODS

1. History
2. Physical examination
3. X-rays of flat plate of abdomen—shows presence and location of intestinal gas or fluid
4. Upper GI series
5. Barium enema
6. Laboratory studies—electrolytes, WBC count, amylase

Planning

1. Safe, effective care environment
   A. Prevent avoidable injury and/or infection.
   B. Increase client's and family's knowledge of disease process, diagnostic procedures, and treatment.
2. Physiological integrity
   A. Promote comfort.
   B. Maintain adequate hydration and electrolyte balance.
   C. Maintain NG drainage.
   D. Maintain effective breathing.
3. Psychosocial integrity
   A. Reduce anxiety and fear.
4. Health promotion and maintenance
   A. Increase client's and family's knowledge of home care and follow-up.

Implementation

1. Assess, record, and report signs and symptoms and reactions to treatment.
2. Provide emotional support.
3. Maintain NPO.
4. Monitor vital signs at least every 4 hours; report changes immediately.
5. Assist with gastric or intestinal decompression to decrease nausea and vomiting.
6. Monitor decompression tube; check and report amount and characteristics of drainage.
7. Monitor patency of decompression tube; irrigate with normal saline, if ordered.
8. Listen for presence or absence of bowel sounds; report presence of flatus or mucus through the rectum.
9. Place client in Fowler's position to facilitate breathing and decrease respiratory distress from abdominal distention.
10. Monitor for signs of metabolic alkalosis—changes in consciousness, slow, shallow respirations, hypertonic muscles, tetany.
11. Monitor for signs of metabolic acidosis—shortness of breath, disorientation; later—deep, rapid breathing, malaise, weakness.
12. Monitor urinary output—assessment of circulating blood volume, renal function, possible urinary retention due to bladder compression by distended intestine.
13. Administer and monitor IV therapy and electrolyte supplements.
14. Provide mouth and nose care.
15. Monitor for signs of dehydration.
16. Administer medications as prescribed.
17. Prepare client and family for surgery to relieve mechanical obstruction caused by adhesions and hernias.
18. Provide postoperative care.
    A. Encourage coughing, turning, and deep breathing exercises to promote ventilation.
    B. Monitor bowel sounds (return of peristalsis) and elimination; continue nasogastric drainage.
    C. Monitor fluid and electrolyte balance.
19. Administer pain medication as prescribed.
20. Assist with hygienic needs.
21. Provide quiet, restful environment and emotional support for client.
22. Monitor nutritional status; maintain total parenteral nutrition if necessary.
23. Encourage early ambulation.
24. Teach client and family colostomy care, if required.
25. Instruct client and family regarding disease process, diagnostic procedures, treatment, home care, and follow-up.

Evaluation

1. Reports increased comfort, decreased anxiety
2. Maintains adequate hydration and electrolyte balance
3. Maintains adequate nutritional intake
4. Has decreased or no abdominal distention
5. Maintains adequate bowel sounds, normal bowel movement pattern
6. Shows no evidence of abscess formation or drainage of purulent or fecal matter from drain or wound sites
7. Demonstrates understanding of disease process, diagnostic procedures, treatment, home care, and need for follow-up; similar understanding demonstrated by family

Hernias

Description

1. A hernia is a protrusion of an organ or structure through an abnormal opening of the containing wall of its cavity.
2. Categories of hernias
   A. Reducible: Organ or structure can be returned back into its normal position with relative ease.
   B. Irreducible: It cannot be returned into its normal position.
   C. Incarcerated: It cannot be reduced owing to formation of adhesions in hernial sac, causing an obstruction of intestinal flow.

D. Strangulated: Part of herniated intestine becomes twisted or edematous, cutting off blood supply and interfering with peristalsis. (This may lead to intestinal obstruction and necrosis.)

3. Types
   A. Umbilical hernia
      (1) This type of hernia is due to abnormal muscular structures around umbilical cord.
      (2) It is common in infants—often close spontaneously.
      (3) It is a severe congenital hernia in which abdominal viscera protrude—requires immediate repair.
      (4) It may occur in women who are obese or who have had several pregnancies.
   B. Inguinal hernia
      (1) The large or small intestine, omentum, or bladder protrudes into the inguinal canal.
      (2) This type of hernia is due to increased abdominal pressure.
      (3) It may be direct or indirect.
      (4) It is more common in males.
   C. Femoral hernia
      (1) This type of hernia occurs where femoral artery passes into femoral canal.
      (2) It is caused by an increase in abdominal pressure from pregnancy or obesity.
      (3) It is more common in females.
      (4) It usually appears as a swelling or bulge at the pulse point of the femoral artery.
      (5) It usually is a soft, reducible, nontender mass, which may become incarcerated or strangulated.
   D. Incisional hernia
      (1) Intestine or other structure protrudes through a previous incision.
      (2) This type of hernia is due to increased abdominal pressure and weakened abdominal wall.

4. Causes
   A. Congenital weakness in containing wall
   B. Weakness in containing wall due to previous incisional infections, aging process
   C. Increased intra-abdominal pressure—heavy lifting, pregnancy, obesity, or straining
   D. Improper closure of opening in peritoneal sac in males

Assessment

SUBJECTIVE

1. Presence of abdominal or inguinal mass after straining, coughing, or exertion
2. Possible pain
3. Swelling relieved by lying down
4. Sharp, steady pain in groin (inguinal hernia)
5. Severe pain, nausea with strangulated hernia
6. Signs of intestinal obstruction due to strangulated hernia
7. Anorexia

OBJECTIVE

1. Palpable mass in umbilical, inguinal, or femoral area
2. Signs of intestinal obstruction
   A. Vomiting
   B. Irreducible mass
   C. Diminished or absent bowel sounds
   D. Shock
   E. Increased temperature
   F. Bloody stools
3. Undescended testicle or hydrocele in infants

DIAGNOSTIC TESTS AND METHODS

1. History
2. Physical examination

Planning

1. Safe, effective care environment
   A. Increase client's and family's knowledge of disease process, diagnostic procedures, and treatment.
2. Physiological integrity
   A. Increase comfort.
   B. Maintain adequate fluid balance.
   C. Prevent postoperative complications.
3. Psychosocial integrity
   A. Reduce anxiety.
4. Health promotion and maintenance
   A. Increase client's and family's knowledge regarding home care (including activity) and follow-up.

Implementation

1. Assess, record, and report signs and symptoms and reactions to treatment.
2. Monitor vital signs.
3. Restrict activities.
4. Monitor intake and output.
5. Instruct in use of truss, if prescribed to keep hernia in place.
6. Observe for:
   A. Signs of strangulation
   B. Onset of pain
   C. Nausea and vomiting
   D. Abdominal distention
   E. Signs of shock
   F. Presence of blood in stools
7. Prepare client and family for surgical intervention, if required by client.
   A. Report symptoms of sneezing or upper respiratory tract infections prior to surgery. (They may cause tension and pressure on surgical repair site.)
   B. Types of surgical intervention
      (1) Herniorrhaphy—surgical replacement of protruding part into its containing cavity
      (2) Hernioplasty—surgical reinforcement of the containing wall to prevent recurrence
8. Postoperative care
   A. Monitor vital signs.
   B. Apply ice packs as ordered to control pain and swelling.
   C. Monitor urinary output following inguinal hernia repair.
   D. Monitor intake and output.
   E. Encourage deep breathing exercises.
   F. Administer pain medications as prescribed.
   G. Monitor incision site for signs of infection and edema.
   H. Monitor for signs of urinary retention.
   I. Monitor for signs of paralytic ileus.
   J. Assist with ambulation.

9. Instruct client and family regarding disease process, diagnostic procedures, treatment, home care, and follow-up. Include teaching on:
   A. Caring for incision.
   B. Checking for signs of infection.
   C. Restricting driving for at least 2 weeks.
   D. Restricting activities such as heavy lifting, pulling, or pushing for 6 weeks.
   E. Assuring that sexual activity is not affected.

Evaluation

1. Reports increased comfort, decreased anxiety
2. Maintains adequate hydration and nutritional intake
3. Has no signs and symptoms
4. Has no postoperative complications
5. Explains signs and symptoms related to incarceration and strangulation
6. Demonstrates understanding of disease process, diagnostic procedures, treatment, home care (including activity restrictions), and need for follow-up; similar understanding demonstrated by family

Hemorrhoids

Description

1. Hemorrhoids are varicosities or dilated hemorrhoidal veins in the rectal and anal area that interfere with venous return.
2. Condition may occur internally, externally, or both.
3. Incidence is highest in adults between ages 20 and 50 and involves both sexes.
4. Types
   A. First-degree hemorrhoids—may itch due to poor anal hygiene
   B. Second-degree hemorrhoids—may prolapse, usually painless and return to anal canal following a bowel movement
   C. Third-degree hemorrhoids—cause constant discomfort and prolapse due to increased intra-abdominal pressure; must be manually returned to anal canal.
5. Thrombosis of external hemorrhoids causes sudden rectal pain.
6. Severe or recurrent rectal bleeding may lead to secondary anemia with signs of pallor, fatigue, and weakness.
7. Probable cause—increased intravenous pressure in hemorrhoidal vessels.
8. Predisposing factors
   A. Occupation—extended periods of sitting or standing
   B. Pregnancy
   C. Heredity
   D. Straining due to constipation, diarrhea, coughing, sneezing, or vomiting
   E. Congestive heart failure, obstructed venous flow
   F. Hepatic disease, such as cirrhosis, amebic abscesses, or hepatitis
   G. Constipation
   H. Anorectal infections
   I. Loss of muscle tone (aging patterns)
   J. Rectal surgery
   K. Episiotomy
   L. Anal intercourse
   M. Obesity

Assessment

SUBJECTIVE

1. Rectal pain, itching
2. History of prior episodes
3. Painless intermittent rectal bleeding on defecation

OBJECTIVE

1. Prolapsed hemorrhoids
2. Bleeding
3. Thrombosis of hemorrhoid
   A. Edema
   B. Inflammation
   C. Intense pain
   D. Possible ischemia and ulceration

DIAGNOSTIC TESTS AND METHODS

1. History
2. Physical examination
3. Digital examination
4. Proctoscopy

Planning

1. Safe, effective care environment
   A. Increase client's and family's knowledge of disease process, diagnostic procedure, and treatment (particularly surgery).
2. Physiological integrity
   A. Increase comfort.
   B. Prevent constipation.
3. Psychosocial integrity
   A. Provide emotional support.
4. Health promotion and maintenance
   A. Increase client's and family's knowledge of home care and follow-up.

Implementation

1. Assess, record, and report signs and symptoms and reactions to treatment.
2. Provide privacy and time for bowel elimination.
3. Administer topical medications as prescribed to shrink mucous membranes—local anesthetic agents (lotions, creams, or suppositories); astringents; or cold compresses.
4. Administer stool softeners to keep stools soft and to prevent straining.
5. Assist with sitz bath to relieve pain.
6. Assist with comfort measures, supportive care.
7. Provide high-fiber diet to keep stools soft.
8. Assist with injection of sclerosing agent to produce scar tissue.
9. Assist with manual reduction of hemorrhoids as ordered.
10. Instruct client regarding treatment, prevention of constipation, increased fluid intake, high-fiber diet.
11. Provide information regarding surgical interventions such as ligation surgery (constriction impairs circulation; tissues become necrotic and slough off), sclerotherapy, freezing, infrared photocoagulation, or hemorrhoidectomy (surgical excision of hemorrhoids).
12. Postoperative care
    A. Check for signs of prolonged rectal bleeding.
    B. Administer analgesics as prescribed for pain.

C. Assist with sitz baths as prescribed.
D. Promote elimination (check stool).
E. Monitor vital signs.
F. Resume oral feedings as ordered (administer bulk medications following evening meal).
G. Provide meticulous wound hygiene.
13. Instruct client and family regarding disease process, diagnostic procedures, treatment, home care, and follow-up. Include teaching on:
   A. Avoiding stool softeners soon after hemorrhoidectomy—firm stools help to dilate anal strictures and to prevent scar tissue formation
   B. Importance of high-fiber foods, regular bowel habits, and good anal hygiene
   C. Use of medicated astringent pads and white toilet paper—chemicals in colored paper may irritate skin

Evaluation

1. Reports increased comfort, decreased anxiety
2. Reports absence of pain, bleeding, constipation
3. Has no signs of urinary retention
4. Maintains normal bowel elimination
5. Maintains adequate hydration and nutritional status
6. Demonstrates understanding of disease process, diagnostic procedures, treatment, home care (including medication, diet, and hygiene) and need for follow-up; similar understanding demonstrated by family

Appendicitis

Description

1. Appendicitis is an inflammation of the appendix.
2. Condition may result in edema, abscess, necrosis, and rupture causing peritonitis, the most common emergent complication of appendicitis.
3. It can occur at any age and affects both sexes.
4. It is more prevalent in males between puberty and age 30.
5. Incidence and death rate have declined owing to use of antibiotics.
6. Condition is fatal if untreated.
7. Causes
   A. Obstruction to lumen of appendix due to kinking, fecal mass, barium ingestion, viral infections, or foreign bodies
   B. Increased intraluminal pressure
   C. Reduced venous drainage
   D. Thrombosis
   E. Hemorrhage
   F. Edema
   G. Decreased resistance to organisms within body (intestinal flora)
   H. Appendiceal artery becomes occluded due to inflammation and venous stasis
   I. Perforation may result

Assessment

SUBJECTIVE

1. In the majority of cases, the initial pain is most often in epigastric or periumbilical areas.
2. Pain localizes in lower right abdomen (McBurney's point).

3. In other cases, diffuse or lower abdominal pain (referred pain) makes diagnosis more difficult.
4. Anorexia.
5. Nausea.
6. Increased tenderness in area.
7. **NOTE:** Sudden cessation of abdominal pain is indicative of rupture or infarction of appendix.

OBJECTIVE

1. Vomiting
2. Abdominal rigidity
3. Retractive respirations
4. Severe abdominal spasms
5. Rebound tenderness (**NOTE:** Rebound tenderness on left side is indicative of rupture or infarction of appendix.)
6. Constipation
7. Slight fever
8. Decreased bowel sounds
9. Tachycardia
10. Elevated WBC count (12,000–15,000/mm^3)—leukocytosis

DIAGNOSTIC TESTS AND METHODS

1. History
2. Physical examination
3. WBC
4. Routine urinalysis
5. Ruling out illnesses with similar symptoms—gastritis, colitis, diverticulitis, pancreatitis, renal colic, bladder infection, ectopic pregnancy, ovarian cyst, uterine disease, and intestinal obstruction

Planning

1. Safe, effective care environment
   A. Increase client's knowledge of disease process, diagnostic procedures, treatment (particularly surgery).
   B. Prevent postoperative complications.
2. Physiological integrity
   A. Increase comfort.
3. Psychosocial integrity
   A. Reduce anxiety.
4. Health promotion and maintenance
   A. Increase client's knowledge of home care, postoperative care, and follow-up.

Implementation

1. Assess, record, and report signs and symptoms and reactions to treatment.
2. Maintain bed rest.
3. Place client in Fowler's position to decrease pain.
4. Use ice packs to abdomen as prescribed.
5. Keep client NPO.
6. Administer and monitor IV fluids to prevent dehydration.
7. Monitor electrolytes.
8. Administer sedatives and antibiotics as prescribed—remember that narcotics can mask symptoms.
9. Monitor vital signs.
10. Do not apply heat to abdomen—may cause appendix to rupture.
11. Do not administer cathartics or enemas—may cause rupture.

12. Prepare client and family for surgical intervention.
13. If perforation is likely, initiate NG suction if ordered.
14. Provide postoperative care.
    A. Monitor vital signs.
    B. Monitor intake and output.
15. Administer analgesics and antibiotics as prescribed.
16. Monitor, report, and record bowel sounds—sign of return of peristalsis, indicating readiness to resume oral fluid intake.
17. Encourage deep breathing, coughing, and changing position.
18. Monitor dressing and operative site for drainage, signs of infection.
19. Encourage ambulation as soon as possible.
20. Encourage progressive nutrition.
21. Observe for complications.
    A. Continuing pain may be due to intra-abdominal abscess formation or mechanical small-bowel obstruction.
    B. Complaint of "something gave away" may be indicative of wound dehiscence.
    C. Symptoms suggestive of peritonitis.
22. Instruct client regarding disease process, diagnostic procedures, treatment, home care, postoperative care, and follow-up.

Evaluation

1. Reports increased comfort, decreased anxiety
2. Remains free of infection and other complications
3. Demonstrates understanding of disease process, diagnostic procedures, treatment (particularly surgery), home care, postoperative care (including reason for withholding pain medication), and need for follow-up

Peritonitis

Description

1. Peritonitis is an acute or chronic inflammation of the peritoneum (membrane lining the abdominal cavity and covering the visceral organs).
2. Inflammation may extend throughout peritoneum or may be localized.
3. It may affect organs of abdominal cavity—adhesions, abscesses, and obstruction.
4. Intestinal motility decreases resulting in intestinal distention with gas.
5. Mortality is approximately 10%, most often due to bowel obstruction.
6. Mortality was much higher before the advent of antibiotics.
7. Causes
    A. Bacterial inflammation
       (1) Bacterial invasion of peritoneum, usually from inflammation and perforation of GI tract.
       (2) Common causes include appendicitis, diverticulitis, peptic ulcer, ulcerative colitis, volvulus, strangulated obstruction, abdominal neoplasm, or stab wound.
       (3) Common organisms include streptococci, staphylococci, *E. coli*, pneumococci, and gonococci.
    B. Chemical inflammation—rupture of ovarian tube or bladder, perforation of gastric ulcer, or release of pancreatic enzymes.
8. In both bacterial and chemical inflammation, the body's normal immune response results in redness, edema, accumulation of fluids containing protein and electrolytes; adhesions, and abscess.

Assessment

SUBJECTIVE

1. Sudden, severe, and diffuse abdominal pain
2. Nausea
3. Weakness
4. Oliguria
5. Thirst
6. Shoulder pain—due to inflammation of diaphragmatic peritoneum

OBJECTIVE

1. Excessive sweating
2. Vomiting
3. Cold skin—due to excess loss of fluid, electrolytes, and protein into abdominal cavity
4. Decreased or absent bowel sounds—due to effect of bacterial toxins on intestinal muscles
5. Hypotension
6. Signs of dehydration—dry swollen tongue, pinched skin
7. Abdominal rigidity
8. Rebound tenderness
9. Increased temperature (<103°F)
10. Hiccups—due to inflammation of diaphragmatic peritoneum
11. Abdominal distention with upward displacement of diaphragm
12. Decreased respiratory capacity—tendency to breathe shallowly
13. Symptoms of shock
14. Elevated WBC count (>20,000/mm^3)

DIAGNOSTIC TESTS AND METHODS

1. History
2. Physical examination
3. Laboratory tests—WBC count, electrolytes, blood culture
4. Abdominal x-rays
5. Chest x-ray—may show elevated diaphragm
6. Paracentesis—reveals bacteria, exudate, blood, pus, or urine
7. Laparotomy—may be required to identify underlying cause

Planning

1. Safe, effective care environment
    A. Prepare for NG tube insertion.
    B. Increase client's and family's knowledge of disease process, diagnostic procedures, and treatment (particularly surgery).
2. Physiological integrity
    A. Increase comfort.
    B. Maintain adequate fluid and electrolyte balance.
    C. Control, eliminate infection.
    D. Prevent postoperative complications.
3. Psychosocial integrity
    A. Reduce anxiety.

4. Health promotion and maintenance
   A. Increase client's and family's knowledge of home care, postoperative care, and follow-up.

Implementation

1. Assess, report, and record signs and symptoms and reactions to treatment.
2. Maintain bed rest.
3. Place in semi-Fowler position.
4. Assist with intestinal decompression—explain NG tube insertion.
5. Administer and monitor IV and electrolytes.
6. Administer antibiotics as prescribed.
7. Keep client NPO.
8. Monitor fluid intake and output.
9. Monitor amount and characteristics of NG drainage or vomitus.
10. Administer oral hygiene.
11. Explain surgical procedure to family, if surgery is required.
12. Administer preoperative analgesics as prescribed.
13. Perform postoperative care.
    A. Administer postoperative analgesics, antibiotics, and sedatives as prescribed; monitor for side effects.
    B. Monitor IV and electrolytes.
    C. Accurately record and report fluid intake and output, including NG and incisional drainage.
    D. Support patient and allay anxiety.
    E. Observe for disorientation—keep side rails up.
    F. Encourage and assist with ambulation as ordered.
    G. Watch for signs of dehiscence and abscess.
    H. Assess bowel sounds frequently for peristaltic motility (abdomen, soft, distended) to determine peristaltic status.
14. Increase oral fluids as prescribed following return of peristalsis, normal temperature, and pulse rate.
15. Instruct client and family regarding disease process, diagnostic procedures, treatment, home care, postoperative care, and follow-up.

Evaluation

1. Reports increased comfort, decreased anxiety
2. Remains free of infection
3. Remains free of other postoperative complications
4. Demonstrates understanding of disease process, diagnostic procedures, treatment, home care, postoperative care, and need for follow-up; similar understanding demonstrated by family

Colorectal Cancer, Polyps

Description

1. Cancer of the colon and rectum may be in the form of a well-defined tumor or cancerous polyp.
2. It is the second most common neoplasm in the United States.
3. Incidence is equally distributed among males and females.
4. Highest incidence is in adults older than 60 years.
5. Almost always adenocarcinoma. (Approximately 50% are lesions in the rectosigmoid area, and remaining 50% constitute polypoid lesions.)

6. Neoplasm tends to progress slowly and remain localized for a long period of time.
7. It is potentially curable in 80%–90% of patients if diagnosed early.
8. The overall 5-year survival rate is nearing 50% owing to improvements in diagnosis and early treatment.
9. Graded according to cellular differentiation.
   A. Well differentiated
   B. Moderately well-differentiated
   C. Poorly differentiated
   D. Anaplastic
10. Prognosis can be related to the grade, with grade 1 the most favorable in terms of patient survival.
11. Tumor spread occurs in several ways:
    A. Spread within layers of bowel wall
    B. Spread to the lymphatic and lymph nodes
    C. Spread via the bloodstream
    D. Spread across peritoneum
    E. Spread to suture lines, abdominal incisions, or drain sites
12. Secondary effects of tumor growth include:
    A. Occlusion of the lumen of the bowel with accompanying obstruction, ulceration of the bowel, and hemorrhage.
    B. Tumor penetration resulting in perforation with abscess, fistula formation, and secondary tumor deposit to adjacent tissues
13. Dukes' method of staging
    A. Stage A—cancer confined to bowel wall
    B. Stage B—cancer has penetrated the bowel into surrounding rectal tissue with no lymph involvement.
    C. Stage C—lymph node involvement, with possible growth through the bowel wall
    D. Stage D—nonresectable growths
14. Cause—unknown
15. Predisposing factors
    A. Relationship to diet—excess animal fat and low fiber
    B. History of ulcerative colitis, Crohn's disease
    C. History of familial polyps and/or colorectal cancer
    D. Previous history of colorectal cancer
    E. Previous pelvic irradiation

Assessment

SUBJECTIVE

1. Initially vague symptoms
2. Abdominal aching, pressure, or cramps
3. Weakness, fatigue
4. Dizziness
5. Loss of appetite, nausea
6. Change in bowel habits and shape of stool
7. Signs of obstruction in left colon
   A. Intermittent abdominal fullness or cramping
   B. Rectal pressure, dull and constant ache in rectal or sacral region
   C. Relief of pain following passage of gas or stool

OBJECTIVE

1. Black, tarry stools
2. Presence of anemia
3. Exertional dyspnea
4. Diarrhea, obstipation

5. Vomiting
6. Signs of intestinal obstruction
7. Possible palpable tumor—right side
8. Rectal bleeding
9. Ribbon- or pencil-shaped stool
10. Dark red blood and mucus in feces
11. Cachexia

DIAGNOSTIC TESTS AND METHODS

1. History
2. Physical examination
3. Digital examination to palpate abnormalities
4. Hemoccult test (guaiac)—to detect blood in stools
5. Proctoscopy or sigmoidoscopy
6. Flexible fiberoptic sigmoidoscopy
7. Colonoscopy—to permit visual inspection and access for biopsy of tissue
8. Intravenous pyelography—to assess kidney function
9. Barium x-ray—to detect lesions
10. Carcinoembryonic antigen (CEA) (blood test that is helpful in monitoring patients before and after treatment)—to detect metastasis or recurrence
11. Appropriate body scans if CEA is elevated
12. Serum alkaline phosphatase or bilirubin levels if liver involvement suspected
13. Tumor biopsy—to verify disease

Planning

1. Safe, effective care environment
   A. Increase comfort.
   B. Increase client's knowledge of disease process, diagnostic procedures, and treatment (particularly surgery).
   C. Prevent infection.
2. Physiological integrity
   A. Maintain adequate nutrition.
   B. Prevent postoperative complications.
3. Psychosocial integrity
   A. Assist in developing effective coping mechanisms.
4. Health promotion and maintenance
   A. Increase client's knowledge of home care, postoperative care, and follow-up.

Implementation

1. Assess, record, and report signs and symptoms and reactions to treatment.
2. Monitor vital signs at least every 4 hours.
3. Monitor intake and output.
4. Provide emotional support.
5. Administer medications as prescribed; monitor for side effects.
6. Prepare client and family for surgical intervention.
7. Factors involved in choosing appropriate operative procedure include:
   A. Location of tumor
   B. Obstruction or perforation of bowel
   C. Possible metastasis
   D. Fitness of the patient
   E. Surgeon's preferences
8. Procedure for condition without obstruction includes:
   A. Procedure varies with location of tumor
   B. Portion of bowel on either side of tumor is removed

C. End-to-end anastomosis is performed between the divided ends
   D. Amount and extent of bowel resection depends on location and blood supply to the segment involved.
9. Procedure for condition with obstruction of the bowel includes:
   A. One-stage resection with anastomosis
   B. Two-stage resection with either resection and exteriorization of the ends as a temporary colostomy, with closure performed later.
   C. Three-stage resection with a loop colostomy, followed by resection 2–3 weeks later, with closure performed later.
10. Instruct client regarding disease process, diagnostic procedures, treatment, home care, postoperative care, and follow-up.

Evaluation

1. Consumes sufficient nutrients to maintain body weight
2. Is able to make informed decisions about care
3. Verbalizes preferences for pain control methods and expectations of surgery outcome
4. Demonstrates postoperatively an understanding of ostomy care

Cholelithiasis, Choledocholithiasis, Cholangitis, Cholecystitis

Description

1. Cholelithiasis
   A. Cholelithiasis is the presence of stones or calculi (gallstones) in the gallbladder.
   B. Stones are made up of cholesterol, calcium bilirubinate, or a mixture of cholesterol and bilirubin pigment.
   C. Fifth leading cause of hospitalization among adults.
   D. Condition accounts for approximately 90% of all gallbladder and bile duct disease.
   E. Prognosis usually good with treatment unless infection occurs.
   F. If infection occurs, prognosis depends on severity and response to antibiotics.
   G. Causes
      (1) Inflammation of biliary tract resulting in increased absorption of bile salts, which in turn decrease the solubility of cholesterol.
      (2) Metabolic alterations resulting from periods of sluggishness in gallbladder due to pregnancy, diabetes mellitus, oral contraception, celiac disease, cirrhosis of the liver, and pancreatitis.
2. Choledocholithiasis
   A. Choledocholithiasis is the presence of gallstones in the hepatic and bile ducts.
   B. Obstruction of bile flow into duodenum.
   C. Condition leads to elevated bilirubin level, jaundice, and interference with fat and fat-soluble vitamin absorption.
   D. Progress usually good unless infection occurs.
3. Cholangitis
   A. Cholangitis is infection of the bile duct.
   B. It is often associated with choledocholithiasis.

C. It may follow percutaneous cholangiography.
D. Inflammatory process may cause fibrosis and stenosis of common bile duct.
E. Predisposing factors
   (1) Bacterial alteration of bile salts
   (2) Metabolic alteration of bile salts
4. Cholecystitis
A. Cholecystitis is acute or chronic inflammation of gallbladder.
B. It is usually associated with impacted gallstone in the cystic duct.
C. Painful distention of gallbladder.
D. Accounts for 10%–25% of patients needing gallbladder surgery.
E. Acute form common in middle-aged adults.
F. Chronic form common among elderly.
G. Prognosis—good with treatment.

Assessment

SUBJECTIVE

1. Acute abdominal pain in right upper quadrant following meals rich in fats
2. Pain radiating to back, between shoulders, or to front of chest
3. Intolerance to fat
4. Indigestion, flatulence
5. Nausea
6. Chills
7. Weakness, fatigue
8. Pruritus

OBJECTIVE

1. Belching
2. Profuse sweating
3. Vomiting
4. Jaundice
5. Abdominal distention
6. Absence of bowel sounds in severe cholangitis
7. Elevated WBC count
8. Elevated bilirubin level
9. Clay colored stool
10. Dark colored urine
11. Increase in temperature, heart rate, respiration, and blood pressure
12. Stones observed on cholecystogram
13. Prolonged PT due to interference with vitamin K absorption
14. Easy bruising

DIAGNOSTIC TESTS AND METHODS

1. History
2. Physical examination
3. Laboratory studies—WBC, total bilirubin, urine bilirubin, icteric index, alkaline phosphatase, PT
4. Differential diagnosis—to rule out MI, angina, pancreatitis, pneumonia, peptic ulcer, hiatus hernia, esophagitis, and gastritis
5. Serum amylase levels—to differentiate between gallbladder disease and pancreatitis
6. Serial enzyme tests and ECG—to rule out heart disease
7. Oral cholecystography
8. IV cholangiography

Planning

1. Safe, effective care environment
   A. Ensure that surgical client remains free from postoperative complications.
2. Physiological integrity
   A. Ensure that client's fluid and electrolyte levels are balanced.
   B. Ensure that client is free from pain and discomfort.
3. Health promotion and maintenance
   A. Ensure that client observes proper dietary measures to avoid further attacks of cholelithiasis or cholecystitis.

Implementation

1. Nonsurgical
   A. Administer ursodiol orally to dissolve stones.
   B. Assist with endoscopic retrograde cholangiopancreatography (ERCP) or endoscopic papillotomy (EPT)
2. Surgical
   A. Provide postoperative care of the client with laparoscopic laser cholecystectomy.
   B. Provide postoperative care of the client with abdominal cholecystectomy.
      (1) Observe Jackson-Pratt drain or Penrose drain—should produce <50 mL of blood-tinged drainage.
      (2) Observe T-tube drainage—should produce up to 500 cc during first 24 hours.
      (3) Clamp T-tube as directed.

Evaluation

1. Remains pain free after meals
2. Maintains compliance with diet
3. If postoperative, returns to preoperative level of activity

Hepatitis

Description

1. Hepatitis is inflammation of the liver caused by viral agents, bacteria, or exposure to toxic chemicals.
2. Marked liver destruction, necrosis, and autolysis
3. Complications include:
   A. Chronic persistent hepatitis—may be benign
   B. Chronic aggressive hepatitis
      (1) Approximately 25% die from hepatic failure
   C. Fulminating hepatitis
      (1) Life-threatening complication.
      (2) Condition develops in about 1% of patients, causing hepatic failure with encephalopathy.
      (3) It progresses to coma and death in approximately 2 weeks.
4. Preventive measures include:
   A. Enteric precautions
   B. Good hand-washing technique
   C. Vaccination and immune globulin therapy
   D. Avoidance of contact with blood or body fluids
   E. Avoid recapping needles
5. Forms
   A. Hepatitis A
      (1) Highly infectious (short-incubation hepatitis).
      (2) Hepatitis A caused by hepatitis virus A (HAV).
      (3) It is usually transmitted by contact with feces or contaminated water or food.

(4) It is occasionally transmitted parenterally.

(5) Outbreaks often occur following ingestion of contaminated seafood.

(6) Incubation period is 15–50 days.

(7) Condition tends to be benign and self-limiting.

(8) High-risk individuals include children, travelers to developing countries, personnel providing health care to others.

B. Hepatitis B

(1) Serum (long-incubation hepatitis).

(2) Hepatitis B is caused by hepatitis virus B (HBV) DNA virus.

(3) It rarely occurs in epidemics.

(4) It has a higher mortality than type A hepatitis.

(5) It is transmitted:

  (a) Parenterally by blood transfusion or contaminated needles.

  (b) Through contact with mucous membranes.

  (c) Through exposure or direct contact with sexual partners or healthcare workers.

(6) May be spread through contact with human secretions and feces.

(7) Incidence is rising among homosexuals (oral and sexual contact).

(8) Incubation period is 45–160 days.

(9) High-risk individuals include users of parenteral drugs, healthcare workers in contact with contaminated blood or body fluids.

(10) May progress to a chronic form.

6. Hepatitis C

A. Mildest course of all types of hepatitis.

B. Caused by an RNA virus.

C. Transmitted parenterally by blood transfusion or needlestick.

D. Incubation period is 14–150 days.

E. High-risk individuals include those receiving blood transfusions or in contact with contaminated blood.

F. May progress to a chronic form.

7. Hepatitis D—caused by an incomplete RNA virus and occurs as a complication of hepatitis B

8. Hepatitis E—caused by an RNA virus with an incubation period of 2–9 weeks. Occurs mainly in developing countries.

Assessment

SUBJECTIVE—PREICTERIC PHASE (LASTS 1 WEEK)

1. Chills
2. Anorexia, nausea
3. Malaise, weakness, fatigue
4. Headache
5. Photophobia
6. Pharyngitis
7. Cough
8. Respiratory difficulty—especially in type A
9. Arthralgia—especially to type B
10. Alterations in sense of taste and smell
11. Loss of desire to smoke, drink alcohol

SUBJECTIVE—ICTERIC PHASE (LASTS 2–6 WEEKS)

1. Mild weight loss
2. Continuation of anorexia
3. Discomfort and pain in upper abdominal quadrant
4. Increased nausea
5. Increased malaise and weakness
6. Increased respiratory difficulty
7. Pruritus
8. Irritability

SUBJECTIVE—POSTICTERIC PHASE (LASTS 2–6 WEEKS WITH FULL RECOVERY IN 6 MONTHS)

1. Decline in nausea, anorexia, and dyspnea
2. Increased comfort
3. Weakness decreased

OBJECTIVE—PREICTERIC PHASE

1. Dyspnea
2. Vomiting
3. Cough, coryza
4. Elevated temperature
5. Liver and lymph node enlargement

OBJECTIVE—ICTERIC PHASE

1. Dark urine
2. Clay-colored stools
3. Yellow sclera
4. Liver remains tender and enlarged
5. Pain in right upper quadrant
6. Splenomegaly
7. Cervical adenopathy
8. Bile obstruction
9. Onset of jaundice
10. Elevated serum bilirubin levels
11. Elevated bilirubin and urobilinogen in urine
12. Prolonged PT and PTT (partial thromboplastin time)
13. Elevated AST, ALT, alkaline phosphate
14. Decreased serum albumin

OBJECTIVE—POSTICTERIC PHASE

1. Decreased jaundice
2. Decreased dyspnea, anorexia
3. Resolution of abnormal laboratory test results

DIAGNOSTIC TESTS AND METHODS

1. History
2. Physical examination
3. Presence of hepatitis B surface antigens (HB$_s$AG) and hepatitis B antibodies (anti-HB$_s$)—confirms type B hepatitis
4. Presence of anti-HAV antibody—confirms type A hepatitis
5. Absence of anti-HAV, HB$_s$AG, and anti-HB$_s$—confirms hepatitis C
6. PT
7. ALT, AST levels, serum alkaline phosphatase
8. Serum albumin, globulin, and bilirubin
9. Urine bilirubin
10. Cephalin flocculation and thymol turbidity levels
11. Liver biopsy
12. A CT scan of liver

Planning

1. Safe, effective care environment
   A. Prevent further infection.
   B. Prevent injury from prolonged bleeding and fatigue.
   C. Prevent injury to skin.
   D. Maintain enteric isolation precautions.

E. Increase client's and family's knowledge of disease process, diagnostic procedures, and treatment.
2. Physiological integrity
   A. Increase comfort.
   B. Maintain adequate fluid and nutritional intake.
3. Psychosocial integrity
   A. Prevent social isolation.
4. Health promotion and maintenance
   A. Increase client's and family's knowledge of prevention (including available immunizations), home care, and follow-up.

Implementation

1. Assess, report, and record signs and symptoms and reactions to treatment.
2. Provide restful environment.
3. Assist with comfort measures.
4. Provide emotional support.
5. Monitor intake and output.
6. Monitor body weight.
7. Provide and encourage adequate caloric intake (po or IV).
8. Limit visitors and impose isolation precautions.
9. Encourage fluid intake.
10. Observe feces for color, consistency, frequency, and amount.
11. Watch for signs of dehydration, pneumonia, vascular problems, decubitus ulcers, and hepatic coma.
12. Administer prescribed medications such as antiemetics, antibiotics, vitamin K, antihistamines, corticosteroids, fluid and electrolyte replacement.
13. For patients with fulminant hepatitis:
    A. Maintain electrolyte balance.
    B. Maintain patent airway.
14. Control bleeding.
15. Administer prescribed medications to correct hypoglycemia.
16. Provide rest periods.
17. Monitor laboratory results.
18. Monitor for signs of bleeding.
19. Check skin integrity.
20. Instruct client and family regarding disease process, treatment, diagnostic procedures, prevention (such as enteric isolation procedure), home care, and follow-up.

Evaluation

1. Reports increased comfort, decreased anxiety
2. Shows no signs of injury and/or infection
3. Maintains adequate fluid and nutritional intake
4. Demonstrates understanding of disease process, diagnostic procedures, treatment, prevention (such as enteric isolation procedure), home care, and need for follow-up; similar understanding demonstrated by family

Cirrhosis of the Liver

Description

1. Cirrhosis of the liver is a chronic hepatic disease with diffuse destruction and fibrotic regeneration of liver cells.
2. Liver structure and vasculature are altered, resulting in impaired blood and lymph flow leading to hepatic insufficiency.
3. Prevalent among malnourished chronic alcoholics over 50 years of age.
4. Cirrhosis is 50% more common in men than in women.
5. Mortality is high.
6. Five types of cirrhosis exist.
   A. Portal, nutritional, or alcoholic cirrhosis (Laennec's type)
      (1) Most common—30–50% of clients, up to 90% with history of alcoholism
      (2) Liver damage primarily from malnutrition, especially lack of protein
   B. Biliary cirrhosis
      (1) Affects 15%–20% of clients
      (2) Results from bile duct diseases which disrupt bile flow
   C. Postnecrotic (posthepatic) cirrhosis
      (1) Affects 10%–30% of clients
      (2) Results from various types of hepatitis
   D. Cardiac cirrhosis
      (1) Rare condition
      (2) Liver damage caused by right heart failure
   E. Idiopathic cirrhosis
      (1) Affects about 10% of clients
      (2) Has no known cause

Assessment

SUBJECTIVE

1. GI symptoms—anorexia, indigestion, nausea, constipation, flatus, dull abdominal ache
2. Respiratory difficulties
3. CNS—lethargy, mental changes
4. Hematological—easy bruising
5. Endocrine—menstrual irregularities
6. Skin—itching
7. Miscellaneous—fatigue, pain in upper right abdomen

OBJECTIVE

1. GI system—vomiting, diarrhea, or constipation
2. Respiratory system—decreased thoracic expansion due to abdominal ascites
3. Decreased gas exchange—hypoxia
4. CNS—slurred speech, asterixis, peripheral neuritis, hallucinations, unconsciousness, and coma
5. Hematological—nosebleeds, bruising, bleeding gums, anemia, increased bleeding time
6. Endocrine—testicular atrophy, menstrual irregularities, loss of hair on chest and axillary region
7. Skin—pruritus, poor tissue turgor, extreme dryness, spider angiomas, palmar erythema, jaundice
8. Hepatic—jaundice, ascites, edema of legs, enlarged liver, hepatorenal syndrome, hypoglycemia
9. Miscellaneous—enlarged superficial abdominal veins, muscle atrophy, palpable liver or spleen, elevated temperature, bleeding from esophageal varices due to portal hypertension, hypernatremia, hypoalbuminemia
10. Elevated AST, ALT, LDH, bilirubin, ammonia

DIAGNOSTIC TESTS AND METHODS

1. History
2. Physical examination
3. Laboratory studies—WBC count, hemoglobin, hematocrit, albumin, bilirubin, alkaline phosphatase, serum

ammonia, serum electrolytes, globulin, thymol turbidity, AST, ALT, LDH, PT, PTT
4. Bromsulphalein (BSP) excretion test
5. Glucose tolerance test (GTT)
6. Urine bilirubin
7. Fecal urobilinogen
8. Liver biopsy
9. Cholecystography
10. Cholangiography
11. Splenoportal venography
12. Percutaneous transhepatic cholangiography

Planning

1. Safe, effective care environment
   A. Prevent avoidable injury and/or infection.
   B. Increase client's and family's knowledge of disease process, diagnostic procedures, and treatment.
2. Physiological integrity
   A. Increase comfort.
   B. Maintain fluid and electrolyte balance.
   C. Maintain adequate nutritional status.
   D. Prevent alterations in skin integrity.
3. Psychosocial integrity
   A. Provide counseling on alcohol consumption and self-concept.
4. Health promotion and maintenance
   A. Increase client's and family's knowledge regarding home care and follow-up.

Implementation

1. Assess, report, and record signs and symptoms and reactions to treatment.
2. Monitor skin, gums, stools, and emesis for bleeding tendencies.
3. Apply pressure to injection sites to prevent bleeding.
4. Advise client not to take aspirin, blow nose, strain during bowel movement, sneeze.
5. Monitor weight daily.
6. Measure abdominal girth daily.
7. Monitor sacrum, legs, and ankles for presence of dependent edema.
8. Monitor vital signs.
9. Monitor electrolytes and other laboratory results.
10. Monitor intake and output accurately.
11. Assist with comfort measures.
12. Provide emotional support.
13. Provide counseling on alcoholic consumption. Encourage client to refrain from hepatotoxins such as alcohol and acetaminophen.
14. Provide good oral hygiene.
15. Place in high Fowler position to assist in breathing when ascites is present.
16. Prepare patient for paracentesis or surgery for placement of LaVeen shunt, if necessary.
17. Administer prescribed medication such as diuretics, vitamin A, C, K, and folic acid; electrolyte supplements; IV fluids; antiemetics; antihistamines; albumin.
18. Monitor skin integrity; use lubricating lotion in place of soap when giving skin care to prevent skin breakdown in clients who have edema and pruritus.
19. Provide diet with high protein, high carbohydrates, and vitamins. (High-protein diet is contraindicated in presence of portal system encephalopathy because liver is not able to metabolize amino acids or ammonia. Proteins are broken down to amino acids.)
20. Instruct client and family regarding disease process, diagnostic procedures, treatment (including medication), home care, prevention, and follow-up.

Evaluation

1. Reports increased comfort, decreased anxiety
2. Maintains adequate fluid and electrolyte balance
3. Maintains effective breathing pattern
4. Reduced ascites and edema
5. Shows no signs of injury and/or infection
6. Maintains skin integrity
7. Maintains adequate nutrition
8. Demonstrates understanding of disease process, diagnostic procedures, treatment, prevention, home care, and need for follow-up; similar understanding demonstrated by family

Pancreatitis

Description

1. Pancreatitis is inflammation of the pancreas.
2. Forms
   A. Acute—occurs suddenly, one attack or recurrent, but resolves
   B. Chronic—continuous inflammation and destruction of pancreas with proliferations of scar tissue in place of normal pancreatic tissue
3. Inflammation may be due to edema, necrosis, or hemorrhage.
4. It is commonly associated with alcoholism, trauma, or peptic ulcer in men.
5. It is also commonly associated with biliary tract disease in females.
6. Prognosis is poor when condition is due to alcoholism.
7. Prognosis is good when condition is due to biliary tract disease.
8. Mortality rises up to 60% when condition is associated with necrosis and hemorrhage.
9. Causes
   A. Most common causes are biliary tract disease and alcoholism.
   B. Other causes include pancreatic carcinoma, trauma, certain drugs, complication of peptic ulcer, mumps, or hypothermia.
   C. Rare causes include stenosis or obstruction of sphincter of Oddi, metabolic endocrine disorders, vascular diseases, viral infections, and pregnancy.
10. Causes may stimulate activation of autodigestion mechanism of specific enzymes within the pancreas, leading to edema, hemorrhage, coagulation, necrosis, fat and cell destruction.
11. An increased permeability of the vascular bed occurs leading to further edema.
12. Damaged islets of Langerhans can lead to complications including diabetes mellitus.
13. Fulminant pancreatitis causes massive hemorrhage and

destruction of pancreatic tissue, ending in diabetic acidosis, shock, coma and/or death.

Assessment

SUBJECTIVE

1. Abdominal discomfort, pain centered close to umbilicus unrelieved by vomiting
2. Severe attack—causes severe abdominal pain
3. Relief of pain by drawing knees up
4. Malaise
5. Restlessness
6. Nausea
7. History of alcohol intake, previous trauma, surgery, gallbladder disease
8. Chills
9. Weight loss

OBJECTIVE

1. Severe attack—persistent vomiting, abdominal rigidity, diminished bowel sounds, rales at bases of lungs, left pleural effusion
2. Dehydration
3. Elevated temperature
4. Tachycardia
5. Cold, sweaty extremities
6. Elevated enzyme levels
7. Elevated WBC count, bilirubin, blood glucose, serum amylase, serum lipase, hematocrit
8. Decreased serum calcium
9. ECG changes—prolonged QT segment, normal T wave
10. Abdominal x-ray—dilation of small or large intestine
11. GI series—pressure on duodenum or stomach due to edema of pancreas head
12. Paracentesis—exceedingly high amylase levels
13. Positive stool test results for meat fibers, fat
14. Chronic pancreatitis
15. Chronic form—calcification on CT scan or ultrasound

DIAGNOSTIC TESTS AND METHODS

1. History
2. Physical examination
3. Laboratory tests—serum amylase, serum lipase, serum calcium, WBC, serum glucose, hematocrit
4. Routine ECG
5. Abdominal x-ray
6. GI series
7. Chest x-ray
8. Paracentesis
9. Ultrasonography—to identify gallstones, a pancreatic mass, or pseudocyst.
10. CT scan with or without vascular enhancement.
11. Endoscopic retrograde cholangiopancreatography (ERCP)—to diagnose pancreatic cancer. Differentiates inflammation and fibrosis from cancer.

Planning

1. Safe, effective care environment
   A. Assist with self-care needs.
   B. Increase client's and family's knowledge of disease process, diagnostic procedures, and treatment.
2. Physiological integrity
   A. Increase comfort.
   B. Maintain adequate nutrition.
   C. Maintain fluid and electrolyte balance.
3. Psychosocial integrity
   A. Counsel on alcohol intake.
4. Health promotion and maintenance
   A. Increase client's and family's knowledge of home care and follow-up.

Implementation

1. Assess, record, and report signs and symptoms and reactions to treatment.
2. Position client to relieve pain.
3. Keep client NPO—allows pancreas to rest.
4. Explain and assist in insertion of NG tube—allows pancreas to rest.
5. Monitor intake and output.
6. Monitor vital signs continuously.
7. Provide meticulous supportive care.
8. Monitor PAP closely, if present.
9. Monitor CVP line closely, if present.
10. Monitor fluid intake and output hourly.
11. Monitor electrolyte levels, BUN, creatinine.
12. Assist in administration of IV fluids or blood as ordered.
13. Assist in administration of plasma or plasma expanders to maintain blood pressure, if ordered.
14. Assess for rales, decreased breath sounds.
15. Maintain constant NG suctioning to decompress bowel, if required.
16. Provide good mouth care.
17. Provide emotional support.
18. Start client on clear liquids progressing to bland low-fat diet in small feedings daily once oral intake is ordered.
19. Monitor for signs and symptoms of complications, such as hyperglycemia or hypoglycemia, respiratory difficulties.
20. Instruct client and family regarding disease process, diagnostic procedures, treatment, home care, and follow-up. Include teaching on:
   A. Avoidance of alcohol
   B. Maintaining adequate nutrition
   C. Medications

Evaluation

1. Reports increased comfort, decreased anxiety
2. Maintains adequate nutritional intake
3. Maintains fluid and electrolyte balance
4. Demonstrates understanding of disease process, diagnostic procedures, treatment, home care, and need for follow-up; similar understanding demonstrated by family

Integumentary System (Skin)

Description

1. The skin acts as the body's barrier and protector from the environment.
   A. The functions of the skin include temperature regulation, sensation, and excretion of small amounts of water and sodium chloride.

B. It protects the body tissues and organs from external insults such as injury.

C. Melanin in the epidermis absorbs ultraviolet light and decreases its damaging effect on the subepidermal layers.
   (1) Ultraviolet light does have a damaging effect on the germinal layer of the epidermis, especially in those individuals with fair complexions.
   (2) Individuals with fair complexions have less melanin than dark-skinned individuals.
   (3) The risk of damage to the germinal layer of the epidermis is proportional to the intensity and duration of the individual's exposure to the ultraviolet radiation.
   (4) Excretion, although not a primary function of the skin, does contain a variety of waste products; skin odor can give clues as to health status and cleanliness.

D. Proper nutrition, hydration, exercise, rest, and electrolyte balance are required to maintain a healthy integumentary system.

Assessment

SUBJECTIVE

1. History—onset of problem, changes, presence of pain, burning, itching sensations
2. Allergic reactions
3. Changes in lifestyle—diet, medications, environment, detergents, etc.
4. Change in body image
5. Changes in activities owing to disease condition
6. Burning sensation
7. Itching
8. Pruritus
9. Numbness
10. Soreness
11. Tenderness
12. Tingling
13. Eczema
14. Bruising
15. Changes in texture, thinning of hair, and presence of dandruff

OBJECTIVE

1. Skin
   A. Color—deviations from normal such as pallor, jaundice, cyanosis
   B. Temperature—differences in feeling of warmth, coolness
   C. Turgor—elasticity (hydration)
   D. Pressure sores—location, size, odor, color, edema, open wound
   E. Bruises
   F. Lesions
   G. Rash
   H. Insect bites
   I. Cleanliness of skin
2. Hair
   A. Texture—coarse, fine
   B. Lice, parasites
   C. Absence of body hair

3. Nails
   A. Shape
   B. Brittleness

DIAGNOSTIC TESTS AND METHODS

1. History
   A. Medication use, types
   B. Allergies
   C. Injury and surgery—to determine wound and scar sites
   D. Skin cancer, polyps, eczema, acne, and other disease processes
   E. Nutritional and fluid intake
   F. Edema
   G. Assessment of bowel and urinary elimination—important to the elimination of wastes, which can cause skin irritation
2. Physical examination
3. Allergy testing
   A. Patch test
   B. Intradermal skin test
4. Wound, lesion culture
5. Histopathological studies
6. Skin biopsy
7. Scrapings
8. Culture
9. Wood's light—used to directly visualize skin in a darkened room
   A. Certain skin lesions show characteristic color under light.
   B. Some superficial fungal infections appear as a blue-green color.
   C. *Pseudomonas* organisms appear as a yellow-green color.
   D. Cytology.
   E. Immunofluorescence.

Implementation

1. Problems
   A. Pruritus (itching)
      (1) Administer antipruritics and antihistamines as prescribed.
      (2) Advise client to wear cotton gloves while sleeping.
      (3) Have client keep nails short.
      (4) Bathe with tepid water with minimal soap use.
      (5) Use oil or medicated baths as prescribed.
      (6) Use cotton bed linens and clothing.
   B. Seborrhea (oily scalp with shedding of scales)
      (1) Use medicated shampoo as prescribed.
      (2) Advise client to shampoo hair frequently.
   C. Drainage
      (1) Use aseptic technique when cleaning or changing dressings.
      (2) Use dressings only as required (loosely applied and taped with nonallergenic tape).
      (3) Isolate client if infective and use standard precautions.
   D. Disfigurement from trauma
      (1) Check for personality changes, depression.
      (2) Demonstrate acceptance.
      (3) Allow time to have client verbalize feelings.

Psoriasis

Description

1. Psoriasis is a chronic, recurrent disease marked by epidermal proliferation.
2. Patches of inflammation are red and covered with silvery scales that shed.
3. Patches vary widely in severity and distribution—often seen on elbows, knees, lower back, and scalp.
4. Condition can occur at any age, but most common in adults.
5. It is characterized by recurring remissions and exacerbations.
6. Flare-ups may be related to environmental and systemic factors.
7. Cause—unknown.
8. Predisposing factors
   A. Possible autoimmune deficiency
   B. Environmental factors
   C. Trauma—lesions develop at site of injury
   D. Infections (β-hemolytic streptococcus—may cause flare of drop-shaped lesions)
   E. Pregnancy, endocrine changes, environmental (climate) conditions
   F. Emotional stress
   G. Alcoholism

Assessment

SUBJECTIVE

1. Moderate pruritus
2. Pain from dry, encrusted lesions
3. Morning stiffness—associated with arthritis
4. Recent lifestyle changes—environment, stress
5. Recent trauma

OBJECTIVE

1. Erythematous, scaly plaques most commonly on scalp, chest, elbows, knees, back, and buttocks
2. Yellow, thickened nails
3. Inflammation of the joints
4. Elevated serum uric acid level

DIAGNOSTIC TESTS AND METHODS

1. History
2. Physical examination
3. Skin biopsy

Planning

1. Safe, effective care environment
   A. Prevent avoidable injury and/or infection.
   B. Increase client's and family's knowledge of condition, diagnostic procedures and treatment.
2. Physiological integrity
   A. Increase comfort.
   B. Maintain skin integrity.
3. Psychosocial integrity
   A. Facilitate effective coping.
4. Health promotion and maintenance
   A. Increase client's and family's knowledge of prevention, home care, and follow-up.

Implementation

1. Assess, report, and record signs and symptoms and reactions to treatment.
2. Monitor location and appearance of skin lesions.
3. Apply prescribed ointment such as petroleum, salicylic acid preparations to soften scales.
4. Gently remove scales during bath.
5. Administer coal tar agent and ultraviolet light, if lesions are resistant to topical medications.
6. Assist with photochemotherapy—administration of Methotrexate 2 hours prior to exposure to ultraviolet light, if prescribed.
7. Administer steroid cream followed by occlusive dressing or plastic wrap as prescribed.
8. Assist with intralesional steroid injections for small stubborn plaques, if prescribed.
9. Administer low-dosage antihistamines as prescribed for side effects of treatments.
10. Provide oatmeal baths, open wet dressings as ordered.
11. Administer aspirin; apply local heat for pain of psoriatic arthritis.
12. For psoriasis of the scalp: Apply tar shampoo followed by steroid lotion while hair is still wet.
13. Monitor RBC, WBC, and platelet counts for clients receiving methotrexate to check for hepatic or bone marrow toxicity.
14. Prepare client for liver biopsy if required to assess effects of methotrexate.
15. Monitor for side effects of treatment—allergic reactions to medications, burning, itching, nausea.
16. Facilitate effective coping strategies.
17. Watch for psychological problems—depression.
18. Provide for referral to the National Psoriasis Foundation.
19. Promote adequate rest periods.
20. Instruct client and family regarding disease process, diagnostic procedures, treatment, prevention, home care, and follow-up. Include teaching on:
    A. Correct application of prescribed creams and lotions
    B. Refraining from scrubbing skin
    C. Avoidance of situations that exacerbate condition

Evaluation

1. Shows no signs of infection or injury
2. Maintains appropriate skin integrity
3. Reports increased comfort
4. Uses effective coping measures
5. Demonstrates understanding of disease process, diagnostic procedures, treatment, prevention, home care, and follow-up; similar understanding demonstrated by family

Burns

Description

1. A burn is an injury to the skin from dry or moist heat, chemicals, electrical currents, or radiation that destroy the skin's normal protective function.
2. Physiological changes
   A. Depend on the severity of the burn
      (1) Loss of protective barrier against infection
      (2) Decreased sensory perception
      (3) Loss of body fluids and electrolytes

(4) Loss of body temperature regulation

(5) Damage to sweat and sebaceous glands

3. Two stages of physiological changes

A. Emergent/Resuscitative stage

(1) Intravascular fluid shifts into interstitial space around burn, resulting in increased permeability of capillaries and cells, vasodilation.

(2) Leakage of protein and sodium into area with edema, and blister formation.

(3) These changes occur at onset of injury.

(4) Stage lasts for 48–72 hours.

(5) Changes may lead to dehydration of healthy tissue, oliguria, hypoproteinemia, hypovolemic shock, hyperkalemia, hyponatremia, respiratory distress, and metabolic acidosis depending on severity of the burn.

B. Acute stage

(1) Stage begins approximately 48–72 hours after initial injury.

(2) Increase in intravascular volume and restoration of capillary integrity occurs.

(3) These changes result in increased blood volume, increased renal function, and diuresis.

(4) Changes may cause hypokalemia, fluid overload, sodium deficit, metabolic acidosis, anemia, and malnutrition.

C. Rehabilitative; stage begins with wound closure and ends when highest level of functioning is achieved.

4. Classification of burns

A. First degree

(1) Superficial partial-thickness burn is limited to the epidermis.

(2) Presence of erythema (redness), edema, pain.

B. Second degree

(1) Deep partial-thickness burn involving epidermis and part of the dermis.

(2) Presence of blisters, mottled, white, or red skin.

(3) Mild or moderate edema and pain.

(4) Healing occurs with undamaged epithelial cells.

C. Third degree

(1) Full-thickness burn involving both the epidermis and the dermis.

(2) Presence of white, leathery tissue (eschar) and thrombosed blood vessels.

(3) Damage may extend through subcutaneous tissue to muscle and bone (fourth degree).

(4) Presence of charred, white, dark, black, or red skin.

(5) Absence of pain due to total nerve damage.

(6) Skin grafting required to repair injury due to extent of damage.

5. Use of Parkland formula to estimate percentage of burned body surface area, taking into account client's age

A. Measured by percent of body surface area (BSA) covered by burn

B. Allows estimate of size of burn

C. Correlation of size and depth of burn allows estimation of severity

6. Classification of severity of burn

A. Minor

(1) Third-degree burn on < 2% of BSA

(2) Second-degree burn on < 15% of adult BSA (10% in children)

B. Moderate

(1) Third-degree burn on 2%–10% of BSA

(2) Second-degree burn on 15%–25% of adult BSA (>10% in children)

C. Major

(1) Third-degree burn on >10% of BSA

(2) Second-degree burn on >25% of adult BSA (>20% in children)

(3) Burns of eyes, ears, face, hands, feet, or genitalia

(4) Electrical burns

(5) Burns in presence of fractures or with respiratory damage

(6) All burns in poor risk patients

(a) Children under age 4, adults over age 60

(b) Patients with history of complicating medical problems, such as disorders that impair peripheral circulation such as diabetes and coronary artery disease

Assessment

SUBJECTIVE

1. Pain depending on degree of burn
2. Anxiety
3. Confusion

OBJECTIVE

1. Skin appearance—indicative of type of burn
2. Disfigurement
3. Infection
4. Loss of body tissue (protein)
5. Hypoproteinemia (protein shifts into tissue space around injury)
6. Electrolyte imbalance
7. Decreased serum sodium levels
8. Dehydration
9. Edema
10. Oliguria
11. Hypovolemic shock—due to fluid loss or shift
12. Hematuria—due to hemolysis of RBC and decreased blood flow
13. Signs of neurogenic shock
14. Respiratory distress—due to hypovolemic shock, inhalation injury, or airway obstruction

DIAGNOSTIC TESTS AND METHODS

1. History
2. Physical examination

Planning

1. Safe, effective care environment
   A. Prevent infection.
   B. Keep pain at an acceptable level.
   C. Promote healing of burn wound.
2. Physiological integrity
   A. Maintain functioning of body systems (integumentary, cardiovascular, renal, pulmonary, gastrointestinal).

Implementation

1. Assess, record, and report signs and symptoms and reactions to treatment.

2. Anticipate and prevent respiratory distress.
   A. Maintain airway—may be intubated if head and/or neck involved or for inhalation injury.
   B. Monitor breathing every hour, then every 4 hours.
   C. Keep endotracheal tube available. Client must be intubated at first sign of respiratory distress.
3. Keep client NPO for first 24 hours.
4. Monitor vital signs and status of nervous system frequently.
5. Insert catheter and urinary drainage as ordered.
6. Assist in insertion of CVP lines and other IV lines.
7. Assist in administration of rapid fluid replacement as prescribed—Ringer's lactate or colloid solution for first 24 hours, then colloid solutions for the second 24 hours.
8. Monitor intake and output hourly—maintenance of 30–50 mL/hr.
9. Monitor for presence of hematuria.
10. Monitor serum and urine electrolytes, hematocrit.
11. Monitor weights daily. (**NOTE:** Weight gain of 15%–20% is expected in first 72 hours.)
12. Administer analgesics for pain as prescribed.
13. Avoid heavy sedation to prevent respiratory complications.
14. Administer prophylactic tetanus as prescribed.
15. Monitor burn site for appearance, fluid loss, infection, and damage extent.
16. Monitor pulses in all extremities if possible.
17. Monitor O_2.
18. Dressing burned area, changing dressings.
    A. Administer analgesic for pain prior to dressing changes.
    B. Clean and debride burn area with antiseptic agents and prescribed dressing.
    C. Apply appropriate wet dressings as prescribed.
19. Anticipate infection—maintain asepsis, reverse isolation; administer antibiotics; monitor vital signs frequently.
20. Anticipate shock—assess level of consciousness and mental state; monitor vital signs.
21. Prevent complications of immobilization—provide proper alignment to prevent deformities; prevent skin surfaces from touching by use of turning frames, cradles.
22. Anticipate Curling's ulcer (stress ulcer)—assess for GI distress or bleeding.
23. Administer topical agents such as Sulfamylon cream, Silvadene cream, or silver nitrate to prevent infection and assist in the healing process.
24. Monitor for presence of paralytic ileus, impaction.
25. Prepare client for skin grafts, if required.
26. Provide adequate nutritional intake (following acute phase)—diet high in protein, vitamins, carbohydrates, fat, and calories.
27. Administer frequent mouth and skin care.
28. Encourage deep-breathing and coughing exercises.
29. Promote effective coping.
30. Allow client to verbalize feelings regarding condition.
31. Arrange for counseling.
32. Instruct client regarding condition, diagnostic procedures, treatment, home care, and follow-up. Include teaching on:
    A. Care of burn
    B. Skin care
    C. Medications
    D. Protective measures against irritants and infection
    E. Signs of complications

Evaluation

1. Shows no signs of avoidable injury and/or infection
2. Reports increased comfort, decreased anxiety
3. Maintains effective airway and breathing patterns
4. Maintains fluid and electrolyte balance
5. Maintains adequate cardiac output
6. Maintains adequate intake and output
7. Maintains adequate caloric intake to promote healing and maintains ideal body weight as evidenced by maintenance of weight and progressive healing
8. Resumes social interaction
9. Adapts to change in family process
10. Demonstrates understanding of condition, diagnostic procedures, treatment (including medication), home care, and need for follow-up

Neoplasms of the Skin

Description

1. Skin neoplasms are malignant lesions of the skin.
2. They are the most common form of cancer in the United States.
3. Neoplasms may or may not metastasize to other tissues.
4. They may cause destruction of cells.
5. They may result in infection.
6. Types of neoplasms
   A. Basal cell epithelioma
      (1) Slow-growing destructive skin tumor.
      (2) It usually occurs in individuals over age 40.
      (3) It is more prevalent in blond, fair-skinned males.
      (4) Most malignant neoplasm of the skin affecting whites.
      (5) Tumor appears as an opaque light pink or tan nodule.
      (6) Most common sites are sun-exposed areas of face and neck.
      (7) Tumor usually does not metastasize but may become invasive.
      (8) It may become so large that entire nose, lip, or ear must be removed and reconstructed.
      (9) Causes
         (a) Prolonged sun exposure
         (b) Radiation
         (c) Burns
         (d) Vaccinations
         (e) Arsenic ingestion
   B. Squamous cell carcinoma
      (1) Invasive tumor of the epidermal surface with metastatic potential.
      (2) It usually is located on arms or face.
      (3) It appears on sun-exposed areas or on mucous membranes but can occur on nonexposed skin.
      (4) It may develop from pre-existing skin lesions such as keratosis or leukoplakia.
      (5) It appears as a rough, scaly tumor with a wide, thick edge.
      (6) It frequently bleeds or becomes infected.
   C. Therapeutic management of basal cell and squamous cell carcinomas
      (1) Removal or destruction of tumor.
      (2) Type of treatment depends on location of lesion, depth, and level of invasion.

(3) Usual treatments include curettage, electrodesiccation, cryosurgery, surgical excision, radiation therapy, and microscopically controlled excision.

D. Malignant melanoma
(1) Most serious type of skin neoplasm.
(2) It is a cancer affecting the melanocyte cells in the skin.
(3) It is relatively rare—accounts for only 1%–2% of all malignancies.
(4) Peak incidence occurs between ages 50 and 70.
(5) It occurs mostly on skin areas exposed to sunlight.
(6) Color of lesion varies—blue, black, or yellow with irregular shapes and pigmentation.
(7) Tumor spreads through the lymphatic and vascular systems.
(8) It metastasizes to regional lymph nodes, liver, lungs, and CNS (course is unpredictable).
(9) Prognosis varies with thickness of tumor.
(10) Superficial lesions are generally curable; deeper lesions tend to metastasize.
(11) Prognosis is better for involvement on an extremity (drained by one lymphatic network) than for involvement of head, neck, or trunk (drained by several lymphatic networks).

Assessment

SUBJECTIVE

1. History of prior skin tumors or lesions
2. Soreness around site
3. Itching

OBJECTIVE

1. Presence of skin lesions
2. Change in appearance, size, or shape of existing mole or nodule
3. Drainage or bleeding from lesion
4. Positive biopsy of lesion

DIAGNOSTIC TESTS AND METHODS

1. History
2. Physical examination
3. Skin biopsy with histological examination
4. Baseline lab studies—CBC with differential, ESR, platelet count, urinalysis, liver function studies
5. Chest x-rays
6. A CT scan of body

Planning

1. Safe, effective care environment
   A. Prevent injury and/or infection.
   B. Increase client's knowledge of disease process, diagnostic procedures, and treatment.
2. Physiological integrity
   A. Maintain skin integrity.
3. Psychosocial integrity
   A. Reduce anxiety.
4. Health promotion and maintenance
   A. Increase client's knowledge of prevention, home care, and follow-up.

Implementation

1. Assess, report, and record signs and symptoms and reactions to treatment.
2. Monitor skin lesions for appearance, size, shape, color, and drainage.
3. Administer prescribed topical agents such as chemotherapeutic drugs, antibiotics.
4. Provide skin care to lesion.
   A. Avoid use of metal-containing powders or creams.
   B. Use septic technique in cleaning area.
   C. Monitor for local reaction to topical medications.
5. Explain condition and treatments such as:
   A. Biopsy procedure
   B. Surgical excision of lesion and surrounding tissue
   C. Chemotherapy
   D. Chemosurgery—application of prescribed medication on dressing, following by removal of dressing with some malignant cells that adhere to medicated dressing
   E. Irradiation
   F. Curettage with electrodesiccation under local anesthesia—use of a needle with a monopolar current for removal of the lesion, allowing for drying of the lesion with subsequent scraping with a curette
6. Instruct client regarding disease process, diagnostic procedures, treatment, prevention, home care, and follow-up.

Evaluation

1. Reports increased comfort, reduced anxiety
2. Maintains skin integrity
3. Reports excision site is healing properly without infection
4. Understands importance of limiting sun exposure and use of sun screens when outdoors
5. Demonstrates understanding of disease process, diagnostic procedures, treatment, prevention, home care, and need for follow-up

Renal and Urologic Systems

Description

1. The renal system maintains homeostasis through the production and elimination of urine.
   A. The kidneys regulate the volume, acid-base balance, and electrolyte balance of body fluids.
   B. This system also is responsible for detoxification of the blood, elimination of wastes; aids in erythropoiesis; and regulates blood pressure.
   C. Body wastes are eliminated by the kidneys via urine formation, tubular reabsorption, and tubular excretion.
   D. Disorders of these systems affect the body's normal function.
   E. Factors that compromise the integrity of the renal and urinary systems include reproductive alterations, infections, and illnesses or conditions such as hypertension or diabetes mellitus.
   F. Repeated infections may result in formation of renal calculi.
   G. Diabetes mellitus can result in diabetic nephropathy and progress to renal failure.

Assessment

SUBJECTIVE

1. Problems with elimination
2. Changes in voiding habits
3. Discharge from the urethra
4. Pain in the suprapubic area
5. Incontinence
6. Burning sensation on voiding
7. Cloudy, odoriferous urine
8. Lower back pain or discomfort
9. Painful abdominal spasms
10. Flank pain that may radiate to groin or genitals
11. Chills
12. Rectal fullness
13. Perineal heaviness
14. Pain in the glans
15. Nausea
16. Anorexia
17. GI symptoms
18. Weight changes
19. Fluid retention
20. Impaired sensorium

OBJECTIVE

1. Bladder distention—rigid, tender abdomen
2. Urine color, odor, cloudiness, presence of mucus, sediment, blood
3. Genital irritation
4. Amount of urinary output
5. Edema of extremities, scrotum
6. Vital signs—temperature, pulse, respiration, and blood pressure
7. Bruits in aorta and renal arteries
8. Masses and sensitivity of abdominal area on palpation
9. Presence of enlarged right and/or left lumbar areas
10. History of:
    A. Normal urinary habits
    B. Health problems with urinary system and other body systems
    C: Family history of cancer, renal calculi, and anatomical discrepancies
    D. Presence and location of edema
    E. Medications
    F. Food or medication allergies
    G. Spasms, pain in bladder region
    H. Presence of discharge
    I. Symptoms of uremic syndrome
       (1) Itching
       (2) Accumulation of urea on skin surface (uremic frost)

DIAGNOSTIC TESTS AND METHODS

1. Urine examination
   A. Routine urine examination—to assess renal function
   B. Specific gravity—to assess if renal function is adequate and to determine hydration status
   C. Twenty-four-hour urine creatine measurement
   D. Composite urine collections
   E. Urine culture and sensitivity—to determine presence of organisms and sensitivity to specific medications
   F. Phenosulfonphthalein test—decreased excretion is indicative of impaired kidney function

2. Blood serum studies
   A. BUN—Increase in urea is indicative of renal disorder
   B. Albumin—loss of albumin in urine reflects a change from the normal globulin ratio, indicating damage to nephrons with retention of fluid and edema formation
   C. Alkaline and acid phosphatase—increases may be indicative of metastasis to liver or bone
3. X-rays of kidneys, ureters, and bladder
   A. IVP—injection of radiopaque dye to check renal function. Renal pelvis, ureters, bladder, and urethra are outlined on x-ray.
   B. Kidneys, ureter, bladder (KUB)—x-ray of abdomen for information about size and location of the organs and for presence of stones.
   C. Cystoscopy—direct visualization of bladder and urethra via a cystoscope.
   D. Retrograde pyelogram—injection of radiopaque dye through ureteral catheters for visualization of upper GU tract.
4. Renal angiography
5. Renal ultrasonography
6. Voiding cystogram
7. Renal scan
8. Renal biopsy

Implementation

1. Problems
   A. Urinary retention
      (1) Use measures to promote voiding—offering bedpan at scheduled times, pouring warm water over perineum, letting water run from tap, providing privacy.
      (2) Monitor intake and output.
      (3) Force fluids if not contraindicated.
      (4) Keep catheter and urinary drainage equipment patent; wash meatus with prescribed solution or soap and water to decrease potential for infection.
   B. Incontinence
      (1) Provide privacy.
      (2) Wash and thoroughly dry skin.
      (3) Check for signs of skin irritation, breakdown.
      (4) Provide for bladder training.
   C. Hematuria
      (1) Assess urine for presence of blood.
      (2) Report presence of blood clots immediately.
      (3) Maintain patency and gravity drainage of catheter and urinary drainage tubing.
      (4) Check for signs of anemia—weakness; fatigue; hemoglobin, hematocrit studies.
   D. Spasms of the bladder
      (1) Check location and severity.
      (2) Check catheter for patency—obstruction of urine flow may be causing spasms.
      (3) Report condition and irrigate catheter, if ordered.
      (4) Administer antispasmodic as prescribed if catheter is not obstructed.
      (5) Reassure patient.
   E. Uremia: Metabolic wastes are retained resulting in toxicity to the body system
      (1) Check skin for odor and pruritus—urea is excreted through the skin.
      (2) Provide frequent skin care.

(3) Check for nausea and vomiting; provide mouth care.

(4) Check mental status—confusion, disorientation, hallucinations, unconsciousness, coma.

(5) Explain home care and preventive measures.

Renal Calculi (Kidney Stones)

Description

1. The most common area for development of calculi is in the renal pelvis or calyces of the kidney, but calculi may form anywhere in the urinary tract.
2. Calculi formation occurs as a result of precipitation of substances such as calcium oxalate, calcium phosphate, urate, or cystine, which are normally dissolved in the urine.
3. Stones vary in size and may be solitary or multiple.
4. They may stay in renal pelvis or descend into the ureter.
5. They may damage renal and urinary tract tissue.
6. Pressure necrosis may occur from large calculi.
7. They may cause obstruction along urinary tract resulting in hydronephrosis.
8. They tend to recur.
9. More common in males aged 30 to 50.
10. Rare in the black population.
11. More prevalent in southeastern United States ("stone belt"), possibly due to:
    A. Regional dietary habits
    B. Dehydration due to hot climate
12. Cause—unknown
13. Possible causes
    A. The largest number of stones (80%–90%) contain calcium as calcium oxalate, calcium phosphate, or a combination of the two.
    B. Anything that promotes increased calcium levels in urine and blood can predispose the individual to stone formation.
    C. Oxalate stones are the second most common type of renal stone and may be related to diet.
    D. Uric acid, the end product of purine metabolism, may be a source for stone formation.
    E. Struvite stones are caused by the urea-splitting action of certain bacteria, usually Proteus.
    F. Urinary pH influences stone formation.
       (1) Alkaline urine is associated with infection and struvite stones.
       (2) Acid urine is associated with uric acid, cystine, and xanthine calculi.
       (3) Calcium phosphate calculi dissolve in acid urine.
       (4) Calcium oxalate stones are not affected by urinary pH.
14. Predisposing factors
    A. Dehydration: Decrease in urine production allows concentration of calculi-forming substances.
    B. Prolonged immobilization: causes urinary stasis with accumulation of calculus-forming substances.
    C. Infection: pH changes result in a medium favorable for calculus formation.
    D. Obstruction: allows calculi-forming substances to collect, promotes infection and further obstruction.
    E. Metabolic factors: Excessive intake of calcium or vitamin D, hyperparathyroidism, renal tubular acidosis, elevated uric acid, defective metabolism of oxalate.

Assessment

SUBJECTIVE

1. Severe pain in flank area, suprapubic area, pelvis or external genitalia (renal colic)
2. Urgency, frequency of urination
3. Nausea
4. Chills

OBJECTIVE

1. Increased temperature
2. Pallor
3. Hematuria
4. Abdominal distention
5. Pyuria
6. Anuria (from bilateral obstruction)
7. Evidence of urinary tract infection via diagnostic procedures
8. Evidence of presence of calculi via diagnostic procedures

DIAGNOSTIC TESTS AND METHODS

1. Urinalysis and urine culture
2. Retrograde pyelography
3. Twenty-four-hour urine examination—for calcium, uric acid and oxalates
4. Kidney-ureter-bladder (KUB) x-ray
5. Calculi analysis
6. IVP
7. Renal ultrasonography
8. Cystoscopy
9. Serial blood calcium and phosphorous levels—to detect hyperparathyroidism and detect increased calcium level compared to normal serum protein
10. Blood chloride and HCO_3 levels—to detect presence of renal tubular acidosis
11. Blood protein level—to determine level of free calcium unbound to protein
12. Serum uric acid levels
13. CT of the kidney
14. Magnetic resonance imaging (MRI) of the kidney

Planning

1. Safe, effective care environment
   A. Prevent avoidable infection and injury.
   B. Increase client's knowledge of disease process, diagnostic procedures, and treatment.
2. Physiological integrity
   A. Maintain adequate urinary elimination pattern.
   B. Increase comfort.
3. Psychosocial integrity
   A. Reduce anxiety
4. Health promotion and maintenance
   A. Increase client's knowledge of prevention, home care, and follow-up.

Implementation

1. Assess, report, and record signs and symptoms and reactions to treatment.
2. Maintain a 24–48-hour record of urine pH—test with nitrazine paper.
3. Strain all urine.

4. Save all solid material in urine for analysis.
5. Provide and encourage intake of clear fluids for a urinary output of 3–4 L/day.
6. Offer fruit juices, especially cranberry juice, to acidify alkaline urine.
7. Assist with administration of supplemental IV fluids as prescribed.
8. Record intake and output accurately.
9. Weigh client and record weight daily.
10. Have dietician instruct client regarding importance of proper diet.
    A. Calcium stones—acid-ash foods such as whole grains, cranberry juice, prunes, meats. Foods low in calcium and phosphate—these foods assist in acidifying alkaline urine.
    B. Uric acid stones—Decreasing foods high in purine (when metabolized form uric acid). Avoiding foods such as meats, and whole grains. Alkaline-ash foods may assist in decreasing the acidity of the urine.
    C. Cystine stones—foods low in methionine (an essential amino acid that forms cystine), foods high in alkaline-ash such as vegetables and fruit.
11. Instruct client regarding compliance with drug therapy.
12. Prepare client for:
    A. Cystoscopy or passage of ureteral catheter for crushing or dislodging calculi
    B. Transcutaneous shock wave lithotripsy—patient sits in large warm bath as ultrasound waves are delivered to area of stone to disintegrate it
13. Prepare client for surgery to remove ureteral or kidney stone.
    A. Nephrolithotomy—incision through kidney and removal of stone
    B. Pyelolithotomy—removal of stones from renal pelvis
    C. Ureterolithotomy—removal of calculus in the ureter
14. Provide general preoperative and postoperative nursing care.
15. Provide analgesics as needed.
16. Maintain patency of catheters—do *not* irrigate renal or ureteral catheters.
17. Maintain gravity urinary drainage from catheter—do *not* clamp ureteral or nephrostomy catheters.
18. Record output from ureteral and nephrostomy catheters separately; report output from each.
19. Monitor for bleeding, vital signs, and signs of urinary obstruction.
20. Keep NPO if nausea, vomiting, or abdominal distention occur.
21. Assist with comfort measures.
22. Protect against infection.
23. Encourage activity.
24. Instruct client regarding disease process, diagnostic procedures, treatment, prevention, home care, and follow-up.

Evaluation

1. Reports increased comfort, decreased anxiety
2. Shows no signs of infection
3. Maintains adequate urinary elimination pattern
4. Demonstrates understanding of disease process, diagnostic procedures, treatment, prevention, home care, and need for follow-up

Glomerulonephritis

Description

1. Acute glomerulonephritis is a relatively common bilateral inflammation of the glomeruli.
2. Two types
   A. Post-infectious—the most common type
      (1) This type is caused by a group A β-hemolytic streptococcal infection elsewhere in the body.
      (2) It typically occurs 2–3 weeks following a throat infection or a skin infection.
      (3) It is primarily a disease of children and young adults.
      (4) Approximately 95% of children and 50% of young adults will fully recover, whereas the rest will develop chronic glomerulonephritis.
      (5) A small percentage will develop end-stage renal failure requiring dialysis or transplantation.
      (6) This type results in antigen-antibody complexes that destroy glomerular capillary cells and cause cellular inflammation with increased membrane permeability and scarring.
      (7) Damaged glomeruli allow RBCs and protein to filter through into the urine.
      (8) Uremic poisoning may result.
   B. Infectious—caused by infection (bacterial, viral, or parasitic) elsewhere in the body
3. Causes
   A. Immunological disease—streptococcal infection
   B. Vascular disorders such as hypertension
   C. Metabolic disorders such as diabetes mellitus
4. Acute infectious glomerulonephritis is caused by infection elsewhere in body, but the renal symptoms occur within only a few days of the original bacterial, viral, or parasitic infection.
5. Chronic glomerulonephritis may occur, but usually there is no evidence of a previous infection.
   A. It may be overlooked owing to a mild antigen-antibody reaction.
6. Chronic glomerulonephritis usually produces insidious manifestations of the disease.
   A. Hypertension and abnormal findings in urine may be detected during routine physical examination.
   B. Individual may complain of headache, especially in the morning.
   C. Other symptoms include general fatigue or weakness, blurring of vision, and dyspnea on exertion.

Assessment

SUBJECTIVE

1. Headache
2. Weakness, fatigue
3. Visual problems
4. Flank pain
5. Shortness of breath—due to fluid retention
6. Chills

OBJECTIVE

1. Mild to moderate generalized and periorbital edema due to fluid retention.
2. Mild to severe hypertension caused by sodium or water retention due to decreased glomerular filtration rate.

3. Proteinuria, oliguria, azotemia, hematuria (smoky or coffee-colored urine).
4. Elevated specific gravity of urine.
5. Elevated BUN and creatinine levels.
6. Elevated antistreptolysin-O titer.
7. Low serum complement level.
8. CHF from hypervolemia with symptoms of pulmonary edema.
   A. Dyspnea
   B. Orthopnea
9. Clinical manifestations of chronic renal failure may be observed.
10. Dyspnea and edema are most common symptoms in the elderly.
    A. Older person may have hematuria with a history of sore throat with streptococcus cultures.
    B. Reduction in real function may be seen when there is volume depletion, hypotension, or impaired renal perfusion from other causes.

DIAGNOSTIC TESTS AND METHODS

1. History
2. Physical examination
3. Serum electrolytes, BUN and creatinine
4. Urine values—RBCs, WBCs, mixed cell casts, proteins
5. Antistreptolysin-O titers
6. Streptozyme and anti-DNase B titers
7. Low serum complement levels
8. Throat culture
9. KUB x-ray studies
10. Renal biopsy and renal scan
11. Urine creatinine
12. Erythrocyte sedimentation rate (ESR), a general indicator of the inflammatory response
13. Antinuclear antibodies (ANA)—to rule out systemic lupus erythematosus, a common cause of glomerulonephritis

Planning

1. Safe, effective care environment
   A. Prevent avoidable injury and/or infection.
   B. Increase client's knowledge of disease process, diagnostic procedures, and treatment.
2. Physiological integrity
   A. Maintain adequate urinary elimination.
   B. Maintain fluid balance.
   C. Maintain adequate nutritional balance.
3. Psychosocial integrity
   A. Facilitate effective coping.
4. Health promotion and maintenance
   A. Increase client's knowledge of prevention, home care, and follow-up.

Implementation

1. Assess, report, and record signs and symptoms and reactions to treatment.
2. Provide for bed rest.
3. Restrict fluid and dietary sodium.
4. Administer diuretics and antihypertensives as prescribed, to control fluid overload and hypertension.
5. Maintain bed rest, as activity may increase proteinuria and hematuria.

6. Administer non-nephrotoxic antibiotics as prescribed.
7. Monitor, report, and record side effects of medications.
8. Provide emotional support.
9. Monitor vital signs and laboratory test results.
10. Monitor intake and output accurately.
11. Monitor weight daily.
12. Watch for and immediately report signs of acute renal failure.
    A. Oliguria
    B. Azotemia
    C. Acidosis
13. Request dietitian to instruct client regarding diet—high in calories; low in protein, sodium, potassium, and fluids.
14. Monitor for signs of secondary infection.
15. Instruct client to report signs of sore throat immediately.
16. Encourage pregnant clients to have frequent medical examinations—pregnancy stresses the kidneys and increases risk of development of chronic renal failure.
17. Prepare client for plasmaphoresis—helpful in removing immune complexes or antibodies
18. Instruct client regarding disease process, diagnostic procedures, treatment, prevention, home care, and need for follow-up.

Evaluation

1. Reports increased comfort, decreased anxiety
2. Shows no signs of avoidable injury and/or infection
3. Maintains fluid balance
4. Maintains adequate urinary elimination pattern
5. Maintains adequate nutritional intake
6. Demonstrates understanding of disease process, diagnostic procedures, treatment, prevention, home care, and need for follow-up

Polycystic Disease

Description

1. Polycystic disease of the kidneys is an inherited disorder characterized by multiple, bilateral grapelike clusters of cysts filled with fluid.
2. Presence of cysts results in gross enlargement of the kidneys with compression of normal tissue and eventual replacement of functioning kidney tissue.
3. Cysts rupture, causing infection and scar tissue to accumulate.
4. Ischemia to kidney tissue occurs leading to atrophy.
5. End result is nephron damage.
6. Two distinct forms
   A. Infantile form
      (1) This form causes stillbirth or early neonatal death.
      (2) Few infants survive beyond 2 years before succumbing to fatal renal, CHF, or respiratory failure.
   B. Adult form
      (1) Onset is insidious, becoming obvious between the ages of 30 and 50
      (2) This form may not cause symptoms until client is in his or her 70s (rare).
      (3) Renal deterioration is more gradual in adult form than in infant form.
      (4) Condition progresses to fatal uremia.

(5) Prognosis is variable—may be slow even with symptoms of renal insufficiency, usually fatal within 4 years following the appearance of uremic symptoms unless dialysis is used.

Assessment

SUBJECTIVE

1. Chills
   A. Malaise
   B. Fever
2. Signs of respiratory distress
   A. Hypertension
   B. Presence of CHF
   C. Pronounced features—pointed nose; small chin; floppy, low-set ears
   D. Presence of bilateral symmetrical masses on flanks at birth
   E. Symptoms of uremia and renal failure
3. Later symptoms
   A. Lumbar or flank pain
   B. Colicky abdominal pain

OBJECTIVE

1. Nonspecific symptoms
   A. Hypertension
   B. Polyuria
   C. Urinary tract infection (UTI)
2. Later symptoms
   A. Enlarged kidney mass
   B. Presence of UTI with positive urine culture
   C. Positive KUB and IVP
   D. Widening girth
   E. Swollen, tender abdomen
   F. Recurrent hematuria
   G. Retroperitoneal bleeding
   H. Proteinuria
3. Advanced stage symptoms
   A. Renal insufficiency
   B. Renal failure
   C. Uremia

DIAGNOSTIC TESTS AND METHODS

1. History
2. Physical examination
3. Excretory urography of newborn
4. X-rays and tomography
5. Urinalysis and creatinine clearance tests
6. IVP
7. Renal ultrasound

Planning

1. Safe, effective care environment
   A. Increase client's knowledge of disease process, diagnostic procedures, and treatment.
   B. Prevent avoidable injury and/or infection.
2. Physiological integrity
   A. Maintain adequate renal tissue perfusion.
   B. Maintain adequate urinary elimination pattern.
   C. Maintain fluid balance.
   D. Increase comfort.
3. Psychosocial integrity
   A. Facilitate effective coping.
4. Health promotion and maintenance
   A. Increase client's knowledge of home care and follow-up.

Implementation

1. Assess, report, and record signs and symptoms and reactions to treatment.
2. Monitor vital signs.
3. Monitor intake and output.
4. Collect urine for routine analysis and culture.
5. Avoid use of urinary catheters to prevent infection.
6. Administer antibiotic therapy and analgesics as prescribed.
7. Provide emotional support.
8. Provide bed rest in case of ruptured cysts and bleeding.
9. Encourage independence with ADL when appropriate.
10. Assist with ADL when necessary.
11. Obtain information regarding allergy to iodine or shellfish prior to IVP procedure.
12. Monitor for side effects of medications.
13. Explain dialysis procedure, if required.
14. Instruct client regarding transplant procedure, if needed.
15. Explain need for family counseling on inherited disease.
16. Instruct client regarding disease process, diagnostic procedures, treatment (including medication), home care, and follow-up.

Evaluation

1. Reports increased comfort, decreased anxiety
2. Shows no signs of avoidable injury and/or infection
3. Maintains adequate renal perfusion
4. Maintains adequate urinary elimination
5. Demonstrates understanding of disease process, diagnostic procedures, treatment, home care (including need for family counseling) and need for follow-up

Hydronephrosis

Description

1. Hydronephrosis is an abnormal dilation of the renal pelvis and the calyces of one or both kidneys.
2. Fluid accumulates in the renal pelvis, resulting in distention of the renal tubules, calyces, and pelvis.
3. Renal tissue is destroyed from pressure.
4. Uremia results.
5. Cause
   A. Obstruction of urine flow in the GU tract
      (1) Congenital defective drainage due to blockage from stones or scar tissue
      (2) Benign prostatic hypertrophy (BPH) causing backup from obstructed bladder neck
      (3) Urethral strictures
      (4) Strictures or stenosis of ureter or bladder outlet
      (5) Abdominal tumors

(6) Neurogenic bladder

(7) Renal calculi

Assessment

SUBJECTIVE

1. Mild pain and minimal change in urine output in some clients
2. Severe, colicky renal pain, dull flank pain radiating to groin in other clients
3. Nausea and vomiting
4. Abdominal fullness
5. Pain on urination, dribbling or hesitancy

OBJECTIVE

1. Decreased urinary flow
2. Dribbling or hesitancy on urination
3. Hematuria, pyuria, alternating oliguria and polyuria, or anuria
4. Pyelonephritis due to stasis, which exacerbates renal damage
5. Paralytic ileus
6. CT scan
7. Cystoscopy

DIAGNOSTIC TESTS AND METHODS

1. History
2. Physical examination
3. IVP
4. Retrograde pyelography
5. Renal ultrasound
6. Renal function tests

Planning

1. Safe, effective care environment
   A. Increase client's knowledge of disease process, diagnostic procedures, and treatment.
   B. Prevent avoidable injury and/or infection.
2. Physiological integrity
   A. Maintain adequate renal tissue perfusion.
   B. Maintain adequate urinary elimination pattern.
   C. Maintain fluid balance.
   D. Increase comfort.
3. Psychosocial integrity
   A. Facilitate effective coping.
4. Health promotion and maintenance
   A. Increase client's knowledge of home care and follow-up.

Implementation

1. Assess, report, and record signs and symptoms and reactions to treatment.
2. Provide restful environment.
3. Administer medications for pain as prescribed.
4. Check client for allergy to IVP dye.
5. Prepare client for surgical procedures.
   A. Dilation for stricture of urethra, if present
   B. Prostatectomy for BPH
   C. Diet low in protein, sodium, and potassium, if renal function altered

D. Decompression and drainage of kidney with nephrostomy tube for inoperable obstructions

6. Administer antibiotics as prescribed for concurrent infections.
7. Provide postoperative care.
   A. Monitor intake and output, vital signs, fluid and electrolyte status.
   B. Monitor renal function test results daily.
   C. Monitor nephrostomy tube frequently for patency and blood.
   D. Irrigate nephrostomy tube, if ordered; do *not* clamp.
8. Instruct client regarding disease process, diagnostic procedures, treatment (including medications), prevention, home care, and follow-up.

Evaluation

1. Reports increased comfort, decreased anxiety
2. Shows no signs of avoidable injury and/or infection
3. Maintains adequate renal function
4. Maintains adequate urinary elimination pattern
5. Maintains adequate fluid balance
6. Demonstrates understanding of disease process, diagnostic procedures, treatment, prevention, home care, and need for follow-up

Renal Cancer

Description

1. Renal cancer usually occurs in older adults; it accounts for about 85% of all primary kidney cancers.
2. Secondary kidney cancers due to metastases from other primary-site carcinomas.
3. Usually tumors are large, firm, nodular, encapsulated, unilateral, and solitary.
4. Occasionally tumors are bilateral.
5. Histological classification
   A. Clear cell
   B. Granular cell
   C. Spindle cell
6. Prognosis is considered better for cases of clear cell type than other two types.
7. In general, prognosis depends more on stage of disease than on type.
8. Prognosis has improved—5-year survival rate for about 50% of those diagnosed with kidney cancer and 10-year survival rate for 18%–23%.
9. Incidence is increasing—accounts for approximately 2% of all adult cancers.
10. Twice as common in males than in females.
11. Kidney cancer usually strikes after age 40; peak incidence is between 50 and 60 years of age.
12. Four stages
    A. Stage 1—tumor limited to kidney
    B. Stage 2—spread confined to fascia around kidney
    C. Stage 3—spread to renal vein or inferior vena cava; lymph involvement may occur
    D. Stage 4—spread to adjacent organs (except adrenal gland) or metastases to distant lymph nodes, liver, lung, and bones
13. Cause—unknown

14. Predisposing factors
    A. Exposure to environmental carcinogens
    B. Increased longevity

Assessment

SUBJECTIVE

1. Abdominal and flank pain
2. Nausea

OBJECTIVE

1. Microscopic or gross hematuria
2. Palpable mass—smooth, firm, and nontender
3. Increased temperature
4. Hypertension due to compression of renal artery, resulting in ischemia of renal tissues
5. Hypercalcemia
6. Urinary retention
7. Weight loss
8. Anemia and fatigue
9. Vomiting
10. Increased alkaline phosphatase, bilirubin, transaminase, and prolonged prothrombin time (PT)

DIAGNOSTIC TESTS AND METHODS

1. History
2. Physical examination
3. An IVP
4. Retrograde pyelography
5. Ultrasound studies
6. Nephrotomography or renal angiography—to differentiate between cyst and tumor
7. Cystoscopy
8. KUB and chest x-ray studies
9. A CT scan
10. Liver function tests
11. MRI

Planning

1. Safe, effective care environment
   A. Prevent avoidable injury and/or infection.
   B. Increase client's knowledge of disease process, diagnostic procedures, and treatment.
2. Physiological integrity
   A. Maintain adequate urinary elimination pattern.
   B. Increase comfort.
   C. Maintain adequate fluid and electrolyte balance.
3. Psychosocial integrity
   A. Reduce anxiety.
   B. Facilitate effective coping.
4. Health promotion and maintenance
   A. Increase client's knowledge of home care and follow-up.

Implementation

1. Assess, report, and record signs and symptoms and reaction to treatment.
2. Provide nursing care for individual symptoms.
3. Monitor urine output and appearance.
4. Monitor intake.

5. Force oral fluids; administer prescribed IV fluids, medications.
6. Prepare client for radical nephrectomy.
7. Provide postoperative care.
   A. Monitor intake and output.
   B. Monitor appearance of urine output.
   C. Monitor urinary drainage system.
   D. Check dressings.
   E. Administer analgesics for pain.
   F. Provide meticulous skin care around urinary drainage system.
   G. Monitor for signs of infection.
8. Prepare client for radiation procedure
9. Assist in administration of chemotherapeutic regimen.
10. Instruct client regarding disease process, diagnostic procedures, treatment, home care, and follow-up.

Evaluation

1. Reports increased comfort, decreased anxiety
2. Shows no signs of avoidable injury and/or infection
3. Maintains adequate renal perfusion with remaining kidney
4. Maintains adequate urinary elimination pattern
5. Maintains adequate fluid and electrolyte balance
6. Demonstrates understanding of disease process, diagnostic procedures, treatment, home care, and follow-up

Acute Renal Failure

Description

1. Acute renal failure is sudden interruption of kidney function due to obstruction, reduced circulation, or disease of renal tissue.
2. Condition results in retention of toxins, fluids, and end products of metabolism.
3. It is usually reversible with medical treatment.
4. It may progress to end-stage disease, uremic syndrome, and death without treatment.
5. Causes
   A. Prerenal failure associated with decreased blood flow to kidneys
      (1) Hypovolemia
      (2) Shock
      (3) Blood loss
      (4) Embolism
      (5) Pooling of fluid due to ascites, or burns
      (6) Cardiovascular disorders (CHF, arrhythmias)
      (7) Sepsis
   B. Intrinsic (parenchymal) renal failure due to damage to kidneys
      (1) Acute tubular necrosis
      (2) Acute poststreptococcal glomerulonephritis
      (3) Sickle cell disease
      (4) Bilateral renal vein thrombosis
      (5) Nephrotoxins
      (6) Ischemia
      (7) Renal myeloma
      (8) Acute pyelonephritis
   C. Postrenal failure due to bilateral obstruction of urinary outflow
      (1) Renal calculi
      (2) Blood clots

(3) BPH
(4) Urethral edema from catheterization

Assessment

SUBJECTIVE

1. Nausea
2. Loss of appetite
3. Headache
4. Lethargy
5. Tingling in extremities

OBJECTIVE

1. Oliguria phase
   A. Vomiting
   B. Disorientation
   C. Edema
   D. Hyperkalemia
   E. Hyponatremia
   F. Elevated BUN and creatinine
   G. Acidosis
   H. Arrhythmias
   I. CHF, pulmonary edema
   J. Hypertension due to hypervolemia
   K. Anorexia
   L. Sudden drop in urine output
   M. Convulsions, coma
   N. Pruritus
   O. Altered clotting mechanisms
   P. Diarrhea or constipation
   Q. Stomatitis
   R. Hematemesis
   S. Uremic breath
2. Diuretic phase
   A. Increased urine output—4–5 L/day
   B. Gradual decline in BUN and creatinine levels
   C. Hyponatremia
   D. Hypokalemia
   E. Tachycardia
   F. Improved level of consciousness

DIAGNOSTIC TESTS AND METHODS

1. History
2. Physical examination
3. Laboratory blood tests—BUN, serum creatinine, sodium, potassium, arterial blood gasses, hematocrit, and hemoglobin
4. Urine studies—urinalysis, specific gravity, urea, creatinine
5. Ultrasound of kidneys
6. Plain films of abdomen
7. KUB x-rays
8. IVP
9. Renal scan
10. Retrograde pyelography
11. Nephrotomography
12. CT
13. Renal biopsy

Planning

1. Safe, effective care environment
   A. Prevent avoidable injury and/or infection.

   B. Increase client's and family's knowledge of disease process, diagnostic procedures, and treatment.
2. Physiological integrity
   A. Maintain adequate urinary elimination pattern.
   B. Maintain fluid balance.
   C. Maintain adequate nutritional intake.
   D. Maintain skin integrity.
3. Psychosocial integrity
   A. Reduce anxiety.
4. Health promotion and maintenance
   A. Increase client's and family's knowledge of home care and follow-up.

Implementation

1. Assess, report, and record signs and symptoms and reactions to treatment.
2. Monitor fluid intake and output.
   A. Oral fluids
   B. All body fluids such as wound drainage, NG output, diarrhea
3. Monitor laboratory test results.
4. Assist in administering parenteral blood products as ordered.
5. Monitor vital signs.
6. Check for signs of pleuritic chest pain, tachycardia, pericardial friction rub indicative of pericarditis.
7. Monitor electrolyte study results.
   A. Observe for symptoms of hyperkalemia such as malaise, anorexia, paresthesia, or muscle weakness and changes in ECG readings—report immediately.
   B. Watch for signs of hyperglycemia or hypoglycemia in patients receiving hypertonic glucose and insulin infusions.
8. Maintain nutritional status—provide high-caloric, low-protein, low-sodium, and low-potassium diet with vitamin supplements as ordered.
   A. Provide small, frequent meals to clients with anorexia.
9. Provide good mouth care—dry mucous membranes.
10. Check stools for blood.
11. Prevent complications due to immobilization.
    A. Encourage frequent coughing and deep-breathing exercises.
    B. Assist the client to ambulate when ordered.
12. Use safety measures such as side rails for patients who are confused or dizzy.
13. Prepare client for peritoneal dialysis, if ordered.
    A. Elevate head of bed to reduce pressure on diaphragm, to aid respiration.
    B. Monitor for signs of infection—elevated temperature, cloudy drainage.
    C. Monitor blood sugar periodically; administer insulin as ordered.
    D. Monitor for complications such as peritonitis, hypokalemia, pneumonia, and shock.
14. Prepare client for hemodialysis, if ordered.
    A. Check site of arteriovenous shunt, fistula or A-V access device every 2 hours for patency and presence of clot.
    B. Use opposite arm for drawing blood or taking blood pressure readings.
    C. Have clips available at bedside to clamp off shunt in case of disconnection.

D. Monitor vital signs, clotting time, vascular access site, arterial and venous pressures, blood flow during dialysis procedure.
E. Monitor for complications such as embolism, hepatitis, septicemia, and electrolyte loss.
15. Provide posthemodialysis care.
    A. Monitor vital signs.
    B. Monitor vascular access site.
    C. Observe for signs of fluid and electrolyte imbalance.
16. Provide reassurance and emotional support to client and family.
17. Instruct client and family regarding disease process, diagnostic procedures, treatment, prevention, home care, and follow-up.

Evaluation

1. Reports increased comfort, decreased anxiety
2. Shows no signs of avoidable injury and/or infection
3. Maintains adequate renal perfusion
4. Maintains adequate urinary elimination pattern
5. Maintains adequate skin integrity
6. Maintains adequate fluid and nutritional intake
7. Demonstrates understanding of disease process, diagnostic procedures, treatment, prevention, home care, and need for follow-up; similar understanding demonstrated by family

Chronic Renal Failure

Description

1. Chronic renal failure is the result of a gradually progressive loss of renal function.
2. It is occasionally due to rapidly progressive disease of sudden onset.
3. Symptoms become apparent once 75% of glomerular filtration is lost.
4. Progressive destruction of the nephrons occurs resulting in cellular hypertrophy, retention of fluid, and waste products with resultant loss of renal function.
5. Uremic toxins accumulate and produce physiological changes in major organ systems if condition is not treated.
6. Maintenance dialysis and transplantation can temporarily support life.
7. Causes
   A. Recurrent infections, pyelonephritis
   B. Congenital anomalies such as polycystic kidneys
   C. Vascular disorders such as renal nephrosclerosis
   D. Toxic agents such as phenacetin overdose
   E. Endocrine disorders such as diabetic neuropathy
   F. Urinary obstruction such as calculi, strictures
   G. Chronic glomerular disease such as glomerulonephritis
   H. Acute renal failure that does not respond to treatment

Assessment

SUBJECTIVE

1. Anorexia
2. Nausea

3. Lethargy
4. Headache

OBJECTIVE

1. Renal
   A. Hyponatremia
   B. Initially resulting in hypotension, dry mouth, loss of skin turgor
   C. Progressing to confusion, salt overload, accumulation of potassium with muscle irritability and muscle weakness
   D. Fluid overload and metabolic acidosis
   E. Proteinuria
   F. Glycosuria
   G. RBCs, WBCs, and casts
2. Cardiovascular
   A. Hypertension
   B. Dysrhythmias
   C. Pericardial effusion
   D. CHF
   E. Peripheral edema
3. Neurological
   A. Restless leg syndrome with burning, pain, and itching
   B. Paresthesia
   C. Motor nerve dysfunction
   D. Muscle cramping
   E. Shortened memory span
   F. Apathy
   G. Drowsiness
   H. Confusion
   I. Convulsions
   J. Coma
   K. EEG changes
4. GI
   A. Stomatitis, gum ulceration and bleeding
   B. Parotitis
   C. Esophagitis, gastritis, duodenal ulcers
   D. Ulcerative lesions on small and large bowel
   E. Pancreatitis
   F. Ammonia smell to breath (uremic fetor)
   G. Vomiting
   H. Constipation
5. Respiratory
   A. Pulmonary changes with increased susceptibility to infection
   B. Pulmonary edema
   C. Pleural friction rub and effusion
   D. Pleural pain
   E. Uremic pneumonitis
   F. Dyspnea due to CHF
   G. Kussmaul's respiration due to acidosis
6. Endocrine
   A. Stunted growth patterns in children
   B. Amenorrhea and cessation of menses
   C. Impotence in males
   D. Increased aldosterone secretion
   E. Impaired blood glucose levels due to impairment of carbohydrate metabolism
7. Hematopoietic
   A. Anemia
   B. Decrease in RBC survival time
   C. Blood loss from dialysis and GI bleeding
   D. Platelet deficits

E. Bleeding and clotting disorders—purpura, hemorrhage from body orifices, ecchymoses

8. Skeletal
   A. Muscle and bone pain
   B. Bone demineralization
   C. Pathological fractures
   D. Calcifications in blood vessels, myocardium, joints, gums, eyes, brain
9. Cutaneous
   A. Pallid, yellowish-bronze, scaly skin
   B. Pruritus
   C. Purpura
   D. Uremic frost
   E. Thin, brittle fingernails
   F. Dry, brittle hair—may change color and fall out

DIAGNOSTIC TESTS AND METHODS

1. History
2. Physical examination
3. Creatinine clearance test
4. BUN, serum creatinine, potassium levels
5. Arterial blood gasses
6. Hemoglobin and hematocrit
7. Urine specific gravity
8. Urinalysis
9. KUB x-ray
10. IVP
11. Renal scan
12. Renal arteriography
13. Nephrotomography
14. Kidney biopsy

Planning

1. Safe, effective care environment
   A. Prevent avoidable injury and/or infection.
   B. Increase client's knowledge of disease process, diagnostic procedures, and treatment.
2. Physiological integrity
   A. Maintain fluid balance.
   B. Maintain adequate nutrition.
   C. Maintain appropriate urinary elimination pattern.
   D. Maintain skin integrity.
3. Psychosocial integrity
   A. Facilitate effective coping.
   B. Promote positive self-concept.
   C. Provide counseling on sexual dysfunction.
4. Health promotion and maintenance
   A. Increase client's knowledge of home care and follow-up.
   B. Encourage compliance.

Implementation

1. Assess, report, and record signs and symptoms and reactions to treatment.
2. Provide emotional support.
3. Provide meticulous skin care.
4. Provide good perineal care.
5. Pad side rails to prevent ecchymoses.
6. Turn client often—use egg-crate mattress.
7. Provide good oral hygiene.
8. Offer small nutritious meals—high-caloric foods.

9. Instruct client and family to avoid high-potassium and high-sodium foods.
10. Monitor for signs of hyperkalemia—leg and abdominal cramps, diarrhea, muscle irritability, weak pulse rate, ECG changes.
11. Monitor for bone and joint complications such as pathologic fractures.
12. Monitor hydration status.
    A. Check JVD.
    B. Auscultate lungs for rales.
    C. Measure intake and output including all drainage.
    D. Record daily weight.
    E. Assess for thirst.
    F. Monitor for signs of hypertension.
    G. Check for peripheral edema.
    H. Encourage deep breathing and coughing—to prevent pulmonary congestion.
13. Monitor for signs of pulmonary edema—dyspnea, restlessness, rales.
14. Administer diuretics and other prescribed medications.
15. Maintain strict aseptic technique.
16. Watch for signs of infection—increased temperature, leukocytosis, malaise.
17. Monitor for convulsions, coma.
    A. Assist with administration of IV sodium bicarbonate for acidosis.
    B. Administer sedatives or anticonvulsants as ordered.
    C. Keep padded tongue blade and suction at bedside.
    D. Assess neurological status frequently.
    E. Check for Trousseau's and Chvostek's signs—indicate low serum calcium.
18. Monitor for signs of bleeding—ecchymoses, petechiae.
    A. Check IV sites for prolonged bleeding.
    B. Monitor hemoglobin and hematocrit levels.
    C. Monitor stool, urine, and vomitus for blood.
19. Prepare client for hemodialysis, if required.
    A. Instruct client on care of arteriovenous shunt, if present.
    B. Check vascular access site every 2 hours for patency.
    C. Check extremity—temperature, pulse rate, capillary refill, and sensation to determine blood supply and nervous system function.
    D. Check for bright red blood pulsating in tube and listen for bruit on auscultation, if shunt is present.
    E. Notify charge nurse if clotting is suspected.
    F. Avoid using arm with vascular access for drawing blood or taking blood pressure.
    G. Keep clamps attached to A-V access dressing in case of disconnection.
    H. Monitor hemoglobin and hematocrit.
20. Provide posthemodialysis care.
    A. Monitor for disequilibrium syndrome (headache, seizures) due to sudden correction of blood chemistry abnormalities.
    B. Check dialysis site for excessive bleeding.
    C. Apply pressure dressing as ordered.
    D. Monitor blood pressure readings.
21. Prepare client for kidney transplantation, if indicated.
    A. Selection criteria
    B. Immediate postoperative period
    C. Reverse isolation and protection against infection
    D. Fluid balance maintenance
    E. Use of immunosuppressive drugs and their side effects

22. Refer client and family to appropriate counseling for assistance in coping with condition.
23. Instruct client regarding disease process, diagnostic procedures, treatment, prevention, home care, and follow-up.
    A. Diet
    B. Skin care
    C. Medications

Evaluation

1. Reports increased comfort, decreased anxiety
2. Shows no signs of avoidable injury and/or infection
3. Maintains adequate nutritional status
4. Maintains adequate fluid and electrolyte balance
5. Maintains adequate urinary elimination pattern
6. Maintains good skin hygiene
7. Demonstrates understanding of disease process, diagnostic procedures, treatment, prevention, home care, and need for follow-up

Lower Urinary Tract Infection (Cystitis and Urethritis)

Description

1. Cystitis and urethritis are two forms of lower urinary tract infections (UTIs).
2. They usually respond well to treatment.
3. They may reoccur owing to presence of resistant bacteria.
4. They are more common in females than in males.
5. Prevalent disorder in children, especially girls.
6. Conditions are frequently associated with anatomical or physiological abnormalities in children and adult males.
7. Causes
   A. Gram-negative bacterial infection due to organisms such as *Proteus, Enterobacteria, Pseudomonas,* and *E. coli* ascending from the urethra.
   B. Contamination of lower urinary tract during catheterization or instrumentation.
   C. Breakdown in bladder's defense mechanisms allowing bacteria to invade bladder mucosa.
   D. Bacterial flare-up due to resistance of organisms to antimicrobial therapy.
   E. Majority of recurrent UTIs are due to reinfection by same or new pathogen.
   F. Small number of recurrent cases are due to perseverant infection from conditions such as kidney stones or chronic prostatitis.
   G. High incidence in women may be due to shortness of urethra.
   H. Bacterial invasion from vagina, perineum, rectum, or from sexual partner.

Assessment

SUBJECTIVE

1. Urgency
2. Frequency of urination
3. Cramps or bladder spasms
4. Dysuria
5. Itching
6. Nocturia
7. Burning on urination
8. Low back pain
9. Malaise
10. Nausea
11. Abdominal or flank pain
12. Chills

OBJECTIVE

1. Hematuria
2. Increased temperature
3. Vomiting
4. Tenderness over bladder region
5. Purulent urine

DIAGNOSTIC TESTS AND METHODS

1. History
2. Physical examination
3. Routine urine examination
4. Urine culture and sensitivity—to identify pathogen and correct antimicrobial agent to use
5. Culture of discharge from urethra—especially in males
6. Voiding dystourethrography, IVP—to detect congenital abnormalities that may be a cause for recurrent UTIs

Planning

1. Safe, effective care environment
   A. Prevent avoidable injury and/or infection.
   B. Increase client's knowledge of disease process, diagnostic procedures, and treatment.
2. Physiological integrity
   A. Maintain adequate serum glucose level.
   B. Maintain adequate fluid balance.
   C. Maintain adequate nutritional status.
   D. Maintain adequate tissue perfusion.
3. Psychosocial integrity
   A. Facilitate effective coping.
4. Health promotion and maintenance
   A. Increase client's knowledge of prevention, home care (including medication, diet, and activity), and follow-up.

Implementation

1. Assess, report, and record signs and symptoms and reactions to treatment.
2. Force fluids unless contraindicated; avoid cola drinks, coffee.
3. Provide diet that acidifies urine.
4. Monitor temperature; administer antipyretics as prescribed.
5. Administer antimicrobials as prescribed.
6. Monitor results of urine examination, culture.
7. Provide perineal care.
8. Provide sitz baths.
9. Prepare client for dilatation if stricture is present.
10. Provide for isolation for urethritis, if indicated.
11. Prepare client for surgery in cases of recurrent infection due to chronic prostatitis, renal calculi, or structural abnormality.
12. Instruct client regarding disease process, diagnostic procedures, treatment, prevention, home care, and follow-up. Include teaching on:
    A. Medications

B. Diet
C. Activity

Evaluation

1. Reports increased comfort, decreased anxiety
2. Shows no signs of infection
3. Maintains adequate elimination pattern
4. Demonstrates understanding of disease process, diagnostic procedures, treatment, prevention, home care, and need for follow-up

Cancer of the Bladder

Description

1. Bladder cancers are malignant lesions of the bladder.
2. Lesion can develop on surface of bladder wall (papillomas, benign or malignant) or grow within bladder (usually more virulent).
3. Cancer invades underlying muscles.
4. Most bladder tumors (90%) are transitional cell carcinomas.
5. They may result from malignant transformation of benign papillomas.
6. Less common are adenocarcinomas, squamous cell carcinomas, and sarcomas.
7. Bladder cancer more prevalent in individuals over age 50, more common in males than in females.
8. Incidence rises in densely populated industrial areas.
9. Individuals at high risk include rubber workers, weavers, aniline dye workers, hairdressers, petroleum workers, spray painters, and leather finishers.
10. Bladder cancers account for about 2%–4% of all cancers.
11. Predisposing factors
    A. Specific environmental carcinogens such as benzidine tobacco, nitrates—latent period between exposure and development of symptoms is about 18 years.
    B. Squamous cell carcinomas occur with greater frequency in geographic areas where schistosomiasis is endemic, such as Egypt; they are also associated with infection and chronic bladder irritation due to renal calculi and recurrent use of Foley catheters.

Assessment

SUBJECTIVE

1. Urinary urgency, dysuria

OBJECTIVE

1. Signs of cystitis
2. Gross, painless, intermittent hematuria
3. Suprapubic pain after voiding (when invasive lesions occur)
4. Signs of renal failure
5. Positive bladder biopsy
6. Positive cystoscopic examination
7. Urinary frequency, nocturia, and dribbling

DIAGNOSTIC TESTS AND METHODS

1. History
2. Physical examination
3. Cystoscopy

4. Bladder tissue biopsy
5. IVP
6. Urinalysis and urine cytology
7. Excretory urography
8. Pelvic arteriography
9. A CT scan
10. Renal ultrasound

Planning

1. Safe, effective care environment
   A. Increase client's and family's knowledge of disease process, diagnostic procedures, and treatment.
   B. Prevent avoidable injury and/or infection.
2. Physiological integrity
   A. Maintain adequate elimination pattern.
   B. Increase comfort.
3. Psychosocial integrity
   A. Promote effective coping.
   B. Promote positive self-image.
4. Health promotion and maintenance
   A. Increase client's and family's knowledge of home care and follow-up.

Implementation

1. Assess, report, and record signs and symptoms and reactions to treatments.
2. Provide emotional support.
3. Monitor urine output for evidence of bleeding.
4. Obtain urine specimen for culture and sensitivity.
5. Prepare client and family for client's surgical procedure.
   A. Transurethral fulguration or excision—removal of small tumors with little tissue-layer infiltration.
   B. Laser photocoagulation—lowest risk of bleeding or perforation of the bladder wall.
   C. Cystectomy—complete removal of bladder with permanent alteration of urinary elimination. Types are:
      (1) Uterotomy—excision of ureters from bladder and connection of ureters to abdominal wall to form stomas for urinary drainage
      (2) Colonic conduit—excision of the ureters from bladder to a resected portion of the colon, which is passed through abdominal wall to construct a stoma for urinary drainage
      (3) Ileal conduit—similar to the colonic conduit, except a portion of the ileum is used instead of the colon
      (4) Ureterosigmoidostomy—ureters anastomosed to sigmoid colon for urinary drainage through the rectum
      (5) Nephrostomy—insertion of a catheter into kidney for drainage
6. Provide postoperative care.
   A. Monitor urinary drainage and patency of conduits.
   B. Monitor for abdominal distention due to hemorrhage.
   C. Monitor for signs of hemorrhage.
   D. Promote adequate respiratory ventilation.
   E. Provide frequent, meticulous skin care around stomas.
   F. Encourage fluid intake when ordered.
   G. Protect client from infection.
7. Prepare client for radiation treatment and/or chemotherapy.
8. Explain drainage equipment and application.

9. Arrange for visit with ostomy therapist.
10. Provide information regarding local ostomy organization.
11. Instruct client and family regarding disease process, diagnostic procedures, treatment, home care (including stoma and skin care), and follow-up.

Evaluation

1. Reports increased comfort, decreased anxiety
2. Shows no signs of avoidable injury and/or infection
3. Maintains adequate urinary elimination pattern
4. Uses effective coping strategies
5. Demonstrates understanding of disease process, diagnostic procedures, treatment, home care, and follow-up; similar understanding demonstrated by family

Male Genitourinary System

Benign Prostatic Hypertrophy

Description

1. Benign prostatic hypertrophy (BPH) is slow enlargement of the prostate gland with extension into the bladder.
2. Urinary outflow through the urethra is obstructed.
3. Urinary stream becomes smaller with dysuria.
4. Stasis of urine in bladder occurs.
5. Gradual dilation of ureters and kidneys occurs due to the obstruction.
6. Hydronephrosis, calculi formation, or cystitis may occur.
7. Acute urinary retention occurs with complete obstruction.
8. BPH occurs frequently in males older than 50 years of age.
9. Cause—unknown.
10. Possible causes
    A. Link between BPH and hormonal activity—androgenic hormone decreases with age, causing an imbalance between androgen and estrogen levels and high levels of dihydrotestosterone
    B. Neoplasms
    C. Arteriosclerosis
    D. Inflammation
    E. Metabolic or nutritional disturbances

Assessment

SUBJECTIVE

1. Urgency, frequency, burning, and hesitancy on urination
2. Decreased force on urination
3. Nocturia
4. Sensation of incomplete emptying

OBJECTIVE

1. Small amounts on voiding
2. Possible hematuria
3. Urinary retention
4. Infection
5. Enlarged prostate gland on palpation and cystoscopic examination
6. Renal insufficiency secondary to obstruction
7. Hemorrhage
8. Shock

DIAGNOSTIC TESTS AND METHODS

1. History.
2. Physical examination.
3. IVP.
4. BUN, creatinine levels.
5. Urinalysis and urine culture.
6. Cystourethroscopy immediately before surgery.
7. Urodynamics—to evaluate the degree of urine obstruction.
8. Acid phosphatase and prostate specific antigen (PSA) to establish baseline values and rule out prostatic cancer.

Planning

1. Safe, effective care environment
   A. Prevent avoidable injury and/or infection.
   B. Increase client's knowledge of disease process, diagnostic procedures, and treatment.
2. Physiological integrity
   A. Increase comfort.
   B. Maintain adequate elimination pattern.
3. Psychosocial integrity
   A. Promote positive self-concept.
   B. Reduce anxiety.
4. Health promotion and maintenance
   A. Increase client's knowledge of home care and follow-up.

Implementation

1. Assess, report, and record signs and symptoms and reactions to treatment.
2. Monitor urinary elimination pattern, intake and output, and characteristics of urine.
   A. Prepare patient for surgical intervention—transurethral resection, prostate; or suprapubic, retropubic, perineal prostatectomy.
3. Explain postoperative course, including bladder spasms, hemorrhage, pain, and catheter placement.
4. Provide postoperative care—observe post–transurethral resection, prostate syndrome.
   A. Explain reason for sensation of bladder fullness from retention balloon on catheter.
   B. Instruct patient to avoid attempting to urinate around catheter.
   C. Monitor three-way irrigation catheter patency—keep bladder free of clots.
   D. Keep catheter system sterile.
   E. Monitor urine output and characteristics—red to light pink for first 24 hours.
   F. Monitor intake and output—record all drainage tubes separately.
   G. Change dressing around suprapubic catheter frequently.
   H. Administer analgesics or antispasmodics as prescribed.
   I. Avoid use of rectal thermometer.
   J. Administer analgesics for pain as prescribed.
   K. Monitor urinary output, retention, and continence following catheter removal.
   L. Encourage oral fluid intake.
5. Instruct client regarding disease process, diagnostic procedures, treatment, prevention, home care, and need for follow-up.

Evaluation

1. Reports increased comfort, decreased anxiety
2. Shows no signs of avoidable injury and/or infection
3. Maintains adequate urinary elimination pattern
4. Demonstrates understanding of disease process, diagnostic procedures, treatment, home care, and need for follow-up

Cancer of the Prostate

Description

1. Cancer of the prostate is a malignant tumor of the prostate gland.
2. After skin cancer, prostatic cancer is the most common neoplasm found in males over age 50.
3. Seldom produce symptoms until well advanced.
4. Adenocarcinoma is the most common form.
5. Approximately 85% of tumors originate in posterior part of gland; 15% originate near the urethra.
6. Seldom result from BPH.
7. It accounts for 17% of all cancers.
8. Incidence is highest among blacks and in males with blood type A.
9. Incidence is lowest in Orientals.
10. Occurrence unaffected by socioeconomic status or fertility.
11. Five-year survival rate is 70% when cancer is treated in its localized form.
12. Five-year survival rate is under 35% if treatment occurs after metastases.
13. Fatal when widespread bone metastases occurs.
14. Cause—unknown.

Assessment

SUBJECTIVE

1. Early tumor—no symptoms
2. Back pain
3. Symptoms from metastases

OBJECTIVE

1. Difficulty in starting urinary stream
2. Dribbling
3. Urinary retention
4. Unexplained cystitis
5. Hematuria (rare)

DIAGNOSTIC TESTS AND METHODS

1. History
2. Physical examination—rectal examination
3. Biopsy examination
4. Serum acid phosphatase levels
   A. Elevated in prostatic cancer.
   B. Study is used as baseline to determine effectiveness of treatment.
5. Serum alkaline phosphatase levels
   A. Elevated levels point to bone metastasis.
6. Bone scan

Planning

1. Safe, effective care environment
   A. Prevent avoidable injury and/or infection.
   B. Increase client's knowledge of disease process, diagnostic procedures, and treatment.
2. Physiological integrity
   A. Increase comfort.
   B. Maintain adequate elimination pattern.
3. Psychosocial integrity
   A. Promote positive self-concept.
   B. Reduce anxiety.
4. Health promotion and maintenance
   A. Increase client's knowledge of home care and follow-up.

Implementation

1. Assess, report, and record signs and symptoms and reactions to treatment.
2. Provide emotional support to client and family.
3. Explain expected effects of surgery such as possible incontinence, impotence, and treatment of radiation side effects.
4. Encourage patient to express fears.
5. Explain postoperative procedures such as dressing changes, placement of tubes.
6. Teach perineal exercises to decrease incontinence.
7. Provide postprostatectomy care.
   A. Monitor dressing, incision, and drainage system for excessive bleeding.
   B. Monitor client for signs of bleeding—cold, clammy skin; pallor; restlessness; decreasing blood pressure readings; rising pulse rate.
   C. Administer antispasmodics as ordered—control of postoperative bladder spasms.
   D. Monitor for signs of infection—chills, increased temperature, inflamed incisional site.
   E. Maintain adequate fluid intake—minimum of 2000 mL daily.
   F. Provide good skin care—incontinence is a frequent problem.
8. Provide post–suprapubic prostatectomy care.
   A. Encourage family's psychological support of client.
   B. Keep skin around drain clean and dry.
   C. Encourage perineal exercises 24–48 hours after surgery.
   D. Provide meticulous catheter care—check tubing for kinks, mucus plugs, clots.
   E. Explain reason for avoiding pulling on tubes or catheter.
9. Provide post–perineal prostatectomy care.
   A. Avoid taking rectal temperature or inserting rectal tubes.
   B. Provide frequent sitz baths to relieve pain and inflammation.
   C. Use pads to absorb urinary drainage.
10. Provide post–transurethral resection care.
    A. Monitor for abdominal distention—due to urethral stricture or blockage of catheter by blood clot.
    B. Irrigate catheter as ordered.
    C. Monitor for signs of urethral stricture—straining to urinate, dysuria.
11. Monitor for radiation effects such as nausea and vomiting, dry skin, and alopecia.
12. Watch for side effects of diethylstilbestrol (estrogen ther-

apy) such as gynecomastia, fluid retention, nausea and vomiting.
13. Monitor for presence of thrombophlebitis in patients receiving diethylstilbestrol.
14. Teach clients undergoing radiotherapy about diet and skin care while undergoing treatment.
15. Instruct client regarding home care and follow-up.

Evaluation

1. Reports increased comfort, decreased anxiety
2. Maintains adequate urinary elimination pattern
3. Shows no signs of avoidable injury and/or infection
4. Demonstrates understanding of disease process, diagnostic procedures, treatment, home care, and need for follow-up

Female Reproductive System

Basic Information

Nursing care of the gynecological client is a reflection of the interest in improving the quality of health for women. Multiple gynecological abnormalities occur at the same time. For example, a client with vaginitis may also have dysmenorrhea, dysuria, and infertility. There may also be complications associated with the urological disorders, due to the proximity of the reproductive system to the urinary system. Disorders of the reproductive system may interfere with sexuality, conception, and self-image.

Assessment

SUBJECTIVE

1. Lower abdominal pain and cramping
2. Backache
3. Urinary frequency and urgency
4. Stress incontinence
5. Tenderness
6. Tenderness and burning of nipples
7. Itching and burning of external genitalia
8. Burning, itching, tenderness, and pain during intercourse
9. Pain, headache, irritability, depression, and insomnia related to menstrual cycle

OBJECTIVE

1. General appearance
2. Vital signs
3. Weight
4. Breasts
   A. Shape
   B. Skin dimpling
   C. Presence of nodules
      (1) Size
      (2) Consistency
      (3) Fixed or mobile
   D. Nipples
      (1) Asymmetry
      (2) Discharge
      (3) Retraction
      (4) Ulceration
   E. External genitalia
      (1) Irritation
      (2) Redness
      (3) Excoriation
   F. External vaginal orifice
      (1) Irritation
      (2) Redness
      (3) Nodules
   G. Excoriation
      (1) Vaginal discharge
      (2) Color
      (3) Consistency
      (4) Odor

DIAGNOSTIC TESTS AND METHODS

1. Laboratory tests
   A. Follicle-stimulating hormone (FSH)
      (1) FSH stimulates secretion of estrogen.
      (2) Elevated serum levels may cause excessive uterine bleeding.
      (3) Diminished levels may be associated with bleeding between menstrual cycles.
   B. Luteinizing hormone (LH)
      (1) LH stimulates secretion of progesterone.
      (2) Elevated serum levels may be associated with prolonged and heavy menses.
      (3) Diminished serum levels may cause short and scanty menses.
   C. Adrenal function tests
      (1) Tools used to rule out abnormalities of menstruation due to dysfunction of the adrenal cortex.
      (2) Diminished or elevated production of adrenal cortex hormone secretion may cause amenorrhea.
   D. Thyroid function tests
      (1) Tools used to rule out abnormalities of menstruation due to thyroid disorder.
      (2) Diminished secretion of thyroid hormone may result in irregular menstrual cycles, absence of menstrual flow, or bleeding between menstrual cycles.
2. Procedures
   A. Pelvic examination—inspection and evaluation of the condition of the external genitalia, perineal and anal areas, external vaginal orifice, vagina, and cervix
   B. Culdoscopy—visualization of the ovaries, fallopian tubes, and uterus using a lighted instrument inserted into the vaginal tract
   C. Laparoscopy—visualization of pelvic structures using a lighted laparoscope inserted through a small incision in the abdominal wall
   D. Colposcopy—visualization of the cervix using a magnifying instrument
   E. Conization—instrument used to remove cone-shaped tissue from the cervix for analysis of malignant cells
   F. Schiller's test
      (1) Application of a dye to the cervix for detection of malignant cells.
      (2) Abnormal cells will not absorb dye.
      (3) Normal cells will stain a deep brown color.
   G. Biopsy examination—removal of tissue for diagnostic purposes

H. Culture and sensitivity test—tool used to determine causative microorganism and sensitivity of antibiotic to the identified microorganism
I. Ultrasonography—recording device that uses sound frequency to reflect an image of the pelvic structures; it is used to confirm uterine and ovarian tumors
J. Dilatation and curettage (D & C)—a diagnostic and therapeutic procedure in which the cervix is dilated allowing the use of a curette to scrape the lining of the uterine cavity
K. Xerography—an x-ray examination of the breast and skin
L. Mammography—an x-ray examination of the breasts used to detect tumors

Implementation

1. Inadequate knowledge regarding menstruation.
   A. Provide factual information in regard to menstruation.
   B. Describe emotional changes that might occur.
   C. Explain abnormalities that may be associated with menstruation.
   D. Instruct patient in hygiene.
2. Pain associated with menstruation.
   A. Assess location, onset, duration, and severity of pain.
   B. Administer massage to lumbar area.
   C. Apply heating pad to abdomen.
   D. Administer prescribed analgesics—monitor for effects.
3. Breast examination—teach patient how and when to examine breast.
4. Menopause—provide information related to menopause.

Pelvic Inflammatory Disease

Description

1. Pelvic inflammatory disease (PID) is any acute, recurrent, or chronic infection of the ovaries and oviducts and adjacent tissue.
2. Condition includes inflammation of the cervix (cervicitis), uterus (endometritis), fallopian tubes (salpingitis), and ovaries (oophoritis).
3. Inflammation may extend to connective tissue (parametritis).
4. It may result in adhesions, strictures, or sterility.
5. Normally cervical secretions have protective and defensive functions.
6. Early diagnosis and treatment prevents injury to the reproductive system.
7. Untreated PID may lead to septicemia, pulmonary emboli, and shock.
8. Causes
   A. Infection with aerobic or anaerobic organisms
      (1) The gonococcus, an aerobic organism, is the most common cause.
      (2) Staphylococcus or streptococcus.
   B. Any procedure such as conization or cauterization or condition that alters the cervical mucus damages the bacteriostatic mechanism allowing bacteria to ascend into the uterine cavity.
9. Uterine infection can also occur following instrumentation such as an intrauterine device biopsy curette, irrigation catheter by which contaminated cervical mucus is carried into the uterine cavity.

Assessment

SUBJECTIVE

1. Abdominal fullness, pressure, or pain
2. Cramps in the lower abdomen
3. Pelvic pain
4. Low-back pain
5. Nausea
6. Chills
7. Malaise

OBJECTIVE

1. Elevated temperature
2. Vomiting
3. Spotting between menstrual cycles
4. Purulent vaginal discharge
5. Pain and tenderness on abdominal palpation
6. Positive vaginal cultures
7. Positive laparoscopy
8. Elevated WBC count

DIAGNOSTIC TESTS AND METHODS

1. History
2. Physical examination
3. Culture and sensitivity test
4. CBC with differential
5. Gram's stain
6. Ultrasonography
7. Culdocentesis—to obtain peritoneal fluid or pus for culture and sensitivity
8. Laparoscopy

Planning

1. Safe, effective care environment
   A. Prevent avoidable injury and/or infection.
   B. Increase client's knowledge of disease process, diagnostic procedures, and treatment.
2. Physiological integrity
   A. Increase comfort.
   B. Prevent complications.
3. Psychosocial integrity
   A. Reduce anxiety.
4. Health promotion and maintenance
   A. Increase knowledge of prevention, home care, and follow-up.

Implementation

1. Assess, report, and record signs and symptoms and reactions to treatment.
2. Provide nonjudgmental attitude.
3. Place client in mid-Fowler position to facilitate vaginal drainage.
4. Monitor vital signs.
5. Monitor WBC and vaginal cultures.
6. Administer prescribed analgesics, antibiotics, and probenecid (prolongs effects of antibiotics).

7. Apply heat to abdominal area, if ordered (to improve circulation and provide comfort).
8. Allow client to verbalize feelings regarding condition.
9. Provide good perineal hygiene.
10. Explain suggested treatment for sexual contacts and abstinence from sexual intercourse until infection is resolved.
11. Encourage compliance with treatment in order to prevent recurrence.
12. Monitor for signs of abdominal rigidity and distention (possible signs of peritonitis).
13. Instruct client to immediately report signs of infection following gynecological procedures such as a D & C.
14. Instruct client to avoid douching or intercourse for at least 7 days following minor gynecological procedures.
15. Instruct client regarding disease process, diagnostic procedures, prevention, home care, and follow-up. Include teaching on:
    A. Transmission of organisms
    B. Signs and symptoms of recurrence
    C. Medication regimen and compliance
    D. Prevention of vaginal or vulval infections
    E. Appropriate hygienic measures
    F. Recognizing if sexual partner is infected with gonococcus—discharge from penis of whitish fluid with painful urination
    G. Importance of routine examinations because gonococcal infection is asymptomatic in females

Evaluation

1. Reports increased comfort, decreased anxiety
2. Shows no signs of avoidable injury and/or infection
3. Demonstrates understanding of disease process, diagnostic procedures, treatment, prevention, home care, and need for follow-up

Vulvovaginitis

Description

1. Vulvovaginitis is an inflammation of the vulva (vulvitis) and vagina (vaginitis).
2. It is due to the proximity of these two structures; inflammation of one precipitates the inflammation of the other.
3. It is caused by alterations in pH, decreased resistance, and/or increase in number of offending microorganisms.
4. It may occur at any age and affects most females at some time in their lives.
5. Prognosis is good with treatment.
6. Causes of vaginitis:
    A. *Pseudomonas*
    B. *Escherichia coli*
    C. Infection with *Trichomonas vaginalis,* usually transmitted through sexual intercourse
    D. Infection with *Candida albicans* (*Monilia*)
       (1) A fungus that requires glucose for growth.
       (2) It occurs twice as often in pregnant women than in nonpregnant women.
       (3) It commonly affects diabetics, clients receiving broad-spectrum antibiotics, and users of oral contraceptives.
    E. Infection with *Haemophilus vaginalis* (gram-negative bacillus)

F. Viral infection with venereal warts or herpes virus type II, usually transmitted by sexual intercourse
G. Venereal infection (gonococcus)
H. Vaginal mucosa atrophy in menopausal females as a result of decreasing levels of estrogen, which predispose to bacterial invasion
7. Causes of vulvitis
    A. Trauma—skin breakdown may cause secondary infection
    B. Parasitic infection (crab louse)
    C. Chemical irritation or allergic reactions to feminine hygiene products, clothing, or toilet paper
    D. Poor personal hygiene—contamination with urine, feces, or vaginal secretions
    E. Atrophy of the vulva in menopausal females as a result of decreased estrogen levels
8. Factors that may decrease resistance to infection
    A. Stress
    B. Aging process
    C. Drugs
    D. Frequent douching
    E. Malnutrition
    F. Disease

Assessment

SUBJECTIVE

1. Vaginal itching, burning, or irritation
2. Abdominal cramps or feeling of fullness in pelvis
3. Urinary frequency, burning, and pain
4. Painful intercourse

OBJECTIVE

1. Inflammation of vulva and vagina
2. Trichomonal vaginitis—presence of thin, bubbly green-tinged, and malodorous vaginal discharge
3. Candida vaginitis—presence of a thick, white, curd-like discharge
4. Haemophilus vaginitis—presence of a gray, foul-smelling vaginal discharge
5. Gonorrheal vaginitis—asymptomatic or profuse, purulent vaginal discharge
6. Atrophic vaginitis—blood-flecked discharge
7. Simple vaginitis—yellow mucoid discharge
8. Acute vulvitis—mild to severe inflammation (edema, redness, pruritus)
9. Herpes vulvitis—painful ulceration or vesicle formation in active phase
10. Chronic vulvitis—mild inflammation, edema (may involve entire perineum)

DIAGNOSTIC TESTS AND METHODS

1. History
2. Physical examination
3. Diagnosis of vaginitis
    A. Culture and sensitivity
    B. Microscopic examination of vaginal exudate
4. Diagnosis of vulvitis or suspected venereal disease
    A. CBC
    B. Urinalysis
    C. Cytology screening
5. Biopsy of lesions

Planning

1. Safe, effective care environment
   A. Prevent avoidable injury and/or infection.
   B. Increase client's knowledge of disease process, diagnostic procedures, and treatment.
2. Physiological integrity
   A. Increase comfort.
   B. Maintain skin integrity.
3. Psychosocial integrity
   A. Reduce anxiety.
   B. Promote positive self-image.
4. Health promotion and maintenance
   A. Increase knowledge of prevention, home care, and follow-up.

Implementation

1. Assess, report, and record signs and symptoms and reactions to treatment.
2. Administer prescribed vaginal creams or suppositories such as nystatin (Mycostatin) at bedtime to prevent medication loss and promote distribution within the vagina.
3. Instruct client to use sanitary pads with vaginal creams to protect clothing.
4. Administer prescribed systemic antibiotic therapy for clients with gonorrhea.
5. Administer prescribed local antibiotics for *Haemophilus* vaginitis.
6. Explain techniques to relieve vaginal itching or discomfort.
   A. Proper cleansing
   B. Sitz baths
   C. Appropriate creams or lotions
7. Explain techniques to relieve vulvular itching or discomfort.
   A. Cold compresses or cool sitz baths for acute vulvitis
   B. Avoidance of drying soaps
   C. Wearing loose clothing to allow air circulation
   D. Application of prescribed topical corticosteroids to decrease inflammation
   E. Proper hygienic measures
8. Apply topical estrogen ointments for atrophic vulvovaginitis.
9. Instruct client regarding need for good hand washing with each application of vaginal medication, proper cleansing of applicator, and good perineal hygiene.
10. Instruct client on proper use of douches, if prescribed.
11. Administer prescribed medications such as metronidazole for clients with trichomonal vaginitis.
12. Instruct client to abstain from sexual intercourse until infection resolves, or have partner use a condom.
13. Explain need for treatment of partner, if indicated, to prevent recurrence.
14. Offer emotional support and comfort.
15. Instruct client regarding disease process, diagnostic procedures, treatment, prevention, home care, and follow-up. Include teaching on:
   A. Avoidance of douching, unless prescribed, because it can alter vaginal pH
   B. Proper hygienic measures
   C. Compliance with sitz medication regimen
   D. Early recognition of symptoms

Evaluation

1. Reports increased comfort, decreased anxiety
2. Shows no signs of avoidable injury and/or infection
3. Demonstrates understanding of disease process, diagnostic procedures, treatment, prevention, home care, and need for follow-up

Endometriosis

Description

1. Endometriosis is the presence of endometrial tissue outside the lining of the uterine cavity.
2. The endometrial cells bleed into nearby spaces, causing inflammation, adhesions, tumor, or cystic formation as a result of stimulation by ovarian hormones.
3. Condition is usually confined to the pelvic area, most commonly around the ovaries, the cul-de-sac, uterosacral ligaments, and the uterovesical peritoneum, but it can appear anywhere in the body.
4. It usually occurs in adults between the ages of 30 and 40, especially in women who postpone pregnancy; uncommon before the age of 20.
5. Severe endometriosis may have an abrupt onset or may develop slowly over a period of years.
6. Condition is uncovered in approximately 20% of patients who are undergoing gynecological surgical intervention for other disorders.
7. It usually becomes progressively severe during the menstrual years.
8. Treatment varies depending on stage of the disease.
   A. Conservative treatment in stages I and II may be followed for young women who wish to have children.
   B. Surgical intervention is conducted in stages III and IV when ovarian masses are present in order to rule out presence of a malignancy.
   C. Conservative surgical intervention may be conducted to resect cysts and remove adhesions.
   D. For women who do not wish to bear children, or when the condition is in stages III to V, the treatment of choice is a total abdominal hysterectomy with bilateral salpingo-oophorectomy.
9. Condition usually subsides after menopause.
10. Staging of endometriosis
   A. Stage I: One or more small superficial endometrial cell growths implant on the pelvic peritoneum.
   B. Stage II: Larger superficial implants on rectovaginal septum, ovaries, or uterosacral ligaments.
   C. Stage III: Endometriomas appear on the ovary.
   D. Stage IV: Endometriomas change to adenocarcinomas.
11. Cause—unknown
12. Possible causes:
   A. Transportation: Fallopian tubes expel endometrial fragments that implant on the ovaries or pelvic peritoneum during the menstrual period.
   B. Formation in situ: Hormonal change or inflammation triggers changes in epithelium.
   C. Induction: A combination of transportation and formation in situ.
13. Predisposing factors:
   A. Familial susceptibility or recent surgery necessitating opening of the uterus such as cesarean section

Assessment

SUBJECTIVE

1. Abdominal fullness
2. Dysmenorrhea—constant pain in lower abdomen, vagina, posterior pelvis, and back
   A. Begins at approximately 5 days prior to menses; lasts for 2 to 3 days.
3. Different from primary dysmenorrhea, which is more cramplike and located in the midline of the abdomen
4. Affecting ovaries or cul-de-sac—dyspareunia
5. Affecting ovaries and oviducts—profuse menses
6. Affecting cervix, vagina, and perineum—bleeding from endometrial implants
7. Affecting rectovaginal septum and colon—nausea
8. Affecting small bowel—nausea that worsens prior to menses, abdominal cramps
9. Irregular menses
10. Menorrhagia

OBJECTIVE

1. Infertility
2. Nodular, tender uterosacral ligaments, enlarged uterus per pelvic examination
3. Positive findings on laparoscopy

DIAGNOSTIC TESTS AND METHODS

1. History
2. Physical examination
3. Pelvic examination
4. Palpation
5. Laparoscopy
6. Cul-de-sac aspiration
7. Barium enema—to rule out disorders of the bowel

Planning

1. Safe, effective care environment
   A. Prevent injury and/or infection.
   B. Increase client's and family's knowledge of disease process, diagnostic procedures, and treatment.
2. Physiological integrity
   A. Increase comfort.
3. Psychosocial integrity
   A. Promote effective coping mechanisms.
4. Health promotion and maintenance
   A. Increase client's and family's knowledge of prevention, home care, and follow-up.

Implementation

1. Assess, report, and record signs and symptoms and reactions to treatment.
2. Allow client to verbalize feelings regarding condition.
3. Administer prescribed medication that suppresses ovulation, such as danazol or oral contraceptives.
4. Advise adolescents to use sanitary napkins in place of tampons—assist in prevention of retrograde (backward) flow in girls who have a narrow vagina or small introitus (external vaginal orifice).
5. Reassure client that condition is not life threatening.
6. Prepare client and family for surgical intervention (laparotomy or laparoscopy) such as hysterectomy, salpingec-tomy, or oophorectomy, if required by client to remove endometrial implants or to lyse adhesions.
7. Provide appropriate postoperative care.
   A. Monitor vaginal packing.
   B. Monitor for signs of hemorrhage.
8. Monitor urinary output—dysuria.
9. Instruct client and family regarding disease process, diagnostic procedures, treatment, prevention, home care, and need for follow-up. Include teaching on:
   A. Medications
   B. Hygiene
   C. Activity
   D. Estrogen therapy if premenopausal
   E. Need for an annual pelvic examination and Pap smear for early diagnosis and more effective treatment

Evaluation

1. Reports increased comfort, decreased anxiety
2. Shows no signs of avoidable injury and/or infection
3. Uses effective coping strategies
4. Demonstrates understanding of disease process, diagnostic procedures, treatment, prevention, home care, and need for follow-up; similar understanding demonstrated by family

Dysmenorrhea

Description

1. Dysmenorrhea is painful menstruation or menstrual cramps.
2. The most common gynecological complaint; leading cause of absenteeism from work and school.
3. It affects approximately 10% of high-school girls each month.
4. An estimated 140 million work hours are lost per year.
5. It may occur as a primary or secondary disorder.
6. Prognosis for primary dysmenorrhea is good, it is self-limiting.
7. Prognosis for secondary dysmenorrhea depends on the underlying disorder.
8. The condition is generally secondary after age 20.
9. Predisposing factors
   A. Hormonal imbalances and psychogenic factors
   B. Increased prostaglandin secretions, which increase uterine contractions
   C. Underlying disorders such as endometriosis, PID, pelvic tumors, and malposition of the uterus

Assessment

SUBJECTIVE

1. Sharp, intermittent cramps
2. Lower abdominal pain radiating to back, thighs, groin, and vulva with or just prior to menstruation
3. Breast tenderness, headache, nausea, vertigo, and palpitations
4. Chills
5. Irritability, headache, and fatigue

OBJECTIVE

1. Vomiting and diarrhea
2. Urinary frequency
3. Abdominal distention (bloating)
4. Elevated temperature

DIAGNOSTIC TESTS AND METHODS

1. History
2. Physical examination
3. Pelvic examination
4. Psychological examination, if necessary
5. For secondary dysmenorrhea to diagnose underlying disorders:
   A. Laparoscopy
   B. D & C
   C. X-rays
   D. CT
   E. FSH and LH levels, to assess pituitary function
   F. Progesterone and estradiol levels, to assess ovarian function

Planning

1. Safe, effective care environment
   A. Increase client's knowledge of disease process, diagnostic procedures, and treatment.
2. Physiological integrity
   A. Increase comfort.
3. Psychosocial integrity
   A. Promote effective coping.
   B. Reduce anxiety.
4. Health promotion and maintenance
   A. Increase client's knowledge of home care and follow-up.

Implementation

1. Assess, report, and record signs and symptoms and reactions to treatment.
2. Administer analgesics such as aspirin for mild pain.
3. Administer prescribed opioids for severe pain.
4. Administer prescribed prostaglandin inhibitors such as ibuprofen to relieve pain (decreases uterine contractions).
5. Apply heat to lower abdomen. (Caution: Heat is not recommended for young girls because appendicitis may mimic dysmenorrhea.)
6. Instruct client to drink warm fluids prior to onset of pain.
7. Identify factors that increase or alleviate pain.
8. Provide measures such as rest, massage, exercise, balanced diet.
9. Allow client to verbalize feelings; assist with development of coping strategies.
10. Encourage a positive attitude toward menstruation.
11. Instruct client regarding disease process, diagnostic procedures, treatment, home care, and follow-up.

Evaluation

1. Reports increased comfort, decreased anxiety
2. Uses effective coping strategies
3. Demonstrates understanding of disease process, diagnostic procedures, treatment, home care (including measures to alleviate pain and discomfort), and need for follow-up

Uterine Displacement or Prolapse, Cystocele, and Rectocele

Description

1. Uterine displacement or prolapsed uterus is protrusion of vaginal mucosa downward through the vaginal opening.

   A. First-degree prolapse: Cervix protrudes inside vagina.
   B. Second-degree prolapse: Cervix protrudes below the vagina.
   C. Third-degree prolapse: Uterus protrudes below vaginal opening.
2. Cystocele—herniation of the bladder into the vagina
3. Rectocele—protrusion of posterior vaginal wall with anterior wall of rectum through the vagina
4. Cause
   A. Weakness of supporting muscles and pelvic ligaments due to:
      (1) Congenital weakness
      (2) Close frequent pregnancies
      (3) Laceration of pelvic muscles
      (4) Improper bearing down during childbirth

Assessment

SUBJECTIVE

1. Back or pelvic pain—may increase with ambulation
2. Stress incontinence or application of pressure to lower abdomen (Credé's maneuver) in order to void
3. Dysmenorrhea
4. Backache
5. Fatigue
6. Pelvic pressure
7. Dyspareunia

OBJECTIVE

1. Urinary stasis
2. Evidence of prolapse (prolapsed uterus)
3. Displacement of uterus on pelvic examination
4. Constipation or incontinence of feces and flatus (rectocele)
5. Cystitis or residual urine after voiding (cystocele)
6. Hemorrhoids (rectocele)
7. Ulcerations in third-degree prolapse

DIAGNOSTIC TESTS AND METHODS

1. History
2. Physical examination
3. Pelvic examination

Planning

1. Safe, effective care environment
   A. Prevent avoidable injury and/or infection.
   B. Increase client's and family's knowledge of disease process, diagnostic procedures, and treatment.
2. Physiological integrity
   A. Increase comfort.
   B. Maintain adequate elimination pattern.
   C. Maintain tissue integrity.
3. Psychosocial integrity
   A. Reduce anxiety.
   B. Promote effective coping.
4. Health promotion and maintenance
   A. Promote positive self-image.
   B. Increase client's and family's knowledge of prevention, home care, and follow-up.

Implementation

1. Assess, report, and record signs and symptoms and reactions to treatment.

2. Cover prolapsed uterus with saline compresses.
3. Discuss specific treatments.
   A. Pelvic exercises for prolapsed uterus
   B. Pessary to hold uterus in place if surgical intervention is contraindicated
   C. Hysterectomy for prolapsed uterus
   D. Anterior colporrhaphy for repair of cystocele
   E. Posterior colporrhaphy for repair of rectocele
4. Prepare client and family for client's surgical intervention.
5. Provide appropriate postoperative care.
   A. Prevent pressure on suture line—maintain patent Foley catheter so that bladder is emptied; administer stool softeners to prevent constipation; avoid Valsalva's maneuver.
   B. Place patient in low Fowler position or flat in bed to prevent pressure on suture line.
   C. Administer catheter care twice daily and as other-wise needed.
   D. Use heat lamp, anesthetic spray, or ice packs to perineum, if ordered.
   E. Clean perineum with warm water and soap; rinse and pat dry anterior to posterior.
   F. Use Sitz bath once sutures are removed.
   G. Administer prescribed analgesics for pain.
6. Provide postoperative care for abdominal hysterectomy.
   A. Chart number of perineal pads used in 8-hour period following hysterectomy.
   B. Monitor for signs of hemorrhage.
   C. Monitor vaginal discharge other than serosanguineous fluid.
   D. Monitor for return of bowel sounds.
   E. Monitor for signs of urinary retention.
7. Instruct client and family regarding disease process, diagnostic procedures, treatment, home care, and follow-up. Include teaching on:
   A. Avoidance of heavy lifting after surgery.
   B. Use of pelvic exercises.
   C. Avoidance of constipation, use of laxatives.
   D. Use of stool softeners.
   E. Prescribed hygienic measures.
   F. Abstinence from sexual intercourse until medically safe.

Evaluation

1. Reports increased comfort, decreased anxiety
2. Maintains adequate elimination pattern
3. Uses effective coping strategies
4. Maintains tissue integrity
5. Develops positive self-image
6. Ensure that client and family demonstrate understanding of disease process, diagnostic procedures, treatment, home care, and need for follow-up

Carcinoma of the Cervix

Description

1. Cervical carcinoma is a malignant lesion of the cervix, classified as either preinvasive or invasive.
2. Preinvasive carcinoma
   A. Ranges from minimal cervical dysplasia to carcinoma in situ
      (1) Three stages of cervical dysplasia (cervical intraepithelial neoplasia [CIN])
         (a) CIN I—mild to moderate dysplasia
         (b) CIN II—moderate to severe dysplasia
         (c) CIN III—severe to malignant
   B. Is curable 75%–90% of the time with early detection and proper treatment
   C. May progress to invasive cervical cancer if untreated
3. Invasive carcinoma
   A. Cancer cells can spread directly to adjacent pelvic structures or to distant sites via lymphatic system.
   B. It is responsible for approximately 8000 deaths per year in the United States.
   C. About 95% of all cases are squamous cell carcinomas; only 5% are adenocarcinomas.
   D. It generally occurs in adults between ages 30 and 50; rarely under age 20.
4. Mortality has declined with early detection and Pap smear examinations.
5. Condition is asymptomatic in early stages, and treatment depends on stage of disease, health status, age, and presence of complications.
6. Related risk factors
   A. Sexual intercourse at an early age
   B. Multiple sexual partners
   C. Lower socioeconomic status
   D. Contact with herpes virus type II and certain types of human papilloma virus (HPV) infection
   E. Cigarette smoking

Assessment

SUBJECTIVE

1. Mild bleeding after intercourse or between menstrual cycles
2. Back pain
3. Pelvic pain
4. Anorexia
5. Weight loss

OBJECTIVE

1. Watery discharge
2. Foul vaginal discharge with disease progression
3. Leakage of urine and feces from a fistula
4. Evidence of malignancy via Pap (Papanicolaou) smear—CIN III
5. Evidence of dysplasia via Pap smear—CIN I or CIN II, indicating need for follow-up studies

DIAGNOSTIC TESTS AND METHODS

1. History
2. Physical examination
3. Pap smear
4. Culposcopy and biopsy examination
5. Conization
6. Schiller's test
7. MRI or CT of pelvis and abdomen or bones, to determine metastasis
8. Cystoscopy

Planning

1. Safe, effective care environment
   A. Prevent avoidable injury and/or infection.
   B. Increase client's and family's knowledge of disease process, diagnostic procedures, and treatment.

2. Physiological integrity
   A. Increase comfort.
   B. Prevent complications.
   C. Maintain tissue integrity.
3. Psychosocial integrity
   A. Reduce anxiety and fear.
   B. Facilitate effective coping.
   C. Promote positive self-image.
4. Health promotion and maintenance
   A. Increase client's and family's knowledge of prevention, home care, and follow-up.

Implementation

1. Assess, report, and record signs and symptoms and reactions to treatment.
2. Allow client to verbalize feelings regarding condition.
3. Prepare client for appropriate treatment such as hysterectomy, cryosurgery, radiotherapy, and/or chemotherapy.
4. Provide appropriate postoperative care for simple or radical hysterectomy.
   A. Monitor intake and output, patency of Foley catheter.
   B. Monitor for postoperative complications such as thrombophlebitis and abdominal distention, vaginal hemorrhage, or vaginal discharge other than serosanguineous.
   C. Monitor for urinary retention if Foley catheter is not used.
   D. Change perineal pads every 3–4 hours and as otherwise needed.
   E. Monitor for return of bowel sounds.
5. Provide the following nursing interventions for patients who receive an internal radium implant:
   A. Provide isolation.
   B. Instruct client to maintain a side-lying or supine position to prevent displacement of implant.
   C. Provide perineal hygiene.
   D. Monitor for radiation sickness—nausea, vomiting, malaise, fever, diarrhea.
   E. Administer prescribed medications including antiemetics.
   F. Provide a high-protein, low-residue diet to avoid straining during defecation.
   G. Encourage high fluid intake—2000–3000 mL daily.
   H. Explain to client, family, visitors that time spent with client will be limited in order to avoid overexposure to radiation.
   I. Provide emotional support for feelings of alienation.
   J. Monitor patency of Foley catheter, intake and output.
   K. Monitor vaginal packing used to protect bladder and rectum from radiation.
   L. Monitor for complications such as cystitis, hemorrhage, vaginal fistula.
6. Instruct client and family regarding disease process, diagnostic procedures, home care, treatment, and need for follow-up. Include teaching on:
   A. Avoidance of heavy lifting for approximately 2 months.
   B. Avoidance of sexual intercourse for 4–6 weeks following surgery.
   C. Checking for vaginal discharge or bleeding that may appear after irradiation.
   D. Engage in activities that do not cause straining.
   E. Keeping follow-up appointment.

Evaluation

1. Reports increased comfort, decreased anxiety
2. Has no complications
3. Shows no signs of avoidable injury and/or infection
4. Maintains skin integrity
5. Develops a positive self-image
6. Demonstrates understanding of disease process, diagnostic procedures, treatment, home care, and need for follow-up; similar understanding demonstrated by family

Ovarian Cancer

Description

1. Primary ovarian cancer is the fifth most common cause of cancer deaths among women in the United States, after cancer of the breast, colon, and lung.
2. Metastatic ovarian cancer is more common than cancers at other sites in women who have had previously treated breast cancer.
3. Spread rapidly by local extension, surface seeding, and occasionally via the lymph system and the bloodstream.
4. Prognosis is generally poor because of rapid spread.
5. About 25% of women survive for 5 years.
6. Incidence is higher in women who are:
   A. Between 40 and 65
   B. In upper socioeconomic groups
   C. Single
7. Three main types:
   A. Primary epithelial tumors—account for 90% of all ovarian cancers
   B. Germ cell tumors
   C. Sex cord (stromal) tumors
8. Exact causes are unknown.

Assessment

1. Symptoms vary with size of tumor.
2. In early stage:
   A. Vague abdominal discomfort
   B. Dyspepsia
   C. Other mild GI disturbances
3. In later stage:
   A. Urinary frequency
   B. Constipation
   C. Pelvic discomfort
   D. Abdominal distention
   E. Weight loss
   F. Palpable mass
   G. Bleeding between periods in premenopausal women with sex cord (granulosa cell) tumors
   H. Masculine characteristics in premenopausal women with sex cord (arrhenoblastoma cell) tumors
4. In advanced stage:
   A. Ascites
   B. Symptoms relating to metastatic sites such as symptoms of pleural effusion
   C. Rarely postmenopausal bleeding or pain

DIAGNOSTIC TESTS AND METHODS

1. History
2. Physical examination
3. X-rays of abdomen

4. Chest x-ray—to detect distant metastasis and pleural effusion
5. CBC, blood chemistry, and ECG
6. Culdoscopy
7. Ultrasonography
8. Lymphangiography—to determine lymph node involvement
9. Mammography—to rule out primary breast cancer
10. Liver function tests or liver scan for patients with ascites
11. Ascites fluid aspiration—to identify cells by histology
12. Biopsy examination
13. Barium enema for patients with GI symptoms—to determine presence of obstruction and size of tumor
14. Exploratory laparotomy, including tumor resection and lymph node evaluation—to make accurate diagnosis
15. Histologic studies
16. CA125 antigen level: highly specific tumor marker used to detect epithelial ovarian cancer

Planning

1. Safe, effective care environment
   A. Prevent avoidable injury and/or infection.
   B. Increase client's knowledge of disease process, diagnostic procedures, and treatment.
2. Physiological integrity
   A. Increase comfort.
   B. Prevent complications.
   C. Maintain tissue integrity.
3. Psychosocial integrity
   A. Reduce anxiety and fear.
   B. Facilitate effective coping.
   C. Promote positive self-image.
4. Health promotion and maintenance
   A. Increase client's knowledge of home care and follow-up.

Implementation

1. Assess, report, and record signs and symptoms and reactions to treatment.
2. Prepare client for surgical intervention.
   A. Explain all preoperative tests.
   B. Explain expected course of treatment.
   C. Explain surgical and postoperative procedures.
   D. Explain the effects of bilateral oophorectomy to premenopausal women (artificial menopause with hot flashes, headaches, palpitations, insomnia, sweating, and depression).
   E. Provide emotional support; allow time for verbalization of feelings.
3. Provide appropriate postoperative nursing care (oophorectomy, panhysterectomy).
   A. Monitor vital signs frequently.
   B. Monitor IV fluid therapy.
   C. Monitor intake and output.
   D. Maintain patent Foley catheter.
   E. Check dressings for excessive bleeding or drainage.
   F. Observe for signs of infection.
   G. Provide abdominal support—check for signs of abdominal distention.
   H. Administer prescribed analgesics for pain.

I. Administer prescribed chemotherapeutic drugs—monitor for side effects.
J. Reposition client at least every 2 hours.
K. Encourage deep breathing and coughing.
L. Encourage and assist with ambulation as necessary.
4. Monitor and treat side effects of radiation and chemotherapy, if applicable.
   A. Provide psychological support for client and family.
   B. Discourage "smothering" of client by family.
   C. Request supportive care from chaplain, social worker, and other healthcare team members as appropriate.
   D. Assist client in dealing with changes of body image.
   E. Assist client in developing coping strategies.
5. Instruct client regarding disease process, diagnostic procedures, treatment, home care, and follow-up.

Evaluation

1. Reports increased comfort, decreased anxiety
2. Has no complications
3. Shows no signs of avoidable injury and/or infection
4. Maintains skin integrity
5. Develops a positive self-image
6. Demonstrates understanding of disease process, diagnostic procedures, treatment, home care, and need for follow-up

Breast Mass

Description

1. Breast mass refers to a nodule or mass in the breast that may or may not be malignant.
2. Nonmalignant breast lesions
   A. Fibroadenomas
      (1) Epithelial and fibroblastic cell tumors.
      (2) Nodule round, encapsulated, movable, firm, and nontender on palpation.
   B. Dysplasia
      (1) Thick, nodular lumps within the breast.
      (2) Associated with pain during menses.
      (3) Nodule is soft, movable, and tender on palpation.
      (4) There may be multiple nodules.
      (5) It occurs most often in women between 30 years of age and menopause.
3. Malignant breast tumors
   A. Most common form of cancer in women.
   B. Incidence increases with age.
   C. It affects whites more than blacks.
   D. High-risk factors
      (1) Women who have not breastfed
      (2) Presence of fibrocystic breast disease
      (3) Family history
      (4) Early menarche
      (5) Prolonged menstrual history
      (6) First pregnancy after age 25 or women who have never had children
   E. Tumor may be firm, nonmovable, tender, and nontender on palpation.
   F. It is most frequently located in upper outer portion of the breast.
   G. Metastasis occurs early, transported by lymph system, spreading to lung, bone, and/or brain.

Assessment

SUBJECTIVE

1. Small mass felt during breast self-examination.

OBJECTIVE

1. Palpable mass in breast tissue
2. Presence of tumor on mammography
3. Nipple retraction or elevation
4. Skin dimpling
5. Nipple discharge
6. Abnormal findings on thermography
7. Positive xeroradiography results
8. Positive benign or malignant breast biopsy through needle aspiration or surgical removal of tumor and microscopic examination for malignant cells

DIAGNOSTIC TESTS AND METHODS

1. History.
2. Physical examination.
3. Mammography—x-ray of breast tissue.
4. Thermography—method that measures heat from breast tissue.
5. Xerography—type of mammography using an electrically charged aluminum plate with a selenium layer. It has ability to detect carcinoma 1–2 years prior to formation of a palpable 1-cm lesion.
6. Hormonal reception assay tests—conducted on tumor tissue to determine if tumor is estrogen or progesterone dependent. Useful in determining therapeutic strategies.

Planning

1. Safe, effective care environment
   A. Prevent avoidable injury and/or infection.
   B. Increase client's and family's knowledge of disease process, diagnostic procedures, and treatment.
2. Physiological integrity
   A. Increase comfort.
   B. Maintain adequate mobility.
   C. Maintain tissue integrity.
3. Psychosocial integrity
   A. Reduce anxiety and fear.
   B. Facilitate effective coping mechanisms.
   C. Promote positive self-concept.
4. Health promotion and maintenance
   A. Increase client's and family's knowledge of prevention, home care, and need for follow-up.

Implementation

1. Assess, report, and record signs and symptoms and reactions to treatment.
2. Allow client to verbalize feelings.
3. Provide emotional support.
4. Provide frequent client contact and encouragement in illness adjustment.
5. Provide for visit of individuals from Reach to Recovery.
6. Prepare client for biopsy procedure.
7. Prepare client for surgical intervention, if required. (See intraoperative section.)

8. Provide appropriate postoperative nursing care.
   A. Administer prescribed analgesics.
   B. Monitor dressing and drainage and/or drainage system; check client's back for pooling of blood.
   C. Empty drainage system and measure drainage every 8 hours.
   D. Elevated affected arm above level of right atrium of heart to prevent edema.
   E. Monitor circulatory status of affected arm.
   F. Measure upper arm and forearm of affected arm twice daily to detect presence of edema.
   G. Avoid drawing blood, administering parenteral fluids, or taking blood pressure in affected arm.
   H. Encourage exercises of affected arm; avoid abduction.
      (1) Squeezing ball
      (2) Brushing hair
      (3) Feeding self
      (4) "Climbing" wall with fingertips
      (5) Rope pull
      (6) Elbow spread
      (7) Arm swing
   I. Encourage adequate nutritional intake when appropriate.
9. Provide appropriate nursing care for patients receiving radiation therapy.
   A. Apply prescribed lotion to skin.
   B. Monitor for skin problems such as radiation burns.
10. Administer adjuvant chemotherapeutic agents, if prescribed.
11. Explain and assist with potential side effects for patients receiving radiation and chemotherapy.
    A. Nausea, vomiting, and diarrhea
    B. Anorexia
    C. Stomatitis
    D. Malaise
    E. Hair loss
    F. Itching
    G. Reduced energy
    H. Heartburn
    I. Cough
    J. Bone marrow depression
    K. Anemia
12. Prepare patient for breast reconstruction, if indicated.
13. Instruct client and family regarding disease process, diagnostic procedures, treatment, prevention, home care, and follow-up. Include teaching on:
    A. Correct technique for breast examination
    B. Arm exercises and activity level
    C. Resumption of sexual activity
    D. Medication
    E. Information on community resources such as Reach for Recovery

Evaluation

1. Reports increased comfort, decreased anxiety and fear
2. Shows no signs of avoidable injury and/or infection
3. Maintains adequate mobility
4. Develops a positive self-image
5. Demonstrates understanding of disease process, diagnostic procedures, treatment, home care, and follow-up; similar understanding demonstrated by family

Endocrine System

Basic Information

Together with the nervous system, the endocrine system regulates and integrates the metabolic activities of the body. The hypothalamus controls endocrine organs by hormonal and neural pathways. Hormones are chemical transmitters that are released from certain type cells in the bloodstream and then carried to organ-receptor cells responding to the specific hormone.

The pathways of the nervous system connect the hypothalamus to the posterior pituitary gland. Neural stimulation causes the posterior pituitary gland to secrete two hormones: antidiuretic hormone (ADH) and oxytocin.

The hypothalamic hormones stimulate the anterior pituitary to emit the following tropic hormones: corticotropic hormone (ACTH), thyroid-stimulating hormone (TSH), follicle-stimulating hormone (FSH), and luteinizing hormone (LH). The hypothalamic hormones are also responsible for the release or inhibition of the human growth hormone (HGH) and prolactin. The tropic hormones in turn stimulate the adrenal cortex, thyroid, and gonads.

Additionally, the endocrine system is regulated by a negative simple or complex feedback system. In a simple feedback system, the level of one substance regulates the secretion of a hormone. For example, high serum calcium inhibits the secretion of the parathyroid hormone (PTH), whereas low serum calcium levels stimulate the secretion of PTH. An example of the complex feedback system is that of the stimulation of the release of ACTH due to the secretion of the hypothalamic corticotropin-releasing hormone (CRH). ACTH then stimulates the adrenal gland to secrete cortisol. Once serum cortisol rises, it inhibits the secretion of ACTH by decreasing CRH.

Careful evaluation of each level of the endocrine system is necessary in clients whose clinical condition suggest endocrine dysfunction due to the involvement of the complex hormonal sequence. A disturbance in one of the secreting endocrine glands can affect the regulation of another gland. The client with an endocrine dysfunction may experience multiple problems.

Assessment

SUBJECTIVE

1. Pain—skeletal, back, abdominal, muscle spasms, headache
2. Weakness, lethargy
3. Numbness
4. Mood swings
5. Tingling
6. Intolerance to cold or heat
7. Polyuria, dysuria, nocturia
8. Impotence, infertility, decreased libido
9. Menstrual disturbances
10. Anorexia or polyphagia
11. Frequent infections
12. Nausea

OBJECTIVE

1. General appearance
2. Skin color
   A. Flushed
   B. Pale
   C. Bronze pigmentation
   D. Yellow pigmentation
3. Skin temperature
   A. Excess perspiration
   B. Dry
   C. Moist
4. Poor wound healing
5. Nails
   A. Thin, brittle, or dry
6. Hair
   A. Brittle, thin, dry, or patchy
7. CNS
   A. Alterations in consciousness
      (1) Decreased cognition
      (2) Seizures
      (3) Confusion, stupor, coma
   B. Personality changes
   C. Abnormal reflexes—Chvostek's or Trousseau's sign
   D. Slowed, sluggish speech
8. Eyes
   A. Protruding eyeball (exophthalmos)
   B. Drooping eyelids (ptosis)
   C. Edema around eyes (periorbital)
9. Respiratory system
   A. Kussmaul's respirations
   B. Acetone breath
   C. Tachypnea
10. Cardiovascular system
    A. Tachycardia, bradycardia
    B. Hypertension
    C. Hypotension
11. GI system
    A. Anorexia
    B. Polyphagia
    C. Polydipsia
    D. Diarrhea
    E. Constipation
12. Renal system
    A. Oliguria
    B. Anuria
    C. Polyuria
13. Musculoskeletal system
    A. Weight loss or gain
    B. Stature—excessive or delayed growth

DIAGNOSTIC TESTS AND METHODS

1. Thyroid function tests
   A. Laboratory tests
      (1) Thyroid-releasing hormone (TRH) stimulation test
      (2) Iodine 131 (^{131}I) uptake
      (3) (T_3) and (T_4) tests
      (4) Free thyroid assay (FT_4)
      (5) Free thyroid index (FTI)
      (6) TSH assay
      (7) Thyroglobulin level
   B. Thyroid scan
   C. Thyroid ultrasonography
   D. Fine needle aspiration
   E. Basal metabolic rate (BMR)
   F. Serum thyroid antibodies (TA)
2. Parathyroid Function Tests
   A. Laboratory tests
      (1) Serum calcium
      (2) Serum phosphorus

(3) Chloride-phosphate ratio
(4) PTH assay
(5) Adenosine 3′,5′-monophosphate assay, urine (cyclic AMP)
(6) Glucosteroid suppression—cortisone administration test, Dent test
B. Skeletal x-rays
3. Adrenal function tests
    A. Laboratory tests
        (1) Cortex plasma cortisol
        (2) Urine-free cortisol test
        (3) 17-hydroxycorticosteroids urinary assay; 17-ketosteroids urinary assay (17-OCHS; 17-KS)
        (4) Serum ACTH
        (5) ACTH suppression test
        (6) Standard dexamethasone suppression test
        (7) ACTH stimulation test
        (8) Corticotropin-releasing factor (CRF) in ACTH stimulation
        (9) Metyrapone test (metyrapone pituitary reserve test)
        (10) Aldosterone assay; plasma and urine
        (11) 18-Hydroxycorticosterone (18-OHB)
        (12) Plasma renin activity
        (13) Furosemide test for renin release
        (14) Plasma catecholamines
        (15) Urine catecholamines
    B. A CT scan
    C. Adrenal Arteriography
    D. Adrenal venography
    E. Scintigraphy
4. Pituitary function tests
    A. Laboratory tests
        (1) Serum growth hormone (GH)
        (2) Insulin tolerance test
        (3) GH suppression test
        (4) Somatomedin-c assay
        (5) Serum prolactin (lactogen)
        (6) Serum testosterone
        (7) Serum estradiol
        (8) Plasma progesterone
        (9) Gonadotropins—FSH, LH
        (10) ADH (vasopressin)
        (11) Urine and serum osmolality
        (12) Water deprivation and vasopressin injection test
        (13) Water loading test
    B. X-ray of hand-wrist
    C. X-ray of sella turcica
5. Hypoglycemia assessment
    A. Serum insulin
    B. C-Peptide
    C. Prolonged fast
6. Tests for diabetes mellitus
    A. Fasting blood glucose
    B. Two-hour postprandial glucose test
    C. Glycosylated hemoglobin test
    D. Glucose tolerance test
7. Pneumonencephalography
8. Cerebral angiography
9. Cholesterol, carotene, triglycerides
10. Alkaline phosphatase
11. Blood and urine pH
12. ABGs
13. ECG
14. ESR

Implementation

1. Problems
    A. Symptoms of toxic effects of iodine
        (1) Swelling of buccal mucosa
        (2) Swelling of neck glands
    B. Signs of noncoping related to altered body image
        (1) Unwillingness to discuss body image
        (2) Disinterest in self
        (3) Depression
    C. Symptoms of potential seizures precipitated by low serum calcium
        (1) Numbness
        (2) Tingling
    D. Symptoms of hypoglycemia caused by insulin dosage
        (1) Headache
        (2) Hunger
        (3) Vertigo
        (4) Diaphoresis
        (5) Nervousness
        (6) Tachycardia
        (7) Weakness
        (8) Coma

Hyperpituitarism (Acromegaly or Gigantism)

Description

1. Hyperpituitarism is a chronic, progressive disease condition characterized by oversecretion of growth hormone (GH).
2. It is usually due to a secreting pituitary tumor.
3. Gigantism occurs before puberty, prior to epiphyseal closure, causing proportional overgrowth of all body tissues.
4. Acromegaly occurs after epiphyseal closure, causing bone thickening, visceromegaly, and transverse growth.
    A. Oversecretion of HGH results in atrophy of skeletal muscle and formation of new bone and cartilage after closure of the epiphyses.

Assessment

SUBJECTIVE—ACROMEGALY

1. Headache
2. Weakness
3. Visual disturbances
4. Joint pain

OBJECTIVE—ACROMEGALY

1. Characteristic hulking appearance
2. Thickened ears, nose, lips, tongue, and jaws
3. Broad hands, fingers, and feet
4. Enlarged supraorbital ridge
5. Galactorrhea in female, gynecomastia in male
6. Disturbance in carbohydrate metabolism
7. Clinically apparent diabetes mellitus
8. Disturbances in menstruation and libido
9. Increased GH levels

DIAGNOSTIC TESTS AND METHODS

1. History
2. Physical examination
3. Radioimmunology
4. Glucose suppression test
5. Skull x-rays
6. A CT scan
7. Arteriography
8. Pneumoencephalography
9. Skeletal x-rays
10. MRI scans

Planning

1. Safe, effective care environment
   A. Increase client's and family's knowledge of disease process, diagnostic procedures, and treatment.
   B. Prevent avoidable injury and/or infection.
2. Physiological integrity
   A. Increase comfort.
   B. Maintain adequate mobility.
3. Psychosocial integrity
   A. Reduce anxiety.
   B. Maintain effective coping.
   C. Promote positive self-image.
4. Health promotion and maintenance
   A. Increase client's and family's knowledge of prevention, home care, and follow-up.

Implementation

1. Assess, report, and record signs and symptoms and reactions to treatment.
2. Assess for skeletal manifestations.
3. Assist with ROM exercises to promote joint mobility.
4. Provide emotional support to aid patient in coping with altered body image.
5. Administer medications as prescribed; monitor for side effects.
6. Assess muscular weakness—check handclasp strength.
7. Provide meticulous skin care—keep skin dry and avoid use of oily lotions.
8. Assess for signs of hemianopia—stand where client can see you.
9. Test urine for presence of glucose; check for signs of hyperglycemia—profuse sweating, polyuria, polydipsia, fatigue.
10. Assess for mood swings.
11. Prepare client and family for hypophysectomy.
12. Provide postoperative care.
13. Instruct client and family regarding disease process, diagnostic procedures, treatment, prevention, home care, and follow-up.

Evaluation

1. Reports increased comfort, decreased anxiety
2. Has no complications
3. Recognizes and reports visual and neurological changes immediately
4. Shows no evidence of injuries or accidents related to sensoriperceptual defects

5. Maintains adequate breathing pattern and tissue oxygenation
6. Maintains a normal blood pressure
7. Recognizes symptoms of fluid volume excess
8. Able to tolerate daily activities without becoming fatigued
9. Demonstrates acceptance of body image
10. Ensure that client and family demonstrate understanding of disease process, diagnostic procedures, treatment (including surgery), home care (including monitoring of hormone replacement therapy), and need for follow-up

Hypopituitarism (Panhypopituitarism and Dwarfism) Syndrome

Description

1. Hypopituitarism is a complex syndrome marked by metabolic dysfunction, growth retardation in children, and sexual immaturity due to a deficiency of hormones secreted by the anterior pituitary gland.
2. A generalized condition, panhypopituitarism is a result of the partial or total deficiency of all of the six vital hormones secreted by the anterior pituitary—ACTH, TSH, FSH, LH, GH, and prolactin. Total loss of all hormones results in death.
3. Causes
   A. Lesion of the anterior pituitary gland—intra- or extrasellar tumor
   B. Congenital defects—hypoplasia or aplasia of gland
   C. Pituitary infarction often caused by postpartum hemorrhage
   D. Partial or total hypophysectomy
   E. Irradiation
   F. Chemical agents
4. A predictable pattern usually occurs with primary hypopituitarism.
   A. It starts with hypogonadism or gonadotropin failure due to decreased FSH and LH.
   B. It causes cessation of menses in adult women and impotence in men.
   C. A deficiency in growth hormone follows—causes short stature in children, delayed growth, sexual immaturity.
   D. Subsequently, a deficiency in thyrotropin occurs, resulting in hypothyroidism.
   E. Finally, decreased secretion of ACTH results in adrenal insufficiency.
5. Damage to the neurohypophysis may result in diabetes insipidus.

Assessment

SUBJECTIVE—HYPOPITUITARISM

1. Impotence, infertility
2. Decreased libido
3. Polyuria, polydipsia
4. Lethargy
5. Sensitivity to cold
6. Menstrual disturbances
7. Loss of visual acuity

OBJECTIVE

1. Symptoms of diabetes insipidus
2. Hypoglycemia
3. Lack of pubic and axillary hair

4. Symptoms of thyroid and adrenocortical failure
5. Dwarfism in children
6. Lack of secondary sex characteristics if disease occurs before puberty
7. Neurological signs—bilateral temporal hemianopia, blindness
8. Hypopituitarism as a result of surgery—increased temperature, hypotension, vomiting, hypoglycemia due to adrenal insufficiency

DIAGNOSTIC TESTS AND METHODS

1. History
2. Physical examination
3. Neurological assessment
4. Tests to rule out disease of target glands (adrenals, thyroid, gonads) or the hypothalamus
5. Radioimmunoassay for plasma levels of pituitary hormones
6. Measurement of GH levels in blood following administration of insulin
7. A CT scan
8. Pneumoencephalography
9. Cerebral angiography
10. T_3 and T_4
11. Urine ketogenic steroids

Planning

1. Safe, effective care environment
   A. Increase client's and family's knowledge of disease process, diagnostic procedures, and treatment.
   B. Prevent avoidable injury.
2. Physiological integrity
   A. Increase comfort.
   B. Assist with alterations in vision.
   C. Counsel on sexual dysfunction.
3. Psychosocial integrity
   A. Maintain effective coping.
   B. Assist with alteration in self-concept.
4. Health promotion and maintenance
   A. Increase client's and family's knowledge of home care (including medication, activity) and follow-up.

Implementation

1. Assess, report, and record signs and symptoms and reactions to treatment.
2. Monitor all laboratory tests for hormonal deficiencies.
3. Check for signs of thyroid deficiency, adrenal deficiency, and gonadotropin deficiency.
4. Administer hormone replacement medications as prescribed.
5. Monitor for weight gain or loss.
6. Monitor vital signs every 4–8 hours.
7. Check eyelids, nailbeds, and skin for pallor—indicative of anemia.
8. Provide emotional support to client and family.
9. Explain hormonal replacement therapy, reversal of altered growth and sexual function with medication, and possible side effects.
10. Provide extra blankets if body temperature is low.
11. Assist client in activities requiring good vision.
12. Monitor for signs of hypoglycemia during insulin testing—initial slow cerebration, tachycardia, and nervousness, progressing to convulsions.

A. Have $D_{50}W$ at bedside for rapid IV administration.
13. Instruct client in self-administration of steroids parenterally in case of emergency.
14. Instruct client in self-administration of hormone replacement drugs.
15. Prepare client and family for surgical procedure (transsphenoidal approach or craniotomy) and/or radiation, if required by client.
16. Provide counseling on sexual concerns.
17. Instruct client and family regarding disease process, diagnostic procedures, treatment, home care, and follow-up.

Evaluation

1. Reports increased comfort, decreased anxiety
2. Uses effective coping strategies
3. Shows no signs of avoidable infection and/or injury
4. Develops a positive self-concept
5. Demonstrates understanding of disease process, diagnostic procedures, treatment (including hormone replacement therapy), home care, and need for follow-up; similar understanding demonstrated by family

Diabetes Insipidus

Description

1. Diabetes insipidus is a water metabolism disorder related to hyposecretion of pitressin (ADH) by the posterior pituitary lobe.
2. It causes increased water loss in the urine and increased plasma osmolality and sodium levels.
3. It is characterized by polyuria and excessive thirst, which stabilizes plasma osmolality and compensates for the increased urinary output.
4. Nephrogenic diabetes insipidus may be inherited as an X-linked dominant trait, or it may be secondary to:
   A. Chronic renal disease
   B. Primary aldosteronism
5. Causes
   A. Familial or idiopathic in origin
   B. Secondary diabetes insipidus due to:
      (1) Metastatic lesions
      (2) Intracranial tumors
      (3) Neurosurgery
      (4) Head trauma
      (5) Infection
      (6) Vascular lesions
      (7) Autoimmune conditions
      (8) Trauma

Assessment

SUBJECTIVE

1. Thirst
2. Nocturia
3. Fatigue
4. Muscular weakness
5. Vertigo

OBJECTIVE

1. Polyuria—4–20 L/day.
2. Signs of dehydration—poor skin turgor, dry mucous membranes, constipation—usually as a result of fluid restriction, anesthesia, or trauma.

3. Hypotension
4. Low specific gravity—1.001–1.005
5. Serum osmolality increased above 280 mOsm/L.
6. Increased fluid intake
7. Electrolyte imbalance

DIAGNOSTIC TESTS AND METHODS

1. History
2. Physical examination
3. Baseline measurement of vital signs, weight, urine, and plasma osmolalities
4. Fluid restriction to evaluate changes in urine volume and concentration
5. Subcutaneous injection of 5 U of aqueous vasopressin—patients with diabetes insipidus respond to vasopressin with a decrease in urine volume and an increase in specific gravity.

Planning

1. Safe, effective care environment
   A. Increase client's and family's knowledge of disease process, diagnostic procedures, and treatment.
2. Physiological integrity
   A. Maintain fluid and electrolyte balance.
3. Psychosocial integrity
   A. Maintain effective coping.
4. Health promotion and maintenance
   A. Increase client's and family's knowledge of home care (including medication, activity) and follow-up.

Implementation

1. Assess, report, and record signs and symptoms and reactions to treatment.
2. Perform hourly measurement of urine volume, specific gravity, osmolality, and plasma osmolality following fluid restriction procedure and subcutaneous injection of aqueous vasopressin.
3. Administer vasopressin medications as prescribed—desmopressin, lypressin, vasopressin tannate, chlorpropamide, clofibrate, carbamazine (Tegretol); monitor for side effects. Administer diuretics as prescribed.
4. Record fluid intake and output as ordered.
5. Maintain adequate fluid intake to prevent dehydration; monitor for signs of dehydration.
6. Monitor blood pressure, heart and respiratory rates on a regular basis.
7. Monitor weight daily.
8. Provide a safe environment—keep side rails up for clients who complain of vertigo and/or weakness.
9. Provide a well-balanced diet.
10. Have orange juice or other carbohydrate on hand to treat potential hypoglycemic attacks, some of which may be triggered by the drug chlorpropamide.
11. Monitor for decreased urinary output and increased specific gravity between medication doses.
12. Monitor laboratory test results for presence of hyponatremia and hypoglycemia.
13. Provide bulk foods and fruit juices to prevent or alleviate constipation.
14. Provide meticulous skin and mouth care.
15. Identify clients with coronary artery disease—explain im-

portance of periodic evaluations due to effect of vasopressin constriction of arteries.
16. Advise client to wear medical identification bracelet and to carry medications with him or her at all times.
17. Instruct client and family regarding disease process, diagnostic procedures, treatment, home care, and follow-up.

Evaluation

1. Reports increased comfort, decreased anxiety
2. Shows no signs of avoidable injury and/or infection
3. Uses effective coping strategies
4. Maintains normal fluid volume status
5. Verbalizes importance of comfort and normal rest, sleep, and elimination patterns
6. Understands importance of recognizing signs and symptoms of polyuria, nocturia, and insomnia and of contacting physician when these occur
7. Demonstrates understanding of disease process, diagnostic procedures, treatments, home care, and need for follow-up; similar understanding demonstrated by family
   A. Self-injection techniques
   B. Need to adequately warm and shake vials of vasopressin tannate suspended in oil, if prescribed
   C. Avoidance of inhaling nasal sprays because of potential pulmonary side effects
   D. Need to increase dosage of nasal sprays when nasal congestion is present
   E. Dangers of medication overdose

Hyperthyroidism (Graves' Disease, Thyrotoxicosis)

Description

1. Hyperthyroidism is a metabolic imbalance due to thyroid hormone overproduction.
2. Most common form is Graves' disease, in which there is an increase in thyroxine production with an enlargement of the thyroid gland, resulting in multiple system changes.
3. Thyroid storm is an acute exacerbation of this condition and may lead to life-threatening cardiac, renal, or hepatic failure if not treated immediately.
4. Causes and predisposing factors
   A. Presence of genetic and immunologic factors
   B. Abnormal iodine metabolism
   C. Other endocrine disorders such as thyroiditis, hyperparathyroidism, diabetes mellitus
   D. Potential defect in suppressor T-lymphocyte function allowing formation of autoantibodies such as long-acting thyroid stimulator
   E. Excessive dietary iodine intake
   F. Stressful conditions, especially in patients with untreated or inadequately treated hyperthyroidism may precipitate thyroid storm—surgery, infection, toxemia of pregnancy, diabetic ketoacidosis

Assessment

SUBJECTIVE

1. Fatigue, weakness
2. Vision problems
3. Intolerance to heat

4. Increased appetite
5. Palpitations
6. Nervousness
7. Menstrual abnormalities
8. Difficulty in concentrating
9. Irritability

OBJECTIVE

1. Enlarged thyroid gland (goiter)
2. Weight loss
3. Profuse diaphoresis
4. Tremors
5. Exophthalmos
6. Shaky handwriting
7. Smooth, warm, flushed skin
8. Fine, soft hair
9. Friable nails
10. Thickened skin
11. Tachycardia
12. Cardiomegaly
13. Paroxysmal supraventricular tachycardia (SVT) and atrial fibrillation especially in the elderly
14. Dyspnea on exertion and at rest
15. Gynecomastia in males due to increased estrogen levels
16. Increased serum T_3 and T_4 concentrations
17. Thyroid storm—extreme irritability, hypertension, tachycardia, vomiting, temperature up to 106°F, delirium, coma

DIAGNOSTIC TESTS AND METHODS

1. History
2. Physical examination
3. Radioimmunoassay
4. Thyroid scan for evaluation of ^{131}I uptake
5. Thyroid suppression test for evaluation of pituitary control of thyroid gland
6. TRH stimulation test for evaluation of TSH levels
7. BMR
8. Serum protein-bound iodine
9. Serum cholesterol and total lipids
10. Ultrasonography to evaluate subclinical ophthalmopathy
11. T_3 and T_4 levels
12. Serum thyroid antibodies (TA)

Planning

1. Safe, effective care environment
   A. Increase client's knowledge of disease process, diagnostic procedures, and treatment.
   B. Prevent avoidable injury and/or infection.
   C. Promote adequate rest pattern.
2. Physiological integrity
   A. Maintain adequate cardiac output.
   B. Increase comfort.
   C. Maintain adequate nutrition.
   D. Assist with self-care needs.
   E. Facilitate activity tolerance.
3. Psychosocial integrity
   A. Promote effective coping.
   B. Facilitate positive self-image.
4. Health promotion and maintenance
   A. Increase client's knowledge of home care and follow-up.

Implementation

1. Assess, report, and record signs and symptoms and reactions to treatment.
2. Monitor vital signs and neurological status.
3. Monitor weight daily.
4. Monitor serum electrolytes.
5. Monitor for signs of hyperglycemia and glycosuria.
6. Monitor cardiac function.
7. Monitor fluid intake and output.
8. Monitor pregnant women for signs of spontaneous abortion—spotting, occasional mild cramps.
9. Mix prescribed iodine medication with milk to prevent GI distress.
10. Administer prescribed iodine medication through a straw to prevent tooth discoloration.
11. Administer other prescribed medications such as digitalis, β-adrenergic blockers, calcium antagonists, thioamides (antithyroid drugs), sedatives, and sleep aids.
12. Encourage adequate intake of high-calorie, high-carbohydrate, protein and vitamin diet.
13. Explain basis for mood swings to client.
14. Monitor for signs of thyroid crisis.
    A. Cardiovascular
       (1) Palpitations
       (2) Tachycardia
       (3) Dyspnea on exertion
       (4) Systolic hypertension
    B. Neuromuscular
       (1) Easy fatigability
       (2) Fine tremors
       (3) Muscle weakness, especially shoulder and pelvic muscles
    C. Neurological
       (1) Elevated temperature
       (2) Restlessness
       (3) Delirium
       (4) Coma
    D. Psychological
       (1) Insomnia
       (2) Difficulty concentrating
       (3) Nervousness, anxiety
       (4) Increased stress level
15. Treat thyroid crisis.
    A. Administer medications as prescribed.
       (1) SSKI or ^{131}I to inhibit thyroid hormone (Instruct patient to expectorate or cough freely after ^{131}I therapy—saliva remains radioactive for 24 hours.)
       (2) Glucocorticoids to inhibit release of thyroid hormone
       (3) β-adrenergic blockers for increased adrenergic stimulation
       (4) Medications for CHF
    B. Provide the following nursing interventions for clients taking methimazole or propylthiouracil:
       (1) Monitor CBC periodically to detect leukopenia, thrombocytopenia, and agranulocytosis.
       (2) Instruct client to take medication with meals to decrease GI distress.
       (3) Instruct client to avoid over-the-counter cough preparations because they may contain iodine.
       (4) Instruct client to report signs of blood dyscrasia

such as enlarged cervical lymph nodes, fever, mouth sores, sore throat, skin rash or eruptions.
C. Monitor blood pressure, cardiac rate and rhythm.
D. Monitor temperature.
E. Administer hypothermic measures for high fever—sponging, hypothermia blankets, and acetaminophen (avoid aspirin because it raises thyroxine levels).
F. Maintain IV line.
16. Provide the following nursing interventions for clients with exophthalmos:
A. Advise use of sunglasses, shields, or eye patches to protect eyes.
B. Moisten conjunctivas with isotonic eye drops.
C. Advise client with severe lid retraction to avoid sudden movement—may cause lid to slip behind eyeball.
D. Monitor for corneal damage.
17. Prepare client and family for surgical procedure, if required by client.
18. Provide appropriate postoperative care (see operative section).
19. Instruct client regarding disease process, diagnostic procedures, treatment (including medications), home care, and follow-up.

Evaluation

1. Reports increased comfort, decreased anxiety
2. Shows no signs of avoidable injury and/or infection
3. Maintains adequate nutritional status
4. Maintains adequate rest and sleep patterns
5. Participates in self-care activities
6. Uses effective coping skills
7. Demonstrates understanding of disease process, diagnostic procedures, treatment (including medications), home care, and need for follow-up

Hypothyroidism (Myxedema)

Description

1. Hypothyroidism is a condition characterized by low serum thyroid hormone resulting from hypothalamic, pituitary, or thyroid insufficiency.
2. It leads to a decline in the metabolic rate and in the development of almost all systems.
3. Clinical effects range from mild fatigue and loss of appetite to life-threatening myxedema coma.
4. Causes
A. Dysfunction of thyroid gland due to
(1) Thyroidectomy
(2) Irradiation therapy, especially ^{131}I
(3) Inflammation
(4) Chronic autoimmune thyroiditis
B. Failure of pituitary gland to produce TSH
C. Failure of hypothalamus to produce TRH
D. Inborn errors of thyroid hormone synthesis
E. Iodine deficiency—usually dietary, resulting in inability to synthesize the hormone
F. Use of antithyroid medications such as propylthiouracil

Assessment

SUBJECTIVE

1. Fatigue
2. Forgetfulness
3. Sensitivity to cold
4. Loss of appetite
5. Decreased libido, oligomenorrhea or menorrhagia
6. Chest pain
7. Headache
8. Drowsiness or apathy
9. Numbness or tingling
10. Decreased mental status
11. Cramps, paresthesias
12. Depression
13. Vertigo

OBJECTIVE

1. Weight gain
2. Decreased bowel sounds
3. Constipation
4. Dry, flaky, cool, coarse inelastic skin
5. Puffy face, hands, and feet
6. Decreased BMR
7. Bradycardia
8. Hoarseness
9. Periorbital edema
10. Dry, sparse, brittle hair
11. Upper eyelid droop
12. Abdominal distention
13. Intention tremor
14. Nystagmus
15. Reflexes—delayed reaction time
16. Decreased urine output
17. Low temperature
18. Decreased T_3, T_4, and ^{131}I
19. Pleural effusion on chest x-ray
20. Elevated serum cholesterol, carotene, alkaline phosphatase, and triglycerides
21. Signs of myxedema coma
A. Progressive stupor
B. Hypoventilation
C. Hypoglycemia
D. Hypotension
E. Hyponatremia
F. Hypothermia
G. Enlarged tongue and slow, slurred speech
H. Increased TSH
I. High-titer thyroid autoantibodies
J. Decreased serum T_3 and T_4

DIAGNOSTIC TESTS AND METHODS

1. History
2. Physical examination
3. Radioimmunoassay—T_3, T_4, and ^{131}I uptake
4. TSH levels
5. Serum cholesterol, carotene, alkaline phosphatase, and triglycerides
6. CBC with differential
7. For myxedema coma:
A. Serum sodium levels—decreased
B. ABGs—decreased pH and elevated P_{CO_2}

Planning

1. Safe, effective care environment
   A. Prevent avoidable injury and/or infection.
   B. Increase client's and family's knowledge of disease process, diagnostic procedures, and treatment.
2. Physiological integrity
   A. Maintain adequate mobility.
   B. Increase comfort.
   C. Maintain skin integrity.
   D. Maintain adequate elimination pattern.
   E. Facilitate thought process.
   F. Maintain adequate cardiac output.
3. Psychosocial integrity
   A. Reduce anxiety.
   B. Promote positive self-image.
4. Health promotion and maintenance
   A. Increase client's and family's knowledge of home care and follow-up.

Implementation

1. Assess, report, and record signs and symptoms and reactions to treatment.
2. Monitor vital signs, respirations, GI functions, neurological status.
3. Orient to environment as needed.
4. Provide safe, warm environment.
5. Provide a high-bulk, low-calorie diet.
6. Encourage activity to promote weight loss and combat constipation.
7. Administer prescribed thyroxine replacement, analgesics for pain, laxatives or stool softeners for constipation, and IV fluids.
8. Monitor for signs of hyperthyroidism due to thyroxine replacement.
   A. Restlessness, nervousness, sweating, excessive weight loss
9. Instruct client to report signs of cardiovascular diseases such as chest pain, tachycardia.
10. Instruct client to report signs of infection immediately.
11. Encourage fluid intake.
12. Encourage use of emollients on dry skin.
13. Provide meticulous skin care; monitor for skin breakdown.
14. Monitor for signs of myxedema coma.
    A. Decreased urinary output—sign of decreased cardiac output.
    B. Decreased temperature—hypothermia.
    C. Monitor intake and output and weight daily.
    D. Turn patient every 2 hours.
    E. Provide meticulous skin care.
    F. Avoid sedation or reduce dosage—hypothermia delays metabolism of many drugs.
    G. Maintain patent IV line.
       (1) Monitor serum electrolytes while patient is receiving IV therapy.
       (2) Monitor vital signs especially if patient is receiving levothyroxine—too rapid correction of hypothyroidism may cause adverse cardiac effect.
    H. Report chest pain or tachycardia immediately.
    I. Monitor elderly clients for hypertension and CHF.
    J. Monitor ABGs for signs of hypoxia and respiratory acidosis.
    K. Monitor for need of ventilatory assistance.
    L. Monitor urine, sputum for sources of infection (blood, urine, sputum) because coma may have been triggered by infection.
15. Instruct client and family regarding disease process, diagnostic procedures, treatment, home care, and follow-up.

Evaluation

1. Reports increased comfort, decreased anxiety
2. Shows no signs of avoidable injury and/or infection
3. Maintains skin integrity
4. Maintains adequate mobility
5. Maintains adequate cardiac output
6. Maintains adequate elimination pattern
7. Demonstrates improvement in thought process
8. Develops positive self-image
9. Complies with thyroid medication routine
10. Demonstrates understanding of disease process, diagnostic procedures, treatment, home care (including medications), and need for follow-up; similar understanding demonstrated by family

Hyperparathyroidism

Description

1. Hyperparathyroidism is a condition characterized by overactivity of one or more of the four parathyroid glands, which results in an abnormal increase in the secretion of PTH.
2. Increased levels of PTH promotes resorption of bone and results in hypercalcemia (elevated serum calcium levels) and hypophosphatemia (diminished levels of phosphorus).
3. As a result, there is an increase in renal and GI absorption of calcium.
4. Classification as either primary or secondary hyperparathyroidism.
   A. Primary type: Increased PTH secretion is due to the enlargement of one or more of the parathyroid glands, which results in increased serum calcium levels.
   B. Secondary type: Increased secretion of PTH is due to a hypocalcemia-producing abnormality excluding the parathyroid gland, which causes resistance to the metabolic action of PTH.

Assessment

SUBJECTIVE

1. Fatigue, weakness
2. Anorexia, nausea
3. Chronic low back pain
4. Bone tenderness
5. Constipation
6. Abdominal pain
7. Pruritus
8. Marked muscle weakness

OBJECTIVE

1. Elevated PTH levels
2. Marked muscle atrophy
3. Elevated serum calcium, chloride, and alkaline phosphatase levels

4. Diminished serum phosphorus levels
5. Elevated urine calcium levels, renal calculi
6. Bone fractures or cysts on x-ray due to osteoporosis
7. Polyuria
8. Polydipsia
9. Dysrhythmias
10. Hypertension
11. Renal calculi and later, renal insufficiency
12. Hematemesis
13. Signs of pancreatitis, peptic ulcer
14. Stupor, coma
15. Cataracts
16. Calcium microthrombi in lungs and pancreas
17. Positive Trousseau's or Chvostek's signs
18. Memory loss
19. Symptoms of secondary hyperparathyroidism—related to underlying conditions of rickets, vitamin D deficiency, chronic renal failure, or osteomalacia due to use of phenytoin or laxative abuse
    A. Decreased serum calcium levels
    B. Variable serum phosphorus levels
    C. Skeletal deformities
    D. Symptoms of underlying condition

DIAGNOSTIC TESTS AND METHODS

1. History
2. Physical examination
3. Radioimmunoassay for PTH
4. Total serum calcium
5. Serum phosphorus
6. Quantitative urinary calcium
7. Uric acid and creatinine levels
8. Basal acid secretion and serum immunoreactive gastrin levels
9. Serum amylase levels—may indicate acute pancreatitis
10. X-ray of skeletal system
11. X-ray spectrophotometry (microscopic examination of bone)
12. Tests for underlying condition in secondary hyperparathyroidism

Planning

1. Safe, effective care environment
   A. Prevent avoidable injury.
   B. Increase client's knowledge of disease process, diagnostic procedures, and treatment.
2. Physiological integrity
   A. Maintain adequate cardiac output.
   B. Increase comfort.
   C. Maintain adequate elimination pattern.
   D. Maintain adequate nutritional status.
3. Psychosocial integrity
   A. Reduce anxiety.
4. Health promotion and maintenance
   A. Increase client's knowledge of prevention, home care, and follow-up.

Implementation

1. Assess, report, and record signs and symptoms and reactions to treatment.

2. Check pretreatment baseline serum calcium, phosphate, magnesium, potassium levels against later laboratory levels.
3. Administer prescribed diuretics and medications to inhibit bone resorption.
4. Provide a safe environment; assist with comfort measures.
5. Administer prescribed analgesics for pain.
6. Record intake and output.
7. Encourage fluid intake of 3000 mL daily—include cranberry juice to acidify urine.
8. Monitor for signs of pulmonary edema in clients receiving large amounts of IV solutions.
9. Monitor clients who are receiving digitalis carefully—elevated calcium levels can result in digitalis toxicity.
10. Provide the following nursing interventions to help prevent spontaneous fractures:
    A. Assist with ambulation.
    B. Lift immobilized client carefully to decrease stress on bones.
11. Administer prescribed antacids, if required.
12. Explain rationale for low-calcium, low-phosphorus diet.
13. Encourage high dietary fiber to prevent constipation.
14. Strain urine to monitor for presence of stones; check for signs of hematuria.
15. Prepare client and family for surgical intervention (parathyroidectomy), if indicated.
16. Provide appropriate postoperative care (see postoperative section).
17. Instruct client regarding disease process, diagnostic procedures, treatment, prevention, home care, and need for follow-up.

Evaluation

1. Reports increased comfort, decreased anxiety
2. Shows no signs of avoidable injury and/or infection
3. Maintains adequate cardiac output
4. Maintains adequate nutritional status
5. Maintains adequate elimination patterns
6. Demonstrates understanding of disease process, diagnostic procedures, treatment, prevention, home care, and need for follow-up

Hypoparathyroidism

Description

1. Hypoparathyroidism is a condition characterized by a deficiency of PTH.
2. It results in decreased bone resorption due to low serum calcium levels (hypocalcemia) and increased levels of phosphorus (hyperphosphatemia).
3. Hypocalcemia produces neuromuscular symptoms, which range from paresthesia to severe tetany.
4. Three classifications and causes
   A. Idiopathic hypoparathyroidism—results from an autoimmune genetic dysfunction or congenital absence of parathyroid glands
   B. Acquired reversible hypoparathyroidism—may result from low levels of serum magnesium, which impairs hormone synthesis, or from delayed maturation of parathyroid function
   C. Acquired irreversible hypoparathyroidism—may result from injury or accidental removal of one or more of the

glands during thyroidectomy or other neck surgery; ischemic infarction of parathyroids during surgery, sarcoidosis, tuberculosis, neoplasms, or trauma

Assessment

SUBJECTIVE

1. Numbness and tingling
2. Dyspnea
3. Depression or irritability
4. Confusion
5. Headache
6. Visual problems, photophobia
7. Muscle cramps, spasms
8. Muscle pain

OBJECTIVE

1. Positive Trousseau's and Chvostek's signs (tetany)
2. Convulsions
3. Laryngeal stridor
4. Arrhythmias
5. CHF
6. Calcification of skull on x-ray
7. Dry, scaly skin
8. Decreased calcium levels
9. Elevated serum phosphorus levels
10. Decreased urine calcium levels
11. Increased bone density on x-ray
12. Increased QT and ST intervals on ECG due to hypocalcemia
13. Cataracts

DIAGNOSTIC TESTS AND METHODS

1. Laboratory serum values—calcium, phosphorus
2. Qualitative urinary calcium test
3. X-rays of skeletal system
4. ECG
5. Trousseau's and Chvostek's tests

Planning

1. Safe, effective care environment
   A. Prevent avoidable injury and/or infection.
   B. Increase client's and family's knowledge of disease process, diagnostic procedures, and treatment.
2. Physiological integrity
   A. Maintain adequate cardiac output.
   B. Maintain effective breathing pattern.
   C. Facilitate thought process.
3. Psychosocial integrity
   A. Reduce anxiety.
4. Health promotion and maintenance
   A. Increase client's and family's knowledge regarding home care and follow-up care.

Implementation

1. Assess, report, and record signs and symptoms and reactions to treatment.
2. Monitor vital signs.
3. Monitor serum calcium and phosphorus levels, urinary calcium levels.
4. Maintain patent IV line; keep calcium IV available.

5. Maintain seizure precautions.
6. Maintain a patent airway.
7. Keep tracheotomy tray and endotracheal tube at bedside (in case of laryngospasm).
8. Assist in administration of diazepam IV—monitor vital signs frequently to ascertain blood pressure and heart rate.
9. Monitor for cardiac rhythm, if indicated.
10. Monitor for signs of tetany—check Trousseau's or Chvostek's sign.
11. Assist in administration of calcium gluconate or calcium chloride and vitamin D and antacids (to bind phosphate) as prescribed.
12. Monitor intake and output.
13. Monitor for signs of heart block and signs of decreasing cardiac output.
14. Provide adequate nutrition with high-calcium, low-phosphate diet.
15. Apply prescribed cream to soften scaly skin.
16. Instruct client and family regarding disease process, diagnostic procedures, treatment, home care (including medication), and follow-up.

Evaluation

1. Reports increased comfort, decreased anxiety
2. Shows no signs of avoidable injury and/or infection
3. Maintains an effective breathing pattern
4. Maintains adequate cardiac output
5. Maintains adequate nutritional and fluid intake
6. Shows improvement in thought process
7. Demonstrates understanding of disease process, diagnostic procedures, treatment, home care, and follow-up; similar understanding demonstrated by family

Addison's Disease (Adrenal Hypofunction)

Description

1. Addison's disease is a condition characterized by hyposecretion of cortisol by the adrenal cortex.
2. Classification as primary or secondary
   A. Primary adrenal hypofunction originates within the adrenal gland; it is characterized by decreased glucocorticoid, mineralocorticoid, and androgen secretion, causing excess sodium excretion and retention of potassium and waste products.
   B. Secondary adrenal hypofunction is a result of a disorder external to the adrenal gland, such as a pituitary tumor with ACTH deficiency—aldosterone secretion frequently is not altered.
3. Adrenal crisis (Addisonian crisis) is a result of extreme deficiency of mineralocorticoids and glucocorticoids due to acute stress in individuals with chronic Addison's disease.
4. Adrenal crisis requires emergency treatment.
5. Causes
   A. Fungal infections such as histoplasmosis
   B. Bilateral adrenalectomy
   C. TB
   D. Adrenal carcinoma
   E. Idiopathic atrophy
   F. Impaired circulation
   G. Autoimmune response—circulating antibodies react against adrenal tissue

Assessment

SUBJECTIVE

1. Weakness, fatigue
2. Nausea
3. Anorexia
4. Inability to concentrate
5. Muscle pain
6. Menstrual changes, impotence
7. Decreased tolerance for minimal stress
8. Craving for salty food

OBJECTIVE

1. Lethargy
2. Bronze coloration to skin
3. Weight loss
4. Vomiting
5. Chronic diarrhea
6. Decreased plasma ACTH
7. Low serum sodium levels
8. High serum potassium and BUN levels
9. Elevated hematocrit, lymphocyte, and eosinophil counts
10. Hypoglycemia (fasting blood sugar)
11. Poor skin turgor, sunken eyeballs, dry mucous membrane due to dehydration
12. Hypotension
13. Weak, irregular pulse
14. Decreased concentration of corticosteroids in plasma or urine
15. Decreased 17-hydroxysteroid, 17-KS, and 17-OHCS in 24-hour urine test
16. Sparse body hair in women
17. Positive response to metyrapone test—increased ACTH serum levels, no change in urinary concentration of 17-OHCS.

DIAGNOSTIC TESTS AND METHODS

1. History
2. Physical examination
3. Plasma and urine corticosteroids levels
4. Serum sodium, potassium, and BUN levels
5. Fasting blood sugar
6. ACTH stimulation test—to differentiate between primary and secondary adrenal insufficiency
   A. In primary type: Plasma and urine cortisol levels do not increase normally in response to ACTH.
   B. In secondary type: Repeated doses of ACTH over several days result in a gradual increase in cortisol levels reaching normal levels.
7. X-rays

Planning

1. Safe, effective care environment
   A. Prevent avoidable injury and/or infection.
   B. Increase client's and family's knowledge of disease process, diagnostic procedures, and treatment.
2. Physiological integrity
   A. Increase comfort.
   B. Maintain fluid balance.
   C. Maintain adequate nutrition.
3. Psychosocial integrity
   A. Facilitate effective coping.
4. Health promotion and maintenance
   A. Increase client's and family's knowledge of home care and follow-up.

Implementation

1. Assess, report, and record signs and symptoms and reactions to treatment.
2. Monitor for electrolyte imbalance and hypoglycemia.
3. Check blood sugar levels of diabetic clients periodically—steroid replacement therapy may require an adjustment of insulin dosage.
4. Provide diet that maintains sodium and potassium balance.
5. Administer prescribed glucocorticoid and mineralocorticoid replacement.
6. Administer antacids to prevent ulcers.
7. Provide safe, calm environment—limit visitors, eliminate stressors.
8. Provide emotional support.
9. Monitor client receiving steroids for cushingoid symptoms such as edema of face and around eyes.
10. Observe client for signs of petechiae.
11. Monitor for facial hair growth and other masculinization signs in females who are on testosterone injections for muscle weakness and decreased libido.
12. Explain need for lifelong steroid therapy and need to watch for symptoms of over- and underdosage.
13. Advise client to avoid infections, injury, or heat, which may precipitate an adrenal crisis.
14. Monitor for signs of Addisonian crisis:
    A. Acute hypotension
    B. Profound weakness
    C. Nausea, vomiting
    D. Vascular collapse
    E. Shock
    F. Renal failure
    G. Coma
    H. Impending death
15. Addisonian crisis:
    A. Assist in administration of prescribed hydrocortisone IV immediately.
    B. Administer prescribed hydrocortisone IM following initial IV therapy, or assist in administration of prescribed hydrocortisone diluted with saline or dextrose IV until condition stabilizes.
    C. Monitor vital signs every 15 minutes.
    D. Monitor urine output hourly.
    E. Monitor weight.
    F. Monitor serum sodium levels.
    G. Monitor fluid intake.
16. Instruct client to carry a medical identification card.
17. Advise client and family to keep hydrocortisone in a prepared syringe for use in case of stress, and instruct how to inject.
18. Provide comfort measures such as back rubs and relaxation techniques.
19. Assist with gradual return to activities.
20. Instruct client and family regarding disease process, diagnostic procedures, treatment, home care, and follow-up.

Evaluation

1. Reports increased comfort, decreased anxiety
2. Shows no signs of avoidable injury and/or infection
3. Maintains adequate fluid balance
4. Maintains adequate nutrition
5. Maintains compliance with treatment regimen
6. Uses effective coping strategies
7. Demonstrates understanding of disease process, diagnostic procedures, treatment, home care, and need for follow-up; similar understanding demonstrated by family

Cushing's Syndrome, Disease

Description

1. Cushing's syndrome is a condition characterized by a cluster of abnormalities due to excessive levels of adrenocortical hormones (especially cortisol), androgens, and aldosterone.
2. It affects:
   A. Protein, carbohydrate, and fat metabolism
   B. Inflammatory and immune response
   C. Mineral and water metabolism
   D. Blood components
   E. Emotional status
3. Prognosis depends on underlying cause—poor in individuals who have not received treatment and in those with metastatic adrenal malignancy or untreatable ectopic ACTH-producing malignancy.
4. Causes
   A. Overproduction of ACTH with resultant hyperplasia of adrenal cortex (Cushing's syndrome)
   B. Overproduction of ACTH from pituitary hypersecretion
   C. ACTH-producing tumor (ectopic ACTH secretion) in another organ external to the adrenal gland such as pancreatic or bronchogenic carcinoma
   D. Administration of synthetic glucocorticoids or ACTH
   E. Cortisol-secreting adrenal tumor—usually benign

Assessment

SUBJECTIVE

1. Fatigue
2. Muscle weakness
3. Irritability
4. Insomnia
5. Poor wound healing
6. Changes in menstrual cycle and libido
7. Bone pain
8. Emotional disturbances

OBJECTIVE

1. Evidence of steroid diabetes—decreased glucose tolerance, glucosuria, and fasting hyperglycemia
2. Moon face—from fat deposits
3. Buffalo hump—fat pads over upper back
4. Fat pads over clavicle
5. Truncal obesity with slender arms and legs
6. Little or no scar formation
7. Acne and hirsutism in women
8. Muscle atrophy due to increased catabolism
9. Pathological fractures due to decreased bone mineral
10. Skeletal growth retardation in children
11. Striae (stretch marks on skin)
12. Evidence of peptic ulcer due to increased gastric secretions and production of pepsin
13. Hypertension due to sodium and water retention
14. Left ventricular hypertrophy
15. Capillary weakness due to protein loss—leads to petechiae and ecchymosis
16. Presence of infections due to suppressed antibody formation and decreased lymphocyte production
17. Sodium and secondary fluid retention
18. Increase in potassium excretion
19. Ureteral calculi due to increased bone demineralization
20. Elevated urine calcium levels
21. Enlargement of breasts in males and clitoral hypertrophy, virilism, and amenorrhea in females

DIAGNOSTIC TESTS AND METHODS

1. History
2. Physical examination
3. Plasma and urinary steroid levels
4. Low-dose dexamethasone suppression test for Cushing's syndrome
5. High-dose dexamethasone suppression test for Cushing's disease
6. Metyrapone test—blocks cortisol production by adrenals; tests to determine if pituitary gland and hypothalamus can correct low levels of plasma cortisol by increasing ACTH production
   A. In Cushing's disease—excess plasma ACTH secreted
   B. In Cushing's syndrome—an adrenal or a nonendocrine ACTH-secreting tumor; the pituitary gland is suppressed by high cortisol levels so steroid levels remain stable or fall
7. Ultrasound, CT scan, angiography—to localize adrenal tumors
8. CT scan of head—to identify presence of pituitary tumors

Planning

1. Safe, effective care environment
   A. Increase client's and family's knowledge of condition, diagnostic procedures, and treatment.
   B. Prevent avoidable injury and/or infection.
2. Physiological integrity
   A. Increase comfort.
   B. Maintain fluid balance.
   C. Prevent infection.
   D. Maintain activity tolerance.
3. Psychosocial integrity
   A. Maintain effective coping.
   B. Promote positive self-image.
4. Health promotion and maintenance
   A. Increase client's and family's knowledge regarding home care and follow-up.

Implementation

1. Assess, report, and record signs and symptoms and reaction to treatment.
2. Monitor vital signs and neurological status every 4 hours.

3. Monitor serum electrolytes, blood glucose, and cortisol levels.
4. Monitor urinary glucose levels.
5. Monitor weight daily; check for edema.
6. Monitor intake and output carefully.
7. Provide diet high in protein and potassium; low in calories, sodium, and carbohydrates.
8. Monitor for signs of infection.
   A. Check temperature every 4 hours.
   B. Check skin, oral cavity, and lungs for signs of infection.
   C. Encourage coughing and deep breathing exercises.
   D. Turn patient frequently.
   E. Provide proper hygienic measures.
   F. Avoid contact with individuals with upper respiratory infections.
9. Assist in reducing stressors.
   A. Maintain continuity of nursing care.
   B. Avoid excessive noise or temperature changes.
   C. Limit visitors.
   D. Provide privacy.
   E. Allow adequate rest periods.
10. Monitor and record instances of emotional lability.
11. Provide a restful environment.
12. Allow client to verbalize feelings regarding condition.
13. Administer prescribed medications such as potassium replacements and inhibitors of cortisol production or release; monitor for side effects.
14. Prepare client and family for surgical intervention, if indicated.
   A. Bilateral adrenalectomy
   B. Total hypophysectomy
   C. Transsphenoidal adenectomy
15. Provide appropriate postoperative care.
   A. Monitor wound drainage or fever immediately.
   B. Use strict aseptic technique in changing dressings when ordered.
   C. Administer analgesics and replacement steroids as ordered.
   D. Monitor urinary output.
   E. Monitor vital signs—check for shock symptoms (decreased blood pressure, increased pulse rate, pallor, cold clammy skin).
      (1) Administer prescribed vasopressors and increase IV flow rate as ordered.
      (2) Monitor for decreased mental alertness and signs of physical weakness.
      (3) Assess neurological and behavioral status.
      (4) Monitor for signs of nausea, vomiting, and diarrhea.
   F. Monitor laboratory reports for signs of hypoglycemia caused by removal of cortisol source—cortisol maintains normal blood glucose levels.
   G. Monitor for signs of adrenal hypofunction indicative of inadequate steroid replacement.
      (1) Orthostatic hypotension
      (2) Apathy, weakness, fatigue
   H. Monitor for signs of abdominal distention and recurrence of bowel sounds.
   I. Monitor and report signs of increased intracranial pressure in clients undergoing pituitary surgery—agitation, changes in level of consciousness, confusion, nausea, vomiting.

16. Advise client to take steroid replacements with antacids or meals to decrease gastric irritation.
17. Advise client to carry a medical identification card.
18. Advise client to monitor for and immediately report signs of inadequate steroid dosage—weakness, vertigo, fatigue.
19. Instruct client and family that discontinuation of the steroid replacement medications may produce a fatal adrenal crisis.
20. Encourage a positive self-image.
21. Instruct client and family regarding disease process, diagnostic procedures, treatment, home care, and follow-up care.

Evaluation

1. Reports increased comfort, decreased anxiety
2. Shows no signs of avoidable injury and/or infection
3. Maintains adequate activity
4. Maintains adequate fluid balance
5. Uses effective coping strategies
6. Develops a positive self-image
7. Maintains adequate nutritional status
8. Maintains compliance to steroid replacement therapy
9. Demonstrates understanding of disease process, diagnostic procedures, treatment, home care, and need for follow-up; similar understanding demonstrated by family

Diabetes Mellitus

Description

1. Diabetes mellitus is a condition characterized by insulin deficiency or resistance with disturbances in carbohydrate, protein, and fat metabolism followed by chronic neuropathies and microvascular changes.
2. Insulin is responsible for transporting glucose into body cells for use as energy and for storing glycogen.
3. Insulin stimulates protein synthesis and free fatty acid storage.
4. A deficiency in insulin jeopardizes the access of body cells to essential nutrients.
5. Three forms
   A. Insulin-dependent diabetes mellitus (IDDM, ketosis-prone, or juvenile diabetes)
      (1) This form usually occurs before age 30 (although it may occur at any age).
      (2) Individual is usually thin; requires endogenous insulin and dietary management.
      (3) Severely diminished insulin production.
      (4) Endogenous insulin secretion is reduced from disease onset and throughout clinical course.
      (5) Peripheral insulin resistance, which is excessive amounts of circulating insulin antibodies that render insulin less effective, may also be present.
      (6) Loss of insulin secretion may be caused by various mechanisms such as:
         (a) Autoimmune mechanisms in which the immune system attacks and destroys the body's insulin-producing β cells
         (b) Insulin autoantibodies resulting from β-cell destruction
   B. Non-insulin-dependent diabetes mellitus (NIDDM, ketosis-resistant, or maturity-onset diabetes).

(1) The most common form of diabetes mellitus (80%) of all diagnosed cases.

(2) It is most prevalent among obese adults (occurs occasionally in children).

(3) The degree of insulin deficiency results from a progressive loss of β-cell responsiveness to glucose.

C. Other types, defined as diabetes secondary to pancreatic disease or drug or chemical agents

(1) Impaired glucose tolerance: In past, individuals were diagnosed as "borderline diabetics."

(2) Gestational diabetes: A type of carbohydrate intolerance with onset during a current pregnancy that usually disappears after childbirth.

6. Majority of clients fall within the IDDM or the NIDDM classification.

7. Effects of insufficient endogenous insulin or action include:

A. Elevated serum blood sugar (glucose) due to impaired intake by liver.

B. High levels of glucose in the blood pulls fluid from body tissues, causing osmotic diuresis.

C. Lipolysis due to changes in fat metabolism causes ketone formation which may lead to ketonuria.

8. Glucose content in epidermis (skin) and urine stimulates bacterial growth.

9. Causes

A. Heredity

B. Environmental

C. Autoimmune factors

D. Precipitating factors:

(1) Obesity—causes resistance to endogenous insulin.

(2) Physiological or emotional stress—causes prolonged increased levels of cortisol, epinephrine, glucagon, and GH, which in turn raise blood glucose levels, thereby increasing demands on the pancreas.

(3) Pregnancy and use of oral contraceptives—increase estrogen and placental hormones, which are antagonists of insulin.

(4) Use of other insulin antagonists such as thiazide diuretics and renal corticosteroids.

Assessment

SUBJECTIVE

1. Fatigue
2. Polyphagia
3. Polydipsia
4. Nocturia, polyuria
5. Visual disturbances due to edema and sugar deposits that cause changes in lens
6. Anxiety
7. Weight loss

OBJECTIVE

1. Lethargy
2. Weight loss (IDDM), obesity (NIDDM)
3. Elevated fasting serum glucose
4. Glycosuria
5. Dehydration
6. Dry mucous membranes
7. Poor skin turgor
8. Long-term effects
   A. Retinopathy
   B. Nephropathy
   C. MI
   D. Stroke
   E. Peripheral neuropathy
   F. Skin infections
   G. UTIs
   H. Vaginitis

DIAGNOSTIC TESTS AND METHODS

1. History
2. Physical examination
3. Fasting blood glucose test
4. Urinalysis
5. Urine tests for glucose and acetone
6. Postprandial blood sugar cortisone glucose tolerance test—to elicit stress-induced diabetes
7. Twenty-four-hour urine quantitative glucose specimen
8. Blood insulin level determination

Planning

1. Safe, effective care environment
   A. Prevent avoidable injury and/or infection.
   B. Increase client's and family's knowledge of disease process, diagnostic procedures, and treatment.
2. Physiological integrity
   A. Maintain adequate fluid balance.
   B. Maintain adequate nutritional intake.
   C. Maintain skin integrity.
   D. Assist with self-care needs.
3. Psychosocial integrity
   A. Counsel on disturbances of self-concept.
   B. Reduce anxiety and feelings of powerlessness.
4. Health promotion and maintenance
   A. Increase client's and family's knowledge of prevention, complications, home care, and follow-up.
   B. Counsel on consequences of noncompliance.

Implementation

1. Assess, report, and record signs and symptoms and reactions to treatment.
2. Stress importance of compliance with prescribed program.
3. Monitor intake and output.
4. Monitor serum glucose, urine glucose, and electrolytes.
5. Monitor vital signs every 4 hours or as condition warrants.
6. Monitor for signs of insulin shock (hypoglycemia—abnormally low blood glucose levels caused by an excess of insulin or oral hypoglycemic medication in relation to activity or dietary intake, or the result of insufficient glucose to supply CNS needs).
   A. Pallor
   B. Weakness, numbness
   C. Confusion or irritability
   D. Fatigue
   E. Vertigo
   F. Blurred vision
   G. Tachycardia
   H. Diaphoresis
   I. Hunger
   J. Seizures
   K. Coma

7. Instruct client and family on high-carbohydrate foods to treat hypoglycemia.
   A. Fruit juice
   B. Hard candy
   C. Honey
   D. Cola
8. Assist in administration of glucagon or dextrose IV if client is unconscious.
9. Monitor neurological status frequently.
10. Monitor nutritional status.
11. Monitor for signs of diabetic coma (ketoacidosis—acute or gradual insulin deficiency precipitated by emotional stress, infection, trauma, or other stressors; occurs in insulin-dependent diabetic patients. Leads to protein catabolism, release of potassium and urea nitrogen, and ketone formation from the breakdown of fat).
    A. Polydipsia
    B. Nausea, vomiting
    C. Abdominal pain
    D. Drowsiness
    E. Headache
    F. Acetone breath (fruity breath odor from respiratory compensation for elevated serum acetone level)
    G. Elevated serum glucose
    H. Elevated serum acetone and osmolarity
    I. Decreased arterial pH and bicarbonate level
    J. Dehydration
    K. Weak, rapid pulse
    L. Kussmaul's respirations
    M. Osmotic diuresis
    N. Electrolyte imbalance
12. Monitor for signs of hyperglycemic nonketotic coma.
    A. Polyuria
    B. Thirst
    C. Neurological abnormalities
    D. Stupor
13. Provide the following nursing interventions for diabetic ketoacidosis and hyperosmolar coma, both of which are hyperglycemic crises.
    A. Assist in administration of:
       (1) Prescribed IV fluids
       (2) Prescribed insulin and electrolyte replacement
       (3) Potassium replacement, if required
    B. Monitor:
       (1) Signs of hypoglycemia as a result of insulin administration
       (2) Vital signs every 4 hours
       (3) Intake and output hourly
       (4) Serum glucose, electrolytes, and ABGs
       (5) Hydration status
       (6) Diabetic effects on the cardiovascular system
       (7) Any symptoms of cerebral vascular disease
       (8) Any symptoms of coronary artery and peripheral vascular disease
    C. Provide a safe, calm environment
14. Monitor for and treat all injuries, cuts, and blisters (especially on lower extremities) as prescribed.
15. Monitor for signs of UTI and renal failure.
16. Monitor for signs of Kimmelstiel-Wilson syndrome (protein and RBCs in urine)—due to vascular destruction in the kidneys.
17. Assess client for diabetic neuropathy.
    A. Numbness
    B. Pain in arms and legs
    C. Footdrop
    D. Neurogenic bladder
    E. Signs of trauma—may injure self unknowingly due to decreased sensation in arms and legs
18. Instruct client and family about insulin and its use to control serum glucose metabolism and thereby control diabetes.
    A. Types of insulin
       (1) Rapid-acting (Regular) Semilente: Action begins within 1 hour, with peak action in 1–4 hours. Solution appears clear.
       (2) Intermediate-acting (NPH) Lente: Initial action begins in 2–4 hours, with peak action in 8–12 hours. Solution appears cloudy.
       (3) Long-acting (Protamine Zinc) Ultralente: Initial action begins in 4–8 hours, with peak action in 16–18 hours. Solution appears cloudy.
    B. Strength or concentration
    C. Source: pork, beef, Humulin insulin
    D. Purity
    E. Regimen prescribed
    F. Rotation sites and subcutaneous injection
    G. Mixing of different types
19. Instruct client in use of oral hypoglycemic agents
20. Instruct client and family regarding disease process, diagnostic procedures, treatment, prevention, complications, home care, care on "sick" days, diet, and follow-up. Include teaching on:
    A. Self-care
    B. Medication
    C. Activity
    D. Use of equipment such as insulin pump

Evaluation

1. Reports increased comfort, decreased anxiety
2. Shows no signs of avoidable injury and/or infection
3. Maintains adequate serum glucose level
4. Maintains adequate fluid and nutritional status
5. Maintains adequate fluid balance and tissue perfusion
6. Maintains skin integrity
7. Develops a positive self-concept
8. Reports reduction in feelings of powerlessness
9. Verbalizes plan for compliance with therapeutic regimen
10. Uses effective coping strategies
11. Demonstrates understanding of disease process, diagnostic procedures, treatment, complications, prevention, home care, and need for follow-up

Musculoskeletal System

Basic Information

The musculoskeletal system is a complex system of bones, muscles, ligaments, tendons, and other connective tissue. This system gives the body shape and form. It also makes movement possible, protects vital organs, provides the site for hematopoiesis, and stores calcium and other minerals.

Muscle tissue has contractility, which makes movement of bones and joints possible. Muscles move food through the intestines, pump blood through the blood vessels of the body, and make breathing possible. The activity of muscles aids in temperature regulation by producing heat. Muscles also assist in maintaining body position, such as standing and sitting.

Muscles are classified as skeletal (attached to bones); visceral (provide function of internal organs); and cardiac (form the wall of the heart). Muscles are also classified as voluntary and involuntary. Voluntary muscles are controlled by deliberate intention and are under the influence of the somatic nervous system. These muscles are classified as skeletal muscles. Involuntary muscles are under the control of the autonomic nervous system. These muscles include the cardiac and visceral muscles. Muscle mass accounts for about 40% of the weight of humans.

The human skeleton has 206 bones composed of organic salts, such as calcium and phosphate, which are imbedded in fibers of collagen. Bones are classified as long, short, flat, or irregular.

Musculoskeletal disorders can be either acute or chronic. Acute problems are usually due to simple injuries. Chronic conditions often result in loss of mobility and changes in self-image.

Assessment

SUBJECTIVE

1. Weakness
2. Pain
3. Complaints of joint stiffness
4. Weight loss
5. Anorexia
6. Limited movement

OBJECTIVE

1. General appearance
2. Abnormal gait
3. Impaired neurovascular status
4. Differences between affected and unaffected sides
5. Absence of extremity
6. Decreased handgrip
7. Abnormal spinal curvature
8. Joint enlargement
9. Presence of edema, redness, warmth over affected area
10. Decreased range of motion (ROM)
11. Changes in vital signs
12. Nonalignment of extremities
13. Inability to move a body part

DIAGNOSTIC TESTS AND METHODS

1. History
2. Physical examination
3. X-rays
4. Myelography—for evaluation of abnormalities of spinal canal and cord
5. Bone scan—for identification of increased bone activity or active bone formation
6. Bone and muscle biopsies
7. Microscopic examination of synovial fluid
8. Multiple laboratory studies of urine and blood—for systemic abnormality identification
   A. WBC count—aids in determining presence of infection
   B. Uric acid—rules out or identifies presence of gout
   C. Erythrocyte sedimentation rate (ESR)—increases in presence of inflammation
   D. Rheumatoid factor (RF)—presence of this protein indicates rheumatoid arthritis
   E. Lupus erythematosus (LE) cell—identifies condition of systemic lupus erythematosus

Implementation

1. Problems
   A. Potential formation of decubitus ulcer
      (1) Inspect skin over bony prominences frequently.
      (2) Keep skin clean, dry, and lubricated.
      (3) Massage over bony prominences.
      (4) Change client's position frequently (every 2 hours).
      (5) Provide sheepskin or other protective devices.
   B. Potential joint contracture due to improper body alignment
      (1) Place sandbags to prevent poor alignment.
      (2) Position extremities in natural position of function.
      (3) Provide trapeze to allow patient to move self.
      (4) Assist in active and passive ROM exercises.
      (5) Do not use knee gatch position.
      (6) Coordinate care with physical therapist.
   C. Bone pain due to disease, fracture
      (1) Support affected part.
      (2) Inspect site—monitor for edema, bruising, redness, tenderness, and warmth.
      (3) Administer analgesics for pain as prescribed—monitor effects.
      (4) Apply warm, moist compresses to site as prescribed.
   D. Potential for respiratory congestion
      (1) Encourage deep breathing and coughing.
      (2) Monitor for coughing, presence of abnormal sputum, and increased temperature.
      (3) Change the client's position frequently.
   E. Potential for formation of thrombi, emboli
      (1) Avoid use of knee Gatch position.
      (2) Encourage movement of lower extremities.
      (3) Do not rub legs—may cause release of emboli.
      (4) Provide adequate hydration.
   F. Limited ROM due to confinement, joint pain, cast, or traction
      (1) Explain reasons for ROM exercises.
      (2) Maintain body alignment.
      (3) Provide ROM exercises to all muscles and joints except if contraindicated—severe pain, inflammation, or recent surgery on or near joint.
   G. Presence of cast
      (1) Massage area around cast.
      (2) Provide a device for scratching.
      (3) Pad rough areas of cast openings.
      (4) Monitor for signs of cyanosis of extremity in cast—color of toes, feet, fingers, etc.
      (5) Inspect skin around cast for irritation.
      (6) Monitor for complaints of tingling or numbness of affected extremity.

Systemic Lupus Erythematosus

Description

1. Systemic lupus erythematosus (SLE) is a chronic inflammatory disorder of connective tissues. It involves the

production of a large variety of autoantibodies against normal body components.

2. Condition usually affects multiple organ systems as well as the skin.
3. It may be fatal.
4. It is characterized by recurring remissions and exacerbations.
5. It affects females 8 times as often as males; incidence increases during childbearing years.
6. It occurs worldwide—most prevalent among Asians and African Americans.
7. Annual incidence averages 75 cases per 1 million individuals.
8. Exacerbations are more common during the spring and summer seasons.
9. Prognosis improves with early detection and treatment.
10. Prognosis is poor for patients who develop complications—severe bacterial infections; renal, neurological involvement.
11. Cause—unknown
12. Possible causes
   A. Autoimmune: Antibodies entering tissue suppress normal immunity response of body.
   B. Drugs induced or aggravated
      (1) Anticonvulsants
      (2) Hydralazine
      (3) Procainamide
      (4) Sulfa drugs
      (5) Penicillin
      (6) Oral contraceptives
13. Predisposing factors
   A. Physical or mental stress
   B. Streptococcal or viral infections
   C. Immunization
   D. Exposure to sunlight or ultraviolet light
   E. Pregnancy
   F. Genetic predisposition

Assessment

SUBJECTIVE

1. Photosensitivity
2. Fatigue
3. Weakness
4. Weight loss
5. Joint pain and stiffness of hands, feet, or large joints
6. Tenderness of affected joints
7. Anorexia
8. Abdominal pain
9. Nausea
10. Irregular menstrual periods
11. Headaches, irritability

OBJECTIVE

1. Nondeforming arthritis
2. Facial erythema (butterfly rash)
3. Oral or nasopharyngeal ulcerations
4. Pleuritis, pericarditis, neuritis, glomerulonephritis, peritonitis
5. Convulsions
6. Hemolytic anemia, thrombocytopenia, leukopenia
7. Positive antinuclear antibody (ANA) or LE cell test
8. Proteinuria
9. UTIs
10. Increased cellular casts in urine
11. Alopecia
12. Repeated false-positive serological test results for syphilis
13. Increased temperature
14. Vomiting
15. Lymph node enlargement
16. Diarrhea and/or constipation
17. Dyspnea

DIAGNOSTIC TESTS AND METHODS

1. History
2. Physical examination
3. CBC with differential
4. Platelet count
5. ESR and serum complement levels
6. Serum electrophoresis
7. ANA and LE cell tests
8. Anti-DNA test—rarely positive in other conditions; however, in remission states, anti-DNA may be reduced or absent.
9. Urine studies
10. Chest x-ray
11. ECG
12. Kidney biopsy
13. U/A

Planning

1. Safe, effective care environment
   A. Prevent avoidable injury and/or infection.
   B. Increase client's knowledge of disease process, diagnostic procedures, and treatment.
2. Physiological integrity
   A. Increase comfort.
   B. Prevent complications related to organ affected.
   C. Maintain skin integrity.
3. Psychosocial integrity
   A. Develop effective coping strategies.
4. Health promotion and maintenance
   A. Increase client's knowledge of home care and follow-up.

Implementation

1. Assess, report, and record signs and symptoms and reactions to treatment.
2. Provide emotional support to patient and family.
3. Monitor for dyspnea, chest pain, and edema of extremities.
4. Note size, type, and location of skin lesions.
5. Monitor urine for signs of hematuria.
6. Monitor scalp for hair loss (alopecia).
7. Monitor skin and oral mucous membrane for bleeding, ulceration, petechiae, and bruising.
8. Provide a well-balanced diet.
9. Provide a low-sodium, low-protein diet if renal disorder is present.
10. Administer and monitor for side effects of prescribed medications such as:
   A. Ointments or creams for rash
   B. Corticosteroids and antimalarials for inflammatory response and renal or neurologic complications

C. Analgesics for arthritic pain
D. Cytoxic drugs, if prescribed

11. Prepare client and family for dialysis or kidney transplant if renal failure occurs.
12. Advise use of protective clothing, screening agent, sunglasses when client is out in sun.
13. Apply heat packs for relief of joint pain and stiffness.
14. Encourage full ROM exercises to prevent contractures.
15. Arrange for physical therapy and occupational counseling.
16. Provide frequent skin and oral care.
17. Monitor vital signs, intake and output, laboratory reports, weight.
18. Monitor GI secretions and stools for presence of blood.
19. Monitor for signs of renal involvement—hypertension, weight gain.
20. Assess for signs of neurological involvement—personality changes, ptosis, double vision, seizures.
21. Explain use of hypoallergenic cosmetics to female patients.
22. Refer client to Lupus Foundation of America and Arthritis Foundation.
23. Instruct client regarding disease process, diagnostic procedures, treatment, home care, and follow-up.

Evaluation

1. Reports increased comfort, decreased anxiety
2. Shows no signs of avoidable injury and infection
3. Maintains skin integrity
4. Uses effective coping strategies
5. Has no organ-specific complications
6. Demonstrates understanding of disease process, diagnostic procedures, treatment, home care, and need for follow-up

Rheumatoid Arthritis

Description

1. Rheumatoid arthritis is a chronic, systemic inflammatory disease that primarily involves peripheral joints and surrounding muscles, tendons, ligaments, and blood vessels.
2. Eventual depletion of joint cartilage results in joint dislocation.
3. Condition is characterized by spontaneous remissions and unpredictable exacerbations.
4. It usually requires lifelong treatment and occasionally requires surgery.
5. Majority of patients carry on with normal activities.
6. Approximately 10% have total disability from severe deformity.
7. Prognosis worsens with development of nodules and high titers of RF.
8. Condition occurs worldwide and affects females three times more than males.
9. It can occur at any age, but most prevalent in women aged 20 to 60, with peak onset period between ages 35 and 45.
10. It affects approximately 6.5 million individuals in the United States.
11. Inflammatory process within joints progresses in four stages if left untreated.
    A. Stage 1: Synovitis develops from congestion and edema of synovial membrane and joint capsule.
    B. Stage 2: Formation of thickened layers of granulation tissue. Thickened layers cover and invade cartilage destroying joint capsule and bone.
    C. Stage 3: Formation of fibrous ankylosis. Fibrous tissue invades thickened layers of granulation tissue with scar formation, which occludes the joint space. Visible deformities occur owing to bone atrophy and malalignment resulting in muscle atrophy and imbalance.
    D. Stage 4: Calcification of fibrous tissue with bony ankylosis, causing total immobility.
12. Cause—unknown.
13. Possible causes:
    A. Susceptibility due to genetic defects impairing autoimmune system
    B. Bacterial or viral infection
    C. Environmental factors
    D. Endocrine, nutritional, and metabolic factors
    E. Occupational and psychosocial influences

Assessment

SUBJECTIVE

1. Morning stiffness of joints
2. Sore, stiff, swollen joint(s)
3. Weakness
4. Fatigue
5. Malaise
6. Numbness; tingling in feet, hands
7. Loss of sensation in fingers, toes
8. Unable to perform usual activities
9. Pain with ROM
10. Loss of appetite

OBJECTIVE

1. Limited ROM of joint
2. Weakened grip
3. Low-grade fever
4. Anemia
5. Weight loss
6. Subcutaneous nodes
7. Enlarged lymph nodes
8. Muscle atrophy
9. Appearance of joints bilaterally
10. Elevated ESR
11. Positive RF or latex fixation test
12. X-ray evidence of joint deterioration
13. Spindle-shaped fingers
14. Flexion deformities of affected joints
15. Skin lesions, leg ulcers due to vasculitis
16. Peripheral neuropathy
17. Complications such as infection, osteoporosis, and temporomandibular disease (impairs chewing and causes earaches)

DIAGNOSTIC TESTS AND METHODS

1. History
2. Physical examination
3. X-rays of joints
4. RF test
5. ANA and LE cell tests
6. Synovial fluid analysis
7. CBC with differential

8. Serum protein electrophoresis
9. ESR

Planning

1. Safe, effective care environment
   A. Prevent avoidable injury from muscular weakness and joint immobility.
   B. Increase client's knowledge of disease process, diagnostic procedures, and treatment.
2. Physiological integrity
   A. Increase comfort.
   B. Facilitate self-care activities.
3. Psychosocial integrity
   A. Counsel on altered body image.
4. Health promotion and maintenance
   A. Increase client's knowledge of home care and follow-up.

Implementation

1. Assess, report, and record signs and symptoms and reaction to treatment.
2. Explain chronic pain medication or surgical treatment—synovectomy, arthrotomy, arthroplasty, or arthrodesis.
3. Provide emotional support.
4. Encourage adequate nutritional intake; assist with meals as needed.
5. Provide undisturbed periods of rest.
6. Administer heat applications such as paraffin dip, hot packs, and warm tub baths or showers for relief of pain and muscle relaxation as ordered.
7. Administer analgesics, anti-inflammatory medications, corticosteroids and immunosuppressive agents as ordered. Monitor for side effects.
8. Allow verbalization of feelings, and support positive body image.
9. Provide ROM exercises within limits of pain tolerance.
10. Provide meticulous skin care—use lotion or cleaning oil in place of soap for dry skin.
11. Apply splints correctly, if ordered; observe for pressure sores.
12. Encourage mobility.
    A. Encourage client to perform ADL with assistance as necessary.
    B. Assist with active ROM exercises.
    C. Instruct client to protect joints and conserve energy.
    D. Encourage client to ambulate with assistance as necessary.
    E. Coordinate care with physical therapy department.
13. Instruct client regarding disease process, diagnostic procedures, treatment, home care, and follow-up.

Evaluation

1. Reports increased comfort, decreased anxiety
2. Participates in ADL
3. Establishes a positive self-image
4. Maintains adequate nutritional intake
5. Shows no signs of avoidable injury and/or infection
6. Demonstrates understanding of disease process, diagnostic procedures, treatment, home care, and need for follow-up

Osteoarthritis

Description

1. Osteoarthritis is the most common form of arthritis, a progressive disorder causing deterioration of the joint cartilage and formation of reactive new bone at margins of joints.
2. Degeneration is due to a breakdown of chondrocytes.
3. Disorder most often affects weight-bearing joints such as the hips and knees.
4. Incidence is rising among the elderly.
5. Earliest symptoms generally begin in middle age, becoming progressively severe with advancing age.
6. Disorder affects both sexes.
7. Prognosis depends on site and severity of involvement—may range from minor limitations involving the fingers to severe disability involving knees and hips. Rate of progression varies.
8. Causes
   A. Primary osteoarthritis results from genetic predisposition and is a normal part of aging.
   B. Secondary osteoarthritis is an acquired form resulting from joint damage caused by trauma, stress, excessive "wear-and-tear" infection, underlying joint disease, and/or metabolic disorders.

Assessment

SUBJECTIVE

1. Pain after exercise or weight bearing
2. Morning stiffness
3. Aching during changes in weather
4. "Grating" of joint during movement

OBJECTIVE

1. Limited ROM
2. Crepitant joint
3. Prominent bony enlargement
4. Hebreden's nodes on distal joints of phalanges and Bouchard's nodes on proximal joint of phalanges—initially painless, then red, swollen, and tender

DIAGNOSTIC TESTS AND METHODS

1. History
2. Physical examination
3. X-rays of affected joints

Planning

1. Safe, effective care environment
   A. Prevent avoidable injury and/or infection.
   B. Increase client's knowledge of disease process, diagnostic procedures, and treatment.
2. Physiological integrity
   A. Increase comfort.
   B. Relieve pain.
3. Psychosocial integrity
   A. Assist with coping.
4. Health promotion and maintenance
   A. Increase client's knowledge of home care and follow-up.

Implementation

1. Assess, report, and record signs and symptoms and reactions to treatment.

2. Allow client to verbalize feelings regarding condition.
3. Provide adequate rest, especially following activity.
4. Assist with physical therapy.
5. Provide care for affected joint.
    A. Hand: Apply hot soaks, paraffin dips to relieve pain as ordered.
    B. Spine (lumbar and sacral): Provide firm mattress or bed board to decrease morning pain.
    C. Spine (cervical): Provide cervical collar for constrictions—monitor for signs of redness.
    D. Hip:
       (1) Apply moist heat pads to relieve pain.
       (2) Administer antispasmodic medications as ordered.
       (3) Assist with ROM and strengthening exercises.
       (4) Check assistive devices such as crutches, braces, and walker for proper fit.
       (5) Advise use of elevated toilet seat and cushions when client is sitting.
    E. Knee:
       (1) Assist with prescribed ROM exercises.
       (2) Encourage exercises to maintain muscle tone.
6. Instruct client regarding disease process, diagnostic procedures, treatment, home care, and follow-up. Include teaching on:
    A. Avoiding overexertion
    B. Taking mild analgesics as prescribed
    C. Obtaining adequate rest
    D. Wearing well-fitting supportive shoes
    E. Using guard rails in bathroom
    F. Minimizing weight-bearing activities

Evaluation

1. Reports increased comfort, decreased anxiety
2. Shows no signs of avoidable injury and/or infection
3. Participates in self-care activities
4. Establishes a positive self-image
5. Demonstrates understanding of disease process, diagnostic procedures, treatment, home care, and need for follow-up

Gout

Description

1. Gout is a metabolic disease resulting in an acute inflammation of synovial tissue characterized by deposits of urate crystals.
2. Increased concentration of uric acid results in urate deposits (tophi) in joints and tissues, causing local necrosis or fibrosis.
3. Primary gout occurs in males, with onset at approximately age 50, and in postmenopausal females.
4. Secondary gout occurs in the elderly.
5. Disease process follows an intermittent course with most clients free of symptoms for years between attacks.
6. It may lead to chronic disability.
7. In rare instances, it can lead to severe hypertension and progressive renal disease.
8. It can affect any joint but is found mostly in joints of feet and legs.
9. Gout develops in four stages—asymptomatic, acute, intercritical, and chronic.

10. Prognosis is good with treatment.
11. Causes
    A. Primary gout
       (1) Exact cause unknown.
       (2) This form is linked to a genetic defect in purine metabolism resulting in an overproduction of uric acid (hyperuricemia), retention of uric acid, or both.
    B. Secondary gout
       (1) Course follows those of other diseases such as polycythemia vera or multiple myeloma.
       (2) This form is due to breakdown of nucleic acid.
       (3) It may also follow drug therapy, such as hydrochlorothiazide, which interferes with urate excretion.

Assessment

SUBJECTIVE

1. Onset of pain in joint of the great toe, feet, ankles, or knees
2. Pruritus
3. Headache
4. Malaise
5. Severe back pain

OBJECTIVE

1. Elevated serum uric acid
2. Normal or elevated 24-hour urinary uric acid
3. Positive monosodium urate crystals in synovial fluid
4. Inflamed joint(s)
5. Elevated WBC count and ESR
6. Asymptomatic stage—increase in serum urate levels with no apparent symptoms
7. Acute stage
    A. Hypertension, kidney stones: Attack is sudden and peaks quickly.
    B. Affected joints are hot, inflamed, dusky red, cyanotic.
    C. Joint of great toe usually affected first, followed by the instep, ankle, heel, knee, or wrist joints.
8. Intercritical stage—symptom-free between gout attacks
9. Chronic stage
    A. Persistent painful polyarthritis
    B. Large, subcutaneous tophaceous deposits in cartilage, synovial membranes, tendons, and soft tissues—urate deposits above earlobe, fingers, hands, knees, feet, and ulnar sides of forearms
    C. Ulcerations over tophi with presence of chalky white exudate or pus
    D. Joint degeneration, deformity and disability
    E. Kidney involvement resulting in symptoms of chronic renal dysfunction
    F. Urolithiasis (urinary calculi)

DIAGNOSTIC TESTS AND METHODS

1. History
2. Physical examination
3. Serum uric acid levels
4. Urinary uric acid levels
5. WBC count
6. ESR
7. Analysis of aspirated synovial fluid or tophaceous material

8. X-rays of joints
9. RF test—to rule out rheumatoid arthritis

Planning

1. Safe, effective care environment
   A. Increase client's and family's knowledge of disease process, diagnostic procedures, and treatment.
2. Physiological integrity
   A. Increase comfort.
   B. Maintain adequate fluid balance.
3. Psychosocial integrity
   A. Reduce anxiety.
4. Health promotion and maintenance
   A. Increase client's and family's knowledge of prevention, home care (including medication), and follow-up.

Implementation

1. Assess, report, and record signs and symptoms and reactions to treatment.
2. Provide bed rest during acute attacks—use bed cradle to keep bedcovers off.
3. Provide adequate fluid to prevent calculi formation—monitor intake and output.
4. Monitor appearance of joints—ROM ability.
5. Administer analgesics such as aspirin or acetaminophen as prescribed to relieve pain of mild attacks.
6. Position affected joint in mild flexion position during acute attack; assist with mobility.
7. Administer prescribed medications such as colchicine and anti-inflammatory drugs such as indomethacin (Indocin), probenecid (Benemid), or sulfinpyrazone (Anturane) to facilitate uric acid excretion; allopurinal (Zyloprim) to decrease formation of uric acid. Watch for side effects. Encourage fluid intake of 3–4 liters/day to maintain urine output of 2 or more liters per day.
8. Administer corticosteroids for resistant inflammation as prescribed.
9. Assist with joint aspiration and injection of intra-articular corticosteroid injection, if needed.
10. Apply hot or cold packs to inflamed joints as ordered.
    A. Monitor serum uric acid levels on a regular basis.
11. Encourage weight loss in obese clients. (Obesity places additional stress on painful joints.)
12. Prepare client for excision and drainage of infected or ulcerated tophi.
13. Monitor for acute gout attacks 24–96 hours following surgery.
14. Instruct client and family regarding disease process, diagnostic procedures, treatment, prevention, home care, and follow-up. Include teaching on:
    A. Checking serum uric acid levels periodically.
    B. Avoiding use of high-purine foods such as anchovies, kidneys, sweetbreads, all yeast breads, lentils, liver, most meat and alcoholic beverages.
    C. Diet to gradually decrease weight in obese patients.
    D. Complying with prescribed medication regimen.
    E. Reporting side effects of medications immediately.

Evaluation

1. Reports increased comfort, decreased anxiety
2. Shows no signs of avoidable injury and/or infection
3. Maintains adequate diet
4. Maintains adequate fluid intake
5. Maintains adequate mobility
6. Demonstrates understanding of disease process, diagnostic procedures, treatment, prevention, home care (including drug regimen), and need for follow-up; similar understanding demonstrated by family

Osteoporosis

Description

1. Osteoporosis is a metabolic bone disorder with an acceleration of bone resorption rate and a slowing down in the rate of bone formation resulting in loss of bone mass.
2. Calcium and phosphate salts are lost from affected bones.
3. Affected bones become brittle and vulnerable to fractures.
4. Two forms
   A. Primary osteoporosis (senile or postmenopausal)
      (1) Most common in elderly, postmenopausal women.
      (2) Sites usually affected are the vertebrae, pelvis, and femur.
      (3) Cause is unknown.
      (4) Predisposing factors
         (a) Prolonged negative calcium balance due to inadequate dietary intake of calcium
         (b) Decline in gonadal adrenal function
         (c) Faulty protein metabolism due to estrogen deficiency and sedentary lifestyle
   B. Secondary osteoporosis
      (1) Causes
         (a) Prolonged therapy with steroids or heparin
         (b) Total immobilization or disuse of bone as with hemiplegia
         (c) Alcoholism—malnutrition
         (d) Lactose intolerance
         (e) Hyperthyroidism

Assessment

SUBJECTIVE

1. Backache
2. Pain radiating around trunk

OBJECTIVE

1. Vertebral compression
2. Kyphosis
3. Loss of height
4. Pathological fractures—neck, femur, hip, Colles' fracture
5. Changes in skull, ribs, and long bones due to severe or advanced osteoporosis as in hyperthyroidism or Cushing's syndrome

DIAGNOSTIC TESTS AND METHODS

1. History
2. Physical examination
3. Skeletal x-rays
4. Serum calcium, phosphorus, and alkaline phosphatase within normal limits
5. Elevated parathyroid hormone
6. Bone biopsy
7. CT to evaluate bone density

Planning

1. Safe, effective care environment
   A. Prevent avoidable injury and/or infection.
   B. Increase client's knowledge of disease process, diagnostic procedures, and treatment.
2. Physiological integrity
   A. Maintain adequate mobility and posture.
   B. Increase comfort.
   C. Maintain adequate nutritional intake.
3. Psychosocial integrity
   A. Reduce anxiety.
4. Health promotion and maintenance
   A. Increase client's knowledge of prevention, home care (including medication and diet) and follow-up.

Implementation

1. Assess, report, and record signs and symptoms and reactions to treatment.
2. Encourage physical activity and exercise to prevent disuse atrophy.
3. Administer estrogen replacement to improve calcium balance.
4. Administer fluoride as ordered to stimulate bone formation.
5. Provide diet high in protein and calcium.
6. Administer vitamin D supplements and calcium as ordered to support normal bone metabolism.
7. Encourage fluid intake of 2000–3000 mL daily to avoid formation of renal calculi (unless contraindicated).
8. Provide support of spine with brace or corset as ordered.
9. Monitor daily for redness, warmth, and new sites of pain.
10. Perform passive ROM exercises as appropriate.
11. Coordinate care with physical therapist.
12. Provide safety precautions such as side rails, moving client gently and carefully.
13. Administer analgesics as prescribed for pain.
14. Encourage use of walker or cane to stabilize balance when ambulating.
15. Provide prescribed treatment for underlying diseases to prevent secondary osteoporosis.
16. Encourage early mobilization following surgical procedure or trauma.
17. Encourage avoidance or decrease of alcoholic consumption.
18. Instruct client and family in importance of following prescribed daily activity.
19. Advise client and family importance of sleeping on a firm mattress and avoiding excessive bed rest.
20. Emphasize need for routine gynecological checkups, including Pap smears, for females on estrogen. Instruct clients to report any abnormal bleeding and presence of lumps in breast.
21. Instruct client on good body mechanics—stoop before lifting; avoid twisting motions and prolonged bending.
22. Instruct client regarding disease process, diagnostic procedures, treatment, prevention, home care, and follow-up.

Evaluation

1. Reports increased comfort, decreased anxiety
2. Shows no signs of avoidable injury or infection
3. Maintains adequate mobility
4. Maintains adequate nutritional intake
5. Maintains adequate fluid intake
6. Participates in self-care activities
7. Demonstrates understanding of disease process, diagnostic procedures, treatment, prevention, home care, and need for follow-up

Herniated Nucleus Pulposus (Slipped or Ruptured Disc)

Description

1. Herniated nucleus pulposus is protrusion of the nucleus pulposus (soft, mucoid central portion of an intervertebral disk) resulting in compression of nerve roots of spinal cord or spinal cord itself.
2. Nucleus pulposus is forced through the disk's weakened or torn outer ring.
3. Compressed nerve roots or spinal cord result in back pain and other signs of nerve root irritation.
4. Condition usually occurs in adults (mostly males) under age 45.
5. It may occur anywhere along the spine; however, sites usually affected are between L4 and L5, L5 and sacrum, C5 and C6, and C6 and C7.
6. Following trauma in lumbosacral area, pain may begin suddenly, subside for a short time, recur at shorter intervals with progressive intensity. Sciatic pain follows. Valsalva's maneuver, sneezing, coughing, or bending magnifies pain accompanied by muscle spasms.
7. May cause sensory and motor loss in area innervated by compressed spinal nerve root followed by weakness and atrophy of affected muscles.
8. Causes
   A. Severe trauma or strain
   B. Intervertebral joint degeneration
   C. Congenitally small lumbar spinal canal

Assessment

SUBJECTIVE

1. Cervical disk
   A. Stiff neck
   B. Shoulder pain descending down arm into hand
   C. Numbness of arm and hand
2. Lumbosacral disk—severe low back pain radiating down buttocks, legs, and feet, usually unilaterally.

OBJECTIVE

1. Cervical disk—sensory disturbances of neck, arm, and hand
2. Lumbosacral disk
   A. LeSegue's signs—pain in back and legs, loss of ankle or knee-jerk reflex. Client lies flat; thigh and knee are flexed to 90 degrees while raising heel with knee straight.
   B. Straight leg-raising test—pain in posterior leg (sciatic pain) while client is lying supine. Examiner places one hand on client's ilium and other hand under ankle, while slowly raising client's leg.
   C. Difficulty in ambulating.
   D. Numbness of leg and foot.

DIAGNOSTIC TESTS AND METHODS

1. History
2. Physical examination
3. Neurological examination
4. X-rays of spine
5. CT scan of spine
6. Peripheral vascular status check—posterior tibial and dorsalis pedis pulses and skin temperature of extremities to rule out ischemic vascular disease
7. Myelography
8. Electromyography

Planning

1. Safe, effective care environment
   A. Prevent avoidable injury and/or infection.
   B. Increase client's knowledge of disease process, diagnostic procedures, and treatment.
2. Physiological integrity
   A. Maintain effective breathing pattern and gas exchange.
   B. Maintain skin integrity.
   C. Maintain adequate bladder and bowel elimination.
   D. Maintain adequate level of mobility.
   E. Assist with alterations in sensory perception.
3. Psychosocial integrity
   A. Reduce anxiety.
   B. Facilitate coping with alterations in self-image and self-concept.
   C. Counsel on alterations in sexual activity.
4. Health promotion and maintenance
   A. Facilitate participation in activities of daily living (ADL).
   B. Increase client's knowledge of prevention, home care (including medication and activity), and follow-up.

Implementation

1. Assess, report, and record signs and symptoms and reactions to treatment.
2. Encourage verbalization of fears and other feelings related to immobility.
3. Assess allergies to iodides prior to myelography. (They may indicate sensitivity to radiopaque dye used in diagnostic test.)
4. Provide postmyelography care.
   A. Have client remain supine in bed and drink plenty of fluids.
   B. Provide increased fluid intake to prevent renal stasis—monitor intake and output.
   C. Monitor for allergic reaction to dye.
   D. Encourage deep breathing, coughing, and use of blow bottles to prevent pulmonary complications.
   E. Provide meticulous skin care.
   F. Assess bowel function—use fracture bedpan when client is on complete bed rest.
   G. Monitor for abnormal neurological signs.
   H. Apply antiembolism stockings as ordered.
   I. Perform these observations for traction—cervical traction for cervical disk involvement; traction to lower extremities for lumbosacral disk involvement:
      (1) Check that weights are hanging free and have not fallen.
      (2) Observe for frayed ropes and loosened knots.

(3) Maintain proper body alignment.
   J. Provide diet high in fiber with adequate fluid intake to prevent constipation and straining.
   K. Encourage client to move legs if allowed.
   L. Provide high-topped sneakers to prevent footdrop.
   M. Coordinate prescribed exercises with physical therapist to ensure consistent regimen.
   N. Prepare client for surgical intervention, if required— laminectomy or spinal fusion.
5. Instruct client to take analgesics and antispasmodics as prescribed.
6. Instruct client regarding disease process, diagnostic procedures, treatment, prevention, home care, and follow-up.

Evaluation

1. Remains free of skin breakdown
2. Reports that pain is well controlled and alleviated
3. Adapts to neurological defects

Degenerative Joint Disease

Description

1. Degenerative joint disease is destruction of the articular cartilage resulting in replacement by bone spurs.
2. Cartilage becomes opaque, soft, weak, yellow, and deteriorated.
3. It usually occurs from age 50 into the 70s.
4. Causes
   A. Primary—unknown
   B. Secondary—fractures, trauma, infections, and obesity

Assessment

SUBJECTIVE

1. Stiffness after resting
2. Pain in hand joints, hips, and/or knees

OBJECTIVE

1. Enlarged, deformed joints
2. Limited ROM
3. Crepitation of joints when moving
4. Presence of Heberden's nodes (bony prominences on back of distal ends of fingers)
5. Presence of Bouchard's nodes (bony prominences on proximal end of fingers)
6. Difficulty in rising up from chair after sitting for a long period of time
7. Narrowed joint space seen on x-ray
8. Cystlike bony deposits in joint spaces and margins seen on x-ray

DIAGNOSTIC TESTS AND METHODS

1. History
2. Physical examination
3. X-rays of joints

Planning

1. Safe, effective care environment
   A. Increase client's and family's knowledge of disease process, diagnostic procedures, and treatment.

2. Physiological integrity
   A. Increase comfort.
   B. Maintain mobility.
   C. Maintain adequate nutritional intake.
   D. Maintain participation in self-care activities.
3. Psychosocial integrity
   A. Reduce anxiety.
   B. Maintain social interaction.
4. Health promotion and maintenance
   A. Increase client's and family's knowledge of prevention, home care and follow-up.

Implementation

1. Assess, report, and record signs and symptoms and reactions to treatment.
2. Administer analgesics, salicylates, anti-inflammatory medications as prescribed to relieve pain.
3. Apply warm, moist packs to joints as ordered.
4. Provide emotional support and reassurance to assist client to cope with limited mobility.
5. Instruct client on control of disease process and prevention (see Rheumatoid Arthritis, p. 320).
6. Encourage use of assistive devices such as canes or walkers to reduce weight bearing on painful joints.
7. Prepare client and family for surgical intervention, if required by client.
   A. Arthroplasty—replacement of a joint with metal or other material (e.g., hip replacement)
   B. Arthrodesis—fusion of a damaged joint
   C. Debridement—removal of broken cartilage or bone
   D. Osteotomy—realignment of bone or joint
8. Provide appropriate postoperative care.
9. Instruct client and family regarding disease process, diagnostic procedures, treatment, prevention, home care, and follow-up. Include teaching on:
   A. Importance of adequate nutritional intake
   B. Importance of weight reduction in obese clients to reduce stress on weight-bearing joints
   C. Activity
   D. Weight bearing

Evaluation

1. Reports increased comfort, reduced anxiety
2. Maintains adequate mobility
3. Participates in ADL
4. Maintains adequate nutritional intake
5. Maintains adequate weight
6. Demonstrates understanding of disease process, diagnostic procedures, treatment, prevention, home care and need for follow-up; similar understanding demonstrated by family

Fractures

Description

1. Fractures are usually due to trauma and often cause substantial muscle, nerve, and other soft tissue damage.
2. Prognosis varies with:
   A. Extent of disablement or deformity
   B. Amount of tissue and vascular damage
   C. Adequacy of reduction and immobilization.
   D. Client's health status, age, and nutritional status.
3. Bones of adults in poor health along with impaired circulation may not heal properly.
4. Severe open fractures, especially those involving the femoral shaft, may cause considerable bleeding and life-threatening hypovolemic shock.
5. Types of fractures
   A. Incomplete: Break extends only partially through the bone.
   B. Complete: Bone breaks into two or more pieces.
   C. Closed (simple): Overlying skin remains unbroken.
   D. Open (compound): Wound is present over fractured area; fractured bone breaks through skin.
   E. Nondisplaced: Fractured bone remains in proper alignment.
   F. Transverse: Break runs transversally (straight across) the bone shaft.
   G. Spiral: Break encircles bone like a coil.
   H. Oblique: Bone is broken at a diagonal angle.
   I. Comminuted: Bone is shattered or compressed into bone fragments.
   J. Impacted: Bone ends are driven into each other.
   K. Compression: Bone collapses (vertebrae) under excessive pressure.
   L. Linear: Break runs the length of the bone.
   M. Greenstick: Bone splinters fibers on one side of bone, leaving other side intact.
   N. Avulsion: Overexertion resulting in tearing of a muscle or ligament from a bone, pulling a small bone fragment with it.
   O. Depression: Bone fragments are driven inward by trauma (usually refers to fracture of the skull).
6. Healing process consists of five stages and is referred to as *callus formation.*
   A. Stage 1—formation of hematoma.
   B. Stage 2—formation of fibrin meshwork. Fibroblasts form fibrin network.
   C. Stage 3—Invasion of osteoblasts. Osteoblasts strengthen fibrin network; blood vessels form.
   D. Stage 4—callus formation. Collagen forms, calcium is deposited.
   E. Stage 5—remodeling. Trabecular bone forms.
7. Complications of fractures of the extremities
   A. Permanent deformity and dysfunction due to failure of bones to heal (nonunion) or heal improperly (malunion).
   B. Hypovolemic shock due to blood vessel damage.
   C. Muscle contractures.
   D. Aseptic necrosis of bone segments due to decreased circulation.
   E. Renal calculi form decalcification due to prolonged immobilization.
   F. Fat embolism.
8. Causes
   A. Most fractures occur from major trauma.
   B. Pathological fractures occur due to underlying conditions of osteoporosis, bone tumors, or metabolic disease.
   C. Prolonged standing, walking, or running may cause stress fractures of foot and ankle—usually seen in postal workers, nurses, soldiers, and joggers.

Assessment

SUBJECTIVE

1. Pain—usually intense, acute, worsens with pressure or movement
2. Loss of movement of affected extremity
3. Loss of sensory perception distal to fracture site
4. Point tenderness
5. Numbness and tingling

OBJECTIVE

1. Pallor
2. Limited motion or paralysis of affected limb distal to fracture site
3. Deformity of affected limb
4. Edema, discoloration
5. Crepitus on movement of limb
6. Warmth over site
7. Possible arterial compromise or nerve damage
   A. Mottled cyanosis
   B. Cool skin at end of extremity
   C. Loss of pulses distal to injury
   D. Signs of shock
   E. Evidence of fracture on x-ray film

DIAGNOSTIC TESTS AND METHODS

1. History
2. Physical examination
3. X-rays of suspected fracture sites and associated joints

Planning

1. Safe, effective care environment
   A. Prevent avoidable injury and/or infection.
   B. Increase client's and family's knowledge of condition, diagnostic procedures, and treatment.
   C. Ensure safe environment.
2. Physiological integrity
   A. Maintain adequate mobility.
   B. Maintain adequate tissue perfusion.
   C. Maintain skin integrity.
   D. Increase comfort.
   E. Prevent infection.
   F. Maintain adequate nutrition.
3. Psychosocial integrity
   A. Reduce anxiety.
4. Health promotion and maintenance
   A. Increase client's and family's knowledge regarding prevention, home care (including activity), and follow-up.

Implementation

1. Assess, report, and record signs and symptoms and reactions to treatment.
2. Splint or immobilize injured area.
3. Monitor vital signs—observe for shock symptoms (rapid pulse, decreased blood pressure; cool, clammy skin; and pallor).
4. Assist in administration of IV fluids as ordered.
5. Administer analgesics and/or muscle relaxants as prescribed.
6. Apply ice compress to injured area as ordered.

7. Discuss use of relaxing techniques.
8. Prepare client for surgical intervention and provide appropriate postoperative care as indicated.
9. Assist with passive and active ROM of unaffected limbs—maintain mobility.
10. Assist with appropriate exercise to affected limb as ordered.
11. Encourage client to participate in self-care activities.
12. Provide a well-balanced nutritional diet—high in protein and vitamins, high in bulk.
13. Encourage adequate fluid intake to prevent bowel and urinary problems.
14. Monitor for signs of fat embolism—apprehension, sweating, fever, tachycardia, pallor, dyspnea, petechial rash on chest and shoulders, pulmonary effusion, tissue hypoxia, cyanosis, convulsions, coma.
15. Turn client, if not contraindicated, every 2 hours, maintaining proper alignment.
16. Encourage use of isometric exercises to prevent muscle atrophy.
17. Explain types of traction.
    A. Buck's traction—used to ease muscle spasm and immobilize limb by maintaining a straight pull on limb with use of weights.
    B. Russell's traction—same rationale as Buck's traction but pulls at knee and foot with use of knee sling.
    C. Skeletal traction—direct application of traction to bone with use of wires or pins (Steinmann pin, Kirschner wire) that are pulled by traction weights.
    D. Crutchfield tongs—tongs inserted into shallow holes in the skull and joined to skeletal traction for fractures of the cervical vertebrae.
18. Provide care for clients requiring long-term immobilization with traction.
    A. Reposition client often to increase comfort and prevent formation of decubitus ulcers.
    B. Assist with ROM exercises to prevent muscle atrophy.
    C. Encourage deep breathing and coughing to prevent pulmonary complications.
    D. Encourage adequate fluid intake to prevent urinary stasis and constipation.
    E. Monitor for signs of renal colic—flank pain, nausea, and vomiting.
    F. Maintain proper body alignment.
    G. Check ropes and weights for proper placement. Weights should hang freely.
    H. Provide meticulous skin care.
    I. Avoid bumping into or manipulating traction device.
    J. Inspect site of pins and affected limb frequently.
    K. Monitor site of cervical tongs—provide meticulous skin care using aseptic technique.
    L. Use footboard to prevent footdrop; use high-topped sneaker on unaffected leg.
    M. Monitor circulation—check for signs of thrombophlebitis.
19. Provide cast care:
    A. Support cast with pillows while still wet.
    B. Observe for skin irritation near cast edges.
    C. Check for foul odors or discharge.
    D. Instruct client to report signs of decreased circulation to the part—skin coldness, tingling, numbness, discoloration of toes or fingers.
    E. Instruct the client to keep cast dry.

F. Instruct client to avoid inserting foreign objects under the cast.
20. Encourage movement as soon as possible.
21. Assist with ambulation.
22. Demonstrate the correct method of walking with crutches—placing weight on hands and not on axillary region to prevent damage to nerves.
23. Refer to physical therapist following cast removal for assistance in restoring limb mobility.
24. Instruct client and family regarding condition, diagnostic procedures, treatment, prevention, home care (including activity), and follow-up.

Evaluation

1. Reports increased comfort, decreased anxiety
2. Shows no signs of avoidable injury and/or infection
3. Maintains safe environment
4. Maintains adequate mobility
5. Maintains skin integrity
6. Maintains adequate elimination pattern
7. Maintains adequate tissue perfusion
8. Maintains adequate nutritional status
9. Demonstrates understanding of condition, diagnostic procedures, treatment, prevention, home care and need for follow-up; similar understanding demonstrated by family

Amputation

Description

1. Amputation is removal of a body part. There are two types of amputation.
   A. Surgical amputation—surgical removal of part or all of an extremity
      (1) The majority of surgical amputations are due to vascular disorders causing an inadequate O_2 supply to the tissue.
      (2) Other reasons for amputation are septic wounds, gas gangrene, malignant tumors, severe trauma, and burns.
   B. Traumatic amputation—accidental loss of a body part such as an arm, a leg, a finger, or a toe
      (1) In complete amputation, the part is completely severed.
      (2) In partial amputation, some soft tissue remains.
      (3) Prognosis has improved due to:
         (a) Improved emergency and critical care management
         (b) New surgical techniques
         (c) New prosthetic designs
         (d) Early rehabilitation
         (e) Innovative limb reimplantation techniques; however, incomplete nerve regeneration limits their usefulness
      (4) Causes include accidents involving farm, factory, motor vehicles, use of power tools, or war.

Assessment

SUBJECTIVE—SURGICAL AMPUTATION

1. Peripheral vascular diseases—pain, tingling
2. Septic wounds and gas gangrene—pain

OBJECTIVE—SURGICAL AMPUTATION

1. Peripheral vascular diseases
   A. Pallor
   B. Edema
   C. Diminished pulses
   D. Cyanosis
   E. Ulcer formation
   F. Hyperpigmentation
2. Septic wounds, gas gangrene
   A. Foul odor
   B. Blackened wound
   C. Edema
   D. Fever
   E. Necrosis

SUBJECTIVE—TRAUMATIC AMPUTATION

1. Pain

OBJECTIVE—TRAUMATIC AMPUTATION

1. Profuse bleeding
2. Hypovolemic shock
   A. Hypotension
   B. Narrowing pulse pressure
   C. Tachycardia
   D. Rapid, shallow respirations
   E. Oliguria
   F. Cold, clammy skin
   G. Metabolic acidosis

DIAGNOSTIC TESTS AND METHODS

1. Both surgical and traumatic amputations
   A. History
   B. Physical assessment
2. Surgical amputations
   A. Arteriography
   B. Oscillometry
   C. X-rays
   D. Skin temperature studies

Planning

1. Safe, effective care environment
   A. Ensure safe environment.
   B. Promote participation in exercise program.
   C. Increase client's knowledge of condition, diagnostic procedures, and treatment.
2. Physiological integrity
   A. Monitor for signs of bleeding, heating of stump.
   B. Explain phantom pain.
3. Psychosocial integrity
   A. Promote coping with altered body image.
4. Health promotion and maintenance
   A. Increase client's knowledge of prevention, home care, and follow-up.

Implementation

1. Surgical amputation:
   A. Assess, report, and record signs and symptoms and reaction to treatment.
   B. Prepare client and family for surgical intervention.

C. Encourage verbalization of feelings.
D. Provide emotional support.
E. Explain possibility of phantom pain (pain in amputated limb).
F. Explain postoperative plan.
    (1) Program of exercises
        (a) Exercises for strengthening upper extremities
        (b) Transferring from bed to chair and vice versa
        (c) Ambulating with walker or crutches
G. Provide postoperative care.
    (1) Provide routine postoperative care.
    (2) Provide reassurance to help client cope with altered body image.
    (3) Apply Ace bandages in a figure-eight pattern only.
    (4) Monitor for signs of bleeding—have a tourniquet at bedside for emergency use.
    (5) Elevate stump 8–12 hours on a pillow.
    (6) Remove pillow after 12 hours to prevent hip contracture.
    (7) Position client in prone position every 4 hours to prevent hip contracture.
    (8) Place trochanter roll along outer side of stump to prevent outward rotation.
    (9) Instruct the client to massage the stump to improve vascularity.
    (10) Instruct client on conditioning of the stump for a prosthesis.
        (a) Push stump against a pillow.
        (b) Progress by pushing stump against a harder surface.
    (11) Instruct client to avoid letting stump hang over edge of bed, chair to avoid stump contracture.
    (12) Use transcutaneous electrical nerve stimulator for relief of phantom pain, if ordered.
H. Instruct client regarding condition, diagnostic procedures, treatment, prevention, home care, and follow-up.
2. Traumatic amputation
    A. Emergency treatment
        (1) Assess, record, and report signs and symptoms and reactions to treatment.
        (2) Monitor vital signs.
        (3) Cleanse wound.
        (4) Administer prescribed tetanus prophylaxis, antibiotics, analgesics.
        (5) Perform the following nursing interventions after complete amputation:
            (a) Preserve extremity in cooled sterile normal saline solution within a sterile plastic bag.
            (b) Notify reimplantation surgeon.
        (6) Perform the following nursing interventions for partial amputation:
            (a) Position limb in normal alignment.
            (b) Drape with sterile towels soaked in sterile normal saline solution.
    B. Preoperative care: Assist with thorough wound irrigation and debridement.
    C. Postoperative care
        (1) Perform dressing changes using sterile technique.
        (2) Provide reassurance to help cope with altered body image.
        (3) Assist with rehabilitation—same as for postoperative care of surgical amputation.
    D. Instruct client regarding condition, diagnostic procedures, treatment, prevention, home care, and follow-up.

Evaluation

1. Reports increased comfort, decreased anxiety
2. Shows no signs of avoidable injury and/or infection
3. Maintains adequate level of mobility
4. Maintains skin integrity
5. Discusses feelings, self-image, and self-concept
6. Copes effectively with altered body image
7. Participates in appropriate level of self-care needs
8. Demonstrates understanding of condition, diagnostic procedures, treatment, prevention, home care, and need for follow-up

Neurological System

Basic Information

The neurological system consists of the communication network responsible for coordinating and organizing the functions of all body systems. There are three main divisions: the CNS, which is the control center of the body (brain and spinal cord); the peripheral nervous system, which includes nerves communicating with distant body parts, relaying and receiving messages from them; and the autonomic nervous system, which regulates involuntary functions of the internal organs.

The pathology involving the CNS arises from injuries, vascular insufficiency, tumors, infections, and disorders from other diseases. Neurological medical problems are due to interference with normal functioning of the affected cells.

Assessment

SUBJECTIVE

History of:
1. Head injury
2. Vertigo
3. Weakness
4. Headache
5. Loss of consciousness
6. Paralysis
7. Seizures
8. Double vision
9. Pain, numbness
10. Difficulty concentrating
11. Memory loss
12. Drowsiness
13. Difficulty with elimination

OBJECTIVE

1. Orientation to person, time, and place
2. Mental status—drowsiness, lethargy
3. Level of consciousness—arousal status to verbal and physical stimuli
    A. Use of Glasgow Coma Scale to describe level of consciousness
        (1) Eye and pupil responses

      (2) Verbal response
      (3) Motor response
4. Emotional response
5. Speech—presence of aphasia, appropriate speech patterns
6. Behavior—appropriate for situation
7. Ability to follow simple instructions
8. Vital signs—temperature, pulse, respirations, and blood pressure
9. Motor function—gait, balance, coordination, strength, posture, and function
10. Eyes
    A. Movement of lids and pupils
    B. Size, configuration, and reaction of pupils to light
    C. Comparison with baseline assessment
11. Ears—drainage
12. Facial symmetry
13. Sensation for pain, smell, and light
14. Bladder and bowel control
15. Other cranial nerve functions

DIAGNOSTIC TESTS AND METHODS

1. Skull and spinal x-ray studies
2. CT scan
3. Cerebral angiography
4. Brain scan
5. MRI
6. Electroencephalography (EEG)
7. Echoencephalography
8. Cerebrovascular flow tests
9. Carotid phonangiography
10. Ultrasound arteriography
11. Myelography
12. Electromyography
13. Nerve conduction velocities
14. Lumbar puncture

Comatose Client and Unconscious Client

Description

1. Comatose and unconscious clients are unresponsive to sensory stimuli and without wakefulness due to brain dysfunction.
2. Level of consciousness is the single most valuable indicator of neurological function.
3. It can vary from alertness (response to verbal stimulus) to coma (failure to respond even to painful stimuli).
4. The Glasgow Coma Scale is used to assess eye opening as well as verbal and motor responses, and provides a quick standardized account of neurological status.
5. Cause is unknown.
6. Possible causes
    A. Head trauma
    B. Cerebral hemorrhage
    C. Infection—meningitis
    D. Neoplasms
    E. Metabolic disorders—hypoglycemia, myxedema, uremia
    F. Toxicity—drugs, carbon monoxide
    G. Hypoxic conditions—COPD, severe anemia, CHF
    H. Seizures
    I. Deficiency conditions—Wernicke's encephalopathy

Assessment

OBJECTIVE

1. Lack of response to painful stimuli, depending on degree of coma
2. Unarousable even with painful stimuli
3. Evidence of head trauma
4. Presence of any of the above possible causes
5. Quality of respirations
6. Cranial nerve and reflex activity
7. Glasgow Coma Scale score

DIAGNOSTIC TESTS AND METHODS

1. History of potential cause—accident, drugs
2. Physical examination
3. Neurological examination
4. Skull x-ray
5. CT scan
6. Brain scan
7. MRI
8. EEG

Planning

1. Safe, effective care environment
    A. Prevent avoidable injury and/or infection.
    B. Increase family's knowledge of disease process, diagnostic procedures, and treatment.
2. Physiological integrity
    A. Maintain skin integrity.
    B. Maintain effective breathing pattern, airway clearance, and gas exchange.
    C. Maintain adequate cardiac output.
    D. Maintain adequate fluid and electrolyte balance.
    E. Maintain adequate elimination pattern.
    F. Provide hygienic needs.
    G. Prevent complications of immobility and contractures.
3. Psychosocial integrity
    A. Reduce anxiety among family.
    B. Promote effective coping among family.
4. Health promotion and maintenance
    A. Increase family's knowledge of prevention, home care (including medication), and follow-up.

Implementation

1. Assess, record, and report signs and symptoms and reactions to treatment.
2. Maintain open airway with artificial airway, endotracheal tube, or tracheostomy.
3. Suction as necessary.
4. Monitor neurological responses frequently.
5. Monitor vital signs frequently.
6. Elevate head of bed.
7. Monitor intake and output.
8. Monitor laboratory data and diagnostic tests.
9. Monitor skin integrity and temperature.
10. Administer prescribed medications, IV fluids, and TPN.
11. Provide hygienic needs frequently, including oral care, skin care, and hair care.
12. Turn every 2 hours.
13. Give urinary catheter care as prescribed.

14. Monitor nutritional intake and response to TPN or NG feedings.
15. Monitor elimination pattern.
16. Provide passive ROM exercises.
17. Provide support and promote effective coping among family.
18. Use footboard, high-top sneakers to prevent footdrop; splints to prevent wrist contractures.
19. Instruct family regarding disease process, diagnostic procedures, treatment, prevention, home care, and follow-up.

Evaluation

1. Maintains effective airway clearance, breathing pattern, and gas exchange
2. Maintains skin integrity
3. Shows no signs of avoidable injury and/or infection
4. Maintains adequate cardiac output
5. Maintains adequate fluid and electrolyte balance
6. Maintains adequate nutritional status
7. Maintains good oral hygiene
8. Has no deformities or contractures
9. Family demonstrates satisfactory coping
10. Family demonstrates understanding of disease process, diagnostic procedures, treatment, prevention, home care, and need for follow-up

Head Injury

Description

1. Head injuries are a leading cause of disability.
2. They can occur at any age.
3. Signs and symptoms may not appear for several days or weeks, especially in the older individual.
4. Three major classifications.
   A. Closed injury
      (1) Nonpenetrating injuries with no break in the integrity of the skull.
      (2) Basal dura may be torn.
   B. Open or penetrating injury
      (1) Break in the integrity of the skull, meninges between the environment and the intracranial vault.
      (2) High-velocity and low-velocity missiles (knife, bullet) can cause open injury.
      (3) Extent of injury varies from focal to diffuse.
5. Specific classification system is commonly used to further classify head injury into mild, moderate to severe, and severe head injury for the purpose of:
   A. Assistance in proper triage
   B. treatment of client
6. Mild head injury.
   A. Momentary loss of consciousness.
   B. No decrease in level of consciousness.
   C. Absence of focal neurological signs on admission to emergency room.
   D. Client generally not admitted to hospital unless headache, nausea, vomiting, fever, or cerebrospinal fluid (CSF) leakage is present.
   E. Family and client are instructed to watch for these signs and symptoms that indicate the need for immediate admission to the hospital.

7. Moderate to severe head injury.
   A. Momentary loss of consciousness.
   B. Alteration of neurological function on admission to the hospital.
   C. This may include altered level of consciousness, lethargy, confusion, or hemiparesis.
   D. Client is admitted to the ICU.
   E. Injury may require emergency surgery.
8. Severe head injury.
   A. Diagnosis follows inability of client to follow simple commands due to decreased level of consciousness.
   B. Client may exhibit signs of severe neurological damage.
      (1) Posturing
      (2) Dilated pupils
   C. Need for rapid assessment and intervention to prevent death.
9. Skull fracture.
   A. May be concomitant with head injury
   B. Types
      (1) Linear fracture (most common type)—no displacement of bone
      (2) Depressed fracture
         (a) Outer table of skull is depressed.
         (b) It may move beneath the inner table of the adjacent skull.
         (c) This type of fracture can occur with either a closed or an open head injury.
      (3) Basal fracture
         (a) This type of fracture occurs at base of skull.
         (b) It extends into ear or orbit of eye.
10. Primary brain injury.
    A. Primary injury to the brain may be due to:
       (1) Concussion
       (2) Contusion
11. Secondary brain injury.
    A. Epidural hematoma
       (1) Occurs between dura and skull.
       (2) It is associated with severe head injury.
       (3) It is potentially fatal owing to rapid onset of symptoms as a result of arterial bleeding.
       (4) Symptoms include:
          (a) Momentary unconsciousness followed by a lucid period of a few hours to a few days.
          (b) A rapid deterioration in level of consciousness.
          (c) Vomiting, hemiparesis, pupillary changes.
          (d) Medical treatment calls for rapid evacuation of the hematoma.
    B. Subdural hematoma
       (1) Occurs under the dura.
       (2) It usually involves lacerations of the veins crossing subdural space.
       (3) Subtypes
          (a) Acute subdural hematoma
             • Symptoms appear within 24–72 hours.
             • Condition deteriorates rapidly.
             • Client becomes comatose.
             • Symptoms of headache, drowsiness, agitation, coma.
          (b) Subacute subdural hematoma
             • Symptoms develop from 72 hours to 2 weeks.
             • Prognosis is better than that for acute type, but with 25%–35% mortality.

- Major symptom is failure to regain consciousness after an injury.
  - (c) Chronic subdural hematoma
    - Gradual clot formation that allows brain to accommodate.
    - Time from injury to development of symptoms may be months.
    - Symptoms may go unnoticed.
    - Common symptoms include headache, grogginess, confusion, and seizures.
- C. Intracerebral hematoma
  - (1) Associated with cerebral lacerations causing edema of surrounding tissues.
  - (2) Most are related to contusions and usually occur in frontal and temporal lobes.
  - (3) Signs and symptoms include headache, decreasing level of consciousness, hemiplegia on opposite side of injury, and dilated pupil on the same side of injury.
  - (4) Surgical excision is treatment of choice.
- D. Potential complications
  - (1) Cerebral edema
  - (2) Syndrome of inappropriate antidiuretic hormone and diabetes insipidus
  - (3) Stress ulcers
  - (4) Convulsive disorders
  - (5) Carotid-cavernous fistula
  - (6) Meningitis
  - (7) Hyperthermia-hypothermia

Assessment

1. Specific clinical manifestations depend on type and location of injury.
2. Major symptoms are specific to the neurological system and include:
   - A. Decreased level of consciousness
   - B. Irritability
   - C. Confusion
   - D. Restlessness
3. Other symptoms include:
   - A. Pupillary abnormalities
   - B. Nausea
   - C. Vomiting
   - D. Vital sign changes
   - E. Evidence of brain-stem injury in severe cases, such as loss of gag reflex or swallowing reflexes
   - F. Evidence of motor and sensory dysfunction

DIAGNOSTIC TESTS AND METHODS

NOTE: Lumbar puncture is generally contraindicated due to possibility of precipitating a brain-stem herniation, but it may be done when meningitis is suspected.

1. Skull x-ray
2. Cervical spine films
3. A CT scan
4. Cerebral angiography on occasion
5. Echoencephalogram on occasion
6. Laboratory tests
   - A. Serum glucose
   - B. Electrolytes
   - C. BUN
   - D. CBC
   - E. Coagulation studies
   - F. Alcohol and drug screening
   - G. ABGs
   - H. Urinalysis

Planning

1. Safe, effective care environment
   - A. Prevent avoidable injury and/or infection.
   - B. Increase client's and family's knowledge of condition, diagnostic procedures, and treatment.
2. Physiological integrity
   - A. Maintain skin integrity.
   - B. Maintain effective breathing pattern, airway clearance, and gas exchange.
   - C. Maintain adequate cardiac output.
   - D. Maintain adequate cerebral perfusion.
   - E. Maintain adequate fluid and electrolyte balance.
   - F. Maintain adequate elimination pattern.
   - G. Provide hygienic needs.
   - H. Prevent complications of immobility and contractures.
3. Psychosocial integrity
   - A. Reduce anxiety among family.
   - B. Promote effective coping among family.
4. Health promotion and maintenance
   - A. Increase client's and family's knowledge of prevention, home care (including medication), and follow-up.

Implementation

1. Assess, record, and report signs and symptoms and reactions to treatment.
2. Maintain patency of airway.
3. Maintain stabilization of cervical injury.
4. Establish baseline assessment for:
   - A. Level of consciousness
   - B. Pupillary response
   - C. Motor responses
   - D. Sensory responses
   - E. Breathing pattern
   - F. Vital signs
   - G. Symptoms of ICP
5. Use Glasgow Scale to assess neurological status; monitor for and report any changes immediately.
6. Monitor for signs of headache.
7. Monitor for other body injuries.
   - A. Likely to have sustained fractures in other areas of body
   - B. Administer tetanus shot within suggested time frames
8. Monitor intake and output.
9. Check urinary catheter for patency.
10. Administer acetaminophen or codeine judiciously if ordered for pain. (Remember that use of opiates and sedatives may interfere with accurate neurological assessment because they depress activities of the nervous system.)
11. Monitor respiratory and cardiovascular status.
12. Position client properly—immobility is a major cause of respiratory infection.

13. Monitor and report any signs and symptoms of infections.
    A. Three major sites
       (1) Any compound fracture site
       (2) Pulmonary system
       (3) Any invasive instrumentation—arterial lines or intracranial monitoring
14. Monitor for leakage fluid from ear or nose.
    A. Obtain specimen for CSF analysis.
    B. Keep dressing clean and dry.
    C. Keep patient in position for free drainage of fluid.
    D. Caution patient to avoid any excessive movement (stress to dura).
    E. Refrain from cleaning the ear or cleaning and suctioning the nose—increases the likelihood of leakage of CSF.
15. Monitor ability to communicate.
16. Administer meticulous hygienic care—oral, skin, hair.
17. Allow family to participate in care.
18. Allow client to participate in self-care to extent possible.
19. Monitor alterations in cerebral tissue perfusion.
20. Monitor laboratory data and other diagnostic test results.
21. Give emotional support to client, family, and significant others.
22. Instruct client and family regarding condition, diagnostic procedures, treatment, prevention, home care, and follow-up.

Evaluation

1. Demonstrates stabilized or improved sensory and motor function
2. Has normal pupillary size and reactivity
3. Maintains normal level of consciousness
4. Has stable vital signs
5. Maintains fluid and electrolyte balance
6. Maintains adequate airway and breathing patterns
7. Shows no signs of avoidable injury and/or infection
8. Has no complications
9. Demonstrates understanding of condition, diagnostic procedures, prevention (including medication), treatment, home care, and need for follow-up; similar understanding demonstrated by family

Cerebrovascular Accident (Stroke)

Description

1. Cerebrovascular accident produces sudden impairment of the circulation in one or more of the blood vessels supplying the brain; blood vessels are occluded, stenosed, or ruptured.
2. O_2 supply to the affected brain tissue interrupted or diminished, often causing severe damage to or necrosis of the involved tissue.
3. Sudden or gradual onset.
4. Symptoms related to location and size of brain area affected.
5. Approximately 50% of survivors are permanently disabled.
6. High proportion experience recurrence within weeks to years.
7. Chance for complete recovery depends on the circulation returning to normal soon after the initial episode.
8. Third most common cause of death in the United States and most common cause of neurological disability.

9. Classification of CVA (least severe to complete stroke)
   A. Transient ischemic attack (TIA)
      (1) "Little stroke": It is due to temporary interruption of blood flow.
      (2) It occurs most often in carotid and vertebrobasilar arteries.
   B. Progressive stroke
      (1) Thrombus in evolution begins with slight neurological deficit.
      (2) Condition exacerbates within 1–2 days.
      (3) Complete stroke: Maximum neurological deficits occur immediately at onset.
10. Causes
    A. Thrombosis
       (1) Obstruction of blood vessels by blood clot formed within vessel.
       (2) Most common cause of CVA in middle-aged and elderly individuals.
       (3) Clot tends to develop while individual is awake or shortly after awakening.
       (4) Individuals at risk include clients with a history of atherosclerosis, diabetes, or hypertension.
       (5) Risk increases with smoking or obesity or both.
    B. Embolus
       (1) Occlusion of blood vessel in brain by a fragmented clot, tumor, fat, air, or bacteria.
       (2) It can occur at any age and is the second most common cause of CVA.
       (3) Individuals at risk include clients with a history of rheumatic heart disease, myocardial fibrillation or other arrhythmias, or endocarditis; or clients who have just undergone open heart surgery, orthopedic surgery, childbirth, infection.
       (4) Embolus usually develops rapidly (10–20 seconds) and without warning.
       (5) It most often affects the middle cerebral artery.
       (6) If embolus is septic, infection may extend beyond blood vessel wall, with development of abscess or encephalitis.
          (a) Infection within blood vessel wall may develop into an aneurysm with potential cerebral hemorrhage.
    C. Hemorrhage
       (1) Sudden rupture of a cerebral blood vessel.
       (2) It can occur at any age and is the third most common cause of CVA.
       (3) Individuals at risk include patients with chronic hypertension or aneurysms, which rupture the cerebral artery.
       (4) Blood supply to the affected brain tissue decreases with accumulation of blood deep within brain substance, with subsequent compression of nerve tissue and further damage.
11. Predisposing factors
    A. History of TIAs
    B. Hypertension
    C. Arrhythmias
    D. Atherosclerosis
    E. Rheumatic heart disease
    F. Myocardial enlargement
    G. Diabetes mellitus
    H. High serum triglyceride levels
    I. Lack of exercise

J. Cigarette smoking
K. Family history

Assessment

1. Specific assessment depends on artery affected, area of brain involved, severity of damage, and extent of collateral circulation that develops to compensate the brain for diminished blood supply.
2. Left hemisphere involvement results in symptoms on right side of body; right hemispheric involvement, in symptoms on left side of body.
3. CVA causes cranial nerve damage, which produces neural dysfunction on same side of the body.

SUBJECTIVE

1. Changes in sensation and strength
2. Headache
3. Dizziness
4. Difficulty in speaking
5. Visual disturbances

OBJECTIVE

1. Middle cerebral artery
   A. Aphasia, hemiparesis, visual field cuts
   B. Hemiparesis more severe in face and arm than in leg
2. Anterior cerebral artery
   A. Numbness, confusion, weakness—especially in lower limbs
   B. Incontinence
   C. Personality changes
   D. Loss of coordination
   E. Impaired motor and sensory function
3. Posterior cerebral artery
   A. Visual field cuts
   B. Dyslexia
   C. Cortical blindness
   D. Sensory impairment
   E. Usually no paralysis
4. Carotid artery
   A. Weakness, paralysis
   B. Sensory changes
   C. Altered level of consciousness
   D. Headache
   E. Aphasia
   F. Ptosis
   G. Visual disturbances on affected side
5. Vertebrobasilar artery
   A. Numbness around lips
   B. Weakness on affected side
   C. Double vision
   D. Slurred speech
   E. Dysphagia
   F. Poor coordination
   G. Vertigo
   H. Amnesia
   I. Ataxia

DIAGNOSTIC TESTS AND METHODS

1. History
2. Physical examination
3. Neurological assessment
4. MRI or PET (Positron emission tomography) scan
5. CT scan
6. Lumbar puncture
7. EEG
8. Cerebral angiography
9. Ophthalmoscopy
10. Ultrasound Doppler studies-to evaluate blood flow through the carotid arteries
11. Baseline laboratory studies
    A. Coagulation studies
    B. Urinalysis
    C. Serum osmolality
    D. CBC
    E. Triglycerides
    F. Serum electrolytes
    G. Creatinine and BUN levels

Planning

1. Safe, effective care environment
   A. Prevent avoidable injury and/or infection.
   B. Increase client's and family's knowledge of disease process, diagnostic procedures, and treatment.
2. Physiological integrity
   A. Maintain skin integrity.
   B. Maintain effective breathing pattern, airway clearance, and gas exchange.
   C. Maintain adequate fluid and electrolyte balance.
   D. Maintain adequate nutrition needs.
   E. Maintain adequate elimination pattern.
   F. Provide hygienic needs.
   G. Prevent complications of immobility and contractures.
   H. Increase comfort.
3. Psychosocial integrity
   A. Reduce anxiety.
   B. Promote effective family coping.
   C. Counsel on self-concept alterations.
4. Health promotion and maintenance
   A. Increase client's and family's knowledge of prevention, home care (including medication), and follow-up.
   B. Counsel on sexual dysfunction or alterations.

Implementation

1. Assess, record, and report signs and symptoms and reactions to treatment.
2. Maintain bed rest, provide complete care.
3. Maintain patent airway and O_2 therapy.
4. Assess quality and type of respirations (Cheyne-Stokes).
5. Keep unconscious client in a lateral position to allow secretions to drain by gravity or use suction as necessary to prevent aspiration of saliva.
6. Monitor vital signs and neurological status.
7. Monitor blood pressure, voluntary and involuntary movements, changes in pupils, level of consciousness, speech, skin color, sensory function, and neck rigidity or flaccidity.
8. Monitor for signs of pulmonary emboli such as chest pain, shortness of breath, increased temperature, and tachycardia; and check ABGs for signs of increased PCO_2 or decreased PO_2.
9. Monitor for signs of increased ICP.
10. Keep precautionary respiratory equipment at bedside.
11. Provide safe environment—elevate side rails.

12. Administer prescribed medications such as antihypertensives, diuretics, and anticoagulants; monitor for side effects.
13. Maintain fluid and electrolyte balance.
    A. Encourage oral fluid intake as ordered.
    B. Assist in IV administration as ordered.
14. Monitor ability to swallow—check gag reflex.
15. Place bedside stand in client's visual field so that client can see what is on stand.
16. Provide meticulous mouth care—clean and care for dentures.
17. Provide meticulous eye care—patch affected eye if client cannot close lid.
18. Ensure adequate nutrition—make sure gag reflex has returned.
    A. Place food in client's visual field so that client can see what is on tray.
    B. Assist in insertion of NG feeding tube if client is unable to ingest food by mouth.
19. Position client, align extremities correctly; use sheet to turn client every 2 hours.
20. Use padded footboard to prevent footdrop and contracture.
21. Assist client with ROM exercises on both affected and unaffected sides.
22. Instruct client how to use unaffected side to exercise affected side.
23. Provide egg-crate, pulsating, or flotation mattress to prevent decubiti.
24. Facilitate communication with client.
    A. Allow client sufficient time to communicate.
    B. Anticipate needs; speak slowly and clearly.
    C. Set up other means of communication, such as drawing, writing, use of pictures, gestures, if client is aphasic.
    D. Assure client that intellect has not been impaired; include family members in communications.
    E. Encourage speech therapy.
25. Involve family members in client care when possible.
26. Monitor elimination pattern.
    A. Offer bedpan frequently for urinary or fecal incontinence.
    B. Assist client as necessary; provide privacy by not exposing client.
    C. Be alert for signs of straining at stool (which increases intracranial pressure).
    D. Check with dietitian to modify diet and to administer stool softener and/or prescribed laxatives.
    E. Encourage adequate fluid intake.
    F. Provide roughage in diet.
27. Begin rehabilitation of client on admission.
    A. Amount of teaching varies depending on neurological deficit present.
    B. Teach client to bathe, comb hair, and dress, if necessary.
    C. Encourage client to begin speech therapy as soon as possible, if needed.
    D. Involve family in all aspects of rehabilitation.
    E. Coordinate care with physical therapy department; encourage client to use walking frames, hand-bars on toilet, and ramps.
28. Instruct client and family regarding disease process, diagnostic procedures, treatment, prevention, home care, and follow-up. Include teaching on:

A. Need to control diseases such as hypertension or diabetes mellitus
B. Importance of eating a low-salt, low-cholesterol diet
C. Need to control weight
D. Need to increase exercise
E. Avoidance of smoking and prolonged bed rest
F. Signs of CVA
G. Need to watch for possible GI bleeding if aspirin is prescribed to reduce risk of embolic stroke

Evaluation

1. Reports increased comfort, decreased anxiety
2. Shows no signs of avoidable injury and/or infection
3. Uses effective communication
4. Maintains effective airway clearance and breathing patterns
5. Maintains effective elimination (bowel and bladder)
6. Maintains skin integrity
7. Maintains adequate cerebral tissue perfusion
8. Demonstrates understanding of disease process, diagnostic procedures, treatment, prevention, home care, and need for follow-up; similar understanding demonstrated by family

Increased Intracranial Pressure
Description

1. Increased intracranial pressure (ICP) is produced by fluid accumulation or a lesion taking space in the cranial cavity.
2. Results in gradual compression of the brain with potential cessation of life-sustaining functions.
3. May progress slowly or occur suddenly.
4. Causes
   A. Edema from trauma and abscesses
   B. Tumors
   C. Hematoma

Assessment

SUBJECTIVE

1. Related to primary disorder
2. Headache, anxiety
3. Blurred or double vision
4. Lethargy
5. Weakness

OBJECTIVE

1. Vomiting—projectile, recurrent, unrelated to nausea
2. Irregular, Cheyne-Stokes, or Kussmaul's breathing
3. Seizures
4. Altered level of consciousness—confusion, slurred speech, decreased level of response
5. Change in pupil response to light
6. Elevation of blood pressure; wide pulse pressure
7. Initial increase in pulse followed by decrease to 40–60 bpm
8. Progressive signs of paralysis
9. Loss of consciousness, coma, and death

DIAGNOSTIC TESTS AND METHODS

1. History
2. Physical examination
3. Neurological assessment

4. Increased ICP monitoring
5. CT scan or MRI
6. Serum osmolality
7. ABGs

Planning

1. Safe, effective care environment
   A. Prevent avoidable injury and/or infection.
   B. Increase client's and family's knowledge of disease process, diagnostic procedures, and treatment.
2. Physiological integrity
   A. Maintain effective breathing pattern, airway clearance, and gas exchange.
   B. Maintain adequate cerebral tissue perfusion.
   C. Maintain stabilization of cervical injuries.
   D. Maintain adequate cardiac output.
   E. Maintain adequate fluid and electrolyte balance.
   F. Maintain adequate elimination pattern.
   G. Maintain skin integrity.
   H. Provide hygienic needs.
   I. Prevent complications of immobility and contractures.
3. Psychosocial integrity
   A. Reduce anxiety among family.
   B. Promote effective coping among family.
4. Health promotion and maintenance
   A. Increase client's and family's knowledge of prevention, home care (including medication), and follow-up.

Implementation

1. Assess, record, and report signs and symptoms and reactions to treatment.
2. Elevate head to semi-Fowler position—do *not* place client in Trendelenburg position.
3. Maintain patent airway—provide O_2 therapy.
4. Prevent aspiration—position client on side.
5. Monitor vital signs every 15 minutes.
6. Monitor neurological responses frequently.
7. Monitor laboratory data.
8. Monitor intake and output.
9. Turn client every 2 hours.
10. Provide hygienic needs frequently, including mouth, skin, and hair care.
11. Provide passive ROM exercises.
12. Use footboard or high-top sneakers for prevention of footdrop and contractures.
13. Monitor pupillary response—usually unequal and may not react to light.
14. Provide a safe environment—elevate side rails.
15. Report any change in level of consciousness immediately.
16. Assist in administration of prescribed medications or devices.
17. Provide usual care and observation for unconscious client or one with seizures.
18. Instruct client and family regarding disease process, diagnostic procedures, treatment, home care, and follow-up.

Evaluation

1. Reports increased comfort, decreased anxiety
2. Shows no signs of avoidable injury and/or infection
3. Maintains adequate cerebral tissue perfusion
4. Maintains adequate airway clearance, breathing patterns, and gas exchange
5. Maintains adequate cardiac output
6. Maintains adequate fluid and electrolyte balance
7. Maintains adequate nutritional status
8. Maintains adequate elimination pattern
9. Has no deformities or contractures
10. Demonstrates understanding of disease process, diagnostic procedures, prevention, treatment, home care, and need for follow-up; similar understanding demonstrated by family

Intracranial Tumors

Description

1. Intracranial tumors are malignant or benign lesions within the brain that may displace or destroy adjacent structures or increase ICP.
2. It may be a primary lesion within brain tissue or a secondary lesion originating elsewhere in the body.
3. Increased ICP is possible owing to displacement of space by tumor, cerebral edema, and vasodilation resulting from impairment of the cerebral blood flow.
4. Tumors are more common in males than females.
5. They may occur at any age; in adults, incidence usually highest between ages of 40 and 60.
6. Classification according to tissue origin
   A. Gliomas—arise in cerebral connective tissue; unencapsulated
      (1) Tumors characterized by rapid growth with infiltration of the brain tissue.
      (2) They are not well defined for surgical removal.
      (3) They occur most often in cerebral hemispheres, especially frontal and temporal lobes.
      (4) Prognosis—mean survival rate 6 months; maximum 1–10 years (depending on stage of tumor)
   B. Meningiomas—originate within meningeal layers
      (1) These tumors constitute 15% of primary brain tumors.
      (2) Peak incidence among 50-year-olds; rare in children; more common in females than males.
      (3) They occur most often in sphenoidal ridge, anterior part of the base of the skull, and spinal canal.
      (4) Tumors are benign, well circumscribed, and highly vascular.
      (5) They compress adjacent underlying brain tissue by invading overlying skull.
      (6) Prognosis—median survival rate ≤ 1–2 years. If treated early, neurological deficits potentially completely reversible.
   C. Neuromas—originate on cranial nerves
      (1) Benign but often classified as malignant due to growth pattern—slow-growing, present for years before symptoms occur.
      (2) These tumors account for approximately 10% of all intracranial tumors.
      (3) Incidence is higher in women.
      (4) Onset of symptoms occurs at approximately 20–60 years of age.
      (5) Tumors affect craniospinal nerve sheath; usually

eighth cranial nerve; also affect fifth and seventh cranial nerves although to a lesser extent.
  (6) Prognosis—if adequately treated, potential for permanent cure.
D. Pituitary tumors—originate most often in anterior pituitary gland
  (1) These tumors account for 10% of intracranial tumors.
  (2) They occur in adults of both sexes, between ages 20 and 50.
  (3) Three types—chromophobe adenoma, basophilic adenoma, and eosinophilic adenoma.
  (4) Tumors are amenable to surgical treatment.
  (5) Prognosis—fair to good, depending on extent of tumor spread beyond sella turcica.
E. Metastatic tumors—originate elsewhere in body, often from lungs
  (1) Prognosis is poor.
7. Gliomas and meningiomas are most common types among adults.
8. Brain tumors are one of the most common causes of death from cancer in children.
  A. Incidence is usually highest in infants under 1 year old and then in children between 1 and 12 years of age.
  B. Astrocytoma (type of glioma), medulloblastomas (rare type of glioma), and brain-stem gliomas are the most common types.
    (1) Cause—unknown

Assessment

SUBJECTIVE

1. Alterations in judgment or personality
2. Visual disturbances
3. Headache
4. Numbness, tingling sensations
5. Difficulty and loss of hearing
6. Family or personal history

OBJECTIVE

1. Vomiting
2. Orientation to person, place, and time
3. Movement and strength of extremities
4. Reaction of pupils to light
5. Changes in vital signs
6. Presence of papilledema
7. Presence of seizures
8. Abnormal cranial nerve reflexes
9. Changes in level of consciousness
10. Signs of increased ICP
11. Presence of protein and decreased glucose and occasional tumor cells in spinal fluid
12. Signs associated with tumor location
    A. Frontal lobe—personality changes, hemiparesis, visual problems
    B. Temporal lobe—visual hallucinations, seizures, changes in sense of taste, odor
    C. Parietal lobe—visual disturbances, jacksonian seizures–related tumor involving precentral gyrus, inability to differentiate between left and right
    D. Occipital lobe—visual problems, convulsions

DIAGNOSTIC TESTS AND METHODS

1. History
2. Physical examination
3. Neurological assessment
4. CT scan or MRI
5. Skull radiograph
6. Brain scan
7. EEG
8. Biopsy of lesion
9. Cerebral angiography
10. Lumbar puncture
11. Pneumoencephalogram and ventriculogram

Planning

1. Safe, effective care environment
   A. Prevent avoidable injury and/or infection.
   B. Increase client's and family's knowledge of disease process, diagnostic procedures, and treatment.
2. Physiological integrity
   A. Maintain skin integrity.
   B. Maintain effective breathing pattern, airway clearance, and gas exchange.
   C. Maintain adequate fluid and electrolyte balance.
   D. Increase comfort.
   E. Maintain adequate elimination pattern.
   F. Provide hygienic needs.
   G. Prevent complications of immobility and contractures.
   H. Assist with mobility.
3. Psychosocial integrity
   A. Reduce anxiety and fear.
   B. Promote effective coping.
   C. Assist with alterations in self-concept.
4. Health promotion and maintenance
   A. Increase client's and family's knowledge of prevention, home care (including medication), and follow-up.

Implementation

1. Assess, record, and report signs and symptoms and reactions to treatment.
2. Monitor and record baseline information regarding neurological status.
3. Check continually for changes in neurological status.
   A. Watch for and immediately report sudden unilateral dilation of pupil with loss of light reflex—indicates transtentorial herniation.
4. Monitor for signs of increased ICP.
   A. Rising systolic pressure
   B. Widening pulse pressure
   C. Decrease in pulse rate
   D. Changes in level of consciousness
   E. Abnormal respiratory patterns
   F. Elevation of temperature
5. Assist with mobility and exercise.
6. Monitor respiratory changes—anoxia, abnormal respiratory rate and depth—which may indicate rising ICP or herniation of cerebellar tissue from expanding mass.
7. Monitor temperature—increased temperature often follows hypothalamic anoxia and might be indicative of meningitis.
   A. Use hypothermia blankets, if prescribed, to decrease

temperature and decrease metabolic demands of brain tissue.

8. Assist client and family to cope with diagnosis, treatment, potential disabilities, and changes in lifestyle.
9. Document seizure activity.
10. Maintain patent airway.
11. Provide a safe and hazard-free environment—elevate side rails.
12. Administer anticonvulsants, diuretics, and steroids as prescribed.
13. Administer and monitor IV therapy.
14. Monitor fluid intake and output and electrolyte balance; restrict fluids as ordered—rapid diuresis may cause heart failure.
15. Prepare client and family for client's surgical intervention.
16. Monitor for side effects of radiation therapy, if ordered—check for wound breakdown, infection, signs of rising ICP.
17. Monitor for side effects of prescribed medication adjuncts to radiotherapy and surgery.
    A. Causes delayed bone marrow depression—watch for signs of infection or bleeding.
18. Begin rehabilitation early; encourage independence in ADL.
19. Provide aids for self-care, if necessary.
20. Arrange for consultation with speech therapist if client is aphasic.
21. Instruct client and family regarding disease process, diagnostic procedures, treatment, home care, and follow-up. Include teaching on:
    A. Importance of complying with drug therapy
    B. Early signs of recurrence

Evaluation

1. Reports increased comfort, decreased anxiety
2. Shows no signs of avoidable injury and/or infection
3. Maintains adequate cerebral tissue perfusion
4. Maintains adequate airway clearance and breathing patterns
5. Participates in rehabilitation therapy—exercise, ambulation, ADL
6. Demonstrates understanding of disease process, diagnostic procedures, treatment (including medication), prevention, home care, and need for follow-up; similar understanding demonstrated by family

Parkinson's Disease

Description

1. Parkinson's disease is characterized by progressive muscle rigidity, akinesia, and involuntary tremor.
2. Condition is due to damage to neurons in the substantia nigra, located within the basal ganglia.
3. Cause is unknown.
4. Predisposing factors
   A. Deficiency in dopamine, which interferes with inhibition of excitatory impulses
   B. May be related to certain viruses, drugs, and arteriosclerosis
5. Progression of deterioration for an average of 10 years.
6. Death usually due to aspiration pneumonia or other infection.
7. More common in males than in females.

Assessment

SUBJECTIVE

1. Drooling
2. Fatigue
3. Intolerance to heat
4. Muscular pain
5. Problems with coordination
6. Changes in emotion and judgment

OBJECTIVE

1. Muscle rigidity—resistance to passive muscle stretching (jerky)
2. Akinesia (loss of movement) causing shuffling gait, loss of posture control, altered reflexes, masklike facial expression, high-pitched monotone voice, and dysphagia
3. Difficulty performing ADL
4. Tremor of fingers (unilateral "pill-roll" tremor) increasing with stress

DIAGNOSTIC TESTS AND METHODS

1. History
2. Physical examination
3. Neurological assessment
4. Urinalysis—dopamine levels
5. EEG
6. Video fluoroscopy (Client swallows barium. Slowed response of the cricopharnygeal muscles when swallowing is noted in Parkinson's disease.)

Planning

1. Safe, effective care environment
   A. Prevent avoidable injury and/or infection.
   B. Increase client's and family's knowledge of disease process, diagnostic procedures, and treatment.
2. Physiological integrity
   A. Maintain skin integrity.
   B. Maintain effective breathing pattern and airway clearance.
   C. Maintain adequate fluid and electrolyte balance.
   D. Maintain adequate elimination pattern.
   E. Provide hygiene needs.
   F. Prevent complications of immobility and contractures.
   G. Assist with ADL.
   H. Increase comfort.
   I. Reduce muscular rigidity.
   J. Control tremors.
3. Psychosocial integrity
   A. Reduce anxiety among family.
   B. Promote effective coping among family.
4. Health promotion and maintenance
   A. Increase client's and family's knowledge of prevention, home care (including medication), and follow-up.

Implementation

1. Assess, record, and report signs and symptoms and reactions to treatment.
2. Encourage client to maintain independence in ADL as much as possible.

3. Assist client while eating—have client use utensils with large handles for easy gripping.
4. Encourage client to continue with previous work, social, and diversionary activities as much as possible.
5. Maintain effective airway clearance.
6. Provide a safe, hazard-free environment.
7. Administer levodopa (dopamine replacement) as prescribed; monitor for side effects.
8. Administer alternate drug therapy such as anticholinergics and antihistamines as prescribed.
9. Assist in establishment of a regular bowel routine—encourage fluid intake, high-bulk foods.
10. Provide emotional support to client and family.
11. Prepare client and family for stereotaxic neurosurgical procedure—electrical coagulation, freezing, radioactivity, or ultrasound to destroy the ventrolateral nucleus of thalamus in order to prevent involuntary movement—if required by client.
12. Monitor for signs of hemorrhage and increased ICP following surgery.
13. Coordinate care with physical therapy department—for maintenance of normal muscle tone and function.
14. Maintain skin integrity.
15. Instruct client and family regarding disease process, diagnostic procedures, prevention, treatment, home care, and follow-up. Include teaching on:
    A. Medication
    B. Prevention of contractures—have client use a firm mattress without a pillow, lie prone to facilitate proper posture during rest
    C. Prevention of decubiti
    D. Establishing long- and short-term goals for process
    E. Providing intellectual stimulation and diversionary activities

Evaluation

1. Reports increased comfort, decreased anxiety
2. Reports reduction in muscular rigidity and tremors
3. Maintains good skin integrity
4. Maintains effective airway clearance
5. Maintains adequate nutritional status and fluid intake
6. Performs some ADL and participates in physical therapy
7. Socializes with others
8. Demonstrates understanding of disease process, diagnostic procedures, treatment, prevention, home care (including medication), and need for follow-up; similar understanding demonstrated by family

Paraplegia

Description

1. Paraplegia is caused by spinal cord trauma or disease resulting in motor or sensory loss in the lower extremities with or without involvement of abdominal and back muscles.
2. Possibly complete or incomplete paralysis, which may be flaccid or spastic, permanent or temporary, and symmetrical or asymmetrical.
3. Complete severing of spinal cord results in permanent paralysis of body parts below the injury.
4. Approximately 50% of spinal cord injuries result in paraplegia.

5. More prevalent in males than in females; incidence highest between ages 16 and 35.
6. Causes
   A. Trauma—automobile, diving, motorcycle, gunshot wounds, fall, other sporting accidents
   B. Nontraumatic lesions such as spinal bifida, spinal tumors, scoliosis, and chordoma

Assessment

SUBJECTIVE

1. Loss of sensation
2. Loss of voluntary movement

OBJECTIVE

1. Immediate phase
   A. Areflexia due to spinal shock
   B. Complete loss of sensation
   C. Complete loss of voluntary (motor) function
   D. Flaccid paralysis below site of injury
   E. Hypotonia
2. Later phase
   A. Spasticity of muscles below site of injury
   B. Hyperreflexia (hyperactive responses)
3. Level of injury
   A. Lower thoracic level
      (1) Loss of movement of bowel, bladder, and lower extremities
      (2) Paralysis of legs
   B. Lumbar and sacral level
      (1) Loss of movement and sensation of lower extremities.
      (2) S-2—S-4 center of micturition: Injury or lesion above this level allows bladder to empty involuntarily; lesions below this level result in bladder contraction without emptying (autonomous neurogenic bladder).
      (3) Injury above S-2 (in males): Injury above this level allows erection to occur without ejaculation, owing to sympathetic nerve damage.
      (4) Injury below S-2 and S-4: Prevention of erection or ejaculation, owing to damaged sympathetic and parasympathetic nerves.
      (5) Associated injuries such as fractures, hemorrhage, shock.

DIAGNOSTIC TESTS AND METHODS

1. History
2. Physical examination
3. Neurological examination
4. Lumbar puncture
5. Laboratory studies—CBC, PT, electrolytes, urinalysis
6. X-rays of the spine
7. CT or MRI
8. EMG or electromyography
9. After stabilization—hip, knee, chest radiographs, IVP to provide baseline information for detection of pathological changes
10. Weekly urine culture and sensitivity tests

Planning

1. Safe, effective care environment
   A. Prevent avoidable injury and/or infection.

B. Increase client's and family's knowledge of condition, diagnostic procedures, and treatment.
2. Physiological integrity
   A. Maintain skin integrity.
   B. Maintain effective breathing pattern, airway clearance, and gas exchange.
   C. Maintain adequate level of mobility.
   D. Assist with alterations in sensory perception.
   E. Assist with alterations in motor function.
   F. Maintain adequate bladder and bowel elimination pattern.
   G. Provide hygienic needs.
   H. Prevent complications of immobility and contractures.
3. Psychosocial integrity
   A. Reduce anxiety.
   B. Promote effective coping.
   C. Facilitate with alterations in self-image and self-concept.
   D. Counsel on alterations in sexual activity.
4. Health promotion and maintenance
   A. Facilitate participation in ADL.
   B. Increase client's and family's knowledge of prevention, home care (including medication), and follow-up.

Implementation

1. Emergency care
   A. Assess for:
      (1) Pain
      (2) Numbness, tingling
      (3) Weakness
      (4) Alterations of sensation and motor function below level of injury
   B. Monitor for signs of shock.
   C. Provide supportive treatment to control for systemic shock and hemorrhage.
   D. Immobilize client—movement may further damage spinal cord.
   E. Stabilize head and spine by strapping client on board.
   F. Place client on stretcher in emergency department without removing him or her from board.
   G. Insert Foley catheter to ensure uninterrupted urinary drainage.
2. Phase following emergency intervention
   A. Assess, record, and report signs and symptoms and reactions to treatment.
   B. Provide meticulous catheter care—use intermittent catheterization to re-establish bladder capacity and prevent infection once spinal shock period is over.
   C. Maintain proper body alignment and position to prevent contractures in immobilized client.
   D. Provide meticulous skin care, inspect pressure areas daily, and have client shift position at least every 15 minutes while sitting in wheelchair.
   E. Administer prescribed medications such as corticosteroids to reduce spinal cord edema and analgesics to minimize pain.
   F. Monitor fluid intake and output; restrict fluids to 2000–2500 mL/day if patient is on intermittent catheterization program. Increase fluids for patients with indwelling Foley catheters to 4000 mL/day.
   G. Assist with active and passive ROM exercises; coordinate care with physical therapist.
   H. Monitor for symptoms of orthostatic hypotension as client progresses from bed rest to wheelchair; use

antiembolism hose to assist in compensation for a sitting position after being restricted to a lying position for a long time.
   I. Establish a bowel elimination routine.
      (1) Provide stool softeners, suppositories, and laxatives as ordered.
      (2) Administer stool softeners and suppositories on a regular timed schedule.
      (3) Use digital stimulation if necessary.
      (4) Teach muscle strengthening.
      (5) Monitor for abdominal distention, flatus, and fullness in rectum, which indicates need to defecate.
      (6) Teach client to use intra-abdominal compression by leaning forward and performing Valsalva's maneuver, unless cardiac problems are present.
   J. Monitor for UTI.
   K. For autonomic or spastic bladder reflex: Instruct client regarding possible stimuli to initiate urination; use external catheters for men. Teach client to report signs of UTI.
   L. For atonic bladder: Instruct client to observe for distention. Use intermittent catheterization. Teach use of Credé's maneuver or abdominal straining to initiate urination.
   M. Provide postoperative wound care if a laminectomy is performed.
   N. Encourage family involvement in rehabilitation.
   O. Monitor for psychological problems—altered body image, loss of self-esteem, denial, anger.
   P. Provide emotional support to client and family.
   Q. Provide counseling on sexual dysfunction or alterations.
   R. Instruct client and family regarding condition, diagnostic procedures, treatment, prevention, home care (including medication), and follow-up.

Evaluation

1. Reports increased comfort, decreased anxiety
2. Shows no signs of avoidable infection and/or injury
3. Is able to cope effectively with alterations in sensory and motor functions
4. Maintains an adequate bowel and bladder elimination routine
5. Verbalizes feelings regarding self-image, self-concept, and sexual concerns
6. Participates in appropriate level of self-care
7. Demonstrates understanding of condition, diagnostic procedures, treatment, home care (including medications and available community resources), and need for follow-up; similar understanding demonstrated by family

Quadriplegia

Description

1. Quadriplegia is the result of a permanent injury that affects all body systems.
2. It is characterized by paralysis of the arms, legs, and body below level of injury to the spinal cord.
3. It affects approximately 150,000 individuals in the United States.
4. Incidence is highest in males aged 20–40.
5. Condition flaccidity of the arms and legs, and loss of movement and sensation below the level of injury.
6. Injury above the fifth cervical vertebra also causes blockage

of the sympathetic nervous system, which allows the parasympathetic system to dominate; complications that may result from this phenomenon include:

A. Hypotension with BP < 90/60 caused by vasodilation allowing blood to pool in veins of extremities, resulting in slowing of the venous blood return to the heart.

B. Bradycardia (decreased heartbeat) due to stimulation of the heart by the vagus nerve and the absence of the inhibiting effects of the sympathetic system.

C. Decrease in body temperature due to lack of ability of blood vessels to constrict effectively, allowing blood vessel to come in contact with body surface; results in heat loss.

D. Respiratory complications due to damage to upper cervical cord.

E. Decreased peristalsis.

F. Autonomic dysreflexia (injuries above the fourth thoracic vertebra): connection between the brain and spinal cord is severed; produces an exaggerated autonomic response to specific stimuli such as a distended bladder or bowel, presence of infection, decubitus ulcers, and/or surgical manipulation; key symptom is severe hypertension.

7. Causes
   A. Spinal cord injury, especially involving the fifth to seventh cervical vertebrae
   B. Vertebral pressure from tumors and degenerative spinal cord lesions

Assessment

SUBJECTIVE

1. Loss of sensation
2. Difficulty breathing
3. Pain
4. Nature of injury
5. Orientation

OBJECTIVE

1. Symptoms of spinal shock
2. Complete loss of sensation below level of injury
3. Complete loss of movement below level of injury
4. Unconsciousness
5. Flaccid paralysis
6. Hypotonia
7. Respiratory difficulty
8. Level of injury
   A. Cervical lesions with paralysis of trunk and all extremities
   B. May have shoulder movement if at C-5 or below
   C. Decreased perspiration
   D. Decrease in touch sensation
   E. Respiratory failure at level of C-4 or above

DIAGNOSTIC TESTS AND METHODS

1. History
2. Detailed history of trauma
3. Physical examination
4. Neurological assessment
5. Spinal radiographs
6. Myelography—to identify fractures, dislocations, subluxation, and blockage in spinal cord

7. Radiographs of head, chest, and abdomen—to rule out underlying injuries
8. Laboratory data—to assess respiratory, hepatic, and pancreatic functions

Planning

1. Safe, effective care environment
   A. Prevent avoidable injury and/or infection.
   B. Increase client's and family's knowledge of condition, diagnostic procedures, and treatment.
2. Physiological integrity
   A. Maintain skin integrity.
   B. Maintain effective breathing pattern, airway clearance, and gas exchange.
   C. Maintain adequate level of mobility.
   D. Assist with alterations in sensory perception.
   E. Assist with alterations in motor function.
   F. Maintain adequate bladder and bowel elimination pattern.
   G. Provide hygienic needs.
   H. Prevent complications of immobility and contractures.
   I. Maintain adequate nutritional status.
   J. Prevent avoidable respiratory and urinary tract infections.
   K. Maintain adequate cardiac output.
   L. Absence of autonomic dysreflexia.
3. Psychosocial integrity
   A. Reduce anxiety.
   B. Promote effective coping of client and family.
   C. Assist with alterations in self-concept.
   D. Counsel on alterations in sexual activity.
4. Health promotion and maintenance
   A. Facilitate participation in ADL.
   B. Increase client's and family's knowledge of prevention, home care (including medication), and follow-up.

Implementation

1. Assess, record, and report signs and symptoms and reactions to treatment.
2. Monitor respirations, chest movement, and vital signs frequently (injury at C-4 or above will require permanent ventilatory support).
3. Monitor PCO_2 and pH for signs of respiratory insufficiency.
4. Administer IV therapy—do not overhydrate if vasodilation and venous pooling are present below level of injury.
5. Insert NG tube, if needed, as ordered.
6. Observe for signs of GI complications such as paralytic ileus, bleeding, and pancreatic dysfunction.
   A. Listen for bowel sounds every 8 hours.
   B. Record amount and type of NG drainage; check for "coffee-ground" secretions.
7. Administer ventilatory support and intubation, if ordered.
8. Connect client to cardiac monitor if bradycardia occurs.
9. Place client in slight Trendelenburg position if signs of hypotension occur—continually assess respiratory function.
10. Use abdominal binder and antiembolism stockings to aid venous return and prevent orthostatic hypotension.
11. Warm client with blankets if hypothermia occurs (temperature ≥ 90°F [32.2°C]). Do *not* use hot water bottles or

mechanical heat devices; these may cause burning owing to sensory deficit.

12. Maintain proper body alignment and immobilization of spine.
13. Monitor neurological status, level of consciousness, sensations, movement, and pupil response frequently.
14. Monitor for severe hypertension, which may lead to heart failure, intracranial bleeding, and retinal hemorrhage—sign of autonomic dysreflexia in client with injury above T-4.
    A. Provide the following nursing interventions in presence of hypertension
       (1) Elevate head of bed to decrease blood pressure.
       (2) Check for bladder distention, obstructed catheter.
       (3) Check for fecal impaction; do not manipulate rectum, as it worsens symptoms.
           (a) Before removal of impaction, apply topical anesthetic ointment, which decreases risk of further increasing the blood pressure.
           (b) Administer a smooth muscle relaxant or antihypertensive if prescribed.
           (c) Administer an adrenergic blocking agent for persistent hypertension as prescribed.
15. Maintain skeletal traction, tongs, or Circloelectric bed or Stryker frame.
16. Prepare client and family for client's surgical intervention (such as spinal decompression).
17. Provide postoperative care.
18. Administer medications as prescribed.
19. Provide frequent skin care to prevent formation of decubitus ulcers and infection.
20. Turn patient every 2 hours.
21. Maintain firm mattress support.
22. Assist with passive ROM exercises; coordinate care with physical therapy department.
23. Assist with urinary elimination.
24. Instruct client and family regarding condition, diagnostic procedures, treatment, home care (including available community resources), and follow-up.

Evaluation

1. Reports increased comfort, decreased anxiety
2. Shows no signs of avoidable injury and/or infection
3. Maintains effective breathing pattern and gas exchange
4. Maintains adequate level of mobility in wheelchair
5. Maintains skin integrity
6. Participates in appropriate level of self-care needs
7. Copes effectively with alterations in sensory perception and motor function
8. Maintains adequate elimination pattern
9. Demonstrates understanding of condition, diagnostic procedures, treatment, home care (including available community resources), and need for follow-up; similar understanding demonstrated by family

Multiple Sclerosis

Description

1. Multiple sclerosis is a condition characterized by exacerbations and remissions caused by progressive demyelination of the white matter of the CNS.

2. Demyelination occurs at various sites in the brain stem, optic nerve, cerebrum, and spinal cord.
3. Demyelination results in both direct damage to the myelin sheath and to the oligodendrocytes (supportive cells that produce and maintain myelin).
4. Condition results in disruption of transmission of nerve impulses.
5. Major cause of chronic disability in young adults.
6. Sporadic patches of demyelination in various parts of CNS induce widely disseminated and varied neurological dysfunction.
7. Prognosis is variable—may progress rapidly, disabling client by early adulthood or causing death within months of onset.
8. Approximately 70% of affected persons lead active, productive lives with prolonged remissions.
9. Incidence: Onset occurs between ages 20 and 40—average age is 27.
10. Cause is unknown.
11. Possible causes
    A. Slow-acting viral infection
    B. Autoimmune response of the nervous system
    C. Allergic reaction to an infectious agent
12. Predisposing factors
    A. Trauma
    B. Anoxia
    C. Toxins
    D. Nutritional deficiencies
    E. Vascular lesions
    F. Anorexia
    G. Genetic factors (possible)
13. Precipitating factors
    A. Emotional stress
    B. Overwork
    C. Fatigue
    D. Pregnancy
    E. Acute respiratory infections

Assessment

SUBJECTIVE

1. Visual problems—double vision, pain
2. Blindness
3. Numbness, tingling
4. Muscular weakness—lack of coordination
5. Decreased temperature perception
6. Frequency, urgency in urination—retention, incontinence
7. Bowel problems—fecal urgency, constipation, incontinence
8. Difficulty in swallowing
9. Mood swings—irritability, euphoria, depression
10. Decreased short-term memory—short attention span
11. Sexual dysfunction
    A. Decreased libido, orgasmic and genital sensation in women
    B. Erectile, orgasmic, and ejaculatory dysfunction in men

OBJECTIVE

1. Tremors
2. Upper respiratory infections
3. Speech impairments

4. Incoordination and altered gait
5. Frequent urination
6. Nystagmus
7. CSF positive for elevated γ-globulin

DIAGNOSTIC TESTS AND METHODS

1. Client and family history
2. Physical examination
3. Complete neurological examination
4. Laboratory tests–CBC, CSF analysis
5. MRI
6. Myelogram
7. Skull and spine x-rays
8. CT scan
9. Urodynamic studies
10. PET scan
11. EEG

Planning

1. Safe, effective care environment
   A. Prevent avoidable injury and/or infection.
   B. Increase client's and family's knowledge of disease process, diagnostic procedures, and treatment.
2. Physiologic integrity
   A. Maintain skin integrity.
   B. Maintain effective breathing pattern, airway clearance, and gas exchange.
   C. Maintain adequate level of mobility.
   D. Assist with alterations in sensory perception.
   E. Assist with alterations in motor function.
   F. Maintain adequate bladder and bowel elimination pattern.
   G. Provide hygienic needs.
   H. Assist with self-care deficit.
   I. Assist with alterations in visual perceptions.
   J. Maintain adequate nutritional status.
3. Psychosocial integrity
   A. Reduce anxiety.
   B. Promote effective coping.
   C. Facilitate with alterations in self-concept.
   D. Facilitate communication and social interaction.
4. Health promotion and maintenance
   A. Facilitate participation in ADL
   B. Increase client's and family's knowledge of prevention, home care (including medication), and follow-up.

Implementation

1. Assess, record, and report signs and symptoms and reactions to treatments.
2. Provide safe and calm environment.
3. Monitor neurological status, respirations, vital signs, muscular strength, ability to swallow, visual problems, and activity tolerance.
4. Administer prescribed medications such as corticosteroids, ACTH, muscle relaxants, immune system-regulating medications, stool softeners (focused on relieving symptoms).
5. Encourage activity with frequent rest periods to conserve energy and avoid fatigue; assist with ROM exercises.
6. Provide eye patch for diplopia.

7. Protect against upper respiratory or urinary tract infections.
8. Establish an elimination routine.
9. Turn every 2 hours and monitor skin for redness and breakdown when client is on bed rest.
10. Assist client in changing positions every 2 hours while in wheelchair or sitting in bedside chair.
11. Allow client to carry out activities or communication as much as possible—avoid rushing.
12. Instruct client in regard to use of assistive devices.
13. Monitor intake and output.
14. Encourage client to eat a proper diet with adequate fluids.
15. Allow client to verbalize feelings, disturbances in self-concept, and concerns about sexual function. Support positive self-image.
16. Encourage social interaction.
17. Encourage return to work and daily activities with assistance as needed.
18. Discuss further counseling and rehabilitation.
19. Explain precautions regarding sensation of temperature.
    A. Avoid hot baths.
    B. Take precautions in hot weather.
    C. Dress appropriately and comfortably.
20. Explain mood swings and emotional disturbances.
21. Instruct client and family regarding disease process, diagnostic procedures, treatment, prevention, home care, and follow-up. Include teaching on:
    A. Social rehabilitation measures
    B. Medication and side effects
    C. Safety factors
    D. Available community resources such as National Multiple Sclerosis Society

Evaluation

1. Shows no signs of avoidable injury and/or infection
2. Reports increased comfort, decreased anxiety
3. Maintains skin integrity
4. Shows no signs of avoidable respiratory or urinary tract infection
5. Participates in self-care with assistance as necessary
6. Maintains adequate bladder and bowel elimination pattern
7. Copes effectively with visual problems
8. Maintains adequate nutritional intake
9. Maintains adequate communication and social interaction
10. Verbalizes feelings regarding self-concept
11. Demonstrates understanding of disease process, diagnostic procedures, treatment, prevention, home care (including medication and available community resources), and need for follow-up; similar understanding demonstrated by family

The Eyes

Description

1. Visual acuity depends on general good health, CNS regulation of movement and conduction, and condition of eye structures.
   A. Disorders of vision are frequently indicative of systemic disease.
   B. Disorders that affect the eye usually lead to impairment or loss of vision.

C. Routine examination of the eye can provide information regarding diseases in other body systems.
D. The incidence of visual impairment and blindness increases with age; however, individuals of all ages can be affected.
E. Vision has recently been the focus of innovative medical and surgical treatment. Routine and early eye examinations along with early treatment are essential.

Assessment

SUBJECTIVE

1. Double vision
2. Blurred or clouded vision
3. Decreased or absent vision
4. Sensitivity to light
5. Spots, halos around lights
6. Flashes of light
7. Problems seeing in dark
8. Itching, pain, tearing, burning, headache

OBJECTIVE

1. Tearing, discharge—clear or purulent
2. Color of sclera—white, yellow, or pink
3. Glasses, contact lenses
4. Accuracy and range of vision
5. Crusts, blinking, rubbing
6. Edema of eyelids, ptosis
7. Squinting or drooping of lid
8. Symmetry
9. History of:
   A. Trauma to eyes
   B. Contact lenses
   C. Eye medications
   D. Changes in vision
   E. Systemic medications in use

DIAGNOSTIC TESTS AND METHODS

1. History
2. Physical examination
3. Neurological assessment
4. Visual assessment—uses ophthalmoscope to inspect interior of eye
5. Fields of vision testing
6. Refraction—measures light refraction and lenses required for visual acuity
7. Tonometer—measures intraocular pressure (increased pressure may indicate early glaucoma)
8. Electroretinography—evaluates the electrical potential between the cornea and retina
   A. It measures changes in the electrical potential in response to alterations in the wavelength and intensity of light and to the state of adaptation on the eye.
   B. Abnormal activity during dark adaptation is indicative of selective degeneration of the rods.
   C. Abnormal activity during light adaptation is indicative of involvement of all cones, as is seen in congenital total color blindness.
9. Intravenous fluorescein angiography—records appearance of blood vessels inside the eye
   A. Useful in evaluating intraocular conditions such as tumors and retinopathy

10. Ocular ultrasonography—involves penetration of eye tissues with high-frequency waves
    A. Sound waves pass through some tissues and are reflected by others.
    B. Sound waves pass through the aqueous humor.
    C. Sound waves are reflected by tissue masses, such as tumors, and cataract lenses.
    D. Reflections are picked up on microfilm and translated into electrical impulses displayed on the oscilloscope.
11. CT—provides three-dimensional visualization of the orbital structures, such as the eye muscles and optic nerve, enabling the identification of space-occupying lesions
12. MRI—permits excellent visualization of soft tissue and is useful in detecting circulatory abnormalities and tumors of the eye

Implementation

1. Problems
   A. Crusts and drainage
      (1) Clean as necessary with normal saline solution.
      (2) Apply compresses to loosen crusts if necessary.
      (3) Use aseptic technique—wipe from inner canthus to outer canthus.
      (4) Dispose of compresses with purulent drainage properly.
   B. Anxiety, frustration, anger
      (1) Disorders of vision can arouse concerns regarding loss of vision, altered lifestyles, employment, ability to function, and altered body image.
      (2) Allow verbalization of feelings.
   C. Photophobia (sensitivity to light)
      (1) Keep room blinds adjusted to avoid glare.
      (2) Keep room dim and evenly lighted.
   D. Corrective lenses
      (1) Keep glass lens clean and in case.
      (2) Keep contact lens in case with R (right) and L (left) to indicate which eye the lens fits.
      (3) Soak contact lens according to directions and with client's permission.

Blindness

Description

1. Legal blindness is the ability to see at no more than 20 ft what normally should be seen at a distance of 200 ft (20/200).
2. This definition may also refer to severe restrictions in the peripheral field of vision with corrective lenses.
3. Condition appears more often in elderly and women.
4. It creates difficulty in mobility, self-care, employment, home maintenance, and cooking.
5. It creates boredom, frustration, anger.
6. Causes
   A. Degeneration, detached retina, glaucoma, diabetic retinopathy
   B. Vascular or hypertensive retinopathy
   C. Inflammation or optic neuritis
   D. Neoplasms of brain or eye
   E. Trauma or laceration
   F. Cataract

Assessment

SUBJECTIVE

1. Decrease in or loss of vision
2. Frustration, anger

OBJECTIVE

1. Visual field is ≤20/200 in visual testing.
2. Corrected vision is ≤20/200 or is 20/200 in better eye.

DIAGNOSTIC TESTS AND METHODS

1. History
2. Physical examination
3. Neurological assessment
4. Examination with ophthalmoscope

Planning

1. Safe, effective care environment
   A. Prevent avoidable injury.
   B. Increase client's and family's knowledge of disease process, diagnostic procedures, treatment, and prognosis.
2. Physiological integrity
   A. Assist with alterations in perception.
   B. Maintain adequate mobility.
3. Psychosocial integrity
   A. Facilitate effective coping.
   B. Facilitate adjustment in communication.
4. Health promotion and maintenance
   A. Increase client's and family's knowledge of home care (including self-care) and follow-up.

Implementation

1. Assess, record, and report signs and symptoms and reactions to treatment.
2. Orient client to room and unit; guide client to obstacles such as windows, doors, furniture, bed, bathroom, call bell, and telephone.
3. Provide safe, hazard-free environment—keep unit uncluttered, bed in low position, floor clean and dry, call bell near, and side rails up as necessary.
4. Collaborate with family to provide social and emotional support.
5. Allow client to verbalize feelings regarding condition.
6. Allow as much independence as possible in daily activities.
   A. Encourage use of any visual aids recommended by physician—special lenses, canes, books with large type.
   B. Assist in use of existing vision.
   C. Provide reading material in Braille for clients who use this method.
7. Announce your presence when entering room; address client by name.
8. Let client know when you are leaving room.
9. Provide and keep needed items in specific places nearby.
10. Encourage client's participation in planning care.
11. Assist client to gradually adjust to blindness—assist client to develop effective coping strategies.
12. Maintain communication.
13. Instruct client and family regarding disease process, diagnostic procedures, treatment, prognosis, home care (including available community resources), and follow-up.

Evaluation

1. Reports increased comfort, decreased anxiety
2. Shows no signs of avoidable injury
3. Uses effective coping strategies
4. Maintains adequate mobility
5. Maintains adequate independence
6. Maintains effective communication
7. Adjusts to altered sensory perception
8. Demonstrates understanding of disease process, diagnostic procedures, treatment, prognosis, home care (including available community resources), and need for follow-up; similar understanding demonstrated by family

Cataract

Description

1. A cataract is clouding or opacity of the lens, which prevents light rays from reaching the retina.
2. Cataracts commonly occur bilaterally, with each progressing independently.
3. Causes
   A. Aging process (senile cataract)
   B. Injury to eye (traumatic cataract)
   C. Another eye disease (secondary cataract)
   D. Inherited trait (congenital cataract)
   E. Metabolic disease such as diabetes mellitus
   F. Infections

Assessment

SUBJECTIVE

1. Progressively blurred vision
2. Haziness
3. Poor reading vision
4. Halos around lights
5. Blinding glare from headlights
6. Poor vision in sunlight
7. Vision improves in dim light when pupils dilate for patients with central opacities
8. Loss of vision

OBJECTIVE

1. Opaque or cloudy white pupil
2. Less than 20/200 on visual testing

DIAGNOSTIC TESTS AND METHODS

1. History
2. Physical examination
3. Examination with ophthalmoscope
4. Slit-lamp examination
5. Ocular ultrasonography

Planning

1. Safe, effective care environment
   A. Prevent avoidable injury and/or infection.
   B. Increase client's knowledge of disease process, diagnostic procedures, and treatment.
2. Physiological integrity
   A. Facilitate sensory perception.
   B. Increase comfort.
3. Psychosocial integrity
   A. Reduce anxiety.

4. Health promotion and maintenance
   A. Increase client's knowledge of home care and follow-up.

Implementation

1. Assess, record, and report signs and symptoms and reactions to treatment.
2. Provide a safe environment; keep necessary items in specific areas within reach.
3. Administer prescribed preoperative eye medication to dilate pupil for surgery.
4. Provide appropriate postoperative nursing care to prevent increased intraocular pressure.
   A. Position client on unoperative side.
   B. Administer prescribed analgesics and medication.
   C. Instruct client to avoid any actions that may increase intraocular pressure, such as straining, bending, or rapid head movements.
   D. Administer stool softener to prevent straining during bowel movement.
   E. Administer prescribed antiemetic to prevent vomiting.
   F. Monitor dressing—check for bleeding.
   G. Provide bed rest for a specified time period.
   H. Keep patient flat or in low Fowler's position.
   I. Protect against infection; administer antibiotic ointment or drops.
   J. Administer prescribed steroids to reduce inflammation.
   K. Monitor eye shield or dressing, if appropriate.
5. Assist with self-care activities and ambulation.
6. Monitor for complications such as prolapse of iris or sudden sharp pain in eye.
7. Instruct client regarding disease process, diagnostic procedures, treatment, home care, and follow-up. Include teaching on:
   A. Avoiding heavy lifting for several weeks
   B. Activity
   C. Use of eye shield
   D. Medications (including correct instillation of eye drops)

Evaluation

1. Reports increased comfort, decreased anxiety
2. Shows no signs of avoidable injury and/or infection
3. Maintains adequate sensory perception
4. Has improved visual acuity
5. Is able to identify auditory and nonstressful visual diversionary activities of interest that can be done during the recovery period
6. Demonstrates ability to care for eye and self
7. Demonstrates evidence of eye tissue healing without complications by 3 months postoperatively
8. Demonstrates adaptation to prescriptive lenses or lens implant with maximum visual acuity within 6 months following surgery
9. Demonstrates understanding of disease process, diagnostic procedures, treatment, home care, and need for follow-up

Retinal Detachment

Description

1. In retinal detachment, the sensory layer of the retina pulls away from the pigmented layer.
2. It usually occurs laterally and most commonly affects males.

3. Classification
   A. Primary retinal detachment
      (1) This form results when there are one or more breaks in the neural layer, allowing vitreous humor to collect between the neural and pigment layers.
      (2) It is the most common type of retinal detachment.
      (3) Causes
         (a) Recent or previous trauma (blunt or penetrating)
         (b) Severe myopia
         (c) Retinal degeneration
         (d) Aphakia (following cataract surgery)
   B. Secondary retinal detachment
      (1) This form results when separation of the layers occurs from pulling or pushing (traction) of the pigment layer from the neural layer.
      (2) Causes
         (a) Pressure from intraocular tumors and hemorrhage
         (b) Scar formation in vitreous humor following vitreous hemorrhage
         (c) Severe hypertension
         (d) Diabetic retinopathy
         (e) Toxemia of pregnancy
         (f) Retrolental fibroplasia
         (g) Chronic glomerulonephritis
         (h) Vascular changes in retina (retinal vein occlusion)
4. New surgical techniques are used to reattach retinal layers in about 90% of clients.
5. Prognosis for good visual acuity is ensured if macular detachment has been prolonged.

Assessment

SUBJECTIVE

1. Floating spots from blood or retina cells as a result of tears
2. Recurrent flashes of light
3. Curtain effect—described as a shade pulled over part of the vision
4. Gradual, painless loss of vision

OBJECTIVE

1. Loss of vision
2. Retina separation on ophthalmoscopic exam

DIAGNOSTIC TESTS AND METHODS

1. History
2. Physical examination
3. Ophthalmoscopy after full pupil dilation

Planning

1. Safe, effective care environment
   A. Prevent avoidable injury.
   B. Increase client's and family's knowledge of disease process, diagnostic procedures, and treatment.
2. Physiological integrity
   A. Increase comfort.
   B. Facilitate sensory perception.
3. Psychosocial integrity
   A. Reduce anxiety.

4. Health promotion and maintenance
   A. Increase client's and family's knowledge of home care and follow-up.

Implementation

1. Assess, record, and report signs and symptoms and reactions to treatment.
2. Provide bed rest; position head to relieve stress on tear.
3. Restrict activity; use eye patch, shield to limit eye movement.
4. Provide emotional support.
5. Provide a safe, calm, relaxing environment—put side rails up; leave call bell within easy reach.
6. Apply cool compresses as ordered to decrease swelling and discomfort.
7. Instruct client to avoid activities that cause sudden movement of head, such as sneezing, coughing, or vomiting.
8. Administer cough medications or antiemetics as ordered.
9. Assist with ADL.
10. Administer prescribed eye medications such as mydriatics, antibiotics, or steroids.
11. Administer prescribed analgesics.
12. Prepare client for surgical intervention.
    A. Wash face with prescribed surgical soap preparation.
    B. Cut off eyelashes to decrease risk of infection.
    C. Administer antibiotics and mydriatic eye drops as prescribed.
13. Explain surgical procedure to client and family.
    A. Type of surgery varies with type and degree of defect.
    B. Some common surgical approaches include:
       (1) Laser, cryotherapy, or photocoagulation—procedure used to seal breaks and holes
       (2) Scleral buckling—suturing a small, inert material such as silicone sponge onto sclera over site of break or hole
       (3) Banding or encirclement—placement of a silicone band or strap under extraocular muscles around the globe
14. Provide postoperative care
    A. Position patient as ordered—usually elevate head of bed about 30 degrees.
    B. Instruct client to avoid bending over, straining, or rubbing eyes.
    C. Assist with ambulation when ordered.
    D. If on prolonged bed rest, encourage leg exercises to prevent thrombophlebitis.
    E. Cleanse eye with warm compresses and instill prescribed ophthalmic medications.
    F. Monitor for possible complications, such as signs of bleeding or retinal detachment.
    G. Instruct client and family how to instill eye drops and ointments.
    H. Advise client to use dark glasses in bright light.
15. Instruct client and family regarding disease process, diagnostic procedures, treatment, home care, and follow-up.

Evaluation

1. Reports increased comfort, decreased anxiety
2. Develops adequate sensory perception
3. Demonstrates understanding of disease process, diagnos-

tic procedures, treatment, home care, and need for follow-up; similar understanding demonstrated by family

Glaucoma

Description

1. Glaucoma is an abnormal increase in intraocular pressure, which may result in severe and permanent visual defects.
2. Intraocular pressure increases due to disturbance in circulation of aqueous humor as a result of an imbalance between production and drainage as the angle of drainage closes.
3. Glaucoma can be secondary to injuries and infections.
4. It is the most preventable cause of blindness.
5. It affects approximately 2% of individuals over 40 years of age in the United States.
6. It affects females more often than males.
7. It accounts for 15% of all cases of blindness in the United States.
8. Normal intraocular pressure ranges from 10–21 mm Hg.
9. Glaucoma requires early diagnosis to prevent damage to the optic nerve and blindness.
10. Prognosis is usually good with early diagnosis and treatment.
11. Three forms
    A. Chronic open-angle (most common)
       (1) It is caused by overproduction of aqueous humor or obstruction to its outflow.
       (2) It is frequently familial in origin—affects 90% of all individuals with glaucoma.
       (3) It is usually bilateral, with insidious onset.
       (4) Symptoms usually appear late in the disease.
    B. Acute closed-angle (narrow-angle glaucoma)—obstruction to outflow of aqueous humor as a result of:
       (1) Anatomically narrow angles between anterior iris and posterior corneal surface.
       (2) Shallow anterior chamber.
       (3) Bulging iris that presses on the trabeculae (fibrous cords of connective tissue), closing the angle.
       (4) Thickened iris causing closure of the angle on pupil dilation.
       (5) Rapid onset produces blindness in 3–5 days if not treated promptly.
       (6) Symptoms may be misinterpreted as GI distress.
    C. Chronic closed-angle
       (1) Result of untreated acute closed-angle glaucoma.
       (2) Mild, recurring, acute attacks resulting in adhesions in the trabeculae.
       (3) Onset is gradual.
       (4) Progresses to absolute glaucoma with pain and blindness.
       (5) Enucleation may be necessary to relieve extreme pain.

Assessment

SUBJECTIVE—CHRONIC OPEN-ANGLE GLAUCOMA

1. Asymptomatic early in disease
2. Mild aching in eyes
3. Loss of peripheral vision
4. Seeing halos around lights

5. Reduced visual acuity especially at night (not corrected with glasses)

SUBJECTIVE—ACUTE OPEN-ANGLE GLAUCOMA

1. Unilateral pain
2. Pressure over eye
3. Blurred vision
4. Decreased visual acuity
5. Seeing halos around lights
6. Nausea

SUBJECTIVE—CHRONIC CLOSED-ANGLE GLAUCOMA

1. Usually produces no symptoms
2. May have blurred vision
3. May see halos around lights
4. Produces severe pain if not treated

OBJECTIVE

1. Elevated intraocular pressure with tonometry
2. Inflammation
3. Decreased peripheral vision with testing
4. Photophobia
5. Optic-disc cupping on ophthalmoscopic exam
6. Vomiting
7. Loss of vision

DIAGNOSTIC TESTS AND METHODS

1. History.
2. Physical examination.
3. Tonometry.
4. Gonioscopy—procedure that differentiates between chronic open-angle and acute or chronic closed-angle glaucoma.
5. Ophthalmoscopy.
6. Slit-lamp examination.
7. Fingertip tension: On gentle palpation of closed eyelids, one eye feels harder than other in acute closed-angle glaucoma.
8. Perimetry or visual field tests: These tests evaluate extent of chronic open-angle, closed-angle deterioration.

Planning

1. Safe, effective care environment
   A. Prevent avoidable injury and/or infection.
   B. Increase client's and family's knowledge of disease process, diagnostic procedures, and treatment.
2. Physiological integrity
   A. Maintain adequate sensory perception.
   B. Increase comfort from eye pain.
3. Psychosocial integrity
   A. Reduce anxiety.
4. Health promotion and maintenance
   A. Increase client's and family's knowledge of prevention, home care, and follow-up.

Implementation

1. Assess, record, and report signs and symptoms and reactions to treatment.
2. Explain condition, diagnostic procedures, and treatment.
3. Explain and administer prescribed eye drops to decrease aqueous humor production or to facilitate drainage— miotic agent, pilocarpine, β-blocker, timolol maleate.

4. Explain the need for lifetime compliance in the use of eye medications to prevent disc changes, loss of vision, and need for surgery.
5. Prepare client and family for surgical intervention, if required by client.
   A. Trabeculoplasty—facilitates drainage of aqueous humor by changing the trabecular meshwork with a laser beam
   B. Trabeculectomy—creates a new opening at the limbus, allowing aqueous humor to drain into subconjunctival spaces
6. Provide postoperative care.
   A. Administer cycloplegic eye drops to affected eye.
      (1) Decrease inflammation and relax ciliary muscle
      (2) Prevent adhesions
   B. Administer prescribed analgesics for eye pain.
   C. Administer prescribed eye medications to dilate pupil.
   D. Administer prescribed steroids to rest the pupil.
   E. Protect eye with eye patch or shield.
   F. Assist with positioning on unoperative side.
   G. Maintain a safe environment—side rails up, call bell within easy reach.
7. Instruct client and family regarding disease process, diagnostic procedures, treatment, prevention, home care, and follow-up. Include teaching on:
   A. Lifetime medication
   B. Type of medication and side effects
   C. Reporting eye pain, changes in vision, halos around lights immediately to physician
   D. Importance of glaucoma screening for early detection and prevention

Evaluation

1. Reports increased comfort, decreased anxiety
2. Shows no signs of avoidable injury and/or infection
3. Maintains sensory perception
4. Demonstrates understanding of disease process, diagnostic procedures, treatment, prevention, home care, and need for follow-up; similar understanding demonstrated by family

The Ear

Basic Information

Hearing is initiated by sound waves reaching the tympanic membrane, causing a vibration of the ossicles in the middle ear. The stapes transmit the vibrations to the perilymphatic fluid in the inner ear by vibrating against the oval window. These vibrations then pass across the cochlea's fluid receptor cells, stimulating movement of the hair cells of the organ of Corti and initiating auditory nerve impulses to the brain. The inner ear structure also maintains the equilibrium and balance of the body. The fluid in the semicircular canals is set into motion by body movement and stimulates nerve cells lining the canal. These cells transmit impulses to the brain via the vestibular branch of the acoustic nerve. Conductive hearing loss is a result of injury, obstruction, or disease that interferes with sound wave conduction to the inner ear, such as wax in the ear canal. Sensory hearing loss is a result of a malfunction of the inner ear, auditory nerve, or the auditory center in the brain. The cause of nerve deafness is often complications from infections, such as mumps, meningitis, and measles; trauma; neuromas; ototoxic drugs; noise; and the aging process. Specific types of sensory hearing loss include fluctuating hearing loss (hearing varying with time), neural hearing loss (loss of hearing starting in the nerve itself), and presbycusis (hearing loss due to the aging process). Another type of hearing loss involves both conductive and sensory hearing loss. Hearing loss due to injury of the brain that affects the acoustic nerve is designated as central hearing loss, such as that noted in CVAs. A hearing loss without known organic explanations is referred to as a *functional* or *psychogenic* hearing loss. Hearing loss can be acquired or congenital and is the most common disability in the United States.

Assessment

SUBJECTIVE

1. Difficulty in hearing
2. Vertigo
3. Pain
4. Blurred vision
5. Headache
6. Itching, pressure or full feeling
7. Ringing, popping, buzzing

OBJECTIVE

1. Drainage
2. Hearing loss
3. Nonresponsive to loud noises
4. Vomiting
5. Tenderness
6. Dried secretions
7. Deformities of ear
8. Presence of hearing aid
9. History of:
    A. Ear infections
    B. Ear surgery
    C. Head injury
    D. Medications

DIAGNOSTIC TESTS AND METHODS

1. History
2. Physical examination
    A. Examination of external ear position, size, shape, and symmetry
    B. Inspection of skin for color, rash, scaling, and lesions
    C. Inspection behind the auricle, including the mastoid area
    D. Inspection for evidence of tophi (uric acid deposits)
    E. Palpitation of auricle, tragus, and mastoid area for evidence of tenderness and elevated local temperature
    F. Assessment of nose, mouth, and throat and surrounding lymph nodes (alterations in jaw and teeth impact on surrounding glands and ear)
3. Otoscopy: Visual examination of the ear canal and tympanic membrane.
4. Audiometry: A test to determine the ability to discriminate between sounds, voices, and degrees of pitch and loudness.
5. Rinne test: A tuning fork is struck and placed on the mastoid process behind ear. The fork is removed, and the client is asked to indicate when the sound can no longer

be heard. The fork, which is still vibrating, is then placed near the external ear canal. Normally the sound will be heard approximately twice as long in this latter position (air conduction) than in the former position (bone conduction).

6. Weber test: A test used to evaluate unilateral hearing loss. A tuning fork is struck and placed on the midline of the client's forehead, and the client is asked where he or she hears the sound. Sounds should be heard equally in each ear.
7. Pure tone audiometry: Production of a series of pure tones of decibels at different frequencies (400–3000 Hz). Both bone and air conduction are measured for each ear; results are plotted on a graph. The line is plotted as zero decibels if hearing is normal.
8. Impedance audiometry: A test used to evaluate middle ear disorders by determining the degree of tympanic membrane and middle ear mobility. One end of the audiometer (probe with three small tubes) is inserted into the external ear canal; the other end is attached to an oscillator. If the tympanic membrane shows decreased mobility, it produces a high-voltage curve, reflecting maximal sound waves.
9. Tympanometry: A test used to determine the degree of negative pressure in the middle ear by measuring tympanic membrane compliance to air pressure variations in the external ear canal.
10. Caloric testing: Instillation of 0.2 mL of ice water into each ear while client is in a semi-Fowler position (head elevated 30 degrees). This test usually produces rotary nystagmus away from the side of the ear being irrigated. If disease of the labyrinth is present, no nystagmus is elicited.
11. Spondee threshold test: A test used to measure the ability to detect and repeat 50% of a set of two-syllable words presented through earphones (useful in measuring degree of hearing loss for speech and for confirming the results obtained from pure tone audiometry).
12. Word recognition test: A test used to assess the ability to distinguish speech sounds at above normal levels and to locate auditory tract and CNS lesions.
13. Romberg test: A test used to assess vestibular function in those who have symptoms of disequilibrium, nystagmus, or vertigo.
14. Past-pointing test: A test used to assess vestibular function.
15. Electronystagmography test: A more sophisticated version of the caloric test that is used to evaluate vestibular function.
16. X-rays: Diagnostic tools useful in visualizing the temporal and mastoid bones, the middle and inner ears, and the eustachian tube.
17. Culture of ear material for diagnosis and treatment of localized lesions and abscesses.
18. Typanocentesis: Aspiration of middle ear fluid often used during a myringotomy.

Implementation

1. Problems
    A. Inability to communicate
        (1) Attract client's attention before speaking.
        (2) Avoid touching client until he or she is aware of your presence.
        (3) Face client when speaking.
        (4) Speak clearly, not too fast or too slow.

(5) Provide the following nursing interventions for client with a hearing aid:
  (a) Encourage client to wear it.
  (b) Make sure hearing aid is switched on.
  (c) Test batteries.
  (d) Instruct client how to care and store hearing aid.
(6) Provide alternate methods of communication.
  (a) Provide magic slate or pad and pencil.
  (b) Check if client is able to use sign language or lip reading.
B. Communication with the older individual
  (1) Reduce distracting background noise prior to starting conversation.
  (2) Begin conversation with casual topics; avoid crucial messages at first.
  (3) Stay with one topic for a while.
  (4) Keep sentences and questions short.
  (5) Allow extra time for responding.
  (6) Give choices to make decision making easier.
  (7) Listen attentively. Look for hints from eye gaze and gestures if unsure of what is being said.
2. Prepare client for surgery, if required.
3. Provide postoperative care:
  A. Give general postoperative care.
  B. Monitor and report drainage immediately.
  C. Advise patient to avoid blowing nose.
  D. Check for inability to pucker lips or close eyes (indication of facial nerve injury).
  E. Monitor for signs of vertigo.
  F. Provide a safe, hazard-free environment.
  G. Provide activity, diet, and positioning as ordered.

Ménière's Disease

Description

1. Ménière's disease is a chronic disease of the inner ear characterized by sudden attacks of vertigo, tinnitus (ringing in the ears), and hearing loss that affects body equilibrium and balance.
2. Attacks can last for a few minutes to several weeks.
3. Condition usually affects men more often than women between the ages of 30 and 60.
4. It can lead to residual tinnitus and hearing loss if attacks continue over time.
5. There may not be any apparent symptoms between attacks, except for tinnitus, which worsens during an attack.
6. Attacks can occur several times per year or may have remissions, which can last for several years.
7. Attacks eventually become less frequent with increasing hearing loss.
8. Attacks may cease entirely with total hearing loss.
9. Surgical destruction of the affected labyrinth may be required to permanently relieve symptoms if disorder persists for more than 2 years of treatment or produces constant vertigo. The result, however, will permanently produce irreversible hearing loss.
10. Causes are unknown.
11. Precipitating factors
  A. Autonomic nervous system dysfunction resulting in a temporary constriction of blood vessels that supply the inner ear
  B. Premenstrual edema
  C. Associated with viral infection

Assessment

SUBJECTIVE

1. Vertigo
2. Nausea
3. Tinnitus, hearing loss
4. Headache
5. History of ear infection
6. Fullness or blocked feeling in ear
7. Loss of balance

OBJECTIVE

1. Nystagmus
2. Vomiting
3. Diaphoresis
4. Sensorineural hearing loss demonstrated with audiometry and vestibular testing

DIAGNOSTIC TESTS AND METHODS

1. History
2. Physical examination
3. Neurological assessment
4. Caloric testing
5. Laboratory tests for sodium, potassium, and glucose levels to determine if vertigo is associated with electrolyte imbalance, diabetes, or dehydration
6. X-rays

Planning

1. Safe, effective care environment
  A. Prevent avoidable injury and/or infection.
  B. Increase client's knowledge of disease process, diagnostic procedures, and treatment.
2. Physiological integrity
  A. Increase comfort.
  B. Assist with alterations in auditory perception.
3. Psychosocial integrity
  A. Facilitate effective coping.
4. Health promotion and maintenance
  A. Increase client's knowledge of home care and follow-up.

Implementation

1. Assess, record, and report signs and symptoms and reactions to treatment.
2. Provide bed rest during attacks.
3. Advise client to avoid reading and exposure to bright lights to minimize vertigo.
4. Provide a safe environment—keep side rails up.
5. Assist with ADL and ambulation.
6. Instruct client to move slowly and to avoid sudden position changes to prevent vertigo.
7. Administer prescribed medications such as diuretics, vasodilators, antibiotics, antiemetics, and steroids.
8. Provide a low-sodium diet.
9. Provide same care as that for client with limited hearing. (See Basic Information.)

10. Prepare client and family for surgical intervention, if required by client.
    A. Labyrinthectomy—removal of the labyrinth to relieve vertigo resulting in permanent hearing loss.
    B. Endolymphatic sac procedures—use of various shunts to decrease labyrinth fluid pressure for the purpose of relieving vertigo and preservation of hearing.
    C. Record fluid intake and output and characteristics of emesis if patient is vomiting.
    D. Administer prescribed antiemetics as necessary.
11. Provide postoperative care:
    A. Give general postoperative care.
    B. Record fluid intake and output.
    C. Advise client to expect vertigo and nausea for 1–2 days.
    D. Administer prophylactic antibiotics and anti-emetics as ordered.
    E. Instruct client to move slowly.
    F. Assist with ambulation while equilibrium is impaired.
12. Assist with coping and comfort measures.
13. Instruct client regarding disease process, diagnostic procedures, treatment, home care, and follow-up.

Evaluation

1. Reports increased comfort, decreased anxiety
2. Describes signs and symptoms of specific problem
3. Is aware of any triggering mechanisms that exacerbate the problem
4. Knows what actions to take at the sudden onset of symptoms
5. Shows no signs of avoidable injury and/or infection
6. Maintains adequate auditory sensory perception
7. Uses effective coping strategies
8. Reports decreased vertigo
9. Demonstrates understanding of disease process, diagnostic procedures, treatment (including effects and common side effects of medication), home care, and need for follow-up

Otosclerosis

Description

1. Otosclerosis is a hereditary degenerative disorder of the middle ear characterized by a slow formation of new spongy bone along the stapes footplate in the oval window niche.
2. The new bone prevents normal movement of the stapes, resulting in disruption of the conduction of vibrations from the tympanic membrane to the cochlea. This causes a progressive hearing loss in the affected ear, which may progress to the unaffected ear.
3. Tympanosclerosis is seen in the tympanic membrane and middle ear mucosa due to untreated middle ear infections. Chalky white plaques can be observed on the tympanic membrane that indicate a progressive problem. Sclerotic changes may occur in the ossicles later in life.
4. Disorder affects approximately 10% of whites between the ages of 15 and 30.
5. Prevalence is 50% higher in females than in males.
6. Disorder is bilateral in 80% of clients.
7. Prognosis is good with surgery.

Assessment

SUBJECTIVE

1. Hearing loss
2. Tinnitus
3. Ability to hear conversation better in a noisy environment than a quiet one (paracusis of Willis)

OBJECTIVE

1. Positive findings on audiometric testing
2. Conductive loss demonstrated by Weber and Rinne tests.

DIAGNOSTIC TESTS AND METHODS

1. History
2. Physical examination
3. Rinne test
4. Weber test
5. Audiometric testing

Planning

1. Safe, effective care environment
   A. Prevent avoidable injury and/or infection.
   B. Increase client's knowledge of disease process, diagnostic procedures, and treatment.
2. Physiological integrity
   A. Increase comfort.
   B. Assist with alterations in auditory perception.
3. Psychosocial integrity
   A. Facilitate effective coping.
   B. Increase comfort.
4. Health promotion and maintenance
   A. Increase client's knowledge of home care and follow-up.

Implementation

1. Assess, record, and report signs and symptoms and reactions to treatment.
2. Monitor for degree of hearing loss.
3. Maintain safe environment, and assist with activities as necessary.
4. Prepare client/family for client's stapedectomy (removal of stapes) and insertion of plastic or stainless steel prosthesis for the purpose of restoring hearing in the middle ear. Laser stapedectomy may also be done.
5. Provide appropriate postoperative care.
   A. Keep client flat with head turned so that affected ear faces upward—assists in maintaining position of the prosthesis.
   B. Instruct client to avoid sneezing, coughing, blowing nose. (If sneezing is unavoidable, instruct patient to keep mouth open in order to equalize ear pressure.)
   C. Administer prescribed antibiotics, analgesics, and antiemetics.
   D. Instruct client to move slowly to decrease vertigo episodes.
   E. Monitor for presence of nausea, vomiting, vertigo, headache, or abnormal ear sensations.
   F. Assist with activities as necessary.
   G. Reassure client that hearing will improve when packing is removed and edema disappears.

6. Prepare client for use of a hearing aid (air conduction aid with molded ear insert receiver) as a substitute procedure if stapedectomy is not possible; the device enables one to hear conversations in normal surroundings, although it is not as effective as a stapedectomy.
7. Myringoplasty or tympanoplasty may be substituted for the stapedectomy, based on decision made by physician and client.
8. Instruct client regarding disease process, diagnostic procedures, treatment, home care, and follow-up. Include teaching on:
    A. Avoiding loud noises and sudden pressure changes (flying or diving) until healing is complete (usually 6 months)
    B. Refraining from blowing nose for at least 1 week to prevent contaminated air and bacteria from entering the eustachian tube
    C. Protecting ears against cold
    D. Avoiding contact with individuals who have upper respiratory infections
    E. Avoiding any activities that produce vertigo, such as bending, heavy lifting, straining
    F. Changing external ear dressing and caring for the surgical incision
    G. Necessity of completing the prescribed antibiotic regimen

Evaluation

1. Reports increased comfort, decreased anxiety
2. Reports ability to hear better
3. Reports decrease or relief of pain
4. Describes and performs procedures necessary to maintain wellness of the middle ear
5. Shows no signs of avoidable injury and/or infection
6. Maintains appropriate auditory perception
7. Demonstrates understanding of disease process, diagnostic procedures, treatment, home care, and need for follow-up

Mastoiditis

Description

1. Mastoiditis is a bacterial infection and inflammation of the air cells of the mastoid process.
2. Usually a complication of a middle ear infection that was not treated or was inadequately treated.
3. Pus accumulates under pressure in middle ear cavity, which results in necrosis of neighboring tissue and extension of the infection into the mastoid cells.
4. A myringotomy is performed if bone damage is minimal. This procedure allows for drainage of purulent fluid and provides specimen for culture and sensitivity testing.
5. A simple mastoidectomy is usually performed for signs of intracranial complications, or recurrent and persistent infection (involves removal of diseased bone and cleansing of the affected area, followed by an insertion of a drain).
6. A radical mastoidectomy is usually performed in case of a chronically infected mastoid (involves excision of posterior wall of the ear canal, tympanic membrane, malleus, and incus, if not already destroyed by infection).
7. Radical mastoidectomy does not drastically affect the client's hearing because significant hearing loss has already occurred prior to surgery.
8. Radical mastoidectomy is seldom necessary if antibiotic therapy is started early.
9. Prognosis is good with early treatment.
10. Possible complications include facial paralysis, meningitis, suppurative labyrinthitis, and brain abscess.
11. Immunosuppression or chronic systemic diseases may be predisposing factors.

Assessment

SUBJECTIVE

1. Dull ache, tenderness in mastoid process area
2. Headache

OBJECTIVE

1. Elevated temperature
2. Thick, purulent drainage, gradually becoming profuse
3. Postauricular erythema
4. Edema
5. Swelling and obstruction of external ear canal
6. Dull, thickened, edematous tympanic membrane
7. Persistent oozing into external ear canal—indicates perforation of tympanic membrane

DIAGNOSTIC TESTS AND METHODS

1. History
2. Physical examination
3. Weber and Rinne tests
4. Gross hearing evaluation
5. Otoscopic examination
6. X-ray of mastoid area
7. Culture and sensitivity testing of drainage

Planning

1. Safe, effective care environment
    A. Prevent avoidable injury and/or infection.
    B. Increase client's knowledge of disease process, diagnostic procedures, and treatment.
2. Physiological integrity
    A. Increase comfort.
    B. Assist with alterations in auditory perception.
3. Psychosocial integrity
    A. Facilitate effective coping.
4. Health promotion and maintenance
    A. Increase client's knowledge of home care and follow-up.

Implementation

1. Assess, record, and report signs and symptoms and reactions to treatment.
2. Assist in administration of parenteral antibiotic therapy.
3. Prepare client for myringotomy, if needed.
4. Prepare client for simple mastoidectomy.
5. Provide appropriate postoperative care for clients who have undergone simple mastoidectomy, if required.
    A. Administer analgesics as prescribed.
    B. Check wound drainage, reinforce dressings. Assist physician in changing dressing and removing drain (usually after 72 hours).

C. Monitor client's hearing
D. Monitor for signs of complications
   (1) Localized infection
   (2) Extended infection to brain
   (3) Facial nerve paralysis with unilateral drooping of face.
   (4) Bleeding
   (5) Vertigo
6. Prepare client for radical mastoidectomy, if required.
7. Provide appropriate postoperative care for clients who have undergone radical mastoidectomy.
  A. Administer analgesics for pain prior to removal of wound packing.
  B. Monitor for signs of vertigo and nausea—usually occurs for several days after surgery due to stimulation of inner ear during surgery.
  C. Provide a safe hazard-free environment—keep side rails up.
  D. Assist with ambulation when ordered.
  E. Administer prescribed antiemetics as needed.
8. Instruct client regarding disease process, diagnostic procedures, treatment, home care, and follow-up. Include teaching on:
  A. Dressing change
  B. Importance of keeping dressing dry
  C. Importance of compliance with prescribed antibiotic regimen and follow-up visits

Evaluation

1. Reports increased comfort, decreased anxiety
2. Shows no signs of avoidable injury and/or infection
3. Maintains appropriate auditory perception
4. Describes and performs procedures necessary to maintain wellness of the mastoid process
5. Demonstrates understanding of disease process, diagnostic procedures, treatment, home care (including need for compliance with treatment), and need for follow-up

Labyrinthitis

Description

Labyrinthitis is an infection or inflammation of the inner ear involving the cochlear and/or vestibular portion of the labyrinth. Bacterial or viral microorganisms may enter the inner ear from the meninges, middle ear, or bloodstream. Infection is classified as either serous or diffuse suppurative labyrinthitis. The serous type usually produces little or no hearing loss, and may be caused by an allergic reaction, excessive alcoholic intake, or drug intoxication. It is usually a nonpurulent inflammatory process with cellular infiltration and a serous or serofibrinous exudate. Diffuse suppurative labyrinthitis is a result of an acute or chronic otitis media that enters the labyrinth through the oval windows or through the erosion of the bony capsule. It can also occur as a complication following middle ear or mastoid surgical procedures. In this type of labyrinthitis there is an infiltration of polymorphonuclear leukocytes combined with destruction of the soft tissue structures resulting in total, permanent hearing loss. Chronic labyrinthitis may occur following an acute siege of

labyrinthitis. In this instance, the internal ear becomes satiated with granulations that change into fibrous tissue and calcify as new bone in the labyrinth space over a period of 6 months to several years. The result is complete deafness.

Assessment

SUBJECTIVE

1. Vertigo (spontaneous and rotational)
2. Tinnitus
3. Pain
4. Fever
5. Nausea
6. Sensorineural hearing loss

OBJECTIVE

1. Sensorineural hearing loss
2. Nystagmus
3. Elevated temperature
4. Vomiting
5. Evidence of beginning nerve deafness

DIAGNOSTIC TESTS AND METHODS

1. History
2. Physical examination
3. Culture and sensitivity if purulent drainage is present
4. Audiometric testing
5. Testing to rule out a brain lesion or Meniere's syndrome if an infectious etiology cannot be ascertained

Planning

1. Safe, effective care environment
  A. Prevent avoidable injury and/or infection.
  B. Increase client's knowledge of disease process, diagnostic procedures, and treatment.
2. Physiological integrity
  A. Increase comfort.
  B. Assist client to adjust to alterations in sensory perception.
3. Psychosocial integrity
  A. Facilitate effective coping.
4. Health promotion and maintenance
  A. Increase client's knowledge of home care and follow-up.

Implementation

1. Assess, record, and report signs and symptoms and reactions to treatment.
2. Provide bed rest with head immobilized between pillows.
3. Administer meclizine po to control vertigo as prescribed.
4. Administer mild sedatives as ordered to relax client.
5. Administer antibiotics as prescribed to combat diffuse purulent labyrinthitis.
6. Administer oral fluids to prevent dehydration from vomiting.
7. Administer IV fluids as ordered if nausea and vomiting are severe.
8. Instruct client not to turn head quickly.
9. Request consultation with an audiologist to evaluate hearing loss.

10. Prepare client for surgical excision of the cholesteatoma and drainage of the infected areas of the middle and inner ear, if required.
11. Keep side rails up to prevent falls.
12. Administer antiemetics as prescribed for severe vomiting episodes.
13. Record intake and output.
14. Reassure client.
15. Instruct client to limit activities in which vertigo may be hazardous, such as climbing or driving a car, during recovery period.
16. Instruct client regarding disease process, diagnostic procedures, treatment (including medication), home care, and follow-up.

Evaluation

1. Reports increased comfort, absence of pain
2. Does not experience tinnitus and vertigo
3. Shows no signs of avoidable injury and/or infection
4. Maintains appropriate auditory perception
5. Demonstrates understanding of disease process, diagnostic procedures, treatment (including medication), home care, and need for follow-up

1. A client with Bell's palsy does not blink the affected eye. The nurse should:

   A. Apply an eye patch to the affected eye at all times
   B. Ask the client to keep both eyes closed
   C. Assess pupil reaction to light and accommodation
   D. Obtain medical orders for eye lubrication

2. A client has Bell's palsy, and the nurse is planning to assess the client's ability to hear. Of the following, which is the *best* way to test for hearing?

   A. Face the client directly and whisper, "Can you hear me?"
   B. Hold a watch to the client's ear and ask, "Can you hear this watch?"
   C. Stand behind the client and say, "Raise your hand."
   D. Use a tuning fork to test lateralization of sound.

3. A client with right hemiplegia is awake and alert. The client is given exercises to do during the day. One afternoon the client seems very discouraged, so the nurse plans to motivate her by:

   A. Reassuring her that there is no need for her to feel discouraged
   B. Reinforcing the small gains she has made
   C. Suggesting that she could rest today and exercise again tomorrow
   D. Explaining that exercise is necessary to get better

4. Pupil checks every hour are ordered for a client with CVA. This is an important assessment because:

   A. Blurred vision is a sign of increasing ICP
   B. Cranial nerve III exits from the brain stem
   C. Dilated and fixed pupils indicate cardiac arrest
   D. Pinpoint pupils result from CNS depressant drugs

5. If a cerebrovascular injury involves the pyramidal tract, the nurse expects to observe:

   A. Intention tremors
   B. Loss of pain and temperature sensation
   C. Loss of equilibrium
   D. Paralysis of voluntary movement

6. A client has had a CVA. When placing the client on the affected side, it is important to have pillows between the entire length of the legs to prevent:

   A. Adduction of the hip
   B. External rotation of the hip
   C. Flexion of the knee
   D. Plantarflexion

7. A client with a CVA has a diminished gag reflex. The nurse will:

   A. Instill artificial tears
   B. Offer small sips of clear liquids
   C. Maintain a side-lying position
   D. Test cranial nerves III, IV, and VI

8. A female client at home with a CVA has become incontinent of urine. The nurse will teach the caregiver to:

   A. Apply powder to client's perineum
   B. Insert an indwelling catheter
   C. Limit client's fluid intake
   D. Place client on a bedpan according to a schedule

9. Nursing actions directed toward restoring bowel function are effective if the home-care client in 8:

   A. Can tell when she feels "constipated"
   B. Finishes her prune juice and cereal every day
   C. Has a soft formed stool each morning
   D. Tolerates 2400 mL of fluid daily

10. A female client with CVA sometimes has difficulty "finding" the words she wants to say. The nurse will encourage the client's visitors to:

    A. Be patient with client while she thinks of a word
    B. End the visit if she becomes frustrated and angry
    C. Finish her sentence for her if they know what she wants to say
    D. Tactfully change the subject when she cannot find the word she wants to use

11. A client has had a CVA with expressive aphasia. When assisting the client to communicate during the early period after the CVA, it is *most* important for the nurse to:

    A. Create signals for client to use
    B. Speak loudly and clearly
    C. Stand directly in front of the client
    D. Write directions in large letters

12. In a client with left hemiplegia, the nurse is applying pain by pressing on the base of the client's fingernail to assess level of consciousness. The client's *best* response is:

    A. Flexion of both arms
    B. Flexion of the unaffected arm and unaffected leg
    C. Grimacing (making a face)
    D. Pulling the hand away

13. To *best* help a female client cope with a change of body image due to hemiparesis, the nurse would:

    A. Ask the client to tell how she feels
    B. Encourage the client to be independent with grooming
    C. Focus on ability rather than disability
    D. Keep her environment free of clutter

14. After head injury, a client's vital signs are stabilized and he is posted for a CT scan. To prepare him for this test, the nurse needs to understand that a CT scan:

    A. Involves injection of a radiopaque contrast medium into an artery, which causes a burning sensation
    B. Is a measure of electrical energy flowing away from the brain
    C. Lasts only a few minutes, but he will have to remain flat for 12 hours after the test
    D. Requires him to lie very still during the examination

15. A male client with herniated nucleus pulposis (HNP) had a myelogram this morning. To prevent headache, the nurse instructs him to remain flat in bed for 6 hours, and the nurse will:

    A. Dim the lights in his room
    B. Force fluids
    C. Offer analgesic medication
    D. Turn him every 2 hours from side to side

16. After a cerebral angiogram, the nurse will encourage the client to:

    A. Ask for assistance with ambulation
    B. Drink fluids
    C. Turn, cough, and breathe deeply
    D. Void

17. To prepare a female client for an MRI, the nurse explains that the client will:

    A. Be asked to lie still during the entire procedure and will hear a humming sound
    B. Have an injection of a radiopaque contrast medium into her vein
    C. Have many small electrodes placed on her scalp
    D. Need to stay in bed with the head of the bed elevated for 6–8 hours after the procedure

18. A client with Guillain-Barré syndrome is going to undergo plasmapheresis and is concerned about what it means. The nurse's response is based on the understanding that plasmapheresis:

    A. Alleviates symptoms by removing autoimmune antibodies from the blood
    B. May cause a mild allergic reaction with generalized itching
    C. Prevents secondary bacterial infection to the nervous system
    D. Reduces the need for O$_2$ while the client is on a respirator

19. To help prevent tonic-clonic–type seizures due to epilepsy, the nurse will teach a client to:

    A. Avoid any situation that produces fatigue
    B. Refrain from participating in competitive sports
    C. Take extra medication if an infection is present
    D. Try to determine factors that consistently precede a seizure

20. Which of the following assessments *most* likely indicates a complication of total hip replacement during the early postoperative period?

    A. Both legs cool to the touch
    B. Calf tenderness when the foot is dorsiflexed
    C. Tenderness at the surgical site
    D. Lightheadedness when standing

21. When teaching a mother not to continually lift her small child by his arms, the nurse hopes to prevent which dangerous complication?

    A. Bursitis
    B. Dislocation

    C. Greenstick fracture
    D. Subluxation

22. To prevent recurrence of pain related to carpal tunnel syndrome, the nurse would encourage the client to:

    A. Avoid activities causing flexion and extension of the wrist joint
    B. Elevate the wrist joint by wearing a sling
    C. Immobilize the wrist and finger joints with a splint
    D. Take aspirin every 4 hours while awake

23. The nurse expects a person with rheumatoid arthritis to have the *most* difficulty with pain and stiffness after:

    A. ADL
    B. Heat applications
    C. Meals
    D. Sleep

24. When caring for a 2-month-old child in Bryant's traction, the nurse observes that his buttocks are resting on the bed. The nurse should:

    A. Elevate the foot of the bed
    B. Increase the weights
    C. Lift his buttocks off the bed
    D. Take no action

25. When counseling women about exercise to prevent osteoporosis, the nurse knows the *best* exercise is:

    A. Isometric exercises of all major muscle groups
    B. Leg raises with the knees bent
    C. Swimming
    D. Walking

26. When helping an 82-year-old woman with advanced osteoporosis to complete morning care, the nurse should:

    A. Avoid bright lights and loud noises
    B. Be gentle when moving her
    C. Keep the head of her bed elevated 30 degrees
    D. Restrict fluids to 1500 mL/day

27. When teaching a woman taking estrogen replacement therapy how to prevent postmenopausal osteoporosis, the nurse teaches the signs and symptoms of:

    A. Deep vein thrombosis
    B. Increased intraocular pressure
    C. Renal calculi
    D. Uterine atony

28. After 10 minutes of pelvic traction for herniated nucleus pulposus (HNP), a client tells the nurse that he has severe pain radiating down one leg. The nurse should:

    A. Apply a warm compress to his lower back
    B. Call the physician
    C. Reassure him that this is expected with pelvic traction
    D. Remove the traction

29. Which of the following should lead the nurse to suspect compartment syndrome after tibial fracture?

    A. Warm, reddened extremity
    B. Cool skin temperature
    C. Decreased capillary refill
    D. Severe pain with burning in the extremity

30. A young girl has a closed reduction of a fractured ulna and has a synthetic cast. She asks if she can take a shower. The nurse should respond:
    A. "It may take a long time for the cast padding to dry."
    B. "It is unsafe for you to shower alone."
    C. "It can lead to a serious infection."
    D. "Warm water could soften the cast."

31. Which of the following assessments is the *best* indication of adequate circulation to the extremities for a child with a hip spica cast?
    A. Blanching of toenails is seen when pressure is applied.
    B. Circulation to toenails returns within 3 seconds after blanching.
    C. The child is wiggling the toes.
    D. Toes on each foot feel warm to the touch.

32. The primary purpose of Buck's extension for the immediate treatment of hip fracture is to:
    A. Eliminate rotation of the femur
    B. Immobilize the fracture
    C. Maintain abduction
    D. Reduce the fracture

33. When assessing a client in Buck's traction, the nurse observes the client's affected foot resting on the foot of the bed. The appropriate intervention is to:
    A. Place a pillow between the affected foot and the foot of the bed
    B. Pull the client up in bed
    C. Take no action
    D. Turn the client to the side

34. The nurse is assessing a 46-year-old man with a fractured pelvis due to an automobile accident. Which of the following signs or symptoms alerts the nurse to a serious complication of pelvic fracture?
    A. Ecchymosis of the perineum
    B. Edema over the symphysis pubis
    C. Hematuria
    D. Discomfort at the fracture site

35. Because a client with a fractured femur is at risk for a fat embolism, the nurse should monitor the client for:
    A. Pulmonary edema
    B. Osteomyelitis
    C. Petechiae
    D. Seizures

36. Which of the following is an early sign of fat embolism and should alert the nurse to the need for medical intervention?
    A. Irritability and confusion
    B. Fat in the stool
    C. Hyperglycemia
    D. Pruritus

37. Following an injury, the nurse should assess for fat embolism:
    A. During the first 12 hours
    B. During the first 48 hours

C. If the client has chronic respiratory disease
D. If the client is in skeletal traction

38. When caring for skeletal traction pin sites, the nurse will:
    A. Apply continuous warm sterile compresses
    B. Cover the site with antibiotic ointment and a dressing
    C. Use a heat lamp twice a day
    D. Remove serous drainage crusts

39. To *best* assess circulation to extremities, the nurse should check:
    A. Capillary refill
    B. Motion and sensation
    C. Pain and pallor
    D. Skin temperature

40. To strengthen muscles in a client's unaffected leg in preparation for crutch walking, the nurse would encourage the client to periodically:
    A. Flex and extend the unaffected knee while prone
    B. Press the back of unaffected knee into the mattress while supine
    C. Squeeze the buttocks together when sitting
    D. Change position frequently

41. A nurse has been summoned to a neighbor's yard to give emergency help to someone who has just sustained a traumatic amputation of his hand. The nurse will attempt to stop the bleeding by:
    A. Applying ice directly to the stump
    B. Applying pressure to the end of the stump
    C. Elevating the stump above the person's heart
    D. Wrapping a tourniquet as close to the end of the stump as possible

42. After an above-the-knee amputation, the nurse will encourage the client to lie prone periodically to:
    A. Extend the client's hip joint
    B. Increase the client's vital lung capacity
    C. Prepare the client by lifting weights for crutch walking
    D. Provide diversion

43. The nurse's primary objective in the immediate treatment of a person who has just sustained a traumatic amputation is to:
    A. Help the person to cope with the loss
    B. Prepare the amputated part for possible reimplantation
    C. Prevent infection at the amputated site
    D. Provide pain relief

44. A young man has tumbled down the ski slope without one of his skis. The nurse finds him at the bottom of the hill complaining of severe pain in his lower leg. The nurse should:
    A. Assess for compartmental syndrome
    B. Cover both legs with a blanket
    C. Elevate his injured leg
    D. Splint his injured leg

45. The nurse is caring for a client in Buck's extension for treatment of an intratrochanteric fracture of the femur. Which of the following signs or symptoms alerts the nurse to possible peroneal nerve damage of the affected side?
    A. Difficulty dorsiflexing the ankle
    B. Pain in the Achilles tendon
    C. Skin breakdown around the ankle
    D. Swelling and redness of the calf

46. Postprocedure nursing care for a client who has had an endoscopic retrograde cholangiopancreatogram (ERCP) includes:
    A. Abdominal binder
    B. Cleansing enema
    C. NPO
    D. Skin care

47. A client is being taught by the nurse about his laboratory and diagnostic test. The nurse explains that an accurate and safe method of detecting gallstones is:
    A. Biopsy
    B. Oral cholecystogram
    C. Radionuclide imaging
    D. Ultrasound

48. When assessing a client with obstructive cholelithiasis, the nurse might expect to find:
    A. Abdominal distention
    B. Dark urine
    C. Diminished bowel sounds
    D. Loose stools

49. In a client with a stone lodged in the cystic duct, the nurse would expect to observe:
    A. Beginning jaundice, dark urine, and clay-colored stools
    B. Burning and frequency in voiding, cloudy urine
    C. Colicky pain after a fatty meal
    D. Petechiae, melena, and possible hematemesis

50. After a cholecystectomy, a client asks why he has to have a nasogastric (NG) tube. The nurse states the purpose of the NG tube is to:
    A. Administer high-caloric liquid feedings
    B. Facilitate collection of gastric secretions
    C. Prevent postoperative distention
    D. Simplify administration of medications

51. A client with cholecystectomy and exploration of the common bile duct has a T-tube and a Jackson-Pratt drain. Because of the location of the incision, an important nursing action is to encourage the client to:
    A. Lie on the unoperative side
    B. Remain in a semi-Fowler position
    C. Splint the incision when moving
    D. Turn, cough, and breathe deeply

52. In a 40-year-old client in whom bone disease has been ruled out, an elevated serum alkaline phosphatase is a sensitive measure of:
    A. Biliary tract obstruction
    B. Enlarged liver

C. Pancreatic insufficiency
D. Splenic enlargement

53. A priority nursing intervention before sending a male client for an endoscopic retrograde cholangiopancreatography (ERCP) is to:
    A. Administer radiopaque tablets
    B. Check his PT
    C. Give him a cleansing enema
    D. Remove his dentures

54. After which diagnostic test would the nurse assess for bleeding from a client?
    A. Cholecystogram
    B. ERCP
    C. IVP
    D. Percutaneous transhepatic cholangiogram (PTC)

55. After a liver biopsy, the nurse will assess the client for:
    A. Allergic reaction to iodine
    B. Elevated serum bilirubin
    C. Hypertension
    D. Peritonitis

56. Twenty-four hours after cholecystectomy, a client's T-tube has drained 500 mL. The nurse will:
    A. Clamp the T-tube
    B. Empty the bag and discard the drainage
    C. Lower the head of the bed
    D. Take no action after documenting the observation

57. The nurse expects which of the following laboratory results for a client with jaundice?
    A. Decreased PT
    B. Elevated serum bilirubin
    C. Elevated serum potassium
    D. Metabolic acidosis

58. Which of the following is *most* likely to put a client with cirrhosis at risk for hepatic encephalopathy?
    A. Anorexia and weight loss
    B. Diarrhea and tenesmus
    C. GI bleeding
    D. Nausea and vomiting

59. About 30 minutes after a Blakemore-Sengstaken tube for bleeding esophageal varices is inserted, an alert client becomes short of breath. The nurse should first:
    A. Check for airway obstruction
    B. Deflate the esophageal part of the tube
    C. Raise the head of the bed and increase the O_2 flow rate
    D. Remove the tube

60. When caring for a client with advanced cirrhosis, the nurse is alert for changes in all of the following. Which change suggests hepatic encephalopathy?
    A. Level of consciousness
    B. Respiratory status
    C. Urine output
    D. Vital signs

61. The nurse is caring for a client at home with advanced cirrhosis of the liver. The client's laboratory reports reveal hypokalemia, anemia, prolonged PT, and normal serum ammonia. The nurse encourages the client to follow a diet that is:

    A. Bland, low protein, low sodium
    B. High calorie, restricted protein, low sodium
    C. High protein, high fat, high potassium
    D. Well balanced, low sodium

62. A person with advanced cirrhosis tells the nurse that he plans to do all of the following. Which one indicates the need for further health teaching?

    A. Avoid contact with infectious people.
    B. Supplement his diet with multivitamins.
    C. Take a sleeping pill at bedtime.
    D. Try his best to avoid alcohol.

63. The nurse will place a client with ascites in which position?

    A. Any position as long as he or she changes it often
    B. Flat with legs elevated
    C. Head of bed elevated
    D. Side lying

64. A client with cirrhosis is on a 1-g sodium diet. Which of the following drugs promotes sodium excretion while conserving potassium?

    A. Ethacrynic acid (Edecrin)
    B. Furosemide
    C. Hydrochlorothiazide (HydroDiuril)
    D. Spironolactone (Aldactone)

65. A client with cirrhosis is receiving 100 mL of 25% serum albumin solution IV. The nurse knows that this treatment is effective if there is:

    A. Decreased anorexia and itching
    B. Easier breathing
    C. Increased serum glucose
    D. Increased urine output

66. A client with cirrhosis is discharged with a prescription for lactulose. Which statement indicates he understands what the nurse has told him about lactulose?

    A. "I'll keep it in the refrigerator."
    B. "I'll mix it with some apple juice."
    C. "I'll take it with a laxative."
    D. "I'll stop taking it if I have loose stools."

67. A client with cirrhosis is asking for a snack. Because his serum ammonia remains elevated, the nurse would recommend:

    A. Applesauce
    B. Cheeseburger
    C. Granola bar
    D. Unsalted peanuts

68. In a client with cirrhosis, which nursing assessment is a probable sign that the serum ammonia level is increasing?

    A. Ask the client about numbness in the extremities.
    B. Assess ability to write clearly.

    C. Look for extreme nervousness.
    D. Take systolic blood pressure.

69. Oral neomycin and neomycin enemas are prescribed for a client with cirrhosis. The nurse explains to the client that the purpose of this order is to:

    A. Help reduce the ammonia level
    B. Increase bowel elimination
    C. Prevent infection
    D. Treat secondary infection

70. Just prior to a paracentesis for tense ascites, the nurse will prepare a client by:

    A. Having him void
    B. Measuring his abdominal girth
    C. Placing him in a recumbent position
    D. Taking his temperature

71. A nursing goal for a client with cirrhosis is to reduce severe itchiness. The rationale for this goal is because this client has:

    A. Folic acid deficiency
    B. Hypokalemia
    C. Increased bilirubin levels
    D. Prolonged PT

72. After a liver biopsy in a client, the priority nursing intervention is to have the client:

    A. Force fluids
    B. Lie on the left side with head of bed elevated
    C. Lie on the right side on a pillow
    D. Wear a pressure dressing until bleeding subsides

73. The nurse suspects bleeding into the upper GI tract if the client with cirrhosis has:

    A. Black stools
    B. Clay-colored stools
    C. Rectal passage of bright red blood
    D. Shortness of breath

74. An expected result when a client is receiving lactulose (Cephulac) 30 mL po qd for elevated serum ammonia is:

    A. Diarrhea
    B. Headache and nasal stuffiness
    C. Increased urine output
    D. Nausea and vomiting

75. During an admission assessment, the nurse notes a client with hepatitis exhibits all of the following signs or symptoms. Which one is not related to hepatitis?

    A. Anorexia
    B. Bloody stools
    C. Dark urine
    D. Yellow sclera

76. To prevent spread of hepatitis A virus (HAV) infection, the nurse is specially careful when:

    A. Disposing of food trays
    B. Changing the IV tubing
    C. Emptying the bedpan
    D. Taking an oral temperature

77. The nurse will teach a client at home with type B hepatitis to include foods in diet that are:

    A. High protein, high carbohydrate, low fat
    B. High protein, high fat, low sodium
    C. Low calorie, small, frequent meals
    D. Low protein, low carbohydrate, vitamin supplements

78. A client with hepatitis B tells the nurse that she expects all of the following outcomes of her illness. Which one indicates the need for further health teaching?

    A. Full recovery occurs about 3–4 months after symptoms subside.
    B. People with severe symptoms are unlikely to become carriers.
    C. It can lead to chronic hepatitis or to cancer.
    D. It is not contagious once symptoms appear.

79. Skin care for a client with hepatitis B should be directed toward:

    A. Decreasing jaundice
    B. Preventing perspiration
    C. Reducing edema
    D. Relieving itching

80. A client with acute pancreatitis asks for a cup of coffee. The nurse's response is based on the understanding that:

    A. Caffeine has a stimulating effect on the CNS
    B. Decaffeinated coffee, in small sips, would be comforting
    C. She is NPO in preparation for surgery
    D. She is NPO to prevent stimulation of pancreatic secretions

81. When taking a nursing history, the nurse notes that a client with acute pancreatitis exhibits all of the following symptoms. Which one is not directly related to pancreatitis?

    A. Abdominal and back pain
    B. Frothy sputum
    C. Nausea and vomiting
    D. Rebound tenderness

82. When obtaining a health history from a client with acute pancreatitis, the nurse should ask about:

    A. Alcohol consumption
    B. Emotional stress
    C. Family history of diabetes
    D. Recent weight gain

83. A client with acute pancreatitis has an NG tube for low, intermittent suction to prevent:

    A. Gastric distention
    B. Gastrocolic reflex
    C. Pancreatic stimulation
    D. Peristalsis

84. To assess for complications of sulfisoxazole therapy for UTI, a client should have which of the following laboratory tests?

    A. ABGs
    B. Blood culture
    C. Serum creatinine
    D. Stool for occult blood

85. The nurse should teach a client with pyelonephritis to:

    A. Avoid upper respiratory infections
    B. Drink 8 oz of orange juice every day
    C. Prevent urethral contamination
    D. Take 1 g aspirin tid for fever and chills

86. Assessment of the client with pyelonephritis reveals all of the following signs or symptoms. Which one is unexpected and should be reported to the client's physician?

    A. Cloudy urine
    B. Flank pain
    C. General malaise
    D. Hypertension

87. Before a client with pyelonephritis is discharged, the nurse instructs the client to seek medical attention at the first signs of UTI. These signs include:

    A. Burning, frequency, and urgency in voiding
    B. Difficulty initiating urine flow, cloudy urine
    C. General malaise, fever, sore throat
    D. Polyuria, low back pain, stress incontinence

88. Nursing assessment of a client with cystitis should include:

    A. Checking for back pain
    B. Monitoring blood gases
    C. Palpating for rebound tenderness
    D. Testing urine for sugar

89. The nurse should teach a client taking a sulfa drug to:

    A. Chew tablets completely before swallowing
    B. Disregard the blue color of her urine
    C. Drink 2–3 qt of liquids daily
    D. Lie down if tinnitus should occur

90. The nurse has administered methenamine hippurate (Hiprex), a urinary antiseptic. The client tells the nurse he plans to do all of the following. Which one is not a nursing implication for methenamine and requires further client teaching?

    A. Avoid over-the-counter antacids containing sodium bicarbonate.
    B. Weigh oneself daily.
    C. Take with meals.
    D. Take with ascorbic acid or cranberry juice.

91. When implementing a solution for a continuous bladder irrigation, the solution must be:

    A. Body temperature
    B. Infused rapidly
    C. Normal saline (0.9%)
    D. Sterile

92. Before a client taking corticosteroid immunosuppressive drugs for a kidney transplant goes home, the nurse should validate that he knows that:

    A. Salt must be avoided
    B. The dosage must be reduced gradually
    C. The drug must be taken daily
    D. Urine must be tested daily for protein

93. One of the nursing diagnoses for a client with end-stage renal disease (ESRD) is: Inadequate tissue perfusion related to anemia. Which of the following is a nursing order for this nursing diagnosis?

    A. Advise against the use of salt substitutes.
    B. Administer antihypertensives as ordered.
    C. Administer erythropoietin as ordered.
    D. Monitor fluid balance.

94. The nurse teaches a person with chronic glomerulonephritis to have which of the following checked regularly?

    A. Blood pressure
    B. Blood sugar
    C. Hematocrit
    D. Serum sodium

95. The nurse is preparing a teaching plan for a client with end-stage renal disease. Which of the following foods is lowest in biological value?

    A. Bread
    B. Eggs
    C. Meat
    D. Milk

96. A client with acute renal failure has gained 1½ lb since yesterday. The nurse anticipates the client's treatment plan will call for reduction in:

    A. Caloric intake
    B. Dietary calcium
    C. Fluid intake
    D. Steroid medication

97. Which of the following assessment findings is not expected in a client in the early stage of acute renal failure?

    A. Acidosis
    B. Diuresis
    C. Hyperkalemia
    D. Hypertension

98. The nurse teaches the family of a client with end-stage renal disease to offer a diet high in:

    A. Carbohydrates
    B. Fluids
    C. Potassium
    D. Protein

99. A client with end-stage renal disease has the following nursing diagnosis: Fluid imbalance related to compromised ability of the kidneys to excrete urine. Of the following, the *most* important nursing order for this diagnosis is:

    A. Increase fluid intake
    B. Monitor urine specific gravity
    C. Measure intake and output
    D. Weigh every day

100. A client with acute renal failure has the following nursing diagnosis: High risk for decreased cardiac output related to arrhythmia due to hyperkalemia. Of the following, the *most* important nursing order for this diagnosis is:

    A. Assess bowel sounds
    B. Avoid KCl salt substitutes

C. Monitor ECG
D. Prepare for dialysis

101. When caring for a client in acute renal failure, it is *most* important for the nurse to call the physician to report changes in:

    A. BUN
    B. ECG
    C. Hematocrit
    D. Weight

102. The nurse should teach a client with recurrent glomerulonephritis to:

    A. Avoid excessive exposure to the sun
    B. Check her urine daily for the presence of protein
    C. Contact her physician should she experience a headache
    D. Have a throat culture done every time she gets a sore throat

103. One of the outcomes of care for a client with acute renal failure is: Cardiac output is normal. Which of the following is the *most* important evaluation criterion for this outcome?

    A. Blood pressure remains stable.
    B. Pulse is regular in rate and rhythm.
    C. Serum creatinine is within normal limits.
    D. Serum potassium is within normal limits.

104. Prevention of which of the following problems is the *most* important goal when caring for a child taking steroid therapy for nephrosis?

    A. Anorexia
    B. Ascites
    C. Diarrhea
    D. Infection

105. Controlling edema in a child with nephrosis is primarily directed toward preventing:

    A. Potassium retention
    B. Protein loss
    C. Renin production
    D. Sodium loss

106. The nurse is giving prednisone to a 5-year-old child with nephrosis to:

    A. Cause diuresis
    B. Prevent sodium retention
    C. Reduce urinary protein loss
    D. Suppress infection

107. The nurse teaches the parents of a 5-year-old child with nephrosis to offer foods:

    A. High in fat
    B. High in protein
    C. Low in calories
    D. Low in purine

108. The nurse should call the physician to report which of the following assessment findings for a child in the early stage of nephrosis?

    A. Cloudy urine
    B. Oliguria

C. Rising blood pressure
D. Weight gain

109. After transurethral resection, a client has a catheter with continuous bladder irrigation of isotonic saline. The nurse notices his urine has changed from pale red to dark red. The nurse should:

A. Increase the rate of flow of the irrigating solution
B. Notify the surgeon
C. Remove the catheter
D. Take no action

110. A client with benign prostatic hypertrophy (BPH) has difficulty voiding, but he is reluctant to have an operation. The nurse understands that if BPH is not corrected it is *most* likely to result in:

A. Glomerulonephritis
B. Hydronephrosis
C. Nephroptosis
D. Pyelonephritis

111. During the admission assessment of a 57-year-old man in the hospital for a transurethral resection of BPH, the nurse expects to observe:

A. Frequency and burning in micturition
B. Low temperature
C. Narrowed stream of urine flow
D. Pruritus around the urethral meatus

112. A client has just returned from the recovery room after a transurethral resection (TUR). His roommate calls to report blood in the client's urine bag. After promising to check the client, the nurse should:

A. Assure the roommate this is normal
B. Call the surgeon
C. Check the client's vital signs
D. Raise the foot of the client's bed

113. The nurse has taught a client to expect some dribbling for a period of time after TUR. The teaching is effective if the client tells the nurse that he will:

A. Avoid standing for long periods of time
B. Practice perineal exercises
C. Take fluids only with meals
D. Wear plastic protection until dribbling stops

114. Before discharge after TUR, the client should tell the nurse that he will call his physician if he develops:

A. Diminished sexual performance
B. Dark-colored urine
C. Light-colored urine
D. Narrowed stream of urine

115. A client has a traction catheter after a TUR. The nurse finds him in high Fowler position, and he tells the nurse that he is "more comfortable now." The nurse should:

A. Check the patency of the catheter
B. Lower the head of the bed and explain why
C. Observe the color of the urine and document findings
D. Take no action at this time

116. A client's call light is on. He is having severe pain from renal colic. The goal of nursing care right now is to:

A. Collect a urine specimen
B. Prevent hydronephrosis
C. Relieve pain
D. Teach ways of preventing calculi

117. Before discharge, the nurse should ascertain that a client understands that renal calculi are more likely to develop if:

A. He drinks coffee every day
B. He voids frequently
C. His urine contains sugar
D. His urine is concentrated

118. The nurse teaches a man who has passed a calcium phosphate kidney stone to:

A. Alternate an acid-ash diet with an alkaline-ash diet
B. Eliminate all milk products from his diet
C. Have his urine checked each month for infection
D. Maintain a high fluid intake daily

119. When taking a history of a client undergoing a renal evaluation, which of the following would be contraindicated if the client is allergic to shellfish?

A. Cystoscopy
B. IVP
C. Renal scan
D. Ultrasound

120. A postprocedure nursing intervention for a client undergoing extracorporeal shock wave lithotripsy includes:

A. Force fluids
B. Frequent dressing changes
C. Head of bed flat for 4 hours
D. Low-sodium diet

121. Nursing care for a client at home with an indwelling urinary catheter should include:

A. Changing the catheter every month
B. Clamping the catheter for 2 hours a day
C. Continuous bladder irrigation
D. Irrigating the catheter once a week

122. A client who is collecting a 24-hour urine for creatinine clearance tells the nurse that he voided a small amount of urine into the toilet. The nurse should:

A. Call the lab for instructions
B. Restart the test tomorrow
C. Estimate the amount, then add the number of milliliters to the lab report
D. Take no action

123. When assessing a client, the nurse knows it is usually not necessary to test for temperature and vibration if the client:

A. Can discriminate between sharp and dull
B. Has intact cranial nerve function
C. Has weakness or paralysis
D. Is alert and aware

124. When assessing sensory function in an alert client, the nurse:

    A. Includes light touch, pain, temperature, and vibration
    B. Prevents injury when testing for deep pain
    C. Scatters stimuli to cover most dermatomes in the extremities
    D. Squeezes the trapezius muscle to test for central pain

125. The nurse notes normal assessment findings for posture, balance, and gait. This reflects an intact:

    A. Cerebellum and extrapyramidal tract
    B. Cerebrum and pyramidal tract
    C. Occipital lobe
    D. Reticular activating system

126. When assessing the client's cranial nerves, the nurse knows a normal expected finding when testing the function of cranial nerve XII (hypoglossal) is that:

    A. Eyebrows raise symmetrically
    B. Tongue is symmetrical with no fasciculation
    C. Trapezius and sternocleidomastoid muscles have equal strength bilaterally
    D. Uvula is in midline

127. When the nurse is testing the sensory component of cranial nerve V (trigeminal), the nurse does this with client's:

    A. Cheeks puffed out
    B. Eyes closed
    C. Head turned to the side
    D. Teeth clenched

128. When testing cranial nerve II (optic), the nurse should:

    A. Ask the client if she or he wears glasses
    B. Dim the lights in the room
    C. Instruct client to keep both eyes open when visual fields are tested by confrontation
    D. Use an ophthalmoscope to measure pupil size

129. The nurse would use deep pain stimuli, such as squeezing the trapezius muscle, if the client is:

    A. Demonstrating signs of increased ICP
    B. Flaccid on one side of the body
    C. Uncooperative and demanding
    D. Unresponsive to verbal commands

130. The nurse prepares a client for an EEG by:

    A. Administering barbiturate medication
    B. Keeping him NPO
    C. Shampooing his hair and keeping his scalp damp
    D. Withholding fluids containing caffeine

131. A nursing diagnosis for a client with Guillain-Barré syndrome is potential ineffective gas exchange related to:

    A. Increased ICP
    B. Insufficient acetylcholine
    C. Muscle weakness
    D. Sustained seizures

132. A client admitted to the emergency room with a head injury is being hyperventilated with 100% O_2. The nurse explains that the reason for this is to:

    A. Fully aerate the alveoli
    B. Increase PaO_2
    C. Lower $PaCO_2$
    D. Stimulate the reticular activating system

133. The nurse observes for "Battle's sign" or "raccoon sign" in a client with a head injury. The nurse should also look for:

    A. Aphasia
    B. Hemiparesis
    C. Paresthesia of the distal extremities
    D. Spinal fluid leak

134. The nurse is caring for a client with an occipital lobe tumor. All of the following were documented on admission. Which should be documented by the nurse daily?

    A. Difficulty in voiding
    B. Insomnia
    C. Irregular pupil size
    D. Loss of appetite

135. A nursing diagnosis in the emergency treatment of any client with a fractured spine includes high risk for injury related to:

    A. Elevating the legs
    B. External rotation of the hips
    C. Spinal movement
    D. Supine position

136. A teenager dove off a pier into 3 feet of water. During transport to the emergency room, it is most important for the nurse to:

    A. Begin IV therapy with isotonic saline
    B. Assess pupil reaction to light frequently
    C. Prevent spinal movement
    D. Reorient the client to person, place, and time

137. A 28-year-old man has injured his neck in a diving accident. A neurological exam reveals that he has lost sensation and motion of both upper and lower extremities. His family is very concerned and wants to know if he will regain function. The nurse explains to them that:

    A. Full recovery is likely if he has a good rehabilitation program
    B. He probably has spinal shock
    C. His spinal cord will be sutured together
    D. No regain in function is possible

138. Before discharge, a client is scheduled for an EEG. To prepare him for this test, the nurse explains to him that he will feel:

    A. A sensation of warmth during the test
    B. A tiny prickly sensation when the current is turned on
    C. No discomfort during the procedure
    D. Somewhat dizzy after the test is completed

139. After tube feeding, the nurse should irrigate a percutaneous endoscopic gastrostomy tube with:
    A. 30 mL of air
    B. 45 mL of normal saline
    C. 15 mL of sterile solution (saline or water)
    D. 30 mL of tap water

140. The nurse is observing a client with a percutaneous endoscopic gastrostomy tube administer his own tube feeding. He needs further instruction if he:
    A. Checks for residual before the feeding
    B. Instills the feeding at room temperature
    C. Lies down after the feeding
    D. Takes 15 minutes to instill 500 mL of feeding

141. An 86-year-old client is receiving IV lipid emulsions. The nurse gives IV lipid emulsions:
    A. At a rate of 10 mL/min
    B. Through a filter
    C. Warmed to body temperature
    D. Without piggyback additives

142. A serious complication of total parenteral nutrition (TPN) is hyperosmolar diuresis. The nurse evaluates the cause of this as:
    A. Allergy to certain amino acids
    B. Insufficient carbohydrates
    C. Precipitates in the solution
    D. Rapid infusion

143. The nurse evaluates the teaching of a client taking liquid iron medication as effective if he tells the nurse that he will take his medicine with:
    A. Antacid
    B. Milk
    C. Orange juice
    D. Water

144. The nurse evaluates teaching of a client with antrectomy as effective with regard to prevention of dumping syndrome if he tells the nurse that he will:
    A. Avoid concentrated carbohydrates
    B. Ambulate after meals
    C. Eliminate fats from the diet
    D. Take fluids with meals

145. The nurse evaluates discharge teaching of a client with peptic ulcer as effective if she tells the nurse that she will read labels of over-the-counter drugs and will avoid those containing:
    A. Aspirin
    B. Calcium
    C. Magnesium
    D. Sodium

146. The nurse evaluates the teaching of a client with hiatal hernia as effective if the client tells the nurse that she will:
    A. Avoid bending over after eating
    B. Avoid highly concentrated carbohydrates
    C. Lie down after meals
    D. Sleep on her left side

147. The nurse explains to a client that the client is NPO immediately after an esophagogastroduodenoscopy (EGD) because she:
    A. Received topical local anesthesia
    B. Must keep her stomach empty for 4 hours
    C. Must remain flat for 12 hours
    D. Will have a sore throat

148. A client has a history of dumping syndrome following gastric surgery. Anticipated assessment findings for the client with dumping syndrome include:
    A. Bradycardia, perspiration, confusion
    B. Dizziness, tachycardia, palpitations
    C. Pallor, dry skin, constipation
    D. Drowsiness, epigastric burning, flushed skin

149. The nurse evaluates the teaching of an elderly client on a low-sodium diet and taking antacids for peptic ulcer as effective if he tells the nurse:
    A. Aluminum antacids should be avoided
    B. Antacids cause acid imbalance
    C. Chewable antacids are more effective than liquids
    D. Sodium bicarbonate relieves ulcer pain

150. After hemorrhoidectomy, a client asks for a rubber ring to sit on. The nurse's response is based on the understanding that a partially inflated rubber ring may:
    A. Contaminate the operative site
    B. Impede circulation to the operative area
    C. Restrict full mobility in ADL
    D. Rupture, causing trauma to the operative site

151. After total gastrectomy, the nurse encourages the client to turn, cough, and breathe deeply because:
    A. Deep breathing will prevent postoperative vomiting and intestinal distention
    B. Marked changes in intrathoracic pressure will stimulate gastric drainage
    C. The abdominal incision will lead to shallow breathing in an attempt to avoid pain
    D. The phrenic nerve will be stimulated

152. A client was admitted for respiratory infection and had a positive sputum culture for histoplasmosis. He will be treated with amphotericin B IV. To reconstitute the medication, the nurse should mix the drug with which of the following solutions?
    A. Sterile water for injection without preservatives
    B. NaCl for injection
    C. 5% dextrose
    D. NaCl with electrolytes

153. The nurse weighs a client on a bed scale because the client cannot stand and is too weak to sit in a wheelchair. The client weighs 132 lb. The nurse calculates the client's weight in kilograms as:
    A. 129 kg
    B. 0.02 kg
    C. 66 kg
    D. 60 kg

154. Just as in the hospital or clinic, a nurse washes the hands well before caring for a client in her farm home. Which of the following practices contributes *most* to desired asepsis?

    A. Drying with a paper towel
    B. Generous soap lather
    C. Washing nail and finger base areas
    D. Use of warm water

155. When taking a client's blood pressure, the nurse identifies that errors in blood pressure readings are often due to:

    A. Rapid inflation and slow deflation
    B. Using the wrong size cuff
    C. Failure to hear all five Korotkoff sounds
    D. Failure to determine the baseline

156. Two days after surgery, a client has a temperature of 40° Celsius (C). How would you report this in Fahrenheit (F)?

    A. 104°F
    B. 98.6°F
    C. 100.4°F
    D. 99°F

157. A male client has received several IV injections of morphine for complaints of chest pain. The nurse should have resuscitative equipment and which of the following drugs to reduce adverse effects of morphine?

    A. Naloxone (Narcan)
    B. Niacin (Nicobid)
    C. Nitroglycerin
    D. Nitroprusside (Nipride)

158. A client is alert and oriented and knows his name and where he is. The nurse assesses him using the expression "oriented × 3." This means the client is oriented to:

    A. His total surroundings for 3 days in a row
    B. His total surroundings 3 times in a row
    C. Self, hospital, and season
    D. Person, place, and time

159. A 49-year-old client has been under extreme job stress for about 10 years. He is diagnosed as having an enlarged heart. Which of the following factors in his history is a modifiable risk factor?

    A. He has a family history of heart attacks.
    B. He has smoked one pack per day of cigarettes for 1 year.
    C. He exercises 4 times a week.
    D. He uses corn oil margarine and eats beef once a week.

160. A 24-year-old client has diminished popliteal and pedal pulses; his lower extremities are dusky red in the dependent position; and his skin is cool to touch, shiny, thin, and atrophic, with hair loss over the feet and toes. Based on these characteristics, the nurse suspects:

    A. Arterial insufficiency
    B. Venous insufficiency
    C. Varicose veins
    D. Raynaud's disease

161. A client complains of indigestion. The nurse begins an abdominal assessment. When obtaining subjective data (the client's history), the initial priority questions would pertain to:

    A. Diet history, oral care, and bowel patterns
    B. Skin care, sleep patterns, and reproduction
    C. Coping patterns, oral intake, and oral care
    D. Family risk factors, self-care, and exercise patterns

162. A 76-year-old male client slipped and fell when he was alone in the house. He managed to get himself up and into a chair, where he sat for several hours. His son came home later and took him to the hospital, where the client was diagnosed as having a broken right hip. Which of the following is appropriate to check for his lower extremities?

    A. Skin color of both lower extremities
    B. Edema of the right ankle
    C. Passive mobility of the right hip
    D. Sensitivity to temperature changes in both feet

163. A client is admitted for possible respiratory infection. His admission orders include: regular diet, ambulation ad lib, vital signs every 4 hours, ampicillin po 250 mg q6h. While the nurse is collecting a medical history, the client states that he is allergic to penicillin. The nurse should take which of the following actions?

    A. Note the allergy on the chart, and administer medication as ordered.
    B. Withhold the medication and note the allergy on the chart.
    C. Withhold the medication, and notify the physician of the client's allergies.
    D. Administer the medication while closely monitoring the client.

164. A 26-year-old woman is admitted for chemotherapy to treat Hodgkin's disease. Part of her drug therapy includes vincristine 0.01 mg/kg per week. The nurse should counsel the client on which of the following common adverse effects?

    A. Alopecia
    B. Fluid retention
    C. Diarrhea
    D. Polycythemia

165. The nurse should assess a client corticotropic hormone (ACTH) drug therapy for which of the following?

    A. Elevated calcium levels
    B. Dehydration
    C. New infections
    D. Changes in urine color

166. The physician has prescribed aminophylline (theophylline ethylenediamine) 450 mg (continuous release) q6h for a client with bronchial asthma. The medication is available in 225-mg continuous-release tablets. The nurse calculates that the client will receive one tablet every 6 hours. The client states: "I will not skip any doses of this medicine. I will call my doctor if

I have palpitations, vomiting, or trouble sleeping." After double-checking the dosage calculation, the nurse decides to:

A. Not administer the medication as prescribed and calculated
B. Administer two tablets of the medication instead of the dosage calculated
C. Administer the medication as prescribed and calculated, and monitor for theophylline blood levels and cardiorespiratory status
D. Administer the medication as prescribed and calculated, and proceed with further client teaching

167. The nurse instructs a client being discharged after a vaginal hysterectomy 4 days ago. Which of the following statements by the client indicates a need for further health teaching?

A. "I must complete the antibiotics as the physician ordered."
B. "I should not have alcohol while I'm on narcotic pain medications."
C. "I should not douche or have intercourse for 6 weeks."
D. "I should not exercise for 6 weeks."

168. A 64-year-old client is admitted with dyspnea, "heartburn," and pain in the left shoulder. A total history and physical examination should be done, but which immediate miniassessment is a priority at this time?

A. The heart
B. The abdomen
C. Current stressors
D. Recent life changes

169. In assessing a client's apical pulse, you know that the point of maximal impulse (PMI) is usually at which area of the heart?

A. LMCL, 5ICS
B. LMCL, 4ICS
C. LMCL, 2ICS
D. RMCL, 2ICS

170. A client who is considered to be an older adult is believed to be experiencing the developmental crisis (Erikson) of:

A. Ego integrity versus despair
B. Generativity versus stagnation
C. Identity versus role confusion
D. Intimacy versus isolation

171. The nurse palpates a client's left arm as he moves it. The nurse feels a grating sensation and hears a crackling sound. The nurse identifies this as:

A. Pruritus
B. Crepitus
C. Rales
D. Effusion

172. As the nurse inspects a client's skin, the nurse notes and records which of the following factors?

A. The location of any lesions
B. The client's allergies

C. Her family history
D. Her exposure to communicable disease

173. As the nurse continues to assess a client's skin, the nurse finds a blister. This is a serous fluid-filled area less than 1 cm in diameter, rising from below the skin surface. It is also called:

A. Macule
B. Papule
C. Pustule
D. Vesicle

174. A 44-year-old client has had to have both legs amputated because of peripheral vascular insufficiency. He has been told that he can eventually be fitted with prosthetic legs. How may the nurse best help him with his ambulation efforts after he gets his prosthesis?

A. Encourage his adjustment to a changed body image.
B. Allay his feelings of guilt about his injury.
C. Discourage his blaming of others for his plight.
D. Promote safe ambulation.

175. A 60-year-old man has a medical diagnosis of BPH. Which of the following signs and symptoms would the nurse expect to find during this assessment?

A. Urinary hesitancy, frequency, dribbling
B. Nocturia, increased force of the urinary stream
C. Bladder spasms, hematuria
D. Flank pain, hematuria

176. A spry 80-year-old woman has had glaucoma for many years. Even though she instills her eye drops regularly as ordered, the nurse should assess for which of the following complaints?

A. Decreasing visual acuity, eye pain
B. Increased blood pressure
C. Decreased vision at night
D. Nystagmus

177. A construction worker is seen by the occupational health nurse for a piece of glass lodged in his eye from an exploding light bulb. It would be *most* important for the nurse to:

A. Carefully remove the glass from the eye.
B. Offer reassurance that everything is OK.
C. Give a sedative to help relieve pain.
D. Encourage the client to rest in a sitting position.

178. A client with a spinal cord injury is at risk for a phenomenon called autonomic dysreflexia, once reflex activity below the level of the lesion occurs, causing visceral reflex activity. If symptoms occur, the nurse should:

A. Assess for distended bowel or bladder.
B. Assess for urinary continence.
C. Assess for coping behaviors.
D. Promote assessment for skin disruption.

179. A client is receiving rifampin (Rifadin) po for treatment of tuberculosis. The nurse should instruct the client on which of the following?

A. Avoid taking with milk.
B. Avoid taking with alcohol.

C. Avoid breaking capsule.

D. Avoid taking on an empty stomach.

180. An ACE inhibitor is prescribed for a client with hypertension by his physician. The nurse should expect to administer which of the following drugs?

    A. Inderal (propranolol)
    B. Procardia (nifedipine)
    C. Capoten (captopril)
    D. Apresoline (hydralazine)

181. A client with coronary artery disease complains of substernal chest pain. After assessing the client's vital signs, the nurse administers nitroglycerin sublingually (SL) 1/150. After 5 minutes, the client indicates that he is still having chest pain. If his vital signs are stable following the usual dosage regimen (ordered by the physician), the nurse should:

    A. Wait 5 more minutes and then reassess
    B. Apply O$_2$ per nasal cannula
    C. Administer another nitroglycerin tablet SL
    D. Wait 10 minutes, and then administer a second nitroglycerin tablet

182. A client returns to your unit after a coronary angiogram. She complains of fever, itching, and chills. Which of the following drugs should the nurse plan to administer after notifying the physician of the client's complaints?

    A. Diphenhydramine (Benadryl)
    B. Dipyridamole (Persantine)
    C. Dobutamine hydrochloride (Dobutrex)
    D. Droperidol (Inapsine)

183. A client is admitted with a low potassium level and is prescribed parenteral KCl 40 mEq/L stat. Which of the following would be an appropriate method to administer the drug?

    A. IV push
    B. Concentrated IV infusion
    C. Diluted IV infusion
    D. IM

184. A client who has had repeated HIV antibody tests is found to be HIV infected and asymptomatic. Which of these statements about this person's ability to transmit HIV is accurate?

    A. The virus is dormant and the person is not infectious.
    B. The person is infectious only if symptoms are present.
    C. The person is considered infectious for life.
    D. Further laboratory tests are needed to determine infectious state.

185. An oral manifestation of AIDS clients is hairy leukoplakia. The nurse should assess for this manifestation on:

    A. The conjunctiva of the eye
    B. The inner surface of the nares
    C. The lateral margins of the tongue
    D. Posterior chest

186. A client has been diagnosed with AIDS for 3 years. She has been treated for cytomegalovirus retinitis. Discharge instructions by the nurse should include:

    A. Signs of ptosis
    B. Reporting of eye drainage
    C. Signs of exophthalmos
    D. Reporting changes in vision

187. A client with coronary artery disease and hyperlipidemia is prescribed cholestyramine resin (Questran). On discharge, the nurse should caution the client about which of the following side effects of the medication?

    A. Chronic use may cause increased bleeding tendency.
    B. The drug may increase calcium, potassium, and sodium levels.
    C. Chronic use may increase serum low-density lipoprotein.
    D. The drug may cause itching.

188. Dipyridamole and subcutaneous heparin are prescribed for a client by her physician 3 days after a mitral valve replacement. The nurse explains to her that these medications are given together primarily for which of the following reasons?

    A. To prevent angina
    B. To reduce the risk of coronary artery disease
    C. To prevent thromboembolism
    D. To prevent TIAs

189. A client was diagnosed with deep venous thrombosis 2 days ago and is transferred to the cardiology ward with a heparin drip to infuse at 1000 U/hr. On transfer, her physician orders warfarin sodium (Coumadin) po 10 mg daily. The nurse can expect the heparin drip to be discontinued at what time?

    A. After the first dose of oral warfarin
    B. In 2–3 days after oral warfarin is begun
    C. In 2–3 hours after first dose of oral warfarin
    D. Before first dose of oral warfarin

190. In assessing for signs of toxicity with chronic use of azathioprine (Imuran) in a renal transplant client, the nurse should monitor which of the following?

    A. Uric acid levels
    B. Fever, malaise
    C. Vital signs
    D. WBC count

191. A client is admitted to the medical-surgical unit for possible respiratory infection. His admission orders include regular diet, vital signs every 4 hours, ampicillin 250 mg q6h po, and sputum culture. Prior to administering the ampicillin, it would be *most* important for the nurse to:

    A. Allow the client to eat
    B. Collect a sputum specimen
    C. Take the client's pulse
    D. Assess the client's respirations

192. A client has been diagnosed with acute renal failure. She is receiving an IV infusion of mannitol (Osmitrol).

While assessing the client's hourly urine output, the nurse notes that her urine output continues to decline and is now <30 mL/hr for 2 hours. The appropriate nursing action at this time is to:

A. Increase the IV infusion rate
B. Restrict fluid intake
C. Immediately report findings to physician
D. Assess the client for increased ICP

193. A 70-year-old client received morphine (Duramorph) through an epidural line after knee surgery. The nurse should be prepared to act quickly for which of the following life-threatening reactions?

A. Hemorrhagic urticaria
B. Urinary retention
C. Depressed respiration
D. Drowsiness

194. A client is on SC heparin 8000 U daily as an anticoagulant. The nurse will correctly administer this drug by:

A. Pulling back on plunger to observe for blood
B. Using soft-bristle tooth brushes
C. Injecting it in the abdomen between pelvic bone
D. Massage area after injection

195. A client is prescribed isoniazid for treatment of active TB. The nurse should inform this client that therapeutic effects generally appear within which of the following time periods?

A. 2–3 hours
B. 2–3 weeks
C. 2–3 months
D. 2–3 days

196. Isoniazid is prescribed for a client for treatment of tuberculosis. The nurse should instruct the client on which of the following?

A. Decreased niacin stores
B. Increased niacin stores
C. Increased folate stores
D. Decrease in vitamin A

197. A client was admitted to the cardiac unit for congestive heart failure (CHF), and digitalis therapy was initiated. During his hospitalization, he began to complain frequently about many things, including the poor color on his TV and how he has lost his appetite. The client's behavior should alert the nurse to consider which of the following?

A. Digitalis toxicity
B. Anxiety related to CHF
C. Low cardiac output
D. Hypokalemia

198. A client has idiopathic parkinsonism. Her physician prescribed benztropine mesylate (Cogentin) 1 mg po daily. The nurse explains to her that the pathophysiological defect is an imbalance between:

A. Dopamine and acetylcholine
B. Estrogen and progesterone
C. Atherosclerosis and lack of blood supply
D. An autosomal dominant genetic defect

199. A diabetic client is hospitalized for adrenal insufficiency. His drug therapy includes chlorpropamide (Diabinese) po daily and 80 U day IM. Which of the following should the nurse plan to assess?

A. Serum potassium levels increased by ACTH
B. Fluid retention caused by ACTH
C. Requirements of po hypoglycemic agents decreased by ACTH
D. New infections

200. A client has just returned to her room after a cholecystectomy and is complaining of severe abdominal pain. She is scheduled to receive another dose of meperidine (Demerol) IM 7 mg in 20 minutes. Which of the following nursing interventions is not appropriate in this situation?

A. Monitor respiration, heart rate, and blood pressure.
B. Encourage deep breathing and coughing exercises.
C. Avoid aspiration of IM injections.
D. Document client's response to drug.

201. A client is receiving IV gentamicin sulfate (Garamycin) for a severe GI infection. His physician ordered a peak serum gentamicin level to be drawn with the next dose. The nurse should schedule the laboratory procedure at which of the following times?

A. Just before next infusion
B. Immediately after next infusion
C. Thirty minutes after next infusion
D. Thirty minutes before next infusion

202. Cefazolin sodium (Ancef) intravenously is prescribed for a client with a UTI. The nurse should instruct the client to promptly report which of the following?

A. Constipation
B. Becoming fatigued easily
C. Oily skin
D. White patches in mouth

203. A client arrives in the emergency room complaining of weakness. While on the ECG monitor, she develops ventricular ectopy. The nurse should plan to administer which of the following drugs?

A. Bretylium
B. Verapamil
C. Propranolol
D. Lidocaine

204. A 14-year-old girl has come to the obstetric-gynecology clinic for her first pelvic exam. She complains of severe cramping, heavy bleeding with clots, and headache on the first and second day of her menses. The physician orders a nonsteroidal anti-inflammatory drug. Which drugs should the nurse recognize as effective for this problem?

A. Naproxen (Naprosyn)
B. Acetaminophen (Tylenol)
C. Aspirin
D. Lydia Pinkham pills

205. While attending a high school health class, several girls have questions about douching. What

information should the school nurse include in her teaching plan?

- A. Vaginal discharge has a foul odor; douching should be done daily.
- B. Douching during menstruation is safe.
- C. Flavored or perfumed douches are hypoallergenic.
- D. Douching washes away natural mucus and upsets normal vaginal flora.

206. A client decides to use spermicidal foam and condoms as her contraceptive method. She asks the nurse at the clinic for some guidelines. What should the nurse include in her teaching?

- A. Use spermicide before the first and every subsequent act of intercourse.
- B. Positions of coitus are not affected by using spermicide.
- C. Walking and exercising after inserting a spermicide will not affect efficacy.
- D. Douching within 4–6 hours after coitus is acceptable.

207. During the normal menstrual cycle, two hormones predominate. The first part of the cycle is the proliferative phase in which estrogen plays an important role. The second part of the cycle is the secretory phase. In teaching about menstruation to seventh-grade girls, the nurse should include what hormone as the major influence of the secretory phase?

- A. LH
- B. FSH
- C. Progesterone
- D. Chorionic gonadotropin

208. The physician has prescribed 50,000-U SC injection of heparin for a client with pulmonary emboli. The vial contains 20,000 U/mL. The nurse calculates that the client will receive 2.5 mL of heparin. The client states: "This medication will help my blood not to clot." After double-checking the dosage calculation, the nurse decides to:

- A. Not administer the medication as prescribed and calculated
- B. Administer 0.2 mL of the medication instead of the dosage calculated
- C. Administer medication as prescribed and calculated and monitor for bruising, bleeding gums, and blood in urine or stool
- D. Administer medication as prescribed and calculated and proceed with further client teaching

209. The physician has prescribed digoxin 0.2 mg for a client with atrial fibrillation. The medication is available as 0.125-mg tablets. The nurse calculates that the client will receive two tablets of digoxin. The client states: "Every time I get chest pain, I will take an extra one of these heart pills." After double-checking the dosage calculation, the nurse decides to:

- A. Not administer the medication as prescribed and calculated
- B. Administer one-half tablet of the medication instead of dosage calculated

- C. Administer medication as prescribed and calculated, and monitor for untoward effects such as seizures and parkinsonian crisis
- D. Administer medication as prescribed and calculated, and proceed with further client teaching

210. The physician has prescribed meperidine hydrochloride 50 mg IM prn for postoperative pain in a post-hysterectomy client. The medication is available as 25 mg/mL. The nurse calculates that the client will receive 2 mL of the medication. The client states: "I am not having any pain now. I feel much better after walking. I might need a pain shot at bedtime if I have pain then, but I will let you know." After double-checking the dosage calculation, the nurse decides to:

- A. Not administer the medication as prescribed and calculated
- B. Administer 1 mL of the medication instead of dosage calculated
- C. Administer medication as prescribed and calculated, and monitor for bronchospasm and photosensitivity
- D. Administer medication as prescribed and calculated, and proceed with further client teaching

211. The physician has prescribed heparin 1000 U/hr by IV infusion for a client with pulmonary emboli. The IV drip contains 25,000 U of heparin in 500 mL D_5W. The nurse calculates that the client will receive 50 mL of the IV solution per hour. The client states: "I will use a soft-bristle toothbrush when I brush my teeth." After double-checking the dosage calculation, the nurse decides to:

- A. Not administer the medication as prescribed and calculated
- B. Administer 20 mL/hr of the medication instead of dosage calculated
- C. Administer medication as prescribed and calculated, and monitor PTT lab values
- D. Administer medication as prescribed and calculated and proceed with further client teaching

212. The physician has prescribed dexamethasone (Decadron) 3 mg for a client with a collagen disorder. The medication is available as 1.5-mg tablets. The nurse calculates that the client will receive three tablets. The client states: "If I stop this medicine suddenly, I could become very seriously ill." After double-checking the dosage calculation, the nurse decides to:

- A. Not administer the medication as prescribed and calculated
- B. Administer two tablets of the medication instead of dosage calculated
- C. Administer medication as prescribed and calculated, and monitor for nausea, anorexia, dizziness, and fatigue
- D. Administer medication as prescribed and calculated, and proceed with further client teaching

213. The physician has prescribed phenytoin sodium (Dilantin) IV at 50 mg/min for a total dose of 300 mg for a client in the emergency room with a seizure disorder. The medication is available as 10 mg/mL. The nurse calculates that the client will receive the medication

over a period of 6 minutes. The client states: "My urine might look pink." After double-checking the dosage calculation, the nurse decides to:

A. Not administer the medication as prescribed and calculated

B. Administer the medication over 3 minutes instead of over the time calculated

C. Administer the medication as prescribed and calculated, and monitor for respiratory depression and ventricular dysrhythmias

D. Administer medication as prescribed and calculated, and proceed with further client teaching

214. The physician has prescribed two doses of naloxone 0.2 mg IV every 3 minutes for a client in the emergency room with opioid narcotic-induced respiratory depression. The medication is available as 1 mg/mL. The nurse calculates that the client will receive 0.4 mL for each of the two doses. The client's wife states: "He accidentally took too many pain pills. I'm glad you're giving him something to wake him up again." After double-checking the dosage calculation, the nurse decides to:

A. Not administer the medication as prescribed and calculated

B. Administer 0.2 mL for each of the two doses instead of the dosage calculated

C. Administer medication as prescribed and calculated, and monitor for reverse analgesia, tachycardia, and hypertension

D. Administer medication as prescribed and calculated, and proceed with further client teaching

215. The physician has prescribed metoclopramide (Reglan) 20 mg IV in 50 mL NaCl over 15 minutes for a client with gastroesophageal reflux. The infusion bag is to be protected from light with aluminum foil. The medication is available as 5 mg/mL. The nurse calculates that the client will receive 4 mL of the medication. The client states: "When I take this medication at home, I will avoid drinking and driving and take it after my meals." After double-checking the dosage calculation, the nurse decides to:

A. Not administer the medication as prescribed and calculated

B. Administer 2 mL of the medication instead of dosage calculated

C. Administer medication as prescribed and calculated; and monitor for uremia and glucosuria

D. Administer medication as prescribed and calculated, and proceed with further client teaching

216. The physician has prescribed cimetidine 300 mg with meals and at bedtime for a male client with gastric ulcers. The medication is available as 300-mg tablets. The nurse calculates that the client will receive one tablet for each dose. The client states: "This medication will make me temporarily impotent, and my breasts might temporarily enlarge. I can continue to smoke. If I eat spicy foods or foods with black pepper, I will take a double dose of the medicine." After double-checking the dosage calculation, the nurse decides to:

A. Not administer the medication as prescribed and calculated

B. Administer two tablets of the medication instead of dosage calculated

C. Administer medication as prescribed and calculated, and monitor for blurred vision and nasal stuffiness

D. Administer medication as prescribed and calculated, and proceed with further client teaching

217. The physician has prescribed morphine sulfate 100 mg IV for a client in the emergency room with severe chest pain. The medication is available as 10 mg/mL. The nurse calculates that the client will receive 10 mL of the medication. The client states: "This medicine will help to take my pain away. I will let you know when my pain is gone." After double-checking the dosage calculation, the nurse decides to:

A. Not administer the medication as prescribed and calculated

B. Administer 1 mL of the medication instead of dosage calculated

C. Administer medication as prescribed and calculated, and monitor for respiratory depression

D. Administer medication as prescribed and calculated, and proceed with further client teaching

218. The physician has prescribed furosemide 40 mg IV for a client with pulmonary edema. The medication is available as 10 mg/mL. The nurse calculates that the client will receive 0.4 mL of the medication. The client states: "This medicine will take fluid off my lungs so I can breathe better. I will urinate a lot." After double-checking the dosage calculation, the nurse decides to:

A. Not administer the medication as prescribed and calculated

B. Administer 4.0 mL of the medication instead of dosage calculated

C. Administer medication as prescribed and calculated, and monitor for postural hypotension, leg cramps, tachycardia, drowsiness, and restlessness

D. Administer medication as prescribed and calculated, and proceed with further client teaching

219. The physician has prescribed amoxicillin potassium (Augmentin) 500 mg q8h for a client with pneumonia. The medication is available in 250-mg tablets. The nurse calculates that the client will receive two tablets every 8 hours for a total of six tablets in 24 hours. The client states: "I will take the medication with meals. If my pneumonia goes away before I finish my prescription, I can save the rest of the pills for the next time I get pneumonia." After double-checking the dosage calculation, the nurse decides to:

A. Not administer the medication as prescribed and calculated

B. Administer one tablet tid instead of the dosage calculated

C. Administer the medication as prescribed and calculated, and monitor for cardiac studies

D. Administer medication as prescribed and calculated, and proceed with further client teaching

220. The physician prescribes nifedipine 10 mg tid for a client with chronic stable angina pectoris. The medication is available as 10-mg capsules. The nurse calculates

that the client will receive one capsule tid. The client states: "I will change positions slowly as my blood pressure might drop." After double-checking the dosage calculation, the nurse decides to:

A. Not administer the medication as prescribed and calculated

B. Administer two capsules tid instead of dosage calculated

C. Administer medication as prescribed and calculated, and monitor for tachycardia and increased liver function studies

D. Administer medication as prescribed and calculated, and proceed with further client teaching

221. The physician has prescribed lactalose (Chronulac) 20 g/mL qid for a client with portal systemic encephalopathy. The medication is available as 3.33 g 5/mL oral solution. The nurse calculates that the client will receive 30-mL oral solution qid. The client states: "I can take this medication in fruit juice. I should not take other laxatives with it." After double-checking the dosage calculation, the nurse decides to:

A. Not administer the medication as prescribed and calculated

B. Administer 3 mL of the medication instead of dosage calculated

C. Administer medication as prescribed and calculated, and monitor for blood ammonia level

D. Administer medication as prescribed and calculated, and proceed with further client teaching

222. A client has an order for a pulse oximeter. To ensure accuracy of the pulse oximeter reading the nurse would:

A. Place the probe on the radial or temporal artery

B. Place the probe on a finger or earlobe

C. Calibrate at fourth interspace midclavicular line

D. Wait until body temperature is reached by the probe

223. When receiving chemotherapy (Cisplatin) for ovarian cancer, a client develops nausea and vomiting. It would be most important for the nurse to:

A. Assess onset, frequency, and severity

B. Heat foods whenever possible

C. Provide relaxation or distraction

D. Provide a soft, bland diet

224. An insulin-dependent diabetic adult is found unconscious at home. Upon arrival at the emergency room, her blood sugar is 800 mg/dL. The nurse would expect to find:

A. Bradycardia

B. Hypertension

C. Skin warm to the touch

D. Hyperventilation

225. A client with cystitis needs further teaching concerning prevention of recurring cystitis if she states:

A. "I shower rather than take a tub bath."

B. "I try to urinate at least every 2 hours."

C. "I eat lots of eggs, meat, and whole grains."

D. "I begin taking Pyridium (phenazopyridine) if this returns."

226. A client with inflammatory bowel disease receives total parenteral nutrition (TPN). Which outcome of therapy is most desirable for this client?

A. Weight gain of 2 pounds per week

B. Serum albumin level of 1.5 g/dL

C. Serum blood glucose of 180 mg dL

D. BP ranging from 110/80 to 128/88

227. A client is placed on a low-residue diet. Which menu should the nurse encourage the client to consume?

A. Fried fish, corn on the cob, salad, popcorn, tea

B. Pepper steak, french fried potatoes, salad, milk

C. Whole wheat pasta, Swedish meatballs, peaches, coffee

D. Baked chicken, white rice, plain custard, apple juice

228. The home health nurse suspects that a diabetic client is not following the prescribed plan of care. Which test is most appropriate to evaluate compliance with care?

A. Fasting serum glucose

B. Glucosylated hemoglobin

C. Partial thromboplastin time

D. Urine glucose and ketone levels

229. A client with a new ileostomy underwent surgery 2 days ago. Which nursing action is appropriate at this time?

A. Monitor for fluid and electrolyte imbalance

B. Irrigate the ostomy to promote bowel training

C. Change the ostomy appliance when it is full

D. Implement measures to prevent constipation

230. The nurse inserts an indwelling catheter into a female client. Which action is appropriate for this procedure? The nurse:

A. Advances the catheter 4 more inches after urine returns

B. Cleanses the client with antiseptic from anus to clitoris

C. Utilizes medical asepsis through the entire procedure

D. Cleanses directly over the client's meatus prior to insertion

231. A client undergoes a series of diagnostic tests to rule out inflammatory bowel disease. The nurse should schedule the tests in the following order:

A. Barium swallow, colonoscopy, barium enema

B. Barium swallow, barium enema, colonoscopy

C. Colonoscopy, barium enema, barium swallow

D. Colonoscopy, barium swallow, barium enema

232. A client with a history of uric acid kidney stones needs further teaching if he states:

A. "I need to drink about 3 quarts of fluid every day."

B. "I like to take 500 mg of vitamin C every day."

C. "I'm going to try to walk a little every 2 hours."

D. "I will continue taking my allopurinol as prescribed."

233. A patient develops a deep vein thrombophlebitis (DVT) of the left lower leg. During the initial treatment, which intervention is most appropriate?

    A. Maintain strict bed rest
    B. Gentle massage of the calf
    C. Apply ice packs to relieve pain
    D. Encourage active leg exercises

234. The nurse gives discharge instructions to a client who underwent a transurethral resection of the prostate (TURP). Which instruction should the nurse emphasize?

    A. "Restrict fluid intake to prevent urinary retention."
    B. "Maintain soft and regular bowel movements."
    C. "Jog daily to prevent clots in your legs."
    D. "Call your physician if signs of incisional infection develops."

235. Preoperative instruction in leg exercises is mainly intended to prevent which post-op complication?

    A. Infection
    B. Cellulitis
    C. Paralytic ileus
    D. Thrombophlebitis

236. When assessing a client with venous insufficiency, the nurse expects to find:

    A. Edema of the affected extremity
    B. Extreme pain upon ambulation
    C. Extremity is cool to the touch
    D. Pallor of the affected extremity

237. An elderly client has altered arterial peripheral tissue perfusion. The home health nurse encourages the client to assume which position to facilitate peripheral circulation?

    A. Lying in bed with the feet elevated
    B. Sitting in a chair with the feet dependent
    C. Sitting with the feet crossed at ankles
    D. Lying with a pillow under the lower legs

238. A client was diagnosed with a duodenal ulcer. Which medication will promote healing by forming a protective coating over the ulcer?

    A. Ranitidine (Zantac)
    B. Famotidine (Pepcid)
    C. Sucralfate (Carafate)
    D. Cimetidine (Tagamet)

239. Legal responsibility for obtaining informed consent for surgery is the responsibility of the:

    A. Physician
    B. Registered nurse
    C. Admission clerk
    D. Anesthesiologist

240. Which statement describes the correct sequence for assessment of the abdomen?

    A. Palpation, inspection, percussion, and auscultation
    B. Palpation, percussion, auscultation, and inspection
    C. Inspection, palpation, auscultation, and percussion
    D. Inspection, auscultation, percussion, and palpation

241. A client with ulcerative colitis has experienced severe diarrhea for the past 24 hours. The nurse should assess this client for the following conditions at the present time:

    A. Malnutrition
    B. Malabsorption
    C. Metabolic acidosis
    D. Metabolic alkalosis

242. Two days ago a client had surgery to create a colostomy. Which finding is expected when assessing the stoma? The stoma is:

    A. Pale colored
    B. Dark pink or red
    C. Flush with the skin
    D. Dark or bluish purple

243. Which assessment finding is considered within normal limits on a client who underwent a cystoscopy 2 hours ago?

    A. Abdominal pain
    B. Pink-tinged urine
    C. Bladder distention
    D. 35 cc urine output

244. Which is the desired outcome for a client who is taking Levsin (hyoscyamine), an anticholinergic medication? The client:

    A. Voids about 220–250 cc of urine every 2–4 hours
    B. States that bladder spasms have been relieved
    C. Has no complaints of urinary frequency or burning
    D. Has a urine bacterial count below 100,000 microbes/cc

245. A client underwent a hemorrhoidectomy in Ambulatory Surgery. The nurse's discharge instructions should address:

    A. The technique for sitz bath
    B. Restricting fluids for 24 hours
    C. Taking a laxative upon discharge
    D. Lying in the recumbent position

246. The nurse prepares to insert an indwelling catheter into a male client. Which action is appropriate for this procedure?

    A. Test the retention balloon with sterile water before insertion
    B. Cleanse with antiseptic from the base of the penis to the meatus
    C. Use a catheter that is slightly larger than the opening of the meatus
    D. Lubricate one inch of the catheter tip with water soluble lubricant

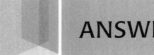

1. **(D)** Client need: physiological integrity, subcategory: reduction of risk potential; content area: med/surg

   RATIONALE

   (A) A client who does not blink must have artificial tears to prevent corneal drying. Applying an eye patch over an open eye also puts the client at risk for corneal abrasion. (B) A client with Bell's palsy who does not blink the affected eye would be unable to close the affected eye. It is not necessary to keep the unaffected eye closed. (C) Pupil reaction to light and accommodation is unaffected by Bell's palsy. (D) Eye lubrication is essential to prevent corneal drying in a client who does not blink.

2. **(C)** Client need: health promotion and maintenance; subcategory: prevention and early detection of disease; content area: med/surg

   RATIONALE

   (A) If the client could read the nurse's lips, this would not actually be a test for hearing. (B) The client could say "yes" even if he or she could not hear the watch. (C) If the client obeys this command, he or she was able to hear it. (D) A tuning fork tests lateralization of sound and assesses the ability to hear longer with air conduction than with bone conduction. A tuning fork does not test hearing.

3. **(B)** Client need: psychosocial integrity; subcategory: psychosocial adaptation; content area: med/surg

   RATIONALE

   (A) The client is discouraged, and she needs to be supported. (B) Positive reinforcement is pleasant and can be a strong motivator. (C) The client needs to be motivated to exercise every day. (D) Telling the client that exercise is necessary is unlikely to make her feel less discouraged.

4. **(B)** Client need: health promotion and maintenance; subcategory: prevention and early detection of disease; content area: med/surg

   RATIONALE

   (A) Blurred vision may be a sign of increasing ICP, but this is not the reason to do a pupil check. (B) Pupils that are equal and react to light and accommodation indicate an intact brain stem. The brain stem functions to maintain cardiorespiratory function. Pupil checks are done to assess brain-stem function. (C) Dilated and fixed pupils may indicate a cardiac arrest, but this is not the reason to do a pupil check. (D) Pinpoint pupils may result from CNS depressant drugs, but this is not the reason to do a pupil check.

5. **(D)** Client need: health promotion and maintenance; subcategory: prevention and early detection of disease; content area: med/surg

   RATIONALE

   (A) Intention tremors are more likely to be associated with a cerebellar lesion. (B) Loss of pain and temperature sensation is due to a lesion of the parietal lobe or the sensory nerves. (C) Loss of equilibrium may be associated with the extrapyramidal tract, the cerebellum, or the inner ear. (D) The pyramidal tract, as well as intact motor pathways, is responsible for voluntary movement.

6. **(A)** Client need: physiological integrity; subcategory: basic care and comfort; content area: med/surg

   RATIONALE

   (A) Hip adduction (moving toward or past midline) should be avoided by properly placed pillows whether the client is on the affected or unaffected side. (B) A trochanter roll prevents external rotation of the hip joint. (C) Knee flexion does not need to be prevented. The client's position does need to be changed frequently. (D) Plantarflexion, with resultant footdrop, can be prevented by using footboards or high-top sneakers.

7. **(C)** Client need: physiological integrity; subcategory: reduction of risk potential; content area: med/surg

   RATIONALE

   (A) Artificial tears are necessary to prevent corneal drying for a client with a diminished or absent corneal reflex. (B) A client with a diminished gag reflex should be NPO to prevent aspiration. (C) A side-lying position helps to prevent aspiration of secretions for a client with a diminished gag or swallowing reflex. (D) The gag reflex is controlled by the sensory function of the glossopharyngeal nerve (cranial nerve IX) and the motor component of the vagus nerve (cranial nerve X).

8. **(D)** Client need: physiological integrity; subcategory: basic care and comfort; content area: med/surg

   RATIONALE

   (A) Powder can be used as a lubricant between dry, opposing skin surfaces. Wet powder becomes irritating to the skin. (B) An indwelling catheter puts any client at risk for UTI. Regaining bladder control is delayed in the presence of UTI. (C) Fluid intake over a 24-hour period should be normal, and the urine output should be of normal concentration. Fluids may be restricted in the evening. (D) Placing the client on a bedpan on schedule and also on demand is a first step in helping the client to regain bladder control. The caregiver should also note the usual times of voiding.

9. **(C)** Client need: physiological integrity; subcategory: basic care and comfort; content area: med/surg

   RATIONALE

   (A) It is good if the client can tell when she feels constipated, but this is not an indication of restored bowel function. (B) Daily prune juice and cereal may be a strategy toward restoring bowel function, but it is not an evaluation. (C) A daily soft formed stool indicates healthy bowel function. (D) A daily fluid intake of 2400 mL may be appropriate for this client. Adequate hydration is important for bowel function, but it does not indicate normal bowel function.

10. **(A)** Client need: psychosocial integrity; subcategory: coping and adaptation; content area: med/surg

    RATIONALE

    (A) The goal for this client is independence with communication. Patience while she thinks of the word she wants to say may be an effective strategy. (B) Ending the visit will not help this client to communicate effectively. (C) Finishing her sentence for her may be necessary, but it will not help her to communicate independently. (D) Changing the subject would serve to increase the client's frustration and may be considered disrespectful by the client.

11. **(A)** Client need: psychosocial integrity; subcategory: coping and adaptation; content area: med/surg

    RATIONALE

    (A) A person who is unable to verbally express needs may be able to communicate by using signals such as picture cards, hand motion, or by pointing to objects. (B) It is necessary to speak loudly and clearly to some people with hearing loss. (C) It is helpful when speaking to some people with hearing loss to stand directly in front of them so they can read lips. (D) Writing directions in large letters may be helpful for people with impaired vision who have difficulty understanding or remembering verbal directions.

12. **(D)** Client need: health promotion and maintenance; subcategory: prevention and early detection of disease; content area: med/surg

RATIONALE

(A) A client with hemiplegia would be unable to flex the affected arm. (B) Flexion of the unaffected arm and unaffected leg indicates a decorticate response to pain. Extension in response to pain indicates a decerebrate response. (C) The client might grimace, but would also pull the hand away. (D) Pulling the hand away is the best response to pain.

13. **(C)** Client need: psychosocial integrity; subcategory: coping and adaptation; content area: med/surg

RATIONALE

(A) The goal for this client is to cope with a change in body image. Asking her to explain how she feels may reinforce a poor body image. (B) Complimenting her when she grooms herself successfully would be a better strategy to strengthen her body image. (C) Focusing on ability rather than on disability is a good strategy for any client in the rehabilitation phase of care. (D) For safety, it is a good idea to keep the client's environment free of clutter.

14. **(D)** Client need: physiological integrity; subcategory: reduction of risk potential; content area: med/surg

RATIONALE

(A) An arteriogram involves injection of a radiopaque contrast medium into an artery, which causes a burning sensation. (B) An EEG is a measure of electrical energy flowing away from the brain. (C) A lumbar puncture, using an oil-based contrast medium, lasts only a few minutes but requires the client to remain flat after the procedure. (D) CT requires the client to lie very still during the examination. Sometimes this test is enhanced with the venous injection of a contrast medium.

15. **(B)** Client need: physiological integrity; subcategory: reduction of risk potential; content area: med/surg

RATIONALE

(A) The goal is to prevent postmyelogram headache. Dimming the lights may help if the client already has a headache. (B) Headache after lumbar puncture is due to loss of CSF. Forcing fluids helps to replace CSF. (C) Analgesic medication may help if the client already has a headache, but it is not a strategy to prevent headache. (D) The client may turn from side to side as long as he keeps the head of his bed flat for 6 hours. Turning will not prevent headache.

16. **(B)** Client need: physiological integrity; subcategory: reduction of risk potential; content area: med/surg

RATIONALE

(A) After a cerebral angiogram, the client should be on bed rest for 12–24 hours. (B) Forcing fluids will help promote the excretion of the contrast medium. (C) The client should not be encouraged to cough. Limited movement is important to prevent arterial bleeding and hematoma at the puncture site. (D) There is no special reason to encourage the client to void after a cerebral angiogram, but he or she may need to void more often because fluids may be forced.

17. **(A)** Client need: physiological integrity; subcategory: reduction of risk potential; content area: med/surg

RATIONALE

(A) During an MRI, it is necessary for the client to lie still during the entire procedure. She should know that she will hear a hum-

ming sound and the pulses of the radiofrequency waves. (B) A radiopaque contrast medium is used with digital subtraction angiogram and enhanced CT. (C) Scalp electrodes are used with EEG. (D) Postprocedure care for a client undergoing a myelogram with a water-based contrast medium includes staying in bed with the head of the bed elevated to prevent headache.

18. **(A)** Client need: physiological integrity; subcategory: reduction of risk potential; content area: med/surg

RATIONALE

(A) Plasmapheresis alleviates symptoms associated with Guillain-Barré syndrome by removing autoimmune antibodies from the blood. (B) Plasmapheresis does not cause an allergic reaction. (C) Plasmapheresis does not prevent bacterial infection. (D) Plasmapheresis does not reduce the need for O_2.

19. **(D)** Client need: physiological integrity; subcategory: reduction of risk potential; content area: med/surg

RATIONALE

(A) For some people with epilepsy, fatigue may be a factor in precipitating seizure. (B) People with epilepsy do not need to refrain from competitive sports, particularly if seizures are under control with medication. (C) Some health problems, such as diabetes or Addison's disease, may require additional medication when infection is present. This is not true with epilepsy. (D) Many people with epilepsy experience an "aura" (visions, feelings, or sounds) immediately preceding a seizure. When experienced, the client may have time to assume a safe position prior to onset of the seizure.

20. **(B)** Client need: health promotion and maintenance; subcategory: prevention and early detection of disease; content area: med/surg

RATIONALE

(A) It is appropriate to assess temperature of an extremity by using the backs of your hands and by comparing one side with the other. Temperature alone, however, is not adequate to assess circulation. (B) Calf tenderness with dorsiflexion of the ankle joint is a sign of deep venous thrombosis, a serious complication after total hip replacement. (C) Tenderness at the surgical site is an expected assessment finding. (D) Dizziness on standing is probably due to postural hypotension. It should be prevented by having the client dangle the legs before standing from a lying position.

21. **(D)** Client need: physiological integrity; subcategory: reduction of risk potential; content area: med/surg

RATIONALE

(A) Inflammation of the bursa can be due to repetitive traumatic injury, but it is not the most dangerous complication. (B) Dislocation of the shoulder can be caused by lifting a small child by the arms. Dislocation, however, is likely to be treated quickly owing to severe pain. (C) Greenstick fracture is possible, but the accompanying severe pain would alert the mother to seek medical treatment. (D) Subluxation of the shoulder joint is a serious complication because it may go unnoticed and therefore untreated. Subluxation is an incomplete dislocation resulting in damage to the articular surfaces of the joint.

22. **(A)** Client need: health promotion and maintenance; subcategory: prevention and early detection of disease; content area: med/surg

RATIONALE

(A) Repetitive flexion and extension of the wrist joint, as in typing, may cause inflammation of the tendons with resultant pressure on the median nerve. (B, C) Elevating the affected wrist, applying a splint, applying ice, and taking nonsteroidal anti-inflammatory drugs may help to alleviate symptoms of carpal tunnel syndrome. To prevent recurrence, it is most important to teach the person to avoid repetitive flexion and extension. (D) Aspirin is an anti-inflammatory drug, but to prevent inflammation of the wrist joint, it is most important to avoid constant flexion and extension.

23. **(D)** Client need: physiological integrity subcategory: physiological adaptation; content area: med/surg

RATIONALE

(A) People with rheumatoid arthritis are likely to have less pain and stiffness after exercise. (B) Heat applications are more likely to reduce the pain of an inflamed joint. (C) Food should not affect the pain and stiffness of rheumatoid arthritis. (D) People with rheumatoid arthritis are likely to experience pain and stiffness after long periods of immobility. They need to plan for sufficient time for grooming and dressing after a night's sleep.

24. **(C)** Client need: physiological integrity; subcategory: reduction of risk potential; content area: med/surg

RATIONALE

(A) Elevating the foot of the bed will not alter the line of pull of Bryant's traction. (B) It is possible that countertraction (the child's weight) is inadequate to maintain traction, but increasing the weight requires a medical order and is not an independent nursing action. (C) Gently lifting the child's buttocks off the bed is usually all that is necessary to restore traction, and this should be the first action. A medical order to increase weight will become necessary if traction cannot be maintained. (D) If the child's buttocks are resting on the bed, Bryant's traction is not being maintained. It is important to restore traction.

25. **(D)** Client need: physiological integrity; subcategory: physiological adaptation; content area: med/surg

RATIONALE

(A) Weight-bearing activities are needed to prevent loss of calcium from the bones. Isometric exercises are appropriate, but they do not prevent osteoporosis. (B) Leg raises help to prepare muscles for crutch walking, but they do not prevent osteoporosis. To prevent lumbar injury, leg raises should always be done with the knees bent. (C) Swimming is good cardiovascular exercise, but weight bearing is essential to prevent osteoporosis. (D) Walking is a weight-bearing exercise. Walking for 1 hour in place is equivalent to walking about a mile.

26. **(B)** Client need: physiological integrity; subcategory: basic care and comfort; content area: med/surg

RATIONALE

(A) Bright lights and loud noises may be annoying to an 82-year-old woman, but they should not compromise her ability to cope with advanced osteoporosis. (B) Clients with advanced bone porosity are at risk for pathological fractures. It is essential to be gentle when moving them. (C) Elevating the head of the bed may assist with respiratory function, but it has no effect on osteoporosis. (D) Unless fluids are contraindicated owing to cardiac or renal disease, people with osteoporosis should have increased fluids to help prevent renal calculi.

27. **(A)** Client need: health promotion and maintenance; subcategory: prevention and early detection of disease; content area: med/surg

RATIONALE

(A) Deep venous thrombosis is a potential complication of estrogen therapy. Women taking estrogen should know to call the physician if they experience redness, pain, or swelling of the legs. (B) Estrogen does not cause increased intraocular pressure. (C) Renal calculi may result from osteoporosis, but estrogen therapy does not cause renal calculi. (D) Estrogen therapy, unopposed by progesterone, puts a woman at risk for endometrial cancer. There is also risk of breast cancer, but estrogen does not cause uterine atony.

28. **(D)** Client need: physiological integrity; subcategory: reduction of risk potential; content area: med/surg

RATIONALE

(A) A warm compress, if ordered, may relieve this client's discomfort, but it is most important to remove the probable source of the pain. (B) The client's physician should be notified of the severe pain after traction was applied, but it is more important to first remove the traction. (C) Severe pain radiating down one leg is not expected after application of intermittent pelvic traction. The client may feel initial discomfort, which should subside as the traction causes the muscles to relax. (D) Severe pain after application of traction is likely to indicate an extension of the lesion with pressure on nerve roots and may have resulted from the traction. Remove the traction, position the client with his hips flexed, and then notify the client's physician.

29. **(D)** Client need: health promotion and maintenance; subcategory: prevention and early detection of disease; content area: med/surg

RATIONALE

(A) A warm, reddened extremity does not indicate compartmental syndrome. (B) With compartmental syndrome, the calf muscles may be hard, but the skin does not feel cool to the touch. (C) A client with compartmental syndrome is likely to have good capillary refill and palpable pedal pulses. (D) Compartmental syndrome is due to pressure from bleeding or edema within an inelastic fibrous compartment. Ischemia due to pressure causes severe pain unrelieved by analgesic medication. Medical and nursing interventions are required immediately to prevent permanent tissue damage.

30. **(A)** Client need: physiological integrity; subcategory: reduction of risk potential; content area: med/surg

RATIONALE

(A) Water does not damage a synthetic cast, but the client should know that it may take a long time for the cast padding to dry. (B) It may be unsafe for the client to shower alone because she may slip and fall, but not because she is wearing a synthetic cast. (C) Osteomyelitis is a serious infection, and the client should call her physician if she experiences discomfort or an odor from her cast, but a shower will not necessarily cause an infection. (D) Water would soften a plaster cast but has no effect on a synthetic cast.

31. **(B)** Client need: physiological integrity; subcategory: reduction of risk potential; content area: med/surg

RATIONALE

(A) Blanching of toenails or fingernails when pressure is applied is expected. (B) Return of circulation within 3 seconds of blanching toenails or fingernails is the best indication of adequate circulation to the extremities. (C) It is important to assess motor function, but wiggling the toes is not the best indication of adequate circulation. (D) Feet that are warm to the touch probably have good circulation, but cool feet may also have good circulation.

32. **(B)** Client need: physiological integrity; subcategory: reduction of risk potential; content area: med/surg

RATIONALE

(A) It is important to prevent further hip rotation after fractured femur, but that is not the reason for Buck's extension. (B) Immediate treatment of any fracture is to immobilize the broken bone to prevent soft tissue injury. (C) Abduction of the affected hip joint is important after open reduction, but it is not the purpose of Buck's extension. (D) Buck's extension does help reduce the fracture, but the primary purpose is to immobilize the broken bone to prevent soft tissue injury.

33. **(B)** Client need: physiological integrity, subcategory: reduction of risk potential; content area: med/surg

RATIONALE

(A) A client in Buck's extension whose affected foot is resting at the foot of the bed is not in traction. Placing a pillow will not restore traction. (B) Pulling the client up in bed will restore traction. Raising the foot of the bed will increase countertraction and may prevent the client from continually sliding down. (C) There is no traction. Action must be taken to restore traction. (D) Turning the client to the side will not restore traction and may cause further soft tissue injury due to movement of the broken bone.

34. **(C)** Client need: health maintenance and promotion; subcategory: prevention and early detection of disease; content area: med/surg

    RATIONALE

    (A) A client with trauma severe enough to fracture his pelvis is likely to have bruises. (B) Any swelling, inflammation, laceration, or bruising should be monitored for change, but they would not alert the nurse to a serious complication of pelvic fracture. (C) Blood in the urine indicates trauma to the kidneys, ureters, or bladder. Any client with a fractured pelvis should be assessed for hematuria. (D) Discomfort at a fracture site is expected and does not necessarily indicate a serious complication. Any discomfort should be monitored for change.

35. **(A)** Client need: health promotion and maintenance, subcategory: prevention and early detection of disease; content area: med/surg

    RATIONALE

    (A) Circulating fatty acids and lipase owing to fat embolism cause an inflammatory reaction in the lungs, with increased capillary permeability leading to pulmonary edema. (B) Clients with multiple fractures and with fractures of long bones are at risk for fat embolism and for infection, but there is not a causative relationship between fat embolism and osteomyelitis. (C) Petechiae due to capillary occlusion may occur with fat embolism, but they are symptoms and not risk factors. (D) Fat embolism is unlikely to cause seizures. It is likely to cause confusion, fever, and pulmonary edema due to irritation to the cerebrum, hypothalamus, and lungs. A fat embolism may also be occlusive in a pulmonary artery, leading to pulmonary embolism.

36. **(A)** Client need: physiological integrity; subcategory: reduction of risk potential; content area: med/surg

    RATIONALE

    (A) Irritability and confusion due to hypoxia and cerebral edema are early signs of fat embolism. (B) With fat embolism, there are circulating fat globules as well as fatty acids and lipase in the bloodstream. Fat in the stool may be caused by diminished pancreatic enzymes in clients with pancreatitis or cystic fibrosis. (C) Hyperglycemia is not expected with fat embolism. Hyperglycemia most commonly occurs with diminished insulin due to diabetes mellitus. (D) Pruritus is not an expected assessment finding and does not require medical intervention.

37. **(B)** Client need: physiological integrity; subcategory: reduction of risk potential; content area: med/surg

    RATIONALE

    (A) Clients should be assessed for fat embolism for at least 48 hours after injury. (B) Fat embolism is most likely to occur 12–48 hours after injury. It rarely occurs later unless there has been further injury. (C) A client with chronic respiratory disease will have more difficulty coping with systemic fat embolism, but all clients with fractures of long bones or multiple trauma are at risk for fat embolism. (D) Skeletal traction does not put a client at risk for fat embolism. It does put a client at risk for osteomyelitis.

38. **(D)** Client need: physiological integrity, physiological adaptation; content area: med/surg

    RATIONALE

    (A) Warm sterile compresses may be used if there is infection at the pin site, but they are not part of routine pin care. (B) Antibiotic ointment may be part of the protocol for pin care, but usu-ally the skin around skeletal traction pins is cleaned with sterile saline or peroxide and left uncovered. (C) A heat lamp would not be effective in keeping pin sites clean, and it would probably be uncomfortable. (D) The purpose of pin care is to maintain free drainage of serous fluid from the pin site. Crusts should be gently removed, and the skin pressed downward around the pins.

39. **(A)** Client need: health promotion and maintenance; subcategory: prevention and early detection of disease; content area: med/surg

    RATIONALE

    (A) Capillary refill within 3 seconds after blanching is the best assessment of circulation to extremities. (B) Motor and sensory assessment is an important part of neurovascular assessment, but it is not the best assessment of circulation to an extremity. (C) The "five P's" of neurovascular assessment include pain, pallor, pulselessness, paresthesia, and paralysis. (D) Skin temperature provides some information about circulation, but temperature alone is insufficient to assess circulation.

40. **(B)** Client need: physiological integrity; subcategory: reduction of risk potential; content area: med/surg

    RATIONALE

    (A) Knee flexion and extension does not strengthen the muscles necessary for crutch walking. (B) Pressing the back of the knee into the mattress while supine (quadriceps setting exercises) as well as straight leg-raising exercises help to strengthen muscles for crutch walking. (C) Perineal exercises do not help with crutch walking. Perineal exercises are useful to help control dribbling of urine after perineal surgery. (D) Everyone should change position at least every 2 hours, but this will not help to prepare a person for crutch walking.

41. **(B)** Client need: physiological integrity; subcategory: physiological adaptation; content area: med/surg

    RATIONALE

    (A) Ice does reduce bleeding, but it should not be applied directly to an amputated stump because it would cause tissue damage, making successful reimplantation unlikely. (B) Gentle, firm, continuous pressure applied to the end of an amputated stump using a clean, dry, bulky, loose material should stop the bleeding. (C) Elevating an amputated stump will help somewhat to control bleeding. Gentle and continuous pressure is required. (D) Unless hemorrhage is life threatening and cannot be controlled by pressure, a tourniquet should not be used because it causes hypoxia and ischemia. The goal of treatment is successful reimplantation.

42. **(A)** Client need: physiological integrity; subcategory: reduction of risk potential; content area: med/surg

    RATIONALE

    (A) People with above-the-knee amputations are at risk for hip flexion contracture because sitting and side-lying positions cause hip flexion and also because flexor muscles are stronger than extensor muscles. Lying prone periodically extends the hip joint. (B) Lying prone does not increase vital capacity. Moving from a lying to a sitting position does increase vital capacity. (C) Leg exercises help to prepare a person for crutch walking. Arm exercises are not necessary. (D) Lying prone may be comfortable, and may even provide a diversion, but hip extension is a more important reason.

43. **(B)** Client need: physiological integrity; subcategory: physiological adaptation; content area: med/surg

    RATIONALE

    (A) It will be important to help a person to cope with loss, but acceptance is not an immediate goal. (B) After airway, breathing, and circulation stabilization, the primary objective after traumatic amputation is reimplantation. Efforts are directed toward protecting the stump and the amputated parts from further injury. (C) Preventing infection is important, but not primary.

Bleeding should be stopped with a clean material, and the amputated parts should be rinsed in water, then double bagged in plastic. (D) Pain relief is very important for the person experiencing traumatic amputation, but not the primary goal of care.

44. **(D)** Client need: physiological integrity; subcategory: physiological adaptation; content area: med/surg

    RATIONALE

    (A) Compartmental syndrome is a potential complication of lower leg fracture, but it is not expected at the time of the accident. (B) The client should be kept warm, but it is most important to prevent further soft tissue injury. (C) If bleeding is a problem, elevating the injured leg and applying pressure would be appropriate. (D) Splinting the injured leg, in the position found, will prevent further trauma to nerves and blood vessels from the broken bone.

45. **(A)** Client need: health promotion and maintenance; subcategory: prevention and early detection of disease; content area: med/surg

    RATIONALE

    (A) Difficulty in active dorsiflexion of the ankle joint should alert the nurse to the possibility of peroneal nerve damage. (B) Decreased sensation in the web space on the anterior foot between the large and second toe is an indication of compromise to the sensory function of the peroneal nerve. (C) Peroneal nerve damage does not cause skin breakdown. (D) Swelling and redness of the calf should alert the nurse to the possibility of deep venous thrombosis.

46. **(C)** Client need: physiological integrity; subcategory: reduction of risk potential; content area: med/surg

    RATIONALE

    (A) An abdominal binder may be necessary for some clients after abdominal surgery, but not after ERCP. (B) A cleansing enema may be necessary if the bowel must be clear for diagnostic studies, or prior to bowel surgery. It is not needed for ERCP. (C) The client is NPO postendoscopy until the gag reflex returns, usually within 2–4 hours. The client is also NPO for about 6 hours before the procedure. (D) Special skin care is not required with endoscopy. The endoscope will be removed after the procedure.

47. **(D)** Client need: physiological integrity; subcategory: reduction of risk potential; content area: med/surg

    RATIONALE

    (A) A biopsy is the surgical removal of a tissue specimen. Gallstones are not biopsied. (B) Oral cholecystography may be done for a client with ascites or extreme obesity if ultrasound is not effective in visualizing gallstones. Oral cholecystography involves ingestion of an iodine contrast medium. (C) With radionuclide imaging, there is injection of a radioactive isotope. This diagnostic procedure is not used to detect gallstones. (D) Ultrasound is the diagnostic procedure of choice to detect gallstones. It is noninvasive and about 95% accurate.

48. **(B)** Client need: physiological integrity; subcategory: reduction of risk potential; content area: med/surg

    RATIONALE

    (A) A client with gallstones could have abdominal distention, but it would not be related to the gallstones. (B) Dark urine is expected when bile flow through the hepatic or common bile duct is obstructed. Bile is reconverted to bilirubin and is excreted in the urine as urobilinogen. (C) A client with gallstones could have diminished bowel sounds, but they would not be related to the gallstones. (D) A client with obstruction to bile flow to the duodenum will have clay-colored stools due to the absence of bile in the stool. Gallstones do not cause the stools to be loose.

49. **(C)** Client need: physiological integrity; subcategory: physiological adaptation; content area: med/surg

    RATIONALE

    (A) Jaundice (often first seen in the sclera), dark urine, and clay-colored stools occur when bile flow to the duodenum is obstructed in the hepatic or common bile duct. Obstruction in the cystic duct does not interfere with bile flow from the liver to the duodenum. (B) Burning, frequency, and urgency are classic signs of UTI. Infected urine may also be cloudy. (C) Biliary colic occurs when the gallbladder contracts in response to a fatty meal, but there is obstruction to bile flow. Biliary colic is very uncomfortable. (D) Petechiae occur with capillary fragility and are not associated with gallstones. Blood in the stool and vomiting of blood occur with GI bleeding.

50. **(C)** Client need: physiological integrity; subcategory: reduction of risk potential; content area: med/surg

    RATIONALE

    (A) After cholecystectomy, the client will have an NG tube to suction to prevent postoperative distention. (B) NG drainage will be measured and discarded, but that is not the reason for placement of the tube. (C) Gastric distention is expected after cholecystectomy due to diminished peristalsis. Gastric decompression prevents pressure on internal suture lines, and also may prevent vomiting. (D) Medications can be administered via an NG tube, but after cholecystectomy, the tube should not be clamped until peristalsis returns.

51. **(D)** Client need: physiological integrity; subcategory: reduction of risk potential; content area: med/surg

    RATIONALE

    (A) After cholecystectomy, the client may lie on the operative or unoperative side. The client may be more comfortable on the unoperative side because of the presence of the Jackson-Pratt drain. (B) The client should lie with the head of the bed elevated in low Fowler position to facilitate drainage of bile through the T-tube. This position is not related to the location of the incision. (C) The client will be more comfortable if he or she splints the incision when turning and coughing, but this is not related to the location of the abdominal incision. (D) Because the surgical incision is high in the abdomen, taking deep breaths and coughing are painful. The client needs to be encouraged to turn, cough, and breathe deeply to prevent postoperative atelectasis.

52. **(A)** Client need: health promotion and maintenance; subcategory: prevention and early detection of disease; content area: med/surg

    RATIONALE

    (A) Serum alkaline phosphatase is normally excreted through the biliary tract. Obstruction to the biliary tree results in elevation of this enzyme. (B) The enzymes AST, ALT, and LDH may be elevated with liver disease, but not because the liver is enlarged. (C) Serum amylase and lipase may be elevated with pancreatitis. Pancreatic insufficiency is not tested by measuring serum enzymes. (D) An enlarged spleen may be palpable, but it is not tested by measuring serum enzymes.

53. **(D)** Client need: physiological integrity, reduction of risk potential; content area: med/surg

    RATIONALE

    (A) Radiopaque tablets are used with oral cholecystography. (B) PT is measured to assess blood coagulability. An ERCP involves passing an endoscope into the duodenum for direct visualization and for injection of contrast medium through the scope. (C) A cleansing enema is needed prior to diagnostic studies or surgery of the colon. An ERCP extends to the duodenum and pancreatic duct. (D) Any client with an endoscope or gastric tube should have dentures removed before the tube is passed.

54. **(D)** Client need: physiological integrity; subcategory: reduction of risk potential; content area: med/surg

RATIONALE

(A) A cholecystogram is an x-ray after ingestion of radiopaque tablets. Bleeding is not expected after a cholecystogram. (B) ERCP involves introducing an endoscope into the esophagus, stomach, and duodenum. Bleeding is unlikely after this procedure, but could occur if complicated by perforation. (C) IVP involves intravenous injection of radiopaque contrast medium for x-ray of the kidneys. Bleeding is unlikely after this test. (D) PTC involves insertion of a long, flexible needle through the abdomen into the biliary tract of the liver. It is important to assess for bleeding and for bile leakage after PTC.

55. **(D)** Client need: physiological integrity; subcategory: reduction of risk potential; content area: med/surg

RATIONALE

(A) A contrast medium containing iodine is not used with liver biopsy. An iodine contrast medium is used to enhance x-rays such as PTC. (B) A client with liver dysfunction is likely to have an elevated serum bilirubin, but this is not related to a liver biopsy. (C) After liver biopsy, a client should be assessed for hypotension due to bleeding or to peritonitis leading to paralytic ileus. (D) Inflammation of the peritoneum after any invasive procedure can lead to paralytic ileus, a neurogenic bowel obstruction that leads to hypovolemic shock.

56. **(D)** Client need: physiological integrity; subcategory: reduction of risk potential; content area: med/surg

RATIONALE

(A) The T-tube is clamped for 1–2 hours before and after meals to allow bile to drain into the duodenum. (B) Biliary drainage should not be discarded. If drainage does not diminish, the bile should be kept cold and may be returned via NG tube. A client going home with a T-tube will discard bile drainage. (C) After cholecystectomy, a client should be in low Fowler's position to promote biliary drainage. (D) Five hundred milliliters of drainage within the first 24 hours is within normal limits.

57. **(B)** Client need: physiological integrity; subcategory: reduction of risk potential; content area: med/surg

RATIONALE

(A) Jaundice is not related to PT. A client with liver dysfunction may have jaundice and also a prolonged PT. (B) Elevated direct bilirubin is due to obstruction to bile flow and results in obstructive jaundice. Elevated indirect bilirubin indicates the liver's inability to conjugate and excrete bilirubin and results in hepatocellular jaundice. (C) Jaundice is not related to serum potassium. A client with jaundice due to liver dysfunction may also have hypokalemia due to the liver's inability to catabolize aldosterone. (D) Jaundice is not related to acid-base balance.

58. **(C)** Client need: physiological integrity; subcategory: reduction of risk potential; content area: med/surg

RATIONALE

(A) A client with cirrhosis may have anorexia, loss of muscle mass, and weight gain due to fluid retention, but these do not contribute to hepatic encephalopathy. (B) A client taking lactulose may have diarrhea, but diarrhea and/or straining at stool do not contribute to hepatic encephalopathy. (C) A client with cirrhosis is at risk for GI bleeding due to portal hypertension and a prolonged PT. For a client with cirrhosis, digested blood is a source of protein in the GI tract. Hepatic encephalitis occurs when the liver is unable to detoxify ammonia, an end-product of protein catabolism. (D) A client with cirrhosis may experience nausea and vomiting, but these do not contribute to hepatic encephalopathy.

59. **(A)** Client need: physiological integrity; subcategory: physiological adaptation; content area: med/surg

RATIONALE

(A) Additional assessment is necessary to determine the cause of shortness of breath. It is likely that the esophageal balloon is pressing on the airway. (B) If shortness of breath is due to airway obstruction, the esophageal balloon must be deflated. Deflating the balloon also reduces the therapeutic function of the tube. (C) If the airway is unobstructed, raising the head of the bed and/or increasing O_2 flow may be effective in alleviating dyspnea. (D) If dyspnea is due to airway obstruction and deflating the esophageal balloon is ineffective, the tube should be removed. The therapeutic function of the tube is to apply pressure to bleeding esophageal varices.

60. **(A)** Client need: physiological integrity; subcategory: physiological adaptation; content area: med/surg

RATIONALE

(A) An elevated serum ammonia is toxic to the brain. Early signs include altered behavior and depressed intellectual function. Later signs include confusion and agitation. Severe hepatic encephalopathy leads to hepatic coma. (B) Respiratory status must be monitored, but a change does not suggest hepatic encephalopathy. (C) Urine output must be monitored, but a change does not suggest hepatic encephalopathy. (D) Vital signs must be monitored, but a change does not suggest hepatic encephalopathy.

61. **(D)** Client need: physiological integrity; subcategory: basic care and comfort; content area: med/surg

RATIONALE

(A) Because serum ammonia is normal, protein need not be restricted. A low-sodium diet helps to limit fluid retention associated with advanced cirrhosis. A bland diet is not necessary because of cirrhosis. (B) If the diet were restricted in protein, it should be supplemented with carbohydrates to reduce the amount of protein being used for energy. (C) Dietary protein may be increased if serum ammonia remains within normal limits. Because bile is insufficient, the diet should not be high in fat. Hypokalemia may be treated with supplements, but not by dietary change. (D) This client's diet should be well balanced and low in sodium. Vitamin supplements and folic acid help to replace deficiencies due to a dysfunctional liver.

62. **(C)** Client need: health promotion and maintenance; subcategory: prevention and early detection of disease; content area: med/surg

RATIONALE

(A) People with a dysfunctional liver have a decreased ability to fight infection. Infection increases metabolic rate and, for a person with cirrhosis, is a source of protein catabolism that should be avoided. (B) The diet should be supplemented with vitamins and folic acid to replace deficiencies due to cirrhosis. (C) All medication should be taken with caution because a dysfunctional liver does not adequately detoxify drugs. (D) Alcohol is a hepatotoxin and should be avoided. This client's plan to try to avoid alcohol should be reinforced.

63. **(C)** Client need: physiological integrity; subcategory: basic care and comfort; content area: med/surg

RATIONALE

(A) Everyone should change position at least every 2 hours, but the client with ascites will be most comfortable if the head of the bed is elevated. (B) Elevating the legs may help to reduce dependent edema, but it is not useful in relieving the discomfort of ascites. (C) With ascites, fluid in the peritoneal space pushes upward on the thoracic cavity and reduces thoracic excursion. Elevating the head of the bed makes breathing easier. (D) A side-lying position is acceptable for a client with ascites as long as the head of the bed is elevated.

64. **(D)** Client need: physiological integrity; subcategory: pharmacological and parenteral therapies; content area: med/surg

    RATIONALE

    (A) Ethacrynic acid is a diuretic, but it does not conserve potassium. (B) Furosemide is a diuretic, but it does not conserve potassium. (C) Hydrochlorothiazide is a diuretic, but it does not conserve potassium. (D) Spironolactone is a diuretic that promotes sodium excretion while conserving potassium. Clients with cirrhosis are at risk for hypokalemia because aldosterone is not adequately catabolized.

65. **(D)** Client need: physiological integrity; subcategory: pharmacological and parenteral therapies; content area: med/surg

    RATIONALE

    (A) Albumin will not relieve anorexia or itching. Anorexia in a client with cirrhosis is probably related to portal hypertension, and itching is probably related to dry skin or to jaundice. (B) Increased fluid output may ease breathing in a client with cirrhosis, but a better way to evaluate the effectiveness of albumin treatment is to measure urine output. (C) Albumin administration does not affect serum glucose. (D) Albumin is a protein that pulls fluid from interstitial to intravascular spaces. The healthy kidney will excrete the excess intravascular fluid. The objective of treatment is to increase fluid output.

66. **(B)** Client need: physiological integrity; subcategory: pharmacological and parenteral therapies; content area: med/surg

    RATIONALE

    (A) Lactulose should be stored at room temperature. It becomes too thick to pour if cold. (B) Juice makes lactulose more palatable and enhances its laxative effect. (C) Lactulose should not be taken with another laxative. The effectiveness of lactulose therapy would be difficult to evaluate. (D) Lactulose causes loose stools. The objective of therapy is to create an acid environment in the colon and to attract ammonium ions to reduce serum ammonia levels. A client with cirrhosis taking lactulose should have several soft bowel movements a day. If lactulose causes diarrhea, the dose should be reduced.

67. **(A)** Client need: physiological integrity; subcategory: basic care and comfort; content area: med/surg

    RATIONALE

    (A) A client with elevated serum ammonia is on a low-protein, low-sodium diet. Applesauce is low in protein and sodium. (B) A cheeseburger is high in protein and probably high in sodium. (C) Granola bars are not low in protein. (D) Peanuts are not low in protein.

68. **(B)** Client need: physiological integrity; subcategory: pharmacological and parenteral therapies; content area: med/surg

    RATIONALE

    (A) Elevated serum ammonia does not cause numbness in the extremities. (B) A change in the ability to write clearly or to calculate numbers correctly is a probable sign that serum ammonia levels are increasing. This should be assessed daily. (C) Extreme nervousness may be a sign of hepatic encephalopathy, but this is not an assessment technique. (D) Blood pressure should be monitored, but it is not an indication of elevated serum ammonia.

69. **(A)** Client need: physiological integrity; subcategory: pharmacological and parenteral therapies; content area: med/surg

    RATIONALE

    (A) Neomycin is an antibiotic that reduces the number of ammonia-producing bacteria in the colon. The objective of treatment is to prevent elevation in serum ammonia. (B) Most enemas help with bowel elimination, but the purpose of a neomycin retention enema is to reduce colonic bacteria that produce ammonia. (C) Neomycin is an antibiotic, and it may be given before

bowel surgery to prevent postoperative infection. (D) Neomycin is poorly absorbed from the GI tract. The medication needs to be in contact with the bacteria.

70. **(A)** Client need: physiological integrity; subcategory: reduction of risk potential; content area: med/surg

    RATIONALE

    (A) Prior to paracentesis, the bladder should be emptied to minimize risk of accidental puncture. (B) The abdominal girth will be reduced after paracentesis. It does not need to be measured. (C) During paracentesis, the client is sitting to facilitate drainage of ascitic fluid. (D) To assess for infection, temperature is monitored after any invasive procedure, but a baseline temperature is not necessary before paracentesis.

71. **(C)** Client need: physiological integrity; subcategory: physiological adaptation; content area: med/surg

    RATIONALE

    (A) Clients with cirrhosis may have folic acid deficiency, but it does not cause pruritus. (B) Clients with cirrhosis may have hypokalemia, but it does not cause pruritus. (C) Increased serum bilirubin causes jaundice, and jaundice causes dry skin and itching. (D) Clients with cirrhosis may have a prolonged PT, but it does not cause itching.

72. **(C)** Client need: physiological integrity; subcategory: reduction of risk potential; content area: med/surg

    RATIONALE

    (A) It is not necessary to force fluids after liver biopsy. Fluids may be forced after lumbar puncture to replace CSF. (B) The liver is on the right side. The head of the bed does not need to be elevated. (C) The client should lie on the right side with a pillow under the liver biopsy site. (D) The liver is a vascular organ and bleeding is a potential complication after biopsy, but a pressure dressing is not applied to the abdomen. The client's weight on the pillow applies pressure to the site to prevent bleeding.

73. **(A)** Client need: health promotion and maintenance; subcategory: prevention and early detection of disease; content area: med/surg

    RATIONALE

    (A) Digested blood causes the stool to be black and tarry. (B) Clay-colored stools occur when insufficient bile reaches the duodenum. A client with cirrhosis may have clay-colored stools, but they are not due to upper GI bleeding. (C) Red blood in the stools is due to bleeding in the lower GI tract. (D) A client with anemia due to GI bleeding may have compensatory increased respiratory and heart rates. Further assessment is required to identify the cause.

74. **(A)** Client need: physiological integrity; subcategory: pharmacological and parenteral therapies; content area: med/surg

    RATIONALE

    (A) Lactulose creates an acidic environment in the colon that attracts ammonia. The osmotic effect of organic acids causes water to move into the colon, which softens the stool and stimulates peristalsis. The dose of lactulose is titrated to enable several soft stools daily. (B) Headache and nasal congestion are not related to lactulose. (C) Lactulose increases fluid output from the colon; it does not affect kidney function. (D) Nausea and vomiting could occur with initial lactulose therapy, along with abdominal distention and discomfort. Nausea is not an expected result, however.

75. **(B)** Client need: health promotion and maintenance, prevention and early detection of disease; content area: med/surg

    RATIONALE

    (A) Anorexia is an expected assessment finding with hepatitis. (B) Rectal bleeding is not related to hepatitis. Further assessment is needed to identify the cause. (C) Dark urine is an expected assessment finding with hepatitis and is a result of increased serum bilirubin being excreted by the kidneys. (D) Yellow sclera is a sign of jaundice and is an expected assessment finding with hepatitis. Jaundice is caused by increased serum bilirubin.

76. **(C)** Client need: safe, effective care environment; subcategory: safety and infection control; content area: med/surg

    RATIONALE

    (A) Care to prevent spread of infection is important when disposing of food trays, but HAV is transmitted through ingestion of contaminated food or water or by contact with contaminated feces. (B) Care to prevent spread of infection is always important when changing IV tubing, but HAV is not transmitted through blood. Hepatitis B virus (HBV) is transmitted through blood or by direct contact. (C) HAV is transmitted through contaminated feces. (D) Care to prevent spread of infection is important when taking an oral temperature, but HAV is not transmitted by saliva.

77. **(A)** Client need: physiological integrity; subcategory: basic care and comfort; content area: med/surg

    RATIONALE

    (A) Protein and carbohydrate are needed for tissue repair. Because bile flow to the duodenum is diminished, the client will feel better with a low-fat diet. (B) The diet should be low in fat. Sodium does not need to be restricted because the client has hepatitis. (C) Calories from protein and carbohydrate are needed. It is good to suggest small, frequent meals because the client with hepatitis has a poor appetite. (D) If serum ammonia is increased due to a dysfunctional liver, the client's diet will be changed to low protein, high carbohydrate. Vitamin supplements are appropriate.

78. **(D)** Client need: health promotion and maintenance; subcategory: prevention and early detection of disease; content area: med/surg

    RATIONALE

    (A) Complete recovery from hepatitis takes a long time. In addition, the client should be taught to abstain from alcohol for a full year after all symptoms subside. (B) People with mild symptoms of HBV are more likely to become carriers than people with severe symptoms. (C) Hepatitis can become chronic and can lead to hepatocellular carcinoma. (D) HBV is contagious during the incubation period before symptoms appear. The incubation period may be as long as 6 months.

79. **(D)** Client need: physiological integrity; subcategory: physiological adaptation; content area: med/surg

    RATIONALE

    (A) Jaundice will subside when serum bilirubin levels return to normal. Skin care does not affect jaundice. (B) Skin care is needed for the client with fever who is perspiring, but it does not prevent perspiration. (C) Edema is not an expected assessment finding with hepatitis, unless the liver becomes dysfunctional. Care is necessary to protect edematous skin, but it does not reduce edema. (D) Jaundice is an expected assessment finding with hepatitis. A client with jaundice has dry, itchy skin. Moisturizing lotions can be used. Antihistamines may help to relieve itching.

80. **(D)** Client need: physiological integrity; subcategory: physiological adaptation; content area: med/surg

    RATIONALE

    (A) Caffeine may stimulate the CNS, but that is not the reason to keep a client with pancreatitis NPO. (B) Decaffeinated coffee may be comforting to the client, but a client with pancreatitis must remain NPO. (C) Pancreatitis may be treated surgically, but there is a more important reason to permit NPO. (D) NPO is maintained to prevent the stimulation of caustic pancreatic secretions when the pancreas is inflamed.

81. **(B)** Client need: health promotion and maintenance; subcategory: prevention and early detection of disease; content area: med/surg

    RATIONALE

    (A) Abdominal and back pain are expected assessment findings with pancreatitis. (B) Frothy sputum is not an expected assessment finding with acute pancreatitis. Further assessment is needed to determine the cause. (C) Nausea and vomiting may occur with pancreatitis. (D) Rebound tenderness is an expected assessment finding with peritonitis. Pancreatitis causes the peritoneum to become inflamed.

82. **(A)** Client need: health promotion and maintenance; subcategory: prevention and early detection of disease; content area: med/surg

    RATIONALE

    (A) Excessive alcohol consumption is one cause of acute pancreatitis. If alcohol consumption is a problem for this client, further counseling is needed. (B) Emotional stress is not a causative factor in pancreatitis. (C) Inadequate insulin may occur with pancreatitis, but diabetes is not a cause. The endocrine part of the pancreas secretes insulin; the exocrine part of the pancreas secretes digestive enzymes. (D) Recent weight gain is not related to pancreatitis.

83. **(C)** Client need: physiological integrity; subcategory: reduction of risk potential; content area: med/surg

    RATIONALE

    (A) An NG tube does prevent gastric distention and is important to prevent pressure on internal suture lines after abdominal surgery. (B) The gastrocolic reflex is the reflexive desire to defecate about one half hour after eating. The client with pancreatitis is NPO. (C) NPO status and gastric decompression are directed toward preventing the acutely inflamed pancreas from secreting digestive enzymes. (D) Gastrointestinal decompression is necessary if a client with pancreatitis develops paralytic ileus (the absence of bowel sounds) due to peritonitis. Suction does not prevent peristalsis.

84. **(C)** Client need: physiological integrity; subcategory: pharmacological and parenteral therapies; content area: med/surg

    RATIONALE

    (A) Sulfisoxazole does not affect ABGs. (B) Sulfisoxazole is a sulfonamide anti-infective. A client with UTI would not have a blood culture unless septicemia were suspected. (C) Sulfisoxazole may be nephrotoxic and hepatotoxic. An elevated serum creatinine indicates compromise to kidney function. (D) Sulfisoxazole may cause GI distress, but it should not cause GI bleeding.

85. **(C)** Client need: health promotion and maintenance; subcategory: prevention and early detection of disease; content area: med/surg

    RATIONALE

    (A) A person with glomerulonephritis should be taught to stay away from people with upper respiratory infections. (B) Orange juice alkalinizes the urine and would be indicated if the client were taking a sulfonamide drug. An acid urine is more likely to prevent cystitis, which could ascend to pyelonephritis. (C) Urethral contamination may lead to cystitis, which could ascend through the ureters to the kidneys. Pyelonephritis is an infection of the kidneys. (D) Aspirin may relieve the discomfort of fever and chills, but the client with a history of pyelonephritis should seek medical attention for these symptoms.

86. **(D)** Client need: health promotion and maintenance; subcategory: prevention and early detection of disease; content area: med/surg

    RATIONALE

    (A) Cloudy urine, due to infection, is expected with pyelonephritis. (B) Costovertebral tenderness is commonly associated with pyelonephritis. (C) General malaise occurs with infections, including pyelonephritis. (D) Hypertension is not expected with pyelonephritis, and its cause needs investigation. Hypertension can be due to a number of health problems, including damaged kidneys.

87. **(A)** Client need: health promotion and maintenance; subcategory: prevention and early detection of disease; content area: med/surg

    RATIONALE

    (A) Urinary burning, frequency, and urgency are classic signs of cystitis, a UTI. (B) Unless scar tissue or congenital stricture is limiting urine flow, the client should not expect difficulty voiding or cloudy urine. Cloudy urine may indicate an infection. (C) General malaise, fever, and sore throat accompany pyelonephritis and should be reported, but they are not the first signs of UTI. (D) Increased urinary output and stress incontinence are not expected with pyelonephritis. Low back pain may signify kidney infection.

88. **(A)** Client need: health promotion and maintenance; subcategory: prevention and early detection of disease; content area: med/surg

    RATIONALE

    (A) Nursing assessment of a client with cystitis should include percussing for costovertebral tenderness. Flank pain indicates extension of infection to the kidneys. (B) Bladder infection does not affect blood gases. (C) Abdominal rebound tenderness occurs with peritonitis. (D) Urine may be tested for protein, indicating compromise to kidney function, but there is no need to test for glycosuria.

89. **(C)** Client need: physiological integrity; subcategory: pharmacological and parenteral therapies; content area: med/surg

    RATIONALE

    (A) Tablets may be crushed and taken with a full glass of water, but they do not need to be chewed. (B) Sulfa drugs do not cause the urine to become blue. (C) To prevent renal crystals, people taking sulfa drugs should drink sufficient fluids to support 1500 mL of urine output daily. (D) Tinnitus and other CNS symptoms could occur with sulfa drugs, but they are not expected. Lying down does not stop ringing in the ears.

90. **(B)** Client need: physiological integrity; subcategory: pharmacological and parenteral therapies; content area: med/surg

    RATIONALE

    (A) To be effective, methenamine requires an acid urine pH of 5.5. Over-the-counter antacids, which alkalinize the urine, should be avoided. (B) Fluid intake should be adequate, but not forced, to prevent diuresis from this drug. It is not necessary for the client to weigh himself daily. (C) To minimize gastric distress, this drug should be taken with meals. (D) Ascorbic acid tablets and foods yielding an acid ash, such as cranberry juice, prunes, and plums, acidify the urine. The client should be taught to limit foods such as citrus fruits, which alkalinize the urine.

91. **(D)** Client need: physiological integrity; subcategory: reduction of risk potential; content area: med/surg

    RATIONALE

    (A) Solution for bladder irrigation should be at room temperature. It is not necessary to warm the solution. (B) The bladder is irrigated to prevent obstruction of urine flow. The irrigation is continuous, but not rapid. (C) Sterile water may be used for bladder irrigation. Normal saline should be used for gastric tube irrigation to prevent losses of electrolytes with the irrigating solution. (D) To prevent UTI, instillation of any solution or insertion of any instrument into the bladder must be sterile.

92. **(C)** Client need: health promotion and maintenance; subcategory: prevention and early detection of disease; content area: med/surg

    RATIONALE

    (A) Because sodium and fluid retention can occur with corticosteroids, salt should not be taken in excess. It does not need to be avoided. (B) Corticosteroid drugs, given to reduce inflammation, are withdrawn gradually to enable the adrenal gland to resume its function. (C) To prevent rejection, immunosuppressive drugs must be taken as prescribed for the life of the transplanted kidney. Forgetting to take the drug 1 day may result in the loss of the kidney. (D) A client with a kidney transplant should know the importance of follow-up medical examinations, but he does not need to test his urine daily for protein.

93. **(C)** Client need: physiological integrity; subcategory: physiological adaptation; content area: med/surg

    RATIONALE

    (A) Clients with ESRD should avoid the use of salt substitutes containing potassium, but this nursing order will not help them cope with anemia. (B) Clients with ESRD may be given antihypertensive medication, but this drug does not affect anemia. (C) Erythropoietin is a hormone, normally produced by the kidney, which stimulates the bone marrow to produce RBCs. (D) Clients with ESRD must monitor fluid balance, but this nursing action does not relieve anemia.

94. **(A)** Client need: physiological integrity; subcategory: physiological adaptation; content area: med/surg

    RATIONALE

    (A) Renal hypertension occurs with progressive kidney dysfunction. Damaged kidneys release the hormone renin, a powerful vasoconstrictor, in a compensatory effort to increase tissue perfusion through the kidneys. (B) Blood sugar does not increase because of glomerulonephritis. (C) Anemia does occur with progressive glomerulonephritis, primarily due to inadequate erythropoietin production. It is more important to periodically assess for renal hypertension. (D) Serum sodium may fluctuate with glomerulonephritis, but it is more important to assess for hypertension.

95. **(A)** Client need: physiological integrity; subcategory: basic care and comfort; content area: med/surg

    RATIONALE

    (A) Bread, fruits, and vegetables contain incomplete proteins because they do not contain all of the essential amino acids, and they are of low biological value. (B) Eggs contain complete proteins because they contain sufficient amounts of all of the essential amino acids and they are of high biological value. (C) Meat, fish, poultry, and cheese contain complete proteins and are of high biological value. (D) Milk contains complete proteins and is of high biological value.

96. **(C)** Client need: physiological integrity; subcategory: physiological adaptation; content area: med/surg

    RATIONALE

    (A) A rapid increase in weight is not due to too many calories. (B) Calcium is not directly related to weight gain. (C) Five hundred milliliters of fluid is equal to 1 lb. This client is most likely retaining fluid. (D) Steroid medication can cause fluid retention, but her treatment plan will most likely call for reduction in fluid intake.

97. **(B)** Client need: health promotion and maintenance; subcategory: prevention and early detection of disease; content area: med/surg

    RATIONALE

    (A) Metabolic acidosis occurs when the kidneys fail to regulate acid-base balance. (B) Oliguria or anuria occurs in the early stages of acute renal failure owing to the kidney's inability to excrete urine. As the client recovers, diuresis is expected. (C) Hyperkalemia occurs when the kidneys fail to maintain electrolyte balance. (D) Hypertension occurs when damaged kidneys secrete renin.

98. **(A)** Client need: physiological integrity; subcategory: basic care and comfort; content area: med/surg
    RATIONALE
    (A) Dietary carbohydrate is increased to spare body protein from being used for energy. Clients with ESRD cannot adequately excrete the toxic end products of protein metabolism. (B) Fluid intake is restricted to equal fluid output. (C) Dietary potassium must be restricted to prevent toxic hyperkalemia. (D) Dietary protein is restricted and should be of high biological value.

99. **(D)** Client need: physiological integrity; subcategory: physiological adaptation; content area: med/surg
    RATIONALE
    (A) Fluid intake should be decreased to equal fluid output. (B) It is not necessary to monitor specific gravity because a low and fixed urine specific gravity is expected with ESRD owing to the kidney's inability to concentrate the urine. (C) It is important to monitor intake and output, but weight is a better assessment of fluid balance. (D) Rapid weight gain is the best indicator of fluid retention. For clients with ESRD, weight should be measured daily.

100. **(B)** Client need: physiological integrity; subcategory: physiological adaptation; content area: med/surg
    RATIONALE
    (A) Increased bowel sounds may indicate hyperkalemia. It is more important to avoid giving potassium. (B) KCl salt substitutes are contraindicated for clients in renal failure. (C) It is important to monitor the ECG for changes characteristic of hyperkalemia. It is more important to avoid giving potassium. (D) It will be important to prepare the client for dialysis if serum potassium is rising. Serum potassium above 6 mEq/L is likely to result in fibrillation or asystole.

101. **(B)** Client need: physiological integrity; subcategory: physiological adaptation; content area: med/surg
    RATIONALE
    (A) BUN is an indicator of kidney function, but a rising serum creatinine is a more accurate measure of dysfunction. (B) ECG changes characteristic of hyperkalemia include: peaked and elevated T wave, widened QRS complex, and flat or absent P wave. It is most important to report these changes because hyperkalemia can lead to cardiac fibrillation or asystole. (C) Changes in hematocrit should be reported. (D) Weight is an important assessment of fluid balance and changes should be reported.

102. **(D)** Client need: physiological integrity; subcategory: physiological adaptation; content area: med/surg
    RATIONALE
    (A) A client with glomerulonephritis does not need to avoid exposure to the sun, only excessive exposure. (B) A client with chronic glomerulonephritis should report cloudy urine, which may indicate proteinuria, but she does not have to test her urine daily for protein. (C) Persistent headache in a person with kidney dysfunction may indicate renal hypertension. (D) It is imperative for a person with recurrent glomerulonephritis to have a culture for sore throat. Glomerulonephritis is a kidney inflammation usually caused by b-hemolytic streptococcus.

103. **(D)** Client need: physiological integrity; subcategory: physiological adaptation; content area: med/surg
    RATIONALE
    (A) A stable blood pressure is one evaluation criterion, but serum potassium is more important. (B) Heart rhythm is important, and it should be monitored continuously because, for a client with acute renal failure, an irregular rhythm may indicate hyperkalemia. (C) Serum creatinine levels monitor kidney function, but they are not indicators of cardiac output. (D)

Clients with acute renal diseases are at high risk for decreased cardiac output related to arrhythmia due to hyperkalemia.

104. **(D)** Client need: physiological integrity; subcategory: pharmacological and parenteral therapies; content area: pediatrics
    RATIONALE
    (A) Children with nephrosis may have a poor appetite when they do not feel well, but anyone taking steroids is more likely to have an increased appetite. (B) Ascites may occur with nephrosis, but it is due to fluid shifts from the intravascular space when proteins are lost through the glomerular filtrate. (C) Everyone taking steroids is at risk for peptic ulcers, but steroids are unlikely to cause diarrhea. (D) Steroids suppress the immune response and therefore compromise the client's ability to resist infection.

105. **(B)** Client need: physiological integrity; subcategory: physiological adaptation; content area: med/surg
    RATIONALE
    (A) Hyperkalemia occurs with renal failure but is not associated with nephrotic syndrome. (B) There is increased glomerular permeability, resulting in the loss of protein from the intravascular space to the urine. Hypoproteinemia causes fluid shifts, resulting in the massive edema of nephrosis. (C) Renal hypertension due to renin secretion occurs with renal failure but is not associated with nephrosis. (D) Nephrosis does not cause sodium loss. The client stays on a sodium-restricted diet to help control edema.

106. **(C)** Client need: physiological integrity; subcategory: pharmacological and parenteral therapies; content area: pediatrics
    RATIONALE
    (A) Diuretics are given to help control edema. (B) Spironolactone, a diuretic that antagonizes aldosterone, may be given to help control fluid imbalance due to sodium retention. (C) Steroids are given to children with nephrosis to reduce glomerular inflammation. The goal is to reduce proteins from being lost owing to increased glomerular permeability. (D) Steroids suppress the inflammatory response, which puts the client at greater risk of infection.

107. **(B)** Client need: physiological integrity; subcategory: basic care and comfort; content area: pediatrics
    RATIONALE
    (A) A healthy diet is not high in fat. (B) Increased protein intake of 2–3 g/k of body weight is essential to replace protein losses. High-protein foods and/or diet supplements should be offered, especially if the child's appetite is poor. (C) Calories are increased to spare protein from being used as energy. (D) A low-purine diet is suggested for someone who has gout and is unable to metabolize purine, but it is not necessary for a child with nephrosis.

108. **(C)** Client need: health promotion and maintenance; subcategory: early detection and prevention of disease; content area: pediatrics
    RATIONALE
    (A) Cloudy urine due to the presence of protein is expected with nephrosis. (B) Reduced urine output is expected in the early stages of nephrosis. As the child recovers, diuresis will restore fluid balance. (C) Blood pressure and heart rate should be within normal limits or slightly higher. Rising blood pressure may indicate kidney damage or CHF and should be reported. (D) Weight gain due to fluid retention is expected in the early stages of nephrosis.

109. **(B)** Client need: physiological integrity; subcategory: reduction of risk potential; content area: med/surg
    RATIONALE
    (A) The client's urine is being diluted with saline. It should not change from pale red to dark red unless there is increased

bleeding. It is necessary to notify the surgeon. (B) The surgeon will cauterize bleeding vessels. (C) The catheter must not be removed. Obstruction to urine flow can cause pressure at the surgical site with risk of severe bleeding. The catheter is anchored with tape to prevent bleeding and must never be repositioned by the nurse. (D) Action is necessary. The change in color indicates active bleeding.

110. **(B)** Client need: physiological integrity; subcategory: physiological adaptation; content area: med/surg

    RATIONALE

    (A) Glomerulonephritis is a kidney inflammation usually caused by b-hemolytic streptococcus, often from a strep throat. (B) Hydronephrosis occurs when obstruction to urine flow causes back pressure on the kidney(s), with eventual destruction of kidney function. (C) Nephroptosis occurs when a kidney prolapses downward. It is not related to urine-flow obstruction. (D) Pyelonephritis is a kidney infection usually due to an ascending pathogen from the bladder.

111. **(C)** Client needs: health promotion and maintenance; subcategory: prevention and early detection of disease; content area: med/surg

    RATIONALE

    (A) Frequency, burning, and urgency are classic signs of UTI. They are not expected with BPH. (B) A client with BPH should have a body temperature within normal limits. (C) Narrowed stream of urine flow and difficulty initiating voiding are expected with BPH due to the obstruction of the enlarged prostate gland. (D) Itching is not expected with BPH.

112. **(A)** Client need: physiological integrity; subcategory: reduction of risk potential; content area: med/surg

    RATIONALE

    (A) Bloody urine is expected immediately after TUR. Assure the roommate that a pink to clear red color is normal, then check the client for excessive bleeding. (B) Excessive bleeding or large clots must be reported to the surgeon. (C) Vital signs should be assessed, and the surgeon called if there is excessive bleeding. (D) If bleeding is within expected limits, it is not necessary to take measures to raise blood pressure.

113. **(B)** Client need: health promotion and maintenance; subcategory: prevention and early detection of disease; content area: med/surg

    RATIONALE

    (A) Position does not help to control dribbling after TUR. (B) Perineal exercises such as squeezing the buttocks together or attempting to stop the stream of urine flow will help to control dribbling. (C) The client should have a normal fluid intake and does not need to limit fluids to mealtimes. (D) Plastic protection may be necessary, but perineal exercises are directed at controlling the problem.

114. **(D)** Client need: physiological integrity; subcategory: reduction of risk potential; content area: med/surg

    RATIONALE

    (A) Sexual performance should not diminish because of TUR. There may be retrograde ejaculation of semen into the bladder. (B) Dark urine after TUR is probably due to increased concentration. The client does not need to call his physician unless the urine stays dark or if he suspects bleeding. (C) Light urine after TUR is probably due to decreased concentration. He does not need to call his physician unless the situation persists. (D) A narrowed stream of urine developing after TUR may be due to obstruction caused by scar tissue. He should call his physician for further investigation.

115. **(B)** Client need: physiological integrity; subcategory: reduction of risk potential; content area: med/surg

    RATIONALE

    (A) It is always important to check the patency of a catheter after TUR, but there is a more important problem. (B) If the client's hips are flexed, the traction catheter is ineffective. Lower the head of the bed and explain why so the client will be better able to comply. (C) It is always important to check urine color after TUR, but there is a more important problem. (D) It is necessary to take action. The purpose of the traction catheter is to apply pressure to the internal surgical site to prevent bleeding.

116. **(C)** Client need: physiological integrity; subcategory: basic care and comfort; content area: med/surg

    RATIONALE

    (A) Urine should be strained for stones, but this is not the immediate goal of care. (B) Hydronephrosis is a serious potential complication of renal calculi, but prevention is not the goal at this time. (C) Renal colic is extremely painful. The goal of care is to relieve pain as soon as possible. (D) It is important to teach the client ways of preventing further calculi formation, but this is not the goal at this time.

117. **(D)** Client need: health promotion and maintenance; subcategory: prevention and early detection of disease; content area: med/surg

    RATIONALE

    (A) Coffee in moderation does not cause renal calculi. (B) The client should void when his bladder is full and he feels the urge. It is not necessary to teach him to void frequently. (C) Health problems causing glucose in the urine are not related to renal calculi. (D) Predisposing factors that may lead to renal calculi include concentrated urine due to dehydration, acid or alkaline-ash diet, immobility, and infection.

118. **(D)** Client need: health promotion and maintenance, subcategory: prevention and early detection of disease; content area: med/surg

    RATIONALE

    (A) Calcium phosphate kidney stones are less likely to form in an acid medium. Foods that acidify the urine include cranberry juice, meat, eggs, whole grains, and prunes. Foods such as citrus fruits, milk, and tomatoes alkalinize the urine and should be limited. (B) Milk should not be taken in excess, but it is not necessary to eliminate milk from the diet. (C) Infection can occur if there is obstruction to urine flow, but it is not necessary to teach the client to test his urine monthly (D) Forcing fluids to 2400–3000 mL daily will help dilute the urine to prevent stone formation and to flush existing stones.

119. **(B)** Client need: physiological integrity; subcategory: pharmacological and parenteral therapies; content area: med/surg

    RATIONALE

    (A) Cystoscopy involves direct visualization of the bladder. Iodine is not used. (B) IVP involves injection of an iodine contrast medium. A client allergic to shellfish is likely to be allergic to iodine. (C) Renal scan involves administration of tracer doses of a radioisotope. Iodine is not used. (D) Ultrasound, used as an initial diagnostic procedure, uses sound waves. Iodine is not used.

120. **(A)** Client need: physiological integrity; subcategory: reduction of risk potential; content area: med/surg

    RATIONALE

    (A) The goal of treatment for extracorporeal shock wave lithotripsy is to break up kidney stones so they can pass into the urine. Forcing fluids will help the client pass the stone fragments. (B) Transient hematuria is expected postprocedure, but a dressing is not necessary. (C) The client should rest after the procedure and may need antispasmodic or urinary analgesics. It is not necessary to keep the head of the bed flat. (D) A regular diet is resumed after the procedure. The client will be advised to include in his diet foods that acidify the urine if calcium phosphate stones are passed.

121. **(A)** Client need: physiological integrity; subcategory: reduction of risk potential; content area: med/surg

RATIONALE

(A) An indwelling catheter should be replaced approximately every 30 days. The client is at risk for UTI. (B) If the goal of care is bladder training, the catheter should be clamped for 4 hours then released. (C) It would be inconvenient for a client at home to have continuous bladder irrigation. (D) Intermittent catheter irrigation is not effective in reducing bacteria.

122. **(B)** Client need: physiological integrity; subcategory: reduction of risk potential; content area: med/surg

RATIONALE

(A) The lab will tell the nurse to restart the test tomorrow. (B) A 24-hour urine requires all urine output for 24 hours. The first voided specimen is discarded; then all urine produced for the next 24 hours is collected. (C) The amount voided is not important because the test requires all urine to be collected. (D) It is necessary to take action. The test has been invalidated because urine was discarded.

123. **(A)** Client need: health promotion and maintenance; subcategory: prevention and early detection of disease; content area: med/surg

RATIONALE

(A) If the client can discriminate between sharp and dull, then temperature and vibration sense are probably intact. (B) Spinal sensory nerves are tested for temperature and vibration. (C) Assessing for weakness or paralysis is a test of motor nerve function. (D) An alert and aware client may have diminished temperature and vibration sense.

124. **(C)** Client need: health promotion and maintenance; subcategory: prevention and early detection of disease; content area: med/surg

RATIONALE

(A) Assessment of touch, discrimination between sharp and dull, temperature, and vibration may be included with an alert client. (B) It is important to prevent injury when testing for deep pain, but deep pain is not tested with an alert client. (C) Scattering stimuli in a circular motion around the extremities will cover most dermatomes and will more likely reveal a spinal cord lesion. (D) Squeezing the trapezius muscle is a test for central pain when a client does not respond to verbal commands owing to a depressed level of consciousness.

125. **(A)** Client need: health promotion and maintenance; subcategory: prevention and early detection of disease; content area: med/surg

RATIONALE

(A) The cerebellum and extrapyramidal tract control posture, balance, and gait. (B) The cerebrum controls thinking and feeling. The pyramidal tract controls voluntary movement. (C) The occipital lobe controls vision. (D) The reticular activating system maintains an awake state.

126. **(B)** Client need: health promotion and maintenance; subcategory: prevention and early detection of disease; content area: med/surg

RATIONALE

(A) Raising the eyebrows symmetrically indicates intact motor function of the trigeminal nerve (cranial nerve V). (B) A symmetrical tongue with no fasciculation indicates an intact hypoglossal nerve (cranial nerve XII). (C) Bilateral strength of the trapezius and sternocleidomastoid muscles indicates an intact spinal accessory nerve (cranial nerve XI). (D) A uvula remaining in midline when the client says "ah" indicates intact motor function of the vagus nerve (cranial nerve X).

127. **(B)** Client need: health promotion and maintenance; subcategory: prevention and early detection of disease; content area: med/surg

RATIONALE

(A) The ability to puff out the cheeks indicates intact motor function of the trigeminal nerve (cranial nerve V). (B) A wisp of cotton is used to test the sensory component of the three branches of the trigeminal nerve bilaterally. The client's eyes should be closed so that he or she cannot see when the cotton is applied. (C) It is not necessary to turn the client's head to the side when testing sensory function of cranial nerve V. (D) The ability to clench teeth indicates intact motor function of the trigeminal nerve (cranial nerve V).

128. **(A)** Client need: health promotion and maintenance; subcategory: prevention and early detection of disease; content area: med/surg

RATIONALE

(A) A client who normally wears glasses should have them on when the optic nerve is tested. This is a test of vision. (B) Room light should be of normal intensity when the optic nerve is being tested. (C) When testing visual fields by confrontation, the examiner's right eye is closed when testing the client's left eye. The procedure is reversed when testing the client's right eye. (D) An ophthalmoscope examines the retina and does not measure pupil size. Pupil size is measured by estimating the size of the pupil on a scale of 1 to 10 or by comparing the pupil size with a gauge.

129. **(D)** Client need: health promotion and maintenance; subcategory: prevention and early detection of disease; content area: med/surg

RATIONALE

(A) Change in level of consciousness is the first sign of increasing ICP. The GCS is used to assess and monitor level of consciousness. (B) Deep pain stimuli are used to assess level of consciousness. They are not used to test motor function. (C) An uncooperative and demanding client does not have a depressed level of consciousness. (D) Deep pain stimuli are an appropriate assessment technique when a client is unresponsive to verbal commands owing to a depressed level of consciousness.

130. **(D)** Client need: health promotion and maintenance; subcategory: prevention and early detection of disease; content area: med/surg

RATIONALE

(A) CNS depressants are usually withheld prior to EEG. (B) It is not necessary for clients to have nothing by mouth prior to EEG. (C) The client's hair should be clean, but his scalp should not remain damp. His hair should be shampooed after the EEG to remove the electrode paste. (D) Stimulants containing caffeine, such as coffee, tea, and colas, should be withheld for 8 hours prior to EEG.

131. **(C)** Client need: physiological integrity; subcategory: physiological adaptation; content area: med/surg

RATIONALE

(A) Increased ICP is not an expected assessment finding for a client with Guillain-Barré syndrome. (B) Insufficient acetylcholine at the myoneural junction is associated with myasthenia gravis. (C) Ascending paralysis associated with Guillain-Barré syndrome may affect muscles required for respiration. (D) Seizures are not associated with Guillain-Barré syndrome.

132. **(C)** Client need: physiological integrity; subcategory: reduction of risk potential; content area: med/surg

RATIONALE

(A) Hyperventilation may fully aerate the alveoli, but this is not the goal of care for this client. (B) O_2 administration will increase

PaO_2, but this is not the goal for this client. (C) Hyperventilation lowers CO_2, a potent vasodilator of cerebral vessels. Dilated cerebral vessels increase ICP due to edema, because hydrostatic pressure causes fluid to leak out of the vessel. The client should be on a mechanical ventilator. (D) Hyperventilation does not stimulate the reticular activating system.

133. **(D)** Client need: health promotion and maintenance; subcategory: prevention and early detection of disease; content area: med/surg

    RATIONALE

    (A) Aphasia, a language dysfunction, is more commonly associated with a CVA of the left hemisphere. (B) Hemiparesis, weakness of one side of the body, is more commonly associated with a CVA. (C) Paresthesia, increased sensation (tingling), is associated with a number of neurological problems affecting the sensory branches of the nervous system. (D) Battle's sign, ecchymosis near the mastoid bone, and raccoon sign, ecchymosis around the eyes, are commonly associated with a basilar skull fracture. The nurse should be alert for spinal fluid leak in a client with a basilar skull fracture.

134. **(C)** Client need: physiological integrity; subcategory: reduction of risk potential; content area: med/surg

    RATIONALE

    (A) Voiding patterns should be monitored, but it is more important to assess pupil size. (B) The client should be helped to sleep restfully, but it is more important to assess pupil size. (C) Because the cranial nerves exit from the brain stem, change in pupil size or reaction to light indicates compromise to the brain stem. The irregular pupil size on admission is a baseline from which to monitor change. (D) Nutrition is important and there are many fundamental nursing measures to help people regain appetite, but for this client it is more important to assess pupil size.

135. **(C)** Client need: physiological integrity; subcategory: reduction of risk potential; content area: med/surg

    RATIONALE

    (A) Elevating the legs may be done to combat hypovolemic shock due to internal bleeding, but it is not done as treatment for spinal cord injury. (B) External rotation of the hip joints has no effect on a fractured spine. (C) Any client with spine fracture must be protected from further injury caused by movement of sharp broken bone fragments. Laceration of the spinal cord results in permanent loss of motion and sensation. (D) A client with a fractured spine will be immobilized in a supine position, but it is most important to protect from further cord injury.

136. **(C)** Client need: physiological integrity; subcategory: reduction of risk potential; content area: med/surg

    RATIONALE

    (A) A venous access site will be established, but it is most important to prevent further cord injury due to movement. (B) It is important to assess for brain-stem dysfunction due to a possible head injury, but it is most important to prevent further cord injury. (C) It is very likely that this client has sustained a cervical fracture and cord injury. Flexion, extension, and rotation of the spine must be prevented to reduce the risk of further cord injury. (D) It is important to assess for disorientation because it may be a sign of a decreasing level of consciousness due to head injury. It is most important to prevent further cord injury.

137. **(B)** Client need: psychosocial integrity; subcategory: coping and adaptation; content area: med/surg

    RATIONALE

    (A) Full recovery is possible if there is no permanent damage to the cord due to laceration or sustained pressure. (B) During spinal shock, pressure on the cord may cause loss of motion and sensation. The goals of medical and nursing management are to prevent further injury, to perfuse the cord with oxygenated blood, and to reduce pressure. (C) Medical technology is not sufficiently advanced to successfully repair a lacerated spinal cord. (D) As spinal shock and pressure subside, the client will regain function if there is no permanent damage. Full function may not be apparent for 6 months to a year.

138. **(C)** Client need: safe, effective care environment; subcategory: management of care; content area: med/surg

    RATIONALE

    (A) An EEG does not cause a sensation of warmth. A cerebral arteriogram may cause a burning sensation. (B) The client will not feel any sensation when the current is turned on. The EEG is a test of brain-wave activity. (C) The client should know that he will feel no discomfort during the procedure. (D) The client will not feel dizzy after an EEG.

139. **(D)** Client need: physiological integrity; subcategory: reduction of risk potential; content area: med/surg

    RATIONALE

    (A) Air may effectively irrigate the tube, but it is likely to cause distention and discomfort. (B) Normal saline instills sodium, which is not appropriate for irrigating a feeding tube. (C) Fifteen milliliters of solution is not enough to fully irrigate the length of the tubing. (D) Sterile irrigating solution is unnecessary unless there are fresh internal suture lines. Thirty milliliters is sufficient to clear the tubing. Tap water does not introduce electrolytes.

140. **(C)** Client need: physiological integrity; subcategory: reduction of risk potential; content area: med/surg

    RATIONALE

    (A) The client should check for residual. The feeding should be withheld if there is more than 50 mL of residual feeding. (B) The feeding should be comfortable at room temperature, or it may be warmed to near body temperature. (C) To aid in digestion and prevent aspiration, the client should sit up for about one-half hour after the feeding. (D) The client should be able to tolerate 300–500 mL of tube feeding over a period of 10–15 minutes.

141. **(D)** Client need: physiological integrity; subcategory: pharmacological and parenteral therapies; content area: med/surg

    RATIONALE

    (A) The initial rate of flow for 10% lipid emulsions is 1 mL/min (0.5 mL/min for 20% emulsion) to monitor safely for allergic reaction. Once established, the maximum flow rate for lipid emulsions should be 2 mL/min (500 mL in 4 hours) for a 10% solution, or 1 mL/min (500 mL in 8 hours) for a 20% solution. (B) Filters can break down emulsions and should never be used. (C) Lipid emulsions need not be refrigerated and should be administered at room temperature. (D) Additives may cause separation of emulsions and should not be used.

142. **(D)** Client need: physiological integrity; subcategory: pharmacological and parenteral therapies; content area: med/surg

    RATIONALE

    (A) Total parenteral nutrition (TPN) solutions do contain amino acids, but proteins do not cause hyperosmolar diuresis. (B) TPN solutions should contain sufficient carbohydrates, but carbohydrates do not cause hyperosmolar diuresis. (C) Any IV solution with precipitates should be discarded, but precipitates do not cause diuresis. (D) Rapid IV infusion of a concentrated solution pulls fluid from less concentrated interstitial spaces. In a compensatory effort to maintain fluid balance, healthy kidneys will excrete the resulting increased intravascular fluid volume, resulting in diuresis and leading to severe dehydration and possibly hypovolemic shock.

143. **(C)** Client need: physiological integrity; subcategory: pharmacological and parenteral therapies; content area: med/surg

RATIONALE

(A) Antacids interfere with the absorption of iron. (B) Milk interferes with the absorption of iron. (C) Acids such as orange juice increase iron absorption. Iron should be given between meals for maximum absorption, but it may be given with meals if GI disturbance occurs. Liquid iron should be taken through a straw to prevent staining of teeth. (D) Iron may be taken with water, but for maximum absorption should be taken with an acid such as orange juice.

144. **(A)** Client need: physiological integrity; subcategory: basic care and comfort; content area: med/surg

RATIONALE

(A) Dumping syndrome occurs because a concentrated solution pulls fluid from intravascular spaces, and also because concentrated carbohydrates stimulate insulin production. The client should avoid concentrated carbohydrates to prevent hypoglycemia, and he should limit sodium to prevent further drawing of fluid. (B) The client should lie down after meals, preferably on his left side to slow gastric emptying. (C) A healthy diet contains some fat. A person who limits carbohydrate intake should increase dietary protein and fat to provide necessary calories. (D) Fluids should be taken between meals. Liquids taken with meals increase gastric emptying into the duodenum.

145. **(B)** Client need: physiological integrity; subcategory: pharmacological and parenteral therapies; content area: med/surg

RATIONALE

(A) Aspirin is damaging to the gastric mucosa and should be avoided by anyone with history of peptic ulcer. (B) Many antacids contain calcium. Calcium antacids may cause constipation. Calcium carbonate antacids may cause gastric acid rebound. (C) Some antacids contain magnesium. Magnesium antacids may cause diarrhea. (D) Local antacids contain sodium, some in significant amounts. Sodium is not contraindicated with peptic ulcer disease. Systemic antacids, such as sodium bicarbonate, should be avoided to prevent systemic alkalosis.

146. **(A)** Client need: physiological integrity; subcategory: physiological adaptation; content area: med/surg

RATIONALE

(A) Bending over allows caustic gastric contents to flow upward to the esophagus, causing pain in a client with hiatal hernia. The esophageal mucosa, unlike the gastric mucosa, cannot defend against strong acid. (B) Concentrated carbohydrates should be avoided for people with dumping syndrome. They do not affect a hiatal hernia. (C) People with hiatal hernia should sit up after meals to prevent gastric reflux to the esophagus. (D) People with hiatal hernia may be more comfortable if they sleep with the head of the bed elevated to prevent gastric reflux.

147. **(A)** Client need: physiological integrity; subcategory: reduction of risk potential; content area: med/surg

RATIONALE

(A) Topical anesthesia, given prior to EGD, eliminates the gag reflex. Any client with a diminished or absent gag reflex must be kept NPO to prevent aspiration. (B) The client is kept NPO prior to EGD, but once the gag reflex has returned, she may resume her diet. (C) It is not necessary to remain flat after EGD. It is necessary to remain flat after lumbar puncture with a water-based contrast medium. (D) When anesthesia wears off after EGD, the client will have a sore throat. She must be kept NPO until her gag reflex returns.

148. **(B)** Client need: health promotion and maintenance; subcategory: prevention and early detection of disease; content area: med/surg

RATIONALE

(A) Symptoms of dumping syndrome are due to hypotension when fluid shifts from the intravascular space, and to hypoglycemia when insulin is secreted in response to rapid absorption of carbohydrates. Compensatory tachycardia occurs with hypotension. Hypoglycemia may cause perspiration. The client should not be confused. (B) Dizziness, tachycardia, palpitations, perspiration, faintness, weakness, feeling of fullness, pallor or flushing, and nausea may occur with dumping syndrome because of hypotension and hypoglycemia. (C) Pallor may occur with dumping syndrome. Perspiration may accompany hypoglycemia. Constipation is not related to hypotension or to hypoglycemia. (D) Drowsiness and flushed skin may occur with dumping syndrome, but epigastric burning is not related to hypotension or to hypoglycemia.

149. **(D)** Client need: physiological integrity; subcategory: pharmacological and parenteral therapies; content area: med/surg

RATIONALE

(A) Aluminum antacids may contain more than 1000 mg of sodium per dose. Aluminum hydroxide and dihydroxyaluminum sodium carbonate antacids are high in sodium. Aluminum carbonate is much lower in sodium. The client should read the labels before switching to a different antacid. (B) Local antacids do not cause acid-base imbalance. (C) Chewable antacids are usually less effective than liquid antacids. For maximum effectiveness, they must be chewed thoroughly. (D) Sodium bicarbonate may relieve gastric pain, but it also causes systemic alkalosis and sodium overload. Any client should know to refrain from taking systemic antacids to relieve pain of peptic ulcer.

150. **(B)** Client need: physiological integrity; subcategory: reduction of risk potential; content area: med/surg

RATIONALE

(A) A rubber ring would not be in direct contact with the operative site, but there is a disadvantage to using a rubber ring after perineal or perianal surgery. (B) A rubber ring may be comfortable to sit on initially, but it causes pressure on tissues surrounding the operative site and may increase edema and pain at the operative site. (C) Sitting on a rubber ring should not restrict mobility. (D) If a rubber ring were to rupture, it probably would traumatize the operative site, but rupture is unlikely.

151. **(C)** Client need: physiological integrity; subcategory: reduction of risk potential; content area: med/surg

RATIONALE

(A) Postoperative vomiting and intestinal distention are minimized by gastric suction. (B) Changes in intrathoracic pressure may increase blood pressure, but they will not stimulate gastric drainage. (C) Any abdominal incision, and especially one high in the abdomen, is painful with breathing. The client may take short, shallow breaths to minimize pain. Turning, coughing, and deep breathing are important to aerate alveoli and to prevent atelectasis. (D) Coughing does not stimulate the phrenic nerve. Gastric distention may stimulate the phrenic nerve and cause hiccough.

152. **(A)** Client need: physiological integrity; subcategory: pharmacological and parenteral therapies; content area: med/surg

RATIONALE

(A) To prevent precipitation during reconstitution, amphotericin B must be mixed with sterile water for injection without bacteriostatic agents or preservatives. (B, C, D) Reconstitution with acidic solutions, sodium chloride, or benzyl alcohol may cause precipitation. After reconstitution, amphotericin B may be further diluted in 5% dextrose with a pH above 4.2.

153. **(D)** Client need: physiological integrity; subcategory: basic care and comfort; content area: med/surg

 RATIONALE

 (A, B, C, D) 1 kg = 2.2 lb

 $$\frac{132 \text{ lb}}{2.2 \text{ kg}} = 60 \text{ kg}$$

154. **(C)** Client need: health promotion and maintenance; subcategory: prevention and early detection of disease; content area: med/surg

 RATIONALE

 (A, B, D) The nurse may not always have paper towels, soap, or warm water available. (C) Regardless of facilities, the fingers and nails are the most important to clean, because they harbor microorganisms and dirt.

155. **(B)** Client need: health promotion and maintenance; subcategory: prevention and early detection of disease; content area: med/surg

 RATIONALE

 (A) Inflate rapidly to avoid collapsing or rolling the artery; deflate slowly to read the manometer. (B) Using the wrong size cuff will cause the reading to be falsely high (cuff too small, thus overcompressing the artery) or falsely low (cuff too large, thus undercompressing the artery). (C) Two or three sounds will ensure accuracy of the reading. (D) The baseline is determined on the first reading and serves only as a guideline for future readings.

156. **(A)** Client need: physiological integrity; subcategory: basic care and comfort; content area: med/surg

 RATIONALE

 Formula

 $$\text{degree Celsius} \times \frac{9}{5} + 32$$

 $$40 \times \frac{9}{5} = \frac{360}{5} = 72 + 32 = 104$$

157. **(A)** Client need: physiological integrity; subcategory: pharmacological and parenteral therapies; content area: med/surg

 RATIONALE

 (A) Naloxone is a narcotic antagonist that is indicated in narcotic overdose to reverse respiratory or narcotic depression. For emergency use in adults, the usual dose is 0.4–2.0 mg at 2–3 minute intervals until 10 mg is given. (B) Niacin is a vitamin. (C) Nitroglycerin is a vasodilator. (D) Nitroprusside is a vasodilator.

158. **(D)** Client need: health promotion and maintenance; subcategory: prevention and early detection of disease; content area: med/surg

 RATIONALE

 (A, B) These responses are incorrect. (C) This response is a way of defining the mental status of the client; the client knows who he is, that he is in the hospital (which information is not in the stem of the question), and what season it is. (D) The phrase "oriented × 3" is an accepted way of noting that the client has intact thought processes in relation to who he is; where he is; and what time of day, month (holiday), or year it is.

159. **(B)** Client need: health promotion and maintenance; subcategory: prevention and early detection of disease; content area: med/surg

 RATIONALE

 (A) Family history is not modifiable. (B) Research reveals a correlation between smoking and heart disease. Smoking is a modifiable behavior. (C, D) These responses are not risk factors.

160. **(A)** Client need: physiological integrity; subcategory: physiological adaptation; content area: med/surg

 RATIONALE

 (A) These are symptoms of arterial versus venous insufficiency because of decreased circulation to the distal parts of the body, especially to the toes of the lower extremities. (B, C) Varicose veins contribute to venous insufficiency, with decreased return of blood to the heart resulting in signs of stasis. (D) Raynaud's disease is a medical diagnosis.

161. **(A)** Client need: health promotion and maintenance; subcategory: prevention and early detection of disease; content area: med/surg

 RATIONALE

 (A) All are important, but some are not priorities in the initial assessment of indigestion. (B) Skin care and self-care are too general; sleep and exercise patterns are relevant, but are not initial priorities; reproduction is relevant, but others in the B response are too general. (C) Coping patterns are not an initial priority, although oral intake and oral care are important assessment questions. (D) Family risk factors may be relevant but must be specific.

162. **(A)** Client need: physiological integrity; subcategory: physiological adaptation; content area: med/surg

 RATIONALE

 (A) Both legs must be assessed and compared, and skin color is directly related to circulation. (B) Edema of the ankle is not a symptom of a fractured hip. (C) This response is incorrect because the right hip must be stabilized to promote healing and prevent further injury. (Toe motion would instead be assessed.) (D) Sensitivity to temperature is assessed only if the client does not respond to local sharp touch.

163. **(C)** Client need: safe, effective care environment; subcategory: safety and infection control; content area: med/surg

 RATIONALE

 (A) Administering a medication that a client is allergic to could result in anaphylactic shock. (B) The client needs an antibiotic for the respiratory infection. (C) Ampicillin is a semisynthetic amino penicillin and is contraindicated in clients with allergies to penicillin-related drugs and cephalosporins. A careful history is important to discover allergic reactions to these two drug groups. The nurse should withhold the medication and obtain a different antibiotic. (D) Administering a medication to which a client is allergic could result in anaphylactic shock.

164. **(A)** Client need: physiological integrity; subcategory: physiological adaptation; content area: med/surg

 RATIONALE

 (A) Alopecia (loss of hair) generally occurs in about 70% of the clients who receive vincristine. It is a reversible adverse effect, and regrowth of hair may begin prior to the end of treatment. (B) Signs of dehydration including poor skin turgor are common. (C) Constipation is a frequent side effect. The nurse should evaluate frequency of stools. (D) RBC, hematocrit, and hemoglobin may be decreased.

165. **(C)** Client need: physiological integrity; subcategory: reduction of risk potential; content area: med/surg

 RATIONALE

 (A, B) Side effects of this drug include a loss of calcium and potassium and water retention. (C) ACTH decreases a person's resistance to fungal or viral organisms. The nurse should assess the client routinely for any signs of infection and report them promptly before they become severe. (D) ACTH has no effect on urine color.

166. **(B)** Client need: physiological integrity; subcategory: pharmacological and parenteral therapies; content area: med/surg

RATIONALE

(A) This is correct, but choice B is best because it is the specific appropriate calculation. (B) Two tablets, not one tablet, will deliver a dose of 450 mg every 6 hours. (C) This choice indicates appropriate nursing considerations, but the medication should not be administered as calculated. (D) Medication should not be administered as calculated, and client has an understanding of the medication.

167. **(D)** Client need: physiological integrity; subcategory: reduction of risk potential; content area: med/surg

RATIONALE

(A) A short course of antibiotics is usually given after gynecological surgery, especially if a bladder repair was included. (B) Many clients do not know that alcohol and narcotics potentiate respiratory depression and unconsciousness. (C) Nothing foreign should be introduced into the vagina for 6 weeks so that healing can take place. (D) Exercise will promote healing.

168. **(A)** Client need: physiological integrity; subcategory: reduction of risk potential; content area: med/surg

RATIONALE

(A) Although these symptoms may be indicative of alteration in the GI tract, the nurse must assess the heart for the possibility of a myocardial infarction, which is an immediate life-threatening condition. (B) Some abdominal disorders such as peptic ulcer and cholecystitis can produce heartburn or pain in the right shoulder. (C) Psychosocial change and stressors could be manifested by similar symptoms and signs, but assessment of the heart would take first priority. (D) Some abdominal disorders such as peptic ulcer and cholecystitis can produce heartburn or pain in the right shoulder, but the heart is a priority.

169. **(A)** Client need: health promotion and maintenance; subcategory: prevention and early detection of disease; content area: med/surg

RATIONALE

(A, B, C, D) LMCL, 5ICS is the approximate location of the mitral valve of the left ventricle; this is the usual PMI. All other locations are incorrect.

170. **(A)** Client need: health promotion and maintenance; subcategory: growth and development through the lifespan; content area: med/surg

RATIONALE

(A) These represent Erikson's theories of developmental stages and crises of the life cycle. (B) This choice refers to middle adulthood. (C) This choice refers to adolescence. (D) This choice refers to early adulthood.

171. **(B)** Client need: health promotion and maintenance; subcategory: prevention and early detection of disease; content area: med/surg

RATIONALE

(A) Pruritus is itching. (B) Crepitus is the crackling sound often heard in movements of joints. (C) Rales are crackling sounds that may be heard over a consolidated lung. (D) Effusion refers to fluid in the joint space.

172. **(A)** Client need: health promotion and maintenance; subcategory: prevention and early detection of disease; content area: med/surg

RATIONALE

(A) The location of lesions is the only factor that can be inspected. (B, C, D) All the other factors are subjective data to be recorded in the history.

173. **(D)** Client need: health promotion and maintenance; subcategory: prevention and early detection of disease; content area: med/surg

RATIONALE

(A) Macules are flat surface lesions. (B) Papules are raised lesions. (C) A pustule contains pus (WBCs). (D) A vesicle is a small blister-like elevation on the skin containing serous fluid. All are under 1 cm in diameter.

174. **(D)** Client need: safe, effective care environment: subcategory: safety and infection control; content area: med/surg

RATIONALE

(A, B, C) Although these answers will promote psychological adjustment, answer D is the only answer that will physically help the client's ambulation. (D) The response is directly related and specific to physical function (ambulation).

175. **(A)** Client need: physiological integrity; subcategory: physiological adaptation; content area: med/surg

RATIONALE

(A) The prostate gland begins to grow at age 45. When it interferes with urinary function, the following can occur: hesitancy, decreased caliber and force of the urinary stream, dribbling, incomplete emptying of the bladder, urgency, frequency, nocturia, and dysuria. (B) Nocturia may occur from sphincter incompetence; the urinary force may decrease. (C) Hematuria may occur from renal damage. Bladder spasms are not a symptom. (D) Flank pain is usually not a symptom of BPH, but may indicate a kidney infection.

176. **(C)** Client need: physiological integrity; subcategory: reduction of risk potential; content area: med/surg

RATIONALE

(A) Decreasing visual acuity or eye discomfort may indicate blockage of drainage channel. Changes in vision may also indicate cataract development. (B) Increased ocular pressure should be assessed, not blood pressure. (C) Night blindness is common in clients with glaucoma, whether or not their pupils are constricted. (D) Nystagmus is not a complication of glaucoma but may indicate neurological disease.

177. **(D)** Client need: safe, effective care environment; subcategory: safety and infection control; content area: med/surg

RATIONALE

(A) The nurse should never attempt to remove a penetrating object such as glass from the eye because it could tear or rupture the internal ocular structure, resulting in permanent damage. (B) The nurse should reassure the client that medical care is on the way and stay with or have the family stay with the client. (C) The nurse cannot give a sedative unless it is ordered by the physician. (D) The nurse should encourage the client to rest until the ophthalmologist arrives to decrease the possibility of further eye damage. Placing the client in a lying position may increase intraocular pressure or cause the glass to advance further into the eye.

178. **(A)** Client need: physiological integrity; subcategory: physiological adaptation; content area: med/surg

RATIONALE

(A) A distended bowel or bladder can cause a noxious stimulus below the level of the injury to produce visceral reflex activity resulting in increased BP, decreased heart rate, and flushing above the level of the injury. (B) Urinary continence depends on the presence of lower or upper motor neuron damage. (C) Coping is important because autonomic dysreflexia is a life-threatening event. (D) Skin integrity is a lifelong assessment, but this situation is an emergency.

179. **(B)** Client need: physiological integrity; subcategory: pharmacological and parenteral therapies; content area: med/surg

RATIONALE

(A) This is incorrect because the capsule can be emptied and mixed with fluids or food if needed. (B) Alcohol increases the risk of hepatotoxicity. (C) This is incorrect because the capsule can be emptied and mixed with fluids or food if needed. (D) Food may delay peak serum levels.

180. **(C)** Client need: physiological integrity; subcategory: pharmacological and parenteral therapies; content area: med/surg

RATIONALE

(A) Propranolol blocks β-adrenergic receptors. (B) Nifedipine blocks influx of calcium during phase 2 of the action potential. (C) Captopril is an ACE inhibitor, causing vasodilation and decreased peripheral vascular resistance. (D) Hydralazine directly affects arteriole smooth muscles.

181. **(C)** Client need: physiological integrity; subcategory: pharmacological and parenteral therapies; content area: med/surg

RATIONALE

(A, C, D) SL nitroglycerin tablets are usually prescribed as one tablet SL for chest pain every 5 minutes, for a total of three doses. Because of the hypotensive effects, the nurse should assess the client's blood pressure response after each dose. (B) A client with coronary artery disease and chest pain should have O_2 therapy started on admission.

182. **(A)** Client need: physiological integrity; subcategory: pharmacological and parenteral therapies; content area: med/surg

RATIONALE

(A) The client's complaints may indicate an allergic reaction to the dye used for the coronary angiogram. Diphenhydramine is an antihistamine used frequently for relief of allergic reactions because it blocks release of histamine. (B) Dipyridamole is a vasodilator and antiplatelet drug. (C) Dobutamine hydrochloride is a β-adrenergic stimulant. (D) Droperidol is an antiemetic and antipsychotic drug.

183. **(C)** Client need: physiological integrity; subcategory: pharmacological and parenteral therapies; content area: med/surg

RATIONALE

(A, D) KCl is never given by IM injection, IV push, or in concentrated amounts by another route in order to prevent life-threatening hypokalemia. (B) An IV infusion >40 mEq/L also increases risk of vascular irritation. (C) KCl should be diluted with appropriate IV solution (usually dextrose) and administered via infusion.

184. **(C)** Client need: physiological integrity; subcategory: physiological adaptation; content area: med/surg

RATIONALE

(A, B) An HIV-infected person has the potential to transmit HIV regardless of the presence of symptoms. (C) HIV infection causes a chronic infectious state. (D) A positive HIV antibody test confirms the presence of HIV. T_4 cell counts do not determine infectious state.

185. **(C)** Client need: health promotion and maintenance; subcategory: prevention and early detection of disease; content area: med/surg

RATIONALE

(A, D) Hairy leukoplakia presents on the oral mucosa, not on the conjunctiva or the chest. (B) *Candida* may present on the nares; hairy leukoplakia presents on the oral mucous membranes. (C) Hairy leukoplakia presents in an immuno-deficiency state as white patches on the lateral margins of the tongue or oral mucosa that cannot be rubbed off by scraping.

186. **(D)** Client need: physiological integrity; subcategory: physiological adaptation; content area: med/surg

RATIONALE

(A) Ptosis is associated with multiple sclerosis. (B) Eye drainage is common with bacterial conjunctivitis. (C) Exophthalmos is associated with hyperthyroidism. (D) Cytomegalovirus virus retinitis presents as blurred vision, floaters, decreased visual fields, and vision loss.

187. **(A)** Client need: physiological integrity; subcategory: pharmacological and parenteral therapies; content area: med/surg

RATIONALE

(A) Chronic use of cholestyramine resin may cause hypoprothrombinemia and increased bleeding tendency. The client should watch for petechiae, abnormal bleeding from the mucous membranes, bruising, and tarry stools. (B) It also inhibits absorption of calcium, potassium, and sodium. (C, D) Cholestyramine resin is used to lower serum cholesterol by decreasing low-density lipoproteins, and to control itching.

188. **(C)** Client need: physiological integrity; subcategory: pharmacological and parenteral therapies; content area: med/surg

RATIONALE

(A) It is also given with aspirin for long-term therapy for angina pectoris. (B) Dipyridamole is given by itself to increase O_2 saturation in coronary tissues and to improve coronary blood flow. (C) Dipyridamole is used in combination with anticoagulant therapy to decrease the risk of thromboembolism after replacement of a cardiac valve. (D) It is also given alone to prevent TIAs.

189. **(B)** Client need: physiological integrity; subcategory: pharmacological and parenteral therapies; content area: med/surg

RATIONALE

(A, C, D) It may take a few days for desired anticoagulation effects to develop with warfarin. (B) Peak anticoagulating effects with warfarin generally occur in 0.5 to 3 days. The heparin IV is usually discontinued when desired prothrombin activity is reached. Duration of heparin may last 8–12 hours depending on the dose, but clotting time returns to normal near 2–6 hours.

190. **(D)** Client need: physiological integrity; subcategory: pharmacological and parenteral therapies; content area: med/surg

RATIONALE

(A) Azathioprine is metabolized in the liver. (B) Fever, chills, and sore throat are signs of serious infection and are important to report. (C) The drug will not affect vital signs. (D) Azathioprine is an immunosuppressant drug that has hematological toxic effects with chronic use. It may cause thrombocytopenia, leukopenia, acute leukemia, and bone marrow depression. The drug should be discontinued if WBCs are <3000 or platelet count is <100,000/mm^3.

191. **(B)** Client need: physiological integrity; subcategory: reduction of risk potential; content area: med/surg

RATIONALE

(A) Ampicillin should be given on an empty stomach. (B) To accurately culture the infectious organism, a sputum specimen should be collected prior to initiating antibiotic therapy. Therapy may be started before culture results are reported. (C, D) Taking the client's pulse and assessing respirations are important nursing actions in terms of the respiratory status, but not in terms of administering the ampicillin.

192. **(C)** Client need: physiological integrity; subcategory: pharmacological and parenteral therapies; content area: med/surg

RATIONALE

(A) The nurse should not decrease or increase an IV rate without a physician's order. (B) The nurse should not restrict fluid intake without a physician's order. The oliguria of acute renal failure may be due to hypovolemia or decreased blood volume. (C) The nurse should immediately report the findings of oliguria. Increasing oliguria is a sign to discontinue mannitol therapy, because accumulation of the drug will occur. (D) Fluid retention leads to edema formation and hypertension and may precipitate CHF and pulmonary edema and metabolic acidosis. Uremic toxins can cause neurological irritability such as headache, seizure, and coma.

193. **(C)** Client need: physiological integrity; subcategory: pharmacological and parenteral therapies; content area: med/surg

RATIONALE

(A) Rash and urticaria are adverse effects of morphine but do not require immediate action. (B) Morphine can cause urinary retention, but it is not a life-threatening problem. The physician should be notified if respirations are <10 /min. (C) The most serious side effect of epidural injection of morphine is respiratory depression, which may last for up to 24 hours after injection. (D) Drowsiness may be caused by morphine, especially if given with other CNS depressants.

194. **(C)** Client need: physiological integrity; subcategory: pharmacological and parenteral therapies; content area: med/surg

RATIONALE

(A) The nurse should not pull back on the plunger. (B) A soft-bristle toothbrush is appropriate for hygiene but does not affect administration of heparin. (C) SC injections should be given in the adipose tissue of the abdomen to avoid excessive pain, to decrease the risk of hematoma, and to enhance duration as compared to shallow subcutaneous injection sites. (D) The nurse should not massage the area or aspirate when giving SC injection; gentle pressure should be applied for 1 minute.

195. **(B)** Client need: physiological integrity; subcategory: pharmacological and parenteral therapies; content area: med/surg

RATIONALE

(A, B, C, D) Therapeutic effects usually appear within the initial 2–3 weeks of drug therapy and include reduced night sweats, fever, coughing, and sputum production and improved appetite and weight gain. More than 90% of clients on appropriate therapy develop a negative sputum culture at 6 months. Even though the client feels better, it is important for the nurse to emphasize that the therapy must be continued for the time period prescribed.

196. **(A)** Client need: physiological integrity; subcategory: pharmacological and parenteral therapies; content area: med/surg

RATIONALE

(A, B, C) Isoniazid drug therapy may cause a decrease in niacin and folate stores. The client should be instructed on dietary replacements. (D) Isoniazid has no known effect on vitamin A.

197. **(A)** Client need: physiological integrity; subcategory: pharmacological and parenteral therapies; content area: med/surg

RATIONALE

(A) Signs of digitalis toxicity include visual disturbances and anorexia. (B) Agitation, among other signs such as confusion, vomiting, diarrhea, headaches, and hallucinations, may occur as a side effect. Anxiety is not related to digitalis therapy. Prompt recognition of digitalis intoxication is important to prevent life-threatening complications. (C) Low cardiac output would cause signs and symptoms such as low urine output, low blood pressure, fatigue, restlessness, syncope, changes in mental status, and dyspnea. (D) Symptoms of hypokalemia include muscle weakness, anorexia, decreased bowel sounds, and arrhythmias.

198. **(A)** Client need: physiological integrity; subcategory: pharmacological and parenteral therapies; content area: med/surg

RATIONALE

(A) Reduced dopamine input from the substantia nigra to the corpus striatum leads to loss of the inhibitory effect of acetylcholine and increased dominance of ACH. (B) Estrogen and progesterone have no effect on Parkinson's disease. (C) Atherosclerosis can cause decreased blood supply to the brain and cause DVAs, but it does not affect the syndrome of nerve cell loss in the basal ganglia of Parkinson's disease. (D) Although Parkinson's disease may have genetic and viral factors, they have not been clearly delineated.

199. **(D)** Client need: physiological integrity; subcategory: pharmacological and parenteral therapies; content area: med/surg

RATIONALE

(A) Side effects of ACTH include a loss of calcium and potassium. (B) ACTH can cause sodium and fluid retention. (C) ACTH increases the requirements of po hypoglycemia agents or insulin in diabetic clients owing to hyperglycemia. Blood glucose should be monitored closely until stabilization occurs. (D) ACTH decreases a person's resistance to fungal or viral organisms. The nurse should assess the client for signs of infection and report them before they become severe.

200. **(C)** Client need: physiological integrity; subcategory: pharmacological and parenteral therapies; content area: med/surg

RATIONALE

(A, B) Meperidine is an opioid analgesic with side effects of respiratory depression and hypotension with reflex tachycardia. (C) Careful aspiration prior to IM injections is suggested to prevent accidental IV administration of an undiluted dose, which could lead to excessive increase in heart rate and syncope. (D) Response to all drug therapy should routinely be assessed and documented.

201. **(C)** Client need: physiological integrity; subcategory: pharmacological and parenteral therapies; content area: med/surg

RATIONALE

(A, B, C, D) Peak serum levels of gentamicin are usually drawn 30 minutes after the IVPB dose has infused completely.

202. **(D)** Client need: physiological integrity; subcategory: pharmacological and parenteral therapies; content area: med/surg

RATIONALE

(A) Constipation and oily skin are not usually side effects of the medication. Anaphylaxis, rash, and urticaria can be side effects of the drug. (B) Fatigue could be a symptom of depressed bone marrow such as thrombocytopenia, neutropenia, leukopenia. (C) Constipation and oily skin are not usually side effects of the medication. Anaphylaxis, rash, and urticaria can be side effects of the drug. (D) Extended administration of cephalosporins may cause nonsusceptible organisms to proliferate, leading to superinfections. Susceptible areas include the mouth, respiratory system, colon, and anus. Personal hygiene (especially mouth care and perineal care) is important. Superinfections of the oral cavity may cause mucosal erosions, black hairy tongue, or white patches inside the mouth.

203. **(D)** Client need: physiological integrity; subcategory: pharmacological and parenteral therapies; content area: med/surg

RATIONALE

(A) Bretylium is used when clients do not respond to lidocaine. (B, C) Verapamil and propranolol have stronger myocardial and hemodynamic depressant effects, and verapamil is indicated in supraventricular tachycardias. (D) IV lidocaine is the first-line drug of choice for ventricular ectopy because it has a rapid onset without myocardial and hemodynamic effects, and therapeutic levels are safely achieved with IV administration.

204. **(A)** Client need: physiological integrity; subcategory: pharmacological and parenteral therapies; content area: med/surg

RATIONALE

(A) Naproxen is the drug of choice for dysmenorrhea because it works as a prostaglandin synthesis inhibitor. (B) The Tylenol may relieve some of the discomfort but will not stop the uterine cramps. (C) Aspirin is too weak to inhibit cramping but might help with the clots. (D) Lydia Pinkham pills are an over-the-counter product that claims "great relief" but is basically less effective than aspirin.

205. **(D)** Client need: health promotion and maintenance; subcategory: prevention and early detection of disease; content area: med/surg

RATIONALE

(A) Normal vaginal secretions have a distinctive but not foul odor. (B) During menstruation, douching can force the blood backward and cause endometriosis. (C) Flavored or perfumed douches can cause irritation, rash, blisters, and tissue damage. Only vinegar or povidone-iodine (Betadine) douches should be used, and as infrequently as possible. (D) The vagina naturally cleanses itself using the vaginal flora.

206. **(A)** Client need: health promotion and maintenance; subcategory: growth and development through the life span; content area: med/surg

RATIONALE

(A) The effects of spermicide last for about 1 hour. If inserted too soon prior to intercourse, and the woman gets up, spermicide will leak out. (B, C) Positions of coitus and walking and exercising are affected because, as the spermicide increases in temperature from body heat, it becomes liquid and can easily be displaced from the vagina. (D) Douching cannot take place for at least 6–8 hours postcoitus for effective contraception. Spermicide must be reapplied prior to each sexual act.

207. **(C)** Client need: health promotion and maintenance; subcategory: growth and development through the life span; content area: med/surg

RATIONALE

(A) LH influences part of the maturation process of the follicle. (B) FSH helps mature the follicle in the proliferative phase before ovulation. (C) After the ovum leaves the follicle, the corpus luteum develops and produces large amounts of progesterone, called the "hormone of pregnancy." (D) Chorionic gonadotropin is the hormone tested for antigenicity in pregnancy testing kits.

208. **(A)** Client need: physiological integrity; subcategory: pharmacological and parenteral therapies; content area: med/surg

RATIONALE

(A) A therapeutic dosage would be 5000 U. A dose of 50,000 U would be unsafe. The nurse should verify dose with physician. (B) This response would be the correct calculation if 5000 U was prescribed, but this dosage was not prescribed. (C) This response indicates appropriate nursing considerations, but the medication should not be administered as prescribed. (D) This response is incorrect as medication should not be administered and the client has an understanding of the medication.

209. **(D)** Client need: physiological integrity; subcategory: pharmacological and parenteral therapies; content area: med/surg

RATIONALE

(A) Medication is indicated, and dosage is safe and appropriate. (B) Two tablets are to be administered, not one half tablet. (C) These are not untoward effects of the medication. (D) Appropriate dosage has been prescribed and calculated. Further client teaching is indicated as this medication is not indicated for treatment of chest pain.

210. **(A)** Client need: physiological integrity; subcategory: pharmacological and parenteral therapies; content area: med/surg

RATIONALE

(A) Medication is not indicated at this time because the client is not in pain. (B) Two milliliters is the appropriate dosage, not 1

mL, and medication is not indicated at this time. (C) These are not nursing considerations for the medication, and medication is not indicated at this time. (D) Medication is not indicated at this time, and the client understands what it is given for.

211. **(B)** Client need: physiological integrity; subcategory: pharmacological and parenteral therapies; content area: med/surg

RATIONALE

(A) This is correct, but response B is best as it is the specific appropriate calculation. (B) There are 50 U of heparin per milliliter. To deliver 1000 U of heparin per hour, the drip would infuse at 20 mL/h (1000 ÷ 50 = 20 mL/hr.) (C) This choice indicates appropriate nursing considerations, but the medication should not be administered as calculated. (D) Medication should not be administered as calculated, and the client has an understanding of the medication.

212. **(B)** Client need: physiological integrity; subcategory: pharmacological and parenteral therapies; content area: med/surg

RATIONALE

(A) This is correct, but choice B is best because it is the specific appropriate calculation. (B) Two of the 1.5-mg tablets equal a total of 3 mg. (C) This choice indicates appropriate nursing considerations (adrenal insufficiency), but the medication should not be administered as calculated. (D) Medication should not be administered as calculated, and the client has an understanding of the medication.

213. **(C)** Client need: physiological integrity; subcategory: pharmacological and parenteral therapies; content area: med/surg

RATIONALE

(A, B) The medication may be administered, and the prescribed dose and calculation are appropriate. (C) At 50 mg/min for 6 minutes, a total of 300 mg would be delivered. The nursing considerations are appropriate. The client would be placed on a cardiac monitor in the emergency room. (D) The medication may be administered as prescribed and calculated, and the client has an understanding of the effect of medication on urine.

214. **(B)** Client need: physiological integrity; subcategory: pharmacological and parenteral therapies; content area: med/surg

RATIONALE

(A) This is correct, but choice B is the best as it is the specific appropriate calculation. (B) The appropriate dosage is 0.2 mL for each of the two doses. (C) Indicates appropriate nursing considerations, but the medication should not be administered as calculated. (D) Medication should not be administered as calculated, and the client's wife has an understanding of the medication.

215. **(D)** Client need: physiological integrity; subcategory: pharmacological and parenteral therapies; content area: med/surg

RATIONALE

(A) Medication is indicated, and dosage is safe and appropriate. (B) Four milliliters are to be administered, not 2 mL. (C) These are not untoward effects of the medication. (D) Appropriate dosage has been prescribed and calculated. Driving until stabilized on the medication and drinking alcohol should be avoided, but further client teaching is indicated as medication should be taken one-half to 1 hour before meals for better absorption.

216. **(D)** Client need: physiological integrity; subcategory: pharmacological and parenteral therapies; content area: med/surg

RATIONALE

(A) Medication is indicated, and dosage is safe and appropriate. (B) One tablet is to be administered, not two tablets. (C) These are not untoward effects of the medication. (D) Appropriate dosage has been prescribed and calculated. Reversible impotence and gynecomastia may occur, but further teaching is indicated as pepper and spices should be avoided. Also, the medication must be taken exactly as prescribed for effectiveness and not doubled. Also, smoking decreases the effectiveness of the medication.

217. **(A)** Client need: physiological integrity; subcategory: pharmacological and parenteral therapies; content area: med/surg
   RATIONALE
   (A) A safe dosage would be 10 mg titrated for pain. A dosage of 100 mg would be unsafe. The nurse should verify dose with physician. (B) This would be the correct calculation if 10 mg was prescribed, but this dosage was not prescribed. (C) This choice indicates an appropriate nursing consideration, but the medication should not be administered as prescribed. (D) Medication should not be administered as prescribed, and the client has an understanding of the medication.

218. **(B)** Client need: physiological integrity; subcategory: pharmacological and parenteral therapies; content area: med/surg
   RATIONALE
   (A) This is correct, but choice B is best because it is the specific appropriate calculation. (B) To deliver a total of 40 mg, 4.0 mL would be administered. (C) This choice indicates appropriate nursing considerations, but the medication should not be administered as calculated. (D) Medication should not be administered as calculated, and client has an understanding of the medication.

219. **(D)** Client need: physiological integrity; subcategory: pharmacological and parenteral therapies; content area: med/surg
   RATIONALE
   (A) Medication is indicated, and dosage is safe and appropriate. (B) Two tablets, not one tablet, are to be administered every 8 hours. (C) In the client, liver, blood, and renal studies should be monitored, not cardiac studies. (D) Appropriate dosage has been prescribed and calculated. Further client teaching is indicated, as medication should be taken on an empty stomach with a full glass of water. Also, the entire course of medication must be completed to ensure organism death.

220. **(C)** Client need: physiological integrity; subcategory: pharmacological and parenteral therapies; content area: med/surg
   RATIONALE
   (A, B) The medication may be administered, and the prescribed dose and calculation are appropriate. (C) The medication may be administered as prescribed and calculated, and the nursing considerations are appropriate. (D) The medication may be administered as prescribed and calculated, and the client has an understanding of the medication.

221. **(C)** Client need: physiological integrity; subcategory: pharmacological and parenteral therapies; content area: med/surg
   RATIONALE
   (A, B) The medication may be administered, and the prescribed dose and calculation are appropriate. (C) The medication may be administered as prescribed and calculated, and the nursing consideration is appropriate. (D) The medication may be administered as prescribed and calculated, and the client has an understanding of the medication.

222. **(B)** Client need: physiological integrity; subcategory: reduction of risk potential; content area: med/surg
   RATIONALE
   (A) The probe is placed on a finger or earlobe. (B) Capillaries are closest to the surface on a finger, toe, or earlobe. (C) The probe does not need to be calibrated. (D) Readings can be obtained immediately.

223. **(A)** Client need: physiological integrity; subcategory: pharmacological and parenteral therapies; content area: med/surg
   RATIONALE
   (A) Assessing the onset, frequency, and severity will help identify patterns of nausea and vomiting and help in scheduling round-the-clock emetic therapy. (B) Cold foods decrease odor formation that may precipitate vomiting. (C) Relaxation and distraction are important but not as important as assessment of nausea and vomiting patterns. (D) Providing a bland diet may decrease nausea and vomiting, but this is not as important as assessing nausea and vomiting patterns.

224. **(D)** Client need: physiological integrity; subcategory: reduction of risk potential; content area: med/surg
   RATIONALE
   (A) Tachycardia, not bradycardia, will result from hypovolemia and dehydration. (B) Hypotension, rather than hypertension, may result from hypovolemia. (C) An elevated temperature will occur only if infection is present. (D) This is a compensatory mechanism of the respiratory system to attempt the elimination of excess carbon dioxide when metabolic acidosis develops.

225. **(D)** Client need: physiological integrity; subcategory: reduction of risk potential; content area: med/surg
   RATIONALE
   (A) Showers rather than tub baths promote better perineal hygiene. (B) Emptying the bladder of urine every 2 hours is desirable for a client with recurring cystitis. (C) This diet will acidify the urine, thus decreasing the likelihood of recurring cystitis. (D) The client should seek attention from her health care provider to confirm the diagnosis, rather than taking an over-the-counter preparation.

226. **(A)** Client need: physiological integrity; subcategory: basic care and comfort; content area: med/surg
   RATIONALE
   (A) The purpose of TPN is to maintain or improve a client's nutritional status, usually resulting in weight gain of less than 3 pounds per week. (B) The normal serum albumin range is 3.2–5.0 g/dL; levels below 2.5 g/dL indicate a need for TPN. (C) The desired serum glucose level while a client receives TPN should not exceed normal upper limits or 120 mg/dL. (D) Although this range is desirable, it is not the primary aim of TPN.

227. **(D)** Client need: physiological integrity; subcategory: basic care and comfort; content area: med/surg
   RATIONALE
   (A, B, C) On a low-residue diet, highly seasoned and fried foods along with raw fruits and vegetables are to be avoided. Coffee and tea are allowed; milk is limited to 2 cups per day. (D) *Baked* chicken, *white* rice (not brown), and plain custard and fruit juices are included on a low-residue diet.

228. **(B)** Client need: physiological integrity; subcategory: reduction of risk potential; content area: med/surg
   RATIONALE
   (A) This test is usually ordered if a client is experiencing hypoglycemia or hyperglycemia. (B) This test reveals the average blood glucose level over approximately the previous 120 days. (C) This test is used to assess bleeding disorders or to monitor the efficacy of heparin therapy. (D) These tests are not as accurate in detecting changes in blood glucose as tests of fasting blood sugar or glycosylated hemoglobin. These tests only reveal a client's recent glucose level.

229. **(A)** Client need: physiological integrity; subcategory: reduction of risk potential; content area: med/surg
   RATIONALE
   (A) Excessive loss of fluid from ileostomy drainage necessitates careful monitoring of fluid intake and output and electrolytes. (B) Stool from an ileostomy drains continuously and is liquid.

A client with a traditional ileostomy will not be continent and does not require bowel training. (C) The appliance should be changed when it is approximately one-third full. (D) A traditional ileostomy continuously drains liquid stool. Constipation should not be a problem.

230. **(D)** Client need: physiological integrity; subcategory: reduction of risk potential; content area: med/surg

RATIONALE

(A) Once urine drains, an indwelling catheter should be advanced another 1–2 inches. (B) The client is cleansed directly over the meatus, using downward strokes. (C) Sterile technique must be maintained throughout the entire procedure. (D) This statement demonstrates the correct technique.

231. **(C)** Client need: physiological integrity; subcategory: reduction of risk potential; content area: med/surg

RATIONALE

(A, B, D) Endoscopic studies such as colonoscopy are done before barium studies, to ensure visualization of the bowel. The barium enema should then be scheduled before the barium swallow because barium retained from the latter test could distort findings from the barium enema. (C) This is the correct sequence.

232. **(B)** Client need: physiological integrity; subcategory: pharmacological and parenteral therapies; content area: med/surg

RATIONALE

(A) This statement does not indicate need for further teaching. Fluid intake of 2500–3000 cc/day is recommended to prevent kidney stones. (B) Indicates that the client needs further teaching, as water-soluble Vitamin C (ascorbic acid) is excreted in the urine. Acidic urine promotes development of uric acid stones. (C) This statement does not indicate need for further teaching. An activity level that prevents urinary stasis is recommended to prevent kidney stones. (D) This statement does *not* indicate need for further teaching. Allopurinol (Zyloprim) inhibits production of uric acid and is indicated for prevention of nephropathy and secondary hyperuricemia.

233. **(A)** Client need: physiological integrity; subcategory: physiological adaptation; content area: med/surg

RATIONALE

(A) Clients are usually placed on bed rest until symptoms of DVT resolve. (B) Massage is contraindicated as it increases the risk of detaching the thrombus from the vein wall. (C) Warm, moist compresses are usually applied to the affected area. (D) Initially, leg exercises are contraindicated, as this could dislodge the clot from the vein wall.

234. **(B)** Client need: physiological integrity; subcategory: reduction of risk potential; content area: med/surg

RATIONALE

(A) Increased fluids are indicated after a TURP to dilute urine and prevent clot formation. (B) Bowel movements should be soft and regular in order to avoid pressure on the prostate area. (C) Physical activity is usually limited for up to 8 weeks postoperatively. (D) There is no abdominal incision in a TURP.

235. **(D)** Client need: physiological integrity; subcategory: reduction of risk potential; content area: med/surg

RATIONALE

(A, B) Postoperative leg exercises will not prevent infection or cellulitis. (C) Although leg exercises may stimulate peristalsis and possibly prevent an ileus, this is not the main reason for encouraging a client to do them. (D) Leg exercises are intended to promote venous return from the extremities, thereby decreasing the client's risk of thrombophlebitis due to immobility.

236. **(A)** Client need: health promotion and maintenance; subcategory: prevention and early detection of disease; content area: med/surg

RATIONALE

(A) Lower leg edema is a common finding with venous insufficiency. (B) Pain upon ambulation is commonly noted in Buerger's disease. (C) The affected extremity will not be cool to touch, unless *arterial* circulation is impaired. (D) The affected extremity will often appear discolored, not pale. Color is noted with arterial thrombosis.

237. **(B)** Client need: physiological integrity; subcategory: physiological adaptation; content area: med/surg

RATIONALE

(A) This position will facilitate venous return. (B) When the extremities are placed in the dependent position, gravity helps the arterial blood to reach the distal portions of the extremity. (C, D) Both of these positions may further impede peripheral tissue perfusion.

238. **(C)** Client need: physiological integrity; subcategory: pharmacological and parenteral therapies; content need: med/surg

RATIONALE

(A, B, D) These medications are histamine H2 antagonists. They inhibit gastric acid secretion. (C) Sucralfate reacts with the gastric acid to form a thick paste, which selectively adheres to the surface of the ulcer.

239. **(A)** Client need: safe, effective care environment; subcategory: management of care; content area: med/surg

RATIONALE

(A) It is the responsibility of the surgeon who performs surgery to obtain informed consent from the client. (B, C, D) These health care workers may provide additional information about the surgical procedure and witness the client's signature. However, it is not their responsibility to obtain the client's informed consent.

240. **(D)** Client need: health promotion and maintenance; subcategory: prevention and early detection of disease; content area: med/surg

RATIONALE

(A, B, C, D) Percussion and palpation may stimulate peristalsis. Therefore, auscultation is done prior to percussion and palpation, after inspection of the abdomen.

241. **(C)** Client need: physiological integrity; subcategory: physiological adaptation; content area: med/surg

RATIONALE

(A, B) These conditions are possible long-term complications of ulcerative colitis; they would not be present after a 24-hour long bout of diarrhea. (C, D) Metabolic acidosis, not alkalosis, stemming from increased bicarbonate loss could result from severe diarrhea.

242. **(B)** Client need: physiological integrity; subcategory: reduction of risk potential; content area: med/surg

RATIONALE

(A) A pale stoma could indicate circulatory compromise. (B) A healthy stoma appears red or pink, much like the mucous membranes in the mouth. (C) This abnormal finding indicates a retracted stoma. The stoma should protrude slightly from the abdomen. (D) A dark or dusky stoma could indicate circulatory compromise.

243. **(B)** Client need: physiological integrity; subcategory: reduction of risk potential; content area: med/surg

RATIONALE

(A) Abdominal pain post-cystoscopy may indicate a complication. (B) Pink-tinged urine is a common finding post-cystoscopy. (C, D) Bladder distention and low urine output are complications, requiring further assessment and/or catheterization.

244. **(B)** Client need: physiological integrity; subcategory: pharmacological and parenteral therapies; content area: med/surg

RATIONALE

(A, C, D) These are incorrect. They do not describe the action/desired outcome of an anticholinergic medication such as Levsin. (B) This is correct.

245. **(A)** Client need: physiological integrity, subcategory: basic care and comfort; content area: med/surg

RATIONALE

(A) Warm, moist heat, such as a sitz bath, is recommended 3–4 times a day for several days post hemorrhoidectomy. (B) A fluid intake of at least 2000 cc/day is recommended. (C) A stool softener may be prescribed by the surgeon. Laxatives may cause diarrhea and increased pain the rectal area. (D) The side lying position reduces pressure on the surgical site and prevents additional discomfort.

246. **(A)** Client need: safe, effective care environment; subcategory: safety and infection control; content area: med/surg

RATIONALE

(A) Catheter retention balloon that does not inflate or that leaks must be replaced before insertion into a client. (B) The glans penis around the meatus is cleaned *toward* the base of the penis. This movement prevents bringing organisms to the meatus. (C) A catheter that is larger than the meatus opening is usually unnecessary and will cause additional discomfort upon insertion. (D) The catheter should be lubricated generously for about 6–7 inches to decrease friction and discomfort upon insertion.

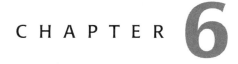

CHAPTER 6

Gerontological Nursing: Content Review and Test

Ola Burns Allen, RNC, DNSc

Integumentary System

Description

The most obvious reflections of age appear in the integumentary system. Hair, skin, nails, body composition, and teeth all undergo change. Integumentary changes are related to internal (genetic) and external causes such as exposure to sunlight and environmental chemicals. About 90% of all older adults have some kind of skin disorder.

Pathophysiology

SKIN

The skin is composed of three layers:
1. **Epidermis:** This skin outer layer prevents the entry of foreign substances and the loss of body fluids. Melanocytes decrease within the epidermis and the dermal-epidermal junction flattens owing to the retraction of papillae. These changes cause the skin to appear thin, pale, and translucent.
2. **Dermis:** The dermis contains blood vessels that provide nutrients to the epidermis and assist in thermoregulation. Nerve fibers serve a sensory perceptual purpose in perception of pain, touch, and other sensations. Collagen, which makes up the major portion of the dermis, is decreased, leading to decreased elasticity and strength. Decreased vascularity and increased vascular fragility lead to skin hemorrhage (purpura) and venous stasis. Decreased regeneration of cells and decreased vascularity make the older adult less resistant to shearing forces and more prone to decubitus ulcers.
3. **Subcutaneous:** This inner layer composed of fat tissue serves as a storage area for calories, as an insulator and regulator for temperature change, and protects the body from trauma. Sebaceous glands and sweat glands are contained within the subcutaneous tissue. With advancing age, function is reduced in these glands due to the loss of hair follicles and impairment in the ability to maintain body temperature homeostasis. There is an increase in body fat due to the atrophy of subcutaneous tissue.

NAILS

Nail growth slows around the third decade with a decrease in lunula size and a decrease in peripheral circulation. The nail plate yellows and thickens, causing the nail to become soft and brittle, and to split easily.

HAIR

Graying of the hair is the result of decline in melanin production. The hair becomes thinner on the head and the body, while there is increased density of nasal and ear hair, particularly in males. Increased facial hair is seen in women as a result of a decrease in estrogen.

Assessment

SUBJECTIVE

1. Risk factors
   A. Positive family history of skin conditions
   B. Exposure to environmental irritants such as strong acids, soaps, sunlight
   C. Diet, obesity, malnutrition
2. History
   A. Past or present skin conditions
   B. Allergies
   C. Use of topical or systemic drugs
   D. Functional status, mobility
3. Psychosocial and cultural assessment
   A. Physical environment and social support systems
   B. Family interactions

OBJECTIVE

Skin

1. Appearance—examine the entire skin surface for symmetry and overall appearance related to grooming and hygiene.
   A. Color, discoloration, irregular pigmentation, texture, general condition
   B. Temperature in extremities and other body areas
   C. Moist, dry, scaly, oily, flaking, clammy
   D. Turgid, supple, pliable
   E. Varicosities or red, brown, or blue discoloration indicating poor circulation or stasis
   F. Bruises or skin tears
   G. Edema
2. Lesions
   A. Moles, sores, scars, or identifying marks
   B. Evidence to suggest falls or abuse
   C. Moisture or drainage
   D. Pain or discomfort
   E. Raised or irregular edges

Hair

1. Color, texture, general condition
2. Distribution pattern
3. Dandruff, scaling, itching, or odor

Nails

1. Color and general condition of nail beds
2. Color, length, splitting, texture, thickness, general condition of nails
3. Edema or accumulation of fluid

Pruritus

Description

Pruritus, or generalized itching, may be caused by internal, external, or emotional conditions. Drying and flaking of the skin due to xerosis is a common cause of pruritus. Excessive scratching may lead to acute or chronic dermatitis. Acute dermatitis is accompanied by redness, high temperature, edema, and pain. Dermatitis in the perianal area due to heat, hemorrhoids, or swelling may occur with chronic illness or confusion. Drugs are the most common cause of allergic dermatitis. Allergic dermatitis is characterized by a generalized maculopapular rash accompanied by itching.

Assessment

SUBJECTIVE

1. Scratching
   A. Most often itching occurs on the lower legs, hands, and forearms, but it may also occur in skin folds and in the genital and anal regions.
2. Psychosocial and cultural assessment
   A. Evidence of anxiety or stressors
   B. Bathing routine
3. History
   A. Risk factors present
      (1) Medications
      (2) Contact with chemical substances

(3) Communicable disease (e.g., scabies caused by a mite that burrows under the skin or shingles caused by the herpes virus)
(4) Medical conditions
   (a) Chronic renal failure
   (b) Hepatitis
   (c) Iron-deficiency anemia
   (d) Hyperthyroidism
   (e) Diabetes mellitus
   (f) Lymphomas

OBJECTIVE

1. Appearance—examine the entire skin surface for symmetry and overall appearance related to grooming and hygiene.
   A. Color, discoloration, irregular pigmentation, texture, general condition
   B. Temperature in extremities and other body areas
   C. Moist, dry, scaly, oily, flaking, clammy
   D. Turgid, supple, pliable
   E. Varicosities or red, brown, or blue discoloration indicating poor circulation or stasis
   F. Bruises or skin tears
   G. Edema
   H. Insect bites
2. Lesions
   A. Moisture or drainage
   B. Pain or discomfort
   C. Raised or irregular edges
   D. Tissue breaks
   E. Insect bites

Planning

Client Needs

1. Safe, effective care environment
   A. Encourage client to wash hands.
   B. Advise client to avoid scratching.
2. Health promotion and maintenance
   A. Maintain optimal fluid status.
   B. Maintain optimal nutritional status to promote tissue integrity.
   C. Monitor drug allergies.
3. Psychosocial integrity
   A. Prevent odor.
   B. Prevent embarrassment.
4. Physiological integrity
   A. Alleviate uncomfortable skin conditions or itching.
   B. Prevent impaired skin integrity.
   C. Prevent infection.

Implementation

1. Perform skin inspection.
2. Identify conditions that may cause drying, itching, or allergic response.
3. Reduce frequency of bathing, if necessary.
4. Use mild, nondetergent soap.
5. Rinse skin carefully in tepid to warm water.
6. Dry skin thoroughly by patting rather than by rubbing the skin surface.
7. Apply emollient lotions at least twice a day and immediately after bathing.

8. Provide a diet that allows an adequate intake of protein, vitamin A, and vitamin C.
9. Provide at least eight glasses of water during the day unless contraindicated.
10. Monitor for signs and symptoms of inflammation or infection.

Outcomes

1. Verbalizes increase in comfort and lack of itching
2. Shows no signs of scratching, redness, temperature, edema, or infection
3. Shows no signs of scaling, flaking, or fissures

Neoplastic Disorders

Description

The neoplastic disorders commonly occurring in older adults are described in the following paragraphs.

Seborrheic keratoses originate in the horny layer of the epidermis, usually in unexposed skin or around the hairline. Lesions are raised and have a wartlike texture. They may have a black or brownish-gray appearance. These are noninvasive and benign.

Actinic keratoses, also known as solar or senile keratoses, are associated with exposure to the sun. They begin as small, reddened areas that become well demarcated with a rough surface and brown or yellowish coloring. Actinic keratoses are potentially malignant and may develop into squamous cell carcinoma.

Epitheliomas: the two most common types of epitheliomas found in the older adult are basal cell epitheliomas and squamous cell epitheliomas. Both are readily treatable when detected early.

Basal cell epithelioma usually appears on the face in cells of the epidermis or hair follicles. A small, smooth, translucent papule appears, through which dilated blood vessels or small black or brown pigments can be seen. The papule enlarges to a mass, which may be dark or pearly in color. Basal cell epitheliomas may become ulcerated and locally invasive and without treatment can lead to death.

Squamous cell epithelioma is found in the epidermis and mucosa of sun-exposed, damaged skin. It appears usually as a small, hard, red, wartlike nodule but may appear as a raised gray-yellow dome-shaped lesion. A deep incision biopsy is required to confirm the diagnosis.

Malignant melanoma is a flat or slightly raised lesion with irregular edges associated with exposure to sunlight or mole irritation. This lesion is often mistaken for rapidly enlarging warts, and biopsy is necessary for definitive diagnosis. Rapid metastasis makes early diagnosis a high priority.

Assessment

SUBJECTIVE

1. Risk factors
   A. Positive family history of skin conditions
   B. Exposure to environmental irritants such as strong acids, soaps, sunlight, etc.
   C. Diet, obesity, malnutrition
2. History
   A. Past or present skin conditions
   B. Allergies
   C. Use of topical or systemic drugs
   D. Functional status, mobility

3. Psychosocial and cultural assessment
   A. Physical environment and social support systems
   B. Family interactions

OBJECTIVE

1. Appearance—examine the entire skin surface for symmetry and overall appearance related to grooming and hygiene.
   A. Color, discoloration, irregular pigmentation, texture, general condition
   B. Temperature in extremities and other body areas
   C. Moist, dry, scaly, oily, flaking, clammy
   D. Turgid, supple, pliable
   E. Varicosities or red, brown, or blue discoloration indicating poor circulation or stasis
   F. Bruises or skin tears
   G. Edema
2. Lesions
   A. Moles, sores, scars, or identifying marks
   B. Moisture or drainage
   C. Pain or discomfort
   D. Raised or irregular edges

Planning

Client Needs

1. Safe, effective care environment
   A. Increase client's knowledge of neoplastic diseases, diagnostic procedures, and treatment (i.e., curette, caustics, cautery, freezing, diathermy, excision, chemotherapy, or radiotherapy).
   B. Promote early detection and intervention.
2. Health promotion and maintenance
   A. Increase client's knowledge related to solar exposure and neoplastic disorders.
   B. Increase client's knowledge related to prevention practices related to solar exposure—clothing, sunscreens, early or late sun exposure.
   C. Increase client's knowledge related to early detection and follow-up care.
3. Psychosocial integrity
   A. Reduce anxiety and fear.
   B. Reduce embarrassment.
4. Physiological integrity
   A. Maintain skin integrity.
   B. Increase client's comfort.

Implementation

1. Perform complete skin assessment.
2. Identify underlying conditions.
3. Palpate skin lesions for size, shape, consistency, texture, temperature, and hydration.
4. Determine onset and characteristics of lesions.
5. Monitor affected areas for changes in color, texture, shape, size.
6. Explain disease process, diagnostic procedures, and treatment.
7. Allow client to verbalize anxieties, feelings, or fears.
8. Provide emotional support.
9. Prepare for appropriate treatment.
   A. Radiation
   B. Chemotherapy
   C. Surgery

10. Protect from infection.
11. Educate on prevention practices and follow-up care.

Outcomes

1. Maintains skin integrity
2. Verbalizes comfort and/or decrease in embarrassment
3. Reports healthy lifestyle behaviors related to prevention of exposure to sunlight
4. Explains disease process, diagnostic procedures, and treatment
5. States reduction in anxiety and fear

Decubitus Ulcers

Description

1. Decubitus ulcers are localized cellular necrosis due to prolonged pressure over a bony prominence that deprives the area of blood supply.
2. Types
   A. Superficial (benign)—reddened areas involving only the outer skin layers
      (1) Caused by friction; shearing forces; irritating agents such as urine, trauma, or infection
   B. Deep—thrombosis of the vessels in deep tissue over a bony area that begins as reddened areas without evidence of necrosis. The area becomes abscessed to reveal a large, deep cavity filled with tissue that may contain infected material.
3. Stages
   A. Stage 1—nonblanching erythema of the intact skin.
   B. Stage 2—superficial ulcer appearing as a blister, abrasion, or shallow crater. It involves the epidermis and dermis.
   C. Stage 3—damage to the subcutaneous tissue that may extend to the fascia. Deep crater may or may not extend to adjacent tissue.
   D. Tissue necrosis with full thickness skin loss. It may extend to the muscle or bone mass.

Assessment

SUBJECTIVE

1. History of skin problems, trauma, or debilitating disease
2. Age
3. Psychosocial and cultural assessment
   A. Ability to perform activities of daily living (ADL)
   B. Mental status
   C. Ability to control bowel or bladder

OBJECTIVE

1. Assessment of the skin—color, elasticity, moisture, sensation, temperature, or breaks in the skin
2. Inspection of each pressure site for erythema, blanching, reactive hyperemia following removal of pressure source
3. Assessment of circulatory status of peripheral pulses
4. Assessment of nutritional status, particularly protein and vitamin C intake
5. Assessment of laboratory values, particularly hematocrit, hemoglobin, and serum albumin to determine protein intake

Planning

Client Needs

1. Safe, effective care environment
   A. Relieve or remove pressure.
   B. Eliminate shearing or friction.
2. Health promotion and maintenance
   A. Turn bedridden clients frequently.
3. Psychosocial integrity
   A. Provide client with opportunity to verbalize feelings.
   B. Provide client with opportunity to socialize.
4. Physiological integrity
   A. Maintain clean, dry skin.
   B. Promote adequate fluid and nutritional intake.
   C. Maintain skin integrity.
   D. Maintain comfort.

Implementation

1. Perform integumentary assessment.
2. Identify client risk for ulcer formation; institute preventative program.
3. Assist with personal hygiene.
4. Observe and remove any source of moisture in contact with the skin.
5. Turn every 1–2 hours.
6. Assess condition of skin over bony prominence.
7. Monitor length of time redness of skin persists.
8. Document assessment findings; maintain dressing changes.
9. Monitor fluid and nutritional intake.
10. Reduce pressure to any bony prominence when indicated—use toe pleat for bed linens; air, water mattress; flotation pads; bridging; egg-crate mattress; specially designed therapeutic beds such as the Clinitron bed.
11. Explain procedures and teach family members as appropriate.

Outcomes

1. Shows no signs of shearing forces or friction
2. Maintains clean, healthy, intact skin free from redness, lesions, or tissue necrosis
3. Maintains adequate nutritional intake
4. Verbalizes understanding of need to change position; to increase activities (if appropriate); to keep area free of moisture, wrinkles, or pressure
5. Maintains hemoglobin and albumin levels within normal limits
6. Shows timely healing of wounds, lesions, or ulcerations

Musculoskeletal System

Description

The primary changes in the musculoskeletal system include:
1. Stature and posture
   A. Decrease in height (1.2–4 cm) mainly due to compression of the spinal column.
   B. Lengthening and broadening of the ears and nose.
   C. Long bones are not affected by aging.
2. Bone mass and metabolism
   A. Changes in body tissue as a result of stress, vitamin D intake, parathyroid hormones, and calcium.

B. Increase in bone absorption within the vertebral bodies, wrist, and hips due to decrease in calcium levels.
3. Muscle mass
   A. Decrease in lean body mass with increase in body fat.
   B. Slowing of muscle tissue regeneration.
   C. Muscles atrophy and become fibrous.
   D. Changes in musculoskeletal and nervous systems lead to slower movement and decrease in strength and endurance.

Assessment

SUBJECTIVE

1. History
   A. Medical history
   B. Prescription and nonprescription medications
   C. Usual body weight
   D. Activity patterns and functional status
   E. Previous injuries, trauma, and falls
2. Psychosocial and cultural assessment
   A. Effect of dysfunction on lifestyle
   B. Past and present coping methods
   C. Family and other support systems

OBJECTIVE

1. Physical assessment—look for symmetry, gait, and balance
   A. Height and weight
   B. Posture and body alignment
   C. Range of motion in all joints
   D. Edema, pain, redness
   E. Ability to perform ADL
   F. Assistive devices
2. Diagnostic tests and methods
   A. Complete blood count (CBC) with differential
   B. Electrolytes
   C. Rheumatoid arthritis factor

Osteoporosis

Description

1. Types of osteoporosis:
   A. Postmenopausal
      (1) Associated with decreasing estrogen levels and low serum calcium levels
      (2) Affects primarily the trabecular bone of the vertebral column
   B. Senile osteoporosis
      (1) Results from an imbalance in the activity of osteoblasts (bone formation) and osteoclasts (bone reabsorption)
      (2) Affects both trabecular and cortical bones of the vertebrae and articulating bones in the hip
2. Causes of osteoporosis
   A. Hormonal
      (1) Decrease in estrogen and androgen
      (2) Imbalance in sex and adrenal hormones
      (3) Increase in parathyroid hormone
   B. Lifestyle behaviors
      (1) Lifelong low calcium intake
      (2) High caffeine intake
      (3) Excessive alcohol intake

(4) Smoking
(5) Sedentary lifestyle
(6) Excessive exercise
(7) Decreased vitamin D utilization
   C. Genetic
      (1) Family history or medical history
         (a) Diabetes
         (b) Cushing's syndrome
         (c) Chronic obstructive pulmonary disease
         (d) Multiple myeloma
         (e) Medications such as anticonvulsants and cortisone
      (2) White, particularly fair skin
      (3) Less than ideal body weight
      (4) Female gender

Assessment

1. History
   A. Family history
   B. Lifestyle behaviors
      (1) Smoking habits
      (2) Use and amount of alcohol intake
      (3) Nutritional intake, particularly calcium and vitamin D
      (4) Exercise habits
      (5) Postmenopausal
   C. Past history of fractures
   D. Menstrual history
      (1) Oophorectomy before age 45
      (2) Age at menopause
   E. Drug history
      (1) Estrogen replacement therapy
      (2) Use of anticonvulsant or glucocorticosteroid
2. Physical assessment
   A. Weight and height
   B. Radiographic evidence of low bone mass
   C. Back pain or point tenderness
   D. Fracture without apparent or adequate cause
   E. Functional assessment

Planning

Client Needs

1. Safe, effective care environment
   A. Increase client's knowledge related to diagnostic procedures.
   B. Promote early detection and intervention.
   C. Effect measures to prevent complications related to severe kyphosis and falls.
2. Health promotion and maintenance
   A. Increase client's knowledge related to cause and preventive measures:
      (1) Proper body mechanics to maintain function
      (2) Proper use of exercise to promote mobility, increase muscle strength and endurance
      (3) Diet modifications and proper nutrition
3. Psychosocial integrity
   A. Reduce anxiety and fear.
   B. Provide support services for client to maintain independent living.

4. Physiological integrity
   A. Increase client's comfort.
   B. Promote optimal mobility.
   C. Provide effective pain management.

Implementation

1. Provide complete musculoskeletal assessment.
2. Identify risk factors.
3. Encourage correct body posture.
4. Initiate an individualized exercise program suited to functional and mobility status (e.g., swimming, walking, biking, tennis, volleyball, etc.).
5. Establish a muscle-strengthening program in collaboration with a physician and physical therapist (e.g., lifting small weights, prone extension, or use of other equipment).
6. Initiate nutritional program to:
   A. Reach ideal body weight
   B. Increase calcium intake to 1000 mg daily
7. Provide estrogen therapy as prescribed—usual dosage is 1.25 mg.
8. Include teaching on:
   A. Smoking cessation
   B. Weight control
   C. Reduction in caffeine and alcohol consumption
   D. Exercise
   E. Prevention of injury

Outcomes

1. Experiences restoration and maintenance of function and joint mobility
2. Verbalizes increased comfort
3. Demonstrates understanding through performance of healthy lifestyle behaviors
4. Maintains proper body posture
5. Ingests diet meeting calcium and mineral needs
6. Shows no signs of breaks and/or injury related to falls
7. Complies with the medical regimen

Joint Diseases

Degenerative Joint Disease

Description

Degenerative joint disease, also known as osteoarthritis, is a noninflammatory disorder of the movable joints, most frequently the weight-bearing joints, knees, hips, and lumbar spine. It is characterized by deterioration of articular cartilage with formation of new bone at the joint surfaces. Heberden's nodes, bony protuberances found at the distal interphalangeal joints, are characteristic of the disease and are often seen in older women. In the later stages, degenerative joint disease produces pain, stiffness, crepitation, and joint hypertrophy. Systemic symptoms are weakness and muscle wasting from immobility. Predisposing factors include older age, joint trauma or injury, excessive joint use, obesity, and familial tendencies.

Physiology

1. Normal cartilage loses its elasticity, splits, and fragments.
2. Cartilage thins and becomes denuded.

3. Subchondral bone becomes sclerotic with thickening and narrowing of the joint spaces accompanied by the formation of bony cysts.
4. A layer of rough, thick, irregular bone develops.
5. Proliferation of new bone and cartilage at the periphery of joints and at sites of tendon and ligament attachments (osteophyte).
6. Osteophytes irritate the periosteum, causing pain.

Assessment

1. History
   A. Familial history of joint disease
   B. History of injury or trauma to joints
2. Physical assessment
   A. Symptoms of pain, stiffness, joint hypertrophy, crepitation, muscle spasms, contracture, or Heberden's nodes
   B. Asymmetry, abnormalities of posture or gait
   C. Range of motion in all extremities
3. Psychosocial and cultural assessment
   A. Activities that produce trauma or injury to weight-bearing joints, such as jogging, active sports
   B. Stress or anxiety

Planning

Client Needs

1. Safe, effective care environment
   A. Minimize weight bearing on affected joints.
   B. Teach proper body mechanics.
2. Health promotion and maintenance
   A. Ensure adequate calcium intake.
   B. Maintain exercise program.
3. Psychosocial integrity
   A. Reduce stress.
   B. Teach nutritional management to lose weight.
4. Physiological integrity
   A. Provide relief from pain.
   B. Encourage participation in mild exercise program to maintain muscle strength and joint mobility.
   C. Prevent further injury.

Implementation

1. Relieve pain.
   A. Drugs
      (1) Analgesics/anti-inflammatory drugs
         (a) Observe for toxicity (e.g., dizziness, hearing loss, drowsiness, hyperpnea, mental confusion and agitation).
      (2) Other drug therapies (i.e., indomethacin [Indocin], ibuprofen [Motrin], and phenylbutazone [Butazolidin])
         (a) Observe for toxic effects (e.g., nausea and vomiting, epigastric distress, bleeding from the gastrointestinal tract, rash, anemia, leukopenia, edema, mental agitation and confusion).
      (3) Other comfort measures
         (a) Dry or moist heat
         (b) Massage over joints and muscles

B. Rest of the affected joint
  (1) Assistive devices
    (a) Cane or crutch walking
      • Place on unaffected side.
      • Advance with unaffected side.
2. Provide preventive, maintenance measures.
  A. Exercise program
    (1) Isometric exercise
    (2) Teaching related to use of exercise, reduction to weight-bearing joints
  B. Nutrition
    (1) Reduction in caloric intake to control weight and prevent obesity
  C. Surgical procedures
    (1) Total joint replacement (arthroplasty)
      (a) Prevention of complication
        • Urinary tract infection—avoiding catheterization if possible, encouraging fluid intake
        • Hemorrhage—close observation of the client and operative site
        • Infection—proper hand washing, dressing changes using sterile technique
        • Injury to implant—teaching related to avoidance of weight bearing for 6–12 weeks, avoidance of excessive activity such as lifting or yard work, and maintenance of an exercise program to promote muscle strength and joint mobility

Outcomes

1. Verbalizes increase in comfort, relief of pain
2. Adheres to diet to control weight and prevent obesity
3. Demonstrates correct posture and body alignment
4. Maintains exercise program to maintain joint mobility and muscle strength
5. Has no complications related to surgical treatment
6. Uses effective stress management and coping strategies

Rheumatoid Arthritis

Description

Rheumatoid arthritis (RA) is a chronic, systemic, progressive disease affecting women more often than men. It is characterized by decrease in joint mobility, pain, swelling, and deformity. In the early stages, symptoms include pain and stiffness of involved joints, which early on may be relieved by rest. RA may occur at any age, and the course of the disease is marked by remissions and exacerbations.

1. Theories related to cause
  A. Condition is believed to be an immunological reaction possibly due to a virus. Associated with rheumatoid factors (antigen-antibody).
  B. Abnormal metabolism of trace metals, particularly gold.
2. Physiology
  A. Inflammation of the synovial membrane due to deposits of rheumatoid factors.
  B. Synovial membrane thickens and forms a mass known as a pannus, containing chronic inflammatory cells.
  C. Pannus destroys the cartilage and underlying bones.
  D. Pain results as naked bones rub against each other in movement.

Assessment

1. History
  A. Onset of pain and stiffness
    (1) Time of day occurring
    (2) Joints involved
  B. Medication history
2. Physical assessment
  A. Range of motion
    (1) Measure and record active and passive range of motion
    (2) Evidence of pain on movement
  B. Musculoskeletal assessment
    (1) Observation and palpation of each joint for swelling, redness, and deformity
    (2) Grip strength
    (3) Ability to perform ADL
    (4) Observation of gait, ability to walk, and ability to enter and exit chair
    (5) Contracture
  C. Accompanying characteristics
    (1) Fatigue, malaise, anemia
    (2) Changes in cardiovascular, respiratory, renal systems
  D. Diagnostic tests and methods
    (1) Increase in erythrocyte sedimentation rate
    (2) Presence of rheumatoid factor
    (3) CBC indicating mild anemia
    (4) Increase in C-reactive protein
    (5) Elevation in lupus erythematosus cell preparation
    (6) Examine the synovial fluid for evidence of high white blood cell count and low viscosity
3. Psychosocial and cultural assessment
  A. Physical or emotional stresses, anxieties, or concerns
  B. Body image
  C. Support systems
  D. Community resources
2. Health promotion and maintenance
  A. Ensure adequate calcium intake.
  B. Maintain exercise program.

Planning

Client Needs

1. Safe, effective care environment
  A. Minimize joint stress that may lead to deformity.
  B. Teach proper body mechanics, and encourage client to change position frequently.
  C. Limit joint use to only necessary tasks if client's joints are warm and swollen.
2. Health promotion and maintenance
  A. Help client to deal with stressors when they occur and do not let them build up.
  B. Ensure that client maintains activity and uses joints when they are not inflamed.
3. Psychosocial integrity
  A. Reduce stress.
  B. Promote positive body image.
  C. Identify support systems.
4. Physiological integrity
  A. Relieve pain and inflammation.
  B. Encourage participation in exercise program to enhance muscle strength in larger muscles.

C. Prevent further injury.

D. Maintain functional ability to carry out ADL.

Implementation

1. Relieve pain.
   A. Drugs
      (1) Analgesics, anti-inflammatory
         (a) Observe for toxicity (e.g., dizziness, hearing loss, drowsiness, hyperpnea, mental confusion and agitation).
      (2) Nonsteroidal anti-inflammatory drugs (e.g., indomethacin, ibuprofen, and phenylbutazone)
         (a) Observe for toxic effects (e.g., nausea and vomiting, epigastric distress, bleeding from the gastrointestinal tract, rash, anemia, leukopenia, edema, mental agitation and confusion).
      (3) Antimalarial (chloroquine [Aralen], hydroxychloroquine sulfate [Plaquenil sulfate])
         (a) Perform ophthalmology examination prior to beginning treatment and at frequent intervals to detect retina or cornea changes.
         (b) Observe for side effects such as blurring of vision and halos around lights.
      (4) Gold salts (aurothioglucose, gold sodium thiomalate)
         (a) Careful monitoring of bone marrow, kidney, and liver function is necessary.
         (b) Observe for signs of toxicity (e.g., pruritus, redness of the skin, inflammation of the mucous membranes of the mouth, stomatitis, or glossitis).
   B. Other comfort measures
      (1) Warm bath or shower
      (2) Warm, moist compresses
      (3) Ice packs during acute episode
      (4) Gentle massage
2. Physical mobility
   A. Assistive devices
      (1) Cane or crutch walking
         (a) Place weight on unaffected side.
         (b) Advance with unaffected side.
      (2) Trapeze bar to assist in bed transfer
      (3) Elevated chair, toilet seats, handrails
      (4) Wheelchair
         (a) Transfer procedure
         (b) Wheel locks
   B. Active and passive range of motion, isometrics
      (1) Resting affected joint during exacerbation
      (2) Maintaining upright and erect posture
   C. Surgical procedures
      (1) Total joint replacement (arthroplasty)
         (a) Prevention of complications
            • Urinary tract infection—avoiding catheterization if possible, encouraging fluid intake
            • Hemorrhage—close observation of the client and operative site
            • Infection—proper hand washing and dressing changes using sterile technique
            • Injury to implant—teaching related to avoidance of weight bearing for 6–12 weeks, avoidance of excessive activity such as lifting or yard work, and maintenance of an exercise program to promote muscle strength and joint mobility
3. Psychosocial and cultural assessment
   A. Monitor for body image disturbance
      (1) Verbal expression related to dependency, change in lifestyle, sexual concerns, negative self-concept
      (2) Giving positive reinforcement
      (3) Teaching effective coping methods
      (4) Monitoring for depression
   B. ADL
      (1) Monitoring functional status
      (2) Identifying community resources
      (3) Identifying support systems
      (4) Allowing independence when possible

Outcomes

1. Verbalizes increase in comfort, relief of pain
2. Performs self-care activities within functional ability
3. Demonstrates correct posture and body alignment
4. Maintains exercise program to maintain joint mobility and muscle strength
5. Has no complications related to surgical treatment
6. Uses effective stress management and coping strategies
7. Uses community and other resources
8. Verbalizes understanding of disease, procedures, and treatment
9. Adheres to drug therapy
10. Shows no evidence of feelings of depression, helplessness, or concern with body image

Cardiovascular System

Pathophysiology

With age, the heart has an increase in lipofuscin deposits in the myocardial fibers. The number of pacemaker cells in the sinoatrial node is decreased, which produces changes in the normal sinus rhythm. An accumulation of lipids combined with a degeneration of collagen and calcification of the valve fibrosa causes the valves to become thick and stiff. The increase in thickness produces cardiac murmurs, which are usual in the older adult. There is an increased amount of calcium deposits in the walls of the aorta and large vessels, leading to increased systolic blood pressure. In addition, the baroreceptors, which regulate blood pressure, are less sensitive in the older adult. Blood volume is reduced owing to the drop in plasma volume, and there is a slight drop in the number of red blood cells and in hemoglobin and hematocrit values. Blood coagulability increases with age.

Hypertension

Description

Hypertension is the most prevalent cardiovascular disease found in the elderly and is the major risk factor for stroke, heart failure, and coronary artery disease.

TYPES

1. Systolic hypertension—systolic BP > 160 mm Hg with a diastolic BP < 90 mm Hg.

2. Systolic-diastolic hypertension—systolic BP > 160 mm Hg with a diastolic ≥ 90 mm Hg.
3. Secondary hypertension—diastolic BP > 115 mm Hg. Condition may be the result of atherosclerosis, hyperparathyroidism, estrogen administration, or renal disease.

Assessment

1. History
   A. Familial risk factors
      (1) Family history of hypertension, atherosclerosis, heart disease, diabetes, renal disease
      (2) Race—black or Southeast Asian
   B. Lifestyle risk factors
      (1) Smoking
      (2) Excessive alcohol consumption
      (3) Sedentary lifestyle with little or no exercise
      (4) Food preferences—high-salt, high-fat, high-calorie, and/or high-cholesterol diet
      (5) Use of birth control pills or other hormones
2. Physical assessment
   A. Serial blood pressure readings (sitting, standing, and prone) include Osler's maneuver (raising the cuff pressure above the systolic pressure while palpating the radial artery to determine the presence of atherosclerosis).
   B. Height and weight.
   C. Pulses—radial, carotid, brachial, jugular, apical, popliteal, femoral, posterior tibial, and pedal.
      (1) Pulse strength
         0 No pulse palpated
         1 Difficult to palpate, weak or thready
         2 Light touch necessary because pulse is difficult to palpate
         3 Normal pulse
         4 Strong and bounding
      (2) Comparison of rate of radial or brachial pulses with femoral pulses; compare rate of apical and radial pulses for pulse deficit
      (3) Rate and rhythm—tachycardia, bradycardia, variations from beat to beat, dysrhythmia
      (4) Evidence of thrills (a vibration similar to the purring of a cat) or bruit (a murmurlike sound) to suggest arterial narrowing
      (5) Examination of bilateral jugular vein pressure with a ruler
3. Psychosocial and cultural assessment
   A. Support systems
   B. Ability to adhere to medical regimen
   C. Functional status
   D. Lifestyle behaviors

Planning

Client Needs

1. Safe, effective care environment
   A. Monitor patient's response to treatment.
   B. Provide teaching related to diet, exercise, and medication.
   C. Monitor for complications related to drugs.
2. Health promotion and maintenance
   A. Encourage healthy lifestyle behaviors.
   B. Encourage adherence to the medical regimen.

3. Psychosocial integrity
   A. Encourage client to verbalize feelings.
   B. Help client to deal with stressors when they occur.
   C. Assess client's sexual functioning.
4. Physiological integrity
   A. Maintain systolic and diastolic blood pressure within acceptable limits.

Implementation

1. Monitor vital signs using correct equipment and procedure.
2. Document pulse discrepancies or abnormalities.
3. Provide instructions related to administration of medications, complications, or precautions.
4. Monitor client's response to medical regimen.
5. Teach the importance of proper diet and exercise regimen.
6. Assess for further cardiovascular symptoms.
7. Monitor for electrolyte disturbance, glucose intolerance, depression, orthostatic hypotension, and impotence.

Outcomes

1. Maintains systolic and diastolic blood pressure within acceptable limits
2. Verbalizes understanding of medications and side effects
3. Demonstrates healthy lifestyle behaviors such as proper diet, regular exercise, cessation of alcohol and tobacco use
4. Verbalizes the importance of follow-up care
5. Shows no signs of adverse reactions to medical treatment or complications of hypertension

Angina

Description

Angina is chest pain resulting from a temporary insufficiency of blood supply to the heart muscle.
1. Symptoms—pressurelike discomfort, feeling of suffocation, strangulation, or crushing sensation. It may be accompanied by pain that radiates to the extremities, neck, or jaw. Older adults may experience only feelings of breathlessness, fatigue, or faintness.
2. Types.
   A. Stable—short duration and easily relieved
   B. Unstable—severe, long lasting, may not be relieved with rest or medication
   C. Variant—no evidence of chest pain, but ECG changes reflect ischemia

Assessment

1. History
   A. Familial risk factors
      (1) Family history of hypertension, atherosclerosis, heart disease, diabetes, renal disease
      (2) Race—black or Southeast Asian
   B. Lifestyle risk factors
      (1) Smoking
      (2) Excessive alcohol consumption
      (3) Sedentary lifestyle with little or no exercise
      (4) Food preferences—high-salt, high-fat, high-calorie and/or high-cholesterol diet
      (5) Use of birth control pills or other hormones

C. Medical history
   (1) Onset of attack
   (2) Duration
   (3) Treatment
   (4) Complications
2. Physical assessment
   A. Serial blood pressure readings (sitting, standing, and prone) include Osler's maneuver (raising the cuff pressure above the systolic pressure while palpating the radial artery to determine the presence of atherosclerosis)
   B. Height and weight
   C. Pulses—radial, carotid, brachial, jugular, apical, popliteal, femoral, posterior tibial, and pedal
      (1) Pulse strength
         0 No pulse palpated
         1 Difficult to palpate, weak or thready
         2 Light touch necessary because pulse is difficult to palpate
         3 Normal pulse
         4 Strong and bounding
      (2) Comparison of rate of radial or brachial pulses with femoral pulses, comparison of rate of apical and radial pulses for pulse deficit
      (3) Rate and rhythm—tachycardia, bradycardia, variations from beat to beat, dysrhythmia
      (4) Evidence of thrills (a vibration similar to the purring of a cat) or bruit (a murmurlike sound) to suggest arterial narrowing
      (5) Examination of bilateral jugular vein pressure using a ruler
   D. Skin changes—observe for brown pigmentation around the ankles suggesting venous insufficiency, and shiny skin with little hair growth for arterial insufficiency
3. Psychosocial and cultural assessment
   A. Support systems
   B. Ability to adhere to medical regimen
   C. Functional status
   D. Lifestyle behaviors

Planning
Client Needs

1. Safe, effective care environment
   A. Provide teaching related to activities that would restrict blood flow (e.g., diet, exposure to cold, use of caffeine and nicotine).
   B. Monitor for complications, side effects, therapeutic effects related to drugs.
2. Health promotion and maintenance
   A. Encourage healthy lifestyle behaviors.
   B. Encourage adherence to the medical regimen.
3. Psychosocial integrity
   A. Encourage client to verbalize stresses.
   B. Control stress and anxiety.
   C. Assess client's body image.
4. Physiological integrity
   A. Maintain systolic and diastolic blood pressure within acceptable limits.

Implementation

1. Monitor vital signs using correct equipment and procedure.
2. Document pulse discrepancies or abnormalities.

3. Provide instructions related to administration of medications, complications, or precautions.
4. Monitor client's response to medical regimen.
5. Teach the importance of proper diet and regular exercise regimen.
6. Assess for further cardiovascular symptoms.
7. Monitor for electrolyte disturbance, glucose intolerance, depression, orthostatic hypotension, and impotence.

Outcomes

1. Maintains systolic and diastolic blood pressure within acceptable limits
2. Verbalizes understanding of medications and side effects
3. Demonstrates healthy lifestyle behaviors such as proper diet, regular exercise, cessation of alcohol and tobacco use
4. Verbalizes the importance of follow-up care
5. Shows no signs of adverse reactions to medical treatment or complications of hypertension

Peripheral Vascular Diseases
Description

Peripheral vascular problems, both arterial and venous, increase in frequency with age and produce changes in both functional status and lifestyle. Peripheral vascular disease is characterized by the vessels becoming filled with a substance usually composed of fatty and fibrofatty tissue, which impedes the blood flow. When arterial blood flow is decreased, ischemia or infarction of the affected organ can result. When venous blood flow is decreased, veins become dilated with incomplete emptying, resulting in permanent impairment of fluid exchange. The only specific symptom of peripheral arterial disease is intermittent claudication, which results from muscle hypoxia. Claudication is pain, tightness, or weakness in an exercising muscle that occurs on walking and is relieved by rest.

Assessment

1. History
   A. Medical history of diabetes mellitus; hyperlipidemia; hypertension; polycythemia; or in women, early hysterectomy or ovariectomy
   B. Family history of homocystinuria (abnormal presence of homocystine, an amino acid, in the blood and urine)
2. Physical assessment
   A. Examination of the peripheral pulses, particularly the posterior tibial, which is always present in healthy individuals
   B. Doppler ultrasound
   C. Skin changes—observe for brown pigmentation around the ankles suggesting venous insufficiency
3. Psychosocial and cultural assessment
   A. Stressors and coping behaviors
   B. Sedentary lifestyle

SUBJECTIVE

1. Cigarette smoking
2. Dietary intake of foods high in lipid content
3. History of prior conditions

OBJECTIVE

1. Intermittent claudication
2. Numbness

3. A sense of coldness to extremities
4. Cyanotic color to lower or upper extremities
5. Foot pain at rest
6. Edema
7. Skin integrity

Planning

Client Needs

1. Safe, effective care environment
   A. Assess extremities regularly.
   B. Monitor bath water temperature.
2. Health promotion and maintenance
   A. Prevent fatigue.
   B. Encourage adherence to current medical regimen.
   C. Encourage participation in regular exercise, particularly walking or swimming.
   D. Prevent injury.
3. Psychosocial integrity
   A. Promote more effective coping or reduction of stressors.
4. Physiological integrity
   A. Maintain optimal nutritional and hydration status.
   B. Maintain environmental stimuli (heat and cold).

Implementation

1. Assist the client to conserve O_2.
2. Encourage the client to adhere to the prescribed medical regimen.
3. Encourage the client to maintain a regular exercise program, particularly walking or swimming.
4. Teach relaxation techniques to decrease anxiety and stressors.
5. Promote knowledge of the medication effects and side effects.
6. Teach nutritional need for increased protein, vitamin C, low-fat diet and need for eight glasses of fluid daily.
7. Prevent extreme exposure of the feet to heat or cold.
8. Promote regular foot care, which includes washing with mild soap, lukewarm water; drying feet carefully, particularly between the toes; use of lanolin lotion to dry, scaly skin; treatment of corns or calluses by podiatrist.
9. Prevent injury to feet by avoiding walking barefoot and by self-inspection of feet for cracks, cuts, or color changes. Test bath water with elbows. Do not use heating pads.
10. Teach client to wear properly fitted shoes and to avoid garters or elastic-top socks or hose.

Outcomes

1. Verbalizes ways of conserving energy and O_2 demand
2. Shows no signs of cuts, abrasions, lesions, cracks, or color changes to feet
3. Adheres to medical and exercise regimen
4. Verbalizes food intake of low-fat, high-protein, high-vitamin content
5. Demonstrates effective coping through use of relaxation techniques

6. Practices healthy lifestyle behaviors
7. Uses family or other support systems

Myocardial Infarction

Description

The following normal changes contribute to myocardial infarction (MI):
1. Slowing of capillary blood flow
2. Tortuosity of vessels
3. Changes in vascular walls
4. Increased adhesiveness of platelets
5. Increased cholesterol and serum lipid levels

Assessment

1. History: The older adult does not generally exhibit typical symptoms of MI, which may lead to misdiagnosis. The following symptoms should indicate to the nurse the need to rule out a MI:
   A. Dyspnea—particularly in an older adult who has had good exercise tolerance and suddenly develops dyspnea
   B. Sudden mental deterioration—particularly of a confused or irritable nature
   C. Dizziness, intense or prolonged weakness or fatigue, fainting or loss of consciousness without pain
   D. Mid- or lower abdominal distress
   E. Vomiting, hiccough, or palpations
   F. Pain (ranging from almost no pain to severe pain) of the anterior chest, neck, shoulder, or mandible occurring during rest or exertion
   G. Extreme anxiety
2. Physical assessment
   A. Vital signs
      (1) Temperature is a less pronounced indicator.
      (2) Pulse increase—may be sudden and rapid with rate up to or over 240 bpm.
      (3) Respiration—dyspnea, rapid, increased rate.
   B. Cardiovascular auscultation for the presence of:
      (1) Arrhythmia
      (2) Gallop rhythm
      (3) Reversed splitting of the S_2
      (4) Paroxysmal atrial or ventricular tachycardia
   C. ECG, 12 lead
      (1) Elevated or depressed ST segment
      (2) Inverted T
      (3) Rapid, irregular rhythm
3. Diagnostic tests and methods
   A. Erythrocyte sedimentation rate (ESR)—may or may not be increased
   B. Aspartate aminotransferase, lactic dehydrogenase, and creatinine phosphokinase—elevated
   C. Blood urea nitrogen, serum and creatinine clearance—elevated
   D. Changes in the color of the urine
4. Psychosocial and cultural assessment
   A. Extreme anxiety
   B. Denial of symptoms
   C. Sudden onset of confusion or irritability
   D. Recent loss of spouse
   E. Change in usual habits

Planning

Client Needs

1. Safe, effective care environment
   A. Relieve pain.
   B. Restore normal breathing.
   C. Relieve anxiety.
2. Health promotion and maintenance
   A. Encourage healthy lifestyle behaviors.
   B. Encourage adherence to the medical regimen.
      Promote return to normal activities.
3. Psychosocial integrity
   A. Assess client's body image.
   B. Provide health teaching related to sexuality.
4. Physiological integrity
   A. Maintain systolic and diastolic blood pressure and heart rhythm within acceptable limits.
   B. Prevent complications related to treatment.
   C. Increase cardiovascular and respiratory function.

Implementation

1. Monitor vital signs and heart rhythm.
2. Document pulse discrepancies or abnormalities.
3. Administer O_2 at 2 liters, elevate head of bed, and monitor lung sounds for rales.
4. Relieve anxiety—give reassurance.
5. Maintain a calm environment.
6. Give simple explanations of care and procedures.
7. Relieve chest pain.
   A. Nitroglycerin
   B. Narcotics—monitor carefully for toxicity
8. Treat arrhythmias.
   A. Ventricular
      (1) Lidocaine—usually given in divided doses over 20 minutes—monitor for confusion as a sign of toxicity
      (2) Pronestyl (Procainamide)—usually given in 100-mg IV doses over 2 minutes at 5-minute intervals
   B. Bradyarrhythmias
      (1) Atropine—usually given in 0.5-mg bolus until heart rate returns to 70–80 bpm
   C. Atrial fibrillation or atrial flutter
      (1) Digoxin—given in 0.25-mg IV doses every 4 hours
   D. Atrial tachycardia
      (1) Verapamil
9. Perform cardioversion.
10. Monitor for complications related to therapy.
    A. Hypotension
    B. Cardiogenic shock
    C. Congestive heart failure
    D. Drug interactions, toxicity
11. Provide teaching related to activities that would restrict blood flow (i.e., diet, exposure to cold, use of caffeine and nicotine).
12. Encourage adherence to the medical regimen.
13. Provide instructions related to administration of medications, dosage, and side effects to report.
14. Provide teaching related to resuming normal activities, especially sexual activities.

Outcomes

1. Reports decrease in pain
2. Maintains vital signs and heart rhythm within normal limits
3. Resumes normal ADL
4. Demonstrates healthy lifestyle behaviors
5. Verbalizes knowledge related to causes of restricted blood flow
6. Adheres to medical regimen

Congestive Heart Failure and Pulmonary Edema

Description

Congestive heart failure is an acute or chronic syndrome that develops as a result of any of many other disorders. Three disorders primarily cause congestive heart failure in about 95% of the cases: coronary artery disease, hypertension, and heart valve damage. The heart's ability to pump blood to the body tissues is impaired, resulting in a reduction of cardiac output. The veins become engorged with blood, and fluid leaks from the venous capillaries and accumulates in the lungs and in the other tissue spaces.

Assessment

1. History
   A. Coronary artery disease
   B. Hypertension
   C. MI
   D. Increased fluid volume or cardiac workload
   E. Medications
      (1) β-adrenergic blockers
         (a) Inderal (propranolol)
         (b) Lopressor (metroprolol tartrate)
      (2) Cardiotonic glycosides
         (a) Digitalis
         (b) Digoxin
2. Physical assessment
   A. Right-sided congestive heart failure
      (1) Orthostatic hypotension
      (2) Edema
      (3) Distended jugular veins
      (4) Liver enlarged and tender
      (5) S_3 gallop
   B. Left-sided congestive heart failure
      (1) Dyspnea
      (2) Tachypnea
      (3) S_3 and S_4 heart sounds
      (4) Displaced point of maximum impact
      (5) Pulsus alternans (alternating loud and soft Korotkoff sounds or doubling of the heart rate heard through a sphygmomanometer as the blood pressure cuff is released to the systolic level and below)
   C. Pulmonary edema
      (1) Cyanosis
      (2) Diaphoresis
      (3) Rales, rhonchi, and wheezing
      (4) Pink frothy sputum
      (5) Verbalizes a feeling of drowning

3. Psychosocial and cultural assessment
   A. Extreme anxiety
   B. Difficulty performing ADL
   C. Presence of cardiovascular stressors

Planning

Client Needs

1. Safe, effective care environment
   A. Decrease cardiac demand.
   B. Decrease stressors.
2. Health promotion and maintenance
   A. Ensure early intervention with beginning CHF.
   B. Carefully assess extremities.
3. Psychosocial integrity
   A. Decrease anxiety.
   B. Provide quiet, calm environment.
   C. Provide emotional support to client and family.
   D. Return to normal activities.
4. Physiological integrity
   A. Restore normal heart rate, vital signs.
   B. Increase tissue perfusion.
   C. Prevent infection.
   D. Increase comfort.
   E. Increased cardiac output.
   F. Improve gas exchange.

Implementation

1. Give O$_2$ at 2 L/min.
2. Elevate head of bed.
3. Monitor intake and output strictly; obtain daily weights.
4. Position with legs dangling.
5. Monitor ECG changes.
6. Monitor heart rate and vital signs carefully.
7. Administer medications as prescribed.
   A. Nitroglycerin.
   B. Cardiac glycosides—monitor for toxicity, which may include ECG changes and slowing of pulses, anorexia, nausea, and vomiting, which indicate early overdigitalization; headache and blurred vision with halos, confusion, or irritability. Take apical and radial pulses for at least 1 minute.
   C. Narcotics—monitor respiratory rate and signs of toxicity.
   D. Diuretics (furosemide [Lasix]—monitor potassium levels, heart rhythm.
   E. Aminophylline.
8. Decrease stressors and maintain quiet, calm environment.
9. Keep family informed of progress.
10. Decrease anxiety.
11. Provide instructions regarding medications, dose, action, and side effects.
12. Increase activity slowly after initial period of bed rest; monitor vital signs and heart rate before and after activity.

Outcomes

1. Verbalizes increased comfort
2. Maintains heart rate, rhythm, and vital signs within normal limits
3. Maintains slow, deep respirations without rales, rhonchi, or wheezing
4. Demonstrates reduced anxiety
5. Verbalizes understanding of medications and side effects
6. Resumes normal ADL

Cerebrovascular Accident

Description

About 75% of cerebrovascular accidents (CVAs), or strokes, occur in persons over the age of 65, and the incidence increases steadily with age. In the elderly, two thirds of those who suffer a stroke will have another stroke within a month. Stroke usually results in mild to significant dysfunction and may cause the individual to be institutionalized. Rehabilitation is a major component of care.

1. Causes
   A. Most common cause—usually arteriosclerotic cerebral infarction, may include a thrombosis or embolism
   B. Subarachnoid hemorrhage
   C. Intracerebral hemorrhage
2. Risk factors
   A. Hypertension
   B. Diabetes mellitus
   C. Lipid abnormalities, especially cholesterol
   D. History of transient ischemic attacks (TIAs)
   E. Coronary artery disease
   F. Obesity
   G. Smoking
   H. Peripheral vascular disease
   I. Use of birth control pills
   J. Polycythemia
3. Signs and symptoms—clear history of sudden, acute neurological deficit with presence of any of the following signs or symptoms of TIA: paresis, paresthesia, binocular vision, vertigo, diplopia, ataxia, dizziness, monocular vision, headache, dysphasia, dysarthria, nausea or vomiting, decreased level or loss of consciousness, visual hallucinations, tinnitus, mental changes, drop attacks, drowsiness, lightheadedness, generalized weakness, convulsion
4. Phases
   A. Acute—lasts about 2 weeks; client concerned with basic survival
   B. Rehabilitation—lasts from 8–12 weeks; client is usually placed in a rehabilitation setting in which assistance is given to help client with restoration of independence and ADL
   C. Final—lasts up to 2 years; client may return home or be placed in an institutional setting where assistance is given to help client return to maximum capability

Assessment

1. History
   A. Presence of risk factors
   B. Sudden, acute onset with acute neurological deficit
   C. Past history of stroke or TIA
2. Physical assessment
   A. Vital signs—elevated
   B. Cardiovascular exam
      (1) Presence of arrhythmias
      (2) Carotid bruits

(3) Irregularity in pulses
C. Neurological exam
   (1) Level of consciousness—note any changes and response to stimuli
   (2) Mental status
   (3) Alterations in speech pattern
      (a) Agnosia—failure to recognize familiar object
      (b) Agraphia—failure to write intelligible words
      (c) Dysarthria—defects in articulation
      (d) Paraphasia—use of the wrong word, word substitution, grammatical errors, or faults in word usage
      (e) Preservation—continued and automatic repetition of word or phrase or activity that is inappropriate
   (4) Cranial nerves—check for intactness
   (5) Presence or absence of voluntary or involuntary movements of the extremities, or muscle tone
D. Laboratory or other diagnostic tests
   (1) ECG
   (2) Chest x-ray
   (3) Electroencephalogram
   (4) CBC with prothrombin time—a high normal hematocrit level is related to cerebral infarction, and prothrombin time is necessary for anticoagulant therapy regulation
   (5) Glucose
   (6) Cholesterol and triglyceride levels
   (7) Computed tomography (CT) scan
3. Psychosocial assessment
A. Lifestyle behaviors—smoking, alcoholism, obesity, diet high in fat or other cholesterol-producing products, lack of exercise
B. Evidence of stressors

Planning

Client Needs

1. Safe, effective care environment
  A. Protect from falls or injury.
2. Health promotion and maintenance
  A. Encourage healthy lifestyle behaviors.
  B. Assist in establishing healthy coping patterns.
3. Psychosocial integrity
  A. Improve verbal communication.
  B. Restore normal ability to perform self-care activities.
  C. Relieve depression.
4. Physiological integrity
  A. Increase tissue perfusion; improve cerebral blood flow and metabolism.
  B. Increase fluid output.
  C. Restore physical mobility.
  D. Maintain cholesterol and triglyceride levels within normal limits.
  E. Prevent contracture.
  F. Relieve pain, especially in the shoulders.

Implementation

1. Acute phase
  A. Maintain a patent airway; administer O_2 at 2 liters.
  B. Explain and prepare client for all procedures.
  C. Monitor vital signs.
  D. Position in lateral or semiprone position; elevate head of bed.
  E. Monitor for pulmonary complications—aspiration, atelectasis, pneumonia.
  F. Change positions every 2 hours.
  G. Reduce anxiety.
  H. Provide support for family.
2. Rehabilitative phase
  A. Provide a sling or position flaccid arm on a table or pillows to prevent shoulder pain.
  B. Provide proper body alignment while client is in bed to prevent contracture and other deformities.
  C. Position flat in bed except during activities.
  D. Use appliances to prevent contracture as follows:
    (1) Footboard—to prevent footdrop
    (2) Splints—to prevent flexion of the affected extremity
    (3) Trochanter roll—to prevent external rotation of the hip
    (4) Pillows—positioned under the axilla—to reduce edema and fibrosis
    (5) Hand rolls—to maintain flexion in the fingers
  E. Assist with passive and active range of motion exercises to all extremities 4–6 times daily.
  F. Assist with balance during sitting and standing.
  G. Encourage client during relearning ambulation.
  H. Teach client proper wheelchair use.
  I. Encourage client to be as independent as possible and to perform self-care activities as improvement is noted.
  J. Start bowel and bladder retraining.
  K. Provide emotional support during speech therapy.
  L. Provide an environment conducive to communication.
  M. Provide emotional support for family.
  N. Assist the family to identify community resources.
  O. Prepare client for discharge to home or institution.
3. Final phase
  A. Monitor progress.
  B. Assist client with exercises to regain strength.
  C. Provide positive reinforcement for achievements.
  D. Encourage client to adhere to exercise, speech, and occupational therapies.
  E. Allow client and family to verbalize concerns, thoughts, and feelings.
  F. Provide nursing care as condition warrants.

Outcomes

1. Verbalizes increased comfort
2. Verbalizes relief of shoulder pain
3. Has no contractures, deformities, or footdrop
4. Is able to ambulate or regain mobility through use of braces or wheelchair
5. Maintains self-care activities
6. Maintains bowel and bladder function
7. Demonstrates improved communication
8. Shows no signs of injuries or falls
9. Reports relief of depression
10. Adheres to exercise, speech, physical, and occupational therapies, and demonstrates positive feelings related to therapies

11. Demonstrates effective coping
12. Uses community resources as needed

Respiratory System

Description

Aging produces changes both within the respiratory system and in other related systems. In addition, changes in other systems affect the respiratory system. Musculoskeletal changes include:

1. Shortening of the thorax, with an anterior-posterior diameter increase
2. Osteoporosis of the ribs and vertebrae
3. Calcification of the costal cartilages
4. Decreased rigidity of the chest wall
5. Weakening of the diaphragm, intercostal muscles, and accessory muscles
6. Muscle atrophy of the pharynx and larynx

Normal internal pulmonary changes:

1. Decreased blood flow to pulmonary circulation
2. Decreased diffusion
3. Shorter breaths with decreased maximum breathing capacity
4. Airway resistance increase, less ventilation at the bases of the lung and more at the apex, impaired gas exchange
5. Bronchus more rigid, decreased ciliary action, impaired cough mechanism

These combined normal age-related changes produce increased stiffness of the chest wall and diminished muscular strength and lead to reduced efficiency of breathing. Maximal inspiratory and expiratory force is reduced, and more work is needed to move air in and out.

The most common respiratory problems in the elderly include:

1. Chronic obstructive pulmonary disease (COPD)
2. Pneumonia
3. Tuberculosis
4. Lung cancer

Chronic Obstructive Pulmonary Disease

Description

Chronic obstructive pulmonary disease is used to describe chronic airway obstruction in the form of chronic bronchitis, chronic emphysema, and asthma. Usually all three conditions are present in the older adult. Although each condition is precipitated by unique risk factors, the interventions are similar in assisting the client to modify or cope with the illness.

Bronchitis—presence of a productive cough at least 3 months out of the year for ≥2 years. Condition is usually caused by cigarette smoking or by environmental or occupational pollutants.

Emphysema—abnormal and permanent dilation of the terminal air spaces of the lungs, combined with destruction of the alveolar wall.

Asthma—hyperactive airways and increased resistance to expiratory flow and hyperinflation of the lungs. Extrinsic asthma is primarily allergic in origin, mediated by antigen-antibody responses. Intrinsic asthma is more common in the elderly and is associated with respiratory infections, dust, cigarette smoking, pollutants, and even change in temperature.

Assessment

SUBJECTIVE

1. Age of onset
2. Allergic history
3. Family history
4. Precipitating stress
5. Smoking

OBJECTIVE

1. Dyspnea—determine grade:
   A. Grade I—can keep pace with a healthy person when walking on the level; unable to do so on stairs or hills
   B. Grade II—can walk 1 mile at own pace without dyspnea; cannot keep up with a healthy person walking on the level
   C. Grade III—becomes breathless after walking 100 yards or a few minutes on the level
   D. Grade IV—becomes breathless when performing simple activities such as bathing or dressing
2. Inspect posture; observe for large, hyperinflated chest.
3. Observe for prolonged expiratory phase.
4. Auscultate breath sounds for rales, rhonchi, and wheezes.
5. Observe for hypoxemia and CO_2 retention (only when complications develop).
6. Monitor anxiety.
7. Determine height and weight—look for thin stature, emaciation.
8. Observe chest x-ray.
9. Inspect site of skin test.

Planning

Client Needs

1. Safe, effective care environment
   A. Prevent avoidable injury.
   B. Prevent respiratory and other infections.
   C. Maintain patent airway.
2. Health promotion and maintenance
   A. Increase client's knowledge of causative factors.
   B. Encourage appropriate lifestyle behaviors.
   C. Encourage active participation in treatment regimen.
3. Psychosocial integrity
   A. Decrease anxiety.
   B. Facilitate appropriate coping behaviors.
4. Physiological integrity
   A. Increase comfort and rest.
   B. Maintain fluid balance.
   C. Support adequate nutrition.
   D. Improve ventilation and oxygenation.
   E. Maintain effective breathing pattern.
   F. Eliminate signs and symptoms of hypoxia.
   G. Maintain arterial blood gas values within normal limits.

Implementation

1. Assess causative and contributing factors.
2. Monitor vital signs.

3. Assist with deep-breathing and coughing exercises.
4. Increase fluid intake to at least 2000 mL/day within cardiac reserve.
5. Give warm rather than cold fluids.
6. Provide opportunities for rest as needed.
7. Observe for signs and symptoms of infection.
8. Provide postural drainage and percussion as indicated to all but asthmatics.
9. Teach pursed-lip or diaphragmatic breathing techniques.
10. Observe for signs and symptoms of respiratory distress.
11. Administer medications as directed.
12. Note response to medication.
13. Provide emotional support and teach relaxation techniques.
14. Assess client's knowledge of disease process and treatment regimen.
15. Instruct in proper use and safety related to home O_2 therapy.

Outcomes

1. Keeps environment free of pollutants and conducive to adequate gaseous exchange
2. Refrains from smoking
3. Demonstrates proper medication management
4. Maintains effective gas exchange with arterial blood gases within normal limits
5. Explains use and side effects of medications and treatment regimen correctly
6. Shows no signs of colds, flu, or other respiratory infections
7. Adheres to preventive measures
8. Maintains mild to moderate anxiety

Pneumonia

Description

Pneumonia due to influenza is the fourth leading cause of death in older adults. Four organisms are primarily responsible for pneumonia in older adults: *Klebsiella pneumoniae* (common in nursing homes), *Haemophilus influenza* or *Streptococcus pneumoniae* (common in the community), and *Legionella pneumophilia*. Because pneumonia may be caused by a variety of organisms, it is important to obtain sputum for Gram's stain and culture.

Assessment

SUBJECTIVE

1. Malaise
2. Altered mental status
3. Assistance with feeding or tube feeding required
4. History of colds, influenza, or pneumonia

OBJECTIVE

1. Increased cough and sputum
2. Fever—may appear later and may not be spiking
3. Tachypnea
4. Dehydration
5. Hyperventilation
6. Chest pain
7. Diagnostic tests and methods
   A. Chest x-ray
   B. CBC
   C. Gram's stain of expectorated sputum

Planning

Client Needs

1. Safe, effective care environment
   A. Prevent adverse reactions to therapy.
2. Health promotion and maintenance
   A. Increase client's knowledge of home care and follow-up.
3. Psychosocial integrity
   A. Reduce anxiety
4. Physiological integrity
   A. Maintain effective breathing pattern and airway clearance.
   B. Maintain comfort, rest.
   C. Maintain functional status.
   D. Maintain nutrition and fluid balance.

Implementation

1. Assess for risk factors.
   A. Especially aspiration
   B. CVAs
   C. Parkinson's disease
   D. Swallowing dysfunctions
   E. Impaired cough or gag reflex
   F. Depressed sensorium
   G. Nasogastric tube feedings
   H. Immobility
2. Assess level of consciousness.
3. Monitor vital signs.
4. Teach importance of immunizations for influenza and pneumonia.
5. Maintain adequate nutrition and fluid balance.
6. Administer antibiotic therapy as ordered.
7. Assist client to perform cough, turn, and deep-breathing exercises every 2 hours.
8. Initiate comfort measures.
9. Monitor O_2 therapy.
10. Teach exercises to strengthen muscles used in swallowing.
11. Administer cimetidine 1 hour before meals to assist in swallowing.

Outcomes

1. Shows no signs of confusion, fever, malaise, or respiratory distress
2. Maintains effective airway clearance with improved oxygenation
3. Verbalizes increased comfort and relief of chest pain
4. Shows no evidence of infiltrate on chest films
5. Demonstrates knowledge of preventive strategies
6. Is able to perform usual ADL

Tuberculosis

Description

Tuberculosis is an acute or chronic infection caused by the tubercle bacillus organism that leads to inflammation and formation of a permanent nodule containing the bacillus. The infected person harbors the bacillus for life. It may remain dormant or become active during physical or emotional stress. The organism is transmitted by airborne droplets. The incidence of tuberculosis is rising and drug-resistant strains of bacillus are developing.

Assessment

SUBJECTIVE

1. Weight loss
2. Anorexia
3. History of risk factors
   A. Malnutrition
   B. Alcoholism
   C. Diabetes
   D. Use of immunosuppressive drugs
   E. Renal dialysis
   F. Cancer

OBJECTIVE

1. Positive findings of infiltrate on chest x-ray
2. Positive acid-fast bacilli in the sputum
3. Tuberculin skin test
   A. If initial skin test is negative, a repeated test is given in 1 week.
4. Increased fever
5. Hemoptysis
6. Night sweats

Planning

Client Needs

1. Safe, effective care environment
   A. Prevent adverse reaction to medical regimen.
2. Health promotion and maintenance
   A. Increase client's knowledge of disease process and medical regimen.
   B. Encourage adherence to long-term medical therapy.
3. Psychosocial integrity
   A. Reduce anxiety.
4. Physiological integrity
   A. Maintain rest and comfort.
   B. Prevent skin breakdown due to moisture.
   C. Maintain adequate nutritional and fluid balance.
   D. Maintain functional status.

Implementation

1. Teach client and family about:
   A. Disease process
   B. Hygienic measures
   C. Drugs and their side effects
   D. Need for adherence to long-term medical therapy
   E. Need to test others in the household
2. Monitor liver function studies, bilirubin, serum creatinine, platelet count for signs of drug toxicity or adverse effects.
3. Monitor vital signs and respiratory function.
4. Provide emotional support and sense of psychological well-being.
5. Allow client to verbalize negative feelings toward self related to disease.
6. Provide nutritional consultation.
7. Monitor adherence to long-term drug therapy.

Outcomes

1. Maintains normal liver function values, bilirubin, creatinine clearance
2. Shows no signs of hepatitis, jaundice, peripheral neuropathy
3. Has negative sputum test within 3 months of medical therapy
4. Adheres to long-term therapy
5. Demonstrates healthy lifestyle behaviors
6. Shows evidence of positive self-concept and body image

Cancer of the Lung

Description

Lung cancer is a major disease of the elderly and is the most common fatal malignancy in men. The disease is extremely lethal, with an average 5-year survival rate of less than 10%.

Assessment

SUBJECTIVE

1. History of exposure to carcinogenic pollutants
   A. Smoking
   B. Asbestos
   C. Uranium
   D. Nickel
   E. Chlormethyl ether
   F. Chromium
2. Family history

OBJECTIVE

1. Medical history
   A. Cough
   B. Hemoptysis
   C. Wheezes and stridor
   D. Dyspnea from obstruction
   E. Pneumonitis
2. Pain from pleural or chest wall involvement
3. Diagnostic tests and methods
   A. Chest x-ray

Planning

Client Needs

1. Safe, effective care environment
   A. Maintain comfort and rest.
   B. Prevent injury or other complications.
2. Health promotion and maintenance
   A. Prepare client for surgical procedures.
   B. Increase client's knowledge of community resources.
3. Psychosocial integrity
   A. Promote positive mental attitude.
   B. Allow client to verbalize feelings related to pain, surgery, or death.
   C. Identify support network.
4. Physiological integrity
   A. Provide optimal nutrition.
   B. Maintain effective airway clearance.
   C. Maintain functional status.

Implementation

1. Allow client to verbalize feelings regarding condition or death.
2. Provide preoperative teaching.
   A. Turn, cough, and deep-breathing exercises
   B. Chest tubes and drainage
   C. Pain management
   D. Radiation therapy
3. Administer medications for pain, nausea, and comfort.
4. Assist to identify community resources such as hospice care.
5. Encourage adequate nutrition and fluid balance.
6. Provide emotional support.

Outcomes

1. Demonstrates knowledge of disease process and treatment
2. Reports relief of pain and discomfort
3. Verbalizes feelings related to disease or death
4. Demonstrates knowledge of community and other support systems
5. Participates in postoperative care
6. Maintains anxiety at mild to moderate level
7. Maintains functional status at optimal level

Gastrointestinal System

The gastrointestinal (GI) system of the older adult may be characterized by decreased secretion, absorption, and motility. Constipation is a frequent complaint among older people, but it is most likely caused by decreased fluid intake, insufficient bulk, and lack of exercise. After the age of 50, the liver begins to shrink and enzyme production is decreased. Changes in the liver are particularly important when considering drug therapy, especially those drugs that are metabolized by the liver. Lower drug dosage in the elderly is a common rule. The elderly may have decreased absorption of iron, vitamin B_{12}, and folate resulting in anemia.

Abdominal Pain

1. Causes
   A. Cholecystitis
   B. Cholelithiasis
   C. Cancer
   D. Intestinal obstruction
   E. Peptic ulcer
   F. Diverticulitis
   G. Hernia
   H. Pancreatitis
   I. Appendicitis
   J. Dissecting aneurysm
   K. Ischemic colitis
   L. Urinary retention

Signs and Symptoms

1. Cholecystitis (most common GI problem in the elderly)
   A. Pain in right upper quadrant
   B. Marked abdominal tenderness
   C. Vomiting
   D. Jaundice
   E. Low-grade fever
   F. Leukocytosis
   G. Normal bowel sounds
2. Cancer
   A. Abdominal distention
   B. Dull sound on percussion
   C. Constipation
   D. Occult blood in stool
3. Intestinal obstruction
   A. Intermittent abdominal cramps
   B. Vomiting
   C. Abdominal distention
   D. High-pitched bowel sounds
   E. Hyperactive bowel activity
   F. Inability to pass flatus
   G. Constipation
4. Hernia
   A. Abdominal pain
   B. Abdominal swelling
   C. Tenderness
5. Pancreatitis
   A. Pain in the left lower quadrant or midline
   B. Nausea and vomiting
   C. Lack of bowel sounds
6. Appendicitis
   A. Vague complaints of diffuse pain
   B. Twelve to 18 hours later pain moves to right lower quadrant
   C. Low-grade fever
   D. Anorexia
   E. Abdominal distention
   F. Nausea and vomiting
   G. Hypoactive or absence of bowel sounds
   H. Constipation
7. Diverticulosis
   A. Lower abdominal pain
   B. Complaint of fullness
   C. Bloating and abdominal distention
8. Peptic ulcer
   A. Epigastric discomfort
   B. Atypical, poorly localized pain
   C. Anorexia
   D. Weight loss
   E. Vomiting
   F. Ulcer may lead to these major complications if untreated:
      (1) Severe anemia
      (2) Hemorrhage
9. Ischemic colitis
   A. Acute left-sided abdominal pain
   B. Low-grade fever
   C. Rectal bleeding

Assessment

SUBJECTIVE

1. History
   A. Oral hygiene patterns
   B. Dietary habits
   C. Elimination habits

2. Family medical history
3. Pain
   A. Location
   B. Severity

OBJECTIVE

1. Physical assessment

   NOTE: Assessment of the GI system requires a deviation in technique: inspection, auscultation, percussion, with palpation being completed last.

   A. Inspection
      (1) Scars, striae, lesions, masses, tautness
      (2) Symmetry, pulsation, peristalsis
      (3) Swelling, rigidity
   B. Auscultation
      (1) Bowel sounds, bruits, rubs
   C. Percussion
      (1) Tympany (normal abdominal sounds)
      (2) Dullness
   D. Palpation
      (1) Rebound tenderness
      (2) Pain
      (3) Organomegaly
2. Diagnostic tests and methods
   A. CBC, serum amylase, bilirubin levels
   B. Urinalysis
   C. Stool guaiac, occult blood
   D. Chest x-ray—to rule out pneumonia
   E. ECG—to rule out MI
   F. Plain-film x-ray of abdomen
   G. Kidney, ureter, bladder x-ray
   H. Ultrasound
   I. Other GI studies
3. Psychosocial and cultural assessment
   A. Anxiety, stressors
   B. Family or community support systems

Planning

Client Needs

1. Safe, effective care environment
   A. Provide increased comfort and rest.
   B. Prevent complications.
2. Health promotion and maintenance
   A. Increase client's knowledge of nutritional needs, normal elimination patterns, exercise.
   B. Reduce use of laxatives.
3. Psychosocial integrity
   A. Facilitate effective coping behaviors.
   B. Ensure lack of somatic complaints.
   C. Reduce anxiety.
   D. Increase client's knowledge of procedures and treatment.
4. Physiological integrity
   A. Maintain nutrition and fluid balance.

Implementation

1. Assess oral cavity.
2. Promote oral hygiene and refer to dentist, if necessary.
3. Teach role of nutrition and exercise in regular bowel elimination.

4. Assess abdomen and bowel sounds.
5. Prepare client for diagnostic tests.
6. Administer medications and/or other treatments in preparation for diagnostic tests.
7. Relieve anxiety.
8. Teach effective coping behaviors.
9. Support family to promote self-care by client.
10. Monitor results of diagnostic tests.

Outcomes

1. Verbalizes increased comfort
2. Verbalizes knowledge of appropriate nutrition and normal bowel elimination
3. Demonstrates lifestyle changes to aid in elimination
4. Expresses concern or anxiety related to diagnostic tests
5. Shows no signs of fullness, bloating, or rigid abdomen
6. Demonstrates evidence of soft, formed bowel movement every 2–3 days

Genitourinary System

Description

Age-related changes in the genitourinary system include a decreased filtration surface area with a progressive loss of renal mass and kidney weight. Renal blood flow progressively decreases from 1200 mL/min to 600 mL/min by age 80. Glomerular filtration rate declines with age owing to nephron loss and decrease in proximal tubular function. Changes in the tubules decrease tubular transport mechanisms, causing diminished ability to concentrate or dilute urine in response to excess or loss of salt and water. Creatinine clearance decreases with age and should be carefully monitored before administration of drugs dependent on renal function. The diurnal rhythm of urine production is lost, with urine production remaining relatively the same over 24 hours, with nocturia as the outcome. Drugs excreted in an unchanged form are likely to be excreted more slowly. In addition, renal disease may cause an accumulation of drugs while low serum albumin levels provide fewer binding sites, making more free drug available. Drugs commonly taken by the elderly (e.g., digitalis, aminoglycosides, and antibiotics) should be calculated using the creatinine clearance. Because creatinine clearance requires a 24-hour urine collection, an estimation can be calculated using the person's age, sex, weight, and serum creatinine level. The formula is:

$$\text{Estimated Creatinine} = \frac{(140 - \text{age}) \times \text{Body Weight in Kilograms}}{72 \times \text{Serum Creatinine Level}}$$

*Value is 15% less for women

Acute and Chronic Renal Failure

Description

1. Acute and chronic renal failure is a condition caused by a multitude of pathological processes that lead to derangement and insufficiency of renal excretory and regulatory functions.
2. Causes
   A. Prostatic hypertrophy
   B. Cancer
   C. Atherosclerosis

D. Multiple myeloma
E. Drug related
F. Azotemia from heart failure
G. Diabetes
H. Urinary tract infection

Assessment

SUBJECTIVE

1. Medical history
   A. Evidence of disease predisposing to renal failure
   B. Drug history
   C. Past urinary function
      (1) Change in urinary stream
      (2) Difficulty starting stream
      (3) Dribbling
      (4) Feeling of fullness after voiding
      (5) Symptoms of infection, frequency, urgency, burning
      (6) History of nocturia

OBJECTIVE

1. Rectal examination
2. Assessment of reproductive organs
   A. Women
      (1) Muscle tone
      (2) Uterine prolapse
      (3) Cystocele
      (4) Cervix
      (5) Palpate for masses
   B. Men
      (1) Foreskin of penis
      (2) Benign prostatic hypertrophy
      (3) Urinary stream and output
3. Urinalysis

Planning

Client Needs

1. Safe, effective care environment
   A. Prevent secondary infections from:
      (1) Bladder catheterization
      (2) IV lines
   B. Prevent pruritus.
2. Health promotion and maintenance
   A. Increase client's knowledge of disease process and treatment.
   B. Encourage adherence to treatment protocol.
3. Psychosocial integrity
   A. Maintain anxiety at mild to moderate levels.
   B. Provide emotional support.
4. Physiological integrity
   A. Maintain electrolyte levels within normal limits.
   B. Maintain nutritional and fluid balance.
   C. Administer medications as ordered.
   D. Prepare client for procedures such as dialysis.

Implementation

1. Keep skin clean and dry.
2. Apply moisturizers.
3. Monitor electrolyte levels.
4. Monitor nutritional intake, particularly potassium.
5. Perform strict intake and output recording.
6. Use strict hand-washing and aseptic technique.
7. Allow client to verbalize concerns and anxiety.
8. Administer medications as ordered.
9. Explain all procedures.
10. Provide health teaching related to dialysis and maintenance care.
11. Provide emotional support.
12. Provide follow-up care.

Outcomes

1. Keeps skin smooth and free from flaking, itching, or dryness
2. Shows no signs of secondary infections
3. Maintains electrolyte levels within normal limits
4. Has no anxiety related to treatment
5. Demonstrates knowledge of disease process, cause, and treatment
6. Adheres to the treatment protocol

Incontinence

Description

Incontinence is the loss of urine sufficient in quantity and/or frequency to be a social or health concern.

1. Types
   A. Urge—a sudden need to void and urinate before reaching the toilet due to urethral sphincter inefficiency. The bladder contracts without the person initiating micturition.
      (1) Causes
         (a) CVA
         (b) Dementia
         (c) Parkinson's disease
         (d) Multiple sclerosis
      (2) Signs
         (a) Sudden or strong urge to urinate
         (b) Urinating more frequently than normal
         (c) Getting up more at night to urinate
         (d) Urinating small amounts
      (3) Treatment
         (a) Drugs to decrease contractions
         (b) Treating underlying condition
            Urinary infection
            Prostate or uterine problems
            Bladder retraining
         (c) Wearing disposable shields
   B. Stress incontinence—accounts for half of all incontinence; occurs mostly in women who have borne children. Muscles that control pressure in urethra get weak and are unable to resist the pressure from the bladder muscle, with resulting leakage.
      (1) Cause
         (a) Childbearing
         (b) Urinary tract infections
         (c) Tumors
         (d) Surgery to urinary tract
         (e) Damage due to radiation
      (2) Signs
         (a) Grade 1—leakage occurring due to coughing, sneezing, laughing, or straining

(b) Grade 2—leakage occurring as a result of running, jogging, or walking

(c) Grade 3—total incontinence

(3) Treatment

(a) Pelvic floor (Kegel) exercise

(b) Surgery
Bladder suspension
Vesicourethral suspension

(c) Protective undergarments

(d) Treatment of other conditions

C. Overflow—develops when the bladder cannot create enough pressure to overcome resistance at bladder neck.

(1) Cause

(a) Weakened bladder muscle

(b) Faulty signals from nervous system

(c) Enlarged prostate

(d) Spinal cord damage

(e) Diabetes

(f) Muscle-relaxing drugs

(2) Signs

(a) Swollen bladder

(b) Tenderness over pubic area

(c) Decreased urinary stream

(3) Treatment

(a) Medication
To treat diabetes
To decrease edema in bladder

(b) Surgery
Prostatectomy
Relieving blockage to nervous system

(c) Intermittent catheterization

D. Functional incontinence—inability to get to the bathroom due to functional ability

(1) Cause

(a) Decreased mobility

(b) Decreased dexterity

(c) Improper clothing

(2) Signs

(a) Wetness of clothing

(b) Body odor

(3) Treatment

(a) Keep a record in order to anticipate when urination will occur.

(b) Use Velcro closures rather than buttons or zippers.

(c) Use bedside commode.

Assessment

SUBJECTIVE

1. History

A. Medical history that might contribute to cause

B. Medication history

C. Childbearing and reproductive history

D. Verbalized report of incontinence

E. Mental status examination

OBJECTIVE

1. Physical assessment

A. Rectal examination, including prostate gland

B. Vaginal examination

C. Pattern of incontinence

2. Psychosocial and cultural assessment

A. Lifestyle behaviors

B. Reaction to incontinence

C. Environmental assessment

Planning

Client Needs

1. Safe, effective care environment

A. Encourage client to perform self-care activities of toilet hygiene.

2. Health promotion and maintenance

A. Increase client's and family's knowledge of condition.

B. Increase client's knowledge of incontinent undergarments, bladder training, and Kegel exercises.

C. Identify support system and pattern of family dynamics.

3. Psychosocial integrity

A. Help client to reestablish social network.

4. Physiological integrity

A. Decrease or alleviate incontinent episodes.

B. Establish bladder routine.

C. Maintain skin integrity.

Implementation

1. Review history for evidence of cause and type of incontinence.

2. Perform Clinitest of urine for glucose, which can cause polyuria.

3. Determine the difference between the time it takes to get to the bathroom and when urination occurs.

4. Identify environmental conditions that may affect incontinence.

5. Determine the frequency of incontinence.

6. Measure intake and output.

7. Perform urinalysis to detect infection and/or bacteriuria.

8. Administer and teach administration of diuretics during morning hours.

9. Reduce use of medications, which might alter sensorium.

10. Adapt clothing for quick removal.

11. Provide night light.

12. Provide bedside commode.

13. Establish a schedule of voiding every 3 hours.

14. Restrict fluids after 6 PM.

15. Instruct in pelvic floor (Kegel) exercise.

16. Implement bladder training program.

17. Restrict coffee and other diuretic-type beverages.

Outcomes

1. Demonstrates understanding of condition and treatment

2. Establishes pattern of urination

3. Alters environment to accommodate individual needs

4. Shows no signs of complication from incontinence (e.g., falls, skin breakdown, etc.)

5. Shows no evidence of embarrassment or isolation due to incontinence

Endocrine System

Description

There is little decrease in hormone secretion in aging, with the exception of estrogen and testosterone. The most common disorders associated with the endocrine system are thyroid dysfunctions and diabetes mellitus.

The thyroid gland is a butterfly-shaped gland located in the neck anterior to the trachea. The thyroid gland produces thyroxine (T_4) and triiodothyronine (T_3). The three most important conditions of the thyroid are hypothyroidism, hyperthyroidism, and nodules. The signs and symptoms of these disorders may not be typical in the older adult and may go undiagnosed and untreated.

Hypothyroid: The most common symptoms of hypothyroidism in the older adult may be attributed to normal aging changes and thus go undiagnosed. Among these symptoms are fatigue, loss of initiative, depression, myalgia, constipation, and dry skin. In addition, some frail older adults may develop mental confusion, anorexia, weight loss, decreased mobility, falling, incontinence, and arthralgia.

Hyperthyroid: Hyperthyroidism in the elderly may go undiagnosed because the symptoms are vastly different than in the younger population. Common atypical presentations in the elderly are weakness and apathy, weight loss, congestive heart failure with atrial fibrillation, angina, bowel disturbance such as diarrhea or constipation, dyspepsia, abdominal distress, mental confusion and depression.

Assessment

1. History
   A. Complaints of fatigue, weight loss, confusion, decreased mobility or falls, constipation, incontinence, intolerance to cold or heat, puffiness of the eyes
2. Diagnostic tests and methods
   A. Vital signs
   B. Palpation of the thyroid gland
   C. T_3, T_4, free T_4 index, and thyroid-stimulating hormone
   D. Thyroid scan
3. Psychosocial and cultural assessment
   A. Depression, loss of motivation, apathy
   B. Confusion, disorientation, mental and physical slowing

Planning

Client Needs

1. Safe, effective care environment
   A. Prevent injury or other complications.
   B. Return to optimal level of functioning.
   C. Maintain thyroid levels within normal range: T_3 = 90–130 ng/dL, T_4 = 5–13.5 mg/dL, free T_4 = 0.8–3.3 ng/dL, thyroid-stimulating hormone = 0–15 μIU/mL.
2. Health promotion and maintenance
   A. Increase client's knowledge of normal aging and pathological manifestations of thyroid disorders.
   B. Encourage early detection, referral, and treatment.
   C. Increase client's knowledge of medications and their side effects.
3. Psychosocial integrity
   A. Promote positive self-concept and body image.
   B. Relieve depression and mental confusion.
   C. Encourage use of support systems and resources.
4. Physiological integrity
   A. Monitor thyroid function.

Implementation

1. Assess for atypical signs and symptoms.
2. Promote referral and treatment.
3. Encourage adherence to the medical regimen.
4. Instruct regarding medication actions and side effects.
5. Monitor thyroid levels.
6. Teach stress reduction techniques such as relaxation therapy.
7. Monitor for cardiovascular functions and other complications of treatment.
8. Allow client to verbalize feelings regarding body image, sexuality, and lifestyle changes.

Outcomes

1. Verbalizes typical and atypical signs and symptoms of thyroid disorders
2. Adheres to the medication and other medical regimens
3. Shows no signs of injury or other complications
4. Maintains skin integrity
5. Maintains adequate nutrition and hydration
6. Maintains lab values within normal range
7. Verbalizes feelings and anxieties related to condition
8. Returns to optimal level of functioning
9. Uses community and family support

Diabetes Mellitus

Description

Diabetes increases in frequency in the older adult group. Some diabetes specialists suggest that high results of glucose tolerance tests in older adults should be considered normal and that treatment should be initiated only when plasma glucose levels are elevated as much as 10 mg/dL per decade after age 50. Diabetes has two components: a metabolic and a vascular component. The metabolic component of diabetes is due to absent or diminished insulin secretion and is characterized by hyperglycemia. The vascular component consists of abnormalities of the small and large blood vessels. These vascular abnormalities, diabetic neuropathy, and retinopathy lead to visual defects with blindness, severe renal disease, hypertension, peripheral vascular problems, cerebral vascular accidents, and sexual dysfunction.

Pathophysiology

Insulin is produced by the pancreatic cells in the islets of Langerhans. The actions of insulin are threefold: it provides for glucose storage, it prevents fat breakdown, and it increases protein synthesis. Insulin lowers blood sugar by facilitating its transport into skeletal muscle and adipose tissue. Insulin release is regulated by blood glucose levels, increasing as blood sugar levels rise and decreasing when blood sugar levels decline. The actions of glucagon are diametrically opposed to those of insulin. Glucagon stimulates glycogenolysis and gluconeogenesis, enhances lipolysis in adipose tissue, and increases the breakdown of proteins into amino acids. Theoretically, glucagon secretion is unopposed in the diabetic because of lack of insulin. This leads to increased production of glucose by the liver.

The incidence of diabetes in the older adult is further complicated by poor nutrition, physical inactivity, decreased amounts of lean body mass in which to store ingested carbohydrates, impairment in insulin secretion, and insulin antagonism. There are two forms of diabetes: Type I, or insulin-dependent diabetes mellitus, and Type II, or non–insulin-dependent diabetes mellitus. The latter type comprises 85%–90% of the diabetic population and is the most common form observed in the elderly.

Assessment

1. Medical history
   A. Family history of diabetes
   B. Polyuria, polydipsia, polyphagia (increased hunger)
   C. Complaints of blurred vision or other visual disturbance
   D. Delayed wound healing
   E. Recurrent vaginal or yeast infection
2. Diagnostic tests and methods
   A. Random plasma glucose concentrations $\geq$ 200 mg/dL
   B. Fasting plasma glucose concentrations $\geq$ 124 mg/dL
   C. Plasma glucose concentrations $\geq$ 200 mg/dL 2 hours after oral glucose
3. Psychosocial and cultural assessment
   A. Lifestyle behaviors related to nutritional and dietary intake
   B. Stressors or anxieties
   C. Self-concept and body image
   D. Sexual functioning

Planning

Client Needs

1. Safe, effective care environment
   A. Increase client's knowledge of the need for diet high in carbohydrates and low in fat.
   B. Maintain skin integrity intact.
   C. Prevent infection.
   D. Increase client's knowledge of signs and symptoms of hypoglycemia or hyperglycemia.
   E. Increase client's knowledge of glucometer use and care.
   F. Increase client's knowledge of medical regimen to control diabetes.
2. Health promotion and maintenance
   A. Encourage exercise.
   B. Maintain nutritional status.
   C. Prevent infections.
   D. Encourage foot care.
3. Psychosocial integrity
   A. Establish and maintain optimal exercise program.
   B. Promote positive self-concept and body image.
   C. Maintain community and family activities of daily living.
   D. Maintain minimal stress and anxiety.
   E. Use family and community resources.
4. Physiological integrity
   A. Maintain lab values within normal limits.
   B. Maintain body weight within normal range for height.
   C. Relieve signs and symptoms of congestive heart failure or peripheral vascular disease.
   D. Maintain vital signs within normal limits.
   E. Prevent neuropathy or retinopathy.
   F. Maintain normal sexual functioning.

Implementation

1. Assess feet and skin daily.
2. Monitor for signs and symptoms of infection and other complications.
3. Monitor blood glucose levels.
4. Teach patient how to use the glucometer.
5. Teach proper foot and skin care.
6. Provide education regarding medication actions and side effects.
7. Provide nutritional education and monitor for adherence.
8. Teach exercise regimen appropriate for age and functional status and the need for daily exercise.
9. Teach client signs and symptoms of hypoglycemia and hyperglycemia.
10. Identify community resources.
11. Allow client to verbalize feelings and anxieties regarding body image, sexuality, and lifestyle changes.
12. Encourage communication with family members.
13. Provide mental health, sexual counseling as needed.

Outcomes

1. Shows no signs of infection and maintains intact skin integrity
2. Verbalizes signs and symptoms of hypoglycemia or hyperglycemia and means of controlling
3. Adheres to medical regimen
4. Maintains weight appropriate for height
5. Adheres to dietary intake high in carbohydrates, low in fat
6. Practices a daily exercise program
7. Demonstrates correctly the use of glucometer
8. Maintains plasma glucose levels within normal range
9. Verbalizes satisfaction with sexual performance
10. Verbalizes positive body image and self-concept
11. Communicates openly with family and significant others

Reproductive System

Description

FEMALE

Age-related changes occurring in women include atrophy of the tissues of the external genitalia, decreased elasticity of the vagina wall, and atrophy of the vaginal tissue. The vagina canal shortens, and the vaginal flora become more alkaline in nature. Yeast infections may increase as a result of the change in vaginal flora. In addition, decreased secretion and diminished blood supply may cause discomfort when an older adult is engaged in sexual intercourse. There is also atrophy of the uterus, fallopian tubes, and the ovaries. Dysfunctions most often seen in women include atrophic vaginitis; prolapse of the uterus; and cancer of the uterus, ovary, and breast.

MALE

The male reproductive system is basically unchanged by aging, and reproduction is possible into the ninth decade. The testes decrease in size, and fibrotic changes occur in the tubules and connective tissue. The prostate gland atrophies and stromal connective tissue increases. Blood supply to the prostate also diminishes. Impotence has been associated with sclerotic changes occurring in the arteries and veins of the penis; however, diabetes, prostate surgery, disorders of the vascular or nervous system, and medications can cause the dysfunction.

Assessment

SUBJECTIVE

1. History
   A. Past sexual problems
   B. Conditions that interfere with sexual function
      (1) Arthritis
      (2) Diabetes
      (3) Dementia
      (4) COPD
      (5) Cardiovascular disease
      (6) Surgery to sexual organs
   C. Medication
2. Psychosocial and cultural assessment
   A. Availability of sexual partner
   B. Relationship with spouse or significant other
   C. Feelings of depression, anxiety, or fear

Planning

Client Needs

1. Safe, effective care environment
   A. Encourage verbal expression of sexual concerns.
2. Health promotion and maintenance
   A. Increase client's knowledge related to normal aging changes.
   B. Promote lifestyle changes to enhance physical and mental well-being.
3. Psychosocial integrity
   A. Prevent anxiety related to sexuality.
   B. Increase client's communication related to sexuality.
4. Physiological integrity
   A. Increase client's ability to enjoy and express sexuality.
   B. Increase client's comfort during sexual activity.

Implementation

1. Provide instructions to enhance sexual enjoyment.
2. Teach normal reproductive changes of aging.
3. Encourage open communication between partners.
4. Allow client to verbalize anxiety, fear, or other sexual concerns.

Outcomes

1. Verbalizes sexual needs
2. Verbalizes methods to increase sexual fulfillment
3. Reports increased comfort in sexual activity
4. Reports increased communication with spouse or significant other

Neurological System

Description

There is still much that is unknown about nervous system changes with age. Some experts believe that there is a 10%–12% brain weight decrease due primarily to a progressive loss of neurons. Both gray and white matter are lost. Lipofuscin deposits, neurofibrillary tangles, and neuritic plaques are found increasingly in the cytoplasm of the neurons, brain cells, and brain tissue. In the cerebral cortex, the dendrites shrink, reducing the number of fibers that receive synapses from other cells, resulting in reduced transmitted impulses. Monamine oxidase (MAO) and serotonin increase in the brain, platelets, and blood plasma, while norepinephrine decreases. The increase in MAO and decreased norepinephrine may contribute to depression. There is a slowing of motor neuron conduction, which accounts for slower reaction time. Age-related changes in the autonomic nervous system interfere with the ability of the hypothalamus to regulate heat production and heat loss. Sleep patterns also change with age. Stages 3 and 4 (deep sleep) are greatly decreased, while frequent awakenings and total awake time are increased. Changes in cognition are not a normal aging change and should be investigated.

Dementia

There are more than 70 conditions that can imitate dementia in the older adult, many of which are reversible. For this reason, a major responsibility of the nurse is to assist in careful assessment and in ruling out reversible and irreversible causes of dementia. Senile dementia of the Alzheimer's type (SDAT) accounts for 66% of irreversible dementias, and cerebral infarctions account for the remainder. Although the etiology of SDAT is unknown, environment, hereditary, and immunologic factors are suspected. Neurofibrillary tangles and senile plagues are found within the brain on autopsy. SDAT has a slow, uncertain onset that progresses until the individual becomes bedridden; death is usually the result of respiratory complications. Three stages are noted in SDAT. Stage 1 is marked by memory loss and slight change in affect. Stage 2 shows progressive memory loss, behavioral changes, and loss of language skills. During stage 3, emaciation, inability to communicate, helplessness, and coma are common.

Assessment

1. History
   A. Onset of problems
   B. History of past or present accidents, trauma, or infections
   C. Family history of neurological disease
   D. Current medications
2. Psychosocial assessment
   A. Depression or substance abuse
   B. Mental status examination
   C. Past mood and affect
   D. Family interaction pattern
3. Diagnostic tests and methods
   A. Electroencephalogram
   B. ECG
   C. CT scan
   D. Magnetic resonance imaging

E. Complete physical examination
  (1) Level of consciousness
  (2) Speech and language
  (3) Gait, balance, and coordination
  (4) Reflexes
  (5) Functional status

Planning

Client Needs

1. Safe, effective care environment
   A. Prevent avoidable injury.
   B. Maintain maximum functioning.
2. Health promotion and maintenance
   A. Promote adequate exercise to maintain functional status.
   B. Help family to verbalize anxiety related to role and responsibility changes.
3. Psychosocial integrity
   A. Prevent anxiety, irritability, and undue confusional states.
   B. Maintain family function.
   C. Provide for diversional activities.
   D. Provide supportive family therapy.
   E. Promote use of community support.
   F. Educate family in regard to condition and care.
4. Physiological integrity
   A. Maintain nutritional and fluid requirements.
   B. Maintain ADL.
   C. Prevent complications such as infections, constipation.
   D. Promote rest and sleep.
   E. Monitor drug therapy.

Implementation

1. Assess present physical, mental, and functional ability and maintain baseline data.
2. Provide a safe, structured environment free from hazards.
3. Attempt to determine reason for wandering behaviors.
4. Monitor weight, nutrition, fluid, sleep, and elimination.
5. Develop exercise program to maximize functional ability.
6. Allow independence in self-care activity with assistance.
7. Maintain consistency in routine and healthcare personnel.
8. Alleviate situations that promote frustration.
9. Provide emotional support for client and family.
10. Keep sensory stimulation to a minimum.
11. Provide for educational support to family.
12. Identify community supports and respite services.
13. Practice reminiscent therapy.
14. Provide total care needs as deemed necessary.

Outcomes

1. Shows no signs of bruises, cuts, or abrasions
2. Evidences appropriate behavior
3. Performs ADL according to ability
4. Demonstrates ability to communicate needs and concerns
5. Family verbalizes knowledge of illness
6. Uses family supports
7. Uses community resources
8. Shows no signs of other complications related to dementia (respiratory, decubitus ulcers, etc.)

Parkinson's Disease

Parkinson's disease is the second most common neurological condition in older adults. It is characterized by tremor, rigidity, akinesia, and gait disturbance.

Assessment

1. History of weakness, tiredness, or fatigue
2. Tremor of hands (pill-rolling), which becomes worse when client is stressed
3. Tremor of feet
4. Rigidity, masked facial expression
5. Stooped posture with shuffling of feet, little swinging of arms
6. Slow, monotone voice
7. Excessive salivation and perspiration, with difficulty swallowing

Planning

Client Needs

1. Safe, effective care environment
   A. Prevent respiratory complications or aspiration.
   B. Prevent fatigue.
   C. Prevent falls or injury related to gait disturbance.
2. Health promotion and maintenance
   A. Encourage client to perform ADL slowly.
   B. Maintain health and safety.
3. Psychosocial integrity
   A. Allow client to verbalize anxiety related to swallowing and gait difficulties.
   B. Encourage attendance at support group meetings.
4. Physiological integrity
   A. Encourage maintenance of ADL with assistance.
   B. Ensure compliance with drug and physical therapy programs.
   C. Teach use of assistive appliances.
   D. Maintain nutritional status.

Implementation

1. Assess environment for safety hazards.
2. Provide information related to assistive devices.
3. Provide knowledge related to drug therapy and side effects of medications.
4. Encourage adherence to exercise program.
5. Provide health teaching to assist in swallowing, nutritional maintenance.
   A. Use of medications 30 minutes prior to eating
   B. Sitting in chair
   C. Use of suction plates and other assistive eating utensils
   D. Outpatient physical or speech therapy
   E. Following a well-balanced, high-fiber diet
6. Provide emotional support for client and family.
7. Assist in identifying community resources and support groups.
8. Pace activities to prevent fatigue.

Outcomes

1. Shows no signs of complications related to gait or swallowing difficulties (falls or aspiration)

2. Maintains weight and nutritional status
3. Exhibits no fatigue when performing ADL
4. Has no side effects from drug therapy
5. Attends support group meetings
6. Verbalizes community resources providing assistance
7. Demonstrates knowledge of disease and disease process

Hemolytic Diseases

Anemia

Description

Anemia is a condition in which an abnormally low number of circulating red blood cells, abnormally low hemoglobin, or both occur. There may be excessive loss or destruction (hemolysis) of red blood cells or deficient red cell production. Anemia is not a disease; it is an indicator of a disease process or alteration in body function. Three manifestations of anemia are: impaired O_2 transport, alteration in red cell structure, and a pathological process.

Pathophysiology

There are few hematological changes related to aging. The mean cell diameter may increase slightly after 50 years of age, but blood volume remains constant. There is some question regarding the reduction of hemoglobin levels as a result of the aging process, but there is little evidence to support this concept. Problems resulting from the hematological system occur as a result of anemia, bleeding disorders, or nutritional deficiencies.

Iron-Deficiency Anemia. Iron-deficiency anemia is one of the most common types of anemia in older adults. Iron-deficiency anemia may be caused by blood loss owing to drugs, ulcers, diverticulosis, vascular ectasia of the cecum and ascending colon, peptic ulcer, or cancer of the GI tract. Poor dietary intake also contributes to iron deficiency. Treatment includes correcting the cause and daily oral administration of replacement iron. Iron may irritate the GI tract and should be given during or after meals. Food high in vitamin C should be given in conjunction with iron supplements to enhance absorption.

Pernicious Anemia, Vitamin B_{12}, and Folate Deficiencies. Pernicious anemia is caused by deficiency in intrinsic factor secreted by the stomach. Without this factor, vitamin B_{12}, which is required for red blood cell maturation in the bone marrow, is not absorbed. Pernicious anemia is manifested by weakness, numbness or tingling in the extremities, anorexia, and weight loss.

Vitamin B_{12} and folate deficiencies may occur on a nutritional basis. Older adults who live alone and alcoholics are most likely to have poor nutrition. Poor dietary intake of fresh fruits and vegetables may lead to folate deficiency. Lack of meat, fish, poultry, eggs, and dairy products in the diet may lead to vitamin B_{12} deficiency.

Treatment of pernicious anemia, vitamin B_{12}, and folate disorders typically consists of cyanocobalamin injections, oral folic acid, and iron supplements. Iron may irritate the GI tract and should be given during or after meals. Food high in vitamin C should be given in conjunction with iron supplements to enhance absorption.

Hemolytic Anemia. Hemolytic anemia is characterized by the premature destruction of red cells. The bone marrow is usually hyperactive, resulting in increased numbers of reticulocytes in the circulating blood. Hemolytic anemia results from defects of the red cell membrane, hemoglobinopathies, and inherited enzyme defects. Acquired forms of hemolytic anemia may be caused by drugs, antibodies, trauma, bacteria, and other toxins. Hemolytic anemia is treated by adrenocorticosteroid hormones, surgical removal of the spleen, or correction of the primary disorder.

Assessment

1. History
   A. Current medications, cardiovascular changes, respiratory changes, bleeding disorders, congestive heart failure, renal insufficiency, chronic GI disorders
   B. Family history of cancer or bleeding disorders
   C. Alcohol intake
   D. History of depression, dementia
2. Nutritional history
   A. Food preferences
   B. Usual dietary habits
   C. Usual dietary intake
   D. Food fads
   E. Decreased taste and smell
   F. Dental and periodontal disease
3. Physical assessment
   A. Vital signs
   B. Pallor, fatigue, weakness, tarry stools, bleeding gums, conjunctivitis, shortness of breath
   C. Skin fold and upper arm circumference measures; weight, height
   D. Functional status
4. Diagnostic tests and methods
   A. Serum iron, total iron-binding capacity, transferring saturation, ferritin, CBC
   B. Upper GI series
   C. CT scan, magnetic resonance imaging
5. Psychosocial and cultural assessment
   A. Isolation, living alone, family support
   B. Socioeconomic status

Planning

Client Needs

1. Safe, effective care environment
   A. Monitor for early detection of fatigue, cardiovascular and respiratory abnormalities.
   B. Prevent injury, falls.
   C. Monitor for early detection of bleeding.
   D. Restore optimal physical and psychosocial functioning.
2. Health promotion and maintenance
   A. Encourage nutritious diet including iron.
   B. Advise client to decrease alcohol intake.
3. Psychosocial integrity
   A. Encourage optimal social interaction.
   B. Identify sources of nutrition problems.
   C. Ensure adequate intake of foods high in vitamins, particularly vitamin B.
   D. Promote abstinence from or minimal intake of alcohol.
   E. Encourage optimal interaction with friends and family.

4. Physiological integrity
    A. Regain and maintain optimal weight for height and age.
    B. Maintain vital signs within normal limits.
    C. Maintain functional status.
    D. Maintain optimal dentition.
    E. Restore and maintain blood levels within normal limits.

Implementation

1. Assess and monitor for presence of bleeding.
2. Assess and monitor all food intake.
3. Assess gums and teeth for proper dentition.
4. Assess and monitor cardiovascular and respiratory function.
5. Provide opportunities to verbalize thoughts, feelings, fears, concerns.
6. Monitor lab reports.
7. Explain all procedures.
8. Identify community and social resources.
9. Provide nutritional education.

Outcomes

1. Maintains weight and nutritional status
2. Maintains hematology lab values within normal range
3. Reports no black, tarry stools
4. Shows no signs of fatigue, dyspnea, or cardiovascular dysfunction
5. Shows no signs of lesions, cuts, bruises
6. Verbalizes dietary intake of low-calorie, high-vitamin foods
7. Uses community resources
8. Reports no stress, anxiety, or fear
9. Maintains optimal family relationships

Sensory Changes

VISUAL

Presbyopia

Presbyopia is rigidity and loss of elasticity to the crystalline lens and decrease in ciliary muscle prevent the accommodation for near vision. Diagnosis can be made during eye examination and glasses usually correct the problem.

Cataracts

Description

Senile cataracts are the most common cause of adult blindness. Clouding or opacity of the crystalline lens is due to changes in lens protein, which causes swelling within the lens capsule. Clouding of the lens results in blurred vision and also causes light rays to scatter, producing a glare. Cataracts are visible in dark pupils. Diagnosis is made by fundoscopic eye examination, and the problem is corrected surgically.

Assessment

1. History
    A. Complaints of intolerance to glare
    B. Complaints of yellow halos around lights
    C. Complaints of double vision
    D. Progressive loss of vision not corrected with prescription change
2. Ophthalmic examination
    A. Observation of lens opacity in the red reflex of the retina and choroid with pupil dilation and use of a 110 diopter lens. Lens opacity shows as a black area.
3. Psychosocial and cultural assessment
    A. Changes in ADL
    B. Changes in social interaction patterns
    C. Support systems
    D. Environmental assessment for safety—elevation or changes in floor level, lighting, color contrast to walls and entryways

Planning

Client Needs

1. Safe, effective care environment
    A. Increase client's awareness of visual impairment and ways to correct.
2. Health promotion and maintenance
    A. Maintain a safe environment.
    B. Advise client to avoid driving at night.
3. Psychosocial integrity
    A. Encourage verbalization of anxieties and fears concerning vision loss or surgical intervention.
    B. Encourage continued engagement in the community and social activities.
4. Physiological integrity
    A. Prevent accident or injury.
    B. Prevent complications or discomfort.
    C. Restore to optimal level of functioning.

Implementation

1. Assess visual acuity and visual fields bilaterally, and report deficits.
2. Refer for professional eye examination.
3. Encourage to wear glasses or corrective lens.
4. Use bright contrasting colors in the environment.
5. Provide for adequate light to read and perform ADL.
6. Provide large-print reading materials, books, calendars, and clocks.
7. Allow time to adapt from dark to light and light to dark environments.
8. Place call light and personal items within reach.
9. Encourage involvement in performing activities of daily living.
10. Monitor for inflammation or other complications after cataract repair.
11. Encourage social interaction.

Outcomes

1. Verbalizes knowledge of sensory changes and appropriate resources to correct these
2. Makes informed decision regarding surgical intervention
3. Shows no signs of injury, inflammation, or other postoperative complications
4. Demonstrates appropriate compensatory mechanisms for visual impairment

5. Uses adaptive equipment as prescribed
6. Maintains hobbies, interests, and social activities
7. Uses community or social support systems

Hearing

Presbycusis

Presbycusis is a sensorineural loss of hearing, particularly of consonant, high-pitched sounds. Hearing loss may be gradual, and the older adult adapts by reading lips or cupping the less affected ear. Diagnosis is made from a hearing examination. Implants, surgery, or assistive hearing devices may correct or improve the problem. The nursing goal is aimed at preventing social isolation and increasing self-esteem and social interaction.

QUESTIONS
Ola Burns Allen, RNC, DNSc

1. A 79-year-old woman has been diagnosed with osteoarthritis. She has been active in the community and is otherwise in good health. The physician recommends a hip replacement, and after much consideration, the client agrees. In the preoperative teaching, the nurse instructs the client that the physician will most likely begin ambulation on the 3rd postoperative day. The rationale for early ambulation following joint replacement is:

   A. Prolonged inactivity in an older adult increases the chance of venous thrombosis.
   B. Prolonged bed rest increases the chance of developing decubitus ulcers.
   C. Late ambulation fosters dependence on the nursing staff.
   D. Early ambulation ensures that the client will return to the baseline functional status.

2. A 79-year-old woman who has undergone hip replacement begins physical therapy for the first time on the 3rd postoperative day. Although she has been resting for 45 minutes after the active physical therapy session, she continues to have an elevated blood pressure (162/92) and pulse rate (94). The nurse's most appropriate nursing action would be to:

   A. Do nothing and reevaluate her in an hour
   B. Order a stat ECG
   C. Call the physician
   D. Call physical therapy and see if an error was made in therapy

3. The physician writes an order to change the operative site dressing of a hip replacement client 4 days postoperatively. In preparing to change the dressing, the nurse knows that the most important nursing action is:

   A. The need to prevent pain
   B. The need to prevent infection
   C. The need to be supportive
   D. The need to explain the procedure to the client

4. A post–hip replacement client successfully completes the physical therapy program and is scheduled to be discharged soon. The nurse begins discharge teaching. The *most* important area to assess before discharge is:

   A. The ability to take medications as prescribed
   B. The ability to manage ADL
   C. Support from family and friends
   D. The ability to properly use the ambulatory aid (walker)

5. When assisting an older adult with her meal choices, the nurse would help the client choose:

   A. Broiled pork chop, green peas, and cantaloupe
   B. Boiled ham, spinach, and banana
   C. Beef liver, carrots, and orange slices
   D. Fried chicken, rice, and strawberries

6. When assessing a 75-year-old client, the nurse would recognize that normal age-related changes in vision could result in:

   A. Difficulty in nighttime driving
   B. Seeing halos around lights
   C. Inability to see a dark color against a yellow wall
   D. Ignoring objects placed in the center of the visual field

7. A nurse's friend asks for advice concerning her 75-year-old grandmother. She states, "Grandmother goes to bed at 9 PM, but I can hear her walking around the house and preparing snacks in the kitchen at 4 AM." She asks for advice on how to help her grandmother. The nurse's best response based on nursing knowledge of the older adult would be:

   A. "Give your grandmother a protein-rich snack immediately before going to bed."
   B. Obtain a comprehensive physical and mental examination to determine the cause of insomnia.
   C. "Give her a glass of warm milk and a sleeping pill at bedtime."
   D. "Do nothing unless it worries your grandmother."

8. A general rule of thumb for nurses to remember when administering medications to an older adult is:

   A. Except for cardiac drugs, some medications should be prescribed in greater amounts.
   B. Drugs are less effective in the older adult and must be given more frequently.
   C. Most medications do more harm than good.
   D. Most medications should be given in lower dosages.

9. An 87-year-old man attends a community health center during the week and receives a health screening monthly. He relates to the nurse during the health screening that he has recently been troubled with impotence. The most appropriate nursing action at this time is to:

   A. Listen and respond empathetically
   B. Do nothing as this is normal
   C. Do a complete health history, including medications
   D. Refer him to a physician

10. An 87-year-old male client complains of abdominal cramping shortly before lunch. The nurse questions him to obtain data related to the abdominal pain and then palpates the abdomen for constipation. The action by the nurse was:

   A. Appropriate because constipation is a common problem for older adults
   B. Inappropriate because palpation in the GI assessment is performed following percussion
   C. Inappropriate because the client did not complain of constipation
   D. Appropriate because abdominal pain is the first symptom of constipation

11. The nurse refers an 87-year-old male client to his physician because she fears that he has an intestinal obstruction. The nurse bases this decision on the following assessment data:

    A. Abdominal cramps and high-pitched bowel sounds
    B. Diffuse pain with low-grade fever
    C. Absence of bowel sounds with hyperactivity
    D. Nausea with marked abdominal tenderness

12. An 87-year-old male client is admitted to the hospital with a diagnosis of intestinal obstruction, and initial laboratory tests and x-rays are ordered. The nurse notices that he has urinary incontinence. The most likely reason for his incontinence is:

    A. Frequency due to normal aging changes
    B. Inability to get to the bathroom in time
    C. Stress related to all the treatments during hospitalization
    D. Pressure from the intestinal obstruction

13. The nursing action most appropriate in assisting an 87-year-old male client who is incontinent of urine at night to remain dry would be to:

    A. Place an absorbent garment, such as Depends, on him
    B. Provide him with a bedside commode and leave the night light on
    C. Talk to him to determine the stressors in his life
    D. Insert a Foley catheter

14. An 87-year-old male client has surgery to relieve intestinal obstruction. He returns to the unit with the following physician's orders: meperidine (Demerol) 50 mg IM q4h prn for pain, diphenhydramine (Benadryl) 25 mg po q hs prn for sleep, and gentamicin 75 mg IM 8 hr. The nurse notes that his creatinine clearance is 70 mL/min. The *most* appropriate action by the nurse should be to:

    A. Give his medicine as scheduled
    B. Do nothing as the values are within the normal limits
    C. Hold the gentamicin and inform the physician of the creatinine results
    D. Call the lab to see if this is in error

15. A client has been in a nursing home for 2 weeks. She seems to be having more difficulty hearing a conversation, and conversations must be repeated several times before she can hear them. The admission nursing history indicates the client was able to hear a watch ticking. Her medications include carbamazepine (Tegretol) 300 mg twice daily and aspirin 325 mg once daily. The initial nursing action by the nurse should be to:

    A. Talk louder so that she can hear
    B. Inspect the ear canals for blockage
    C. Sit facing her so she can more effectively lip read
    D. Call the physician as this is related to CVA

16. A 68-year-old female client is scheduled to receive carbamazepine at 9 AM. In checking the lab reports, the nurse notes her carbamazepine level to be 8 mg/mL. The action by the nurse should be to:

    A. Administer the carbamazepine as prescribed
    B. Call the physician before administering the carbamazepine

    C. Give a reduced dose of carbamazepine
    D. Withhold the carbamazepine until level returns to 3 mg/mL

17. In planning priority nursing care for a 78-year-old client with a CVA, the nurse is aware that clients with left hemispheric infarctions may have:

    A. Dramatic mood swings
    B. Impaired judgment
    C. Labile affect
    D. Aggressive potential

18. The nurse correctly identifies that the most important need at this time for a client who has had a recent CVA involving the left hemisphere is:

    A. Maintenance of nutritional status
    B. Need for diversional activities
    C. Prevention from injury
    D. Need for psychological counseling

19. Which nursing plan *best* demonstrates the nurse's knowledge of caring for CVA clients?

    A. Allow clients to make decisions about their care.
    B. Provide clients with clock and calendar to maintain orientation.
    C. Encourage clients to attend unit functions.
    D. Provide a structured, consistent environment.

20. A post–CVA client becomes very apathetic and frequently refuses to attend scheduled therapies. The *most* important action by the nurse at this time is to:

    A. Assess the client for depression
    B. Do nothing as this is normal
    C. Ask the client's family to make her attend therapy
    D. Call the physician and request assistance

21. A post–CVA client is discharged but will continue with physical and speech therapy daily. Which statement by the family *best* demonstrates a supportive environment?

    A. "I just don't know if we can manage mother at home."
    B. "We have placed rails in the tub and widened the bathroom doors for the wheelchair."
    C. "We have a sitter who will be staying with mother at night."
    D. "Mother will be back to her old self in no time once we get her home."

22. A 71-year-old client is admitted to the hospital for observation following a fall from a ladder. Vital signs on admission are: BP 170/98; P 92; respirations 22. In performing morning care for the client, the nurse notes a brown pigmentation around both ankles. The nurse correctly identifies this as suggestive of:

    A. Earlier abuse
    B. Aging skin change
    C. Lymphatic disease
    D. Venous insufficiency

23. A 71-year-old man who has fallen from a ladder becomes extremely anxious when the physician tells him

he wants to perform additional tests. The *most* appropriate action by the nurse at this time is to:

A. Leave the room until his anxiety decreases
B. Maintain a calm voice and encourage him to verbalize his feelings
C. Tell him there is nothing to worry about
D. Praise his physician and tell him the physician knows best

24. Following surgery to relieve intestinal obstruction, the nurse recognizes that monitoring the client's creatinine clearance is important because it is a diagnostic indicator of:

A. Respiratory function
B. Cardiovascular function
C. Renal function
D. GI function

25. A 71-year-old male client is diagnosed with right-sided congestive heart failure. Which assessment by the nurse is most reflective of right-sided congestive heart failure?

A. Tachypnea
B. Pink frothy sputum
C. Korotkoff sounds
D. Distended jugular veins

26. A 71-year-old male client with congestive heart failure is placed on furosemide and digoxin. In addition to monitoring of vital signs, which complaint by the client might alert the nurse to digoxin toxicity?

A. "I have to hold on to the wall to keep from falling."
B. "My ears are ringing."
C. "I can't see clearly and the lights have halos."
D. "I am itching all over."

27. Lab values reported this morning for a client who is on digoxin and furosemide for congestive heart failure include serum digoxin level 2.9 mg/mL and potassium 3.2 mEq/L. The *most* appropriate nursing action based on these lab values is to:

A. Give an additional dose of digoxin
B. Do nothing as the digoxin level is within normal limits
C. Give one half the usual dose of digoxin
D. Call the physician and inform him or her of the lab values

28. In addition to potassium supplements ordered by the physician, the nurse would encourage the client to choose which of the following menu items to increase potassium intake?

A. Boiled chicken, baked potato, dried figs
B. Beef tips, rice, banana
C. Roast beef, carrots, fresh peach
D. Fried chicken, broccoli, fresh pear

29. The nursing diagnosis identified for a 68-year-old client is hypokalemia. The nurse should assess the client for which symptoms?

A. Muscle weakness and weak, irregular pulse
B. Diminished deep tendon reflexes
C. Positive Trousseau's sign
D. Positive Chvostek's sign

30. A client's potassium level drops to 2.7 mEg/L. The physician orders potassium bicarbonate 80 mEg in 1000 mL of D_5W over 8 hours. The *most* important nursing action related to IV potassium administration includes monitoring:

A. Respiratory rate
B. Urinary output
C. Oral potassium intake
D. The IV site for edema

31. A client recovers from congestive heart failure and is discharged home. His medications on discharge are KCl (K-Dur) 20 mEq once daily, bumetanide (Bumex) 1 mg once daily. The nurse prepares to teach the client about his medications and has prepared several handouts with pertinent information that he will need to know about each drug. Before beginning discharge teaching, the nurse needs to be aware of:

A. His attitude toward illness
B. His educational level
C. His past compliance with medical regimen
D. His usual pattern of ADL

32. The nurse recognizes the need to evaluate a client's understanding of his medications, which include KCl and bumetanide. Which response by the client *best* demonstrates this knowledge?

A. "I will take K-Dur with my meals."
B. "I will call the doctor immediately if I get a headache."
C. "I will have my cholesterol level checked every 3 months."
D. "I will take Bumex shortly before bedtime."

33. A client visits the physician for a checkup. Which complaint is *most* likely to be associated with an adverse reaction to KCl?

A. "I have had a headache for the past 2 days."
B. "I have trouble remembering things lately."
C. "I noticed my stools were dark and tarry this morning."
D. "I have trouble seeing things up close lately."

34. An 83-year-old female client is admitted to the hospital to determine the cause of her increasing memory loss, irritability, and decreasing interest in the family. Her son reports these symptoms have been present for about 2 years but are slowly getting worse. The nurse explains to the son that normal aging changes of brain tissue include:

A. Increased concentration of acetylcholine
B. Increase gray and white matter
C. Lipofuscin deposits and neurofibrillary tangles
D. Increased MAO

35. The *most* appropriate plan of care for the Alzheimer's client who has difficulty eating is to:

A. Eliminate distractions from the environment
B. Place client in the dining room for meals
C. Offer a variety of nourishing foods and allow him to select
D. Serve hot foods to stimulate appetite

36. The nursing assistant asks the nurse how to get a client with Alzheimer's involved in personal hygiene. The nurse correctly informs the nursing assistant to:

    A. Have her follow the hospital procedure for bathing
    B. Give her short, specific instructions for what to do next
    C. Provide step-by-step written directions
    D. Explain ahead of time what she is expected to do

37. The nursing assistant reports that an 83-year-old client with Alzheimer's has been found incontinent twice this morning. To assist the client to remain continent, the nurse should:

    A. Limit fluid intake to within 1000 mL daily
    B. Insert an indwelling catheter
    C. Set up a toileting schedule based on usual voiding pattern
    D. Label the bathroom door and show the bathroom to her

38. The *most* appropriate nursing action to ensure that an 83-year-old client with Alzheimer's is receiving adequate nutrition is to:

    A. Weigh the client weekly
    B. Have the staff feed her
    C. Offer high-protein liquids between meals
    D. Provide several menus and allow the client to select

39. A client with Alzheimer's is confused during the day, but the confusion becomes much worse at night, and she calls "mama" in a very loud voice. The *most* appropriate nursing action is to:

    A. Restrain her at night
    B. Close the door tightly to keep her from awakening the other clients
    C. Have the physician order a stronger sleeping medication
    D. Leave the lights on in the room

40. The increasing irritability and anxiety experienced by dementia clients during the early evening hours is referred to as:

    A. Agnosia
    B. Apraxia
    C. Sundowner's syndrome
    D. Phase 3 dementia

41. The nurse talks with the son of an Alzheimer's client to help him think of activities that he might engage his mother in when she leaves the hospital. Which response *best* demonstrates the family's understanding of Alzheimer's disease?

    A. "We have a big yard, and she can help us when we rake the leaves."
    B. "She can prepare breakfast during the week for the children."
    C. "She can write notes to all her friends."
    D. "She can walk the dog."

42. A 67-year-old engineer is diagnosed with Parkinson's disease. The nurse recognizes that this disease is:

    A. Normal in persons older than 65 years of age
    B. A neurological disorder

    C. A musculoskeletal disorder
    D. A reversible condition with medical management

43. A 68-year-old client is placed on levodopa-carbidopa therapy for Parkinson's disease. In doing dietary counseling, the nurse correctly instructs the client to avoid:

    A. Caffeine products
    B. Foods high in fats
    C. Foods high in calories
    D. Foods containing vitamin B_6

44. In addition to levodopa-carbidopa, a client also receives digoxin 0.125 mg daily, haloperidol (Haldol) 20 mg hs, and temazepam (Restoril) 25 mg hs. He begins to experience involuntary rhythmic movements of his tongue, face, and extremities. The nurse correctly identifies that these behaviors are the result of:

    A. Levodopa-carbidopa
    B. Digoxin
    C. Tamazepam
    D. Haloperidol

45. A nursing diagnosis related to alteration in nutrition is developed. The plan of care *most* appropriate to assist a client who has Parkinson's disease with a nursing diagnosis of alteration in nutrition is to:

    A. Encourage liquids when chewing
    B. Allow client to feed himself
    C. Place in an upright position for meals
    D. Ask family to bring his favorite foods from home

46. A 76-year-old client who has Parkinson's disease is followed up by a home health nurse. The nurse finds the family willing to learn caregiving tasks, although the wife is the primary caregiver. Which action by the nurse is important in assisting him to remain at home?

    A. Encourage him to perform ADL for himself.
    B. Help him to communicate his needs.
    C. Provide for physical and emotional needs of the caregiver.
    D. Keep him active.

47. A 52-year-old female client regularly attends the center for hypertension. She shares with the nurse the fact that she is concerned about osteoporosis. The nurse informs the client that individuals *most* at risk for osteoporosis are:

    A. Men who have taken steroid therapy
    B. Obese women of Asian or Hispanic origin
    C. Thin, white men
    D. Thin, postmenopausal white women

48. A 50-year-old client's physician prescribes estrogen therapy to decrease the amount of bone loss from osteoporosis. The nurse correctly advises her to:

    A. Take the estrogen with meals
    B. Have a yearly mammogram
    C. Have monthly fasting blood glucose
    D. Monitor blood pressure for hypotension

49. The nurse instructs a 60-year-old female client on the need for calcium for the prevention of osteoporosis. The

client states, "I drink at least three glasses of milk each day." The nurse advises the client:

A. That three glasses of milk does not supply enough calcium
B. To supplement the milk with vitamin C to ensure absorption
C. That dietary intake of calcium is not used by the body
D. To increase daily oral phosphate as well as calcium

50. The nurse further instructs a postmenopausal female client on the preventive measures for osteoporosis. Which statement by the client demonstrates understanding of osteoporosis prevention?

A. "I will include citrus juice in my breakfast menu."
B. "I will begin walking exercises 3–5 times weekly."
C. "I will decrease fat in my diet."
D. "I will start swimming as part of my daily exercise regimen."

51. A 65-year-old female client is diagnosed with presbycusis. The nurse explains to the client that she may have difficulty in:

A. Hearing high-pitched sounds
B. Ambulating without mechanical aids
C. Seeing objects at a distance
D. Distinguishing sweet and sour tastes

52. To assist a client who has presbycusis to remain in his home and add to his feelings of security, the nurse would recommend:

A. Installation of a special chair to facilitate getting into and out of the bathtub
B. Installation of a special telephone that facilitates hearing consonant sounds
C. Installation of antiglare windows
D. Installation of burglar bars on all windows and doors

53. A 60-year-old client complains of blurred vision and difficulty in being outside on sunny days. The nurse identifies this condition to be:

A. Caused by psychotropic drug therapy
B. An excuse to avoid exercise
C. Due to cataracts
D. Caused by diuretic therapy

54. The home health nurse visits a client in her home following discharge from the hospital. The client is found to have several bruises under her right breast. When questioned, she says she does not know what caused the bruises. The *most* appropriate nursing action at this time would be to:

A. Assess the family relationship to rule out abuse
B. Question the family in the client's presence to determine the cause
C. Review the medical record to provide information related to the bruises
D. Do nothing as the client is not concerned

55. A 78-year-old client's daughter discusses her fear that something is wrong with her mother because the mother has recently been short of breath on exertion and has begun sweating. She further states, "If she had chest pain during these episodes, I would think she was having a heart attack." The nurse informs her that MIs in the elderly:

A. May not always be associated with chest pain
B. Seldom occur in the absence of a history of cardiac disease
C. Are always fatal
D. Do not require O_2 therapy

56. The nurse suggests that a 68-year-old female client might have an iron deficiency. On which characteristic exhibited by the client does the nurse base this decision?

A. Paresthesia in the lower extremities
B. Spooning of the nails
C. Gingival hemorrhages
D. Carpopedal spasms

57. A 65-year-old client develops a decubitus ulcer. The nurse identifies this superficial ulcer appearing as a blister as:

A. Stage 1
B. Stage 2
C. Stage 3
D. Stage 4

58. A 70-year-old client has recently been diagnosed with hyperlipidemia. The physician orders niacin 1000 mg daily. In addition to niacin, the client is currently prescribed ASA (aspirin 325 mg), folic acid 1 mg daily, and thiamine 100 mg daily. The client informs the nurse that he is thinking of discontinuing the niacin as he experiences extreme flushing when he takes it. The nurse correctly informs the client to:

A. Avoid direct sunlight as this is a photosensitivity reaction.
B. Inform his physician immediately as this could be life threatening.
C. Take the ASA (aspirin) 30 minutes prior to taking the niacin.
D. Take the niacin in the evening so that he will not be embarrassed by flushing

59. An 80-year-old client tells a home health nurse that her feet are always cold and that she has difficulty sleeping at night because of the pain she experiences in her feet. The nurse recognizes that these signs:

A. Are normal cardiovascular aging changes.
B. Are normal musculoskeletal aging changes.
C. Indicate arterial insufficiency.
D. Indicate venous insufficiency.

60. A 76-year-old client is being prepared for a cholecystostomy (surgical removal of the gall bladder). The client is placed on NPO after midnight. The nurse recognizes that the primary reason NPO is indicated in client receiving general anesthesia for cholecystostomy surgery is:

A. To prevent gastric distention which would lead to poor lung expansion during surgery.
B. To prevent fluid loss during the surgical procedure.
C. To prevent diarrhea following the surgical procedure.

D. To prevent vomiting that would lead to possible aspiration of vomitus during surgery.

61. A 65-year-old client is treated for a rectal polyp by having a polypectomy during a complete colonoscopy. The biopsy report indicated that the polyp was a nonmalignant adenoma. The nurse correctly instructs the client that the key to a good prognosis after adenoma polyp is:

A. Maintenance of a high-fiber, low-fat diet.
B. Maintenance of an adequate bowel program.
C. Maintenance of adequate yearly follow-up.
D. Careful adherence to radiation therapy.

62. A 79-year-old client is admitted to the cardiovascular unit after receiving a demand pacemaker. The nurse recognizes that a demand pacemaker provides:

A. Electrical stimulation to the heart muscle when irregular beats are detected.
B. Electrical stimulation to the heart when the heart rate falls below a prescribed rate.
C. Continuous electrical stimulation to the heart muscle to ensure a predetermined heart rate.
D. Continuous electrical stimulation to the heart muscle when ventricular fibrillation is detected.

63. A client who received a heart pacemaker relates to the nurse that he is apprehensive about discharge because he doesn't fully understand his pacemaker and what to expect once he goes home. The best response by the nurse is:

A. "Tell me what you don't understand about your pacemaker."
B. "Don't worry, I will teach you everything about your pacemaker before you go home."
C. "All people who have pacemakers are concerned at first."
D. "I understand your concern and will provide you with written instructions before you go home."

64. A 76-year-old client is seen by a nurse with complaints of diarrhea, bloody stools, and a recent weight loss of 10 pounds. The nurse collects a stool specimen to be sent to the laboratory for diagnostic purposes. The client tells the nurse that she had a stool test for blood recently and this is being repeated to make sure the results were not false positive. The nurse understands that a false

positive reading for blood in the stool can occur when the client:

A. has a high bilirubin level
B. has taken medication containing iron
C. has failed to add the specimen properly
D. has meat residue in the gastrointestinal tract

65. An 80-year-old client is admitted to the outpatient surgery for cataract repair of the left eye. The nurse reviews the medication orders and finds cyclopentolate hydrochloride (Cyclogy) II gtts OD 30 minutes prior to surgery. The best action for the nurse is:

A. Explain to the client that she will get eye drops prior to surgery.
B. Ensure that all other preoperative orders are completed prior to giving eye drops.
C. Call the physician and clarify the order for cyclopentolate hydrochloride (Cyclogy).
D. Call surgery to determine the time the client is scheduled for surgery.

66. A hospice nurse is providing grief counseling to a family following the death of the client. During counseling one family member says, "I don't know how we will pay our bills. I have no idea of where to start financially." The best response by the nurse is:

A. "Tell me what you mean when you say you don't know where to start financially."
B. "I'll ask the social worker to assist you in paying your bills."
C. "You don't have to be concerned, you will learn how to pay the bills."
D. "You will need a financial advisor, I'll call one to assist you."

67. A home health nurse is teaching a 70-year-old newly diagnosed diabetic about insulin and drug interactions. The nurse correctly informs the client:

A. "There is no drug interaction with insulin and alcohol taken in small amounts."
B. "There is no drug interaction with insulin and Acetaminophen (Tylenol)."
C. "There is no drug interaction with insulin and salicylate preparations (aspirin)."
D. "There is no drug interaction with insulin and thiazide diuretics.

1. **(A)** Client need: health promotion and maintenance; subcategory: prevention and early detection of disease; content area: med/surg

   RATIONALE

   (A) Immobilization or even a relatively sedentary existence favors stasis of blood in the veins and predisposes the elderly client to thrombosis. (B) Although prolonged bed rest does increase the chance of developing decubitus ulcers, this is not the rationale for early ambulation following a hip replacement. (C) There is no evidence to support the statement that late ambulation fosters dependence. (D) Although this is a nursing goal, there is no assurance that early ambulation will return the client to baseline functional status.

2. **(A)** Client need: health promotion and maintenance; subcategory: growth and development through the life span; content area: med/surg

   RATIONALE

   (A) Exercise increases the body's need for O_2 and requires the cardiovascular and respiratory systems to increase the workload to meet this demand. Because of the rigidity of the vessels and the loss of elasticity, the older adult requires a longer time to regain homeostasis. (B) Because of normal aging changes in the cardiovascular and respiratory systems, the older adult requires a longer time to regain homeostasis. The client has no other symptoms associated with increased blood pressure; therefore, this choice is not the most appropriate. (C) Because of normal aging changes in the cardiovascular and respiratory systems, the older adult requires a longer time to regain homeostasis. The client has no other symptoms associated with increased blood pressure; therefore, this choice is not the most appropriate. (D) Because of normal aging changes in the cardiovascular and respiratory systems, the older adult requires a longer time to regain homeostasis. The client has no other symptoms associated with increased blood pressure; therefore, this choice is not the most appropriate.

3. **(B)** Client need: physiological integrity; subcategory: basic care and comfort; content area: med/surg

   RATIONALE

   (A) Pain is not of primary concern at this time because the client is several days postoperative and pain should be diminishing. (B) The skin is the first line of defense in the prevention of infection. The defense is broken owing to an opening from the operative site, and the opening provides a medium for the entry of bacteria. Infection is a primary concern as this could be dangerous to the client. (C) A supportive environment is an important component of care, but its absence is not life threatening. (D) Explanation of procedures is an important component of care, but the failure to explain procedures is not life threatening.

4. **(D)** Client need: health promotion and maintenance; subcategory: prevention and early detection of disease; content area: med/surg

   RATIONALE

   (A) The ability to take medications as prescribed is an important assessment item, but it is not as important as D in relation to safety and prevention of injury when the client is ambulating. (B) The ability to manage ADL is an important assessment item, but it is not as important as D in relation to safety and prevention of injury when the client is ambulating. (C) Support from family and friends is an important assessment item, but it is not as important as D in relation to safety and prevention of injury when the client is ambulating. (D) Prosthetic implants require strict adherence to partial weight bearing for at least 2 months. The older

adult usually begins with a walker to achieve the partial weight bearing and then progresses to a cane. Weight bearing can cause injury to the joint and require hospitalization to repair.

5. **(A)** Client need: health promotion and maintenance; subcategory: growth and development through the life span; content area: med/surg

   RATIONALE

   (A) Diet plans for the elderly should focus on increasing vitamins and minerals and decreasing caloric intake. Broiled pork chop is high in the B vitamins, and the broiling process reduces the fat. Cantaloupe is higher in vitamin C than orange slices or strawberries. (B) Ham is high in sodium, and both spinach and banana are lower in vitamins and minerals, particularly vitamins B and C, both of which the older adult requires. (C) Liver as a menu choice may not be the best selection because many people do not like the taste of liver and, unless prepared properly, it may be difficult for an older adult to chew. Both carrots and orange slices are lower in vitamins B and C, both of which the older adult requires. (D) Fried foods are not recommended for older adults because they increase calories and fats.

6. **(A)** Client need: health promotion and maintenance; subcategory: growth and development through the life span; content area: med/surg

   RATIONALE

   (A) Changes in both the lens and vitreous body result in increased scattering of light in the ocular media, especially at night or in low levels of illumination. Thus, it is not unusual for the older adult to complain of glare from oncoming headlights while driving at night. (B) Seeing halos around lights may represent adverse effects from medications such as digitalis preparations. (C) Inability to see a dark color against a light wall may indicate a serious eye condition. (D) Ignoring an object placed in the center of the visual field may be a result of macular degeneration and is not a normal condition.

7. **(D)** Client need: physiological integrity; subcategory: physiological adaptation; content area: med/surg

   RATIONALE

   (A) A protein-rich snack before bedtime would be filling, but the fullness might interfere with sleep. (B) There is no evidence at this time that a comprehensive physical exam is warranted and, unless the grandmother verbalizes additional complaints, it should not be done. (C) Milk is an effective sedative at bedtime; however, sleeping pills are not recommended for the elderly. (D) Sleep problems are common in older adults, who report spending increased time in bed not sleeping, frequent nocturnal arousals, shortened nocturnal sleep time, and prolonged time falling asleep.

8. **(D)** Client need: safe, effective care environment; subcategory: safety and infection control; content area: med/surg

   RATIONALE

   (A) Greater amounts of medication place the client at high risk for toxicity because of the decreased renal function that is a normal aging change. (B) Administering medications more frequently places the client at high risk for toxicity because of the decreased renal function that is a normal aging change. (C) Medications, when administered properly and individualized to client's needs, are seldom harmful. (D) In clinical practice, the doses of many drugs for the older adult that are excreted primarily by the kidneys are routinely adjusted to compensate for alteration in renal function.

9. **(C)** Client need: psychosocial integrity; subcategory: coping and adaptation; content area: med/surg

RATIONALE

(A) Listening to the client is therapeutic but should follow data collection, which will assist in finding the cause of client's impotence. (B) Impotence is related to physiological or psychological causes and is not a normal aging change. (C) A sexual history, with emphasis on current sexual function, should be part of the general medical evaluation of an older person. When a problem exists, evaluation of drugs being taken, psychological testing, and surgery may be necessary. (D) While the nurse might refer the client to the physician, this would not be done until the nurse has completed assessment data to identify the problem. This data will guide the nurse and client to seek the most effective solution mutually.

10. **(B)** Client need: safe, effective care environment; subcategory: management of care; content area: med/surg

RATIONALE

(A) Constipation is a common experience of older adults, but this question refers to the technique of doing physical examination of the GI system. The technique used by the nurse is inappropriate. (B) Because of the bowel activity that palpation can initiate, the correct assessment technique sequence in the GI examination includes inspection, auscultation, percussion, and lastly, palpation. (C, D) The question refers to the technique used by the nurse in performing physical examination of the GI system. The technique used by the nurse is inappropriate.

11. **(A)** Client need: physiological integrity; subcategory: basic care and comfort; content area: med/surg

RATIONALE

(A) Acute intestinal obstruction is characterized by rapid onset of abdominal cramping, vomiting, and distention. Cramps are associated with high-pitched bowel sounds due to peristalsis. (B) Diffuse pain and low-grade fever are symptoms of appendicitis. (C) Hyperactivity is associated with bowel sounds and is not present in the absence of bowel sounds. (D) Nausea and marked abdominal tenderness are symptoms of cholecystitis. Hyperactivity is noted as bowel sounds and is not present in the absence of bowel sounds.

12. **(B)** Client need: safe, effective care environment; subcategory: management of care; content area: med/surg

RATIONALE

(A) Incontinence is caused by neurological or muscular impairments and is not a normal aging change. (B) Functional incontinence is observed in clients with normal bladder and urethral function. Too often, the diagnosis of functional incontinence is made inappropriately when the real problem is due to the client's restricted mobility and failure to get to the bathroom in time. (C) Stress incontinence is the involuntary loss of urine during physical exertion. (D) There is no evidence to suggest that pressure is causing the incontinence.

13. **(B)** Client need: safe, effective care environment; subcategory: management of care; content area: med/surg

RATIONALE

(A) Absorbent pads do assist in keeping the client dry, but are demoralizing to the client and should not be used unless other approaches prove unsatisfactory. (B) Because the client is incontinent only at night, the use of toilet aids such as a bedside commode, urinal, or bedpan can assist the client in remaining continent. The use of a night light assists the client to orient himself to a new environment more quickly and reduces the chance of accidents. (C) Stress is not known to cause incontinence at night. (D) A Foley catheter allows for the introduction of bacteria and predisposes the client to urinary tract infection.

14. **(C)** Client need: safe, effective care environment; subcategory: safety and infection control; content area: med/surg

RATIONALE

(A, C) Gentamicin is excreted by the kidneys. For men, normal creatinine clearance ranges from 85–125 mL/min; values of 70 mL/min indicate decreased renal function. Continuing to give the gentamicin could result in accumulation and untoward pharmacological effects. (B) Normal creatinine clearance ranges from 85–125 mL/min; values of 70 mL/min indicate decreased renal function. (D) Calling the lab to see if this value is in error is an inappropriate answer in regard to safety in medication administration.

15. **(B)** Client need: safe, effective care environment; subcategory: management of care; content area: med/surg

RATIONALE

(A) Talking louder may increase the pitch of the voice, and normal hearing changes affect the hearing of high-pitched noise. (B) Accumulation of cerumen may be rock hard and cause the client to complain of hearing loss and a feeling of fullness in the ear. Obstruction of the external canal is obvious on examination. (C) To sit facing the client so she can lip read is an appropriate nursing action, but because she is having more difficulty hearing than normally since admission, finding the cause is most important. (D) Hearing loss is not associated with CVA.

16. **(A)** Client need: safe, effective care environment; subcategory: safety and infection control; content area: med/surg

RATIONALE

(A) Carbamazepine is slowly and incompletely absorbed from the GI tract. Therapeutic serum levels are between 4 and 12 mg/mL. This level is within the therapeutic range, and the medication should be given as prescribed. (B, C, D) Therapeutic serum levels are between 4 and 12 mg/mL. This level is within the therapeutic range, and there is no reason to call the physician.

17. **(B)** Client need: safe, effective care environment; subcategory: safety and infection control; content area: med/surg

RATIONALE

(A) CVA clients do not have dramatic mood swings; however, safety is the most important need for the client at this time. (B) Clients with left hemispheric infarctions tend to have poor judgment and to overestimate their physical abilities. In addition, they react quickly and impulsively and are at high risk for injury. Because there is the potential for injury, this is a safety need and thus a priority. (C) CVA clients do have labile affect; however, safety is the most important need for the client at this time. (D) Aggression would be individualized and is not necessarily a problem with CVA clients.

18. **(C)** Client need: safe, effective care environment; subcategory: safety and infection control; content area: med/surg

RATIONALE

(A) While it is important to maintain nutritional status, impaired judgment makes safety the most important need for the client at this time. (B) While diversional activity is important, impaired judgment makes safety the most important need for the client at this time. (C) Clients with left hemispheric infarctions have poor judgment, overestimate their physical abilities, and react quickly and impulsively. These behaviors place them at high risk for injury. (D) While psychological counseling may be part of the treatment plan for a client, impaired judgment makes safety the most important need for the client at this time.

19. **(D)** Client need: physiological integrity; subcategory: basic care and comfort; content area: med/surg

RATIONALE

(A) Making decisions about care is important to emotional health, but it does not demonstrate knowledge specific to care of the CVA client. (B) The use of clock and calendar for orientation purposes is important, but there is no evidence that the client is experiencing disorientation. (C) Attending unit functions is important in clients with a social isolation diagnosis, but there is no evidence that suggests the client is socially isolated. (D) Both left and right hemiplegic clients cope better in a structured, consistent environment.

20. **(A)** Client need: psychosocial integrity; subcategory: coping and adaptation; content area: med/surg

RATIONALE

(A) Depression, characterized by apathy and withdrawal, is common following cerebrovascular accidents. (B) Apathy and withdrawal are common following CVA, but with effective nursing intervention, it is possible to restore psychological integrity. (C) Asking the family to make the client attend therapy would not help the client and might further lower her self-esteem. (D) Calling the physician for assistance in this problem does not allow the nurse to be creative in dealing with a challenge and is inappropriate. A team conference would be a more appropriate solution.

21. **(B)** Client need: psychosocial integrity; subcategory: psychosocial adaptation; content area: med/surg

RATIONALE

(A) This response casts doubt on the ability of the family to function and places feelings of burden on the loved one. (B) This response indicates acceptance of the change in the loved one, and changing the environment so that she can function more easily within the home. (C) This response may be supportive but shows no indication of family interaction. (D) This response may indicate unrealistic expectations.

22. **(D)** Client need: physiological integrity; subcategory: physiological adaptation; content area: med/surg

RATIONALE

(A) Brown pigmentation is not a characteristic symptom of earlier elder abuse. (B) Brown pigmentation is not a characteristic skin change in normal aging. (C) Brown pigmentation around the eyes and nose, not the ankles, is characteristic of lymphatic disease. (D) Chronic venous insufficiency is common in the elderly and is evidenced by distended, tortuous veins; hair loss; brown pigmentation around the ankles, cool skin; and pedal edema that worsens during the day.

23. **(B)** Client need: psychosocial integrity; subcategory: coping and adaptation; content area: med/surg

RATIONALE

(A) Leaving the room is only appropriate when the client's anxiety level is escalating quickly and allows the client to regain control. (B) A calm voice will aid in decreasing the client's anxiety level, while encouraging him to verbalize his feelings will assist the nurse in helping him to identify the cause of the anxiety and to find measures to cope more effectively. (C) Telling him there is nothing to worry about is false assurance, which is nontherapeutic. (D) Praising the doctor does little to assist the client in managing the anxiety or finding its source.

24. **(C)** Client need: physiological integrity; subcategory: reduction of risk potential; content area: med/surg

RATIONALE

(A) Creatinine clearance is not an indicator of respiratory function. (B) Creatinine clearance is not an indicator of cardiovascular function. (C) An excellent diagnostic indicator of renal function, the creatinine clearance test determines how efficiently the kidneys are clearing creatinine from the blood. (D) Creatinine clearance is not an indicator of GI function.

25. **(D)** Client need: physiological integrity; subcategory: physiological adaptation; content area: med/surg

RATIONALE

(A) Tachypnea is a symptom of left-sided congestive heart failure. (B) Pink frothy sputum indicates pulmonary edema. (C) Korotkoff sounds are a symptom of left-sided congestive heart failure. (D) Symptoms of right-sided congestive heart failure include orthostatic hypotension, edema, distended jugular veins, liver enlargement, and S_3 gallops.

26. **(C)** Client need: safe, effective care environment; subcategory: management of care; content area: med/surg

RATIONALE

(A) Holding on to the wall may indicate dizziness, which is not a sign of digoxin toxicity in older adults. (B) Ringing of the ears is usually a result of aspirin toxicity, not digoxin toxicity. (C) The clinical manifestations of digitalis toxicity are different in the elderly. GI disturbances, disorientation, agitation, hallucinations, color vision changes such as halos around the light, and changes in behavior are frequently seen. (D) Itching can be an adverse reaction to a medication, but it is not a symptom of digoxin toxicity.

27. **(D)** Client need: physiological integrity; subcategory: pharmacological and parenteral therapies; content area: med/surg

RATIONALE

(A) Normal serum digoxin levels are 0.5–2.0 mg/mL. Giving an additional dose of digoxin is not a nursing decision, and the client could quickly become digoxin toxic. (B) The value given is above normal serum digoxin levels of 0.5–2.0 mg/mL. (C) The value given is above normal serum digoxin levels of 0.5–2.0 mg/mL. Giving one half the dose of digoxin is not a nursing decision, and the client could quickly become digoxin toxic. (D) The value given is above normal serum digoxin level of 0.5–2.0 mg/mL. Hypokalemia further disposes the client to digoxin toxicity, and the physician should be notified.

28. **(A)** Client need: health promotion and maintenance; subcategory: prevention and early detection of disease; content area: med/surg

RATIONALE

(A, B, C) Chicken is higher in potassium than beef. The baked potato and figs are both higher in potassium than any of the other menu selections. (D) Fried foods are inappropriate for the cardiovascular client.

29. **(A)** Client need: physiological integrity; subcategory: reduction of risk potential; content area: med/surg

RATIONALE

(A) Weakness, muscle fatigue, decreased muscle tone, and weak, irregular pulse are early symptoms of hypokalemia. (B) Diminished deep tendon reflexes indicate hypermagnesemia. (C) A positive Trousseau's sign is a symptom of hypocalcemia. (D) A positive Chvostek's sign is a symptom of hypocalcemia.

30. **(B)** Client need: physiological integrity; subcategory: basic care and comfort; content area: med/surg

RATIONALE

(A) Monitoring respiratory rate is important, but it is not critical in providing care to the client. (B) Monitoring urinary output is critical when administering IV potassium because diminished urine flow can rapidly lead to hyperkalemia. (C) Monitoring oral potassium intake is important, but it is not critical at this time. (D) Monitoring the IV site for edema is important, but it is not critical at this time.

31. **(B)** Client need: health promotion and maintenance; subcategory: prevention and early detection of disease; content area: med/surg

RATIONALE

(A) Attitude toward illness is important for the nurse to be aware of, but it is not the key component in preparing handouts and other educational material. (B) Because the nurse has prepared written information regarding the client's medication, these instructions should reflect his educational level. (C) Past compliance with medical regimen is important information, requiring follow-up, but it is not a key component of the teaching plan. (D) Patterns of ADL are not important with regard to daily dosage of medications. A daily dosage schedule allows flexibility in administration.

32. **(A)** Client need: health promotion and maintenance; subcategory: prevention and early detection of disease; content area: med/surg

RATIONALE

(A) KCl should not be taken on an empty stomach because of its potential for gastric irritation. (B) Headache may be important to monitor, but it is not associated with the discharge medications ordered. (C) Cholesterol may be important to monitor, but it is not associated with the discharge medications ordered. (D) Bumetanide is a rapid-acting diuretic and should be taken during waking hours.

33. **(C)** Client need: physiological integrity; subcategory: pharmacological and parenteral therapies; content area: med/surg

RATIONALE

(A) Headaches are not normal occurrences but are not indicative of adverse reactions to KCl. (B) Impairment in cognition is not a normal occurrence, but it is not indicative of adverse reactions to KCl. (C) Tarry stools may indicate gastrointestinal bleeding due to gastric irritation from the KCl and also can represent an adverse reaction to bumetanide. (D) Difficulty seeing things close up (presbyopia) is a normal aging change.

34. **(C)** Client need: health promotion and maintenance; subcategory: growth and development through the life span; content area: med/surg

RATIONALE:

(A) Decreased concentrations of acetylcholine are found normally in the aging brain. (B) There is a decrease in both gray and white matter in the aging brain. (C) Lipofuscin deposits are normal findings in both cardiac and brain tissues of the older adult. Neurofibrillary tangles are formed in the normal aging brain, but in Alzheimer's disease, there is increased accumulation of both lipofuscin deposits and neurofibrillary tangles. (D) Increased MAO is indicative of depression.

35. **(A)** Client need: safe, effective care environment; subcategory: management of care; content area: med/surg

RATIONALE

(A) A quiet environment with no more than one or two people is necessary to reduce distraction and allow the client to complete a task. (B) The dining room will be filled with distractions, which will further increase the client's frustration and irritability. (C) Offering a choice of food items may produce frustration as the client may be unable to make decisions. (D) Hot foods may produce a burn if dropped or thrown.

36. **(B)** Client need: psychosocial integrity; subcategory: coping and adaptation; content area: med/surg

RATIONALE

(A) Following hospital procedure for bathing is appropriate for nursing staff to remember, but it does little to get the client involved in personal hygiene. (B) Giving the client short, specific instructions of what to do allows the client to process the information and aids her in following directions. (C) Step-by-step written instructions may be difficult for the client to comprehend and may produce frustration. (D) Explaining what is expected ahead of time requires increased cognitive ability and will not assist to get the client involved in personal hygiene.

37. **(C)** Client need: safe, effective care environment; subcategory: safety and infection control; content area: med/surg

RATIONALE

(A) Limiting fluids to 1000 mL daily could cause the client to be at risk for electrolyte imbalance, dehydration, and infections. (B) An indwelling catheter provides a medium for urinary tract infections and is inappropriate for incontinence associated with dementia. (C) A regular schedule of toileting provides an environment that decreases anxiety and frustration. (D) While labeling the door may help the client to find the bathroom, there is no assurance that this will increase continence.

38. **(A)** Client need: physiological integrity; subcategory: reduction of risk potential; content area: med/surg

RATIONALE

(A) Weighing the client weekly will provide data that best indicate whether the client is receiving adequate nutrition. (B) Having the staff feed her decreases the ability of the client to perform self-care. While this may be easier than allowing the client to feed herself, it will not provide a means by which nutritional status can be consistently measured. (C) Selection of a menu requires cognitive ability and may increase the client's frustration. (D) Providing high-protein liquids is an appropriate nursing action, but it will not provide a means by which nutritional status can be consistently measured.

39. **(D)** Client need: physiological integrity; subcategory: basic care and comfort; content area: med/surg

RATIONALE

(A) The use of restraints is not recommended for dementia clients because complications such as increased confusion and injury are attributed to restraints. (B) Closing the door may help the other clients to rest, but it does little to help the client and may increase agitation as she tries to gain orientation in an unfamiliar environment. (C) Strong medications for sleep are not recommended for dementia clients because complications such as increased confusion and injury are attributed to strong medications. (D) Leaving the lights on assists the client to gain orientation to the environment, and research suggests that light decreases irritability, which is often seen in the later evening hours.

40. **(C)** Client need: psychosocial integrity; subcategory: psychosocial adaptation; content area: med/surg

RATIONALE

(A) Agnosia is a disturbance in the recognition of objects. (B) Apraxia is the inability to carry out a learned movement voluntarily. (C) Sundowner's syndrome is a condition seen in dementia clients in the early evening hours and is characterized by insomnia, restlessness, agitation, wandering, and increased confusion. (D) Irritability is not seen in phase 3 dementia. This phase is characterized by emaciation, and the client is often bedridden.

41. **(A)** Client need: health promotion and maintenance; subcategory: prevention and early detection of disease; content area: med/surg

RATIONALE

(A) Raking leaves is a repetitive, nonthreatening activity that allows both exercise and range of motion to the extremities. (B) Cooking might be a dangerous activity, and the client could be burned if cooking utensils are not used appropriately. (C) Writing notes to friends requires cognitive ability and could increase frustration if the client is unable to complete the task. (D) The mother might become lost when walking the dog, even in a familiar neighborhood.

42. **(B)** Client need: physiological integrity; subcategory: physiological adaptation; content area: med/surg

RATIONALE

(A) Parkinson's disease is a progressive, degenerative process of the nerve cells in the extrapyramidal system. Although many persons over the age of 65 are affected, it is not a normal aging change. (B) Parkinson's disease is a progressive, degenerative process of the nerve cells in the extrapyramidal system, which is neurological in nature and irreversible. (C) Although the musculoskeletal system is affected, the cause is neurological. (D) Parkinson's disease is progressive and irreversible.

43. **(D)** Client need: physiological integrity; subcategory: pharmacological and parenteral therapies; content area: med/surg

RATIONALE

(A) Caffeine products may not be a therapeutic dietary need in the older adult, but they do not affect the drug therapy. (B) Foods high in fat are not recommended for the older adult, but they do not affect the drug therapy. (C) Foods high in calories are not recommended for the older adult, but they do not affect the drug therapy. (D) Vitamin B_6 promotes the conversion of levodopa to dopamine, thereby inhibiting the effects of levodopa.

44. **(D)** Client need: physiological integrity; subcategory: pharmacological and parenteral therapies; content area: med/surg

RATIONALE

(A) These behaviors are extrapyramidal symptoms and are not the result of levodopa-carbidopa. (B) These behaviors are extrapyramidal symptoms and are not the result of digoxin. (C) These behaviors are extrapyramidal symptoms and are not the result of temazepam. (D) These behaviors are extrapyramidal symptoms and are the result of haloperidol.

45. **(C)** Client need: safe, effective care environment; subcategory: safety and infection control; content area: med/surg

RATIONALE

(A) Adding liquids while the client is chewing might cause the client to aspirate. (B) Allowing the client to feed himself may increase the desire to eat and contribute to psychological well-being, but it does little for the difficulty in swallowing experienced by the Parkinson's disease client. (C) Placing the client in an upright position minimizes facial and pharyngeal muscle rigidity and decreases the possibility of choking on food. (D) Favorite foods brought from home by the family may stimulate the appetite and taste better than institutionally prepared menus, but do little for the difficulty in swallowing experienced by the Parkinson's disease client.

46. **(C)** Client need: psychosocial integrity; subcategory: coping and adaptation; content area: med/surg

RATIONALE

(A) Encouraging the client to perform ADL for himself is important, but it is not the most important action in keeping the client in his home. (B) Finding ways for the client to communicate his needs may decrease some frustration, but communication is not essential for the Alzheimer's client to remain at home. (C) Attending to the physical and emotional needs of the caregiver is the most important nursing intervention in keeping the client at home. Providing for these needs decreases frustration, burnout, and feelings of social isolation, all of which contribute to physical illness of the caregiver and make it necessary to institutionalize the client. (D) Keeping the client active may not be possible as the disease progresses and is not a key factor in his remaining in the home.

47. **(D)** Client need: health promotion and maintenance; subcategory: growth and development through the life span; content area: med/surg

RATIONALE

(A) Men are at lower risk for osteoporosis than are women. Steroid therapy does not interfere with bone processes. (B) Thin white women are more at risk than obese Asian or Hispanic women. (C) Men are at lower risk for osteoporosis than are women. (D) Persons at high risk for osteoporosis are thin, sedentary, white women who are experiencing estrogen loss as a result of menopause.

48. **(B)** Client need: physiological integrity; subcategory: pharmacological and parenteral therapies; content area: med/surg

RATIONALE

(A) There is no evidence of the need to take the drug with meals. (B) It is especially important that women receiving estrogen therapy undergo yearly mammography because estrogen increases the risk of breast cancer. (C) Estrogen has not been associated with glucose tolerance. (D) Estrogen has not been associated with hypotension.

49. **(A)** Client need: physiological integrity; subcategory: reduction of risk potential; content area: med/surg

RATIONALE

(A) Recommended calcium intake for premenopausal women is 1000 mg/day. Each glass of milk contains about 300 mg of calcium. (B) Vitamin D, not vitamin C, is necessary for calcium absorption. (C) Dietary calcium intake is used by the body; however, the average dietary intake of calcium is less than half that recommended. (D) Oral phosphate has not been proved to reduce osteoporosis.

50. **(B)** Client need: health promotion and maintenance; subcategory: prevention and early detection of disease; content area: med/surg

RATIONALE

(A) Including juice or food containing vitamin C in the diet is not a preventive measure for osteoporosis. (B) A regimen of moderate weight-bearing exercise for 45–60 minutes 3–5 times/wk is effective to enhance calcium absorption and prevent osteoporosis. (C) Elimination of fat in the diet is therapeutic but is not effective in the prevention of osteoporosis. (D) Although a good exercise, swimming is not a weight-bearing exercise and is not beneficial to calcium absorption.

51. **(A)** Client need: physiological integrity; subcategory: basic care and comfort; content area: med/surg

RATIONALE

(A) Presbycusis is a bilateral, symmetrical sensorineural hearing loss affecting one's ability to hear very high frequencies. (B) Presbycusis is not difficulty in ambulating without mechanical aids. (C) Inability to see objects at close distance is presbyopia. (D) Although the ability to taste sweet and sour is diminished in the older adult, it is not known as presbycusis.

52. **(B)** Client need: psychosocial integrity; subcategory: coping and adaptation; content area: med/surg

RATIONALE

(A) A special chair to facilitate getting into and out of the bathtub might benefit the client, but there is no evidence that he has need of a special chair at this time. (B) Presbycusis causes difficulty hearing high-pitched consonant sounds such as ch and st. Telephones that facilitate the hearing of these sounds allow persons to remain independent in the home while providing a sense of security by enabling them to call for help and to meet their communication needs. (C) Antiglare devices are necessary for presbyopia, but blinds and other means are less expensive than antiglare windows. (D) Burglar bars may add to feelings of security, but they may also increase the potential for injury if a fire occurs and the client cannot get out quickly.

53. **(C)** Client need: health promotion and maintenance; subcategory: prevention and early detection of disease; content area: med/surg

RATIONALE

(A) Psychotropic drug therapy may cause dizziness but generally is not associated with vision disturbance. (B) There is no evidence to suggest that the client is using visual disturbance as an excuse to avoid exercise. (C) An early symptom of posterior sub-capsular cataracts is the complaint of glare from bright lights during the day or at night; the glare is the result of rays of light being scattered by the opacities. (D) Diuretic therapy may cause dizziness, but it generally is not associated with vision disturbance.

54. **(A)** Client need: psychosocial integrity, subcategory: psychosocial adaptation; content area: med/surg

    RATIONALE

    (A) Assessment of family relationship and communication patterns will provide the nurse with insight into the potential pattern for abuse. (B) When assessing for potential abuse, the client and family members are always questioned separately to pick up discrepancies in what occurred. (C) Review of the medical record is timely and may not provide insight into the present condition. (D) Further assessment is necessary because physical and emotional safety is a primary goal of nursing, and professional accountability calls for immediate action in cases of abuse.

55. **(A)** Client need: physiological integrity; subcategory: physiological adaptation; content area: med/surg

    RATIONALE

    (A) MIs in the elderly may appear as dyspnea, syncope, weakness, vomiting, or confusion, rather than as chest pain. MIs are often silent in the elderly. (B) Generally, a diagnosis of MI may be confirmed with family history or prior history of cardiac disease. (C) MI does not have to be fatal if treatment can be initiated early. (D) Treatment for MI does include the use of O_2, although the amount may be reduced to accommodate for the impaired ventilation system of the older adult.

56. **(B)** Client need: health promotion and maintenance; subcategory: growth and development through the life span; content area: med/surg

    RATIONALE

    (A) Paresthesia in the lower extremities is indicative of vitamin B_{12} deficiency. (B) Spooning of the nails should alert the practitioner to an iron deficiency. (C) Gingival hemorrhage reflects a vitamin C deficiency. (D) Carpopedal spasms indicate a magnesium deficiency.

57. **(B)** Client need: physiological integrity; subcategory: basic care and comfort; content area: med/surg

    RATIONALE

    (A) Stage 1 decubitus is a nonblanching erythema. (B) Stage 2 decubitus appears as a superficial ulcer, which may be a blister, abrasion, or shallow crater. (C) Stage 3 decubitus ulcer formation extends into the deeper subcutaneous tissue. (D) Stage 4 decubitus extends into the deep subcutaneous tissue and ends in full-thickness skin loss.

58. **(C)** Client need: health promotion and maintenance; subcategory: prevention and early detection of disease; content area: med/surg

    RATIONALE

    A) Photosensitivity is not an adverse reaction to niacin. (B) This is a common reaction to niacin and does not warrant immediate medical attention. (C) Taking aspirin 30 minutes prior to taking niacin is recommended to decrease the adverse effects of flushing. (D) Flushing will occur even in the evening hours and there is no indication that embarrassment is an issue.

59. **(C)** Client need: physiological integrity; subcategory: physiological adaptation; content area: med/surg

    RATIONALE

    (A) Pain in the feet and coldness are not normal aging changes but suggest an abnormal cardiovascular occurrence. (B) Pain in the feet and coldness are not normal musculoskeletal aging-

related changes. (C) Arterial insufficiency is characterized by intermittent claudication, pain at rest, and pale, cool extremities. (D) Venous insufficiency is characterized by dull ache, venous stasis with resulting edema, and brown pigmentation around the ankles.

60. **(D)** Client need: safe, effective environment; subcategory: management of care; content area: med/surg

    RATIONALE

    (A) There is no indication that NPO prevents gastric distention during surgery. (B) NPO is restriction of fluids but this does not prevent fluid loss during surgery. (C) NPO is not used to prevent diarrhea following surgery. (D) The primary reason that clients are NPO prior to any surgery is to decrease the chance of vomiting and aspiration.

61. **(B)** Client need: health promotion and maintenance; subcategory: prevention and early detection of disease, content area: med/surg

    RATIONALE

    (A) While a high-fiber, low-fat diet is important, early detection is the key to a good prognosis. (B) Maintenance of an adequate bowel program may be important, but early detection is the key to a good prognosis. (C) The key to a good prognosis is adequate follow-up through a yearly colonoscopy. (D) There is no need for radiation therapy in a nonmalignant adenoma.

62. **(B)** Client need: physiological integrity; subcategory: physiological adaptation; content area: med/surg

    RATIONALE

    (A) A demand pacemaker provides electrical stimulation only when the heart rate falls below a prescribed rate, not when irregular beats are detected. (B) Demand pacemakers function only when the heart rate falls below a prescribed rate. (C) Continuous stimulation of the heart muscle is provided by a fixed-rate pacemaker, not by a demand pacemaker. (D) Same as C.

63. **(A)** Client need: psychosocial integrity; subcategory: coping and adaptation; content area: med/surg

    RATIONALE

    (A) The nurse needs to fully assess what the client's concerns are and this open-ended statement allows verbalization of feelings. (B) Although this response may seem supportive, it minimizes the client's feelings and may decrease the teaching of what the client needs by closing communication. (C) This response minimizes the client's feelings and decreases the change for additional verbalization of real concerns. (D) Same as C.

64. **(D)** Client need: physiological integrity; subcategory: basic care and comfort; content area: med/surg

    RATIONALE

    (A) High bilirubin levels do not influence the detection of blood in feces. (B) Iron medications may cause the feces to be dark but do not cause false-positive readings for blood in the stool. (C) Failure to add a preservative does not lead to false-positive readings for blood in the feces. (D) Meat residue, particularly from rare meat, may lead to false-positive readings for blood in the feces.

65. **(C)** Client need: safe, effective environment; subcategory: management of care; content area: med/surg

    RATIONALE

    (A) While explanation of all pre- and postoperative procedures is important, clarification of the order for eye drops is a priority at this time. (B) There is no indication that all orders should be carried out prior to administering eye drops. (C) Cyclopentolate hydrochloride (cyclogy) paralyzes the ciliary muscle so that there is a decrease in eye movement during surgery. The cataract extraction is scheduled for the left eye and the order is for drops to be instilled into the right eye. The best action is to clarify the site for instillation of drops. (D) The time of surgery may be important to know, but clarification of the doctor's order is a priority.

66. **(A)** Client need: psychosocial integrity; subcategory: coping and adaptation; content area: med/surg

RATIONALE
(A) This allows verbalization to clarify what the client's concerns are. (B) Although a social worker may be needed to assist the client, the nurse must first clarify that the real issue is the financial concern. (C) This response minimizes the client's concerns and restricts communication. (D) This response minimizes the client's concerns and restricts communication.

67. **(B)** Client need: physiological integrity; subcategory: pharmacological and parenteral therapies; content area: med/surg

RATIONALE
(A) Alcohol may antagonize the hypoglycemic effects of insulin. (B) There is no documented evidence of drug interaction with insulin and acetaminophen (Tylenol). (C) Salicylate preparations (aspirin) may antagonize the effects of insulin. (D) Thiazide diuretics may antagonize the effects of insulin.

CHAPTER 7

Psychiatric Nursing: Content Review and Test

Carol Farley-Toombs, MS, RN, CS
Diane B. Hamilton, PhD, RN

Role of the Psychiatric Nurse

1. Agent of change
2. Primary, secondary, and tertiary prevention
3. Independent, dependent, and interdependent functions
4. Psychotherapy intervention to assist individuals, families, and communities
5. Health teaching
6. Collaboration in other healthcare procedures
7. Maintaining a therapeutic environment
8. Formulating nursing care goals, plan, and implementation
9. Evaluation
10. Documentation

Conceptual Modes of Psychiatric Care

Biological Model

The biological model emphasizes the role of genetic and chemical factors. It produces behavioral change through alteration of the central nervous system.
1. Diagnostic inquiry
   A. Assist with medical exam.
   B. Coordinate diagnostic tests, lab studies, x-ray, magnetic resonance imaging, positron emission tomography, etc.
   C. Comprehend diagnostic typology *Diagnostic and Statistical Manual of Mental Disorders (DSM-IV)*.
2. Psychopharmacology
   A. Psychotropic medications relieve physical or behavioral symptoms.
   B. Types
      (1) Antianxiety agents—depress subcortical levels of the central nervous system.

   (2) Antidepressants—work to increase the concentration of norepinephrine and serotonin in the body.
   (3) Antipsychotic (neuroleptics) agents—used in the treatment of acute and chronic psychoses. Exact mechanism of action is unknown.
   (4) Lithium—used in the prevention of manic or depressive episodes associated with bipolar disorder. Alters sodium metabolism in nerve and muscle cells and enhances reuptake of norepinephrine and serotonin in the brain, lowering levels in the body resulting in decreased motor activity.
   (5) Antiparkinsonian agents—used in the treatment of parkinsonian symptoms caused by degenerative, toxic, infective processes or induced by drugs such as some antipsychotic agents.
   (6) Sedative-hypnotic agents—used in the short-term management of various anxiety states and for insomnia.
   C. Nursing role
   (1) Know the actions of psychotropic medications.
   (2) Know the side effects of psychotropic medications.
   (3) Focus on prevention of side effects of drug therapy.
   (4) Report and document side effects.
   (5) Teach the client about the action and side effects of medication.
   (6) Evaluate and document response to medication.
3. Electroconvulsive therapy (ECT)—a series of controlled electrical currents applied to the brain to produce grand mal seizures; given under anesthesia and/or muscle relaxants
   A. Preoperative care—keep NPO, remove dentures, empty bladder.
   B. Obtain informed consent.

C. Give anticholinergic agent (if ordered) prior to ECT to decrease secretions.
D. Assist in starting IV line.
E. Prevent aspiration; suction as needed.
F. Observe for complications of fractures, dislocation.
G. Anticipate client's amnesia, memory impairment.
H. Document recovery.
I. Educate client and family before and after procedure.

Psychoanalytical Model

Early childhood experiences mold personality. Model produces behavioral change through life conflicts.

1. Structural components
   A. Superego, ego, and id
   B. Fixation of libido
   C. Electra and Oedipus complexes
   D. Unconscious, preconscious, conscious
2. Defense mechanisms
   A. Purpose: Defense mechanisms serve as a psychic barrier against anxiety.
      (1) Protect one from feelings of inadequacy
      (2) May be adaptive or maladaptive
      (3) Can distort reality
      (4) Can interfere with interpersonal relationships
      (5) Can limit productivity
      (6) Can promote ego disintegration instead of ego integrity
      (7) Operate on an unconscious level
   B. Types
      (1) **Suppression:** voluntary and intentional exclusion from conscious level of ideas and feelings. For example, a student receives a poor report card and forgets to give it to his parents.
      (2) **Sublimation:** replacement of an unacceptable need, attitude, or emotion with one more acceptable. For example, an adolescent with strong aggressive drive becomes a successful, competitive athlete.
      (3) **Rationalization:** an attempt to make unacceptable feelings and behavior acceptable by using reasonable explanations that may or may not be valid. For example, a student who fails an exam complains that the lectures were disorganized.
      (4) **Identification:** an attempt to change oneself to resemble an admired person by imitating or taking on his or her attributes. For example, a child who dresses like her mother.
      (5) **Introjection:** intense identification in which one incorporates values of another into self. For example, a child scolds her doll for spilling milk.
      (6) **Displacement:** transferring an emotional feeling from one idea, person, or object to another. For example, a frustrated nurse goes home and screams at her cat.
      (7) **Projection:** attributing one's own thoughts or impulses to another. For example, a male physician denies his sexual feelings about a nurse and accuses her of flirting with him.
      (8) **Regression:** retreating to an earlier stage of functioning in order to avoid the tension and demands of a later stage. For example, a 6-year-old girl begins wetting her pants when her new baby sister comes into the family.
      (9) **Repression:** involuntary exclusion from conscious awareness of a painful thought, impulse, or memory. For example, after the loss of a spouse, a man cannot remember his wedding date.
      (10) **Reaction formation:** development of conscious attitudes and behaviors opposite to what one really feels. For example, hostile feelings toward an older parent may be expressed by behaviors that are excessively kind and loving.
      (11) **Intellectualization:** excessive reasoning to avoid feeling. For example, a battered wife who talks about approach-avoidance themes constantly but remains with her husband.
      (12) **Conversion:** expression of intrapsychic conflict through physical symptoms. For example, a student about to leave home for college for the first time develops debilitating headaches.
      (13) **Compensation:** process by which a person makes up for a perceived deficiency. For example, a 5-foot tall neurosurgeon becomes aggressive, forceful, and controlling at work.
      (14) **Denial:** disowning of consciously intolerable thoughts, feelings, or impulses. Dealing with loss often begins by denying the reality of the loss. For example, a terminal client tells her husband the biopsy result was negative.
      (15) **Undoing:** an effort to cancel out certain actions, real or imaginary, through repeated apologies, atonement, or rituals. For example, an adolescent who masturbates may try to undo the behavior by repeated, ritualistic hand washing.
      (16) **Splitting:** viewing people or situations as either all good or all bad. This ego defense mechanism is frequently used by persons experiencing a disruption in self-concept. It reflects the individual's inability to integrate the positive and negative aspects of self.
3. Psychoanalytic therapeutic process
   A. Free association
   B. Dream analysis
   C. Interpretation
   D. Transference
   E. Countertransference
4. Nursing role
   A. Increase or decrease environmental stimuli to promote client interactions.
   B. Protect client.
   C. Enhance the strength of client's personality.
   D. Offer uncritical acceptance.

Behavioral Model

The behavioral model produces behavioral change through a therapeutic approach based on learning and conditioning theories.

1. Structural components
   A. Stimulus
   B. Response
   C. Reinforcement
   D. Behavior as anxiety reducer

2. Behavioral therapeutic process—therapy viewed as an educational process focused on action
   A. Reciprocal inhibition—substitutes a more adaptive behavior for the symptom through learning an alternative means of reducing the anxiety
   B. Desensitization—a process to assist client to cope with anxiety, phobia by gradually exposing the client to a hierarchy of anxiety-producing experiences (low to high) while teaching the client relaxation techniques
   C. Assertiveness training
   D. Aversion therapy
3. Nursing role
   A. Focus on behavior and actions.
   B. Reduce behavior to steps that the client can be taught to master.
   C. Incorporate modeling to demonstrate steps of behavioral change.
   D. Choose positive reinforcement, reinforce immediately, then repeat intermittently.
   E. Avoid punishment or negative reinforcement.

Existential Model

The existential model produces behavioral changes through increased self-awareness and sensitivity to environment.
1. Existential therapeutic process
   A. Emphasizes authentic awareness of being
   B. Emphasizes choices in life
   C. Focuses on genuine presence and on the here and now
   D. Helps client to confront meaning of his or her life
   E. Focuses on encounters and appreciation of self and others
   F. Employs the following therapeutic modalities:
      (1) Rational emotive therapy
      (2) Reality therapy
      (3) Gestalt therapy
2. Nursing role
   A. Serve as a guide.
   B. Develop relationship based on trust, caring, and authenticity.
   C. Emphasize client's responsibility.

Social Model

The social model produces behavioral changes through analysis of social environment's impact on person and his or her life experience.
1. Social therapeutic process
   A. Emphasizes client's responsibility for behavior
   B. Views client as consumer of health care
   C. Avoids labeling
   D. Promotes therapist's participation in community
2. Nursing role
   A. Collaborate with client on treatment.
   B. Strengthen coping mechanisms and social supports.
   C. Provide home visits.
   D. Practices community involvement and consultation.

Interpersonal Model

The interpersonal model produces behavioral changes through alteration of interpersonal relationships.

1. Interpersonal therapeutic process
   A. Emphasizes early life experiences
   B. Emphasizes self-acceptance
   C. Focuses on security and satisfaction sources
   D. Encourages growth, trust, empathy
2. Nursing role
   A. Provide health information.
   B. Assist client to grow, learn, and experience.
   C. Help client to integrate feelings.
   D. Teach client to learn from experiences.

Nursing Model

The nursing model produces behavioral changes through integrative process of modifying biopsychosocial, cultural, and spiritual stressors.
1. Nursing therapeutic process
   A. Fosters nurse-client relationship based on mutuality
   B. Emphasizes client's strengths
   C. Stresses individual client care plan
   D. Includes various psychotherapeutic modalities
   E. Calls for continual assessment and evaluation of interventions
   F. States goals in behavioral terms
   G. Considers the biological, cultural, social, and spiritual needs of the client
   H. Emphasizes growth potentials
   I. Uses North American Nursing Diagnosis Association (NANDA) diagnoses
   J. Enhances the effectiveness of multidisciplinary treatments

Nursing Strategies

Therapeutic Communication

Communication is a shared process of transmitting facts, feelings, and meanings by words, gestures, and actions.
1. Verbal communication
   A. Sender—transmitter of message
   B. Message—verbal or nonverbal meaning
   C. Receiver—recipient of message
   D. Feedback or response—behavior of receiver in relation to message received
   E. Medium—channel or way in which a message is sent
   F. Context—attributes and constraints of physical and psychosocial setting
2. Nonverbal communication
   A. Body language
   B. Proxemics
   C. Territoriality
   D. Neurolinguistics
   E. Kinesthetic
   F. Emblems
   G. Analogical communication—tone, pitch, volume, rate of speech
   H. Metacommunication
3. Communication can be blocked by:
   A. Omission in content of message
   B. Failure to listen
   C. Prejudice, stereotyping

D. Lack of validation
E. Cultural or language barriers
F. Noise
G. Anxiety, fear
H. Using poor, inappropriate, or high-level terminology
I. Incongruent verbal and nonverbal messages
J. Limitation of receivers—therapy, comprehension ability

4. Concepts in therapeutic communication
   A. Client centered
   B. Goal directed
   C. Empathy
   D. Genuineness
   E. Respect
   F. Acceptance
   G. Confidentiality

5. Communication techniques
   A. Facilitating client expression
      (1) Active listening
      (2) Questioning
      (3) Open-ended questions
      (4) Silence
   B. Understanding client expression
      (1) Restating
      (2) Reflecting
      (3) Clarifying
      (4) Validating
   C. Assisting development of self-awareness
      (1) Summarizing
      (2) Focusing
      (3) Confronting
      (4) Connecting behavior to feelings
      (5) Identifying themes
   D. Helping clients to control behavior
      (1) Providing feedback about behavior
      (2) Limit setting
      (3) Positive reinforcement

6. Therapeutic communication methods
   A. Become aware of and monitor own verbal and non-verbal communication patterns. Recognize that one's own cultural and subcultural values and customs influence perception and interpretation of another's behavior.
   B. Select environment that provides privacy, comfort, and minimal distraction.
   C. Allow sufficient time—avoid a hurried approach.
   D. Communicate openness and willingness to trust client and to share a nurse-client relationship.
   E. Demonstrate acceptance of client.
      (1) Remain objective in assessing client's behavior.
      (2) Demonstrate concern, understanding, and respect.
      (3) Remain genuine and nonjudgmental.
   F. Use therapeutic communication techniques.
   G. Operate on facts, not assumptions. Make what is implied explicit.
   H. Focus on strengths of client.
   I. Express empathy by accurately perceiving client's feelings and state of being. Your answers should reflect an awareness and sensitivity to his culture, values, and experiences.
   J. Do not give false reassurance.
   K. Use confrontation appropriately to assist the client to become more fully aware of an aspect of his be-havior or problem. Confrontation should be constructive and should assist the client to grow.
   L. Validate perceptions and interpretations of client's behavior with client or with other professionals.
   M. Use secondary sources of information (e.g., chart, family, physician).

Group Therapy

Collection of individuals (6–12) formed for purposes of psychotherapy (group therapy) or accomplishing interpersonal, cognitive, or behavioral change (therapeutic group).

1. Concepts
   A. Stages of group
      (1) Initial or orientation phase
      (2) Middle or working phase
      (3) Final or termination phase
   B. Group roles
   C. Group content and group process
   D. Therapeutic effects of groups
      (1) Permit information sharing
      (2) Instill hope
      (3) Give sense of universality (client not alone)
      (4) Promote socialization
      (5) Enhance interpersonal skills
      (6) Encourage catharsis
      (7) Provide opportunity for client to help others
      (8) Provide opportunity for corrective re-enactment of original family experience

2. Leadership styles
   A. Autocratic
   B. Democratic
   C. Laissez-faire

3. Types
   A. Task group
   B. Teaching group
   C. Supportive group
   D. Psychodrama

4. Nursing role
   A. Give information about type of group and work of group.
   B. Be knowledgeable about group process and group roles.
   C. Make observations.
   D. Encourage interactive communication.
   E. Teach problem-solving and new skills.

Crisis Intervention Therapy

Brief treatment to help individuals or families reestablish equilibrium. After 6 weeks, a crisis becomes an identified problem.

1. Provide treatment that is immediate, supportive, and directly responsive to immediate crisis.
2. Identify precipitating event and client's perception of event.
3. Identify support systems.
4. Alter environment, give support.
5. Help client to identify options.

Relaxation Therapy

Relaxation therapy involves teaching relaxation exercises to counteract anxiety related to stress-inducing internal or external stimuli. Specific techniques include:

1. Deep-breathing exercises

2. Progressive relaxation
3. Meditation
4. Mental imagery
5. Biofeedback

Family Therapy

Family therapy is a method of addressing human relationship problems through an understanding and interpretation of family dynamics. It is based on the premise that emotional dysfunction of one family member may be evidence of a disruptive family system or of dysfunction in other individuals within the family.

1. Provides interventions that may be supportive, directive, or interpretive
2. May require referral to family therapist

Milieu Therapy

1. Provides a therapeutic environment
2. Capitalizes on client's strengths
3. Sets limits and teaches social skills of orientation, assertion, occupation, and recreation
4. Focuses on action and problem solving
5. Emphasizes involvement
6. Communicates expectations, norms, and standards clearly to clients
7. Requires high staff involvement

Activities Therapy

1. Used as adjunct to psychiatric care
2. Includes music therapy, recreational therapy, pet therapy, art therapy, plant therapy, dance therapy, and occupational therapy

Nursing Interventions for Specific Behaviors

Anger

1. Be aware of own response to anger.
2. Assume a calm manner.
3. Recognize early signs of anger and/or abusive behavior; protect self and others.
4. Assist client to identify anger.
5. Encourage verbal expression.
6. Give permission for angry feelings; set limits on aggressive actions.
7. Decrease environmental stimuli by isolating client from source of anger.
8. Do not escalate client's anger.
9. Explore alternative ways to express anger such as exercise, punching bag, modeling clay.
10. Define the consequences for failure to observe limits.
11. Explore reasons for acting out.
12. Give positive feedback for adherence to limits.
13. Give antianxiety or antipsychotic medication for agitation.
14. Restrain or seclude, if necessary.
15. Act as a role model for constructive management of anger.

Anxiety

1. Identify the feeling and explore situations that create client's anxiety.
   A. Be genuine, caring, and aware of own feelings.
   B. Establish a trusting relationship wherein client can speak freely.
   C. Focus on strengths.
   D. Allow for privacy, and provide a calm environment.
   E. Encourage decision making within limits.
   F. Do not negate client's perceptions of experience.
   G. Use open-ended questions to focus on feelings.
   H. Respond by accurately reflecting client's state of being.
   I. Convey a constructive, interested, caring, and respectful attitude when using confrontation.
   J. Promote clear, consistent, and open communication.
2. Examine client's patterns of coping with anxiety.
3. Help client to learn new methods of coping.
4. Assess client for a pattern of unreasonable self-expectation, fear of failure, self-doubt, and guilt.
5. Examine sources of client's fear.
6. Promote the use of relaxation techniques.
7. Provide for physical exercise.
8. Administer medications that decrease client's discomfort.

Altered Self-Concept

1. Expand client's self-awareness.
2. Focus on meaning of experiences.
3. Facilitate the expression of strong emotion.
4. Encourage self-disclosure.
5. Respond with empathy.
6. Prevent client from isolating self.
7. Reinforce client's positive self-statements.
8. Encourage self-care.
9. Encourage family communication.

Perceptual Alteration

1. Attend to basic physiological needs.
2. Demonstrate accessibility.
3. Assess client need underlying delusions or hallucinations.
4. Avoid arguing about the reality of the delusion or hallucination.
5. Stay with the client; give support and structure.
6. Speak slowly and clearly.
7. Limit choices.
8. Stay alert to client's nonverbal communication.
9. Assign same personnel to give care.
10. Assess potential for self-harm.

Dependence

1. Assess client's limitations, assets.
2. Encourage self-sufficiency; gradually and firmly encourage client to make decisions on his or her own.
3. Avoid rewarding dependent behavior.
4. Initiate activities that allow client to succeed independently.
5. Explore meaning of dependency.
6. Plan regularly scheduled contacts.

7. Share responsibility for treatment planning.
8. Set limits as required in a clear and consistent manner.

Hopelessness, Depression

1. Assess potential for self-harm.
2. Allow client to express feelings.
3. Arrange for circumstances that produce success for client.
4. Attend to physiological integrity, and encourage self-care in ADL.
5. Show client that you expect success.
6. Prevent isolation; encourage activity.
7. Personalize nursing care as a way of indicating the value of the client's preferences.
8. Convey belief in client's recovery; offer hope.
9. Mobilize social support system for the client.

Suspiciousness

1. Be reliable.
2. Plan brief, frequent contacts.
3. Respect the client's need for control of personal space.
4. Attend to physiological needs.
5. Aid the client in modifying his or her negative cognitive set.
6. Be open, honest, and genuine.
7. Provide prescribed medications.

Withdrawal

1. Attend to physiological needs.
2. Be predictable.
3. Respond to client's stated needs.
4. Allow client to set the pace.
5. Limit choices.
6. Communicate expectations clearly.
7. Encourage activities.
8. Provide external controls and safety.

Manipulation

1. Hold client responsible for behavior.
2. Clearly and consistently set limits.
3. Include significant others.
4. Provide structure.
5. Recognize behavior; avoid involvement in intellectualization.
6. Support client's strengths.
7. Clarify and diagnose source of conflicts.

Somatization Behavior

1. Focus on person, not physical symptom.
2. Rule out any physical basis for symptoms.
3. Assist client to identify stressful situations.
4. Encourage relaxation and privacy.
5. Provide structure.
6. Assist client to develop new methods of coping.
7. Mobilize client's resources and support system.
8. Use therapeutic communication.
9. Empathize with client.
10. Teach methods of stress reduction.

Mental Status Assessment

Appearance

1. Age, apparent age
2. Grooming
3. Stature—height and weight
4. Posture—rigid, slumping
5. Health status—skin turgor, skin color, swelling, bruises, condition of hair, diaphoresis, tremor

General Behavior

1. Ability to engage—cooperative, hostile, withdrawn, apathetic, suspicious, compliant, dramatic and histrionic
2. Level of motor activity—agitated, relaxed, fidgety, inability to sit still, psychomotor retarded, nail biting, chain smoking, clenching hands, covering face with hands
3. Level of eye contact—no eye contact, occasional fleeting eye contact, sustained intense eye contact
4. Speech—very rapid, very slow, hesitant, slurred
5. Voice—loud, whisper, high pitched

Affect and Mood

1. Mood is the inner emotional state of the client—sad, angry, enraged, elated, fearful, hopeless, suicidal, homicidal.
2. Affect is the outward expression of mood—tearful, blushing, angry.
   A. Appropriate or inappropriate to thought content
   B. Range—flat, blunted, constricted
   C. Labile, intense

Thought Processes

1. Content of thought—ideas, subject matter. Logical, obsessive, ruminative, phobic.
2. Suicidal, homicidal ideation.
3. Form of thought—organized, coherent, loose, tangential, circumstantial, blocked, dissociated, incoherent.
4. Neologism, rhyming.
5. Confabulation—client fills in details of the past that he cannot recall because of memory loss.
6. Word salad—mixture of words and phrases that have no meaning and are illogical in sequence.
7. Flight of ideas—rapid progression from one thought to another.
8. Echolalia or repetitive imitation of a person's speech.
9. Illusions—misrepresentation of a sensory stimulus.
10. Hallucinations—false sensory perceptions unassociated to real external stimuli; can be associated with any of the five senses.
11. Delusions—false belief maintained despite absence of factual evidence; not consistent with client's intellectual or cultural background.

Cognitive Functions

1. Level of consciousness
2. Orientation to time, place, and person
3. Attention and concentration
4. Memory (recent, remote)

5. Capacity for abstract thought
6. Intellectual function
7. Judgment and insight

Ethical and Legal Issues

Ethical Principles

Ethical principles provide guidance and clarification of intention in decision making.
1. Autonomy—the duty to respect individual's right to make own decisions
2. Beneficence—the duty to promote good for others
3. Nonmaleficence—the duty to do no harm
4. Justice—the duty to treat all people fairly and equally

Clients' Rights

Clients' rights are based on clients' constitutional civil rights. The rights of clients obtaining mental health care are defined by state laws, which vary. Clients' rights involve ethical issues in psychiatric nursing.
1. Client's right to refuse treatment and to be informed of medical and legal consequences (i.e., a legal competency hearing, discharge from hospital)
   A. This right includes right to refuse medications and ECT.
   B. This right may be waived if the client demonstrates an acute danger to self or others that can be ameliorated with medication.
   C. A client can be deemed mentally incompetent to make a decision by a court proceeding in some states and can be treated against his or her will.
2. Client's right to least restrictive treatment
   A. Seclusion and restraints can be used only when less restrictive treatment cannot maintain client safety—when client is imminently in danger of harming self or others.
3. Right to informed consent
4. Right to privacy and confidentiality
5. Right to access to medical record

Nursing Role

1. Be knowledgeable about client's rights.
2. Assist clients to understand their rights.
3. Recognize ethical issues and identify ethical principles involved to guide decision making.
4. Respect client's individuality.
5. Be aware of state mental health laws and institutional policies and procedures in caring for patients in seclusion or restraints.
6. Keep accurate and concise nursing records.
7. Maintain client's confidentiality.
8. Promote the use of least restrictive treatment methods with potentially violent clients by focusing on prevention and early intervention.

Legal Status

The legal status of clients admitted to psychiatric hospitals or units are determined by state laws, which vary. The general categories of admitting status are:

1. Informal voluntary
   A. No formal application needed, similar to admission to medical hospital floors.
   B. Discharge is initiated by the client at any time.
   C. Client retains all civil rights.
2. Formal voluntary
   A. Formal application must be completed by the client or by a parent if the client is younger than 16 years old.
   B. Discharge is initiated by the client, usually by written notice. However, the client may be detained an additional 48 hours to 15 days, depending on state laws, if the psychiatrist deems the client imminently dangerous to self or others if discharged.
   C. Client retains all civil rights.
3. Involuntary
   A. Application is not initiated by the client.
   B. Discharge is initiated by hospital or court, not the client.
   C. Client may retain all, some, or none of his civil rights depending on the state.
   D. Criteria for admission based on client posing clear danger to self or others or on clear need for treatment.
   E. Types
      (1) Emergency—time limited, varies by state. Client is acutely ill and dangerous to self or others.
      (2) Observational—commitment for diagnostic reasons or for short-term therapy without emergency situation.
      (3) Indefinite—formal commitment. Indeterminate time.

Nursing Role

1. Know client's legal status.
2. Assist client to know and understand his or her legal status.
3. Be knowledgeable about hospital and community resources available to client if he or she has questions or concerns about his or her status.

Psychiatric Disorders

Anxiety Disorders

Description

Anxiety disorders are characterized by a generalized fear and/or anxiety that threatens one's physical and emotional integrity for any one or more of the following reasons:
1. Intrapsychic conflict caused by fear of rejection (interpersonal model)
2. Conflict between the id and superego (psychoanalytic model)
3. Interference with a specific goal or behavior (behavioral model)
4. Biological imbalance of neurotransmitters (biological model)
5. Ineffective defense mechanisms
6. Maladaptive coping mechanisms
7. Current traumatic experiences

8. Conflicting cultural messages
9. Chronic feelings of being overwhelmed

Anxiety states may be classified as panic disorders, generalized anxiety disorders, phobias, posttraumatic stress disorders, or obsessive-compulsive disorders. Posttraumatic stress disorders may be acute, chronic, or delayed.

Assessment

PHYSICAL ASSESSMENT

Physical symptoms will vary based on whether anxiety reaction is acute or chronic or whether it is a mild, moderate, severe, or panic attack. Assess for the following clinical manifestations:

1. Increased or decreased heart rate, elevated or decreased blood pressure, chest pain
2. Rapid breathing, vertigo, pain
3. Increased reflexes
4. Perspiration, sweaty palms
5. Headaches, flushed face
6. Nausea, vomiting, anorexia, diarrhea, heartburn
7. Pressure to urinate
8. Chronic fatigue, sleep disturbances
9. Tics, twitching, sneezing, tremors, tight muscles
10. Lump in throat
11. Hot and cold spells
12. Clumsy movements
13. Restlessness, irritability

PSYCHOSOCIAL AND CULTURAL ASSESSMENT

1. Restlessness
2. Aggressive, angry outbursts
3. Depression, withdrawal
4. Anxious, suspicious
5. Lethargic
6. Emotionally labile
7. Critical of self and others, avoidance of people
8. Preoccupied, forgetful, poor judgment
9. Poor concentration
10. Frightening visual images
11. Phobic, fear of losing control
12. Reduced creativity
13. Accident-prone
14. Loss of objectivity
15. Fear of injury or death
16. Inability to effectively accomplish activities of daily living or work
17. Disruption of relationships and activities

Planning

1. Safe, effective care environment
   A. Provide therapeutic nonanxiety-producing environment.
2. Physiological integrity
   A. Reduce or eliminate physiological symptoms.
3. Psychosocial integrity
   A. Demonstrates diminished feelings of anxiety and gains insight into cause of the anxiety.
   B. Demonstrates alternative methods of coping with anxiety.
4. Health promotion and maintenance

A. Resumes activities of daily living (ADL) at baseline level.
B. Resumes work, social, civic activities.

Implementation

1. Establish a trusting relationship.
2. Be aware of own anxiety.
3. Administer anxiolytics, if ordered—benzodiazepines such as lorazepam (Ativan), alprazolam (Xanax), clonazepam (Klonopin).
4. Reassure client of safety, and protect defense mechanisms.
5. Identify nature of anxiety.
6. Assess for accompanying physiological symptomatology.
7. Identify stressors in client's life.
8. Identify client's coping mechanisms.
9. Encourage client's interest in activity outside self.
10. Be supportive of client's self-expression.
11. Encourage client to participate in prescribed treatments.
12. Help client to recognize source of anxiety.
13. Help client to identify and describe underlying feelings.
14. Explore how client reduced anxiety in the past.
15. Promote the relaxation response by instructing client in:
    A. Progressive relaxation
    B. Imaging
    C. Visualization
16. Encourage family members to be supportive of client during treatment and follow-up.
17. Role-play alternative methods of communicating.

Evaluation

1. Recognizes feelings and source of anxiety
2. Remains free of abnormal physiological and psychological symptoms of anxiety
3. Identifies acceptable ways to cope with anxiety
4. Resumes ADL

Phobias and Panic Disorders

Description

A phobia is a persistent fear of an object or situation that presents no actual danger to the person. Examples: **claustrophobia**—fear of closed spaces; **agoraphobia**—fear of open spaces; **social phobia**—fear of scrutiny of others; and **simple phobia**—fear of a specific object or situation. Some causes may be:

1. Displacement of anxiety onto an object or situation, with reinforcement from the environment.
2. Neurochemical imbalance.
3. Family studies show that panic disorders run in families.

Assessment

PHYSICAL ASSESSMENT

1. Physical symptoms are similar to those for anxiety.
2. Nurse should obtain history of hyperthyroidism, hypoglycemia, dietary deficiencies.

PSYCHOSOCIAL AND CULTURAL ASSESSMENT

1. Family history of phobias or panic disorders
2. Low self-esteem

3. Fear of success
4. Avoidance of relationships with family and friends
5. Cumulative stressors in past year
6. Secondary gain from the sick role

Planning

1. Safe, effective care environment
   A. Provide a structured, supportive environment.
   B. Reduce or eliminate anxiety related to phobic situation.
2. Physiological integrity
   A. Reduce or eliminate physiological sequelae.
3. Psychosocial integrity
   A. Decrease disruption of lifestyle due to phobic symptoms.
4. Health promotion and maintenance
   A. Encourage compliance with medical therapy.

Implementation

1. Administer neuroleptic or anxiolytic agents, if ordered (e.g., benzodiazepines or antidepressants).
2. Establish an open, trusting relationship.
3. Encourage client to participate in anxiety-reducing treatment.
4. Modify the environment.
   A. Help client to identify the source of phobia or anxiety.
   B. Use thought stopping, desensitization, and reciprocal inhibition.
   C. Offer support and presence.
5. Encourage outpatient follow-up treatment.
   A. Successful treatment often depends on consistent, congruent follow-up.

Evaluation

1. Demonstrates decreased fear of object or situation as evidenced by ability to confront object or situation
2. Demonstrates decreased disruption of lifestyle due to phobic symptoms
3. Complies with medical therapy

Obsessive-Compulsive Disorder

Description

Obsessive-compulsive disorder is an increased preoccupation with anxiety-producing thoughts (obsessions) and/or impulses (compulsions) designed to prevent or control dreaded consequences. The five major categories are: (1) dirt, (2) aggressive behavior, (3) orderliness, (4) sexual behaviors, and (5) religion.
1. Effort to control anxiety arises from displacement of unconscious conflicts onto unrelated acts.
2. Compulsive behavior helps to minimize obsessions and to control guilt and anxiety.
3. Disorder often displays a familial pattern.
4. Onset is often secondary to depression.

Assessment

PHYSICAL ASSESSMENT

Medical workup should rule out depression, psychosis, alcohol abuse, and organic mental disorder (Tourette's disorder).

PSYCHOSOCIAL AND CULTURAL ASSESSMENT

1. Persistent and recurrent thinking and behavior patterns
2. Ignoring or suppressing thoughts and impulses
3. Inability to tolerate anxiety, depression, and/or frustration
4. Difficulty expressing thoughts and feelings
5. Difficulty being self-reflective
6. Feelings of guilt
7. Need to control environment
8. Ambivalence and difficulty making decisions
9. Strong tendency toward negativism
10. Dependent behavior
11. Performing repetitive acts, such as continually washing hands
12. Participation in time-consuming ritualistic behavior to avoid relating to people

Planning

1. Safe, effective care environment
   A. Keep safe within environment.
2. Physiological integrity
   A. Decrease or eliminate repetitious performance of ritualistic acts.
3. Psychosocial integrity
   A. Return to productive level of functioning.
   B. Provide new methods of anxiety reduction.

Implementation

1. Coordinate diagnostic studies.
2. Assess threats to health caused by compulsive acts (e.g., malnutrition due to compulsive vomiting; fatigue related to excessive exercise).
3. Provide nonthreatening, supportive environment.
   A. Allow specific time for client to complete compulsions, then redirect.
   B. Encourage verbalization of anxiety.
   C. Assist client to see relationship between anxiety and rituals.
4. Promote expression of genuine feelings—fear, guilt, anxiety.
5. Establish a therapeutic relationship with client.
   A. Give positive feedback when feelings are expressed.
   B. Help client use humor.
   C. Reinforce short, succinct conversation.
   D. Use thought stopping, desensitization, and flooding to extinguish behavior and thoughts.
   E. Discuss the compulsion following an episode.
   F. Provide detailed, consistent care.
   G. Assure client that compulsions will not get out of control.
6. Promote self-esteem and pleasure by stimulating creativity.
   A. Refer to occupational therapy, recreational therapy, group therapy.
   B. Encourage client to establish relationships with others.

Evaluation

1. Evidences no loss of physical health due to compulsive behavior
2. Complies with treatment program
3. Minimizes obsessive-compulsive behavior
4. Becomes comfortable with new activities and relationships

Posttraumatic Stress Disorder

Description

Posttraumatic stress disorder (PTSD) is characterized by re-experiencing a traumatic event in either daytime reveries or dreams. Natural or man-made disasters (outside the range of common experiences) are usually the stress experience.

Assessment

PHYSICAL ASSESSMENT

Symptoms of anxiety, depression, and organic mental disorders are common. Assess for the following:
1. Substance abuse
2. Headaches
3. Memory, attention deficit
4. Pain

PSYCHOSOCIAL AND CULTURAL ASSESSMENT

1. Feelings of detachment, guilt
2. Inability to feel emotions
3. Impulsive behavior
4. Anxiety or depression
5. Nightmares
6. Emotional lability
7. Acting out, reliving traumatic experience

Planning

1. Safe, effective care environment
   A. Keep safe within environment.
2. Physiological integrity
   A. Reduce or eliminate physiological symptoms of stress.
   B. Encourage compliance with treatment program.
3. Psychosocial integrity
   A. Return to productive, functioning state.

Implementation

Patient generally follows four stages:
1. Recovery: Assist client to realize he is safe.
2. Avoidance: Offer support while client attempts to suppress thoughts of traumatic experience.
3. Reconsideration: Offer support, listen, assist client to cope with feelings while client reflects on experience.
4. Adjustment: Assist patient to alter environment, if needed, and use support system.

Evaluation

1. Displays no self-destructive behavior
2. Is able to conceptualize future
3. Has no anxiety, depressive symptoms
4. Functions in work and play

Dissociative Disorders

Description

Dissociative disorders are the result of overwhelming anxiety that results in a disturbance in the normally integrative functions of identity, memory, and consciousness. Dissociative disorders include depersonalization disorder, amnesia, fugue, multiple-personality disorder. Causes may be:
1. Family disturbances, sexual abuse
2. Substance abuse
3. Psychosocial anxiety or traumatic experience

Assessment

PHYSICAL ASSESSMENT

The specific physical and psychosocial and cultural symptoms depend on the type of dissociative disorder. Assess for the following clinical manifestations:
1. Absence of abnormal neurological signs (if present, obtain neurological consult)
2. Absence of delusions or hallucinations (if present, diagnosis may be schizophrenia or psychosis)
3. Recent history of head injury

PSYCHOSOCIAL AND CULTURAL ASSESSMENT

1. Amnestic syndrome is characterized by:
   A. Periods of short-term and long-term memory loss.
   B. Sudden onset in psychogenic amnesia.
   C. Amnesia may be localized, in which there is failure to recall all events during a circumscribed period of time.
   D. It may be selective, in which there is a failure to recall some events during a circumscribed period of time.
   E. It may be generalized, in which failure to recall encompasses the individual's total life.
   F. It may be continuous, in which the individual cannot recall events up to a specific time.
   G. During ongoing amnesia, disorientation and wandering may be present.
2. Psychogenic fugue is characterized by:
   A. Sudden, unexpected travel away from home
   B. Inability to recall one's past
   C. Assumption of a new identity
3. Multiple personality is characterized by:
   A. Existence within person of two or more personalities.
   B. Unexplained distortions in time experience.
   C. Each personality is separate and distinct and takes full control of person's behavior.
   D. Disorder preceded by abuse within the family.

Planning

1. Safe, effective care environment
   A. Keep safe and protect from self-harm.
2. Physiological integrity
   A. Rule out physiological etiology of symptoms.
3. Psychosocial integrity
   A. Help client to identify level and meaning of stress.
   B. Help client to identify anxiety and develop alternative methods of coping with anxiety.
4. Health promotion and maintenance
   A. Encourage client to seek help when anxiety increases.

Implementation

1. Provide safe environment.
2. Observe and describe duration, frequency, and type of dissociative reaction.
3. Assist in diagnostic workup.

4. Avoid transferring anxiety to client.
5. Assist client to identify events and situations that precipitate anxiety.
6. Offer empathy, support, and presence.
7. Refrain from making demands or requiring decisions from client.
8. Help client to analyze consequences of maladaptive coping with anxiety.

Evaluation

1. Identifies and verbalizes feelings of anxiety
2. Copes adaptively with anxiety
3. Resumes life functions
4. Seeks assistance when anxiety escalates

Somatoform Disorders

Description

Somatoform disorders are characterized by multiple and recurrent somatic complaints of months' to years' duration, not due to any organic disorder or validated with physiological evidence. Complaints may be vague, exaggerated, or dramatic. Symptoms are not intentional (unlike malingering and factitious disorders). They are linked to psychological factors or conflicts. Included in this category of disorders are dysmorphophobia, conversion disorder, hypochondriacal, and somatization disorder. Generally the client:
1. Seeks out doctors constantly
2. Is fixated on physical symptoms
3. Has visceral symptoms of conversion disorder (see below), including anorexia, vomiting, hiccups, respiratory tics, and abdominal complaints
4. Experiences frequent anxiety and depressed mood (see Conversion Disorder below)

Conversion Disorder

Description

Conversion disorder is a hysterical reaction characterized by:
1. Physiological dysfunction of symbolic value to the person who sees symptoms as a solution to conflict (blindness, paralysis, loss of speech)
2. "La belle indifférence," or little concern about the incapacity caused by the symptoms
3. Classic conversion symptoms suggestive of neurological disease
4. Symptoms possibly involving automatic or endocrine systems
Essential symptoms are exhibited as a loss or alteration in physical functioning that is an expression of a psychological conflict or need.

Planning

1. Safe, effective care environment
   A. Keep safe, free of falls or self-harm.
2. Physiological integrity
   A. Reduce or eliminate physical symptoms.
3. Psychosocial integrity
   A. Help client to identify life stressors.
4. Health promotion and maintenance
   A. Help client to identify new coping behaviors.

Implementation

1. Assist client to make connections between anxiety and symptoms.
2. Give feedback to client about effects of complaining, demanding behavior.
3. Treat physical symptoms matter-of-factly. Remember, the symptoms are not under voluntary control.
4. Provide client with diversionary activities.
5. Help client to accept anxiety as part of life.

Evaluation

Conversion disorders are often of short duration, with abrupt onset and resolution. Recurrence of an episode suggests a chronic course.
1. Regains normal functioning of dysfunctional part
2. Has no complications from prolonged loss of function, such as contractions
3. Resumes usual life activities and social roles
4. Knows consequences of using physical symptoms to cope with emotional needs

Hypochondriasis

Description

Hypochondriasis is preoccupation with one's health or belief that one has a serious disease. The causes may be:
1. An unconscious desire to be nurtured
2. A defense against depression, guilt, or anger

Assessment

PHYSICAL ASSESSMENT

Symptoms vary, but by definition hypochondriasis evidences no physiological pathology.

PSYCHOSOCIAL AND CULTURAL ASSESSMENT

1. Constantly vigilant for symptoms of illness and over bodily functions.
2. Denial of depressive symptoms.
3. Duration of at least 6 months.
4. Anger with healthcare givers worsens for inability to relieve symptoms.
5. Fear of future illness.
6. Beliefs are fixed and difficult to change.

Planning

1. Physiological integrity
   A. Rule out organic basis for symptoms.
2. Psychosocial integrity
   A. Help client to identify antecedents of anxiety and methods of meeting dependency needs.

Implementation

1. Coordinate diagnostic studies—blood work, x-ray, etc.
2. Promote general health habits.
3. Assist client in identifying affective components of experience.
   A. Teach client to distinguish thought from feeling.
   B. Teach client to describe feelings.
   C. Allow expression of anger.

4. Discuss physical sensations associated with anger.
5. Involve client in establishing goals of care.
6. Respond with interest and empathy.
7. Teach client to be self-nurturing (massage, recreation, etc.).
8. Help client to focus on activities outside self.
9. Involve family in treatment.

Evaluation

1. Experiences decrease in physical symptoms
2. Uses alternative coping strategies
3. Returns to daily activities
4. Assumes responsibility for self

Sleep Disorders

Description

This classification refers to disorders of sleep that are chronic (present for more than a month). In dyssomnia, the predominant disturbance is in the amount, quality, or timing of sleep. In the parasomnias, the predominant disturbance is an abnormal event occurring during sleep. Sleep disorders include sleep-wake disorder, hypersomnia, insomnia, dream anxiety disorder, and sleepwalking disorder.

Assessment

PHYSICAL ASSESSMENT

1. Caffeine, drug, alcohol intake
2. Inadequate nutrition or activity
3. Weight loss or gain
4. Pattern of sleep
5. Possible organic disease or depression

PSYCHOSOCIAL AND CULTURAL ASSESSMENT

1. Psychosocial stressors
2. Support system

Planning

1. Physiological integrity
   A. Re-establish normal sleep patterns.
   B. Prevent exhaustion and other physiological complications.
2. Psychosocial integrity
   A. Identify effective coping behaviors.
3. Health promotion and maintenance
   A. Teach relaxation techniques.

Implementation

1. Coordinate sleep studies.
2. Attend to ADL.
3. Monitor nutritional pattern and activity level.
4. Establish environment conducive to sleep.
5. Teach relaxation techniques.
6. Record sleep patterns.

Evaluation

1. Resumes normal sleep pattern
2. Demonstrates a more positive health status

Sexual Disorders

Description

Sexual disorders are divided into two groups: (1) **paraphilias** are characterized by arousal to objects or situations not part of normative arousal patterns; (2) **sexual dysfunctions** are characterized by inhibitions in sexual desire or psychophysiologic changes that characterize the sexual response cycle. Sexual disorders include pedophilia, voyeurism, exhibitionism, sadism, paraphilia, frotteurism, sexual aversion disorder, sexual desire disorder, dyspareunia, male erectile disorder, female arousal disorder.

Assessment

PHYSICAL ASSESSMENT

1. Symptoms of organic illness
2. Symptoms of psychosis
3. Duration of sexual disorder, sexual history
4. Medication history

PSYCHOSOCIAL AND CULTURAL ASSESSMENT

1. Sexual patterns
2. Family sexual patterns
3. Recent loss
4. Intense loneliness

Planning

1. Physiological integrity
   A. Re-establish normative sexual patterns.
2. Psychosocial integrity
   A. Keep self-esteem intact.
   B. Reduce preoccupation with guilt.
3. Health promotion and maintenance
   A. Maintain normative sexual patterns.

Implementation

1. Explore meaning of client's feelings and behaviors.
2. Teach normal sexual responses.
3. Assess cognitive and affective processes.
4. Clarify relationship between organic problem and sexual functioning.
5. Refer to expert and seek consultation.
6. Analyze own feelings and reactions to client.

Evaluation

1. Understands nature of organic illness
2. Identifies his or her typical level of sexual functioning
3. Distorted perceptions, behaviors cease
4. Develops positive self-esteem.

Personality Disorders

Description

When personal traits are maladaptive and cause significant functional impairments or subjective distress. Personality disorders include paranoid, histrionic, passive-aggressive, schizoid, schizotypal, antisocial, obsessive-compulsive, borderline, avoidant, and dependent.

Paranoid Personality Disorder

Description

The essential feature of paranoid personality disorder is a pervasive and unwarranted tendency to interpret actions of people as deliberately demeaning or threatening.

Assessment

PHYSICAL ASSESSMENT

1. Chemical imbalance of the nervous system may result in mistrustful behavior.
2. History of trauma may contribute to suspiciousness.
3. Nutrition and sleep alterations may result from suspiciousness.

PSYCHOSOCIAL AND CULTURAL ASSESSMENT

1. Rigid interpretation of external events
2. Hypervigilant, attentive to details, unforgiving
3. Reluctant to confide in others; expects to be exploited
4. Views life as unfair
5. Morose, reserved, anxious behavior
6. Grandiosity; sees others, not himself or herself, as having problem
7. Quick to react with rage and anger
8. Craving of recognition
9. Narrowed ability to evaluate reality
10. Fund of information diminished
11. Pervasive mistrust of authority figures

Planning

1. Safe, effective care environment
   A. Keep client and others safe in environment.
2. Psychosocial integrity
   A. Help client to identify situations in which he feels distrustful.
   B. Encourage social interaction.
   C. Teach client skills to validate perceptions.
   D. Promote positive self-concept.
3. Health promotion and maintenance
   A. Increase problem-solving and coping skills.

Implementation

1. Coordinate diagnostic studies such as psychological testing, neurochemical tests, electroencephalogram, magnetic resonance imaging, etc.
2. Administer neuroleptics.
3. Encourage involvement in activities.
   A. Maintain environment where client has some control.
   B. Give feedback when client is dealing with others.
   C. Help client clarify thoughts and feelings.
   D. Teach problem-solving skills, relaxation.
4. Establish a trusting relationship with client.
   A. Maintain an honest, genuine attitude.
   B. Provide short, frequent contacts.
   C. Maintain congruent verbal and nonverbal messages.
   D. Help client to identify behaviors that result in rejection.
   E. Set limits on threatening behavior; identify consequences of unacceptable behavior.
5. Attempt to reframe client's delusional system that threatens further alienation.
6. Assist family to be supportive during treatment process, if appropriate.
7. Encourage hope.

Evaluation

1. Establishes a relationship with the nurse and others
2. Demonstrates diminished social isolation
3. Validates perceptions with a supportive person
4. Has a positive self-concept
5. States situations that result in suspiciousness

Schizotypal and Schizoid Disorder

Description

Schizotypal and schizoid disorder is characterized by a pervasive pattern of strange ideation, appearance, and behavioral deficits in interpersonal relatedness that are not severe enough to meet criteria for schizophrenia.

Assessment

PHYSICAL ASSESSMENT

Negativism and erratic behavior may arise in the limbic system.

PSYCHOSOCIAL AND CULTURAL ASSESSMENT

1. Tendency to withdraw from others and appear sad, brooding, or emotionally vacant
2. Odd beliefs or magical thinking
3. Odd or eccentric behavior or appearance
4. Odd speech—vague, digressive, impoverished
5. Detachment in reaction to conflicts
6. Suspicious
7. Unsatisfying and/or dysfunctional relationships
8. Silly, aloof, constricted affect

Planning

1. Physiological integrity
   A. Encourage independence in ADL.
2. Psychosocial integrity
   A. Encourage social interaction.
   B. Support appropriate behavior and thinking.
3. Health promotion and maintenance
   A. Restore to normal functioning in work and play.

Implementation

1. Coordinate diagnostic studies such as psychological testing, biochemical studies, etc.
2. Initiate nurse-client relationship.
   A. Demonstrate accessibility.
   B. Provide honest feedback.
   C. Support client's strengths.
3. Assist client to identify the meaning of social isolation.
   A. Identify relationship between anxiety and isolation.
   B. Encourage client to express his or her thoughts and feelings.
   C. Demonstrate that a relationship can be nonthreatening.

4. Assist patient to interact with others.
   A. Identify stressful stimuli in relationships.
   B. Role-play social interactions.
   C. Encourage participation in group activities.

Evaluation

1. Demonstrates ability to interact with others
2. Demonstrates self-care activities
3. Has positive self-concept

Antisocial Personality Disorder

Description

Antisocial personality disorder is characterized by impulsive, narcissistic behavior patterns that result in a pattern of irresponsible behavior.

1. Patterns begin in childhood. Absence of consistent parental discipline increases likelihood of disorder.
2. Genetic predisposition, particularly common in both males and females who have fathers with the disorder.
3. Those afflicted generally have no guilt or remorse for mistreatment of others.
4. Disorder begins before age 15 and is more common in males.

Assessment

PHYSICAL ASSESSMENT

Pattern of substance abuse often accompanies the disorder.

PSYCHOSOCIAL AND CULTURAL ASSESSMENT

1. Inability to sustain consistent work behavior
2. Failure to conform to social norms with respect to lawful behavior
3. Irritability, aggressiveness; defaults on debts
4. Impulsiveness, no regard for the truth
5. Inability to learn by experience
6. Inability to have monogamous relationships
7. Recklessness regarding safety of self and others
8. Lack of remorse
9. Strong need to manipulate

Planning

1. Safe, effective care environment
   A. Decrease impulsive behavior.
2. Psychosocial integrity
   A. Help client to recognize manipulative, self-destructive patterns.
3. Health promotion and maintenance
   A. Encourage use of problem-solving techniques rather than manipulation in ADL.

Implementation

1. Coordinate diagnostic studies such as psychological testing, etc.
2. Encourage expression of anger and inadequacy.
3. Set limits on manipulation.
4. Explore consequences of behavior.

5. Avoid rejecting client.
6. Be consistent, firm, matter of fact.
7. Reinforce behaviors that indicate sensitivity to others.
8. Promote self-awareness.
9. Foster client's willingness to participate in treatment.
10. Provide a confrontation group for client to learn own manipulative patterns and interact with others who use manipulative behavior.
11. Use behavioral modification, role playing, and group therapy to promote sensitivity.

Evaluation

Many of these symptoms are resistive to treatment and may become chronic. The disorder may result in failure of the client to become an independent, self-supporting adult.

1. Demonstrates ability to live within limits of society by showing decreased impulsive and acting-out behavior
2. Demonstrates consideration for others and recognizes own manipulative behavior patterns
3. Demonstrates that he or she is learning from the past

Obsessive-Compulsive Personality Disorder

See Anxiety Disorders and Obsessive-Compulsive Disorder.

Passive-Aggressive Personality Disorder

Description

Passive-aggressive personality disorder is characterized by passive resistance to demands for adequate performance in both occupational and social functioning.

Assessment

PHYSICAL ASSESSMENT

There are usually no pathological biological symptoms.

PSYCHOSOCIAL AND CULTURAL ASSESSMENT

The behavior has both passive and aggressive characteristics.
1. Passive resistance to demands of social and occupational performance exhibited as:
   A. Procrastination
   B. Stubbornness, sulking
   C. Deliberate slow work pace on tasks that he or she does not want to do
   D. Irritability, argumentativeness
   E. Hostility, provocativeness
   F. Avoidance of obligations
   G. Belief that he or she is more productive than others
2. Resentment of any demands from others
3. Persistent social and occupational ineffectiveness
4. Unreasonable scorn for people in authority

Planning

1. Psychosocial integrity
   A. Promote recognition and verbalization of manipulative behavior.
   B. Demonstrate alternative ways to deal with anxiety and/or hostility.

2. Health promotion and maintenance
   A. Assist to function more effectively in work and play.

Implementation

1. Coordinate diagnostic studies such as psychological testing, etc.
2. Identify hostility and/or anxiety stimuli.
3. Explore past and present interpersonal relationships.
   A. Be straightforward, nonjudgmental, consistent.
   B. Give feedback on behavior.
4. Facilitate expression of anger.
5. Assist client to establish a supportive interpersonal relationship.
   A. Develop a sense of trust and consistency.
   B. Recognize client's need for control in a relationship.
   C. Avoid rejecting client.
6. Help client to meet need for self-respect.
   A. Spend time with client when he or she is not demanding.
   B. Encourage direct communication to get needs met.
   C. Provide confrontation group.
   D. Consistently set limits on behavior.
   E. Support positive behavior.
7. Include family in treatment process.
   A. Instruct family to avoid reinforcing symptoms.
   B. Use role playing and psychodrama.
   C. Encourage family to express their thoughts and feelings.

Evaluation

1. Recognizes passive-aggressive behavior
2. Demonstrates that he or she is learning from past behavior
   A. Uses direct communication to get needs met
   B. Expresses feelings and other thoughts rather than acting them out
   C. Begins to establish satisfying relationships

Borderline Personality Disorder

Description

Borderline personality disorder is marked by an instability in interpersonal behavior, mood, and self-image. The instability is significant to the extent that the client borders on psychosis and neurosis.

Assessment

PHYSICAL ASSESSMENT

Clients with this disorder often manifest recurrent suicidal gestures or self-mutilation; assess physical status and observe for scars, burns, etc.

PSYCHOSOCIAL AND CULTURAL ASSESSMENT

1. A pattern of unstable and intense interpersonal relationships characterized by overidealization and devaluation
2. Interpersonal exploitiveness
3. Impulsive, self-dramatizing behavior—gambling, excessive spending, substance abuse, overeating
4. Affective instability
5. Recurrent self-destructive acts—burning, cutting, slashing
6. Chronic feelings of emptiness
7. Depersonalized feelings
8. Poor reality testing
9. Inappropriate, intense anger
10. Alternating clinging and distancing behaviors

Planning

1. Safe, effective care environment
   A. Keep free of self-harm.
2. Psychosocial integrity
   A. Refine coping mechanisms to control anxiety.
3. Health promotion and maintenance
   A. Encourage compliance with outpatient treatment regimen.

Implementation

1. Observe client's behavior frequently.
2. Keep client's environment safe.
3. Secure verbal contract that client will seek out staff when self-mutilation urge is felt.
4. Care for wounds in matter-of-fact manner if self-mutilation occurs.
5. Encourage client to talk about feelings. Act as role model for expression of angry feelings.
6. Redirect client's angry feelings.
7. Use restraints, seclusion, or one-to-one staffing as needed.
8. Identify client's strengths.
9. Include family in treatment plans.
10. Arrange for outpatient follow-up, and identify community resources.

Evaluation

1. Maintains anxiety at level that reduces need for aggression or impulsive acting-out behaviors
2. Reports lessening of self-harm ideation
3. Agrees to use of outpatient services and community resources

Histrionic Personality Disorder

Description

Histrionic personality disorder is characterized by a pattern of excessive emotionality and attention-seeking behavior.

Assessment

PHYSICAL ASSESSMENT

Client may have multiple physical complaints.

PSYCHOSOCIAL AND CULTURAL ASSESSMENT

1. Constantly seeking reassurance, approval, praise
2. Inappropriate sexual seductiveness
3. Overconcern with physical appearance
4. Exaggerated emotions
5. Uncomfortable when not the center of attention
6. Rapid mood swings
7. Style of speech is impressionistic and lacks detail

Planning

1. Psychosocial integrity
   A. Increase overall social functioning.
   B. Decrease physical symptoms.

Implementation

1. See client frequently for brief periods.
2. Assist to identify strengths.
3. Encourage independent behavior.
4. Set limits on changing behavior.
5. Involve in group activities and milieu.
6. Promote optimal level of functioning.
7. Give honest feedback on inappropriate behavior.
8. Promote decision making skills.
9. Help client to set limits on acting-out behavior.
10. Encourage family involvement, outpatient treatment follow-up, and use of community resources.

Evaluation

1. Returns to adequate social functioning

Eating Disorders

Description

Eating disorders are characterized by gross disturbance in eating behaviors, including anorexia nervosa and bulimia nervosa. Causes include:
1. Family dysfunction
2. Expectations of perfection
3. Ambivalence regarding independence and adulthood
4. Stressful life situation

Assessment

PHYSICAL ASSESSMENT

1. Body weight 15% below normal
2. Absence of three consecutive menstrual cycles
3. Vomiting, bingeing, or vigorous exercise
4. Signs of malnutrition—electrolyte imbalance, poor skin turgor, lanugo, brittle hair and nails
5. History of dieting
6. Cardiac arrhythmias, bradycardia
7. Esophageal tears
8. Gastric rupture

PSYCHOSOCIAL AND CULTURAL ASSESSMENT

1. Persistent concern with body shape and weight
2. Recurrent episodes of bingeing, purging, taking diuretics, or exercising to maintain low weight
3. A feeling of lack of control over food
4. Family history of eating disorder
5. Depressed mood
6. Social isolation, secretiveness, introversion

Planning

1. Physiological integrity
   A. Restore to normal weight and eating patterns.
2. Psychosocial integrity
   A. Increase awareness of feelings; reduce or eliminate self-destructive behaviors—bingeing, purging, overly vigorous exercise.
   B. Help to resolve or improve family conflict.

Implementation

1. Monitor eating and bathroom activities.
2. Protect from self-harm.
3. Administer antidepressants or anxiolytics.
4. Assist in self-care activities.
5. Coordinate activities and psychological therapies.
6. Encourage participation in family therapy.

Evaluation

1. Maintains normal weight
2. Returns to high-level functioning

Schizophrenia Disorders

Description

Schizophrenia disorders compose a clinical syndrome in which thought content, form, affect, identity, and relationships are severely impaired. The schizophrenias are psychotic disorders. Causes for all types of schizophrenia (paranoid, catatonic, disorganized, undifferentiated, residual) may be:
1. Genetic predisposition
2. Biochemical imbalances (e.g., dopamine, serotonin, γ-aminobutyric acid)
3. Inadequate ego development based on unsatisfying parent-child relationship
4. Family dysfunction
5. Poverty, stress, lack of support systems, traumatic events

Assessment

PHYSICAL ASSESSMENT

Assess for the following clinical manifestations:
1. Disturbed eating, sleeping, and self-care patterns.
2. Self-destructive or violent thoughts.
3. Onset during or after puberty.
4. Six-month period of decline includes a prodromal phase, an active phase, and a residual phase.
5. Disease may be subchronic, chronic, or in remission.
6. Physical illness secondary to poor self-care, lack of judgment, and cognitive impairment.
7. Organic illness, organic mental disorders.

PSYCHOSOCIAL AND CULTURAL ASSESSMENT

1. Loss of drive, interest, ambition, initiative, energy
2. Poor attention span, delusions, hallucinations, illusions
3. Form of thought—loose, tangential, circumstantial
4. Faulty perceptions
5. Indifference to relationships, fearful of closeness
6. Affect—blunted, bland, inappropriate
7. Lack of interest in work, inability to work (volition impairment)
8. Sense of self disturbed, loss of ego boundaries
9. Psychomotor retardation

10. Poor judgment, impaired social functioning
11. Magical thinking, depersonalization, and religiosity

Planning

1. Safe, effective care environment
   A. Protect from self-harm.
2. Physiological integrity
   A. Maintain normal eating and sleeping patterns, activities of self-care.
3. Psychosocial integrity
   A. Decrease apathy and indifference.
   B. Increase ability to tolerate self and others.
   C. Improve clarity of thought processes.
4. Health promotion and maintenance
   A. Encourage compliance with outpatient treatment regimen.

Implementation

1. Coordinate diagnostic studies such as psychological testing, biochemical screening.
2. Administer neuroleptic medications.
3. Decrease environmental stimuli.
   A. Institute room program (i.e., 10 minutes out of room, 50 minutes in).
   B. Initiate group activities.
4. Keep client and others safe; observe frequently.
5. Avoid physical contact.
6. Assist in self-care functions.
7. Use consensual validation and therapeutic communication techniques.
8. Provide short, frequent visits by same staff member.
9. Encourage client to resume regular eating and sleeping patterns.
   A. Identify preferences for eating and sleeping.
10. Encourage family to be supportive.
    A. Assist family to recognize symptoms as part of behavioral pattern.
11. Use community agencies to enhance follow-up treatment.

Evaluation

1. Participates in activities, relationships, and follow-up clinic visits
2. Resumes self-care activities and is able to ask for assistance
3. Refrains from responding to hallucinatory voices
4. Knows where to receive assistance after discharge

Disorganized Schizophrenia

Description

Disorganized schizophrenia is marked by incoherence, grossly disorganized behavior, thematic hallucinations and delusions, or grossly inappropriate affect.

Assessment

PHYSICAL ASSESSMENT

Assess for the following clinical manifestations:
1. Impaired ADL
2. Hypochondriacal complaints

PSYCHOSOCIAL AND CULTURAL ASSESSMENT

1. Childlike behavior, silly, laughing for no apparent reason
2. Extreme social withdrawal
3. Flat or inappropriate affect
4. Bizarre makeup and clothing
5. Odd behavior or mannerisms
6. Hallucinations, delusions
7. Echolalia, echopraxia, word salad, loose associations
8. Disregard for social norms—masturbates openly, urinates and defecates anywhere

Planning

1. Safe, effective care environment
   A. Protect from self-harm.
2. Psychological integrity
   A. Encourage cooperation during medical workup.
   B. Promote optimal nutrition and sleep.
3. Psychosocial integrity
   A. Support appropriate behavior.
   B. Maintain contact with reality.
4. Health promotion and maintenance
   A. Encourage compliance with outpatient treatment regimen.

Implementation

1. Administer neuroleptic drugs such as Haldol (haloperidol), fluphenazine, or thiothixene orally or IM as ordered for acute psychoses.
2. Coordinate diagnostic studies such as psychological testing, etc.
3. Assist with ADL.
4. Identify nature of hallucinations and delusions.
5. Initiate milieu, group, family, and/or individual psychotherapy as client tolerates.
6. Encourage positive behavior, and discourage negative behavior.
7. Establish a therapeutic alliance.
   A. Spend time with client, and maintain calm, consistent manner.
   B. Provide private place for client if he or she is unwilling to discontinue inappropriate behavior publicly.
8. Assist client to decrease hallucinations and delusions.
   A. Help client to identify feelings of anxiety.
   B. Explore client's feelings about hallucinations.
   C. Provide tasks and structure to refocus client.
   D. Avoid conveying belief that hallucinations are real.
9. Teach social skills and encourage appropriate social activities.

Evaluation

1. Assumes responsibility for personal hygiene
2. Decreases inappropriate behavior and replaces with socially acceptable behavior
3. Explores needs served by hallucinations and delusions
4. Improves social skills and increases ability to relate to others
5. Demonstrates compliance with follow-up office or clinic visits

Catatonic Schizophrenia

Description

Catatonic schizophrenia is characterized by disturbed psychomotor behavior such as stupor, negativism, posturing, and excitement. Mutism and labile patterns are common.

Assessment

PHYSICAL ASSESSMENT

Assess for the following clinical manifestations:
1. Remaining immobile or assuming bizarre positions when standing or sitting
2. Malnutrition, dehydration
3. Self-inflicted injury
4. Waxy rigidity of muscles
5. Exhaustion, weight loss
6. Hyperpyrexia

PSYCHOSOCIAL AND CULTURAL ASSESSMENT

1. Alternating between catatonic stupor (motor retardation) and catatonic euphoria (hyperactivity)
2. Negativism
3. Emotional blunting
4. Mute or incoherent speech
5. Posturing and/or rigidity
6. Inability to perform ADL
7. Hallucinations and delusions
8. Marked ambivalence

Planning

1. Safe, effective care environment
   A. Improve contact with reality.
2. Physiological integrity
   A. Encourage personal hygiene care.
3. Psychosocial integrity
   A. Increase social interaction.
4. Health promotion and maintenance
   A. Help client to resume activities of daily living.

Implementation

1. Administer neuroleptics as ordered.
2. Coordinate diagnostic studies such as psychological testing, biochemical testing, etc.
3. Observe frequently—client may require a one-to-one relationship.
4. Keep client safe (remove sharp objects, monitor environment).
5. Attend to biological needs, and monitor eating, sleeping, and elimination patterns.
6. Encourage activities as tolerated; monitor environmental stimuli.
7. Establish a therapeutic relationship.
   A. Assume a kind, firm, consistent, undemanding approach.
   B. Be aware of both client's and own verbal and nonverbal communication. Although stuporous, the client is usually aware of the environment and will be able to verbalize events that occurred during stupor.
   C. Enhance self-esteem by supporting positive behaviors.

8. Assist client to decrease stuporous withdrawal and/or hyperactive behavior.
   A. Encourage participation in the therapeutic environment to decrease isolation (persons, objects, activities).
   B. Speak concisely and in simple terms to avoid sensory overload.
   C. Focus and orient client frequently.
   D. Set limits on behavior, and reinforce appropriate behavior in kind, consistent manner.
9. Assist client to decrease hallucinations and delusions.

Evaluation

1. Interacts successfully and more frequently with others
2. Demonstrates ability to perform personal hygiene
3. Takes medication
4. Shows no signs of withdrawal and/or hyperactive behavior
5. Verbalizes understanding of need for follow-up treatment

Paranoid Schizophrenia

Description

An essential feature of paranoid schizophrenia is preoccupation with one or more systematized delusions with auditory hallucinations related to one theme.

Assessment

PHYSICAL ASSESSMENT

Assess for the following clinical manifestations:
1. Refusal to eat or drink for fear of being poisoned
2. Incoherence, loose associations of other types of schizophrenia
3. Onset often later in life (after 30 years of age)
4. Capacity for independent living higher than in other types of schizophrenia

PSYCHOSOCIAL AND CULTURAL ASSESSMENT

1. Preoccupation with systematized delusions—persecutory, grandiose, jealous, somatic, erotomanic
2. Hallucinations—auditory, visual, tactile
3. Ideas of reference
4. Stilted, intense interpersonal relations
5. Suspiciousness, distrustfulness, resentfulness
6. Unfocused anger, anxiety, and argumentativeness
7. Unpredictable violence
8. Perceived as frightening or hostile by coworkers

Planning

1. Safe, effective care environment
   A. Improve contact with reality.
   B. Help client to identify situations in which he or she feels distrustful.
2. Physiological integrity
   A. Promote optimal nutrition and sleep.
3. Psychosocial integrity
   A. Teach skills to validate perceptions.
   B. Promote positive self-concept.
4. Health promotion and maintenance
   A. Increase social interaction.

B. Increase compliance with outpatient treatment regimen.

Implementation

1. Administer neuroleptic drugs as ordered.
2. Coordinate diagnostic studies such as psychological testing, biochemical testing, etc.
3. Be aware of potential for violence.
4. Encourage participation in activities where client will do well.
5. Help client to decrease suspicious behavior.
   A. Maintain matter-of-fact attitude and avoid touch.
   B. Explore situations where client feels suspicious.
   C. Problem-solve alternatives to suspiciousness.
   D. Help client to clarify thoughts.
   E. Assist client to analyze belief system.
6. Let client know what is acceptable and unacceptable behavior and consequences of each.
7. Provide short, frequent contacts; avoid whispering; avoid arguing; give clear, concise information.
8. Help client to identify community resources for socialization and follow-up treatment.

Evaluation

1. Is able to verbalize situations that result in suspiciousness
2. Demonstrates decreased suspicious behavior
3. Has positive self-concept
4. Verbalizes plan to return to social and work activities

Affective Disorders

Bipolar Disorders

Bipolar disorders are classified as mixed, manic, or depressed.

Description

Behavior characterized by a disturbance in mood involving depression and/or elation. Causes may be:
1. Genetic predisposition
2. Biochemical—due to imbalance in dopamine, serotonin, other biogenic amines
3. Malfunction in response to attempts to control anger or depression. (This section focuses on the manic phase only.)

Assessment

PHYSICAL ASSESSMENT

Assess for the following clinical manifestations:
1. Sleep disturbances—difficulty sleeping, decreased rapid eye movement (REM) sleep and dream time
2. Abnormal cortisol, human growth hormone, and thyroid-stimulating hormone laboratory results
   A. Euphoria may be associated with right-side brain damage.
   B. Abnormal EEG.
3. Psychomotor agitation
4. Side effects of lithium, carbamazepine (Tegretol)
5. Exhaustion, malnourishment

PSYCHOSOCIAL AND CULTURAL ASSESSMENT

1. Emotional lability, grandiose delusions, irritability
2. Lack of judgment, insight
3. Short attention span
4. Uninhibited sexuality
5. Flight of ideas; changing, pressured speech
6. Unrealistically inflated self-esteem
7. Theatrical or dramatic behavior
8. Buying sprees, reckless driving
9. Strange, flamboyant dress
10. Unselective enthusiasm for interaction with people

Planning

1. Safe, effective care environment
   A. Protect from physical injury during hospitalization.
   B. Meet basic physical needs.
2. Physiological integrity
   A. Prevent untoward effects of lithium.
   B. Encourage compliance with lithium regimen.
3. Psychosocial integrity
   A. Decrease hyperactive behavior.
   B. Increase cognitive congruence.
4. Health promotion and maintenance
   A. Restore social and occupational functioning.

Implementation

1. Administer lithium as ordered.
2. Administer neuroleptic drugs as ordered.
3. Observe and document side effects.
4. Monitor lithium level.
5. Remove hazardous objects and substances from environment.
6. Decrease environmental stimuli.
7. Help client to decrease manic behavior.
   A. Provide calm, consistent behavior by staff.
   B. Encourage solitary activities to limit distractions.
   C. Encourage large motor activities and avoidance of competitive activities.
8. Encourage client to comply with a structured schedule of activities.
   A. Monitor patterns of eating, sleeping, and elimination.
   B. Provide small, frequent meals and rest periods.
   C. Provide physical activity as substitution for purposeless activity.
   D. Limit group activities.
9. Promote client's motivation and willingness to participate in treatment.
   A. Explain action and importance of medication.
   B. Educate patient about illness.
   C. Teach family about illness, its course, and treatment.
10. Help client to exhibit appropriate behavior with others.
   A. Help client to identify and express painful feelings.
   B. Help client to identify feelings of being overwhelmed.
   C. Offer feedback about influence on others in succinct manner.
   D. Listen to feeling tone rather than to content only.
   E. Reinforce positive behavior.
   F. Provide materials for client to write or draw.

Evaluation

1. Understands nature of illness
2. Verbalizes understanding of need for medical regimen
3. Is able to control behavior
4. Identifies painful feelings and the way they affect behavior
5. Makes realistic self-appraisals

Major Depression (Dysthymic Disorder)

Description

Major depression is characterized by a depressed mood or persistent loss of interest or pleasure in almost all life activities. Causes may be:

1. Unresolved loss and grief
2. Unresolved anger
3. Biochemical imbalance
4. Genetic predisposition
5. Childbirth

Assessment

PHYSICAL ASSESSMENT

The manifestation of specific symptoms depends on the severity of the depression. Assess for the following clinical manifestations:

1. Sleep disturbances—initial insomnia, middle insomnia, terminal insomnia, or hypersomnia
2. Lowered levels of norepinephrine, serotonin, and steroid output as evidenced by laboratory results
3. Anorexia, weight loss, constipation, chest pain, gastrointestinal complaints
4. Decreased muscle tone
5. Immobile face, sunken eyes, wrinkled forehead, dejected appearance
6. Feelings of fatigue, lethargy, slowed speech, or muteness
7. Possible elevated dexamethasone suppression test results

PSYCHOSOCIAL AND CULTURAL ASSESSMENT

1. Feelings of despondency, helplessness, hopelessness, poor self-esteem, guilt, shame, anxiety, indecisiveness
2. Anhedonia (unable to experience or express pleasure)
3. Psychomotor agitation or retardation
4. Somatic complaints
5. Difficulty in concentrating, indecisiveness, slowed thinking
6. Paranoid ideation, memory deficit, delusions, rumination
7. Thoughts of death and/or suicide attempts
8. Poor self-concept, need to be loved, unexpressed rage, powerlessness

Planning

1. Safe, effective care environment
   A. Protect from self-harm.
2. Physiological integrity
   A. Encourage performance of ADL.
3. Psychosocial integrity
   A. Help client to develop a realistic, positive perception of self.
   B. Enhance client's self-esteem, acceptance of others, and sense of belonging.
4. Health promotion and maintenance
   A. Help client to resume ADL.
   B. Encourage efforts to establish satisfying relationships.

C. Encourage compliance with follow-up care and medical regimen.

Implementation

1. Administer antidepressants such as tricyclics, MAO inhibitors, tetracyclics.
2. Assist with ECT, if necessary.
3. Assist client in ADL.
   A. Encourage cleanliness.
   B. Protect against self-destructive tendencies.
   C. Relieve physical symptoms.
4. Encourage expression of feelings associated with depression.
5. Assist client to identify source of negative feelings about self.
6. Decrease suicidal preoccupation.
   A. Remove potentially harmful objects.
   B. Observe closely.
   C. Assess suicide potential.
7. Encourage client to accept responsibility for own feelings.
8. Provide structured environment and activities.
9. Provide information about characteristics of depression.
10. Encourage brief, frequent interaction.
11. Encourage client to participate in activities (group therapy, recreational therapy, occupational therapy, etc.).
12. Encourage client to indulge in pleasant sensations such as those derived from music, art, massage.
13. Teach communication skills.
14. Teach relaxation skills.
15. Encourage client to receive feedback from others.
16. Assist family to participate in treatment process. Encourage family members to verbalize their thoughts and feelings and understanding of illness and to support client in treatment process.

Evaluation

1. Is more animated, energetic, and positive
2. Verbalizes resolution of loss or grief
3. Has positive self-concept
4. Is able to interact with others in work and play
5. Complies with medical treatment

Psychoactive Substance Abuse Disorders

Description

Psychoactive substance abuse disorders are characterized by a cluster of cognitive, behavioral, and physiological symptoms indicating that a person has impaired control of psychoactive substance use (alcohol, nicotine, other drugs) and continues use of substance despite adverse consequences. (See Alcoholism below.)

Alcoholism

Description

Alcoholism is manifested by physical and psychological dependence and/or tolerance to alcohol with resulting impairment of life. Predisposing factors may be:

1. Genetic
2. Availability of alcohol

3. Social, cultural, and family acceptability of alcohol use and abuse
4. Allergic response to alcohol
5. Oral-dependent personality

Assessment

PHYSICAL ASSESSMENT

Assess for the following clinical manifestations:
1. Nausea, vomiting, anorexia, diarrhea
2. Diaphoresis
3. Restlessness, tremors, weakness
4. Convulsions
5. Visual and tactile hallucinations, paranoid delusions
6. Ulcers, gastroenteritis, esophagitis, colitis
7. Impaired food and hydration pattern
8. Tachycardia, hyperpnea
9. Tachycardia, hypertension
10. Peripheral nerve and brain damage
11. Liver disease
12. Sexual dysfunction
13. History of blackouts

PSYCHOSOCIAL AND CULTURAL ASSESSMENT

1. Feelings of anger, resentment, depression, helplessness
2. Distracted perception
3. Impaired communication skills
4. Denial of dependence, impaired memory, disorientation
5. Poor decision making
6. Poor self-concept
7. Mistrust of self and others
8. Inappropriate attention-seeking behaviors
9. Poor occupational functioning
10. Social isolation
11. Family dysfunction

Planning

1. Safe, effective care environment
   A. Keep safe in environment.
2. Physiological integrity
   A. Support client during detoxification process.
   B. Encourage independence in ADL.
3. Psychosocial integrity
   A. Help client to identify the causes of dependence.
   B. Assist client to live free of alcohol.
   C. Encourage resolution of conflicts that surround unmet needs.
4. Health promotion and maintenance
   A. Provide outpatient support system and treatment.

Implementation

1. Intervene as needed for acute alcoholism and/or withdrawal.
   A. Assess vital signs, physical and mental status, and for grand mal seizures.
   B. Be calm, consistent, and nonjudgmental.
   C. Administer medications according to detoxification schedule (benzodiazepines—lorazepam, chlordiazepoxide [Librium]; β-blockers—atenolol).
   D. Coordinate relevant diagnostic studies, such as blood alcohol levels.
   E. Provide physical care—nutrition, hydration, and seizure precaution.
2. Identify and assess social support system available to client.
3. Assist client to identify causes of dependence.
4. Assist client to deal with feelings associated with dependence. Encourage activities, Alcoholics Anonymous (AA) attendance.
5. Help client to set attainable goals.
6. Help client to deal with loss of substance abuse.
7. Enhance client's sense of choice of lifestyle.
8. Intervene directly with denial.
9. Explore methods of improving social skills.
10. Promote decision making skills.
11. Investigate family dynamics.
12. Help family work through tendency to promote substance abuse.
13. Assist client and family to verbalize thoughts and feelings about substance abuse experience.
    A. Identify stressors that influence abuse.
    B. Discuss secondary gains of substance abuse.
14. Enhance client's self-esteem.
    A. Help client develop realistic occupational goals.
    B. Refer client to self-help groups.

Evaluation

1. Identifies his or her dependent behavior
2. Understands risks involved in use of substance
3. Functions independently and interdependently
4. Involved in follow-up program (e.g., AA)
5. Stops abusing substance

Organic Mental Syndromes and Disorders

Description

Organic mental syndrome refers to a constellation of psychological or behavioral signs and symptoms without reference to etiology (e.g., organic anxiety syndrome, dementia). **Organic mental disorder** designates a particular mental syndrome in which the etiology is known (e.g., Parkinson's disease, Huntington's chorea, multi-infarct dementia). Causes of organic mental disorders include:
1. CNS infection
2. Head trauma
3. Intracranial lesion
4. Hepatic disease
5. Subarachnoid hemorrhage
6. Cerebral hypoxia
7. Thyroid, parathyroid, or adrenal dysfunction
8. Down syndrome—predisposes to Alzheimer's disease (genetic)
9. Hypertension

Assessment

PHYSICAL ASSESSMENT

Symptoms vary depending on the nature of the disease. Acute conditions have a sudden onset of symptoms due to disturbance in brain function. Impairment may be reversible with treatment or may become permanent, progressive, and chronic. Assess for the following clinical manifestations:

1. Weakness of limbs
2. Reflex asymmetries
3. Dysarthria
4. Extensor plantar responses
5. Unstable shuffling gait
6. Tremors, slow speech
7. Hyperactivity
8. Seizures

PSYCHOSOCIAL AND CULTURAL ASSESSMENT

1. Dementia (cognitive defects, e.g., memory, orientation, impulse control)
2. Personality changes
3. Delirium (rapid onset of clouding of consciousness, incoherent speech, disorientation, hallucinations)
4. Amnestic syndrome (impairment of long-term and short-term memory, confabulation, flat affect)
5. Organic hallucinosis (persistent hallucinations)
6. Organic affective syndrome (mania or depression)
7. Organic anxiety syndrome (panic attacks or severe anxiety)
8. Rage reactions
9. Impaired social judgment, apathy
10. Tangential, circumstantial speech
11. Inability for self-care
12. Frequent falls, mobility impairment
13. Repetitive movements

Planning

1. Safe, effective care environment
   A. Keep safe in environment.
2. Physiological integrity
   A. Maintain intact physiological functioning.
   B. Encourage client to complete ADL.
   C. Assist in identification (or correction) of etiology of disease.
3. Psychosocial integrity
   A. Teach prospective caregivers principles and methods of care.

4. Health promotion and maintenance
   A. Mobilize community resources.

Implementation

1. Attend to client's safety, well-being.
   A. Remove dangerous objects.
   B. Pad siderails.
   C. Use neuroleptic drugs for agitation, as ordered.
   D. Reorient frequently.
   E. Attend to ADL.
   F. Encourage self-care.
   G. Prevent iatrogenic illness.
2. Organize environment.
   A. Provide calm, well-lighted, simple environment.
   B. Limit number of people caring for client.
   C. Provide external signs of orientation (e.g., calendars, clocks).
   D. Provide stimulation to senses (e.g., balloons, rocking chairs, flowers, pictures).
3. Administer medications as needed (e.g., neuroleptic drugs, vitamins).
4. Coordinate diagnostic studies.
5. Assess and document for behavioral changes often (e.g., every 4 hours).
6. Provide a feeling of security and safety.
   A. Short, frequent visits
   B. Simple explanations
   C. Speak face to face in a low voice.
   D. Give positive feedback when client accomplishes task.
7. Include caregivers in nursing care plan.
8. Collaborate and consult with personnel in other disciplines.

Evaluation

1. Remains safe
2. Functions at highest possible level
3. Caregivers comprehend disease and care
4. Caregivers and client receive support
5. Follow-up care coordinated

1. A 5-year-old girl admitted to the hospital for arm fractures and multiple bruises is a reported victim of child abuse by her mother. The nurse observes the child's behavior after she is hospitalized. Which of the following psychosocial characteristics would the nurse be likely to see her exhibit?

   A. Her behavior is appropriate to the social situation.
   B. She seeks frequent parental contact.
   C. She has accelerated achievement of developmental tasks.
   D. She has minimal socialization with peers.

2. The nurse is caring for a 6-year-old girl admitted for burns to her arms and back. Her case is being investigated as child abuse by authorities. The child is mute during routine care procedures and is often later found crying. An important goal in providing care to this client would be to:

   A. Provide a variety of stimulation by having several nurses take care of the child
   B. Provide a nonthreatening, nurturing environment
   C. Discourage the child from expressing thoughts and feelings about the abuse
   D. Have the child's parents present during care activities

3. The nurse is discussing family history and family dynamics with the parent of a child who may be abused. Which of the following information would increase the nurse's suspicion of potential child abuse?

   A. The parent has a high energy level.
   B. The parent has several children.
   C. The parent's childhood was characterized by abuse.
   D. The parent has a low socioeconomic status.

4. A 7-year-old boy is hospitalized with a diagnosis of autism. The nurse observes the child on admission. Which of the following information regarding his behavior would confirm that he is an autistic child?

   A. Lack of interest in inanimate objects
   B. Dislike of routine
   C. Unresponsive to others
   D. Below average intelligence

5. A 6-year-old boy is admitted to the hospital with the diagnosis of autism. The nurse is interested in helping the child to feel more secure on the unit. The *most* appropriate intervention for the nurse would be to:

   A. Have the same nurses provide care
   B. Administer Ritalin to control hyperactivity
   C. Discourage peer contact
   D. Allow him to control his own eating and sleeping patterns

6. A 6-year-old boy who was recently admitted to the hospital with a diagnosis of autism grabs a toy and hits another child. The *most* appropriate response to the child's attempts to hurt himself or others is to:

   A. Isolate him for 24 hours
   B. Encourage him to explain his angry thoughts

   C. Assume a nonpunitive attitude and stop the attempt to hurt himself or others
   D. Call his parents to get their input

7. An 8-year-old boy has recently been diagnosed with attention-deficit hyperactive disorder by his pediatrician. He and his parents come to the pediatric clinic together. Which of the following behaviors would the nurse be *most* likely to observe from the child?

   A. Lethargy
   B. Preoccupation with body parts
   C. Very poor verbal skills
   D. Short attention span

8. In providing care to a school-age child with attention-deficit hyperactive disorder, the *most* effective intervention would be to:

   A. Increase environmental stimulation and peer interaction
   B. Administer drug therapy (i.e., methylphenidate [Ritalin]) and use behavior modification techniques
   C. Provide parental education and diet therapy
   D. Encourage delayed achievement of normal developmental tasks

9. A 6-year-old girl is recently diagnosed as mildly retarded. An important aspect in the nursing care of a mildly mentally retarded child is to:

   A. Encourage her parents to concentrate on the child rather than on the family at this time
   B. Delay extensive diagnostic studies until the child is older
   C. Modify the child's environment to promote independence and impulse control
   D. Provide 1:1 tutorial education and minimize peer interaction

10. The nurse realizes that the *most* effective way to promote positive behavioral change in a 30-year-old man with severe mental retardation is:

    A. Provide simple, concrete explanations of behavior to be learned
    B. Have client role play new behaviors with the nurse
    C. Provide systematic habit training
    D. Encourage independence

11. A 13-year-old boy has a history of conduct disorder. In obtaining a nursing history, which of the following would not be a characteristic of this disorder?

    A. Reports incidences of fire setting
    B. Has a best friend of several years
    C. Displays physically aggressive behavior toward others
    D. Manipulates others for own gain

12. A nurse conducts an assessment of the dynamics in the family of a young man with a conduct disorder. Which of the following patterns would be considered a predisposing factor in the development of the disorder?

    A. The parents have very high expectations of their children.

B. There is inconsistent limit setting with harsh discipline.
C. The parents are overinvolved with the child.
D. The parents have no other children.

13. A 14-year-old girl is being evaluated for anorexia nervosa. Which of the following would indicate to the nurse that the teenager displays symptoms of anorexia nervosa?

A. She has episodes of overeating and excessive weight gain.
B. She expresses a positive body image.
C. She has had severe weight loss due to self-imposed dieting.
D. She refuses to discuss food.

14. The nurse is obtaining a history from a 16-year-old girl. Which of the following might indicate that the client has symptoms of bulimia?

A. Binge eating and self-induced vomiting
B. Severe weight loss due to metabolic dysfunction
C. Hypertension and hyperglycemia
D. Diaphoresis and vasodilation

15. The nurse is caring for a 13-year-old girl with a diagnosis of anorexia nervosa. The nurse uses her understanding of psychodynamic and family influences in the development of anorexia nervosa to guide her planning. That understanding is reflected in which of the following goals?

A. Client will be able to interact effectively with peer group.
B. Client will be able to interact with staff using appropriate behaviors.
C. Client will demonstrate ability to cope with issues of control in a more adaptive manner.
D. Client will articulate high expectations for herself.

16. The nurse is evaluating the progress of a 17-year-old girl admitted with a diagnosis of bulimia. Which of the following behaviors would indicate that the client had progressed?

A. Her conversations focus on food.
B. She identifies healthy ways of coping with anxiety.
C. She spends time alone in her room after each meal.
D. Family contact around food times is minimal.

17. The nurse is caring for a newly admitted 19-year-old man with a history of abuse of street drugs. She observes that he is restless and irritable shortly after having received a visit from friends. The nurse suspects the client may have taken drugs brought in by the friends. Information that is a priority for the nurse to assess in a client suspected of use of drugs is:

A. Characteristics of his feces
B. His hemoglobin
C. His level of consciousness
D. The color of his nail beds

18. The nurse interviews an 18-year-old woman in the mental health clinic who has a history of drug use and asks for help. In planning treatment, the *most* important information for the nurse to obtain initially is:

A. How the client pays for the drug(s) being used
B. Her current height and weight

C. Her family's response to her drug use
D. The types, quantity, and frequency of the drug(s) used

19. A nurse is obtaining an admission history on a 22-year-old man admitted for a major depressive episode and alcohol abuse. The nurse learns that the client had been drinking 2–3 six-packs of beer a day for the last year and recently lost his job. His wife and 5-month-old son moved into her mother's home 2 weeks ago. In further discussing his alcohol abuse the client states: "I wouldn't drink so much if my wife hadn't nagged me constantly about getting a better job, making more money. I was never good enough for her." The nurse recognizes that this statement *most* likely suggests:

A. A dysfunctional family
B. The client is in denial about his alcohol problem
C. The stressors were too much for this man
D. The client will have a better prognosis if he remains separated from his wife

20. A 7-year-old girl with a diagnosis of separation anxiety disorder has been admitted to an inpatient psychiatric adolescent unit for further evaluation. Which of the following behaviors would the nurse recognize as a common characteristic of this disorder?

A. She isolates herself in her room and has minimal interaction with adults.
B. She adjusts quickly to the unit and exhibits deep attachment to her primary nurse.
C. She becomes acutely anxious whenever her mother visits but is relaxed after her mother leaves.
D. She is preoccupied and anxious on the unit, clings to her mother when she visits, and becomes agitated and out of control when her mother leaves.

21. A primary intervention in caring for a school-age girl with a diagnosis of separation anxiety disorder who requires hospitalization would be:

A. Do not allow the child to verbalize her fears and worries.
B. Establish trust by interacting with the child in a calm manner communicating genuine positive regard.
C. Discourage peer interaction because it contributes to her anxiety.
D. Discourage the mother from visiting because it is too upsetting when she leaves.

22. In an initial interview with a 24-year-old man with a diagnosis of generalized anxiety disorder, the nurse could expect to observe which of the following behaviors?

A. Irritability, difficulty concentrating on the interview
B. Future orientation
C. Increased assertiveness
D. Grandiose ideation

23. The nurse is caring for a 24-year-old man with a generalized anxiety disorder. In assisting the client to be less anxious, which of the following nursing actions would be *most* appropriate?

A. Maintaining a calm and supportive manner while interacting
B. Encouraging the client to cry

C. Administering major tranquilizing drugs

D. Beginning intensive psychotherapy

24. Medication is sometimes needed with clients who have a generalized anxiety disorder. Which of the following would be a likely drug that the nurse would administer?

A. Thorazine (chlorpromazine)

B. Lorazepam

C. Tofranil (imipramine)

D. Noctec (chloral hydrate)

25. The nurse is caring for a 35-year-old woman with agoraphobia. Which of the following behaviors would the nurse expect to observe in the client?

A. The client is afraid of talking to other people.

B. The client is afraid to leave her home.

C. The client is afraid of pain.

D. The client is afraid of fire.

26. In implementing treatment for a client with a phobic disorder, nursing actions include:

A. Insight-oriented psychotherapy

B. Administering lithium

C. Desensitization treatment

D. Crisis intervention

27. In providing care to a client with an obsessive-compulsive disorder, the nurse recognizes that the client's frequent, intensive, and extensive hand washing is an attempt to:

A. Relieve underlying anxiety

B. Give herself a sense of control over her life

C. Increase her self-esteem

D. Reduce the possibility of infection

28. The goals of nursing care for a client admitted to a psychiatric unit with obsessive-compulsive disorder should be that he will:

A. Demonstrate frequent decision making

B. Experience a variety of environmental stimuli

C. Have time and opportunity to complete rituals

D. Demonstrate improvement in behavior within 1 week

29. The nurse is caring for a 30-year-old woman admitted with a diagnosis of PTSD. Three months ago, the client had found the body of her husband, who had hung himself, in their basement. The nurse could expect her to exhibit all but which of the following behaviors:

A. Recurrent distressing dreams

B. Irritability and outbursts of anger

C. Inability to look at husband's picture

D. Discussing plans to remarry someday

30. The nurse is caring for a client admitted 1 week ago with a diagnosis of PTSD. Today he begins to describe the traumatic event that occurred in his life 6 months ago. The best response by the nurse would be to:

A. Allow the client to describe the event and listen empathically

B. Change the subject because the topic is clearly upsetting the client

C. Tell the client that the event was not as bad as he remembers it

D. Encourage the client to share his experience in the therapeutic group meeting

31. The nurse is caring for a 55-year-old client with a diagnosis of somatoform disorder. He has had a thorough physical exam and has been told he does not have cardiac pathology. The client complains of chest pain. His electrocardiogram is fine with no changes noted. The nurse should expect that somatoform disorders will be characterized by:

A. Preoccupation with sexuality

B. Fear of high places

C. Preoccupation with inanimate objects

D. Preoccupation with own health

32. A 45-year-old man is recently admitted with a diagnosis of somatoform disorder. He is convinced he has a serious heart problem. He takes his pulse frequently. One of the primary goals of his nursing care is to:

A. Challenge the validity of his physical symptoms.

B. Coordinate diagnostic testing to rule out an organic basis for the symptoms.

C. Encourage his dependency needs.

D. Discourage family participation in treatment.

33. The morning she is to leave for college, a client finds her legs suddenly paralyzed. After an extensive diagnostic workup, no organic basis is found for the paralysis, which does not conform to neurological pathways as the cause. She is diagnosed as having conversion disorder and admitted to the psychiatric unit. Which of the following nursing actions is *most* appropriate in caring for the client?

A. Promote her dependence to decrease her anxiety.

B. Explain to her that her paralysis is not real.

C. Encourage her to discuss her feelings about losing the use of her legs.

D. Avoid reinforcing or focusing on her paralysis.

34. A 20-year-old client is newly admitted to a psychiatric unit for conversion disorder. The nurse does an admission assessment and finds that he shows little emotion about his sudden inability to feel sensations in both arms. The nurse recognizes this as a common characteristic in clients with the conversion disorder known as:

A. La belle indifférence

B. Fugue state

C. Secondary gain

D. Akathesia

35. A 24-year-old woman is brought to the crisis clinic. Her family states that she cries all the time, and does not leave the house very often. She is evaluated for a depressive episode. The nurse could expect to observe which of the following behaviors if the client is depressed?

A. Sexual preoccupation

B. Psychomotor retardation

C. Hyperexcitability

D. Excessive talking

36. The nurse is developing a care plan for a severely depressed 35-year-old woman with four small children.

Which of the following would not be an appropriate goal for this client?

A. Client will not harm self.
B. Client will be able to verbalize positive aspects about herself.
C. Client will participate in unit activities.
D. Client will focus on self and not family.

37. The nurse administers nortriptyline (Aventyl) 75 mg a day to a client admitted with major depression. After 4 days, the client states that the medication is not helping her. The *best* nursing response to this client would be:

A. "It can take up to 4 weeks for the medication to bring about an improvement in symptoms."
B. "Cheer up. You need to try to have a more positive attitude toward the medicine."
C. "I'll tell the doctor. She may need to change the medicine."
D. "Try not to dwell on the symptoms. It's time for group."

38. A 60-year-old woman who is hospitalized with pneumonia is due to be discharged tomorrow. The nurse notices that she has not touched her food. The client states, "I don't feel hungry. I don't know what the point is. I don't know why God spared me. I don't have the energy to keep going on." The *best* nursing response would be:

A. "Now don't talk like that. You'll feel better when you go home."
B. "It's normal to feel sad leaving the nurses after we've been so good to you."
C. "You sound very sad today. Tell me a little more about how you're feeling."
D. "I'll tell the doctor that you've lost your appetite and feel weak. It might be the medicine."

39. A 55-year-old woman is scheduled for ECT the next morning. The nurse knows that ECT is *most* commonly prescribed for:

A. Disorganized schizophrenia
B. Major depression
C. Antisocial personality disorder
D. Dissociative disorder

40. A male client is scheduled for ECT in the morning. He asks, "What am I going to be like after the treatment?" The *best* nursing response would be:

A. "You will go to the intensive care unit. But if all goes well you should return to our psychiatric unit in a day or two."
B. "You will be in the ECT recovery room for about an hour until the anesthesia wears off, and you will be awake and oriented and can get out of bed. You may experience some confusion, which is temporary."
C. "You will be in the ECT recovery room for about an hour until the anesthesia wears off. When you awake you'll feel much better than you have been feeling."
D. "It must be frightening to be getting ECT. Tell me more about your fears."

41. A 38-year-old man is diagnosed with a paranoid personality disorder. He has been coming to the mental health clinic since his wife divorced him. He thinks that his wife left him because her coworkers demanded it. The nurse is aware that paranoid personality disorders are *most* frequently characterized by:

A. Hearing voices
B. Rigid, hypersensitive, and suspicious behavior
C. Engaging social skills
D. Motivation to seek treatment

42. One nursing goal in the care plan for a client with a paranoid personality disorder is promoting consensual validation of reality. Which of the following nursing actions would be *most* appropriate to achieve this goal?

A. Reinforce reality but avoid arguing with the client about his perceptions.
B. Use humor to challenge his perceptions.
C. Discourage him from verbalizing his perceptions.
D. Administer antidepressant drugs to decrease his depression.

43. The nurse is developing a care plan for a client with a paranoid personality disorder. He has been hospitalized after repeatedly yelling and calling police day and night on his neighbors, whom he suspects of plotting to have him removed from his home. The nurse wishes to assist the client to be less socially isolated. Which of the following goals would be *most* applicable?

A. Share his belongings with others.
B. Engage in group activities and share his feelings freely.
C. Have as much control as possible over his environment.
D. Participate in solitary activities.

44. A 22-year-old woman has been diagnosed with a schizoid personality disorder. Her frequent problems with family and employer have brought her to the crisis clinic. She states that her employer is a real tyrant. The nurse knows that a common characteristic of schizoid personality disorder is:

A. Lethargy
B. Sexual preoccupation
C. Two personalities
D. Tendency to withdraw from others

45. The nurse wishes to establish a supportive therapeutic relationship with a 22-year-old woman with a diagnosis of schizoid personality disorder. In developing a plan of care, it is *most* important for the nurse to:

A. Allow the client's need for distance in a relationship
B. Minimize affiliative needs
C. Encourage her to participate in intensive group therapy
D. Assign different nurses each day until she finds one to whom she can relate

46. A 22-year-old woman is admitted with a diagnosis of schizoid personality disorder. The nurse assesses that her family does not seem interested in being involved in her care. Which of the following behaviors would the nurse want to promote in the family?

A. Challenge her "loner" behavior.
B. Encourage her to continue in treatment because her condition is long-term.

C. Expect a full recovery within the near future.
D. Have weekly family meetings in which the family discusses her behavior.

47. A 21-year-old man has frequent problems with the local police. He is admitted to the psychiatric unit following an attempted hanging while in jail awaiting trial on burglary charges. The nurse is aware that clients with antisocial personality disorders are frequently characterized by:

A. Below average intelligence, high sexual needs
B. Religious preoccupation, grandiose ideas
C. Need for immediate gratification, low tolerance for frustration
D. Ability to learn from experience, criminal records

48. A 28-year-old male client with a history of antisocial personality disorder is admitted to the psychiatric unit because of a suicide attempt while in jail awaiting trial for assault. The client acts very disinterested in treatment and has developed a rapport with several clients whom he is influencing in negative ways. In evaluating his progress, the nurse recognizes that he:

A. Could make behavioral changes within a short time if motivated
B. May not be motivated to change his behavior or lifestyle
C. Manipulates others but does not manipulate family members
D. Usually requires intensive psychotropic drug therapy, which he refuses

49. The nurse is planning the care of a 30-year-old man admitted to the psychiatric unit for court-mandated treatment for alcohol dependence. The client has a diagnosis of antisocial personality disorder as documented in previous court-mandated psychiatric evaluations. The nurse recognizes that an important part of this client's plan will be to:

A. Encourage him to set limits on his own behavior.
B. Establish clear, consistent limits on acting-out behaviors.
C. Minimize peer interactions.
D. Expect full family participation in effective treatment.

50. A 29-year-old client has been admitted to the psychiatric unit with a diagnosis of paranoid schizophrenia because of strange behaviors that alarmed his neighbors. The nurse would expect him to exhibit which behavior?

A. Psychomotor retardation and posturing
B. Regressed, childlike behavior
C. Euphoric mood and sexual acting out
D. Extreme suspiciousness, delusions, and hallucinations

51. A 30-year-old man with a diagnosis of paranoid schizophrenia is admitted to the psychiatric unit with an acute exacerbation of his illness. He had stopped taking his medication and ceased his bimonthly visits to the outpatient department. He is restarted on his medication. The drug *most* commonly ordered for his illness is:

A. Lorazepam
B. Haldol

C. Amitriptyline (Elavil)
D. Isocarboxazid (Marplan)

52. A 22-year-old client with a diagnosis of undifferentiated schizophrenia is being treated with haloperidol 5 mg bid. He was estranged from his father for several years. Recently he has been spending some time with his father. His father comes with him to an appointment at the mental health clinic and asks the nurse what the haloperidol is for. The nurse explains that haloperidol is given to:

A. Reduce extrapyramidal symptoms
B. Prevent neuroleptic malignant syndrome
C. Decrease psychotic symptoms
D. Assist with sleep

53. A 20-year-old woman has recently been diagnosed with paranoid schizophrenia. She has been started on Haldol and seems to be responding less to hallucinations. She has begun to attend an art group for brief periods each day. In planning care to assist the client to be more connected to reality, the nurse should:

A. Reinforce perceptions and thinking that are in touch with reality.
B. Challenge her expressions of distorted thinking.
C. Use peer pressure to discourage delusions.
D. Ignore distorted thinking and bizarre behavior.

54. The nurse is providing care for a client who is taking haloperidol 2 mg bid and has an order for benzotropine (Cogentin) 1 mg bid prn. Which of the following nursing assessments would indicate a need for benzotropine?

A. The client's level of agitation increases.
B. The client develops tremors and drooling.
C. The client complains of a headache.
D. The client has difficulty falling asleep.

55. A 23-year-old female client has been admitted to the inpatient psychiatric unit with a diagnosis of catatonic schizophrenia. She appears weak and pale. The nurse would expect to observe which behaviors in this client?

A. Scratching, catlike motions of the extremities
B. Exaggerated suspiciousness, excessive food intake
C. Stuporous withdrawal, hallucinations, and delusions
D. Sexual preoccupation, word salad

56. The nurse is collecting data to plan the care of a 21-year-old woman with a diagnosis of catatonic schizophrenia. The nurse would likely observe that this client:

A. Has excessive weight gain
B. Appears overhydrated
C. Is hyperreactive to stimuli
D. Stands, sits, or lies immobile

57. The nurse is providing care to a 25-year-old woman experiencing an acute phase of catatonic schizophrenia. One nursing goal is to decrease the client's isolated behavior. Which of the following nursing actions would *best* contribute to that goal?

A. Provide a colorful environment.
B. Speak in concise, simple terms to prevent sensory overload.

C. Avoid setting limits on her behavior.
D. Encourage participation in group therapy.

58. A 23-year-old woman is experiencing an acute phase of catatonic schizophrenia that is not responding to psychopharmacological treatment. She is scheduled for ECT in the morning. A preoperative drug that the nurse would *most* likely administer prior to the treatment would be:

   A. Atropine
   B. Inderal (propranolol)
   C. Lithium
   D. Dalmane (flurazepam)

59. A 42-year-old woman has been admitted to the psychiatric unit with a diagnosis of bipolar disorder, manic phase. She had discontinued her medication as an outpatient and has experienced a significant increase in dysfunctional behavior. On admission, the client is dressed in very colorful clothes with heavy makeup. During the manic phase, the nurse would anticipate assessing which behavior in the client?

   A. Bizarre thoughts
   B. Intense, labile mood
   C. Extreme suspiciousness
   D. Auditory hallucinations

60. The nurse is collecting data on a 42-year-old woman admitted to the psychiatric unit with bipolar disorder, manic phase. The nurse looks through the client's chart. Which of the following information in the chart would reflect a common characteristic of a client with bipolar disorder, manic phase?

   A. Increased REM sleep
   B. Lithium level of 0.15 mEq/L
   C. High intracellular sodium levels
   D. Hypotension

61. The symptoms the nurse would expect to observe in clients experiencing lithium toxicity would be:

   A. Skin rash, photosensitivity
   B. Urinary retention, orthostatic hypotension
   C. Dystonia, akathesia
   D. Ataxia, persistent nausea and vomiting, severe diarrhea

62. The nurse realizes that clients with bipolar disorder who are unable to tolerate therapeutic doses of lithium to prevent decompensation will *most* likely be treated with:

   A. Moban (molindone)
   B. Carbamazepine (tegretol)
   C. Halcion (triazolam)
   D. Sinequan (doxepin)

63. The nurse is developing a plan of care for a 42-year-old woman who is experiencing an acute manic phase of her bipolar disorder. The nurse wants to assist the client to decrease her hyperactive behavior. An appropriate nursing action would be:

   A. Allowing her to set her own limits on her behavior
   B. Encouraging activities that require concentration
   C. Providing a stimulating environment
   D. Providing calm, consistent behavior by staff

64. The nurse is planning the care of a client in the acute manic phase of bipolar disorder. A nursing goal is for the client to meet her nutritional needs. The *most* appropriate nursing action to meet this goal would be to:

   A. Engage the client in frequent conversations at meal times
   B. Encourage the client to eat small, frequent meals
   C. Have the client keep detailed records of intake and output
   D. Provide the client with literature on the four food groups

65. A 62-year-old man has been admitted to the inpatient psychiatric unit with a diagnosis of unipolar major depression. He has a history of two previous suicide attempts. During the nursing admission interview, the client sits with his eyes downcast. The nurse is aware that these behaviors are signs and symptoms of:

   A. Labile mood swings from euphoria to depression
   B. Minimal sleep and appetite disturbance
   C. Persistent feelings of hopelessness and worthlessness
   D. Auditory hallucinations

66. A 68-year-old man is admitted to the psychiatric unit with unipolar major depression after a suicide attempt with carbon monoxide poisoning. He tells the nurse that he has been thinking of taking an overdose. Nursing actions to decrease his suicidal preoccupation should focus on:

   A. Using seclusion to reassure him of his safety
   B. Encouraging him to make decisions
   C. Developing a supportive relationship so he can express his thoughts and feelings
   D. Reminding him frequently that he is on suicide precautions

67. A client was diagnosed with a unipolar major depression and has been receiving a tricyclic antidepressant. The nurse has been assisting him to grieve for the death of his wife 3 months ago. He states, "I don't think I'll ever get over losing Elizabeth." The *best* nursing response would be:

   A. "Don't be so hard on yourself. You'll get over this before you know it."
   B. "You must be feeling very sad and lonely right now."
   C. "You need to focus on today, and forget the past."
   D. "The antidepressant medication will help you get over losing your wife."

68. The nurse is conducting an admission history on a 28-year-old man. If the client is diagnosed with pedophilia, the nurse should expect that he:

   A. Derives sexual pleasure through window peeking
   B. Derives sexual pleasure from children
   C. Derives sexual pleasure from animals
   D. Exposes genitals to others

69. The nurse is a co-leader of a therapy group for men with paraphilias. The men in the group may have different types of paraphilias, but persons with this diagnosis have the following in common:

   A. Repetitive or preferred sexual fantasies or behaviors that are maladaptive and that may be harmful to themselves or others

B. Phobias that contribute to their inability to function
C. Difficulty sustaining erections through intercourse
D. Guilt-ridden feelings, active seeking of treatment

70. The nurse is assessing a 21-year-old man who presented with several lacerations to his chest and back. The client admits to the nurse that the lacerations were part of a sexual act and that he finds it difficult to become sexually aroused unless he submits to aggression. The nurse recognizes this behavior as characteristic of a paraphilia known as:

A. Sadism
B. Masochism
C. Frotteurism
D. Fetishism

71. In assessing a 32-year-old man with a diagnosis of pedophilia, the nurse observed that he appears to have low self-esteem. An additional common characteristic of psychosexual disorders is:

A. Little attachment to others
B. Feelings of guilt
C. Clear understanding of behavior
D. Above-average intelligence

72. A 58-year-old professional man has been admitted to the inpatient substance abuse unit with a diagnosis of alcohol dependence. His plan of care should be based on the rationale that alcoholism is:

A. Excessive social drinking
B. Drinking resulting in increasingly severe hangovers
C. Physiological and psychological dependence with impaired health
D. Increased periods of forgetfulness

73. A client has been admitted to an inpatient substance abuse clinic with alcoholism. He is a professional man who is in danger of losing his job of 30 years because of his drinking and states, "Look, I know I've had a little trouble lately, but this is a mistake. I can quit any time I want. I don't belong here. I don't need this kind of help." The *best* nursing response would be:

A. "You probably could do this as an outpatient. I'll call your family to discuss it."
B. "Why do you think you are here?"
C. "You're an alcoholic, and it's time to admit it."
D. "You are here because your drinking is jeopardizing your job."

74. The nurse is approached by the wife of a 62-year-old man who has just been admitted to the inpatient substance abuse unit for alcoholism. He is in danger of losing his position as an engineer because of his drinking. She states, "This is all my fault. I told my husband I was tired of lying to his boss every week to cover his absences. Now he might lose his job. I should never have let him go to work that day." The best nursing response would be:

A. "Why didn't you call in for him?"
B. "Your husband needs to experience the consequences of his behavior."
C. "You've done too much to protect your husband."

D. "What's happened has happened. It's best we deal with the present."

75. The nurse is caring for a client who has been admitted for routine surgery. The client's history of alcoholism was not known and he experienced abrupt withdrawal from alcohol after chronic consumption. The serious physiological symptom that resulted was:

A. Blackouts
B. Delirium tremens
C. Hypocalcemia
D. Constricted pupils

76. A 33-year-old man who is completing his inpatient stay in a substance abuse unit for alcoholism begins to go to AA meetings. He tells the nurse that he thinks he is coming to acceptance of step 1 in the AA Program. The nurse understands the client to mean that:

A. He is ready to be a sponsor for other alcoholics seeking help
B. He wants to ask his family for forgiveness
C. He is ready to admit that he is powerless over alcohol and that he needs help
D. He is ready to make a searching and fearless moral inventory of himself

77. A 73-year-old man is admitted to the inpatient psychiatric unit from a local nursing home with a diagnosis of dementia, etiology unknown. He mumbles when he talks. The nurse is aware that the client may have other characteristics of dementia, which are:

A. Stuporous withdrawal and muteness
B. Extreme suspiciousness and inability to trust
C. Confusion and impaired cognitive functioning
D. Hypochondriasis and irritability

78. The nurse conducts a mental status exam on a 73-year-old man with dementia, etiology unknown. Which of the following characteristics would the nurse *most* likely find in the mental status exam of a client with this syndrome:

A. Euphoric mood
B. Decreased ability for abstract thinking
C. Auditory hallucinations
D. Echolalia

79. A 73-year-old man is admitted to a psychiatric unit for evaluation of dementia, etiology unknown. During his hospitalization, tests will be conducted to rule out a reversible condition that is contributing to his symptoms. The nurse expects that these tests will include:

A. Serum electrolytes
B. Rorschach Test
C. Minnesota Multiphasic Personality Inventory
D. Vital signs 4 times a day for 10 days

80. The nurse recognizes the importance of controlling the environment for a 73-year-old client who has been diagnosed with primary degenerative dementia (Alzheimer's). Which of the following would be an appropriate nursing action?

A. Changing furniture placement to enhance variety
B. Minimizing lighting

C. Encouraging a variety of visitors
D. Providing external signs of orientation (e.g., clocks and calendars)

81. A primary goal in developing a plan of care for a client with an organic brain syndrome is:

A. The client will maintain social skills.
B. The client will complete all ADL independently.
C. The client will be safe from injury.
D. The client will maintain nutritional status.

82. A 43-year-old mother of three school-age children is dying of metastasized breast cancer. She has been an elementary school teacher for 20 years and has many friends and a close family. In caring for her, the nurse expects to observe changes in behavior. The nurse is aware that the first behavior an individual who is dying usually exhibits is:

A. Shock
B. Denial
C. Avoidance
D. Acceptance

83. A 43-year-old mother of three children who is dying of metastasized breast cancer is still able to communicate. A nursing action to promote optimum care would be to:

A. Provide her with opportunities to have some control over her environment
B. Encourage her to try experimental treatments
C. Discourage her making decisions about treatment
D. Encourage her to verbalize her regrets

84. In interacting with clients on the psychiatric inpatient unit, the nurse demonstrates congruence between what she feels and what she expresses. This characteristic, which is important in establishing a therapeutic relationship, is known as:

A. Trust
B. Respect
C. Genuineness
D. Empathy

85. The nurse leads a goal-setting group on the inpatient psychiatric unit twice a week. A depressed and withdrawn client is listening intently to another depressed client hesitantly verbalize a goal for herself. The group is respectful and acknowledges the client's contribution. Toward the end of the group session, she also verbalizes a goal for the first time since her admission. Which therapeutic effect of group did she demonstrate?

A. Altruism
B. Group cohesiveness
C. Imitative behavior
D. Catharsis

86. The nursing staff members of an inpatient psychiatric unit for acute, short-term admissions use the concepts of therapeutic community (therapeutic milieu) to organize their unit. Which of the following is *not* characteristic of a therapeutic community:

A. The staff clearly and consistently communicates to client what are acceptable and unacceptable behaviors and the consequences if limits are violated.

B. Every interaction with a client is understood by the nurse as an opportunity for a therapeutic intervention.
C. Individual client care is directed by an interdisciplinary team of psychiatrist, psychiatric nurse, social worker, activities therapist, etc.
D. Behavior modification is the only treatment modality used.

87. A 45-year-old woman has recently been divorced after 25 years of marriage. Her ex-husband is planning to marry the woman with whom he has been having an affair for 5 years. The wife comes to the mental health clinic for help. She has never required psychiatric care in the past. She describes feeling enraged and betrayed. She states, "I just don't know where to turn or what to do." The nurse realizes that the *most* appropriate treatment approach for her would be:

A. Intensive psychotherapy
B. Crisis intervention
C. Relaxation therapy
D. ECT

88. A client in a mental health facility tells the clinical nurse specialist that his employer encourages all employees to join the newly implemented healthcare policy under managed care, which includes a mental health reimbursement portion. The nurse explains to the client that a form of financing mental health care under managed care separates mental health services from medical benefits. Which one of the following represents this form of care?

A. Fee-for-service
B. Symptom management
C. Carve-out system
D. Retrospective payment

89. In planning care for a group of psychiatric clients in a partial hospital setting, the nurse has an essential role in providing and directing care. Which one of the following statements accurately reflects the principle role of the nurse case manager?

A. Coordinates care and services.
B. Promotes planned physical health care.
C. Provides partial advocacy role on behalf of clients.
D. Reduces fragmentation of the mental healthcare system.

90. In delivering healthcare services to psychiatric mental health clients in an inpatient setting, the nurse is aware that many current healthcare issues and changes affect the care provided by professional nurses. Which one of the following conditions, would be beneficial to assist nurses in delivering safe and quality patient care?

A. A proactive workplace advocacy program
B. The use of unlicensed assistive personnel (UAP)
C. A decrease in wage growth
D. The collection and integration of detailed healthcare outcomes

91. Mr. A. is referred for psychiatric mental health care because of noncompliance with his medications. The nurse case manager acknowledges the provisions and requirements of his health insurance policy. Which of the following correctly relates to managed care provisions and cost control measures?

A. Long-term hospital stay focusing on charismatic cure is preferred.

B. The medical providership implements pre-admission certification for inpatient care.

C. Pre-certification for crisis and high-risk behaviors is required.

D. Client's selection of a personal psychiatrist or therapist is guaranteed.

92. Ms. S. seeks assistance from the mental health clinic to help her resolve a crisis situation. Because of the access problems that apply to the entire healthcare system, Ms. S. was assessed and referred to another agency, causing the nurse great concern. Which approach would best help the nurse assist the client with changes in the healthcare system?

A. Seek stability, parity, and equilibrium.

B. Seek a nursing position that will ensure financial maintenance and job security.

C. Develop cultural competence and be able to negotiate complex systems.

D. Obtain control of the environment.

93. The psychiatric home care nurse visits a 55-year-old client with multiple physical and mental healthcare needs. Prior to the weekend visit, the client telephones the nurse and requests that the nurse arrange for transportation to Sunday church service and the nurse complies. One problem associated with using case management in psychiatric home care is that:

A. Many time-consuming tasks performed by the case manager occur outside the home visit and are not reimbursable.

B. The nurse case manager works closely with healthcare insurance providers to employ strategies and interventions aimed at increased cost savings for the payer.

C. A responsibility of the nurse case manager is soliciting multiple healthcare providers that will agree to provide a variety of services for the client at any cost.

D. It allows treatment-resistant, chronically mentally ill individuals to increase dependency on others.

94. During the assessment phase of a newly admitted emergency room client, he exhibited severe aggression and hostility and assaulted the nurse. Violence against healthcare workers is one of the problems that has increased and is associated with the restructuring of health care. Which one of the following negatively affects the safety of delivery of nursing care in psychiatric-mental healthcare settings?

A. Inadequate staffing levels

B. Proper utilization of staff

C. Utilization of advanced security technology

D. Training for nurses on violence and self-defense.

95. Ms. J. has been prescribed an atypical antipsychotic agent. Which one of the following is an expected outcome of atypical antipsychotic medications?

A. Increased libido

B. Small effect on negative symptoms of schizophrenia

C. Vastly remote dramatic effects

D. Controls positive, negative and the overall symptoms of psychosis

96. Mr. R., whose only available support system is the staff at the mental health clinic, states that he is compliant with his medications but then admits he takes his medication whenever he needs it. Which of the following suggestions made by staff members reflects the best potential solution to the problem of client noncompliance?

A. Implement the commitment process.

B. Explore alternative treatment modalities with the client.

C. Tell the client that he has no other choice but to comply with the medication regimen.

D. Discharge the client, escort him from the premises and explain that because he is noncompliant he is costing the clinic extra healthcare dollars.

97. When planning care for a client, the nurse acknowledges that the interdisciplinary team has an advocacy role to play. Which of the following is an integral part of the role of nurse advocate?

A. Demanding that the client choose the interdisciplinary team's recommendations for health care.

B. Assisting the client to increase his abilities to make sound personal healthcare decisions.

C. Assuming full responsibility for customizing the client's care

D. Maintaining vigilance regarding the client in a dependent role

98. A small county local hospital, with the cooperation of the nursing staff, implemented the shared governance concept. Which one of the following would be beneficial in assisting the nursing staff to provide safe, effective care to all clients?

A. Defined boundaries

B. Increased input into unit function

C. Decrease control of the environment

D. Increased cost and lengths of stay for selected patients

99. Mr. Z., a client who is being treated for alcohol withdrawal symptoms and episodes of acute depression, has been prescribed clonazepam (Klonopin). Which of these characteristics associated with clonazepam (Klonopin) makes it a drug of choice for treating alcohol withdrawal symptoms?

A. It reduces sedative effects in the central nervous system.

B. It can be given orally or intravenously.

C. It decreases seizure threshold.

D. It is a shorter-acting agent.

100. The nurse's assignment as a discharge planner in an outpatient clinic uses which one of the following techniques that would effectively help substantiate the nurse's ability to provide prevention-focused health services for clients?

A. Participating in state and national nursing organizations

B. Relying on the competency of peers and unlicensed assistive personnel

C. Involvement in interdisciplinary team meetings and grand rounds

D. Documenting when clients take an active role in their own care through the nurse's interventions

101. Mr. K., a 40 year old, states that he suffers from angina pectoris (for which he is currently taking nitroglycerin), erectile dysfunction, and severe depression. He suggests to the clinical nurse specialist that a prescription for Viagra would help his sexual dysfunction and his depression. Which one of the following statements by the nurse would be most therapeutic?

A. "The prescription will be an out-of-pocket expense."
B. "Yes, Mr. K., Viagra will absolutely take care of your sexual dysfunction."
C. "Viagra may temporarily relieve your depression that is possibly caused by sexual dysfunction, but it is contraindicated for persons using organic nitrates."
D. "Viagra potentiates hypertensive effects of nitrates."

102. Mr. R. has been admitted to the psychiatric inpatient unit because he is aggressively psychotic and out of control. Which one of the following medications could be safely used for the acute-treatment phase?

A. Risperidone (Risperadol)
B. Lorazepam (Ativan)
C. Haloperidol (Haldol Deconoate)
D. Valproic acid (Depakene)

103. The nurse interviews a 30-year-old woman in the emergency room who has a history of being physically abused during her 8-year marriage. She has multiple bruises over her body and a broken nose. She stated that she has endured this reign of terror for the sake of her two children but is now motivated to escape the abusive relationship. Which one of the following statements would indicate to the nurse that the patient is ready to leave the situation and seek help through other resources?

A. "Where would I go? I want to protect my children from psychological harm but I perceive little support."
B. "If other women have made it, so can I."
C. "During the first year of marriage there were no signs of rage or bitterness."
D. "I can't make it alone without him."

104. Ms. T., a long time mental health clinic client, is concerned about the rapid changes in the health care system. Which one of the following statements by the nurse may alleviate her concerns?

A. "Your concerns about changes in the healthcare system are unfounded."
B. "If you were concerned about the healthcare system you would contact your legislative representative."
C. "Why would you be concerned? It is beyond your control."
D. "There are other treatment options that may help you take an active role in your care."

105. The nurse typically establishes which of the following guidelines for polypharmacy when working with a client using concurrent medications?

A. Increase patient adherence in the aftercare setting when medication regimen is complex.

B. Recognize that addictive side effects are diminished
C. Be aware of decreased cost of treatment
D. Patient education programs regarding polypharmacy must be particularly clear, organized, and effective.

106. After a recent discharge, Mr. L., who has had an extensive history of multiple psychiatric hospitalizations, continued to direct aggressive, harassing behaviors and written threats of harm toward a staff nurse. Which one of the following strategies is recommended?

A. Implement a change in work schedule.
B. Contemplate a change of residence.
C. File charges against Mr. L.
D. Examine societal changes of increased violence.

107. Ms. P., a Hispanic American who was a devout Catholic, suffered from a major depressive episode. The clinical nurse specialist prescribed an antidepressant and made an appointment for Ms. P. to return to the clinic in 1 week. Ms. P. told her daughter that she was not depressed, refused to take the medication, and would not return to the clinic. In 6 weeks, Ms. P. experienced an increase in the number of depressive episodes but denied suicidal ideation. Which one of the following is an important issue for the treating clinical nurse specialist?

A. Involuntary admission
B. Knowledge about spiritual healers
C. Knowledge about and sensitivity to the client's culture
D. Fluency in the client's language

108. Ms. T., a Hispanic American, sought treatment at the mental health clinic for weight loss, insomnia, back and neck pain. The therapist's initial diagnosis was depression. Prior to building trust and a therapeutic alliance, the best approach for the nurse therapist would be to focus on which one of the client's problems?

A. Medical
B. Psychological
C. Cultural resistance
D. Societal

109. Ms. B., a 35 year old, was diagnosed as having bipolar disorder with psychotic features. Her medical history cited hypertension. Her current medications include lithium carbonate (Lithane), benazepril (Lotensin) and carbamazepine (Tegretol). Because of nausea, diarrhea, and hand tremors, Ms. B. was being tapered off Lithane and onto Zyprexa. Which one of the following statements best describes the rationale for tapering the client's Lithium medication?

A. The client's psychotic behavior is less evident.
B. Diuretics may have increased the concentration toxicity of lithium carbonate.
C. Carbamazepine (Tegretol) is ineffective for the treatment of bipolar illness.
D. Olanzapine (Zyprexa) is preferred over lithium carbonate (Lithane)

110. N. is a 13 year old diagnosed as having attention deficit hyperactivity disorder and conduct disorder. The

client was prescribed guanfacine (Tenex) 5 mg bid to be taken at bedtime to minimize daytime sedation. In the past, N. had been prescribed methylphenidate (Ritalin) 10 mg at breakfast and lunch for attention-deficit hyperactivity, buspirone 5 mg bid (Buspar) for anxiety and haloperidol (Haldol) 1 mg bid for severe behavioral problems. Which one of the following would be the most appropriate nursing action?

A. Set firm and consistent limits.
B. Monitor the blood pressure.
C. Assess the side effects of methylphenidate (Ritalin).
D. Allow the client to express anger by acting out in a physical manner.

111. Ms T., a 42-year-old woman with a history of panic disorder, continued to have daily panic attacks with limited phobic avoidance. As an adjunctive use in patients with panic disorder, the client was prescribed gabapentin (Neurontin) 100 mg daily and titrated to 300 mg tid. over a 2-week period. Ms. T. experienced a marked reduction in panic frequency and a reduction in phobic avoidance within 5 weeks of taking the medication. When teaching the client about gabapentin (Neurotin) the nurse should include which one of the following?

A. Advise the client to take an antacid prior to each dose of the medication to prevent heartburn.
B. Discontinue medication immediately if the client feels emotionally distraught.
C. Alcohol use is acceptable with gabapentin (Neurotin).
D. Continue on the medication regimen along with your other concurrent medications.

112. Mr. S. was admitted to the emergency room because his wife complained of his delusional behavior. Mr. S. demanded to know the purpose of his admission. The psychiatric clinical nurse specialist is aware that she is accountable to the client. Which one of the following statements describes the nurse's accountability requirements?

A. The nurse is responsible for the success of treatment.
B. The nurse must disclose to the client the purpose of nursing activities.
C. The nurse must disclose to the client the expected medical outcomes.
D. The nurse is not expected to keep the client informed regarding the purpose of the work to be done.

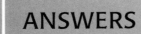

1. **(D)** Client need: psychosocial integrity; subcategory: psychosocial adaptation; content area: psychiatric

   RATIONALE

   (A) The abused child often has behavior inappropriate to social situations. (B) The abused child often exhibits fear and withdrawal in the presence of parents and avoids parental contact. (C) The abused child may exhibit delayed achievement of developmental tasks due to fear of socialization, inconsistent parental response to achievement, and overwhelming anxiety. (D) A common psychosocial characteristic of an abused child is withdrawal and minimal socialization with peers.

2. **(B)** Client need: safe, effective care environment; subcategory: management of care; content area: psychiatric

   RATIONALE

   (A) Having several nurses take care of the child would decrease feelings of security and make it difficult to establish trust in care providers. (B) Providing a nonthreatening, nurturing environment is an important part of the nursing plan of care for a hospitalized abused child. The child has come from an unpredictable, abusive environment and cannot begin the healing process unless exposed to a more positive setting. (C) The child needs opportunities to express her feelings and receive comfort. Not allowing the child to express her thoughts and feelings would prevent important catharsis. (D) Abused children are often afraid of their parents. Their presence during care activities would intensify the child's fear and interfere with the nurse's attempts to promote a nurturing environment for care.

3. **(C)** Client need: health promotion and maintenance; subcategory: growth and development through the life span; content area: psychiatric

   RATIONALE

   (A) A high energy level in a parent is not necessarily linked to child abuse. (B) Having several children is not necessarily linked to child abuse. (C) People abused as children have a much higher likelihood of becoming abusive parents. (D) Child abuse is found in all socioeconomic strata.

4. **(C)** Client need: psychosocial integrity; subcategory: psychosocial adaptation; content area: psychiatric

   RATIONALE

   (A) An autistic child is often very interested in inanimate objects. (B) The autistic child likes routine and is disturbed by lack of routine. (C) Unresponsiveness to others is a common characteristic of an autistic child. Lack of responsiveness to others can be identified by observing behavior. (D) The autistic child is usually of average or above-average intelligence.

5. **(A)** Client need: psychosocial integrity; subcategory: psychosocial adaptation; content area: psychiatric

   RATIONALE

   (A) Having the same nurses provide care is an important intervention with an autistic child. This will meet the child's need for routine. Moreover, there is an increased likelihood of his interacting with one or two nurses rather than with several. (B) Administering methylphenidate has not been shown to be effective in treating the sometimes hyperactive behavior of an autistic child. (C) Discouraging peer contact could lead to further withdrawal from socialization. (D) The child needs external controls on eating and sleeping patterns. An external routine is generally reassuring to an autistic child.

6. **(C)** Client need: psychosocial integrity; subcategory: psychosocial adaptation; content area: psychiatric

   RATIONALE

   (A) Isolating the child would only increase his withdrawal. (B) The autistic child has minimal verbal skills and could not be expected to be able to explain his angry thoughts or feelings. (C) The nurse must intervene to protect the child physically while assuming a nonpunitive approach. The autistic child cannot be expected to limit his own behavior. (D) Getting parental input could be helpful from a preventative standpoint but is not an appropriate intervention at the time when the behavior is occurring.

7. **(D)** Client need: psychosocial integrity; subcategory: psychosocial adaptation; content area: psychiatric

   RATIONALE

   (A) A hyperactive child exhibits constant psychomotor activity, not lethargy. (B) Children with this disorder are very distracted by environmental stimuli and would not be focused on self. (C) Very poor verbal skills are not characteristic of this disorder. (D) Short attention span is a common characteristic of hyperactive children due to their distractibility and restlessness. They have difficulty concentrating.

8. **(B)** Client need: psychosocial integrity; subcategory: psychosocial adaptation; content area: psychiatric

   RATIONALE

   (A) Increasing environmental stimulation and peer interaction might lead to increased hyperactivity. (B) Drug therapy (e.g., methylphenidate) and behavior modification are effective implementations with a hyperactive child. Ritalin decreases hyperactivity, and behavior modification reinforces positive behaviors. (C) Parental education is important, but not the most effective intervention. Diet modification to decrease the amount of sugar may assist in decreasing hyperactivity but is not the most effective means. (D) The nurse should encourage the achievement of normal developmental tasks as much as possible.

9. **(C)** Client need: psychosocial integrity; subcategory: psychosocial adaptation; content area: psychiatric

   RATIONALE

   (A) It is important that parents focus on the welfare of the total family and not just the affected child. The nurse should encourage the parents to integrate the child into family life as much as possible. (B) The sooner diagnostic studies are begun, the sooner appropriate treatment and planning for care can begin. (C) An important goal in the nursing care of a mentally retarded child is to modify the child's environment to promote independence and impulse control. The child's strengths should be accentuated. (D) Increased peer interaction is important for assisting a retarded child to learn socialization skills.

10. **(C)** Client need: psychosocial integrity; subcategory: psychosocial adaptation; content area: psychiatric

    RATIONALE

    (A) The client with severe mental retardation has an IQ range of 20–34 and has minimal verbal skills. The client with this degree of mental retardation typically uses behavior to communicate. Strictly verbal explanations would be meaningless. (B) The severely mentally retarded person does not have the necessary ability to interact at the level required to role play. (C) Systematic habit training is the most effective method of teaching simple self-care behaviors to a severely mentally retarded client. (D) This client would require close supervision and is unable to perform most tasks independently in a safe manner.

11. **(B)** Client need: psychosocial integrity; subcategory: psychosocial adaptation; content area: psychiatric

RATIONALE

(A) Fire setting is one of a list of behaviors that can be used to diagnose conduct disorder in the *DSM-III-R*. (B) Children and adolescents with conduct disorder typically demonstrate the inability to have close sustained relationships with peers. (C) Physically aggressive behavior that violates the rights of others is a classic characteristic of conduct disorder. (D) Children and adolescents with conduct disorder use maladaptive ways to get needs met, including manipulation and coercion.

12. **(B)** Client need: health promotion and maintenance; subcategory: growth and development through the life span; content area: psychiatric

RATIONALE

(A) Family dynamics that contribute to a predisposition of conduct disorder include parental neglect or rejection. Parents often have very little expectations of their children. (B) Inconsistent limit setting with harsh, angry discipline is a common characteristic in families of children with conduct disorder. Consequences do not match behavior. (C) Parental rejection or neglect is a family dynamic identified as a contributor to predisposition of conduct disorder. (D) Large family size is a family factor identified as a contributor to the predisposition of conduct disorder.

13. **(C)** Client need: physiological integrity; subcategory: basic care and comfort; content area: psychiatric

RATIONALE

(A) Clients with anorexia nervosa have poor food intake and are obsessed with thinness. (B) Clients with anorexia nervosa express a distorted body image, believing themselves "fat" or feeling "fat," despite emaciated appearance. (C) Clients with anorexia nervosa have body weight at least 15% below minimal normal weight for their age. Weight loss is accomplished through severe reduction in food intake, concentration of fiber and low-calorie food in the diet, and excessive exercising. (D) Clients with anorexia nervosa often display an obsession with food, talking about food and recipes at great length and making elaborate meals for others.

14. **(A)** Client need: physiological integrity; subcategory: basic care and comfort; content area: psychiatric

RATIONALE

(A) Binge eating and self-induced vomiting are characteristics of bulimia. The client often binges on high-carbohydrate foods and induces vomiting to purge herself of the excess calories. (B) Most clients with bulimia are within normal weight range or slightly above or below. (C) Vomiting can lead to hypotension and hypoglycemia. (D) Excessive vomiting and laxative and diuretic use can lead to dehydration, with dry skin and vasoconstriction.

15. **(C)** Client need: psychosocial integrity; subcategory: psychosocial adaptation; content area: psychiatric

RATIONALE

(A) Poor relationship with peers is not a characteristic of anorexia nervosa. (B) Inappropriate behavior in interacting with authority figures is not a characteristic of anorexia nervosa. (C) The issue of control is often a central one for the client with anorexia nervosa. Symptoms are thought to be triggered by a stressor that the adolescent perceives as a loss of control in some aspect of her life. Often at least one parent is very controlling, with high expectations for the client. Controlling food intake and weight gain is a way the client establishes a sense of control over her life. (D) Clients with anorexia nervosa often exhibit obsessive attempts at perfectionism and are often high achievers in academic and social arenas.

16. **(B)** Client need: psychosocial integrity; subcategory: psychosocial adaptation; content area: psychiatric

RATIONALE

(A) Focusing conversations on food would not indicate progress for this client. (B) Identifying healthy ways to cope with anxiety would be evaluated as a positive change in the client with an eating disorder. The client would need to be able to identify ways that she would use to lower anxiety level without using food to cope. (C) This behavior would indicate the possibility of secret purging after meals. Being able to engage in social behaviors after meals for at least 1 hour would be an indication of progress. (D) Family meals are useful to discourage binge eating and purging.

17. **(C)** Client need: physiological integrity; subcategory: reduction of risk potential; content area: psychiatric

RATIONALE

(A) The characteristics of feces are normally not markedly affected by drug use. (B) Hemoglobin level is not markedly affected by drug use and would not be a priority. (C) Consciousness level is an important nursing assessment of a client suspected of substance abuse, because most drugs affect the central nervous system and the consciousness level. Both the client's behavior and verbalizations and the nurse's subjective and objective data collection would yield this data. (D) Nail bed color is not affected by drug use.

18. **(D)** Client need: physiological integrity; subcategory: physiological adaptation; content area: psychiatric

RATIONALE

(A, B) This information is not a priority for planning treatment in this client. (C) Although this is an important area to explore, it is not the initial priority for planning treatment. (D) The type, quantity, and frequency of drugs, including time of last use, must be determined in assessing the client's pattern of drug use and in planning treatment. The nurse will use these data to determine the potential for serious withdrawal symptoms and the type of related health problems for which the client is at risk (i.e., HIV, hepatitis, cellulitis, GI).

19. **(B)** Client need: psychosocial integrity; subcategory: psychosocial adaptation; content area: psychiatric

RATIONALE

(A) The nurse does not have enough data from this one statement to make assessments about the family. (B) Denial is a common initial response in clients with alcohol abuse problems. The client projects blame onto others, usually a spouse or parent, because his or her ego is not strong enough to accept responsibility for his or her own behavior. (C) This client's statement is a subjective view of his relationship with his wife. The stressors in his life (job loss, loss of wife and son) occurred after the alcohol abuse started. (D) The statement is a reflection of the use of denial to protect his fragile ego from recognizing his own responsibility for the events in his life. It is not an accurate picture of his true feelings for his wife or of their relationship.

20. **(D)** Client need: psychosocial integrity; subcategory: psychosocial adaptation; content area: psychiatric

RATIONALE

(A, B, C) This behavior is not a characteristic of separation anxiety disorder. (D) This behavior is characteristic of separation anxiety disorder. The child exhibits excessive anxiety concerning separation from those to whom the child is profoundly attached. The child is preoccupied with worry that he or she will be permanently separated from the attachment figure by a disastrous event and has difficulty tolerating being away from that person.

21. **(B)** Client need: psychosocial integrity; subcategory: coping and adaptation; content area: psychiatric

RATIONALE

(A) The child needs opportunities to verbalize her fears and worries and receive reassurance. (B) A safe, effective care environment would be one where the child experiences calm, nonjudgmental, reassuring caregivers. This type of environment provides a place where the child can begin to learn coping mechanisms to manage her acute anxiety more effectively. (C) Generally peer relationships are not affected by separation anxiety disorder, and peer interaction could actually provide diversion from anxiety. (D) Nursing interventions should promote less traumatic separations between parent and child, not discourage visits.

22. **(A)** Client need: psychosocial integrity; subcategory: coping and adaptation; content area: psychiatric

    RATIONALE

    (A) Irritability and difficulty concentrating are psychological characteristics of clients with generalized anxiety disorder. As anxiety increases, the ability to attend to external stimuli decreases. (B) Clients with anxiety disorders tend to be focused on the present and frightened about the future. (C) Increased aggressiveness, not assertiveness, is a characteristic of clients with anxiety disorder. (D) Grandiose ideation is not a characteristic of anxiety disorder. Clients with anxiety disorder are often critical of themselves and have low self-esteem.

23. **(A)** Client need: psychosocial integrity; subcategory: psychosocial adaptation; content area: psychiatric

    RATIONALE

    (A) The nurse's maintenance of a calm and supportive manner while interacting is an appropriate implementation with clients with anxiety disorders. (B) The client may not necessarily need to cry, so encouraging him to cry is not the most therapeutic choice. (C) Minor rather than major tranquilizing drugs are usually used with anxiety disorders. (D) Intensive psychotherapy is not the treatment of choice for a highly anxious person.

24. **(B)** Client need: physiological integrity; subcategory: pharmacological and parenteral therapies; content area: psychiatric

    RATIONALE

    (A) Chlorpromazine is a major tranquilizing drug (neuroleptic) used more commonly in psychotic disorders. (B) Lorazepam is a common minor tranquilizing drug that a nurse might give a client with anxiety disorder. (C) Imipramine is an antidepressant used for treatment of depression. (D) Chloral hydrate is a medication for insomnia.

25. **(B)** Client need: psychosocial integrity; subcategory: psychosocial adaptation; content area: psychiatric

    RATIONALE

    (A) Fear of talking with people is not a characteristic of agoraphobia. (B) Clients with agoraphobia are afraid to leave their homes for fear of being trapped without the ability to escape. (C) The fear of pain is called algophobia. (D) The fear of fire is called pyrophobia.

26. **(C)** Client need: physiological integrity; subcategory: reduction of risk potential; content area: psychiatric

    RATIONALE

    (A) Insight-oriented psychotherapy is not a usual treatment for clients with phobic disorders. (B) Lithium carbonate is used in the treatment of bipolar disorder, not phobias. (C) Desensitization treatment is an appropriate part of the nursing care plan for phobic clients. By gradually exposing these clients to the phobic stimulus, such as leaving their homes or the hospital unit, anxiety can gradually be decreased, and the clients can begin to function more effectively. (D) Treatment of clients with phobic reactions is generally long-term, and crisis intervention is not an appropriate treatment modality.

27. **(A)** Client need: psychosocial integrity; subcategory: psychosocial adaptation; content area: psychiatric

    RATIONALE

    (A) The client with obsessive-compulsive disorder uses the rituals to cope with intense anxiety related to aggressive impulses and guilt. (B) Clients with obsessive-compulsive disorder often recognize that they have little control over their obsessions and compulsions and that they are interfering with their ability to function. (C) The rituals do not contribute to a sense of self-esteem for clients with this disorder. They often recognize that the rituals are unreasonable and excessive. (D) The excessive hand washing contributes to the risk of infection because it threatens skin integrity.

28. **(C)** Client need: psychosocial integrity; subcategory: coping and adaption; content area: psychiatric

    RATIONALE

    (A) The client should not feel pressured to make frequent decisions because this would contribute to anxiety and the need to use maladaptive methods of coping with the anxiety. (B) Environmental stimuli contribute to anxiety. Goals would involve decreasing anxiety while developing new coping skills. (C) A goal for a client with an obsessive-compulsive reaction is that the client will have the time and opportunity to complete rituals. Until the client learns to cope with the underlying cause of the overwhelming anxiety, he must be allowed to complete his anxiety-reducing rituals. (D) Improvement takes a much longer period of time.

29. **(D)** Client need: psychosocial integrity; subcategory: psychosocial adaptation; content area: psychiatric

    RATIONALE

    (A) Recurrent distressing dreams related to the traumatic event are a common characteristic of PTSD. (B) Irritability and angry outbursts are symptoms of persistent increased arousal and anxiety characteristic of the clients with this disorder. (C) Efforts to avoid stimuli that arouse recollection of the traumatic event is characteristic of clients with PTSD. (D) Clients with PTSD often experience a sense of a foreshortened future. They often do not expect to live a normal, long life.

30. **(A)** Client need: psychosocial integrity; subcategory: psychosocial adaptation; content area: psychiatric

    RATIONALE

    (A) Part of the healing process is the reconsideration phase when the client reflects on the traumatic experience in an effort to integrate the experience into his life. It is important for the nurse to give the client the opportunity to share the experience. (B) To change the subject might meet the needs of the nurse, because it is difficult to hear about the traumatic event, but this strategy would not meet the needs of the client. (C) Telling the client the event was not as bad as he remembers it devalues the client's experience, conveys lack of understanding, and could discourage the client from sharing his experiences in the future. (D) Although he may benefit from eventually sharing his experience in a group setting where he could get more support, the best nursing response is to listen and convey empathy.

31. **(D)** Client need: psychosocial integrity; subcategory: psychosocial adaptation; content area: psychiatric

    RATIONALE

    (A) Preoccupation with sexuality is not a characteristic of somatoform disorder. It may be seen in the manic phase of bipolar disorder. (B) Fear of high places is a phobia, not a characteristic of somatoform disorder. (C) Preoccupation with inanimate objects is not a characteristic of somatoform disorder. (D) Somatoform disorders are characterized by preoccupation with one's own health.

32. **(B)** Client need: safe, effective care environment; subcategory: management of care; content area: psychiatric

    RATIONALE

    (A) Challenging the validity of his physical symptoms before doing diagnostic testing would result in denial in the client. (B) One of the primary aims is to coordinate the diagnostic testing to rule out an organic basis for the symptoms. (C) The client should be encouraged to be as independent as possible. (D) The family should be encouraged to participate in treatment.

33. **(D)** Client need: psychosocial integrity; subcategory: coping and adaptation; content area: psychiatric

    RATIONALE

    (A) It is important not to allow the client to use her symptoms to avoid independent activities. This would only reinforce the use of conversion symptoms to cope with anxiety generated by fear of independence. (B) Clients with conversion disorder are usually not aware of the psychological implications of the disorder. (C) Encouraging her to discuss her feelings about the paralysis would reinforce the maladaptive coping mechanism. She needs assistance to connect the symptoms with her severe anxiety about leaving home. (D) The appropriate nursing action is to withdraw attention if the client continues to focus on physical limitations.

34. **(A)** Client need: psychosocial integrity; subcategory: psychosocial adaptation; content area: psychiatric

    RATIONALE

    (A) A lack of concern inappropriate to the severity of the impairment experienced is a common characteristic of conversion disorder known as "la belle indifférence." (B) Psychogenic fugue is a sudden, unexpected travel away from home, inability to recall one's previous identity, and taking on a new identity, with an accompanying unawareness of having forgotten the past. (C) Secondary gain is the gratification of psychological needs obtained through maladaptive responses to stress, for example, having all dependency needs met by a caregiver. (D) Akathesia is a type of extrapyramidal side effect of some neuroleptic drugs.

35. **(B)** Client need: psychosocial integrity; subcategory: psychosocial adaptation; content area: psychiatric

    RATIONALE

    (A) Sexual preoccupation is more characteristic of sexual disorders. Depressed clients usually have decreased libido. (B) Psychomotor retardation, a significant slowing of physical movements, including speech, is a characteristic of severe depression. (C) Hyperexcitability might be seen in a manic phase of bipolar disorder. (D) Excessive talking would be seen in a manic phase of bipolar disorder and some personality disorders.

36. **(D)** Client need: psychosocial integrity; subcategory: psychosocial adaptation; content area: psychiatric

    RATIONALE

    (A) A depressed client is at high risk for suicide attempts or self-inflicted harm because of depressed mood, feelings of worthlessness and hopelessness. (B) Preoccupation with feelings of worthlessness, guilt, and helplessness contribute to a significant disturbance in self-esteem. Assisting the client to develop a more positive self-image is appropriate. (C) Depressed clients exhibit self-isolating behaviors and impaired social interaction. Integrating the client into unit activities is appropriate. (D) Depressed clients are often preoccupied with their own self-deprecating thoughts and feelings. They often exhibit dysfunctional interactions with family. It would be inappropriate to reinforce this.

37. **(A)** Client need: psychosocial integrity; subcategory: coping and adaptation; content area: psychiatric

    RATIONALE

    (A) Nortriptyline is a tricyclic medication used in the treatment of depression. It can take up to 4 weeks before positive response to the medication is experienced. It is important that the client receive this information so she does not become discouraged. (B) The client's attitude will not have an impact on the effectiveness of the medication. (C) It is inappropriate to consider changing a tricyclic antidepressant after 4 days. (D) This is an opportunity to teach or reinforce previous teaching about medications.

38. **(C)** Client need: physiological integrity; subcategory: pharmacological and parenteral therapies; content area: psychiatric

    RATIONALE

    (A) This response is an example of failure to listen, which blocks communication and requires further evaluation. (B) This response is an example of making an assumption without gathering adequate data and belittling expressed feelings, which block communication. (C) The nurse uses the therapeutic communication skills of reflecting observations and encouraging clarification to further assess the client's mood. (D) This response is an example of making an assumption without gathering adequate data.

39. **(B)** Client need: physiological integrity; subcategory: reduction of risk potential; content area: psychiatric

    RATIONALE

    (A) ECT is not commonly used for treatment of schizophrenia. Major tranquilizers are most commonly used. (B) ECT is commonly used for treatment of major depression in clients who have not responded to antidepressants, who have medical problems that contraindicate the use of antidepressants. (C) ECT is not commonly used in treatment of personality disorders. (D) ECT is not the treatment of choice for clients with dissociative disorders.

40. **(B)** Client need: psychosocial integrity; subcategory: psychosocial adaptation; content area: psychiatric

    RATIONALE

    (A) This answer is incorrect information. Intensive care is not necessary after ECT. (B) The nurse provides accurate information about what he can expect from the treatment to the client. (C) The client will not experience a significant change of mood after one ECT. (D) The client is asking for information that the nurse can provide. It is inappropriate for the nurse to make assumptions and explore feelings without providing the information the client seeks.

41. **(B)** Client need: psychosocial integrity; subcategory: psychosocial adaptation; content area: psychiatric

    RATIONALE

    (A) Hearing voices is more characteristic of paranoid schizophrenia. (B) A client with a paranoid personality disorder is frequently characterized by rigid, hypersensitive, and suspicious behavior. (C) The client with paranoid personality disorder usually avoids interpersonal relationships and is usually distant and reclusive. (D) Clients with paranoid personality disorders usually see others as having the problem. They are usually not motivated to seek treatment.

42. **(A)** Client need: psychosocial integrity; subcategory: psychosocial adaptation; content area: psychiatric

    RATIONALE

    (A) An effective implementation for promoting consensual validation of reality is to reinforce reality, but the nurse should avoid arguing with the client about his perceptions. Arguing about his suspicions will reinforce them. (B) These clients often interpret the use of humor in others as a personal assault—that they are the intended focus of the joke. (C) Interventions include assisting these clients to clarify thoughts and feelings. They need opportunities to discuss their perceptions. (D) Antidepressant medications are used frequently for clients with depressive disorder, not paranoid personality disorder.

43. **(C)** Client need: psychosocial integrity; subcategory: coping and adaptation; content area: psychiatric

    RATIONALE

    (A) Sharing his belongings with others may be a long-term goal but may never be achieved in this client, who constantly feels vulnerable to exploitation by others. (B) Engaging in group activities and freely sharing his feelings may also be a long-term goal that may never be achieved. (C) Feelings of helplessness and lack of control can reinforce this client's suspicions and pattern of social isolation. The client and nurse must work jointly toward the goal of ensuring that the client has as much control as possible. (D) The client should not be encouraged to engage in solitary activities because such activities promote social isolation.

44. **(D)** Client need: psychosocial integrity; subcategory: psychosocial adaptation; content area: psychiatric

    RATIONALE

    (A) Lethargy is more characteristic of a client with depression. (B) Sexual preoccupation is more characteristic of a sexual disorder. (C) Two or more personalities are characteristic of multiple personality disorder. (D) A client with a schizoid personality disorder is characterized by a tendency to withdraw from others. She is often described by others as a loner.

45. **(A)** Client need: psychosocial integrity; subcategory: psychosocial adaptation; content area: psychiatric

    RATIONALE

    (A) The nurse must recognize the client's need for distance in a relationship. Trying to become too close or too friendly will cause the client to feel threatened and withdraw. (B) The client's affiliation needs should be considered and planned for in an individualized manner. (C) Intensive group therapy would be too threatening to this client and contribute to further withdrawal from social interactions. (D) Consistent interactions by a few nurses would be more therapeutic for this client.

46. **(B)** Client need: health promotion and maintenance; subcategory: growth and development through the life span; content area: psychiatric

    RATIONALE

    (A) Challenging the client could result in a power struggle in the family. (B) The family would be contributing to effective treatment for the client with schizoid personality disorder if they encouraged the client to continue in treatment, because the condition may be long term. Lack of encouragement could result in the client discontinuing treatment. (C) These expectations would be unrealistic and could result in disillusionment in, and discontinuance of, treatment. (D) This intensive family focus on a regular basis would be threatening and contribute to her isolating herself from her family.

47. **(C)** Client need: psychosocial integrity; subcategory: psychosocial adaptation; content area: psychiatric

    RATIONALE

    (A) Clients with antisocial personality disorder may have above average intelligence but an inability to form permanent sexual relationships. (B) Clients with antisocial personality disorder have few, if any, religious values or concerns. (C) The need for immediate gratification and low tolerance for frustration are characteristics of clients with antisocial personality disorder. These characteristics often lead to criminal and other dangerous behaviors. (D) Clients with this disorder do not learn from experience and may have criminal records.

48. **(B)** Client need: psychosocial integrity; subcategory: psychosocial adaptation; content area: psychiatric

    RATIONALE

    (A) Quick behavioral change is not a realistic expectation for a client with antisocial personality disorder. (B) The nurse must realize that the client with an antisocial personality disorder may not be motivated to change behavior or lifestyle. Not sharing the same moral code as society in general often results in the client feeling there is nothing wrong with his behavior. (C) The client with antisocial personality disorder uses manipulation to get his needs met with all

people with whom he interacts. (D) Psychotropic drug therapy is not effective with clients with antisocial personality disorder.

49. **(B)** Client need: psychosocial integrity; subcategory: psychosocial adaptation; content area: psychiatric

    RATIONALE

    (A) Clients with antisocial personality disorder reject social norms as limits and exhibit poor impulse control. This client cannot be expected to monitor his own behavior effectively. (B) Establishing clear, consistent limits on behavior will contribute to this client's ability to interact appropriately on the unit. (C) Peer interaction offers the opportunity for the client to receive feedback about his interactions with others. Encouraging peer interaction also helps model social norms. (D) Clients with antisocial personality disorder come from dysfunctional families and have poor, often volatile, interpersonal relationships. The nurse cannot expect these families and significant others to participate effectively with the client in treatment.

50. **(D)** Client need: psychosocial integrity; subcategory: psychosocial adaptation; content area: psychiatric

    RATIONALE

    (A) Psychomotor retardation and posturing are more characteristic of clients with catatonic schizophrenia. (B) Regressed, childlike behavior is more characteristic of clients with disorganized schizophrenia. (C) Euphoric mood and sexual acting-out behavior are characteristic of clients with bipolar disorder, manic. (D) Clients with paranoid schizophrenia are most often characterized by extreme suspiciousness, delusions, and hallucinations. Common themes of the delusions are of being poisoned or followed. Hallucinations involve hearing threatening voices.

51. **(B)** Client need: physiological integrity; subcategory: pharmacological and parenteral therapies; content area: psychiatric

    RATIONALE

    (A) Lorazepam is an antianxiety drug. It is not the drug of choice for schizophrenia. (B) Haloperidol is a major tranquilizing drug that is frequently used to treat the psychotic symptoms of schizophrenia. It is an effective antipsychotic medication and has fewer side effects than some of the other neuroleptic drugs. (C) Amitriptyline is an antidepressant used in treatment of some symptoms of depression. (D) Isocarboxazid is also an antidepressant.

52. **(C)** Client need: physiological integrity; subcategory pharmacological and parenteral therapies; content area: psychiatric

    RATIONALE

    (A) Side effects of neuroleptic drugs are extrapyramidal symptoms. (B) Neuroleptic malignant syndrome is a rare, potentially fatal complication of treatment with neuroleptic drugs. (C) Neuroleptics such as haloperidol are effective in decreasing psychotic symptoms so that clients with psychotic disorders may interact more functionally with their environment. (D) Although neuroleptic drugs such as haloperidol may make a client drowsy, it is not given to promote sleep.

53. **(A)** Client need: physiological integrity; subcategory pharmacological and parenteral therapies; content area: psychiatric

    RATIONALE

    (A) The plan should focus on reinforcing perceptions and thinking that is in touch with reality. (B) Challenging the client's hallucinations and delusions is not effective and can impede the development of a trusting therapeutic relationship. (C) Using peer pressure to discourage distorted thinking and bizarre behavior is not therapeutic. It could contribute to further social isolation. (D) Ignoring distorted thinking and bizarre behavior is not therapeutic in assisting this client to become more connected to reality.

54. **(B)** Client need: physiological integrity; subcategory: pharmacological and parenteral therapies; content area: psychiatric

RATIONALE

(A) Benzotropine does not have any effect on agitation. (B) Benzotropine prevents and treats extrapyramidal effects of neuroleptic drugs. These symptoms may include drooling, akathesia, shuffling gait, and acute dystonic reaction. (C) Benzotropine would not be used for a headache. (D) Benzotropine does not induce sleep.

55. **(C)** Client need: psychosocial integrity; subcategory: psychosocial adaptation; content area: psychiatric

RATIONALE

(A) This is not a characteristic of catatonic schizophrenia. (B) This is a characteristic of paranoid schizophrenia that is not generally seen in catatonic schizophrenia. The symptoms can result in an unwillingness or inability to eat. (C) Stuporous withdrawal, hallucinations, and delusions are characteristics of catatonic schizophrenia. (D) Sexual preoccupation is more a characteristic of sexual disorders and the manic phase of bipolar disorder. Word salad is a speech pattern in which words do not make sense and is not characteristic of catatonic schizophrenia.

56. **(D)** Client need: physiological integrity; subcategory: reduction of risk potential; content area: psychiatric

RATIONALE

(A) A client with catatonic schizophrenia tends to lose weight because of inability or unwillingness to eat secondary to symptoms of stuporous withdrawal and distorted perceptions. (B) This client would most likely exhibit symptoms of dehydration secondary to poor fluid intake. (C) The client with catatonic schizophrenia has diminished ability to deal with environmental stimuli and withdraws. (D) The client with catatonic schizophrenia can be observed standing, sitting, or lying immobile. The immobility can last for minutes, hours, or days.

57. **(B)** Client need: psychosocial integrity; subcategory: psychosocial adaptation; content area: psychiatric

RATIONALE

(A) The client with catatonic schizophrenia has a diminished ability to deal with external stimulation. (B) As part of the plan to decrease the catatonic client's withdrawn behavior, the nurse should speak in simple, concise terms to avoid sensory overload of the client. (C) These clients need to have limits set on their behavior to promote safety. (D) In the acute phase of catatonic schizophrenia, clients are unable to participate in group therapy.

58. **(A)** Client need: physiological integrity; subcategory: pharmacological and parenteral therapies; content area: psychiatric

RATIONALE

(A) Atropine is given prior to ECT because it acts to prevent airway complications from excessive secretions during the treatment. (B) Propranolol is a β-blocker not used in conjunction with ECT. (C) Lithium is used in the treatment of bipolar disorders. (D) Flurazepam is used for insomnia.

59. **(B)** Client need: psychosocial integrity; subcategory: psychosocial adaptation; content area: psychiatric

RATIONALE

(A) Bizarre thoughts are more characteristic of clients with schizophrenia. (B) Intense, labile mood is characteristic of clients in the manic phase of bipolar disorder. These clients may be euphoric and elated, then suddenly become very irritable and hostile. Behaviors must be closely monitored to maintain safety because these clients often experience poor impulse control with their labile mood. (C) Extreme suspiciousness is more characteristic of clients with paranoid personality disorder or paranoid schizophrenia. (D) Auditory hallucinations are not a common characteristic of clients with bipolar disorder.

60. **(B)** Client need: physiological integrity; subcategory: pharmacological and parenteral therapies; content area: psychiatric

RATIONALE

(A) Clients in the manic phase of their bipolar illness are usually unable to sleep and experience decreased REM sleep. (B) The therapeutic blood level of the psychotropic drug lithium required to prevent manic or depressive episodes of bipolar disorder is between 0.7 and 1.2 mEq/L. A serum level of 0.15 mEq/L would be inadequate to prevent a manic episode. (C) Although high intracellular levels of sodium have been correlated with bipolar disorder, it is not diagnostically definitive. (D) Hypotension is not a definitive characteristic of clients in the manic phase of bipolar disorder.

61. **(D)** Client need: physiological integrity; subcategory: pharmacological and parenteral therapies; content area: psychiatric

RATIONALE

(A) Skin rash and photosensitivity can be side effects of antipsychotic medications, but they are not symptoms of lithium toxicity. (B) Urinary retention and orthostatic hypotension can be side effects of antidepressant medications, but they are not symptoms of lithium toxicity. (C) Dystonia and akathesia are extrapyramidal symptoms that can occur with antipsychotic medications, but they are not symptoms of lithium toxicity. (D) Early symptoms of lithium toxicity include ataxia, persistent nausea and vomiting, severe diarrhea, tinnitus, and blurred vision. More serious symptoms include increasing muscle tremors and mental confusion. The most serious symptoms include nystagmus, delirium, arrhythmias, and cardiovascular collapse.

62. **(B)** Client need: physiological integrity; subcategory: pharmacological and parenteral therapies; content area: psychiatric content area: psychiatric

RATIONALE

(A) Molindine is a dihydroindolone compound used in the treatment of psychotic symptoms. (B) Carbamazepine has been found to be effective in the treatment of clients who develop toxicity to lithium. (C) Triazolam is a hypnotic used to induce sleep. It is not used to control bipolar disorder. (D) Doxepin is an antidepressant. It could precipitate a manic episode. It would not be used instead of lithium.

63. **(D)** Client need: psychosocial integrity; subcategory: psychosocial adaptation; content area: psychiatric

RATIONALE

(A) The client with bipolar disorder in the acute manic phase would not be able to set limits safely on her own behavior. (B) The client in the acute manic phase has great difficulty concentrating for a period of time and would likely become more agitated if encouraged to do so. (C) The client in the acute manic phase is easily overstimulated and overreacts to environmental stimuli. (D) A calm, consistent approach by staff would promote a calm, consistent environment that would assist the client to exhibit less hyperactive behavior resulting from overstimulation.

64. **(B)** Client need: physiological integrity; subcategory: basic care and comfort; content area: psychiatric

RATIONALE

(A) Conversations at mealtime would be too stimulating for the client in the acute manic phase. She is easily distracted. (B) Encouraging small, frequent meals would be the most therapeutic nursing action for a client who has difficulty sitting still long enough for regular meals. (C) Having the manic client keep detailed records is unrealistic. (D) Expecting a manic client to read literature in a meaningful way is unrealistic.

65. **(C)** Client need: psychosocial integrity; subcategory: coping and adaptation; content area: psychiatric

RATIONALE

(A) A client with major depression exhibits a persistent mood of despondency. Labile mood swings are characteristic of clients with bipolar disorder. (B) Significant sleep and appetite disturbance are characteristic of a major depression. (C) Persistent feelings of hopelessness and worthlessness are characteristic of clients with major depression and contribute to the clients' risk of suicide attempts. (D) Auditory hallucinations are more characteristic of schizophrenia.

66. **(C)** Client need: psychosocial integrity; subcategory: coping and adaptation; content area: psychiatric

    RATIONALE

    (A) Placing the client in seclusion would increase his isolation and would violate his right to the least restrictive treatment possible. (B) A client with major depression and suicidal ideation usually has great difficulty making decisions, and the expectation that he do so would decrease his fragile sense of self-worth. (C) A plan to decrease a depressed client's suicidal preoccupation should focus on providing a supportive relationship in which to express his thoughts and feelings. Suppressing thoughts and feelings can result in an internalization of hostility and depression. (D) The client should be on suicide precautions; however, frequent reminders are not therapeutic.

67. **(B)** Client need: psychosocial integrity; subcategory: coping and adaptation; content area: psychiatric

    RATIONALE

    (A) Giving false reassurance may discourage the client from further expression of feelings if he perceives others do not want to hear what he has to say. (B) This response is an example of a therapeutic communication technique known as translating words into feelings. It communicates that the nurse is actively listening and encourages the client to continue. (C) Giving advice implies the nurse knows what is best and invalidates the client's experience. (D) The antidepressant medication will assist in decreasing some of the symptoms of his depression, such as low energy, sleep and appetite disturbance, so that he can grieve more effectively.

68. **(B)** Client need: psychosocial integrity; subcategory: psychosocial adaptation; content area: psychiatric

    RATIONALE

    (A) Deriving sexual pleasure through window peaking is called voyeurism. (B) Pedophilia is a psychosexual disorder in which the client derives sexual pleasure from children. The behavior includes touching and fondling, as well as having sexual intercourse with children. (C) Deriving sexual pleasure from animals is called zoophilia. (D) Exposing genitals to others is exhibitionism.

69. **(A)** Client need: psychosocial integrity; subcategory: psychosocial adaptation; content area: psychiatric

    RATIONALE

    (A) Paraphilia is a term used to diagnose clients who have repetitive sexual fantasies or behaviors that may involve preference for nonhuman objects, for children, for sexual activity with humans that involve real or simulated suffering or humiliation, or for repetitive sexual activity with nonconsenting adults. (B) Phobias are a type of anxiety disorder. (C) Erectile dysfunction is a type of sexual dysfunction called male sexual arousal disorder. (D) Clients with a paraphilia often deny that they have a problem and generally seek treatment only if mandated by the court or if discovered by family or friends.

70. **(B)** Client need: psychosocial integrity; subcategory: psychosocial adaptation; content area: psychiatric

    RATIONALE

    (A) Sadism involves inflicting suffering on a sexual partner as part of the arousal process. (B) Masochism is the psychosexual disorder in which the client obtains sexual pleasure from submitting to aggression from a partner. This can include the infliction of pain. Engaging in these behaviors is dangerous and deaths have occurred. (C) Frotteurism is the psychosexual disorder that involves

intense sexual urges or fantasies to touch or rub against a nonconsenting adult. (D) Fetishism involves recurrent, intense sexual urges involving the use of nonliving objects such as undergarments or other clothing, generally in the process of masturbation.

71. **(A)** Client need: psychosocial integrity; subcategory: psychosocial adaptation; content area: psychiatric

    RATIONALE

    (A) In addition to low self-esteem, clients with psychosexual disorders usually have little attachment to others. Clients with psychosexual disorders have difficulty establishing or maintaining interpersonal relationships. (B) Clients with this disorder often do not have feelings of guilt. (C) Clients with this disorder often do not demonstrate the ability to view their behavior in a clear manner from the perspective of social and ethical norms. (D) Clients with different levels of intelligence can have this disorder.

72. **(C)** Client need: psychosocial integrity; subcategory: psychosocial adaptation; content area: psychiatric

    RATIONALE

    (A) Excessive social drinking may be seen in the pre-alcoholic phase when the person would use alcohol to relieve stress. The alcoholic drinks regardless of the social situation, and a drink is no longer a source of stress relief or a social activity. (B) Drinking resulting in severe hangovers is an indication of problem drinking, but not necessarily of alcoholism. (C) Alcoholism is best defined as physical and psychological dependence with impaired health related to the effects of alcohol consumption. (D) The alcoholic experiences blackouts, which are periods of amnesia about experiences while intoxicated. These are different from forgetfulness.

73. **(D)** Client need: psychosocial integrity; subcategory: coping and adaptation; content area: psychiatric

    RATIONALE

    (A) This response would reinforce the client's denial about the seriousness of his alcoholism. (B) This response is an example of a nontherapeutic communication called "requesting an explanation." Asking "Why" can be intimidating and encourages the client to become defensive. (C) This response does not assist the client to connect his behavior with his illness or separate the behavior from the client. It sounds judgmental. (D) This response is therapeutic because it assists the client to connect his personal problems with his drinking. A nursing goal for a client with alcoholism is to assist the client to acknowledge the association between his drinking and his personal problems.

74. **(B)** Client need: psychosocial integrity; subcategory: coping and adaptation; content area: psychiatric

    RATIONALE

    (A) This is an example of a nontherapeutic communication technique called requesting an explanation. It reinforces the wife's maladaptive guilt. (B) This response is an appropriate nursing action. It provides family teaching and is directed toward the nursing goal of assisting the client to accept responsibility for his own behavior. (C) This is judgmental, communicates disapproval, and is not a therapeutic response. (D) This belittles the family member's concerns and is not therapeutic.

75. **(B)** Client need: physiological integrity; subcategory: pharmacological and parenteral therapies; content area: psychiatric

    RATIONALE

    (A) Blackouts occur with drinking in clients who are alcoholic. (B) Delirium tremens is a serious sequel to abrupt withdrawal from alcohol. It includes disorientation, confusion, visual and tactile hallucinations that are very disturbing to the client; agitation; tachycardia; tremor; diaphoresis; and fever. Prevention involves obtaining nursing history of alcohol use on admission, observing for early symptoms of withdrawal, and administering benzodiazepines as ordered. (C) Hypocalcemia is not a symptom of severe alcohol withdrawal. (D) Constricted pupils are not a serious symptom of withdrawal.

76. **(C)** Client need: psychosocial integrity; subcategory: psychosocial adaptation; content area: psychiatric

    RATIONALE

    (A) This is the last of AA's Twelve Steps. (B) This is the fifth step of the Twelve Steps. (C) This is the first step in the Twelve Step program. It reflects that the client is ready to give up the use of denial in dealing with his alcoholism. (D) This is the fourth step.

77. **(C)** Client need: psychosocial integrity; subcategory: psychosocial adaptation; content area: psychiatric

    RATIONALE

    (A) Stuporous withdrawal and muteness indicates that more serious pathology is present. (B) Extreme suspiciousness and inability to trust is associated with paranoia. (C) The client with organic brain syndrome usually manifests confusion and impaired cognitive functioning. The degree of impairment depends on the cause and stage of the organic brain syndrome. (D) Hypochondriasis is a somatic disorder.

78. **(B)** Client need: psychosocial integrity; subcategory: psychosocial adaptation; content area: psychiatric

    RATIONALE

    (A) A euphoric mood might be found in an organic mood disorder. It is not a common characteristic of dementia. (B) Nursing assessment of the client with dementia frequently reveals decreased ability for abstract thinking. (C) Auditory hallucinations are characteristic of schizophrenia. (D) Echolalia is a characteristic of schizophrenia.

79. **(A)** Client need: physiological integrity; subcategory: reduction of risk potential; content area: psychiatric

    RATIONALE

    (A) Electrolyte imbalance would be a reversible cause of an organic brain syndrome like dementia. (B) The Rorschach Test is a psychological test that has the individual interpret a series of inkblots. The client's interpretations would reveal basic attitudes and conflicts. They would not reveal reversible causes of organic brain syndrome. (C) The Minnesota Multiphasic Personality Inventory is a personality test. It would not reveal reversible causes of organic brain syndrome. (D) Frequent vital signs would not reveal reversible causes of organic brain syndrome.

80. **(D)** Client need: psychosocial integrity; subcategory: psychosocial adaptation; content area: psychiatric

    RATIONALE

    (A) Furniture placement should be uncluttered and stay the same to prevent unnecessary confusion. (B) Lighting should be good. (C) A variety of visitors would cause excessive stimulation and confusion. (D) The use of external signs to help in orientation is an important part of the care for this client.

81. **(C)** Client need: psychosocial integrity; subcategory: psychosocial adaptation; content area: psychiatric

    RATIONALE

    (A) The nurse would want to promote social interaction, but it is not the priority goal for this client. (B) A more appropriate goal would be that the client accomplishes ADL to the best of his or her ability. (C) The priority nursing goal for clients with organic brain syndrome is the maintenance of client safety. Clients with this disorder have impaired cognitive and psychomotor functioning that put them at risk for injury. (D) Maintaining nutritional status is important for this client, but not the priority nursing goal.

82. **(A)** Client need: psychosocial integrity; subcategory: psychosocial adaptation; content area: psychiatric

    RATIONALE

    (A) The first stage an individual usually goes through when told she is dying is shock. The client's behavior may range from verbal denial to immobility. (B, C, D) Denial, avoidance, and acceptance are later steps.

83. **(A)** Client need: psychosocial integrity; subcategory: coping and adaptation; content area: psychiatric

    RATIONALE

    (A) In planning to assist the dying client to have optimum quality of life during her remaining time, the nurse should provide the client with opportunities to have some control over her environment. This would decrease feelings of helplessness and dependence, which could contribute to the development of depression. (B) The client should be provided with information about available treatments, but the decision should be the client's. (C) The client should be encouraged to make decisions about treatment. (D) The client should be encouraged to express her thoughts and feelings. The nurse should not direct the expression to particular topics but be open to listening if they come up.

84. **(C)** Client need: psychosocial integrity; subcategory: psychosocial adaptation; content area: psychiatric

    RATIONALE

    (A) Trust involves a sense of confidence that another person is interested in one's welfare and has a desire to be of assistance. (B) Respect involves the unconditional acceptance of another person as a worthwhile and unique person. (C) When a nurse is aware of internal experiences while interacting with a client and responds to the client with honesty and openness, the nurse is demonstrating genuineness. In the client, this promotes a feeling of being connected to others in a meaningful way. (D) Empathy is the ability to accurately perceive and understand what another person is feeling or experiencing.

85. **(C)** Client need: psychosocial integrity; subcategory: psychosocial adaptation; content area: psychiatric

    RATIONALE

    (A) Altruism is a therapeutic benefit of a group that relates to genuine concern for others. (B) Group cohesiveness is the sense of belonging that meets client's affiliative needs. (C) The client demonstrated imitative behavior. She observed a client with similar problems take a risk and speak in a group with a positive response from the group. She then imitated that behavior and experienced an achievement. (D) Catharsis is the experience of expressing emotionally laden material in a nonthreatening atmosphere.

86. **(D)** Client need: psychosocial integrity; subcategory: psychosocial adaptation; content area: psychiatric

    RATIONALE

    (A) The setting of limits on behavior is communicated clearly in both written forms and community meetings of clients and staff. The focus is reinforcing adaptive behavior in dealing with anxiety. (B) The focus is the therapeutic relationship that promotes the development of trust between the nurse and the client. The nurse conveys acceptance, respect, empathy, and genuineness to promote adaptive behavior. The nurse clearly identifies responses to the behavior while demonstrating unconditional acceptance of the client. (C) A therapeutic community is guided by the input of all disciplines involved in client care as well as clients themselves. (D) Although there is a focus on behavior in a therapeutic community, many treatment modalities are used in individual client treatment.

87. **(B)** Client need: psychosocial integrity; subcategory: psychosocial adaptation; content area: psychiatric

    RATIONALE

    (A) The client is experiencing difficulty coping with a severe crisis after coping effectively previously. Intensive psychotherapy is not indicated. (B) Crisis intervention is the most appropriate treatment approach. The client's coping mechanisms are overwhelmed by the stressor, and she needs assistance to identify resources and work through the problem-solving process. (C) Relaxation therapy may be used in conjunction with crisis intervention to assist her in coping with anxiety. (D) ECT is used to treat major depression if psychopharmacological treatment is ineffective. It is not indicated in this situation.

88. **(C)** Client need: safe, effective care environment, subcategory: management of care; content area: psychiatric

    RATIONALE

    (A) Fee-for-service is a traditional cost-based delivery system in which the insurer pays for whatever the hospital or the private practitioner charges. (B) Symptom management is a stage of treatment and not a form of financing mental health care. (C) Carve-out refers to separating mental health services and substance abuse benefits from the overall medical benefits package. (D) Retrospective payment is the same as fee-for-service.

89. **(A)** Client need: safe, effective care environment; subcategory: management of care; content area: psychiatric

    RATIONALE

    (A) The principle role of the nurse case manager is coordinator of care and services. The nurse assesses client needs, develops treatment plans, allocates resources, and supervises the care provided by others. (B, C, and D) are all goals of the nurse case manager.

90. **(A)** Client need: safe, effective care environment; subcategory: management of care; content area: psychiatric

    RATIONALE

    (A) A proactive workplace advocacy program assists nurses in developing a positive work environment and provides a means of submission of complaints by professional nurses regarding workplace issues. (B) Supervision is required by the professional nurse to oversee the unlicensed assistive personnel because they do not have the education or training to care for patients. (C) A decrease in wage growth would be no incentive for the professional nurse to improve job performance. (D) Collection and integration of detailed healthcare outcomes data may not be beneficial in delivery of quality care.

91. **(B)** Client need: safe, effective care environment, subcategory: management of care; content area: psychiatric

    RATIONALE

    (A) Long-term care is not an option with the managed care providers. Insurance companies place limits on the amount of coverage for an individual's lifetime. (B) Insurance companies pre-certify inpatient care. (C) General criteria for the medical necessity of admission to psychiatric services has been established to accommodate crisis and high risk behaviors. The primary provider must approve access to specific services. (D) There is no guarantee that the client's personal psychiatrist or therapist will be associated with the managed care health plan network.

92. **(C)** Client need: safe, effective care environment; subcategory: management of care; content area: psychiatric

    RATIONALE

    (A) Chaos within the health care arena has replaced stability, parity, and equilibrium. (B) Restructuring, reorganizing, and job redesign have become synonyms for layoffs and using different skill mixes, making job security an impossibility. (C) With the rapid changes in health care and with the responsibility of mental health advocacy, the culturally competent nurse who is able to negotiate complex health care systems will thrive while assisting the client with changes in the health care system. (D) Controlling the environment is an unlikely feat.

93. **(A)** Client need: safe, effective care environment; subcategory: management of care; content area: psychiatric

RATIONALE

(A) Because of the varied nature of nursing that incorporates the concept of caring and attempting to help the client with problems of daily living, the nurse case manager performs tasks outside the home visit that are not reimbursable. Reimbursable nursing services include teaching, assessment, skilled management of the care plan, and direct care costs. (B) Case management acts on behalf of the client as advocates. Interventions include negotiating for services on behalf of the client, and ensure continuity of care. (C) The nurse case manager is responsible for negotiating with multiple healthcare providers to obtain a variety of services for the client but not at any cost. Case management was implemented as a cost-saving measure and fiscally accountable for the health outcomes of the insured. (D) Psychiatric home care allows treatment-resistant, chronically mentally ill individuals to remain at home and enhances functioning by increasing the person's ability to solve problems, and endeavors to diminish dependency on others.

94. **(A)** Client need: psychosocial integrity; subcategory: psychosocial adaptation; content area: psychiatric

    RATIONALE

    (A) Changes in staffing levels and skill mix increase violent behavior toward healthcare providers and negatively affect the delivery of nursing care. (B) Improper utilization of staff increases the incidence of workplace violence. (C) An increase in security technology helps prevent violence in the workplace. (D) Adequate training for nurses on violence prevention and self-defense may assist the nurse when clients exhibit violence in the healthcare setting.

95. **(D)** Client need: psychosocial integrity; subcategory: pharmacological and parenteral therapies; content area: psychiatric

    RATIONALE

    (A) Decreased libido. (B) Effective in treating the negative symptoms of schizophrenia. (C) In many instances the dramatic effects are highly plausible. (D) Because of their efficacy in treating the positive and negative symptoms of schizophrenia and their lower side effect profile, the atypical drugs are coming to be considered the first line of choice in the treatment of psychosis.

96. **(B)** Client need: physiological integrity; subcategory: physiological adaptation; content area: psychiatric

    RATIONALE

    (A) Implementing commitment is not appropriate for this client because he does not pose a threat to his own safety or that of others. (B) The nurse's role is to support clients and educate them about alternative treatments. It may be either another medication or a nonmedication therapy. (C) Mental health clients have the right to refuse any treatment modality except in an emergency or permitted by law. (D) A nurse or staff member who touches a client without the client's consent can be charged with battery.

97. **(B)** Client need: safe, effective care environment; subcategory: management of care; content area: psychiatric

    RATIONALE

    (A) The client has the right to participate in decision making and other appropriate care and services that are provided by the institution. (B) The goal of nursing is to promote wellness and maximize integrated functioning. (C) Together the client and the nurse develop the plan of care. (D) One of the most important nursing actions is to assist the client in maximizing his level of independence.

98. **(B)** Client need: safe, effective care environment; subcategory: management of care; content area: psychiatric

    RATIONALE

    (A) Obscured boundaries are one of the liabilities in the shared governance concept. (B) One of the positive aspects of shared governance is increased input into unit function. (C) Using the shared governance concept, there is increased control of the environment. (D) Shared governance is cost-neutral after planning and implementation costs, and reduced lengths of stay for selected patients.

99. **(C)** Client need: psychosocial integrity; subcategory: pharmacological and parenteral therapies; content area: psychiatric

    RATIONALE

    (A) Clonazepam (Klonopin) produces sedative effects in the central nervous system. (B) Clonazepam (Klonopin) is given orally, not intravenously. (C) It decreases the seizure threshold level and is useful in the prevention of seizures. (D) Clonazepam (Klonopin) has a long half-life.

100. **(D)** Client need: psychosocial integrity; subcategory: psychosocial adaptation; content area: psychiatric

    RATIONALE

    (A, B C) These are all activities that may benefit the nurse but do not substantiate the nurse's ability to provide prevention-focused health services for clients. (D) Documenting the outcomes of the client's progress substantiates the nurse's ability to provide prevention-focused health services.

101. **(C)** Client need: psychosocial integrity; subcategory: pharmacological and parenteral therapies; content area: psychiatric

    RATIONALE

    (A) Half of the clients picking up prescriptions for the impotence-treatment drug are being reimbursed by insurers. (B) Do not give the client false reassurance. (C) The administration of Viagra to patients with heart problems within 24 hours of using Viagra may result in a potentially life-threatening situation because nitroglycerin can cause blood pressure to drop and Viagra greatly increases that effect. (D) Viagra potentiates the hypotensive effects of nitrates.

102. **(B)** Client need: physiological integrity; subcategory: pharmacological and parenteral therapies; content area: psychiatric

    RATIONALE

    (A) Antipsychotic drugs take 1 to 3 weeks to work, which is not a useful time frame for treatment in the acute situation. (B) One advantage of using a benzodiazepine as the first line of therapy for the aggressive psychotic patient is its sedating and hypnotic effect, which allows the patient to relax and, possibly, even to sleep. (C) Haldol decanoate is slowly absorbed, which is not a useful time frame for treatment in the acute situation. (D) Valproic acid is an anticonvulsant and may be used in manic episodes associated with bipolar disorder.

103. **(B)** Client need: psychosocial integrity; subcategory: coping and adaptation; content area: psychiatric

    RATIONALE

    (A) The patient is concerned about her children and at the same time ambivalent about the situation. (B) The patient is reinforcing constructive coping mechanisms that may enhance self-worth. (C) There exists an underlying attachment to her husband, despite the traumas. (D) The patient is exhibiting erroneous, conflicting thought patterns that hinder constructive decisions.

104. **(D)** Client need: psychosocial integrity; subcategory: coping and adaptation; content area: psychiatric

    RATIONALE

    (A) This statement belittles the client and does not provide enough information to alleviate the client's concerns. (B) This statement places the responsibility on the client. However, it may be perceived as a threat and may cause the client to be fearful of the system. (C) A "why" question causes a defensive response by the receiver of the message. (D) It is important to provide clients with the knowledge base, treatment options, and future possibilities that may empower them to take an active role in their care.

105. **(D)** Client need: physiological integrity; subcategory: pharmacological and parenteral therapies; content area: psychiatric

    RATIONALE

    (A) The side effects of medications, and complexity of the medication regimen, can cause decreased patient adherence in the aftercare setting. (B) Consider the possibility of addictive side effects. (C) Concurrent use of drugs increases the cost of treatment. (D) Patient education programs regarding concomitant drug regimens must be clear, organized, and effective.

106. **(A)** Client need: psychosocial integrity; subcategory: psychosocial adaptation; content area: psychiatric

    RATIONALE

    (A, B) Unfortunately, some clients continue to focus their aggressive behavior on the treatment staff even after discharge. Therefore when placing safety first, it is wise for the nurse to change work schedule and if possible change place of residence. A change in the work schedule may disrupt the nurse's lifestyle but it may separate the nurse from the source of the threats. (C) Filing charges will not necessarily help the situation, but may only aggravate the problem. (D) Examining the societal changes will increase knowledge but does not provide safety.

107. **(C)** Client need: psychosocial integrity; subcategory: psychosocial adaptation; content area: psychiatric

    RATIONALE

    (A) Involuntary admission status means that the client did not request hospitalization. It may be implemented when a client acts in a manner that indicates being mentally ill and due to the illness, likely to be dangerous to self or others. (B) Religious leaders may provide significant support. (C) Culture plays a major role in physical and mental health care. (D) It is not necessary for the treating clinical nurse specialist to be fluent in the client's language.

108. **(A)** Client need: psychosocial integrity; subcategory: psychosocial adaptation; content area: psychiatric

    RATIONALE

    (A, B) Focusing on the medical rather than concentrating on the psychological or emotional problems tends to be better accepted among Hispanic American patients. (C) Cultural resistance may not play a role in the therapeutic process. (D) Societal changes are a challenge to the psychiatric-mental health therapist and must be considered. However, these considerations are not the best approach with a new client.

109. **(B)** Client need: physiological integrity; subcategory: pharmacological and parenteral therapies; content area: psychiatric

    RATIONALE

    (A) The client's psychotic features may be more evident due to possible Lithane toxicity. (B) Lotensin is prescribed for hypertension and may increase the risk of Lithane toxicity due to its diuretic effect. (C) Carbamazepine (Tegretol) is effective for the treatment of bipolar disorder. (D) Olanzapine (Zyprexa) is prescribed for psychotic disorders not for bipolar disorders.

110. **(B)** Client need: physiological integrity; subcategory: pharmacological and parenteral therapies; content area: psychiatric

    RATIONALE

    (A) Setting firm and consistent limits is an important nursing action but is not the priority action. (B) The client has been prescribed a medication that lowers the blood pressure, which needs monitoring both sitting and standing frequently during the initial dosage adjustment. (C) Methylphenidate (Ritalin) has a short half-life. Side effects are minimal. (D) Allowing the client to act out in a physical manner will affect the client's ability to interact effectively with others around him.

111. **(D)** Client need: physiological integrity; subcategory: pharmacological and parenteral therapies; content area: psychiatric

RATIONALE

(A) Advise the patient not to take gabapentin (Neurontin) within 2 hours of an antacid. (B) Do not discontinue medication abruptly; the action may cause an increase in frequency of seizures. (C) Avoid alcohol use. (D) Instructions to the patient should emphasize the importance of following the medication regimen.

112. **(B)** Client need: psychosocial integrity; subcategory: psychosocial adaptation; content area: psychiatric

RATIONALE

(A) The nurse is not accountable for or responsible for the success of the treatment. (B) Accountable means that the nurse accepts responsibility for providing quality care and discloses to the client the purpose of the nursing activities. (C) The nurse is responsible for disclosing to the client the expected outcomes of nursing activities not the outcomes of medical treatment. (D) It is important for the nurse to keep the client informed regarding the purpose of the work to be done.

Related Sciences
Review Tests

Nursing Leadership and Management: Content Review and Test

Tommie L. Norris, RN, DNSc
Virginia Kay Rogers, RN, C, MS, MED

1. Leadership and management
   A. Definition of leadership: the ability of an individual to accomplish goals by leading via motivation, rousing confidence, taking risks, and anticipating the future
   B. Definition of management: the ability of an individual to meet goals of an organization via planning, organizing, and balancing resources
   C. Distinguish between a leader and manager
      (1) Similarities
         (a) Both focus on goals
         (b) Both direct followers
      (2) Differences
         (a) Managers have legitimate power
         (b) Leaders inspire followers by interpersonal charisma and may not have an assigned position of power within the organization
         (c) Managers' outcomes focus on the organization or unit goals
         (d) Leaders' outcomes focus on their peers, which ultimately may accomplish the organization's goals if not in direct conflict
      (3) The most valuable assets to an organization are people who have developed both leadership and management qualities, since their influence often extends beyond their own units or organizations, thus encouraging professional networking
2. Leadership and management styles
   A. Use of different types of management and leadership may attain goals
   B. Authoritative style: uses coercion to motivate followers who have no input into decision making process
      (1) Advantage: useful in emergency situation when one person needs to direct chaos (i.e., industrial explosion with thousands injured)
      (2) Disadvantage: suppresses creativity and encourages dependency

   C. Democratic style: based on group decision making with leader/manager encouraging
      (1) Advantage: participative governance decreases hostility and encourages creativity
      (2) Disadvantage: process is slower than authoritative since all members must reach consensus
   D. Laissez-faire: followers and leaders/mangers equally share in decision making with little or no intervention by leaders
      (1) Advantage: Autonomous workers enjoy the flexibility and freedom to shape work environment. Bureaucratic rigidity is not an issue and petitions are encouraged
      (2) Disadvantage: A distinct decision may not be reached
3. Nursing care delivery systems
   A. Private duty/primary nursing: private duty (1 RN: 1 client) was precursor of primary nursing
      (1) Advantage: continuity of care
      (2) Disadvantage: cost effectiveness is questioned
   B. Functional: assignment of staff to specific tasks (giving medications, baths, vital signs)
      (1) Advantages: focus on completing tasks; effective with large numbers of clients; employees can be assigned to task in which they are most proficient
      (2) Disadvantages: fragmented care, low job satisfaction, little team effort
   C. Team: care of group of patients by a team of health care providers who are lead by a knowledgeable nurse
      (1) Advantages: Sense of contribution to team nurtured
      (2) Disadvantages: Need skilled leader, some members may be underutilized
   D. Primary care: 24-hour accountability by a nurse for specific clients from admission to discharge; holistic care of client; primary nurse plans, implements, and evaluates care; accountability is fundamental

(1) Advantages: positive patient outcomes, continuity of care, higher nurse satisfaction

(2) Disadvantages: accountability may eventually result in burnout, novice nurses may feel threatened

E. Case management: service-delivery system that is a cost-saving process and is outcome-oriented.

(1) Advantages: numerous services needs of clients are met; focus is on entire episode of illness; crosses all settings in which care is given; care directed by case manager.

(2) Disadvantages: many tasks are performed outside of the client visit and are nonreimbursable; morale problem and burnout are frequent occurrences; case managers find themselves overworked, poorly paid, and unable to change the system.

4. Communication

A. Communication is the capability of forming and sending a message so that another can receive and interpret its true meaning.

B. Communication is an essential component of the leadership/management process.

C. Five commonly used communication networks

(1) Wheel: the leader/manager is the hub or center, staff are the spokes. All communication goes through the center or leader/manager.

(2) Y: communication is linear until it branches off into different division of nursing units. As in the wheel, all communication going upward and downward passes though the manager who disseminates information or prevents it from moving to other levels.

(3) Chain: information passes along a continuum, which may be directional or nondirectional.

(4) Circle: information passes through all members and resembles the democratic leadership style. This is considered to be the least effective communication method.

(5) All channel: has no communication restrictions. It is effective with problem solving.

D. Feedback is essential to all communication

E. Characteristics of communication

(1) Formal or informal: formal is information upheld by the organization; informal is unofficial information, also known as "grapevine"

(2) Vertical or horizontal: vertical information passes from management to employees; horizontal information passes between peers

(3) Personal or nonpersonal: interdependent influences may occur; nonpersonal information has no shared influences

(4) Instrumental or expressive: instrumental information is essential to perform the task; expressive information may be considered trivial or nonessential

F. Multicultural communication

(1) The demographic profile of registered nurses does not match the demographic profile of the general population.

(2) With cultural diversity of employees comes diversity of opinions.

(3) Managers use many techniques to handle workforce diversity.

(a) Denial: manager simply ignores the diversity since the manager believes it does not affect the organization

(b) Minimize: manager sees diversity as negatively impacting the organization so attempts are made to maintain a homogeneous workforce

(c) Energize: managers views diversity as both negatively and positively influencing the organization so attempts are made to control the negative and increase the positive influences

G. Communication must be clear, simple, and precise with sender being responsible for making sure the message is understood

H. Assertive vs. aggressive communication

(1) Assertive communication

(a) Does not violate another person's rights

(b) Verbal and nonverbal communication are congruent

(c) Uses straightforward honest ways for expression

(2) Aggressive communication

(a) Often involves hostile manner of expression

(b) Does not consider the rights of the other person

(c) "I want to win at all costs"

(3) Passive communication: individual has powerful feelings about an issue but does not verbalize those feelings.

(4) Passive aggressive: an aggressive message delivered in a passive way. Often verbal and nonverbal are not congruent.

5. Quality Improvement and Risk Management

A. A standard is the predetermined "yardstick" for measuring quality care.

(1) Must be established by authority

(2) Must be measurable and achievable

(3) Must be accepted by those who are affected by standards

(4) Standards for Nursing Practice

B. Audits are measurement tools to determine quality of care delivered.

(1) Outcome audits: end results of care or change in health related to care (i.e., morbidity and mortality)

(2) Process audit: measures the process of care or how care was implemented

(3) Structure audit: determines if setting was safe and effective

(4) Retrospective: measures taken after the service rendered

(5) Concurrent: measures taken while receiving services

C. Leaders must define quality and incorporate into the organizational mission statement.

D. Quality improvement is everybody's business.

E. Focus of quality improvement is directed at work process not toward evaluation of individual employees.

F. Steps of quality improvement.

(1) Determine standard: must be known by all.

(2) Collect information to determine if standard is met.

(3) Analyze the information.

(4) Compare information collected to the standard.

(5) Educate or take corrective action if standard not met.

(6) Disseminate results.

G. Threshold: acceptable level

H. Sentinel event: unusual adverse happening (i.e.: maternal death)

I. Indicator: quantitative signal developed by experts that may suggest further evaluation is needed

J. Commonly used tools to illustrate causes of indicator results

    (1) Flow chart: graphical representation of events

    (2) Cause and effect diagram: "Ishikawa": resembles a fish with an outcome being the head and the fish spines representing all major causes (i.e., staff, equipment, methods)

    (3) Pareto chart: exhibits data in rank order

    (4) Histogram: exhibits a summary of how frequently something occurs

    (5) Scatter diagram: shows the relationship between two variables

6. Time Management

A. An important part of leading or managing is the effective use of one's time.

B. Biorhythms play an important part since they affect an individual's energy levels.

    (1) Early bird: wakes up early in the morning and to bed early

    (2) Owl: prefers to sleep late and to bed late

C. To increase and maintain energy levels, alternate physical and mental tasks

D. Dominant brain.

    (1) Left brain dominant: tackle a project by the rules, on a time schedule, and with order. Results: projects usually finished on time but suffer stress.

    (2) Right brain dominant: tackle a project with creativity and resist time schedules. Results: projects may not be finished on time and suffer guilt.

    (3) Mixed brain dominant: use both sides of brain by using a time-frame to organize their creativity.

E. The person who makes the most of their time analyzes their type of biorhythms and determines if they are right, left, or mixed brain dominant and proceeds to plan activities around the findings.

F. Balance time between family and professional obligations.

G. Develop an organized environment

    (1) If you don't use something in a year, toss it out

    (2) Color code files to quickly determine what you need

    (3) Place frequently used items up front

    (4) Keep stock on hand to prevent running to store and wasting time

    (5) Limit social phone calls until project is finished

H. Break large projects into small projects that can be completed

I. Don't procrastinate

J. The first step in time management is to begin each and every shift or project with a planning period and prioritize

K. Lists are wonderful time organizers but they must be flexible and prioritized

L. Delegation can organize your time and increase productivity

    (1) Delegate to lowest practicable level.

    (2) State Boards of Nursing identify the legal aspects of delegation.

    (3) Accountability of task remains with the registered nurse who delegated the task.

    (4) It is imperative to know the skill level of the person to whom you are delegating; as well as the condition of the patient.

        (a) Even simple task such as bathing may not be delegated if patient's condition is critical.

    (5) Reoccurring and simple task are the best to delegate.

    (6) Provide the delegatee with all necessary information.

    (7) Unlicensed personnel such as a nursing assistant may complete an organization's training program or gain certification, which enables them to perform limited tasks.

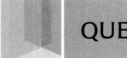

1. The nurses on a nursing unit are experienced and need minimal direction to achieve the nursing care outcomes. A decision must be made promptly to determine which type of work schedule will be utilized on the next rotation. Which leadership style would be effective on this unit?

   A. Authoritative
   B. Democratic
   C. Laissez-faire
   D. Bureaucratic

2. An emergency code (Resuscitative Efforts) has been called on a nursing unit. Which leadership style is most effective in this situation?

   A. Authoritative
   B. Democratic
   C. Laissez-faire
   D. Bureaucratic

3. A nurse is assigned to do dressing changes to all the patients for an entire shift. This is an example of which type of nursing delivery system?

   A. Primary
   B. Team
   C. Functional
   D. Case management

4. When participating in team nursing, which member is assigned the task of ensuring that all patient care was completed appropriately?

   A. Nurse manager
   B. Team leader
   C. Individual staff member
   D. Unit director

5. A nurse who admits a patient in congestive heart failure assumes 24-hour responsibility for the patient throughout the patient's discharge. The nurse is participating in which type of nursing care delivery system?

   A. Primary
   B. Team
   C. Functional
   D. Case management

6. Communication related to the possibility of a pay increase, which occurs between two staff nurses on a nursing unit, is termed which type of information?

   A. Formal
   B. Horizontal
   C. Instrumental
   D. Vertical

7. Successful communication is most likely to occur when the information is:

   A. Clear and detailed from managers.
   B. A memorandum with all information related to the organization.
   C. Simple, clear, and relevant
   D. Irrelevant and all-inclusive

8. A nurse who manages workforce diversity by trying to socialize those of different backgrounds into one similar type of workforce is using which technique of handing workforce diversity?

   A. Denial
   B. Minimize
   C. Energize
   D. Classify

9. The primary characteristic of aggressive communication is:

   A. Attempting to achieve one's goals without consideration of others
   B. Communication of one's needs using empathy
   C. Having strong feelings but choosing to keep them to one's self
   D. Using honest appropriate means to communicate

10. A physician requests a nurse to give an additional dose of digoxin. The nurse explains that the patient's heart rate is only 40 bpm and the potassium level is extremely low. The physician states, "Give the digoxin or I'll have you fired!" An assertive response by the nurse would be:

    A. "I'll give the medication but the patient will die."
    B. "I refuse to listen to anyone like you."
    C. "Don't ever yell at me again or I'll have you fired."
    D. "I think we need to discuss this with the pharmacist or the unit manager."

11. The **first** step in quality improvement is to:

    A. Collect data to determine if standards are met
    B. Implement a plan to correct the problem
    C. Determine the standard
    D. Determine if the findings warrant correction

12. Who should be involved in quality improvement measures?

    A. Everyone
    B. Professional staff
    C. Management staff
    D. Consumers

13. A local hospital reported the unexplained death of a young child admitted for a routine cast application. This is an example of a/an:

    A. Indicator
    B. Sentinel event
    C. Threshold
    D. Outcome

14. Prior to beginning a continuous improvement project, the nurse should determine the minimal safety level of care by referring to the:

    A. Procedure manual
    B. Nursing care standards
    C. Litigation proceeding of a similar case
    D. Job descriptions for the organization

15. The nurse audits charts to determine how many patients discharged over the past year had a positive tuberculin skin test with a negative chest x-ray. This type of audit is termed:

A. Concurrent
B. Process
C. Retrospective
D. Outcome

16. The nurse manager notices an unusually high number of medication errors being reported on her unit. Data collected revealed that prn medications were not being evaluated for pain relief, medications were not being charted after administration, and some medications were not arriving to the floor on time. Using a cause-and-effect/Ishikawa diagram, identify the outcome.

A. Prn medications not being followed up
B. Medications not being charted after administration
C. Medications not arriving on unit in timely manner
D. Unusually high number of medication errors

17. The **first** step in time management is to:

A. Take a break and energize with high carbohydrates
B. Complete the most difficult task first
C. Allow a period of time for planning and prioritizing
D. Delegate all unpleasant tasks

18. When completing a daily list, the nurse must remember that a list:

A. Should be structured with little variability
B. Should not be changed, so that time is not wasted
C. Must be flexible
D. Should include all items that need to be completed

19. The most effective way to manage a large task is to:

A. Not stop until entire task is completed
B. Delegate the task to someone else
C. Break it down into smaller more manageable pieces
D. Put it off until you have adequate time

20. Nurses can increase their own efficiency and energy level by:

A. Keeping a handy supply of candy for quick energy
B. Quickly reacting to all interruptions
C. Agreeing to complete new projects so not to waste time explaining why they're too busy
D. Alternating between mental and physical tasks

21. A nurse will be delegating patient care tasks to other staff on the nursing unit. The nurse should **first**:

A. Refer to organization's procedure manual
B. Review the state Nurse Practice Act
C. Determine if the individual likes to perform the tasks
D. Delegate the most time-consuming task

22. Which person can be delegated the task of completing the history and physical on patients newly admitted to a nursing unit?

A. Registered nurse
B. Licensed practical (vocational) nurse
C. Nursing assistant
D. All levels of personnel are permissible since information is related to the past and cannot change

23. When the nurse delegates a task, who is responsible for ensuring that it was completed correctly?

A. The person to whom it was delegated
B. The nurse who delegated the task
C. The patient
D. The nurse manager

24. Which task may be delegated to a Licensed Practical Nurse if the patient is stable?

A. Administering a warm tap water enema
B. Injecting potassium into an existing IV
C. Determining the nursing care plan
D. Teaching the patient to administer insulin

25. The **first** step in delegation is to:

A. Ask the patient if another nurse can help with their care
B. Informing the delegatee who is in charge
C. Determine the skill level of the person to whom the nurse is delegating
D. Perform the task and allow delegatee to follow-up and evaluate the results

26. Which of the following managed care structures represent an arrangement between employers and insurance companies that provide member services from a selected group of providers?

A. Direct contact Health Maintenance Organizations
B. Preferred Providers Organizations
C. Network Health Maintenance Organizations
D. Exclusive Provider Organization

27. The consequences of how an organization elects to structure itself are significant in that the structure identifies authority and control relationships that have a profound impact on the nurse manager and the provisions of care. At what level are nurse managers identified within the organization?

A. Middle-level managers
B. First-level managers
C. Top-level managers
D. Interim-level managers

28. In a health care environment emphasizing the need for efficient and effective operations, it is essential that nurse managers have the authority necessary to make decisions. An organization that allows for increased responsibility and decision making is referred to as:

A. Centralized
B. Decentralized
C. Apportioned
D. Compartmentalized

29. A professional practice system that manages clinical care of patients across a continuum using managed care concepts and tools is called:

A. Differentiated practice
B. Modular nursing
C. Primary nursing
D. Case management

30. What has nursing research validated about clinical care management by professional nurses?
    A. It diminishes collegiality between health care providers
    B. It decreases patients' length of stay
    C. It increases cost of hospitalization
    D. It contributes to duplication of services

31. Which statement indicates effective communication of ideas?
    A. "We need to discuss ways to make it easier to meet patient needs while using less money."
    B. "Stop using so many supplies since complex budget issues are affecting our delivery of care."
    C. "We're going to have to cut back on nursing staff."
    D. "The work is going to have to improve or else top management will be asked to deal with the outcomes."

32. Which words best describe a nurse who expresses job satisfaction?
    A. Autonomous, credulous, enthusiastic, empowered
    B. Autonomous, challenged, euphoric, empowered
    C. Arduous, challenged, enthusiastic, empowered
    D. Autonomous, challenged, enthusiastic, empowered

33. During a staff meeting, the nurse manager presents his/her own analysis of problems and proposals for actions to the staff, inviting critique and comments. The nurse manager then analyzes the comments and makes the final decision. Which answer indicates the manager's leadership style?
    A. Laissez-faire
    B. Participative leadership
    C. Autocratic
    D. Democratic

34. A newly hired nursing employee is needed to perform patient care before orientation is completed. Which practice would meet Joint Commission on the Accreditation of Health Care Organizations (JCAHO) requirements?
    A. Do not allow the nurse to perform any duties
    B. Allow the nurse to practice since he or she is already licensed and competent to provide patient care
    C. Provide self-learning educational materials, then allow the nurse to proceed with patient care
    D. Place the nurse with a peer to assist with care while assessing competency

35. What is the most frequently neglected area in management?
    A. Managerial knowledge
    B. Successful communications
    C. Clinical skills
    D. Professional development

36. Decision making occurs at many levels. Which level is considered the most empowering to staff members?
    A. The leader makes a decision without consulting anyone and assumes full accountability
    B. The leader asks direct reports to decide on a solution and agrees to support the decision

C. The leader makes a decision after convening a task force to analyze the problem
    D. The leader makes a decision with direct reports

37. A critical component of the supervisory process is delegation. Which of the following is the most empowering to staff?
    A. Delegation starts at top-management
    B. Delegation frees the manager to do other tasks while empowering staff
    C. Effective delegation requires nurse managers to know the abilities, strengths, and weaknesses of their staff
    D. Delegation fosters responsibility of staff while increasing professional growth

38. What is a major characteristic of negotiation?
    A. It is not important to get anything in writing since the truth will prevail in oral communications
    B. Resources tend to involve too many individuals in the decision-making process
    C. Be positive in your approach since optimism goes further than negativism
    D. Harmony is possible even when strategies are not well planned

39. What is the primary purpose of supervision and delegation?
    A. To improve staff compliance to policy and procedure
    B. To influence the organization's approach in recruitment, promotion, and personnel evaluation
    C. To enhance the delivery of quality nursing care
    D. To assign appropriate work tasks to the best-qualified individual

40. According to the National Council of State Boards of Nursing, delegation involves the transfer of care to an individual who has the following characteristic:
    A. Adaptability
    B. Flexibility
    C. Competent
    D. Responsible

41. What is implied when delegating decision-making authority to other staff members?
    A. Trust
    B. Exemplary clinical competency
    C. Solidarity
    D. Confidentiality

42. Effective communications, both verbal and nonverbal, are essential to an understanding of and participation in the workplace. According to Mehrabian (1972), communication research indicates that the nonverbal elements contribute heavily to the significance of the social content of a message. What percentage of the communication process is nonverbal?
    A. 07%
    B. 25%
    C. 52%
    D. 93%

43. Nursing staff is empowered through effective communications. Select the most assertive response made by the nurse manager.

A. "Not getting to work on time has really caused a lot of problems for all of us."

B. "I understand that you are having some difficulty in getting to work on time."

C. "Please try harder to be on time for work."

D. "If you continue being late for work, other measures will have to be taken."

44. What type of negotiation strategy focuses on issues discussed by their merits rather than through a haggling process?

   A. Soft negotiation
   B. Hard negotiation
   C. Principled negotiation
   D. Equity negotiations

45. Effective communication techniques are essential for group leaders. Which is an example of an open-ended question?

   A. "It sounds like you are having difficulty responding to my comment."
   B. "You look very puzzled, Ms. Jones. Would you like to talk about it?"
   C. "Yes, please continue what you were saying."
   D. "How did you feel when you didn't receive the promotion you thought you deserved?"

46. Unfreezing and refreezing are commonly used terms that reflect a type of theory used in everyday practice.

   A. Communication theory
   B. Theory X
   C. Change theory
   D. Theory Y

47. What is the ethical decision-making principle that directs the healthcare professional never to produce harm even during times when it is not possible to directly benefit the patient?

   A. Respect for autonomy
   B. Beneficence
   C. Nonmaleficence
   D. Justice

48. Recognition of the stages of group formation is essential to the nurse manager in terms of effective communications. What example describes the state of performing?

   A. Group members are active and accepting of their roles and responsibilities.
   B. Group members have established trusting relationships and are able to identify the roles and responsibilities of one another.
   C. Group members are beginning to trust each other, yet the ability to be open leads to vulnerabilities with possibilities of conflict.
   D. Group members are learning about each other through verbal and nonverbal communications, decision making, and problem solving.

49. Managing culturally diverse issues in the workplace requires an understanding of terminology used within organizations. Which of the following terms is commonly associated with discrimination control?

   A. Resistance to change
   B. Neutralization to resistance
   C. Dispersing blame
   D. Smoothing

50. A nurse manager's particular uniqueness and strengths determine the roles he or she models most frequently. A builder of communication networks is considered to be which role of the nurse manager?

   A. Spokesperson
   B. Liaison
   C. Resource allocator
   D. Monitor

1. **(B)** Client need: safe, effective care environment; subcategory: management of care

   RATIONALE

   (A) Authoritative style would probably induce hostility. (B) Democratic style would allow workers to have input while reaching a decision within time frame. (C) Laissez-faire style often does not reach a distinct answer and a time frame is indicated. (D) Bureaucratic style infers the use of rules/laws of which an appeal is useless.

2. **(A)** Client need: safe, effective care environment; subcategory: management of care

   RATIONALE

   (A) Authoritarian leaders would take charge and organize the situation rapidly. (B) and (C) Emergency situations require quick decision making and one person to take charge; both democratic and laissez-faire require more time to reach a decision. (D) Bureaucratic styles refers to rules/law and no appeal is appropriate during this time.

3. **(C)** Client need: safe, effective care environment; subcategory: management of care

   RATIONALE

   (A) Primary nursing requires the nurse to be responsible for all the nursing care needs of a patient, not just dressing changes. (B) Team nursing would have staff assigned only to a limited number or group of patients. (C) Functional nursing is concerned with tasks. (D) Case management would consider all aspects of care.

4. **(B)** Client need: safe, effective care environment; subcategory: management of care

   RATIONALE

   (A) In usual circumstances, the nurse manager would not evaluate the care. (B) The team leader assumes the responsibility of evaluating care given by all its members. (C) The individual staff member is under the supervision of the team leader. (D) The unit director is in a higher level of the hierarchy and usually only evaluates care that is seen as being unsafe.

5. **(A)** Client need: safe, effective care environment; subcategory: management of care

   RATIONALE

   (A) Primary nursing assumes 24-hour accountability for patient care. (B) In team nursing a group of individuals assume care for a designated number of patients; however, they do not assume 24-hour responsibility. (C) Functional nursing does not assume 24-hour responsibility. (D) Although case management is concerned with 24-hour care, it is more concerned with coordination of services.

6. **(B)** Client need: safe, effective care environment; subcategory: management of care

   RATIONALE

   (A) Formal information would be transmitted officially by management. (B) Horizontal information passes between two peers of equal status. (C) Instrumental information is necessary to do the job; whereas a pay raise is nice it is not considered necessary. (D) Vertical information is transmitted from management to employees and not between employees.

7. **(C)** Client need: safe, effective care environment; subcategory: management of care

   RATIONALE

   (A) Although information should be clear it does not need to be detailed; instead it should be concise. (B) A memorandum with unnecessary information is not likely to be successful since reader may not be able to assimilate all the facts. (C) A simple clear message containing only relevant information is more likely to be correctly understood. (D) Information that is irrelevant and includes everything may result in the receiver being confused.

8. **(B)** Client need: safe, effective care environment; subcategory: management of care

   RATIONALE

   (A) Managers using denial would not see a need to socialize those of diverse backgrounds since they perceive them as having no impact on the organization. (B) Managers who use the minimizing technique are attempting to maintain a similar workforce. (C) Managers using energize would not attempt to change the workforce but simply put forth the positive influences while downplaying the negative influences. (D) Managers who classify employees into cultural groups are not using any specific management technique.

9. **(A)** Client need: safe, effective care environment; subcategory: management of care

   RATIONALE

   (A) Achievement of one's own goals is the desired outcome regardless of its potential negative effect on others. (B) Empathy is not part of aggressive communication; others are not taken into consideration. (C) Feelings are often forcefully projected onto others. (D) Any means are used regardless of their appropriateness or truthfulness.

10. **(D)** Client need: safe, effective care environment; subcategory: management of care

    RATIONALE

    Options A, B, and C are examples of aggressive communication. (D) does not infringe on the physician's rights, and is an open expression of what needs to be done.

11. **(C)** Client need: safe, effective care environment; subcategory: management of care

    RATIONALE

    (A) Data is collected after the standard has been determine and the outcome is established. (B) The plan is implemented after data collected does not meet the standard previously set. (C) The standard must be determined prior to any quality improvement actions. (D) Findings are compared after the standard has been set.

12. **(A)** Client need: safe, effective care environment; subcategory: management of care

    RATIONALE

    All the answers are correct; however, (A) "Everyone" is most conclusive.

13. **(B)** Client need: safe, effective care environment; subcategory: management of care

    RATIONALE

    (A) An indicator alerts that a problem may need further investigation. (B) A sentinel event is an undesirable happening. (C) The threshold is the acceptable standard. (D) In quality improvement, outcome is the desired result.

14. **(B)** Client need: safe, effective care environment; subcategory: management of care

    RATIONALE

    (A) The procedure manual outlines steps in performing a procedure. (B) Nursing care standards are the means by which we judge all care. (C) Legal cases may identify lack of ethical or legal appropriate care but cannot be used to determine standard by which to judge. (D) Job descriptions are based on the state boards of nursing requirements, which is a standard.

15. **(C)** Client need: safe, effective care environment; subcategory: management of care

    RATIONALE

    (A) A concurrent audit is completed while the patient is still hospitalized. (B) A process audit determines how care was implemented. (C) Retrospective audits are performed after care has been rendered. (D) An outcome audit measures changes in health due to care, this scenario does not imply care changed health.

16. **(D)** Client need: safe, effective care environment; subcategory: management of care

    RATIONALE

    (A) Prn medications not being evaluated is an indicator, as is: (B) Medications not being documented, and (C) Medications not arriving to unit on time. (D) The effect on the indicators is the outcome with the result being a high number of medication errors.

17. **(C)** Client need: safe, effective care environment; subcategory: management of care

    RATIONALE

    (A) Although nutrition is important, the break should be scheduled prior to beginning task and at intervals when energy is waning. (B) It is best to break difficult tasks into smaller manageable pieces. (C) A period of planning and prioritizing can organize each day or project to make the most of time. (D) Delegation is a time management tool but simple repetitive tasks should be delegated.

18. **(C)** Client need: safe, effective care environment; subcategory: management of care

    RATIONALE

    (A) List should be flexible due to changes in patient's conditions and situations. (B) List must be changed as need arises. (C) List is a planning tool and must be adaptable to current situations. (D) List should include important items that are prioritized.

19. **(C)** Client need: safe, effective care environment; subcategory: management of care

    RATIONALE

    (A) Many tasks take days or weeks to complete so this is not feasible. (B) The task may be complicated or if related to a patient, their condition may not make it possible to delegate. (C) By breaking it down, you can accomplish one part and see your progress. (D) Procrastination will result in the task never being completed.

20. **(D)** Client need: safe, effective care environment; subcategory: management of care

    RATIONALE

    (A) Candy can provide for quick energy but does not ensure efficiency. (B) React only to emergencies; others can wait. (C) Agreeing to new projects will just frustrate you and the person delegating the new project when you are not able to complete it. (D) Alternating between physical and mental tasks provides the needed break to increase efficiency and energy.

21. **(B)** Client need: safe, effective care environment; subcategory: management of care

    RATIONALE

    (A) The procedure manual lists steps to complete a skill. (B) A state's Nurse Practice Act defines the legal limitations for delegation. (C) Delegation is not based on an individual's likes or dislikes but on his or her ability. (D) Simple repetitive tasks are best delegated.

22. **(A)** Client need: safe, effective care environment; subcategory: management of care

    RATIONALE

    (A) The registered nurse is responsible and should not delegate this task. (B) State nursing practice acts define the duties of the LPN, which do not include admission assessment. (C) Nursing assistants are not licensed and are not trained to evaluate care needs. (D) Although history is related to the past, it contains important information that can contribute to current health status.

23. **(B)** Client need: safe, effective care environment; subcategory: management of care

    RATIONALE

    (A) The person to whom the task was delegated is responsible for completing the task to the best of their ability or informing the RN that they are not able to complete the task. (B) The nurse who delegated the task is responsible for ensuring that the delegatee has needed information and completes the task appropriately. (C) The patient is not qualified to judge and may have emotional feelings related to the situation. (D) The nurse manager may indeed be qualified to evaluate the completion of the task but may not be familiar with the situation.

24. **(A)** Client need: safe, effective care environment; subcategory: management of care

    RATIONALE

    (A) Most state nursing practice acts allow LPNs to administer enemas that do not contain additives or medications. (B) Administration of IV medications is usually limited to an RN. (C) Planning care is the duty of the RN. (D) Teaching is limited to the RN.

25. **(C)** Client need: safe, effective care environment; subcategory: management of care

    RATIONALE

    (A) The patient is not qualified to determine who can perform care. (B) Although the delegatee needs to know who to ask questions of, this is not the first step. (C) Determining the skill level will ensure the task has a high probability of being completed correctly. (D) Performing the task yourself does not use effective time management.

26. **(B)** Client need: safe, effective care environment; subcategory: management of care

    RATIONALE

    (A) Direct contact HMOs enter into contractual arrangements with a variety of individual physicians to provide services. Physician compensation varies from a predetermined fee to capitation. (B) PPOs represent an arrangement between employees and insurance companies that provide member services from a selected group of providers. (C) Network HMOs contract with more than one group of physicians for medical services. Physician's compensation is determined on a capitated basis. (D) The EPO model parallels the preferred provider organization, with one major exception. Beneficiaries are limited to those providers that are participating physicians for any required health care services. Primary care physicians serve as gatekeepers.

27. **(A)** Client need: safe, effective care environment; subcategory: management of care

    RATIONALE

    (A) Middle level managers serve primarily to coordinate activities between the upper and lower levels of the hierarchy and represent the main channel of communication between levels. These managers (assistant vice-presidents, department heads, shift supervisors, case managers, nurse managers) are focused on the day-to-day operation of nursing functions and frequently play a major role in developing the policies and procedures that guide nursing and organizational activities. (B) First-level managers are focused primarily on the activities of their own work units (assistant nurse managers, primary nurses, unit case managers, team leaders, charge nurses). (C) Top-level managers or the executive group activities are focused on providing direction in the formulation of goals and objectives, achievement of fiscal performance targets and defining and controlling operational policy. Examples are Chief Executive Officer (CEO), President, Director, and those responsible for major divisions such as directors/chiefs of human resources, medical affairs, nursing service, etc. (D) Interim-level managers are not considered a level of management.

28. **(B)** Client need: safe, effective care environment; subcategory: management of care

    RATIONALE

    (A) In centralized organizations decisions are made by a limited number of individuals at the top of the organization or by the managers of a department or unit, and thereafter communicated to the employees. (B) In a decentralized organization authority is distributed throughout the organization to allow for increased responsibility and delegation in decision making. (C) An apportioned organization is not documented in the literature as a type of organization. (D) A compartmentalized organization is not documented in the literature as a type of organization.

29. **(D)** Client need: safe, effective care environment; subcategory: management of care

    RATIONALE

    (A) Differentiated practice is a philosophy that focuses on the structuring of roles and functions of nurses according to education, experience, and competence. (B) Modular nursing occurs when a RN accompanied by one or two nursing personnel provides care for a group of patients located in a particular geographic area. (C) Primary nursing occurs when a single RN is responsible and accountable for providing comprehensive nursing care for a group of patients during their entire hospital stay, delegation of tasks to non-RN personnel is reduced but not eliminated. (D) Case management is a professional practice system that manages clinical care of patients across a continuum. Case management has been described as an alternative care delivery model that expands the concept of primary nursing to include preadmission care, outpatient care, inpatient care, and postdischarge home care.

30. **(B)** Client need: safe, effective care environment; subcategory: management of care

    RATIONALE

    (A) Case managed care enhances collegiality between providers by increasing an environment that fosters a professional practice system. Collaborating with other healthcare providers can reduce fragmentation of care. (B) Numerous research admission and inpatient stays are reduced when registered nurses function as case managers. (C) A considerable advantage of case management is that it can be matrixed over or used in conjunction with a primary, team, or functional nursing model with the case manager providing the management and direction of care. Matrixing this model provides significant cost savings, as the entire nursing practice does not have to be changed. Costs are also reduced due to a decrease in fragmentation of patient care and enhanced job satisfaction for nursing case managers and for patients. (D) Monitoring a patient's response to treatment and services to prevent complications as well as facilitating access to various community-based services and support groups can reduce duplication and fragmentation of care.

31. **(A)** Client need: safe, effective care environment; subcategory: management of care

    RATIONALE

    (A) This statement implies collaboration for the purpose of problem solving. (B) This is a demanding statement that implies that the staff is not using discretion in the use of supplies. It does not offer an explanation about the complex budgetary issues. (C)

This statement implies that staff efforts are not being valued and that the workload will increase. (D) This is a threatening statement that implies that staff is not competent.

32. **(D)** Client need: safe, effective care environment; subcategory: management of care

    RATIONALE

    (A) Autonomous, enthusiastic, and empowered descriptive of job satisfaction. (B) Credulous means gullible or to believe too readily. This is not a characteristic of job satisfaction. (C) Challenged, enthusiastic, and empowered are descriptive of job satisfaction. Arduous means demanding great care, effort, or labor or strenuous. This is not a characteristic of job satisfaction. (D) These words are characteristic of a nurse who expresses job satisfaction. Autonomous is a condition or a quality of being self-governed. Challenged and enthusiastic refer to being positively stimulated and inspired by the environment, which encourages creative thinking and activity. Empowered refers to the facilitation of employee professional growth, by increasing knowledge and decision-making power and providing increased control over ones practice. Empowerment fosters commitment and accountability. It enables staff to perform to their fullest potential.

33. **(B)** Client need: safe, effective care environment; subcategory: management of care

    RATIONALE

    (A) Laissez-faire is a leadership style in which the leader abdicates leadership responsibilities, allowing staff to work without assistance, direction, or supervision. Staff members plan, implement, and evaluate their work in any way they see fit. (B) Participative leadership suggests a compromise between the authoritarian and the democratic styles. The leader presents his or her own analysis of problems and proposals for actions to members of the team, inviting critique and comments. (C) An autocratic style of leadership is task-oriented and directive. The leader uses his or her own power or position in an authoritarian manner to set and implement organizational goals. (D) In the democratic style of leadership, the leader uses personal and positional power to create ideas and input from staff and subordinates. Democratic leaders like to set their own goals and plan their own work in an effort to control their practice. This style empowers staff.

34. **(D)** Client need: safe, effective care environment; subcategory: management of care

    RATIONALE

    (A) Not allowing the nurse to perform will not provide opportunity for staff to observe performance and competency. (B) Licensure does not insure competency. (C) Self-learning modules may identify the nurse's knowledge concerning various aspects of care, but they do not assess issues related to performance and clinical competency. (D) JCAHO suggests that an orienting nurse be placed with a preceptor while assisting with care. The preceptor would then have the opportunity to assess and evaluate clinical competency and to identify further learning needs.

35. **(B)** Client need: safe, effective care environment; subcategory: management of care

    RATIONALE

    (A) Managerial knowledge is a key quality of a motivational leader. A knowledge base is empowering for the professional growth of nursing staff. (B) Successful communications is frequently neglected in the area of management since the means by which a message is sent determines success or failure. The element of time, the affective and subjective components of communication also affect whether or not one will be successful in communications. (C) Clinical skills are achieved by encouraging creativity and supporting continuous improvement and involvement in peer review and self-governance. Critical evaluation of performance with strategies for improving skills is important in reinforcing skills. Clinical skills are measurable. (D) Professional development includes a continuous growing body of practice-oriented knowledge established through research and analysis unique to the work group, collaboration with all service groups and individuals, strong colleagueship demonstrated by licensing and practice laws, autonomy, and a code of ethics.

36. **(B)** Client need: safe, effective care environment; subcategory: management of care

    RATIONALE

    (A) This level of decision making is considered the least empowering to staff according to the Vroom and Velton Decision Tree Model. (B) This level of decision making is the most empowering to staff according to the Vroom and Velton Decision Tree Model. (C) This level of decision making indicates some degree of empowerment. (D) This level of decision making indicates some degree of empowerment.

37. **(D)** Client need: safe, effective care environment; subcategory: management of care

    RATIONALE

    (A) The nurse manager delegates work to immediate nurse practice coordinators, who in turn redelegate all or part of the work to their staff. The components of delegation may include participation on organizational task forces and committees and the assignment of duties and responsibilities of patient care with the authority needed to complete the tasks. (B) Delegation generates greater commitment and fosters professional growth and pride. (C) Supervisors must also trust the judgment of staff who makes decisions. (D) Delegation empowers staff, thereby fostering independence.

38. **(C)** Client need: safe, effective care environment; subcategory: management of care

    RATIONALE

    (A) Always get the final results in writing, not only for your benefit, but also for clarification of the process and solution. (B) Identification and knowledge of resources enhances the negotiation process. Discuss each other's perspective. Do not assume that the opponent's values are the same as yours. Research pertinent information to be prepared. (C) Develop positive coalitions quickly. Negativism prevents focusing on the issues and creates an attitude of defeat. (D) Strategies and alternative strategies or solutions should be well planned during the negotiation process.

39. **(C)** Client need: safe, effective care environment; subcategory: management of care

    RATIONALE

    (A) Improving staff compliance to policy and procedure is not the primary purpose of supervision and delegation, but it is an important component of supervision and delegation. (B) Influencing the organization's approach in recruitment, promotion, and personnel evaluations is an important component of supervision, but it is not the primary purpose of delegation and supervision. (C) Enhancing the delivery of quality nursing care is the ultimate purpose of supervision and delegation. Improving staff compliance to policy and procedure, influencing the organization's approach in recruitment, promotion, and personnel evaluations, and assigning appropriate work tasks to the most qualified individual are examples of supervision and delegation that enhance the delivery of quality nursing care. (D) Assigning appropriate work tasks to the most qualified individual is an important component of supervision and delegation but it is not the primary component.

40. **(C)** Client need: safe, effective care environment; subcategory: management of care

    RATIONALE

    (A) Adaptability is not a characteristic of delegating transfer of care according to the National Council of State Boards of Nursing. Transfer if care requires a competent individual with au-thority to do a selected nursing task in situations. (B) Flexibility is not a characteristic of delegating transfer of care according to the National Council of State Boards of Nursing. Transfer of care requires a competent individual with authority to do a selected task in situations. (C) According to the National Council of State Boards of Nursing, delegation involves the transfer of care to a competent individual with authority to do a selected nursing task in situations. If the registered nurse delegates to a nursing assistant, the nursing assistant is responsible for performing the task; however, the nurse retains responsibility and accountability for the total nursing care of the client. (D) Responsibility, according to the National Council of State Boards of Nursing, is retained by the registered nurse who delegates tasks to an individual. The individual providing the care should be responsible in practice, however, the RN is ultimately responsible.

41. **(A)** Client need: safe, effective care environment; subcategory: management of care

    RATIONALE

    (A) Trust is implied when delegating decision-making authority. Trust fosters an increased exchange of open communication, interpersonal influence, and self-control. (B) Exemplary clinical competency is an outcome of leaders who are committed to providing staff with opportunities for education, critical thinking, and new experiences. (C) Delegating decision-making authority does not include solidarity. Solidarity is defined as a community of interests, objectives, or standards in a group. (D) Confidentiality implies trust yet confidentiality may not always be necessary when decision-making authority is delegated.

42. **(D)** Client need: safe, effective care environment; subcategory: management of care

    RATIONALE

    (A) According to Mehrabian (1981), only 7% of communications are from uttered words. (B) 25% is an arbitrary number chosen for an answer. (C) 52% is an arbitrary number chosen for an answer. (D) According to Mehrabian (1981), 93% of communications is nonverbal.

43. **(B)** Client need: safe, effective care environment; subcategory: management of care

    RATIONALE

    (A) This is an aggressive response. (B) This is an assertive response. (C) This is a passive response. (D) This is an authoritative and threatening response.

44. **(C)** Client need: safe, effective care environment; subcategory: management of care

    RATIONALE

    (A) Soft negotiators want to avoid personal conflict so they make concessions to reach an agreement quickly, even though they may end up feeling bitter and exploited. Soft negotiators want to avoid personal conflict so they make concessions to reach an agreement quickly, even though they may end up feeling bitter and exploited. (B) Hard negotiators look at any situation as a contest of personal wills. They believe that the person who takes the extreme position and holds out the longest does better in negotiating. (C) Principled negotiation is a combination of soft and hard. Issues are discussed on their merits rather than through a haggling process focused by what each party says it will and will not do. This method allows people to be fair while protecting themselves against others who take advantage of them. (D) Equity negotiations are not considered a negotiation strategy.

45. **(D)** Client need: safe, effective care environment; subcategory: management of care

    RATIONALE

    (A) This is a reflective response, noting content only. (B) This is a closed-ended question. This type of question is answered with a "yes" or "no" response. (C) This response is called a general lead. This tells the person that you are listening and want him or her to continue the conversation. (D) This is an open-ended question that allows a person to provide more information concerning the subject that was addressed.

46. **(C)** Client need: safe, effective care environment; subcategory: management of care

RATIONALE

(A) Communication is a process that has been identified as a sequence of activities that are in some way connected. Each activity is required, whether it is face-to-face communications or by a computer. Behavioral components of communications are identified as perceptions, verbal, and nonverbal. (B) Theory X is a human resources model that describes an approach that managers take to motivate employees based upon their assumptions about employee behavior. (C) Lewin suggests that there are three phases in the change process. They are unfreezing, changing, and refreezing. During unfreezing, the process of developing awareness to a need or problem is started and change is seen as the only solution. During the changing phase, a new way of behaving is presented to the group and they are allowed to discuss and assimilate the change into their way of doing business. During the refreezing phase, the change is consolidated into the regular operations of the organization and eventually becomes routine. (D) Theory Y is a type of human resources model in which workers are seen as being able to derive satisfaction from the work itself and make commitments to organizational goals.

47. **(C)** Client need: safe, effective care environment; subcategory: management of care

RATIONALE

(A) Respect for autonomy is an ethical decision-making principle that refers to the inherent respect owed patients to maintain control of their decision-making capacity even when this may differ from what the physician or others may see as in the client's best interest. (B) Beneficence is an ethical decision-making principle that refers to the healthcare professional being obligated to act in a manner that is of benefit to the client, to produce good and not harm. (C) Nonmaleficence is an ethical decision-making principle counter to beneficence that directs healthcare professionals to never produce harm even during times when it is not possible to directly benefit the client. (D) Justice is an ethical decision-making principle that guides ethical thinking to consider the fairness of actions and to attempt a just distribution of healthcare goods.

48. **(A)** Client need: safe, effective care environment; subcategory: management of care

RATIONALE

(A) The stage of performing occurs when group members are active and accepting of their roles and responsibilities. The leader begins to function like the other group members. Each member begins to accept a leadership role. (B) The stage of norming occurs when group members have established trusting relationships and are able to identify the roles and responsibilities of one another. Attention is given to content and process. Problem solving starts to result in recommendations. The leader is supportive of members. (C) During the stage of storming, members are beginning to trust each other, yet the ability to be open leads to vulnerabilities with possibilities of conflict. The leader begins to become less directive and starts assigning goal-directed tasks to the members. (D) During the stage of forming, members are learning about each other through verbal and nonverbal communications. Courtesy, caution, confusion, and commonality characterize forming. The leader's style is directive.

49. **(C)** Client need: safe, effective care environment; subcategory: management of care

RATIONALE

(A) The major reason given for resisting change is threatened self-interest. The individual or group senses that the personal costs involved with changing are greater than the personal benefits that could be gained from the change. Resistance to change is not a term that is commonly associated with discrimination control. (B) Neutralization of resistance is a strategy used to facilitate an effective change. An example of neutralization would be introducing change gradually, providing education and providing extra support. The term is not associated with discrimination control but with the change process. (C) Dispersing blame is a term associated with discrimination control. Dispersing blame results from inaccurate perceptions about someone that usually results in some type of mistreatment such as ignoring the individual. (D) Smoothing is a term associated with conflict management. Smoothing tends to minimize a conflict and informs everyone that everything will be all right. This strategy usually tones down the conflict temporarily but does not solve the underlying conflict.

50. **(B)** Client need: safe, effective care environment; subcategory: management of care

RATIONALE

(A) A spokesperson is a representative speaker for the area of responsibility. (B) A liaison is a builder of communications networks. (C) A resource allocator is a distributor of resources. (D) A monitor is a scanner of the environment to keep abreast of changes pertinent to the job.

CHAPTER 9

Growth and Development Test

MOCK NCLEX-RN BOARD REVIEW TEST QUESTIONS

1. A 14-year-old boy with cystic fibrosis is hospitalized for treatment of a respiratory infection. His mother says that he has been masturbating and that she disapproves. Which of these comments by the nurse would be *most* useful?

   A. "It results in nocturnal emissions."
   B. "It is not normal for 14 year olds."
   C. "It provides sexual experience without invoking risk or harm."
   D. "It suggests a lack of interest in normal sexual expression."

2. A 10-month-old infant is admitted to the pediatric unit for treatment of dehydration after several days of severe diarrhea. His mother also expressed concern about his development. Failure to attain which developmental milestone could indicate a developmental delay?

   A. Says three words other than "mama" and "dada"
   B. Sits without support
   C. Builds a tower of two cubes
   D. Walks well

3. The pediatrician detected a systolic ejection murmur during a routine examination of a 4 year old and referred her to a pediatric cardiologist. She will be admitted to the hospital for a cardiac catheterization. What predominant developmental characteristics of preschoolers should the nurse consider when preparing the child for heart catheterization?

   A. Temper tantrums, separation anxiety
   B. Stranger anxiety, parallel play
   C. Magical thinking, mutilation anxiety, nightmares
   D. Imaginary playmates, peer pressure

4. A 16-year-old girl is admitted from the emergency room to the pediatric unit with asthma. She requested information about her diagnosis. When developing her teaching plan, the nurse uses a hallmark of adolescent cognitive development:

   A. Abstract thinking
   B. Concrete thinking
   C. Productive daydreaming
   D. Self-centered ideology

5. A 2 year old is admitted to the pediatric unit newly diagnosed with acute lymphocytic leukemia. The *best* way for the nurse to facilitate growth and development in the acutely ill toddler is to:

   A. Direct efforts of preparation and teaching toward parents to minimize anxiety over parenting of the child.
   B. Tell the toddler well in advance of a procedure what is to take place.
   C. Separate the toddler from the parent, especially if there are temper tantrums.
   D. Encourage the child to regress to a previous developmental level for familiarity and comfort.

6. A 7-month-old infant is being discharged from the pediatric unit after 24 hours of observation because of a fall and loss of consciousness. His birth weight was 6 lb 10 oz. His mother asks how much he will weigh on his first birthday. The nurse responds that by age 12 months, he should weigh about:

   A. 10 lb, 14 oz
   B. 12 lb, 2 oz
   C. 15 lb, 4 oz
   D. 19 lb, 14 oz

7. A 6-month-old child is at the health unit for examination and immunizations. As a part of routine health education and anticipatory guidance, the nurse includes information addressing principles of growth and development.

Which of the following is accurate regarding growth patterns?

A. Gross motor skills develop after fine motor skills.
B. Differences among each age group are unusual.
C. Growth and development occurs in an orderly sequence.
D. Developmental tasks must be achieved during specific time periods.

8. An 11-month-old infant is brought to the emergency room for a third time with complaints of a fever and pulling at his right ear. His mother thinks he has another ear infection. The nursing assessment would include:

A. Checking for onset of presbycusis
B. Inspecting the position of the ears in relation to the inner and outer canthus of the eyes
C. Pulling the ear lobe gently down and out
D. Using a vibrating tuning fork for the Rinne test

9. A common phenomenon noted in normal pre-school children during nursing assessment of cardiac status is:

A. A large discrepancy in arm and leg blood pressures
B. The point of maximal impulse (PMI) is located at the fifth intercostal space, 7–9 cm from midsternum.
C. The pulse increases with inspiration and decreases with expiration.
D. A systolic click heard at the sternal border

10. A 7-month-old infant is admitted to the hospital. During the initial assessment, he has good head control, can roll over, and reaches for toys but cannot sit up without support nor transfer objects from one hand to the other. Based on these facts, the nurse concludes that the infant is developmentally about what age:

A. 2–3 months
B. 3–4 months
C. 4–6 months
D. 6–8 months

11. The nurse is assessing a 3 month old's abdomen after a hospitalization for diarrhea associated with severe gastroenteritis. Which of the following would be resolved?

A. Absent bowel sounds
B. Ascites
C. Hyperactivity
D. Protuberance

12. A 2-day-old infant was diagnosed as having congenital hip dysplasia. The problem was identified during the admission physical assessment. An early sign of congenital hip dysplasia that could be observed by the nurse in the nursery is:

A. Asymmetry of gluteal folds
B. Depressed Dance's sign
C. Lengthening of the leg on the affected side
D. Limitation in adduction of leg

13. A 65-year-old client has enrolled in an exercise program at a local health center. In planning a personalized program for her, the nurse reviews developmental concerns. One of the major developmental tasks for this age group is:

A. Accepting one's sexuality
B. Achieving a sense of personal independence
C. Adjusting to alterations in health
D. Promoting creativity and independence in children

14. A 14-year-old girl is seen at the clinic for prenatal care. The *greatest* psychological risk for a pregnant adolescent is:

A. Decreased self-esteem
B. Failure to establish a stable family
C. Inability to accept the parenting role
D. Interruption of work on the developmental tasks of adolescence

15. A 4-year-old boy has a diagnosis of severe croup. His treatment required hospitalization and O_2 therapy. A preschooler's concept of illness must be considered in planning care. A preschooler thinks about illness in terms of:

A. Concerns about privacy
B. External causes for body illnesses
C. Punishment for wrongdoing
D. Separation from a favorite toy or blanket

16. A 2-year-old boy is in respiratory distress with a diagnosis of croup but refuses to stay in his mist tent. His mother wants the nurse to help. A developmentally appropriate response by the nurse would be:

A. Giving him a toy and spanking him if he keeps crying
B. Having his mother sit with him under the tent and read a favorite story
C. Telling him it is a spaceship that will take off if he cries
D. Using strong sedation to put him to sleep

17. A 6-year-old boy was admitted with partial- and full-thickness third-degree burns. The first time that he goes to the playroom, he has bandages on both arms. The other children are playing and ignore him. The nurse's response should be to:

A. Act as a role model and bring the child in and play at a table
B. Leave the child alone in the room and hope it gets better
C. Take the child back to his room so he can watch TV
D. Tell the child to find a game and ask someone to play with him

18. A 16-year-old boy wants to get his driver's license so he can go to all the football games. Based on Erikson's stages of psychosocial development, the teenager is in the stage of:

A. Identity versus role confusion
B. Industry versus inferiority
C. Initiative versus guilt
D. Intimacy versus isolation

19. A mother listens carefully when the nurse reviews guidelines for beginning solid foods for a 5-month-old infant. Feeding guidelines would include:

A. Adding egg whites to the diet at about 9 months of age

B. Encouraging self-feeding with grapes, hot dogs, and such
C. Mixing cereal with whole milk at 6 months of age
D. Starting with soft food like processed cheese

20. After a 73-year-old man moved from his home of 40 years, his children became concerned that he was not calling them nor playing bridge with his friends on Thursdays. When his daughter asks the nurse what might be wrong, the nurse's initial interpretation would be that:

A. Cataracts may impair his ability to see for bridge.
B. Presbycusis may impair his ability to hear, and he may need a special telephone at his new house.
C. He could be ill and should see his cardiologist.
D. These are signs of depression, and he might be missing his home.

21. A mother says she knows that her baby is in the stage called "trust versus mistrust." She wants to know more about how children grow and learn. The nurse explains that trust versus mistrust is the first developmental stage described by Erikson, whose theory:

A. Describes eight developmental tasks all people face
B. Is based on deriving pleasure from different parts of the body
C. Outlines the development of logical thinking
D. Parallels that of Selye's adaptation theory

22. A 23-year-old new mother was diagnosed with cancer. When planning teaching, the nurse considers that developmentally the stress of such a diagnosis could precipitate feelings of:

A. Guilt and depression
B. Isolation and loneliness
C. Shame and doubt
D. Stagnation and despair

23. A 15-month-old infant arrives at the well-baby clinic for immunizations with a "runny" nose, which he has had for over a week. The only problem identified during the assessment is a mild upper respiratory infection. His immunization card indicates that his last visit was at 9 months of age when he received diphtheria-pertussis-tetanus (DPT) 2, oral poliovirus (OPV) 2, and *Haemophilus influenzae* type B (HIB) 2 vaccines. The nurse's plan would be to:

A. Administer DPT 3, OPV 3, HIB 3, and hepatitis B vaccines
B. Administer DPT 3, OPV 3, HIB 3, hepatitis, and measles-mumps-rubella (MMR) vaccines
C. Refer him to a physician
D. Schedule a return visit in 2 weeks to see if the upper respiratory infection (URI) has resolved

24. When the nurse stroked the lateral aspect of the soles of a newborn's feet during a newborn physical assessment, his toes flared outward. Which reflex would be considered normal?

A. Babinski's
B. Landau
C. Plantar
D. Stepping

25. A 56-year-old man was involved in a motor vehicle-pedestrian accident. The emergency room nurse assesses pupillary reaction to light and his ability to follow an object when it is moved up, down, left, and right. Which cranial nerve is being assessed?

A. Facial
B. Oculomotor
C. Optic
D. Vagus

26. A 19-month-old child has acute otitis media with an increased temperature. The nurse would anticipate the child's increase in respiration as:

A. Apnea
B. Crepitus
C. Kussmaul's
D. Tachypnea

27. When the physician tells a male client that he has acquired immunodeficiency syndrome (AIDS), he begins to cry. The next day, however, he phones his supervisor from the nurses' station to say that he will be back at work in 2 days. The nurse recognizes this behavior as:

A. Anger
B. Anxiety
C. Denial
D. Depression

28. An 8-year-old boy is learning the rules of how to play ball. According to Erikson, his developmental stage would be that of industry versus inferiority. The nurse plans activities around the developmental tasks identified by which theory?

A. Adaptative
B. Psychodynamic
C. Psychosexual
D. Psychosocial

29. The mother of a 5-year-old girl calls the nurse because five of her child's classmates have the chickenpox. The nurse explains that if the child develops chickenpox, she will have:

A. Macules
B. Nodules
C. Tumors
D. Vesicles

30. A 5-year-old child has recently recovered from a URI. The nurse anticipates a change in which of the following to support the recovery from a URI?

A. Flattening of nasal bridge
B. Hypertelorism
C. Nasal creases
D. Nasal discharge

31. A baby boy was born weighing 7 lb 5 oz at term (40 weeks' gestational age). At his initial physical examination, the nurse locates his urethral opening on the ventral side of his penis. This condition would be referred to as:

A. Cremasteric
B. Epispadias

C. Hypospadias
D. Phimosis

32. The school nurse is reviewing a school-health form for a 5-year-old girl. Her heart rate is 65 bpm. This would be a normal pulse if the child were in what age group?

A. Adolescent
B. Infant
C. School age
D. Toddler

33. The nurse palpates a 2-year-old child's head to assess suture lines and the size of any fontanelles. The nurse recognizes a palpable anterior fontanelle as abnormal because the anterior fontanelle is generally closed by what age?

A. 2 months
B. 6 months
C. 18 months
D. 24 months

34. A 9-month-old infant is in the nurse's office for her checkup. She has been teething and her mother wants to know when she will have her top and bottom teeth. The nurse tells her that a child who follows the usual pattern is expected to have 20 teeth by what age?

A. 6 months
B. 18 months
C. 2 years
D. 6–7 years

35. A mother brings her 6-month-old daughter to the health unit for her immunizations. Knowing that the next visit will not be scheduled until the infant is 9 months old, the nurse prepares the mother for the possibility of the infant experiencing stranger anxiety. This is associated with which stage in the development of logical thinking?

A. Sensorimotor
B. Preoperational
C. Concrete operations
D. Formal operations

36. A mother and father both wear glasses. The school nurse is using the Snellen chart to screen their child for problems as a part of the prekindergarten assessment. The mother wants to know if she has 20/20 vision. The nurse tells her mother that most children do not develop 20/20 vision until what age?

A. 6 months
B. 4 years
C. 7 years
D. 15 years

37. A mother is concerned that her 12-month-old infant is not walking yet. At what age should the child initially be walking well?

A. 9 months
B. 12 months
C. 15 months
D. 24 months

38. The nurse is preparing a class focusing on growth and development for the new employees at a day-care center and plans to include information about developmental principles. Which of the following would be included?

A. Body systems develop simultaneously.
B. Distal motor skills develop the most rapidly.
C. Growth proceeds from the specific to the general.
D. Newly learned skills predominate.

39. A 48-year-old woman complains of irregular menses during her health checkup. She has numerous other signs and symptoms that can be related to the climacteric. One area, however, does not relate to decreased estrogen production and merits another explanation. This complaint would be identified by the nurse as:

A. Atrophic changes in the vagina
B. Epithelium becomes thicker
C. Headaches and palpitations
D. Nervousness and mood swings

40. A father brought his 18-month-old son to a sibling preparation class so he could visit his sister after she was born. After changing his son's diaper for the second time, the father asks the nurse about toilet training. The nurse explains that each child is different and needs to set his or her own pace. The nurse suggests that the father be alert for signs of readiness such as:

A. Ability to dress without help
B. Ability to say "mama" and "dada" appropriately
C. Discomfort with soiled diapers
D. Walking and running for at least a year

41. A 15-year-old client is in the school nurse's office because she is concerned about her nutritional status and how much she weighs. The nurse explains that the *most* common nutritional deficiency for females during adolescence is:

A. Calcium
B. Fat
C. Iron
D. Protein

42. In talking with a group of high-school football referees during their season orientation, the nurse includes information about developmental tasks of adolescence. The nurse would include which of the following as appropriate tasks for adolescents?

A. Accepts community responsibilities
B. Develops self-awareness through reflective activity
C. Interacts appropriately with peers
D. Strengthens commitment to partner

43. In evaluating care for a 65-year-old client, the nurse considers activities related to the achievement of developmental tasks of mature adults. The nurse's evaluation would be based on?

A. Autonomy versus shame
B. Ego integrity versus despair
C. Generativity versus stagnation
D. Identity versus role diffusion

44. A 4-year-old girl has been hospitalized for leukemia several times this year. Her 8-year-old brother has been able to visit the hospital, and the nurses have discussed with the parents ways to help the older child to adjust. Developmental tasks for the 8 year old have been outlined. These include which of the following:

    A. Accepts body changes
    B. Actively participates in group events
    C. Begins to tolerate frustration
    D. Develops a sense of autonomy

45. Play is the work of a child. To promote achievement of school-age child development, the nurse would suggest activities such as:

    A. Pat-a-cake
    B. Pull toys
    C. Simon says
    D. Shopping

1. **(C)** Client need: health promotion and maintenance; subcategory: growth and development through the life span

   RATIONALE

   (A) Masturbation does not cause nocturnal emissions. (B) Masturbation is normal behavior for 14 year olds. (C) Masturbation provides for sexual relief without requiring a sexual relationship for which the adolescent may not be ready. (D) Masturbation is considered normative behavior during adolescence.

2. **(B)** Client need: health promotion and maintenance; subcategory: growth and development through the life span

   RATIONALE

   (A) Ninety percent of children attain the ability to say three words other than "mama" and "dada" between the ages of 11 and 18 months. (B) Ninety percent of children attain the ability to sit without support between the ages of 5 and 7 months. (C) Ninety percent of children attain the ability to build a tower of two cubes between the ages of 13 and 21 months. (D) Ninety percent of children attain the ability to walk well between the ages of 11 and 15 months.

3. **(C)** Client need: psychosocial integrity; subcategory: coping and adaptation

   RATIONALE

   (A) These behaviors are characteristic of infants and toddlers. (B) Parallel play characterizes the 2 year old. (C) Preschool children aged 3–6 are characterized by large capacity for magical thinking, heightened fear of bodily mutilation or harm, and fear expressed through nightmares. (D) Although a 4 year old may have imaginary playmates, peer pressure is not a feature until school years and becomes a characteristic of the adolescent.

4. **(A)** Client need: psychosocial integrity; subcategory: coping and adaptation

   RATIONALE

   (A) Piaget determined that adolescence is the period in which abstract thinking is first demonstrated. (B) Concrete operations, the ability to classify, order, and sort facts, appears in the 7–11 year old according to Piaget. (C) Magical thinking is characteristic of the 2–4 year old. (D) The predominant characteristic of the toddler and preschool period is egocentricity.

5. **(A)** Client need: psychosocial integrity; subcategory: coping and adaptation

   RATIONALE

   (A) Toddlers benefit most from having parents who are not overtly anxious and who trust the hospital personnel. (B) A toddler's thinking is concrete and tangible, and the toddler cannot think beyond the observable. She should be prepared immediately before the procedure. (C) Temper tantrums are a normal developmental characteristic of a 2 year old, and the toddler's parents should be encouraged to hold her to help alleviate fear. (D) Regression may occur with hospitalization but will not increase the toddler's comfort level.

6. **(D)** Client need: health promotion and maintenance; subcategory: growth and development through the life span

   RATIONALE

   (A) Birth weight usually doubles by age 6 months, triples by 1 year, and quadruples by 2 years. This weight would be expected by about 4–5 months of age. (B) This weight would be expected by about 6 months of age. (C) This weight would be expected by about 8 months of age. (D) This weight would be expected by about 12 months of age.

7. **(C)** Client need: health promotion and maintenance; subcategory: growth and development through the life span

   RATIONALE

   (A) Growth and development progress from the general to the specific—refining large muscle use before small muscle use. (B) Usual patterns and timing of growth and development have been identified. (C) Growth and development occur in an orderly, predictable sequence. (D) Although there are critical, sensitive, or optimal periods when certain skills are learned more readily, developmental tasks are not necessarily mastered for life and may be experienced earlier or later, or revisited.

8. **(C)** Client need: physiological integrity; subcategory: physiological adaptation

   RATIONALE

   (A) Presbycusis is the hearing loss that occurs with advancing age during middle to mature adulthood. (B) Low-set ears may reflect other deformities (e.g., renal); however, this would not be a primary focus at this visit. (C) Because of the direction of the ear canals, the ear lobe is pulled down and out for young children and up and back for older children and adults. (D) A vibrating tuning fork is used for the Rinne test to test air conduction versus bone conduction. The client must be able to report accurately when sounds are heard. An 18 month old could not be assessed in this way.

9. **(C)** Client need: physiological integrity; subcategory: physiological adaptation

   RATIONALE

   (A) A large discrepancy in arm and leg blood pressures is indicative of congenital heart defects such as coarctation of the aorta or other obstruction disorders. (B) This location is the PMI for an adult; for a child the PMI is between the fourth and fifth intercostal spaces at the midclavicular line. (C) This phenomenon describes a sinus arrhythmia, which occurs normally in many children and can be differentiated from a truly abnormal arrhythmia by having the child hold his breath. (D) A midsystolic click indicates mitral insufficiency and is not normal in children.

10. **(C)** Client need: physiological integrity; subcategory: growth and development through the life span

    RATIONALE

    (A) This infant has several skills beyond those normally achieved at the 2–3 month age. (B) Twenty-five percent of children begin to reach for a toy at about 4 months of age. (C) Twenty-five percent of children begin to sit with no support between 5–6 months of age. (D) Twenty-five percent of children begin to pass toys from one hand to another at about 5 months of age, and 95% can do this by 7 months of age.

11. **(C)** Client need: physiological integrity; subcategory: physiological adaptation

    RATIONALE

    (A) Absent bowel sounds would be associated with gastrointestinal obstruction or decreased motility. (B) Ascites refers to the presence of serous fluid in the peritoneal cavity most commonly seen with heart failure. (C) Hyperactivity refers to the very active bowel sounds heard with gastritis or gastroenteritis. (D) The abdomen of most infants and toddlers appears protuberant, but this anatomical finding diminishes with age as the child begins to walk.

12. **(A)** Client need: physiological integrity; subcategory: physiological adaptation

    RATIONALE

    (A) Uneven gluteal creases are often the first clue to congenital hip dislocation. (B) Dance's sign is a depression in the right iliac fossa, which is a sign of intussusception. (C) An infant with congenital hip dislocation often exhibits shortening of the femur on the affected side. (D) Abduction of an affected hip is limited; adduction is usually not affected initially.

13. **(C)** Client need: health promotion and maintenance; subcategory: prevention and early detection of disease

    RATIONALE

    (A) This is a developmental task of adolescence. (B) This is a developmental task of school-age children. (C) Tasks of the mature adult developmental stage include the following: manages with decreasing physical strength and health, adjusts to retirement and change in income, adjusts to disability or death of partner, exhibits flexibility in social roles, and supports social and civic activities. (D) This is a developmental task of the middle adult.

14. **(D)** Client need: health promotion and maintenance; subcategory: growth and development through the life span

    RATIONALE

    (A) Pregnancy and motherhood can increase a female's self-esteem. (B) With a supportive family and boyfriend, this risk is decreased. (C) This would be a risk after the delivery. (D) The developmental tasks of pregnancy are added to the developmental tasks of adolescence, creating a tremendous amount of psychological work.

15. **(C)** Client need: psychosocial integrity; subcategory: coping and adaptation

    RATIONALE

    (A) The adolescent thinks about concerns for privacy. (B) The school-age child thinks about external causes for body illness. (C) The preschooler associates illness with fear of being hurt, pain, and bleeding and often considers illness as a punishment for wrongdoing. (D) The infant focuses on separation from significant others and favorite belongings.

16. **(B)** Client need: health promotion and maintenance; subcategory: growth and development through the life span

    RATIONALE

    (A) Young children often fear being enclosed in the mist tent because it physically separates them from their loved ones and deprives them of comforting touch. Anxiety and crying increase respiratory distress. Providing a toy is appropriate, but spanking is not. (B) This response provides physical closeness and a familiar quiet activity. (C) This response might be a good idea for a child if he wants to be an astronaut, but imagination is more common with the preschooler. Threatening him with further separation is not appropriate. (D) Strong sedation can mask respiratory problems.

17. **(A)** Client need: health promotion and maintenance; subcategory: growth and development through the life span

    RATIONALE

    (A) A child who has been separated from other children may need help, especially if he has bandages and looks scary. When the child appears comfortable with the game, invite another child to play with the two of you. The other children may be more willing to play with him if they see the nurse playing too. (B) This response does not promote interactions with others. (C) This response also avoids the areas of concern. (D) This response is not the best with a 6 year old.

18. **(A)** Client need: health promotion and maintenance; subcategory: growth and development through the life span

    RATIONALE

    (A) Identity versus role confusion is the developmental task of adolescence (13–18 years), when peer influence to conform to group norms peaks and adolescents are struggling to integrate their concepts and values with those of society. (B) Industry ver-

sus inferiority is the developmental task of school-age children (6–12 years). (C) Initiative versus guilt is the developmental task of preschool-age children (3–6 years). (D) Intimacy versus isolation is the developmental task of early adulthood (19–34 years).

19. **(A)** Client need: physiological integrity; subcategory: basic care and comfort

    RATIONALE

    (A) Egg whites may be added to the diet at 9 months of age, but the whole egg should not be introduced until 12 months of age because the yolk frequently evokes an allergic response. (B) Foods such as wieners, grapes, or nuts should be avoided owing to hazards of choking. (C) Only breast milk or formula should be used until a child is about 12 months of age because of the fat and protein composition of whole milk and the infant's immature gastrointestinal development. (D) Highly processed foods such as processed cheese should be avoided for infants because they are usually high in salt or sugar and because they are combination foods.

20. **(D)** Client need: psychosocial integrity; subcategory: coping and adaptation

    RATIONALE

    (A) Cataracts are very common for mature adults; however, there is no indication that the client has this problem. (B) Presbycusis is a loss of hearing associated with aging; however, there is no indication that the client has this impairment. (C) Decreased ability to tolerate physical stress is a result of cardiovascular changes associated with aging; however, the lack of contact with family and friends would not be indicative of cardiac problems. (D) Grieving is a normal and necessary response to a loss such as a familiar home. Depression is one of the phases of the grief and mourning process.

21. **(A)** Client need: health promotion and maintenance; subcategory: growth and development through the life span

    RATIONALE

    (A) Erikson describes eight stages, or crises, of psychosocial development centered on an individual relationship with the social environment. (B) Freud's theories of psychosexual development are characterized by focusing on and deriving pleasure from different body parts. (C) Piaget's theories concentrate on cognitive development. (D) Hans Selye described adaptation as one's response to stress, but this theory is not related to Erikson's theories.

22. **(B)** Client need: psychosocial integrity; subcategory: coping and adaptation

    RATIONALE

    (A) The developmental tasks confronting the 5–9 year old are characterized by initiative verses guilt. (B) The developmental tasks confronting the young adult (18–25 years old) are characterized by intimacy verses isolation. Although developmental stages are not necessarily mastered for life and although issues may be experienced earlier or later than the ages typically identified, this is the most plausible response for a young adult. (C) The developmental tasks confronting the preschooler aged 3–5 years are characterized by autonomy versus shame and doubt. (D) The developmental tasks confronting the mature adult are characterized by generativity versus stagnation; and those confronting the older adult are characterized by ego integrity versus despair.

23. **(B)** Client need: health promotion and maintenance; subcategory: prevention and early detection of disease

    RATIONALE

    (A) Healthcare providers are responsible for updating immunization status at any contact. At this age, however, the MMR vaccination is also recommended. (B) DPT 3, OPV 3, HIB 3, hepatitis type B, and MMR immunizations should each be administered at this visit and a return visit scheduled in 2 months to complete the basic immunization series. (C) There is no indication for a physician referral. (D) A mild URI is not a contraindication to the administration of any vaccination in an otherwise healthy child.

24. **(A)** Client need: health promotion and maintenance; subcategory: growth and development through the life span

    RATIONALE

    (A) The Babinski reflex is elicited by gently stroking the lateral surface of the infant's foot. The toes fan out. (B) The Landau reflex is elicited by holding the infant in a prone position while supporting the trunk. The infant responds by raising the head and extending the legs and spine. (C) The plantar reflex is elicited by gently applying steady pressure with a finger on the sole against the balls of the feet. The toes curl inward. (D) The stepping reflex is elicited by holding the infant with the examiner's hands around the chest to support the infant's trunk and touching the infant's feet to a flat surface. Stepping is observed in the lower extremities.

25. **(B)** Client need: physiological integrity; subcategory: physiological adaptation

    RATIONALE

    (A) The facial nerve is assessed by asking the client to smile, frown, close both eyes, puff cheeks, and raise eyebrows. The client is also asked to differentiate between sweet and sour tastes. (B) The oculomotor nerve is assessed by observing pupillary reaction to light, raising the eyelids, and observing extraocular movements in all six cardinal fields of gaze. (C) The optic nerve is assessed by observing peripheral vision, visual acuity, and color vision. (D) The vagus nerve is assessed by asking the client to repeat a phrase and swallow, and checking that the uvula is midline.

26. **(D)** Client need: physiological integrity; subcategory: physiological adaptation

    RATIONALE

    (A) Apnea refers to the cessation of respiration. (B) Crepitus refers to the grating sensation felt over tissue containing beads of air as found with conditions such as subcutaneous emphysema. (C) Kussmaul's respirations refer to severe dyspnea occurring in paroxysms as with diabetic acidosis. (D) Tachypnea refers to an increased rate of respirations.

27. **(C)** Client need: psychosocial integrity; subcategory: coping and adaptation

    RATIONALE

    (A) Anger is usually the second stage of grief and mourning according to Kübler-Ross. (B) Anxiety, a feeling of apprehension, could manifest with physiological signs such as palpitations. (C) Denial is an expected reaction to grief. (D) Depression, usually a later phase of grief, could manifest with reactions such as extreme sadness or withdrawal.

28. **(D)** Client need: health promotion and maintenance; subcategory: growth and development through the life span

    RATIONALE

    (A) Piaget describes the development of intellectual capabilities in four stages: sensorimotor, preoperational, concrete operations, and formal operations. (B) Psychodynamic theory refers to emotions and behaviors that are governed by unconscious impulses. (C) Psychosexual theory described by Freud progresses through five stages: oral, anal, phallic, latency, and genital. (D) Eric Erikson described psychosocial development as a continuum from infancy to late adulthood and divided the life span into eight stages, each characterized by specific developmental tasks.

29. **(D)** Client need: physiological integrity; subcategory: physiological adaptation

    RATIONALE

    (A) A macule is a flat lesion with a different color but no change in skin surface, such as a freckle. (B) A nodule is a well-circumscribed solid lesion such as a wart. (C) A tumor is a solid lesion, usually larger than 2 cm. (D) A vesicle is a raised lesion containing serous fluid that appears in successive crops on different parts of the body with chickenpox.

30. **(D)** Client need: physiological integrity; subcategory: physiological adaptation

    RATIONALE

    (A) A flattened nasal bridge may indicate a cleft palate or Down syndrome. This is an anatomical feature that would not change with illness. (B) Hypertelorism refers to wide-set eyes, another anatomical feature that would not change with illness. (C) Nasal creases refer to an anatomical change that may be associated with allergic rhinitis. (D) Nasal discharge may reflect a URI, which would be expected to resolve with recovery from the URI.

31. **(C)** Client need: physiological integrity; subcategory: physiological adaptation

    RATIONALE

    (A) The cremasteric reflex refers to retraction of the testis in response to stimulation of the skin on the anterior and inner surface of the thigh. (B) Epispadias refers to a urethral opening on the dorsal side of the penis. (C) Hypospadias refers to a urethral opening on the ventral side of the penis. (D) Phimosis refers to tight foreskin.

32. **(A)** Client need: health promotion and maintenance; subcategory: growth and development through the life span

    RATIONALE

    (A) The normal range for an adolescent is 55–115 bpm. (B) The normal range for an infant is 100–160 bpm. (C) The normal range for a school-age child is 75–115 bpm. (D) The normal range for a toddler is 80–130 bpm.

33. **(C)** Client need: health promotion and maintenance; subcategory: growth and development through the life span

    RATIONALE

    (A) The posterior fontanelle averages 1 by 1 cm at birth and is closed by 2 months. (B) At 6 months of age the suture lines where cranial bones are joined should not be palpable. The anterior fontanelle is usually small but remains open for several more months. (C) At 18 months the anterior fontanelle is generally closed. (D) An open anterior fontanelle would be considered abnormal.

34. **(B)** Client need: health promotion and maintenance; subcategory: growth and development through the life span

    RATIONALE

    (A) Lower central incisors are the first teeth to erupt, usually between 4–6 months. (B) The child who follows the normal pattern of dental development usually has the full complement of deciduous teeth (10 upper and 10 lower) by 18 months of age. (C) Upper and lower cuspids (canine teeth) erupt between 18 months and 24 months of age. (D) Shedding of primary teeth begins between 6 and 7 years of age.

35. **(A)** Client need: health promotion and maintenance; content area: growth and development through the life span

    RATIONALE

    (A) During the sensorimotor stage (0–2 years old), the child is learning to recognize object permanence. (B) During the preoperational stage (2–7 years of age), the child is learning to think in terms of past, present, and future. (C) During the concrete operations stage (7–11 years of age), the child is developing the ability to classify, order, and sort facts. (D) During the formal operations stage (12 years to adulthood), the child is developing the ability to think abstractly and logically.

36. **(C)** Client need: health promotion and maintenance; subcategory: growth and development through the life span

RATIONALE

(A) Visual acuity changes markedly with age, being very immature at birth and gradually improving with age. At 6 months, the child usually adjusts posture to see an object. (B) Large-print books are suggested for children younger than 6 years old because they are usually farsighted and it is difficult for them to focus on close objects. (C) Visual acuity reaches 20/20 by age 7 in most children. (D) The eyeball reaches adult size by about 14 years of age, and nearsightedness is often discovered because of the growth.

37. **(C)** Client need: health promotion and maintenance; subcategory: growth and development through the life span

RATIONALE

(A) Between 10 and 12 months, most infants walk by holding on to furniture. (B) Between 12 and 13 months, most infants are able to take a few steps without falling. (C) Between 14 and 15 months, most infants are able to walk alone. (D) At 24 months, a child should be able to walk up steps, and many can balance on one foot.

38. **(D)** Client need: health promotion and maintenance; subcategory: growth and development through the life span

RATIONALE

(A) All body systems do not develop at the same rate. (B) Growth is proximal-distal, advancing more rapidly near the trunk and then proceeding to the distal portions of the body, and cephalocaudal, advancing more rapidly at the head and slowly progressing to the lower body. (C) Growth and development progress from the simple to the complex and from the general to the specific. (D) Newly learned skills predominate. For example, when a child starts to walk, other skills such as speech may not progress.

39. **(B)** Client need: physiological integrity; subcategory: physiological adaptation

RATIONALE

(A) Atrophic changes occur in the vagina; it becomes shorter and narrower. (B) The epithelium becomes thinner and drier; there is increased wrinkling of the skin. (C) Headaches, palpitations, numbness, tingling, and coolness of the extremities are associated with decreased estrogen production. (D) Anxiety, nervousness, and mood swings are symptoms of menopause.

40. **(C)** Client need: health promotion and maintenance; subcategory: growth and development through the life span

RATIONALE

(A) The son needs to be able to take off his pants but does not need to be able to dress without help. (B) The ability to communicate the need to go to the potty is generally a prerequisite to potty training the child, which usually follows the ability to say "mama" and "dada" by some months. (C) Becoming uncomfortable with soiled diapers is considered a sign of readiness for toilet training. It indicates both the ability to communicate and the neurological integrity to identify the need. (D) Presence for 5–6 months of the ability to walk, maybe run, and to stoop and recover [sit on potty chair, take off pants] are considered readiness signs for potty training.

41. **(C)** Client need: physiological integrity; subcategory: physiological adaptation

RATIONALE

(A) Calcium is especially needed during the adolescent growth spurt, and deficiency may be a problem associated with dieting. However, it is not a common problem for adolescents. (B) Most adolescents consume approximately 40% of their diet as fat (30%–50% is recommended). (C) Iron deficiency is the most common nutritional deficiency in female adolescents related to the adolescent growth spurt, menstruation and exacerbated with dieting. Organ meats, green vegetables, whole-wheat flour, bread, and nuts are suggested sources of iron. (D) Protein intake in female adolescents is usually higher than the recommended minimum.

42. **(C)** Client need: health promotion and maintenance; subcategory: growth and development through the life span

RATIONALE

(A) Acceptance of community responsibilities is a developmental task of adulthood reflected by the activities of the adults in this stage. (B) Development of self-awareness through reflective activity is a developmental task of later maturity, promoted through the use of life stories as an assessment technique. (C) Appropriate interaction with peers is a developmental task of adolescents that the referees can promote during games. (D) Strengthening of commitment to partner and maintaining a satisfactory sexual relationship are tasks of the middle adult years. Establishing a close personal relationship with another and accepting one's own sexuality are tasks of adolescents.

43. **(B)** Client need: health promotion and maintenance; subcategory: growth and development through the life span

RATIONALE

(A) Autonomy versus shame and doubt is the focus of psychosocial development for the toddler (ages 1–3). (B) Ego integrity versus despair is the focus of psychosocial development for the mature adult. (C) Generativity versus stagnation is the focus of development during middle adult years (ages 35–60). (D) Identity versus role diffusion is considered an adolescent task (ages 12–18).

44. **(B)** Client need: health promotion and maintenance; subcategory: growth and development through the life span

RATIONALE

(A) Acceptance of body changes is a task of adolescence (12–19 years old), when the body is developing secondary sex characteristics and growing rapidly. (B) Participation in group activities is a task of school-age children (6–11 years old). (C) Beginning ability to tolerate frustration is a task of infancy. (D) Developing a sense of autonomy versus shame and doubt is a task of toddlers (1–3 years old).

45. **(C)** Client need: health promotion and maintenance; subcategory: growth and development through the life span

RATIONALE

(A) Pat-a-cake promotes imitation and the development of the infant (0–1 year old). (B) Pull toys promote gross motor activities and the development of autonomy during the toddler years (1–3 years old). (C) Simon Says is an appropriate activity to recommend for school-age children. It promotes cooperation with some competition, refines communication skills, and is a group activity. (D) Shopping is often suggested for adolescents as an approach to promote increasing financial responsibility.

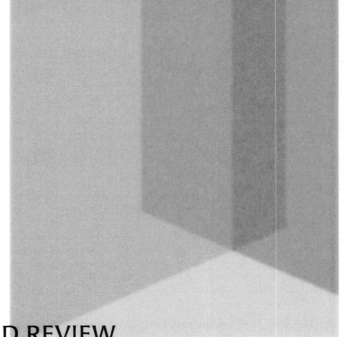
Nutrition Test

MOCK NCLEX-RN BOARD REVIEW TEST QUESTIONS

1. A 22-year-old primigravida is 5 ft 5 inches and weighed 128 lb at the beginning of pregnancy. The expected outcome at term gestation for her weight would be:

   A. 143 lb
   B. 148 lb
   C. 155 lb
   D. 167 lb

2. A client who is a native of the Middle East normally wears a long robe that covers her arms and body, along with a shawl that covers her head and neck. Because she is pregnant, the nurse is aware that she will need a supplement of:

   A. Vitamin D
   B. Calcium
   C. Vitamin C
   D. Zinc

3. A client experiences morning nausea early in her pregnancy. The nurse advises her to:

   A. Eat a small amount of dry, carbohydrate-containing food upon awakening
   B. Increase her intake of fluids in the early morning
   C. Increase her intake of fat in order to provide enough calories
   D. Restrict her intake of fluids throughout the day for a few weeks

4. If an iron supplement is prescribed for a pregnant woman, which point should the nurse emphasize in her teaching?

   A. She should take the supplement with food to avoid stomach upsets.
   B. She should take the supplement with milk to improve absorption.
   C. As long as she takes the supplement, she does not have to worry about including iron sources in her diet.
   D. She should include food such as citrus fruits, melons, broccoli, or strawberries in her diet each day.

5. In a teaching plan for a pregnant woman, the nurse would advise her on the need to avoid:

   A. Cholesterol
   B. Sodium
   C. Alcohol
   D. Saturated fat

6. A 55-year-old man has liver failure due to cirrhosis and is in impending hepatic coma. The nurse is assisting him with his diet selection and would not recommend:

   A. Fruit salad
   B. Cooked buttered carrots
   C. Boiled potato
   D. Cream of chicken soup

7. In evaluating a 10-year-old boy's understanding of his diet for celiac disease, the nurse would expect him to have ordered which of these foods for breakfast?

   A. Corn flakes
   B. Buckwheat pancakes
   C. Oat bran muffins
   D. Wheat germ

8. An 18-year-old female client is admitted to the hospital with acute renal failure. She is oliguric, hypertensive, and hyperkalemic. The nurse would not expect to see which of the following on her meal tray?

   A. Canned, drained pears
   B. Whole wheat bread

C. Fresh orange
D. Unsalted butter

9. A 12-year-old girl has been newly diagnosed with insulin-dependent diabetes mellitus. The nurse advises the client that some carbohydrate needs to be included in her diet because it:

A. Insulates the body to prevent heat loss
B. Furnishes the body with energy
C. Builds and repairs new tissue
D. Provides a source of dietary fiber

10. In evaluating a client's understanding of the exchange diet, the nurse would expect the client to state that part-skim mozzarella cheese is:

A. A milk exchange
B. A meat exchange
C. A fat exchange
D. Either a milk or a meat exchange

11. In teaching a newly diagnosed diabetic the exchange diet, the nurse would explain that potatoes are:

A. A vegetable exchange
B. A starch-bread exchange
C. A fruit exchange
D. Either a vegetable or a starch-bread exchange

12. A 57-year-old client underwent resection of the ileum and much of the jejunum. Postoperatively, he experienced diarrhea and steatorrhea. The nurse would expect his diet to be restricted in:

A. Protein
B. Fluid
C. Sodium
D. Fat

13. A client complains of constipation. The nurse teaches the client to add fiber to diet. The teaching was effective if she has:

A. Carrot raisin salad
B. Hamburger on sesame seed bun
C. Mashed potatoes with gravy
D. Canned fruit cocktail

14. A 44-year-old client with Crohn's disease is receiving total parenteral nutrition (TPN) via a central venous catheter. The nurse should teach the client to:

A. Inhale deeply while the administration tubing is being changed
B. Exhale forcefully with a closed airway while the administration tubing is being changed
C. Hold his breath while the administration tubing is being changed
D. Act normally while the administration tubing is being changed

15. Of the following laboratory tests performed on a client who is receiving TPN, the one which would usually be assessed *most* frequently would be?

A. Serum iron
B. Serum magnesium
C. Serum zinc
D. Serum sodium

16. The nursing practice *most* likely to result in a TPN-related infection would be:

A. Maintaining an occlusive dressing over the catheter insertion site
B. Using an in-line filter in the administration tubing
C. Adding insulin to the bag of TPN fluid after it arrives in the client care area
D. Wearing sterile gloves while changing the administration tubing

17. A 68-year-old woman is receiving a nasogastric tube feeding. Tube placement is known to be correct if:

A. A loud "whoosh" can be heard over the left upper quadrant of the abdomen when air is injected through the tube
B. No air bubbles appear when the free end of the tube is held under water during exhalation
C. The client experiences no gagging or respiratory distress
D. An abdominal x-ray shows the tube to be in the body of the stomach

18. A client who undergoes a gastric resection is *most* likely to require supplementation with:

A. Magnesium
B. Folic acid
C. Chloride
D. Vitamin B_{12}

19. A 14-year-old boy has third-degree burns over 50% of his body. He is in stable condition. The *best* snack for him would be:

A. Peanut butter sandwich and milkshake
B. Buttered popcorn and soft drink
C. Orange juice and fresh vegetables with dip
D. Milk and crackers

20. To promote wound healing in a burn client, the nurse would expect which vitamin or mineral to be supplemented?

A. Folic acid
B. Zinc
C. Iron
D. Vitamin K

21. The nurse would offer which food to a client on a clear liquid diet?

A. Tea
B. Orange juice
C. Sherbet
D. Vegetable soup

22. A client on a full liquid diet received the following foods on his tray. Which food should be removed?

A. Chicken noodle soup
B. Ice cream
C. Cream of tomato soup
D. Custard

23. In teaching a client about a low-fat diet, the nurse explains that a food without any limits is:

    A. Avocado
    B. Blueberry muffin
    C. Chocolate bar
    D. Angel food cake

24. A neonate was diagnosed with phenylketonuria. Which of the following statements by her mother informs the nurse that more education is needed?

    A. "I must read the ingredient listing on foods before I give them to the baby."
    B. "As the baby grows, her diet will change."
    C. "The baby will need a special infant formula."
    D. "After she becomes a teenager, the baby will not need a special diet any longer."

25. Which food would the nurse select for a toddler on a low-phenylalanine diet?

    A. Boiled potato
    B. Macaroni
    C. Corn
    D. Applesauce

26. Which food would the nurse select for a child on a galactose-free diet?

    A. Sherbet
    B. Buttered popcorn
    C. Egg noodles
    D. Pancakes

27. A 4-month-old infant is to begin on solid foods. The following are good reasons for starting with infant rice cereal except that:

    A. Rice cereal is the most economical infant food
    B. An infant of this age has developed the ability to digest the carbohydrate provided by the cereal
    C. Infant cereals are fortified with iron
    D. Rice cereal is not often associated with allergic reactions

28. A mother of a 9-month-old infant gave a diet history of feeding the baby the following foods. Which food indicates the mother needs further teaching?

    A. Infant formula
    B. Scrambled egg
    C. Toast strips
    D. Cottage cheese

29. A client who has essential hypertension is following a 2-g sodium diet restriction. The nurse would expect the client to avoid:

    A. Fresh flounder
    B. Hard rolls
    C. Peanut butter
    D. Milk

30. When evaluating a client's understanding of a low-sodium diet, the nurse would expect her to state she uses which seasoning?

    A. Worcestershire sauce
    B. Garlic salt
    C. Catsup
    D. Lemon juice

31. A client was found to have very high blood cholesterol levels. In regard to his diet, the nurse implements a teaching plan and encourages him to reduce his intake of:

    A. All types of fats
    B. Saturated fats
    C. Polyunsaturated fats
    D. Monounsaturated fats

32. The nurse would encourage a client on a low-cholesterol diet to drink:

    A. Whole milk
    B. Two percent low-fat milk
    C. Skim milk
    D. Acidophilus milk

33. A client states that she is a strict vegetarian (consuming no animal products). What food could the nurse recommend as a source of calcium?

    A. Strawberries
    B. Raisins
    C. Mustard greens
    D. Corn

34. A 34-year-old female bus driver comes in to the clinic to begin a weight loss program. The nurse finds that she weighs 188 lb and is 5 ft 4 inches tall. Using the rule of thumb, approximately how much should the client weigh?

    A. 135 lb
    B. 120 lb
    C. 108 lb
    D. 100 lb

35. In teaching a weight loss class, the nurse emphasizes the *most* effective way for people to achieve and maintain weight loss:

    A. Low-calorie liquid formula diet
    B. Increased exercise combined with a low-calorie diet
    C. Increased exercise
    D. Low-calorie diet selected from common foods

36. The mother of a 7-lb 6-oz newborn is trying to decide whether to breast-feed or bottle-feed. In discussing the decision with her, the nurse can say that:

    A. Growth is better in formula-fed infants
    B. Formula feeding is less expensive than breast-feeding
    C. Breast-fed infants are more likely to have colic than formula-fed ones
    D. Breast-fed infants are less likely to develop allergies

37. A client would like to breast-feed her newborn son. The nurse knows that he will need a supplement to provide:

    A. Zinc
    B. Vitamin E
    C. Fluoride
    D. Thiamine

38. At a baby's 2-week checkup in the clinic, his mother asks if it is time to start him on solid foods. The nurse can tell her that:

A. It is best to start solid food soon because the baby will be more likely to accept them now than when he is older

B. Solid foods should not be started until the infant is at least 4 months old, when they will be less likely to cause allergies

C. It is a good idea to start foods now because doing so will help the baby to sleep through the night at an earlier age

D. Solid foods should be started before 2 months of age, because doing so will help to prevent the baby from becoming obese

39. A mother intends to wean her child from breast-feeding at 8 months of age. She asks what he should receive in place of the breast milk. The nurse explains that:

A. Whole cow's milk is an economical and nutritious substitute for breast milk for an infant of this age

B. An infant of this age can be weaned to skim milk because this helps to reduce the risk of his developing heart disease later in life

C. Formula without iron is the best choice for a child of this age because it is less likely to cause constipation than a formula with iron

D. Iron-fortified formula should be used until the infant is 12 months old

40. A client comes to the clinic when he is 3 years old. His mother reports that he drinks several cups of milk daily but dislikes most other foods except peanut butter and French fries. The nurse would suspect that the child would be *most* likely to have a deficiency of which nutrient?

A. Calcium
B. Phosphorus
C. Protein
D. Iron

41. A client with acute pancreatitis is receiving a low-fat diet. The *best* breakfast for her would be:

A. Orange juice, corn flakes with skim milk, biscuits with jam, coffee

B. Grape juice, bran flakes with skim milk, toast with honey, tea

C. Tomato juice, poached eggs on toast, coffee

D. Grapefruit sections, blueberry muffins, and tea

42. During a healthcare visit, the client states that "sometimes his gums bleed." The nurse in diet teaching explains that bleeding gums is usually a sign of inadequate intake of:

A. Vitamin C
B. Vitamin D
C. Vitamin E
D. Vitamin A

43. When presenting a class on nutrition, the nurse should emphasize that in the United States, the *most* likely cause of anemia is deficiency of:

A. Iron
B. Folic acid

C. Vitamin B_{12}
D. Intrinsic factor

44. A client has an esophageal tumor obstructing his esophagus. He has a gastrostomy. Which type of diet would be *best* for him?

A. Full liquid
B. Soft
C. Low residue
D. Tube feeding via gastrostomy

45. A client develops pneumonia. The nurse encourages his wife to select which nutrient to assist in producing adequate antibodies to resist the infection?

A. Protein
B. Fat
C. Thiamine
D. Riboflavin

46. The nurse might expect the physician to write orders for a low-residue diet for a client 2–3 days before undergoing:

A. Oral surgery
B. Gastrointestinal (GI) surgery
C. Head and neck surgery
D. Any surgery

47. A client undergoes gastric surgery and postoperatively experiences difficulty with symptoms of dumping syndrome. The food that would be most likely to worsen her symptoms is:

A. Fried fish
B. Hard-cooked egg
C. Plain bagel
D. Fruit gelatin

48. A client is experiencing symptoms of the dumping syndrome. The nurse advises him to drink fluids:

A. Just before meals
B. Only with meals
C. Before and during meals
D. After meals

49. A client notes that he experiences cramping, bloating, and watery stools when he drinks milk. A plan of care for the client would be to encourage him to reduce his intake of:

A. Milk protein
B. Lactose
C. Sucrose
D. Galactose

50. A client reports that the following is typical of his usual daily eating habits: 1 cup oatmeal, 2 slices whole-grain toast, 1 cup orange juice, 1 cup 2% fat milk, 5 oz lasagna, 1 cup steamed broccoli, 2 bean tacos, 1 cup tossed salad with olive oil and vinegar, and 30 oz of beer. According to the Food Pyramid and the Dietary Guidelines for Americans, it would be *most* important for him to:

A. Decrease his intake of cholesterol
B. Decrease his alcohol intake

C. Increase his fiber intake

D. Increase his vegetable intake

51. In developing a teaching plan for weight control, the nurse is aware that obesity is usually defined as having a body weight that is at least _____% greater than the desirable body weight.

A. 5

B. 20

C. 40

D. 55

52. A client is found to be obese. The nurse includes diet teaching and makes him aware of risk factors for other diseases, which is/are:

A. Peptic ulcers

B. Periodontal disease

C. Scleroderma

D. Hypertension

53. A 6-ft-tall football player who weights 300 lb has been diagnosed with a hiatal hernia and complains of burning chest pain after eating. Which of the following statements by the client indicates a need for further dietary teaching?

A. "I should be lying down and resting after eating."

B. "I should not snack before I go to bed."

C. I should reduce my weight."

D. "I can use an antacid to relieve the burning."

1. **(C)** Client need: health promotion and maintenance; subcategory: growth and development through the life span

RATIONALE

(A, B) Her weight before pregnancy was appropriate for her height, and a gain of 15–20 lb would be inadequate; inadequate gains increase the risk of delivering low-birth-weight infants. (C) A gain of 25–30 lb would be associated with the best pregnancy outcome. (D) A gain of 39 lb would provide no additional advantage to the infant, and excessive weight gained during pregnancy may be hard for the mother to lose afterward.

2. **(A)** Client need: physiological integrity; subcategory: basic care and comfort

RATIONALE

(A) The client receives little sun exposure. Unless her diet history indicates that she consumes a quart of milk daily or other good sources of vitamin D, a supplement is indicated. (B) There are no data to indicate the need for a calcium supplement. (C) There are no data to indicate the need for a vitamin C supplement. (D) There are no data to indicate the need for a zinc supplement.

3. **(A)** Client need: physiological integrity; subcategory: basic care and comfort

RATIONALE

(A) Plain, dry, carbohydrate-containing foods (e.g., dry toast, crackers) on awakening help to alleviate the nausea experienced by some women. (B) Increased intake of fluids during the morning, when nausea is most common, may worsen the symptoms. (C) Fatty foods may worsen nausea, and carbohydrates can supply most of her calorie needs. (D) Reducing intake of fluids in the early morning may help to reduce nausea, but restricting fluids altogether is inadvisable, because the pregnant woman needs increased fluids for expansion of plasma volume, synthesis of amniotic fluid, excretion of wastes, and other vital bodily processes.

4. **(D)** Client need: physiological integrity; subcategory: pharmacological and parenteral therapies

RATIONALE

(A) The presence of food in the stomach is likely to inhibit absorption of iron. (B) Milk is an inhibitor of iron absorption. (C) "Heme" iron from meats is better absorbed than iron from most supplements, and thus enhances iron nutrition. Moreover, pregnancy is often a time when the woman is highly interested in nutrition and motivated to eat well, and this is a good time to emphasize the principles of a sound diet. (D) Vitamin C sources such as these enhance the absorption of iron from the supplement.

5. **(C)** Client need: health promotion and maintenance; subcategory: growth and development through the life span

RATIONALE

(A) Cholesterol intake has no known deleterious effect on the fetus. (B) Pregnant women without hypertension have no need to restrict sodium unduly. (C) Alcohol consumption during pregnancy may result in congenital malformations and learning disabilities. (D) Saturated fat has no deleterious effect on the fetus.

6. **(D)** Client need: physiological integrity; subcategory: basic care and comfort

RATIONALE

(A) Fruit is low in protein and sodium and thus would not exacerbate liver failure and fluid retention. (B) Carrots are low in protein, and butter would help to provide needed calories. (C) Boiled potato is low in sodium and protein. (D) Unless low-sodium products are used, soup is high in sodium. In addition,

the soup could only be included in the diet if the milk products and poultry contained in soup were included within the daily protein allowance.

7. **(A)** Client need: physiological integrity; subcategory: basic care and comfort

RATIONALE

(A) Corn contains no gluten. (B) Buckwheat is believed by many authorities to contain gluten. In any event, buckwheat pancakes are normally made with added wheat flour, which would be a gluten source. (C) Oats contain gluten. (D) Wheat germ contains gluten.

8. **(C)** Client need: physiological integrity; subcategory: basic care and comfort

RATIONALE

(A) Canned pears, drained of their juice, are almost free of sodium and are low in fluid and potassium. (B) Bread is low in water content and potassium. (C) Oranges are rich in potassium. (D) Unsalted butter is almost free of sodium and will provide needed calories.

9. **(B)** Client need: physiological integrity; subcategory: basic care and comfort

RATIONALE

(A) Fat deposits insulate the body to prevent heat loss. (B) The primary role of carbohydrate is to provide energy. Some cells, particularly red blood cells and the central nervous system cells, rely primarily on carbohydrate to meet their energy needs. (C) Proteins (amino acids) are the primary building blocks for new tissue. (D) Some complex carbohydrates do provide fiber, but fiber is not the major reason for consuming dietary carbohydrate.

10. **(B)** Client need: physiological integrity; subcategory: basic care and comfort

RATIONALE

(A) Cheese is made from milk, but its protein and fat contents are more similar to those of meat than to the items on the milk exchange list. (B) The protein and fat contents of cheese are similar to those of meat. (C) Items in the fat exchange list are primarily composed of fat, and cheese is a good source of protein. (D) The protein and fat contents of cheese are more similar to those of meat than to the items on the milk exchange list.

11. **(B)** Client need: physiological integrity; subcategory: basic care and comfort

RATIONALE

(A) Starchy vegetables such as potatoes are more similar in carbohydrate and protein contents to most foods on the starch-bread exchange list than to other vegetables. (B) Potatoes are similar in carbohydrate and protein contents to foods on the starch-bread exchange list. (C) Potatoes contain more protein than most foods on the fruit exchange list. (D) Starchy vegetables such as potatoes are more similar in carbohydrate and protein contents to most foods on the starch-bread exchange list than to other vegetables.

12. **(D)** Client need: physiological integrity; subcategory: reduction of risk potential

RATIONALE

(A) Protein can be absorbed in the upper portion of the small intestine. Adequate protein is needed to promote healing and hypertrophy (enlargement) of the remaining bowel. (B) Fluid is largely absorbed in the colon. Adequate fluid is needed to replace diarrheal losses. (C) Sodium is lost in diarrhea and needs to be replaced by dietary intake. (D) The ileum is the primary site for fat absorption. After resection of the ileum, a fat restriction often reduces the volume of stools and improves client comfort.

13. **(A)** Client need: physiological integrity; subcategory: basic care and comfort

    RATIONALE

    Fresh and dried vegetables and fruits are among the best dietary sources of fiber, which adds bulk to the stools and helps to prevent constipation. (B) Sesame seeds provide some fiber, but the number included on the bun would be inadequate to add bulk to stools. (C) Mashed potatoes contain starch but little fiber. (D) The heating required in the canning process reduces the fiber content of canned fruits and vegetables.

14. **(B)** Client need: physiological integrity; subcategory: pharmacological and parenteral therapies

    RATIONALE

    (A) Inhaling during tubing changes is likely to draw air into the catheter and the client's blood vessel. (B) Performing the Valsalva maneuver during tubing changes reduces the risk of air embolism. (C) Holding the breath is the second best answer, because it would be less likely than inhalation to allow air entry into the system, but the positive pressure provided by the Valsalva maneuver makes air entry even less likely. (D) Breathing normally during tubing changes entails the risk that the client will inhale and draw air into the circulation.

15. **(D)** Client need: physiological integrity; subcategory: reduction of risk potential

    RATIONALE

    (A) Serum iron levels are not always good indicators of tissue stores, nor are low levels likely to cause the client acute problems. (B) Magnesium is a vital mineral and should be assessed regularly, but acute changes are less likely to occur than changes in serum electrolytes. (C) Zinc levels do not usually change rapidly, and changes are not likely to be associated with sudden, life-threatening events, as may be the case with serum electrolytes. (D) Because sodium is the major extracellular cation, its levels change in response to what is administered in the TPN. Electrolyte levels are closely monitored, especially during the initial period of TPN, to ensure that no imbalances occur.

16. **(C)** Client need: physiological integrity; subcategory: reduction of risk potential

    RATIONALE

    (A) An occlusive dressing over the insertion site helps to prevent bacterial contamination (particularly in the case of clients with draining wounds or tracheostomy sites in the vicinity). (B) A 22-mm in-line filter removes most bacteria that may have contaminated the fluid or administration set (but will not remove endotoxin). (C) If at all possible, medications, electrolytes, or other components should be added to TPN solutions in the pharmacy, where the addition can be made under a laminar air-flow hood and under the strictest of aseptic conditions. (D) Wearing sterile gloves helps to reduce the risk of contaminating the fluid path with skin flora.

17. **(D)** Client need: physiological integrity; subcategory: reduction of risk potential

    RATIONALE

    (A) An in-rush of air can sometimes be heard over the upper left abdominal quadrant even when the tube is positioned in the bronchus or pleural space. (B) If the tube is in the pleural space or lodged against the wall of the bronchus, air bubbles may not be emitted during exhalation. (C) New "nonreactive" (polyurethane, silicone rubber, and similar substances) tubes are less irritating than the harder tubes previously used and may not cause gagging or respiratory distress even when located in the

pulmonary system. In any event, an obtunded client would be unlikely to display these signs. (D) Radiographic evidence is the most certain method of confirming appropriate tube placement.

18. **(D)** Client need: physiological integrity; subcategory: pharmacological and parenteral therapies

    RATIONALE

    (A) Magnesium absorption is not affected by a gastrectomy. (B) Folic acid absorption can be affected, but vitamin B_{12} is a greater concern because of its neurological and RBC formation effects. (C) Chloride is a principal body anion in the extracellular fluid whose absorption is not affected by a gastrectomy. (D) Hydrochloric acid, produced in the stomach, is required to split vitamin B_{12} away from the proteins to which it is bound in food. Intrinsic factor, produced by the gastric mucosa, must be bound to vitamin B_{12} for the vitamin to be absorbed in the ileum. Adults generally have vitamin B_{12} stores sufficient to last approximately 3 years, but after that time, parenteral vitamin B_{12} will be required.

19. **(A)** Client need: physiological integrity; subcategory: basic care and comfort

    RATIONALE

    (A) The client needs a high-protein, high-calorie diet for tissue healing and replacement of blood and tissue proteins lost as a consequence of the burn. This choice provides the most protein and is also rich in calories. (B) These choices are good sources of calories, which the client needs to meet his energy needs, but they provide little protein. (C) Orange juice and vegetables are low in calories and protein. (D) This choice is lower in protein and calories than a peanut butter sandwich and a milk shake.

20. **(B)** Client need: physiological integrity; subcategory: pharmacological and parenteral therapies

    RATIONALE

    (A) Folic acid is necessary for forming red blood cells, which are lost in burns, but zinc is especially important for increasing the strength of healing wounds. (B) Zinc increases the tensile strength (the force needed to separate the edges) of healing wounds. (C) Iron is needed to replace blood losses, but zinc is especially necessary for wound healing. (D) Vitamin K is required for formation of clotting factors.

21. **(A)** Client need: physiological integrity; subcategory: basic care and comfort

    RATIONALE

    (A) Tea is the only choice that is a clear liquid. (B, C, D) are not clear liquids.

22. **(A)** Client need: physiological integrity; subcategory: basic care and comfort

    RATIONALE

    (A) Neither noodles nor chicken chunks would be liquid at room temperature, which is the criterion for including a food in a full liquid diet. (B) Ice cream is liquid at room temperature. (C) Cream of tomato soup is a liquid at room temperature. (D) Custard is a liquid at room temperature.

23. **(D)** Client need: physiological integrity; subcategory: basic care and comfort

    RATIONALE

    (A) Eighty-eight percent of the kilocalories in avocados are derived from fat. (B) Muffins and other "quick breads" (unless specially prepared) contain oil, butter, or margarine, as well as fat from egg yolk. (C) Chocolate candies contain cocoa butter or other fats. (D) Angel food cake contains no egg yolk or other sources of fat.

24. **(D)** Client need: physiological integrity; subcategory: basic care and comfort

RATIONALE

(A) It is essential to read labels to determine whether foods contain proteins (because proteins provide phenylalanine) or are sweetened with aspartame. (B) Infants are initially fed a low-phenylalanine formula or breast milk. As children mature, they eat a wider variety of foods, which requires more vigilance by the family. (C) With careful supervision, it is possible for infants with PKU to be breast-fed. If the mother chooses not to breast-feed, the baby will require a special low-phenylalanine formula. (D) Individuals with PKU display improved mental function if they continue the phenylalanine-restricted diet indefinitely. It is especially important that women who wish to have children ensure that their phenylalanine levels are controlled before they conceive and during pregnancy.

25. **(D)** Client need: physiological integrity; subcategory: basic care and comfort

    RATIONALE

    (A) Starchy vegetables such as potatoes contain some protein and thus supply phenylalanine. (B) Pasta and other grain products are sources of protein. (C) Corn contains some protein and thus supplies phenylalanine. (D) Fruits, which are generally low in protein, provide little phenylalanine.

26. **(C)** Client need: physiological integrity; subcategory: basic care and comfort

    RATIONALE

    (A) Sherbet generally contains milk and therefore contains galactose. (B) Butter contains traces of lactose. (C) Noodles are made without milk or lactose (and therefore are galactose-free). Food labels or the product manufacturer should be consulted if there is any question about a product's lactose content. (D) Unless specially prepared, pancakes are made with milk.

27. **(A)** Client need: physiological integrity; subcategory: basic care and comfort

    RATIONALE

    (A) Infant cereals from all types of grains are usually equivalent in price. (B) Pancreatic amylase activity increases from low levels at birth to relatively normal levels at 4 months, and this prepares the infant to digest the starch in cereal grains. (C) Infant cereals are a good choice for a first food because they are fortified with iron. Iron stores deposited in utero and in the postnatal period begin to be depleted between 3 and 6 months of age. (D) Rice is considered the least allergenic cereal grain for infants; wheat is among the foods that are most likely to cause allergies in infants.

28. **(B)** Client need: physiological integrity; subcategory: basic care and comfort

    RATIONALE

    (A) Iron-fortified infant formula, rather than cow's milk, is recommended until 12 months of age because the infant needs good sources of iron and because cow's milk is likely to cause GI blood loss. (B) Egg white is not recommended for infants younger than 12 months because it is commonly associated with allergy when started earlier. (C) The 9 month old enjoys finger foods such as toast strips. (D) Cottage cheese provides high protein.

29. **(C)** Client need: physiological integrity; subcategory: reduction of risk potential

    RATIONALE

    (A) Fish contains some sodium, but unless it is prepared with added salt, there is no need to avoid it on a 2-g sodium diet. (B) Hard rolls and most other yeast breads are relatively low in sodium and can be included in a 2-g sodium diet. (C) Peanut butter is prepared with salt unless a special salt-free product is used. (D) Milk contains sodium, but at this level of sodium restriction, there is no need to limit its intake unduly.

30. **(D)** Client need: physiological integrity; subcategory: basic care and comfort

    RATIONALE

    (A) Worcestershire sauce, as well as many other seasonings and condiments, is prepared with salt. (B) Garlic salt, as well as many other seasonings and condiments, is prepared with salt. (C) Catsup, as well as many other seasonings and condiments, is prepared with salt. (D) Lemon juice is virtually sodium free.

31. **(B)** Client need: health promotion and maintenance; subcategory: prevention and early detection of disease

    RATIONALE

    (A) Polyunsaturated and monounsaturated fats do not elevate serum cholesterol. (B) Excessive intake of saturated fats is associated with elevations of serum cholesterol. (C) Polyunsaturated fats tend to reduce cholesterol levels. (D) Monounsaturated fats in the diet tend to reduce serum cholesterol or have a neutral effect on it.

32. **(C)** Client need: health promotion and maintenance; subcategory: prevention and early detection of disease

    RATIONALE

    (A) Whole milk is rich in milk fat, which is saturated, and contains cholesterol. (B) Two-percent milk contains saturated fat and cholesterol. (C) Skim milk is virtually devoid of saturated fat. (D) Sweet acidophilus milk is usually whole or 2% milk. It contains bacterial cultures, but they do not change the fat content.

33. **(C)** Client need: health promotion and maintenance; subcategory: prevention and early detection of disease

    RATIONALE

    (A) Strawberries (and most other fruits) are low in calcium. (B) Raisins are low in calcium. (C) Deep green leafy vegetables, with the exception of spinach and Swiss chard, are fair sources of calcium. Spinach and chard contain calcium but also contain so much oxalic acid that absorption of their calcium is prevented. (D) Corn is a poor calcium source.

34. **(B)** Client need: health promotion and maintenance; subcategory: prevention and early detection of disease

    RATIONALE

    (A) A weight of 135 lb is too heavy for the client, according to the rule of thumb. (B) Based on the rule of thumb, the client's weight should be 120 lb (that is, 100 lb for 5 feet, 5 lb for every inch over 5 ft (5×4) = 20 lb; $100 + 20 = 120$. (C) The rationale for the correct answer explains why 100–108 lb is too little for the client. (D) The rationale for the correct answer explains why 100–108 lb is too little for the client.

35. **(B)** Client need: physiological integrity; subcategory: basic care and comfort

    RATIONALE

    (A) Rapid weight loss often occurs with use of liquid-formula diets, but the weight is usually regained. (B) A low-calorie diet plus an increase in activity is the most effective way to promote lasting weight loss. (C) Exercise alone tones the body and increases the muscle mass but rarely results in substantial weight loss. (D) A low-calorie diet alone will result in gradual weight loss, but the addition of exercise to the regimen often helps to curb the appetite and take the dieter's mind off food.

36. **(D)** Client need: health promotion and maintenance; subcategory: prevention and early detection of disease

    RATIONALE

    (A) Growth in infants receiving breast milk is comparable to growth in those receiving commercial formulas. (B) Breast-feeding is often less expensive than formula feeding. The only real cost of breast feeding (other than a one-time expense for nursing bras) is that resulting from the mother's need for a modest increase in her calorie and protein intake. If she chooses foods wisely, she can meet these increased needs very inexpensively. (C) There is no increase in colic in breast-fed infants. (D) Young infants are especially prone to development of allergies. Breast milk is much less likely to cause an allergic reaction than cow's milk or soy, the protein sources used in most infant formulas.

37. **(C)** Client need: physiological integrity; subcategory: reduction of risk potential

    RATIONALE
    (A) Human milk is adequate in zinc to meet the needs of term infants. (B) Human milk is adequate in vitamin E to meet the needs of term infants. (C) Human milk provides little fluoride, so the breast-fed infant usually needs a supplement at an early age to ensure proper tooth formation. (D) Human milk is adequate in thiamine to meet the infant's needs.

38. **(B)** Client need: health promotion and maintenance; subcategory: growth and development through the life span

    RATIONALE
    (A) Early initiation of solid foods does not improve later acceptance of foods. (B) The young infant is prone to development of allergies, and exposure to a wide variety of antigens from foods is apt to result in allergy. (C) Research has shown that infants begin to sleep through the night when they reach approximately 11 lb, and introducing solid foods early does not accelerate the process. (D) Early introduction of solid foods will not reduce the risk of obesity. Very young infants are less able to communicate their satiety and may be overfed by zealous caregivers. Older infants communicate by turning their heads away, withdrawing eye contact, drooling out food, or refusing to open the lips.

39. **(D)** Client need: health promotion and maintenance; subcategory: growth and development through the life span

    RATIONALE
    (A) Cow's milk is not recommended for infants younger than 12 months because it is a poor source of iron and often causes GI blood loss. (B) Infants are rapidly growing and need the kilocalories provided by fat; use of skim milk may impair growth. There is no evidence that use of skim milk in infancy has any beneficial effects on later heart disease. (C) A reliable source of iron, such as iron-fortified formula, is needed by rapidly growing infants. Use of formula without iron is likely to result in iron-deficiency anemia. (D) Iron-fortified formula is recommended until 12 months of age because it provides a reliable source of iron and helps to prevent iron-deficiency anemia.

40. **(D)** Client need: health promotion and maintenance; subcategory: growth and development through the life span

    RATIONALE
    (A, B, C) Milk is a good source of calcium, phosphorus, and protein. (D) Milk is an extremely poor source of iron. Excessive milk consumption by toddlers results in "milk anemia."

41. **(B)** Client need: physiological integrity; subcategory: basic care and comfort

    RATIONALE
    (A) Biscuits are prepared with shortening. (B) This meal is almost fat-free. (C) Poached eggs contain 5 g of fat each. (D) Muffins are prepared with oil or margarine and eggs.

42. **(A)** Client need: physiological integrity; subcategory: basic care and comfort

    RATIONALE
    (A) Vitamin C is necessary for maintaining capillary walls; thus deficiency often results in bleeding. (B) Vitamin D is involved primarily in regulation of calcium and phosphorus metabolism. (C) Vitamin E is an antioxidant and is important in maintaining red cell membranes and preventing anemia. (D) Vitamin A deficiency is commonly associated with deterioration of vision, roughening of the skin, and atrophy of the mucous membranes.

43. **(A)** Client need: physiological integrity; subcategory: basic care and comfort

    RATIONALE
    (A) Iron-deficiency anemia is the most common nutritional anemia in the United States in virtually all age groups. (B) Deficiency of folic acid may occur in malnourished individuals; pregnant women and infants are also at risk, but it is not so widespread as iron deficiency. (C) The only individuals at serious risk of dietary deficiency of vitamin B_{12} are strict vegetarians; also, impaired absorption is likely in individuals with gastric or ileal resection, but this is a limited group of people. (D) Impaired production of intrinsic factor occurs spontaneously in some individuals and also following gastric resection, but this problem affects a limited number of people.

44. **(D)** Client need: physiological integrity; subcategory: basic care and comfort

    RATIONALE
    (A, B, C) If the esophagus is obstructed, no oral feedings would be able to bypass the obstruction. (D) Gastrostomy feedings would bypass the obstruction.

45. **(A)** Client need: health promotion and maintenance; subcategory: prevention and early detection of disease

    RATIONALE
    (A) Amino acids derived from proteins are components of antibodies. (B) Fat is not a component of antibodies. (C) Thiamine is not a component of antibodies. (D) Riboflavin is not a component of antibodies.

46. **(B)** Client need: physiological integrity; subcategory: reduction of risk potential

    RATIONALE
    (A) There is no need to prepare the client with a low-residue diet for oral surgery. (B) Some physicians use a low-residue diet before GI surgery to decrease the fecal content of the GI tract during surgery. (C) There is no need for a low-residue diet prior to head and neck surgery. (D) A low-residue diet is not indicated for any surgery except surgery of the GI tract.

47. **(D)** Client need: physiological integrity; subcategory: reduction of risk potential

    RATIONALE
    (A) The fat and protein provided by the fish would be slowly digested and might reduce symptoms of dumping syndrome. (B) The fat and protein provided by the egg would be slowly digested and might reduce symptoms of dumping syndrome. (C) The starch provided by the bagel would be less likely than simple carbohydrates to cause dumping, because it would be gradually hydrolyzed and would not increase the osmolality of the small bowel as rapidly as simple carbohydrates. (D) Simple carbohydrates such as the sucrose in fruit gelatins enter the small bowel quickly after ingestion and rapidly increase the osmolality of the bowel content. Thus, they are the nutrients most likely to cause symptoms in the person with dumping syndrome.

48. **(D)** Client need: health promotion and maintenance; subcategory: prevention and early detection of disease

    RATIONALE
    (A, B, C) Fluids present in the stomach at the same time as food increase the speed of gastric emptying and thus increase the likelihood of dumping syndrome. (D) Avoiding fluids until at least one-half to one hour after meals reduces the speed with which foods are emptied from the stomach.

49. **(B)** Client need: health promotion and maintenance; subcategory: prevention and early detection of disease

RATIONALE

(A) It is unusual to experience maldigestion of milk protein. (B) Many adults lack lactase, the enzyme required to digest lactose (milk sugar). The undigested carbohydrate passes into the colon, where it draws fluid into the feces and often causes cramping and diarrhea. (C) Inability to digest sucrose is relatively uncommon. (D) Malabsorption of galactose (by itself, as opposed to being a part of the lactose molecule) is uncommon.

50. **(B)** Client need: health promotion and maintenance; subcategory: prevention and early detection of disease

RATIONALE

(A) The client's intake of animal products (which are the only sources of cholesterol) is limited to one serving of milk and the meat and cheese contained in the lasagna, so his cholesterol intake should not be excessive. (B) The Dietary Guidelines for Americans recommends only a moderate alcohol intake, defined as no more than 2 drinks per day. A 12-oz glass of beer is equivalent to one drink, so the client's intake is excessive. (C) Whole-grain breads, oatmeal, legumes (beans), and vegetables provide good sources of fiber in the diet. (D) The broccoli and salad are equivalent to three vegetable servings; three to five are recommended.

51. **(B)** Client need: health promotion and maintenance; subcategory: prevention and early detection of disease

RATIONALE

(A) Individuals within 5% of the desirable weight are usually described as "normal weight." (B) Although there are exceptions, a person whose weight is at least 20% over the ideal or desirable weight for his or her height is usually considered to be obese. (C and D) Individuals whose weights are at least 20% more than the ideal or desirable weight are usually considered obese.

52. **(D)** Client need: health promotion and maintenance; subcategory: prevention and early detection of disease

RATIONALE

(A) Obesity does not increase the risk of peptic ulcers. (B) Obesity does not increase the risk of periodontal disease. (C) Obesity does not increase the risk of scleroderma. (D) Obesity is a risk factor for development of hypertension.

53. **(A)** Client need: health promotion and maintenance; subcategory: prevention and early detection of disease

RATIONALE

(A) Although rest can be important, lying down immediately after eating increases the reflux of acid gastric contents. (B) Snacking at bedtime may cause reflux when lying down to sleep shortly afterwards. (C) Obesity is often a precipitating cause of reflux and subsequent pain. (D) Use of antacids may help control the symptoms.

CHAPTER 11

Dosage Calculation Test

MOCK NCLEX-RN BOARD REVIEW TEST QUESTIONS

1. Maalox 15 mL has been ordered. How many tablespoons would the nurse give?
   - A. 3 tsp
   - B. 2 tbsp
   - C. 1 tsp
   - D. 1 tbsp

2. Nitroglycerin 0.4 mg has been ordered. The drug label states gr ⅟₁₅₀ equals 1 tablet. How many tablets would the nurse give?
   - A. 1 tablet
   - B. ½ tablet
   - C. 2 tablets
   - D. 1½ tablets

3. Cephalexin monohydrate (Keflex) 0.5 g has been ordered. The drug comes in 250 mg per capsule. How many capsules would the nurse give?
   - A. 5 capsules
   - B. 4 capsules
   - C. 2 capsules
   - D. 1 capsule

4. Penicillin V potassium (Pen-Vee K) suspension 0.75 g has been ordered. The drug is available as 250 mg/5 mL. How many milliliters would the nurse give?
   - A. 10 mL
   - B. 15 mL
   - C. 3 mL
   - D. 20 mL

5. Cyclophosphamide (Cytoxan) 4 mg/kg per day po has been ordered. The client weighs 154 lb. How much would the nurse give each day?
   - A. 100 mg
   - B. 120 mg
   - C. 240 mg
   - D. 280 mg

6. Cephalexin monohydrate 3 g over the next 24 hours, divided into six equally spaced doses, has been ordered. How much would the nurse give for each dose?
   - A. 3000 mg
   - B. 500 mg
   - C. 1000 mg
   - D. 2000 mg

7. Aspirin is available as gr V per tablet. Aspirin 300 mg has been ordered. The amount of drug to be administered is:
   - A. ½ tablet
   - B. 1 tablet
   - C. 2 tablets
   - D. 1½ tablets

8. Vitamin K is available as 1 mg/0.5 mL. Vitamin K 0.5 mg has been ordered. The amount of vitamin K to be administered is:
   - A. 2.5 mL
   - B. 0.50 mL
   - C. 0.25 ML
   - D. 1 mL

9. Digoxin is available as 0.125 mg per tablet. Digoxin 0.25 mg has been ordered. The amount of drug to be administered is:
   - A. 1 tablet
   - B. ½ tablet
   - C. 2 tablets
   - D. 1½ tablets

10. Meperidine (Demerol) is available as 75 mg/mL. Meperidine 50 mg has been ordered. The amount of drug to be administered (in adults) is:

A. 0.5 mL
B. 0.6 mL
C. 0.7 mL
D. 1.5 mL

11. Codeine is available as gr 1 tablet. Codeine 30 mg has been ordered. The amount of drug to be administered is:

A. 1 tablet
B. ½ tablet
C. 1.2 tablets
D. ¾ tablet

12. Hydroxyzine (Vistaril) is available as 25 mg/mL. The amount ordered is 100 mg po q4–6h prn. How many milliliters would the nurse give per as-needed dose?

A. 0.25 mL
B. 2.50 mL
C. 4 mL
D. 40 mL

13. The amount of solution and amount of aminophylline received by a client IV each hour when there is 500 mg of aminophylline in 250 mL given every 24 hours is:

A. 12.5 mL/hr and 0.33 mg/hr
B. 10 mL/hr and 21 mg/hr
C. 21 mL/hr and 20 mg/hr
D. 20 mL/min and 40 mL/hr

14. The amount of solution and amount of aminophylline received by a client IV each minute when there is 250 mg of aminophylline in 250 mL given over 16 hours is:

A. 0.5 mL/hr and 0.4 mg/mL
B. 10 mL/hr and 5 mg/mL
C. 0.26 mL/min and 0.26 mg/min
D. 1 mL and 1 mg/min

15. The amount of solution and amount of aminophylline received by a client IV each hour when there is 500 mg of aminophylline in 500 mL over 12 hours is:

A. 21 mL/hr and 20 mg/hr
B. 20 mL/min and 40 mL/hr
C. 50 mL/hr and 21 mg/mL
D. 42 mL/hr and 42 mg/hr

16. The amount of solution and amount of dopamine received by a client IV each hour when there is 400 mg of dopamine in 500 mL over 24 hours is:

A. 21 mL/hr and 17 mg/hr
B. 12.5 mL/hr and 0.33 mg/hr
C. 20 mL/hr and 34 mg/hr
D. 21 mL/hr and 34 mg/min

17. If the client is ordered to receive insulin at 3 U/hr with a solution of 50 U/100 mL in normal saline, the rate of infusion in milliliters would be:

A. 4 mL/hr
B. 12 gtt/mL
C. 10 mL/hr
D. 6 mL/hr

18. Morphine sulfate 10 mg SC has been ordered. The drug label reads 15 mg/mL. How many milliliters would the nurse give to an adult?

A. 0.5 mL
B. 0.6 mL
C. 0.7 mL
D. 1.5 mL

19. Hydroxyzine 25 mg IM has been ordered. The vial reads 100 mg in 2 mL. How many milliliters would the nurse give?

A. 5 mL
B. 4 mL
C. 0.5 mL
D. 1.4 mL

20. The order reads 5000 U heparin SC every 6 hours. The vial reads 20,000 U/mL. How many milliliters would the nurse give?

A. 4 mL
B. 0.4 mL
C. 0.25 mL
D. 2.5 mL

21. The physician orders Ringer's lactate 1000 mL to infuse over 8 hours. Drops per milliliter equal 15. How many drops per minute would the nurse give?

A. 30 gtt/min
B. 31 gtt/min
C. 15 gtt/min
D. 16 gtt/min

22. The nurse is to infuse D_5W 150 mL over 1 hour. Drops per milliliter equal 10. How many drops per minute would the nurse give?

A. 25 mL/min
B. 26 gtt/min
C. 25 gtt/min
D. 50 gtt/min

23. A hypertonic solution of $D_{10}W$ is to infuse over 10 hours via a 16-gauge IV needle. The total amount of fluid is 1000 mL and the drop factor is 10. How many drops per minute would the nurse give?

A. 16 mL/hr
B. 16 gtt/min
C. 17 gtt/min
D. 17 mL/hr

24. The nurse is to infuse 100 mL of IV fluid in 2 hours using a set with a calibration of 60 gtt/mL. How many drops per minute would the nurse give?

A. 50 mL/hr
B. 50 gtt/min
C. 60 gtt/min
D. 60 gtt/mL

25. The nurse is to infuse 900 mL of IV fluid in 2 hours. The set calibration is 20 gtt/mL. How many drops per minute would the nurse give?

A. 90 gtt/min
B. 45 gtt/min
C. 150 gtt/min
D. 45 gtt/min

26. The nurse is to infuse 1000 mL of IV fluid in 8 hours. Set calibration is 10 gtt/mL. How many drops per minute would the nurse give?

    A. 20 gtt/min
    B. 21 gtt/min
    C. 125 gtt/min
    D. 12.5 gtt/min

27. The nurse is to administer IV fluid at 150 mL/hr using a 60 gtt/mL set. How many drops per minute would the nurse give?

    A. 75 gtt/min
    B. 75 mL/min
    C. 150 gtt/min
    D. 150 mL/min

28. The nurse is to infuse 50 mL of antibiotic in 30 minutes. The set calibration is 60 gtt/mL. How many drops per minute would the nurse give?

    A. 100 gtt/min
    B. 50 gtt/min
    C. 150 gtt/min
    D. 10 gtt/min

29. The nurse is to infuse 15 mL of medication over 15 minutes, using a 60 gtt/mL set. How many drops per minute would the nurse give?

    A. 15 gtt/min
    B. 60 gtt/min
    C. 5 gtt/min
    D. 6 gtt/min

30. The nurse is to infuse 600 mL of intravenous fat emulsion (Intralipid) over 8 hours with a 10 gtt/mL set. How many drops per minute would the nurse give?

    A. 10 gtt/min
    B. 60 gtt/min
    C. 13 gtt/min
    D. 600 gtt/min

31. The nurse is to infuse 150 mL of fluid over 2 hours using minidrip (minidrip equals 60 gtt/mL). How many drops per minute would the nurse give?

    A. 150 gtt/min
    B. 60 gtt/min
    C. 75 gtt/min
    D. 7.5 gtt/min

32. The client is to receive 1000 mL D_5 in one-half normal saline with 20 mEq KCl over 10 hours. Drip factor is 15. How many drops per minute would the nurse give?

    A. 15 gtt/min
    B. 25 gtt/min
    C. 2.5 gtt/min
    D. 25 mL/hr

33. Ringer's lactate 100 mL has been ordered to infuse over 2 hours. The set calibration is 10 gtt/mL. How many drops per minute would the nurse give?

    A. 8 gtt/min
    B. 80 gtt/min
    C. 10 gtt/min
    D. 20 gtt/min

34. The nurse is to infuse 15 mL of an antibiotic over 30 minutes using a 60 gtt/mL set. How many drops per minute would the nurse give?

    A. 30 gtt/min
    B. 30 mL/min
    C. 30 mL/hr
    D. 3.0 gtt/min

35. The client is to receive 1800 mL of fluid over 10 hours. The set calibration is 10 gtt/mL. How many drops per minute would the nurse give?

    A. 30 gtt/min
    B. 10 gtt/min
    C. 10 mL/min
    D. 30 mL/min

36. The physician orders Ringer's lactate 1000 mL to infuse over 6 hours. Drops per milliliter equal 15. How many drops per minute would the nurse give?

    A. 4.4 gtt/min
    B. 44 gtt/min
    C. 42 gtt/min
    D. 41 gtt/min

37. The nurse is to infuse D_5W 250 mL over 1 hour. Drops per milliliter equal 15. How many drops per minute would the nurse give?

    A. 62 gtt/min
    B. 63 gtt/min
    C. 52 gtt/min
    D. 53 gtt/min

38. A hypertonic solution of $D_{10}W$ is to infuse over 12 hours. The total amount of fluid is 1000 mL, and the drop factor is 15. How many drops per minute would the nurse give?

    A. 20 gtt/min
    B. 28 gtt/min
    C. 21 gtt/min
    D. 208 gtt/min

39. The nurse is to infuse 300 mL of IV fluid in 2 hours using a set with a calibration of 60 gtt/mL. How many drops per minute would the nurse give?

    A. 15 gtt/min
    B. 150 gtt/min
    C. 75 gtt/min
    D. 300 gtt/min

40. The nurse is to infuse 900 mL of IV fluid in 2 hours. The set calibration is 10 gtt/mL. How many drops per minute would the nurse give?

    A. 450 gtt/min
    B. 750 gtt/min
    C. 75 gtt/min
    D. 7.5 gtt/min

41. The nurse is to infuse 1500 mL of IV fluid in 8 hours. Set calibration is 10 gtt/mL. How many drops per minute would the nurse give?

    A. 31 gtt/min q8h
    B. 32 gtt/min

C. 3.2 gtt/min

D. 3 gtt/min

42. The nurse is to administer an IV infusion of 250 mL of D$_5$W at 100 mL/hr using a 60 gtt/mL set. How many drops per minute would the nurse give?

A. 10 gtt/min

B. 100 gtt/min

C. 25 gtt/min

D. 25 mL/min

43. The nurse is to infuse 60 mL of antibiotic in 15 minutes. The set calibration is 10 gtt/mL. How many drops per minute would the nurse give?

A. 40 gtt/min

B. 60 gtt/min

C. 20 gtt/min

D. 30 gtt/min

44. The nurse is to infuse 20 mL of medication over 30 minutes using a 60 gtt/mL set. How many drops per minute would the nurse give?

A. 40 gtt/min

B. 80 gtt/min

C. 30 gtt/min

D. 60 gtt/min

45. The nurse is to infuse 800 mL of intravenous fat emulsion over 6 hours with a 20 gtt/mL set. How many drops per minute would the nurse give?

A. 44 gtt/min

B. 45 gtt/min

C. 46 gtt/min

D. 47 gtt/min

46. The nurse is to infuse 105 mL of fluid over 2 hours using a minidrip of 60 gtt/min. How many drops per minute would the nurse give?

A. 53 gtt/min

B. 50 gtt/min

C. 60 gtt/min

D. 62 gtt/min

47. The client is to receive 1000 mL D$_5$ in one-half normal saline with 20 mEq KCl over 8 hours. Drip factor is 10. How many drops per minute would the nurse give?

A. 20 gtt/min

B. 21 gtt/min

C. 22 gtt/min

D. 60 gtt/min

48. Ringer's lactate 100 mL has been ordered to infuse over 2 hours. The set calibration is 10 gtt/mL. How many drops per minute would the nurse give?

A. 17 gtt/min

B. 16 gtt/min

C. 8 gtt/min

D. 8.5 gtt/min

49. The nurse is to infuse 30 mL of an antibiotic over 30 minutes using a 60 gtt/mL set. How many drops per minute would the nurse give?

A. 30 gtt/min

B. 45 gtt/min

C. 60 gtt/min

D. 6 gtt/min

50. The client is to receive 1000 mL of fluid over 10 hours. The set calibration is 15 gtt/mL. How many drops per minute would the nurse give?

A. 100 gtt/min

B. 115 gtt/min

C. 25 gtt/min

D. 125 gtt/min

MOCK NCLEX-RN BOARD REVIEW TEST ANSWERS

1. **(D)** Client need: physiological integrity; subcategory: pharmacological and parenteral therapies

   RATIONALE
   (D) Memorization: 1 tbsp = 15 mL; 3 tsp = 15 mL; 1 tsp = 5 mL. The question asks for tablespoons, however.

2. **(A)** Client need: physiological integrity; subcategory: pharmacological and parenteral therapies

   RATIONALE
   (A) Gr 1/150 = 0.4 mg. (B) One-half tablet would be 0.2 mg. (C) Two tablets would be 0.8 mg. (D) One and one-half tablets would be 0.6 mg.

3. **(C)** Client need: physiological integrity; subcategory: pharmacological and parenteral therapies

   RATIONALE
   0.5 g = 500 mg
   500 mg:x:250 mg:1 capsule
   250x = 500
   x = 2 capsules
   Math calculation explains incorrect answers.

4. **(B)** Client need: physiological integrity; subcategory: pharmacological and parenteral therapies

   RATIONALE
   50 mg:1 mL::750 mg:x
   750 mg:x::50 mg:1 mL
   50x = 750
   x = 15 mL
   Math calculation explains incorrect answers.

5. **(D)** Client need: physiological integrity: subcategory: pharmacological and parenteral therapies

   RATIONALE
   1 kg = 2.2 lb
   154 kg ÷ 2.2 lb = 70 kg
   70 kg × 4 mg/kg = 280 mg
   Math calculation explains incorrect answers.

6. **(B)** Client need: physiological integrity; subcategory: pharmacological and parenteral therapies

   RATIONALE
   24 hr ÷ 4 times = 6 doses
   3000 mg ÷ 6 = 500 mg
   Math calculation explains incorrect answers.

7. **(B)** Client need: physiological integrity; subcategory: pharmacological and parenteral therapies

   RATIONALE
   1 gr = 60 mg
   60 mg × 5 gr = 1 tablet
   300 mg:1 tablet::300 mg:x
   300x = 300 mg
   x = 1 tablet
   Math calculation explains incorrect answers.

8. **(C)** Client need: physiological integrity; subcategory: pharmacological and parenteral therapies

   RATIONALE
   1 mg:0.5 mL::0.5 mg:x
   x = 0.25 mL
   Math calculation explains incorrect answers.

9. **(C)** Client need: physiological integrity; subcategory: pharmacological and parenteral therapies

   RATIONALE
   0.125 mg:1 tablet::0.25 mg:x
   0.125x = 0.25
   x = 2
   Math calculation explains incorrect answers.

10. **(C)** Client need: physiological integrity; subcategory: pharmacological and parenteral therapies

    RATIONALE
    75 mg:1 mL::50 mg:x
    75x = 50
    x = 0.66 or 0.7 mL
    Math calculation explains incorrect answers.

11. **(B)** Client need: physiological integrity; subcategory: pharmacological and parenteral therapies

    RATIONALE
    1 gr = 60 mg
    60 mg:1 tablet::30 mg:x
    60x = 30
    x = 0.5 tablet
    Math calculation explains incorrect answers.

12. **(C)** Client need: physiological integrity; subcategory: pharmacological and parenteral therapies

    RATIONALE
    25 mg:1 mL::100 mg:x
    25x = 100
    x = 4 cc
    Math calculation explains incorrect answers.

13. **(B)** Client need: physiological integrity; subcategory: pharmacological and parenteral therapies

    RATIONALE
    500 mg ÷ 24 hr = 20.8 or 21 mg/hr
    250 mL ÷ 24 hr = 10.4 or 10 mL/hr
    Math calculation explains incorrect answers.

14. **(C)** Client need: physiological integrity; subcategory: pharmacological and parenteral therapies

    RATIONALE
    250 mg ÷ 16 hr = 15.6 mg/hr ÷ 60 min/hr = 0.26 mg/min
    250 Ml ÷ 16 hr = 15.6 mL/hr ÷ 60 min/hr = 0.26 mL/min
    Math calculation explains incorrect answers.

15. **(D)** Client need: physiological integrity; subcategory: pharmacological and parenteral therapies

    RATIONALE
    500 mL ÷ 12 hr = 41.6 or 42 mL/hr
    500 mg ÷ 12 hr = 41.6 or 42 mg/hr
    Math calculations explain incorrect answers.

16. **(A)** Client need: physiological integrity; subcategory: pharmacological and parenteral therapies

    RATIONALE
    400 mg ÷ 24 hr = 16.6 or 17 mg/hr
    500 mL ÷ 24 hr = 20.8 or 21 mL/hr
    Math calculations explain incorrect answers.

17. **(D)** Client need: physiological integrity; subcategory: pharmacological and parenteral therapies

    RATIONALE
    50 U = 100 mL
    1 U = 2 mL
    3 U = 6 mL
    Math calculation explains incorrect answers.

18. **(C)** Client need: physiological integrity; subcategory: pharmacological and parenteral therapies

    RATIONALE

    10 mg:x mL::15 mg:1 mL

    15x = 10

    x = 0.66 or 0.7 mL

    Math calculation explains incorrect answers.

19. **(C)** Client need: physiological integrity; subcategory: pharmacological and parenteral therapies

    RATIONALE

    25 mg::x::100 mg::2 mL

    100x = 50

    x = 0.5 mL

    Math calculation explains incorrect answers.

20. **(C)** Client need: physiological integrity; subcategory: pharmacological and parenteral therapies

    RATIONALE

    20,000:1 mL::5000::x

    20,000 × 5000x

    x = 0.25 mL

    Math calculation explains incorrect answers.

21. **(B)** Client need: physiological integrity; subcategory: pharmacological and parenteral therapies

    RATIONALE

    $$\frac{1000 \text{ mL} \times 15 \text{ gtt/mL}}{60 \text{ min/hr} \times 8 \text{ hr}} = \frac{15,000}{480} = 31.2 \text{ or } 31 \text{ gtt/min}$$

    Math calculation explains incorrect answers.

22. **(C)** Client need: physiological integrity; subcategory: pharmacological and parenteral therapies

    RATIONALE

    $$\frac{150 \text{ mL} \times 10 \text{ gtt/mL}}{60 \text{ min/hr} \times 1 \text{ hr}} = \frac{1500}{60} = 25 \text{ gtt/min}$$

    Math calculation explains incorrect answers.

23. **(C)** Client need: physiological integrity; subcategory: pharmacological and parenteral therapies

    RATIONALE

    $$\frac{1000 \text{mL} \times 10 \text{gtt/mL}}{10 \text{hr} \times 60 \text{ min/hr}} = \frac{10,000}{600} = 16.7 \text{ or } 17 \text{ gtt/min}$$

    Math calculation explains incorrect answers.

24. **(B)** Client need: physiological integrity; subcategory: pharmacological and parenteral therapies

    RATIONALE

    $$\frac{100 \text{ mL} \times 60 \text{ gtt/mL}}{60 \text{ min/hr} \times 2 \text{ hr}} = \frac{6000}{120} = 50 \text{ gtt/min}$$

    Math calculation explains incorrect answers.

25. **(C)** Client need: physiological integrity; subcategory: pharmacological and parenteral therapies

    RATIONALE

    $$\frac{900 \text{ mL} \times 20 \text{ gtt/mL}}{60 \text{ min/hr} \times 2 \text{ hr}} = \frac{18,000}{120} = 150 \text{ gtt/min}$$

    Math calculation explains incorrect answers.

26. **(B)** Client need: physiological integrity; subcategory: pharmacological and parenteral therapies

    RATIONALE

    $$\frac{1000 \text{ mL} \times 10 \text{ gtt/mL}}{8 \text{ hr} \times 60 \text{ min/hr}} = \frac{10,000}{480} = 20.8 \text{ or } 21 \text{ gtt/min}$$

    Math calculation explains incorrect answers.

27. **(C)** Client need: physiological integrity; subcategory: pharmacological and parenteral therapies

    RATIONALE

    $$\frac{150 \text{ mL} \times 60 \text{ gtt/mL}}{60 \text{ mL}} = \frac{9000}{60} = 150 \text{ gtt/min}$$

    Math calculation explains incorrect answers.

28. **(A)** Client need: physiological integrity; subcategory: pharmacological and parenteral therapies

    RATIONALE

    $$\frac{50 \text{ mL} \times 60 \text{ gtt/mL}}{30 \text{ min}} = \frac{3000}{30} = 100 \text{ gt/min}$$

    Math calculation explains incorrect answers.

29. **(B)** Client need: physiological integrity; subcategory: pharmacological and parenteral therapies

    RATIONALE

    $$\frac{15 \text{ mL} \times 60 \text{ gtt/mL}}{15 \text{ min}} = \frac{900}{15} = 60 \text{ gtt/min}$$

    Math calculation explains incorrect answers.

30. **(C)** Client need: physiological integrity; subcategory: pharmacological and parenteral therapies

    RATIONALE

    $$\frac{600 \text{ mL} \times 10 \text{ gtt/mL}}{60 \text{ min/hr} \times 8 \text{ hr}} = \frac{6000}{480} = 12.5 \text{ or } 13 \text{ gtt/min}$$

    Math calculation explains incorrect answers.

31. **(C)** Client need: physiological integrity; subcategory: pharmacological and parenteral therapies

    RATIONALE

    $$\frac{150 \text{ mL} \times 60 \text{ gtt/mL}}{60 \text{ min/hr} \times 2 \text{ hr}} = \frac{9000}{120} = 75 \text{ gtt/min}$$

    Math calculation explains incorrect answers.

32. **(B)** Client need: physiological integrity; subcategory: pharmacological and parenteral therapies

    RATIONALE

    $$\frac{1000 \text{ mL} \times 15 \text{ gtt/mL}}{60 \text{ min/hr} \times 10 \text{ hr}} = \frac{15,000}{600} = 25 \text{ gtt/min}$$

    Math calculation explains incorrect answers.

33. **(A)** Client need: physiological integrity; subcategory: pharmacological and parenteral therapies

    RATIONALE

    $$\frac{100 \text{ mL} \times 10 \text{ gtt/mL}}{2 \text{ hr} \times 60 \text{ min/hr}} = \frac{1000}{120} = 8.3 \text{ or } 8 \text{ gtt/min}$$

    Math calculation explains incorrect answers.

34. **(A)** Client need: physiological integrity; subcategory: pharmacological and parenteral therapies

    RATIONALE

    $$\frac{15 \text{ mL} \times 60 \text{ gtt/mL}}{30 \text{ min}} = \frac{900}{30} = 30 \text{ gtt/min}$$

    Math calculation explains incorrect answers.

35. **(A)** Client need: physiological integrity; subcategory: pharmacological and parenteral therapies

    RATIONALE

    $$\frac{1800 \text{ mL} \times 10 \text{ gtt/min}}{60 \text{ min/hr} \times 10 \text{ hr}} = \frac{18,000}{600} = 30 \text{ gtt/min}$$

    Math calculation explains incorrect answers.

36. **(C)** Client need: physiological integrity; subcategory: pharmacological and parenteral therapies

    RATIONALE

    $$\frac{1000 \text{ mL} \times 15 \text{ gtt/mL}}{60 \text{ min/hr} \times 10 \text{ hr}} = \frac{15,000}{600} = 25 \text{ gtt/min}$$

    Math calculation explains incorrect answers.

37. **(B)** Client need: physiological integrity; subcategory: pharmacological and parenteral therapies

    RATIONALE

    $$\frac{250 \text{ mL} \times 15 \text{ gtt/mL}}{60 \text{ min/hr} \times 1 \text{ hr}} = \frac{3750}{60} = 62.5 \text{ or } 63 \text{ gtt/min}$$

    Math calculation explains incorrect answers.

38. **(C)** Client need: physiological integrity; subcategory: pharmacological and parenteral therapies

    RATIONALE

    $$\frac{1000 \text{ mL} \times 15 \text{ gtt/mL}}{12 \text{ hr} \times 60 \text{ min/hr}} = \frac{15,000}{720} = 20.8 \text{ or } 21 \text{ gtt/min}$$

    Math calculation explains incorrect answers.

39. **(B)** Client need: physiological integrity; subcategory: pharmacological and parenteral therapies

    RATIONALE

    $$\frac{300 \text{ mL} \times 60 \text{ gtt/mL}}{60 \text{ min}} = \frac{18,000}{120} = 150 \text{ gtt/min}$$

    Math calculation explains incorrect answers.

40. **(C)** Client need: physiological integrity; subcategory: pharmacological and parenteral therapies

    RATIONALE

    $$\frac{900 \text{ mL} \times 10 \text{ gtt/mL}}{60 \text{ min/hr} \times 2 \text{ hr}} = \frac{9000}{120} = 75 \text{ gtt/min}$$

    Math calculation explains incorrect answers.

41. **(A)** Client need: physiological integrity; subcategory: pharmacological and parenteral therapies

    RATIONALE

    $$\frac{1500 \text{ mL} \times 10 \text{ gtt/mL}}{60 \text{ min/hr} \times 8 \text{ hr}} = \frac{15,000}{480} = 31.25 \text{ or } 31 \text{ gtt/min}$$

    Math calculation explains incorrect answers.

42. **(B)** Client need: physiological integrity; subcategory: pharmacological and parenteral therapies

    RATIONALE

    $$\frac{100 \text{ mL} \times 60 \text{ gtt/mL}}{60 \text{ min/hr} \times 1 \text{ hr}} = \frac{6000}{60} = 100 \text{ gtt/min}$$

    Math calculation explains incorrect answers.

43. **(A)** Client need: physiological integrity; subcategory: pharmacological and parenteral therapies

    RATIONALE

    $$\frac{60 \text{ mL} \times 10 \text{ gtt/mL}}{15 \text{ min}} = \frac{600}{15} = 40 \text{ gtt/min}$$

    Math calculation explains incorrect answers.

44. **(A)** Client need: physiological integrity; subcategory: pharmacological and parenteral therapies

    RATIONALE

    $$\frac{20 \text{ mL} \times 60 \text{ gtt/mL}}{30 \text{ min}} = \frac{1200}{30} = 40 \text{ gtt/min}$$

    Math calculation explains incorrect answers.

45. **(A)** Client need: physiological integrity; subcategory: pharmacological and parenteral therapies

    RATIONALE

    $$\frac{800 \text{ mL} \times 20 \text{ gtt/mL}}{60 \text{ min/hr} \times 6 \text{ hr}} = \frac{16,000}{360} = 44.4 \text{ or } 44 \text{ gtt/min}$$

    Math calculation explains incorrect answers.

46. **(A)** Client need: physiological integrity; subcategory: pharmacological and parenteral therapies

    RATIONALE

    Minidrip = 60 gtt/mL

    $$\frac{105 \text{ mL} \times 60 \text{ gtt/mL}}{60 \text{ min/hr} \times 2 \text{ hr}} = \frac{6300}{120} = 52.5 \text{ or } 53 \text{ gtt/min}$$

    Math calculation explains incorrect answers.

47. **(B)** Client need: physiological integrity; subcategory: pharmacological and parenteral therapies

    RATIONALE

    $$\frac{1000 \text{ mL} \times 10 \text{ gtt/mL}}{60 \text{ min/hr} \times 8 \text{ hr}} = \frac{10,000}{480} = 20.8 \text{ or } 21 \text{ gtt/min}$$

    Math calculation explains incorrect answers.

48. **(C)** Client need: physiological integrity; subcategory: pharmacological and parenteral therapies

    RATIONALE

    $$\frac{100 \text{ mL} \times 10 \text{ gtt/mL}}{60 \text{ min/hr} \times 2 \text{ hr}} = \frac{1000}{120} = 8.3 \text{ or } 8 \text{ gtt/min}$$

    Math calculation explains incorrect answers.

49. **(C)** Client need: physiological integrity; subcategory: pharmacological and parenteral therapies

    RATIONALE

    $$\frac{30 \text{ mL} \times 60 \text{ gtt/mL}}{30 \text{ min}} = \frac{1800}{30} = 60 \text{ gtt/min}$$

    Math calculation explains incorrect answers.

50. **(C)** Client need: physiological integrity; subcategory: pharmacological and parenteral therapies

    RATIONALE

    $$\frac{1000 \text{ mL} \times 15 \text{ gtt/mL}}{60 \text{ min/hr} \times 10 \text{ hr}} = \frac{15,000}{600} = 25 \text{ gtt/min}$$

    Math calculation explains incorrect answers.

Comprehensive Integrated Practice Tests

TEST 1

Northwestern State University of Louisiana Division of Nursing Test

MOCK NCLEX-RN BOARD REVIEW TEST QUESTIONS

1. A 25-year-old client believes she may be pregnant with her first child. She schedules an obstetric examination with the nurse practitioner to determine the status of her possible pregnancy. Her last menstrual period began May 20, and her estimated date of confinement using Nägele's rule is:

   A. March 27
   B. February 1
   C. February 27
   D. January 3

2. The nurse practitioner determines that a client is approximately 9 weeks' gestation. During the visit, the practitioner informs the client about symptoms of physical changes that she will experience during her first trimester, such as:

   A. Nausea and vomiting
   B. Quickening
   C. A 6–8 lb weight gain
   D. Abdominal enlargement

3. A client is 6 weeks pregnant. During her first prenatal visit, she asks, "How much alcohol is safe to drink during pregnancy?" The nurse's response is:

   A. Up to 1 oz daily
   B. Up to 2 oz daily
   C. Up to 4 oz weekly
   D. No alcohol

4. A 38-year-old pregnant woman visits her nurse practitioner for her regular prenatal checkup. She is 30 weeks' gestation. The nurse should be alert to which condition related to her age?

   A. Iron-deficiency anemia
   B. Sexually transmitted disease (STD)
   C. Intrauterine growth retardation
   D. Pregnancy-induced hypertension (PIH)

5. A client returns for her 6-month prenatal checkup and has gained 10 lb in 2 months. The results of her physical examination are normal. How does the nurse interpret the effectiveness of the instruction about diet and weight control?

   A. She is compliant with her diet as previously taught.
   B. She needs further instruction and reinforcement.
   C. She needs to increase her caloric intake.
   D. She needs to be placed on a restrictive diet immediately.

6. Pregnant women with diabetes often have problems related to the effectiveness of insulin in controlling their glucose levels during their second half of pregnancy. The nurse teaches the client that this is due to:

   A. Decreased glomerular filtration and increased tubular absorption
   B. Decreased estrogen levels
   C. Decreased progesterone levels
   D. Increased human placental lactogen levels

7. Diabetes during pregnancy requires tight metabolic control of glucose levels to prevent perinatal mortality. When evaluating the pregnant client, the nurse knows the recommended serum glucose range during pregnancy is:

   A. 70 mg/dL and 120 mg/dL
   B. 100 mg/dL and 200 mg/dL
   C. 40 mg/dL and 130 mg/dL
   D. 90 mg/dL and 200 mg/dL

8. When assessing fetal heart rate status during labor, the monitor displays late decelerations with tachycardia and decreasing variability. What action should the nurse take?

   A. Continue monitoring because this is a normal occurrence.

B. Turn client on right side.

C. Decrease IV fluids.

D. Report to physician or midwife.

9. A client has been diagnosed as being preeclamptic. The physician orders magnesium sulfate. Magnesium sulfate ($MgSO_4$) is used in the management of preeclampsia for:

A. Prevention of seizures

B. Prevention of uterine contractions

C. Sedation

D. Fetal lung protection

10. The predominant purpose of the first Apgar scoring of a newborn is to:

A. Determine gross abnormal motor function

B. Obtain a baseline for comparison with the infant's future adaptation to the environment

C. Evaluate the infant's vital functions

D. Determine the extent of congenital malformations

11. Provide the 1-minute Apgar score for an infant born with the following findings:

Heart rate: Above 100
Respiratory effort: Slow, irregular
Muscle tone: Some flexion of extremities
Reflex irritability: Vigorous cry
Color: Body pink, blue extremities

A. 7

B. 10

C. 8

D. 9

12. A pregnant woman at 36 weeks' gestation is followed for PIH and develops proteinuria. To increase protein in her diet, which of the following foods will provide the greatest amount of protein when added to her intake of 100 mL of milk?

A. Fifty milliliters light cream and 2 tbsp corn syrup

B. Thirty grams powdered skim milk and 1 egg

C. One small scoop (90 g) vanilla ice cream and 1 tbsp chocolate syrup

D. One package vitamin-fortified gelatin drink

13. The physician recommends immediate hospital admission for a client with PIH. She says to the nurse, "It's not so easy for me to just go right to the hospital like that." After acknowledging her feelings, which of these approaches by the nurse would probably be best?

A. Stress to the client that her husband would want her to do what is best for her health.

B. Explore with the client her perceptions of why she is unable to go to the hospital.

C. Repeat the physician's reasons for advising immediate hospitalization.

D. Explain to the client that she is ultimately responsible for her own welfare and that of her baby.

14. Which of the following findings would be abnormal in a postpartal woman?

A. Chills shortly after delivery

B. Pulse rate of 60 bpm in morning on first postdelivery day

C. Urinary output of 3000 mL on the second day after delivery

D. An oral temperature of 101°F (38.3°C) on the third day after delivery

15. What is the *most* effective method to identify early breast cancer lumps?

A. Mammograms every 3 years

B. Yearly checkups performed by physician

C. Ultrasounds every 3 years

D. Monthly breast self-examination

16. Which of the following risk factors associated with breast cancer would a nurse consider *most* significant in a client's history?

A. Menarche after age 13

B. Nulliparity

C. Maternal family history of breast cancer

D. Early menopause

17. Which of the following procedures is necessary to establish a definitive diagnosis of breast cancer?

A. Diaphanography

B. Mammography

C. Thermography

D. Breast tissue biopsy

18. The nurse should know that according to current thinking, the *most* important prognostic factor for a client with breast cancer is:

A. Tumor size

B. Axillary node status

C. Client's previous history of disease

D. Client's level of estrogen-progesterone receptor assays

19. When teaching a sex education class, the nurse identifies the most common STDs in the United States as:

A. Chlamydia

B. Herpes genitalis

C. Syphilis

D. Gonorrhea

20. A 30-year-old male client is admitted to the psychiatric unit with a diagnosis of bipolar disorder. For the last 2 months, his family describes him as being "on the move," sleeping 3–4 hours nightly, spending lots of money, and losing approximately 10 lb. During the initial assessment with the client, the nurse would expect him to exhibit which of the following?

A. Short, polite responses to interview questions

B. Introspection related to his present situation

C. Exaggerated self-importance

D. Feelings of helplessness and hopelessness

21. The therapeutic blood-level range for lithium is:

A. 0.25–1.0 mEq/L

B. 0.5–1.5 mEq/L

C. 1.0–2.0 mEq/L

D. 2.0–2.5 mEq/L

22. A client with bipolar disorder taking lithium tells the nurse that he has ringing in his ears, blurred vision, and diarrhea. The nurse notices a slight tremor in his left hand and a slurring pattern to his speech. Which of the following actions by the nurse is appropriate?

    A. Administer a stat dose of lithium as necessary.
    B. Recognize this as an expected response to lithium.
    C. Request an order for a stat blood lithium level.
    D. Give an oral dose of lithium antidote.

23. Which of the following activities would be *most* appropriate during occupational therapy for a client with bipolar disorder?

    A. Playing cards with other clients
    B. Working crossword puzzles
    C. Playing tennis with a staff member
    D. Sewing beads on a leather belt

24. A client diagnosed with bipolar disorder continues to be hyperactive and to lose weight. Which of the following nutritional interventions would be *most* therapeutic for him at this time?

    A. Small, frequent feedings of foods that can be carried
    B. Tube feedings with nutritional supplements
    C. Allowing him to eat when and what he wants
    D. Giving him a quiet place where he can sit down to eat meals

25. Three weeks following discharge, a male client is readmitted to the psychiatric unit for depression. His wife stated that he had threatened to kill himself with a handgun. As the nurse admits him to the unit, he says, "I wish I were dead because I am worthless to everyone; I guess I am just no good." Which response by the nurse is *most* appropriate at this time?

    A. "I don't think you are worthless. I'm glad to see you, and we will help you."
    B. "Don't you think this is a sign of your illness?"
    C. "I know with your wife and new baby that you do have a lot to live for."
    D. "You've been feeling sad and alone for some time now?"

26. Which of the following statements relevant to a suicidal client is correct?

    A. The more specific a client's plan, the more likely he or she is to attempt suicide.
    B. A client who is unsuccessful at a first suicide attempt is not likely to make future attempts.
    C. A client who threatens suicide is just seeking attention and is not likely to attempt suicide.
    D. Nurses who care for a client who has attempted suicide should not make any reference to the word "suicide" in order to protect the client's ego.

27. The physician orders fluoxetine (Prozac) for a depressed client. Which of the following should the nurse remember about fluoxetine?

    A. Because fluoxetine is a tricyclic antidepressant, it may precipitate a hypertensive crisis.

    B. The therapeutic effect of the drug occurs 2–4 weeks after treatment is begun.
    C. Foods such as aged cheese, yogurt, soy sauce, and bananas should not be eaten with this drug.
    D. Fluoxetine may be administered safely in combination with monoamine oxidase (MAO) inhibitors.

28. The day following his admission, the nurse sits down by a male client on the sofa in the dayroom. He was admitted for depression and thoughts of suicide. He looks at the nurse and says, "My life is so bad no one can do anything to help me." The most helpful initial response by the nurse would be:

    A. "It concerns me that you feel so badly when you have so many positive things in your life."
    B. "It will take a few weeks for you to feel better, so you need to be patient."
    C. "You are telling me that you are feeling hopeless at this point?"
    D. "Let's play cards with some of the other clients to get your mind off your problems for now."

29. A long-term goal for the nurse in planning care for a depressed, suicidal client would be to:

    A. Provide him with a safe and structured environment.
    B. Assist him to develop more effective coping mechanisms.
    C. Have him sign a "no-suicide" contract.
    D. Isolate him from stressful situations that may precipitate a depressive episode.

30. After 3 weeks of treatment, a severely depressed client suddenly begins to feel better and starts interacting appropriately with other clients and staff. The nurse knows that this client has an increased risk for:

    A. Suicide
    B. Exacerbation of depressive symptoms
    C. Violence toward others
    D. Psychotic behavior

31. Nursing care for the substance abuse client experiencing alcohol withdrawal delirium includes:

    A. Maintaining seizure precautions
    B. Restricting fluid intake
    C. Increasing sensory stimuli
    D. Applying ankle and wrist restraints

32. A psychotic client who believes that he is God and rules all the universe is experiencing which type of delusion?

    A. Somatic
    B. Grandiose
    C. Persecutory
    D. Nihilistic

33. A client confides to the nurse that he tasted poison in his evening meal. This would be an example of what type of hallucination?

    A. Auditory
    B. Gustatory
    C. Olfactory
    D. Visceral

34. A schizophrenic client has made sexual overtures toward her physician on numerous occasions. During lunch, the client tells the nurse, "My doctor is in love with me and wants to marry me." This client is using which of the following defense mechanisms?

    A. Displacement
    B. Projection
    C. Reaction formation
    D. Suppression

35. Hypoxia is the primary problem related to near-drowning victims. The first organ that sustains irreversible damage after submersion in water is the:

    A. Kidney (urinary system)
    B. Brain (nervous system)
    C. Heart (circulatory system)
    D. Lungs (respiratory system)

36. One of the most dramatic and serious complications associated with bacterial meningitis is Waterhouse-Friderichsen syndrome, which is:

    A. Peripheral circulatory collapse
    B. Syndrome of inappropriate antidiuretic hormone
    C. Cerebral edema resulting in hydrocephalus
    D. Auditory nerve damage resulting in permanent hearing loss

37. An 8-year-old child comes to the physician's office complaining of swelling and pain in the knees. His mother says, "The swelling occurred for no reason, and it keeps getting worse." The initial diagnosis is Lyme disease. When talking to the mother and child, questions related to which of the following would be important to include in the initial history?

    A. A decreased urinary output and flank pain
    B. A fever of over 103°F occurring over the last 2–3 weeks
    C. Rashes covering the palms of the hands and the soles of the feet
    D. Headaches, malaise, or sore throat

38. The *most* commonly known vectors of Lyme disease are:

    A. Mites
    B. Fleas
    C. Ticks
    D. Mosquitoes

39. A laboratory technique specific for diagnosing Lyme disease is:

    A. Polymerase chain reaction
    B. Heterophil antibody test
    C. Decreased serum calcium level
    D. Increased serum potassium level

40. The nurse would expect to include which of the following when planning the management of the client with Lyme disease?

    A. Complete bed rest for 6–8 weeks
    B. Tetracycline treatment
    C. IV amphotericin B
    D. High-protein diet with limited fluids

41. A 3-year-old child is hospitalized with burns covering her trunk and lower extremities. Which of the following would the nurse use to assess adequacy of fluid resuscitation in the burned child?

    A. Blood pressure
    B. Serum potassium level
    C. Urine output
    D. Pulse rate

42. Proper positioning for the child who is in Bryant's traction is:

    A. Both hips flexed at a 90-degree angle with the knees extended and the buttocks elevated off the bed
    B. Both legs extended, and the hips are not flexed
    C. The affected leg extended with slight hip flexion
    D. Both hips and knees maintained at a 90-degree flexion angle, and the back flat on the bed

43. A child sustains a supracondylar fracture of the femur. When assessing for vascular injury, the nurse should be alert for the signs of ischemia, which include:

    A. Bleeding, bruising, and hemorrhage
    B. Increase in serum levels of creatinine, alkaline phosphatase, and aspartate transaminase
    C. Pain, pallor, pulselessness, paresthesia, and paralysis
    D. Generalized swelling, pain, and diminished functional use with muscle rigidity and crepitus

44. When administering phenytoin (Dilantin) to a child, the nurse should be aware that a toxic effect of phenytoin therapy is:

    A. Stephens-Johnson syndrome
    B. Folate deficiency
    C. Leukopenic aplastic anemia
    D. Granulocytosis and nephrosis

45. A six-month-old infant has been admitted to the emergency room with febrile seizures. In the teaching of the parents, the nurse states that:

    A. Sustained temperature elevation over 103°F is generally related to febrile seizures
    B. Febrile seizures do not usually recur
    C. There is little risk of neurological deficit and mental retardation as sequelae to febrile seizures
    D. Febrile seizures are associated with diseases of the central nervous system

46. When assessing a child with diabetes insipidus, the nurse should be aware of the cardinal signs of:

    A. Anemia and vomiting
    B. Polyuria and polydipsia
    C. Irritability relieved by feeding formula
    D. Hypothermia and azotemia

47. The usual treatment for diabetes insipidus is with IM or SC injection of vasopressin tannate in oil. Nursing care related to the client receiving IM vasopressin tannate would include:

    A. Weigh once a week and report to the physician any weight gain of ≥10 lb.
    B. Limit fluid intake to 500 mL/day.

C. Store the medication in a refrigerator and allow to stand at room temperature for 30 minutes prior to administration.

D. Hold the vial under warm water for 10–15 minutes and shake vigorously before drawing medication into the syringe.

48. A child is admitted to the emergency room with her mother. Her mother states that she has been exposed to chickenpox. During the assessment, the nurse would note a characteristic rash:

A. That is covered with vesicular scabs all in the macular stage

B. That appears profusely on the trunk and sparsely on the extremities

C. That first appears on the neck and spreads downward

D. That appears especially on the cheeks, which gives a "slapped-cheek" appearance

49. Discharge teaching was effective if the parents of a child with atopic dermatitis could state the importance of:

A. Maintaining a high-humidified environment

B. Furry, soft stuffed animals for play

C. Showering 3–4 times a day

D. Wrapping hands in soft cotton gloves

50. The priority nursing goal when working with an autistic child is:

A. To establish trust with the child

B. To maintain communication with the family

C. To promote involvement in school activities

D. To maintain nutritional requirements

51. The child with iron poisoning is given IV deforoxamine mesylate (Desferal). Following administration, the child suffers hypotension, facial flushing, and urticaria. The initial nursing intervention would be to:

A. Discontinue the IV

B. Stop the medication, and begin a normal saline infusion

C. Take all vital signs, and report to the physician

D. Assess urinary output, and if it is 30 mL an hour, maintain current treatment

52. As the nurse assesses a male adolescent with chlamydia, the nurse determines that a sign of chlamydia is:

A. Enlarged penis

B. Secondary lymphadenitis

C. Epididymitis

D. Hepatomegaly

53. When teaching a mother of a 4-month-old with diarrhea about the importance of preventing dehydration, the nurse would inform the mother about the importance of feeding her child:

A. Fruit juices

B. Diluted carbonated drinks

C. Soy-based, lactose-free formula

D. Regular formulas mixed with electrolyte solutions

54. The primary reason that an increase in heart rate (>100 bpm) detrimental to the client with a myocardial infarction (MI) is that:

A. Stroke volume and blood pressure will drop proportionately

B. Systolic ejection time will decrease, thereby decreasing cardiac output

C. Decreased contractile strength will occur due to decreased filling time

D. Decreased coronary artery perfusion due to decreased diastolic filling time will occur, which will increase ischemic damage to the myocardium

55. To appropriately monitor therapy and client progress, the nurse should be aware that increased myocardial work and O_2 demand will occur with which of the following?

A. Positive inotropic therapy

B. Negative chronotropic therapy

C. Increase in balance of myocardial O_2 supply and demand

D. Afterload reduction therapy

56. The nurse would need to monitor the serum glucose levels of a client receiving which of the following medications, owing to its effects on glycogenolysis and insulin release?

A. Norepinephrine (Levophed)

B. Dobutamine (Dobutrex)

C. Propranolol (Inderal)

D. Epinephrine (Adrenalin)

57. Which of the following medications requires close observation for bronchospasm in the client with chronic obstructive pulmonary disease or asthma?

A. Verapamil (Isoptin)

B. Amrinone (Inocor)

C. Epinephrine (Adrenalin)

D. Propranolol (Inderal)

58. The following medications were noted on review of the client's home medication profile. Which of the medications would *most* likely potentiate or elevate serum digoxin levels?

A. KCl

B. Thyroid agents

C. Quinidine

D. Theophylline

59. In the client with a diagnosis of coronary artery disease, the nurse would anticipate the complication of bradycardia with occlusion of which coronary artery?

A. Right coronary artery

B. Left main coronary artery

C. Circumflex coronary artery

D. Left anterior descending coronary artery

60. When inspecting a cardiovascular client, the nurse notes that he needs to sit upright to breathe. This behavior is *most* indicative of:

A. Pericarditis

B. Anxiety

C. Congestive heart failure

D. Angina

61. When a client questions the nurse as to the purpose of exercise electrocardiography (ECG) in the diagnosis of cardiovascular disorders, the nurse's response should be based on the fact that:
    A. The test provides a baseline for further tests
    B. The procedure simulates usual daily activity and myocardial performance
    C. The client can be monitored while cardiac conditioning and heart toning are done
    D. Ischemia can be diagnosed because exercise increases O_2 consumption and demand

62. In assessing cardiovascular clients with progression of aortic stenosis, the nurse should be aware that there is typically:
    A. Decreased pulmonary blood flow and cyanosis
    B. Increased pressure in the pulmonary veins and pulmonary edema
    C. Systemic venous engorgement
    D. Increased left ventricular systolic pressures and hypertrophy

63. The cardiac client who exhibits the symptoms of disorientation, lethargy, and seizures may be exhibiting a toxic reaction to:
    A. Digoxin (Lanoxin)
    B. Lidocaine (Xylocaine)
    C. Quinidine gluconate or sulfate (Quinaglute, Quinidex)
    D. Nitroglycerin IV (Tridil)

64. Which of the following ECG changes would be seen as a positive myocardial stress test response?
    A. Hyperacute T wave
    B. Prolongation of the PR interval
    C. ST-segment depression
    D. Pathological Q wave

65. Assessment of the client with pericarditis may reveal which of the following?
    A. Ventricular gallop and substernal chest pain
    B. Narrowed pulse pressure and shortness of breath
    C. Pericardial friction rub and pain on deep inspiration
    D. Pericardial tamponade and widened pulse pressure

66. Clinical manifestations seen in left-sided rather than in right-sided heart failure are:
    A. Elevated central venous pressure and peripheral edema
    B. Dyspnea and jaundice
    C. Hypotension and hepatomegaly
    D. Decreased peripheral perfusion and rales

67. Which classification of drugs is contraindicated for the client with hypertrophic cardiomyopathy?
    A. Positive inotropes
    B. Vasodilators
    C. Diuretics
    D. Antidysrhythmics

68. To ensure proper client education, the nurse should teach the client taking SL nitroglycerin to expect which of the following responses with administration?

A. Stinging, burning when placed under the tongue
B. Temporary blurring of vision
C. Generalized urticaria with prolonged use
D. Urinary frequency

69. When a client is receiving vasoactive therapy IV, such as dopamine (Intropin), and extravasation occurs, the nurse should be prepared to administer which of the following medications directly into the site?
    A. Phentolamine (Regitine)
    B. Epinephrine
    C. Phenylephrine (Neo-Synephrine)
    D. Sodium bicarbonate

70. Which of the following would differentiate acute from chronic respiratory acidosis in the assessment of the trauma client?
    A. Increased $PaCO_2$
    B. Decreased PaO_2
    C. Increased HCO_3
    D. Decreased base excess

71. Which of the following signs and symptoms indicates a tension pneumothorax as compared to an open pneumothorax?
    A. Ventilation-perfusion ($\dot{V}/\dot{Q}$) mismatch
    B. Hypoxemia and respiratory acidosis
    C. Mediastinal tissue and organ shifting
    D. Decreased tidal volume and tachypnea

72. Hematotympanum and otorrhea are associated with which of the following head injuries?
    A. Basilar skull fracture
    B. Subdural hematoma
    C. Epidural hematoma
    D. Frontal lobe fracture

73. A client with a C-3–4 fracture has just arrived in the emergency room. The primary nursing intervention is:
    A. Stabilization of the cervical spine
    B. Airway assessment and stabilization
    C. Confirmation of spinal cord injury
    D. Normalization of intravascular volume

74. In a client with chest trauma, the nurse needs to evaluate mediastinal position. This can best be done by:
    A. Auscultating bilateral breath sounds
    B. Palpating for presence of crepitus
    C. Palpating for trachial deviation
    D. Auscultating heart sounds

75. Priapism may be a sign of:
    A. Altered neurological function
    B. Imminent death
    C. Urinary incontinence
    D. Reproductive dysfunction

76. When evaluating a client with symptoms of shock, it is important for the nurse to differentiate between neurogenic and hypovolemic shock. The symptoms of neurogenic shock differ from hypovolemic shock in that:
    A. In neurogenic shock, the skin is warm and dry
    B. In hypovolemic shock, there is a bradycardia

C. In hypovolemic shock, capillary refill is less than 2 seconds

D. In neurogenic shock, there is delayed capillary refill

77. Which of the following would have the physiological effect of decreasing intracranial pressure (ICP)?

A. Increased core body temperature
B. Decreased serum osmolality
C. Administration of hypo-osmolar fluids
D. Decreased $PaCO_2$

78. A client who has sustained a basilar skull fracture exhibits blood-tinged drainage from his nose. After establishing a clear airway, administering supplemental O_2, and establishing IV access, the *next* nursing intervention would be to:

A. Pass a nasogastric tube through the left nostril
B. Place a 4 × 4 gauze in the nares to impede the flow
C. Gently suction the nasal drainage to protect the airway
D. Perform a halo test and glucose level on the drainage

79. A client with a diagnosis of C-4 injury has been stabilized and is ready for discharge. Because this client is at risk for autonomic dysreflexia, he and his family should be instructed to assess for and report:

A. Dizziness and tachypnea
B. Circumoral pallor and lightheadedness
C. Headache and facial flushing
D. Pallor and itching of the face and neck

80. The initial treatment for a client with a liquid chemical burn injury is to:

A. Irrigate the area with neutralizing solutions
B. Flush the exposed area with large amounts of water
C. Inject calcium chloride into the burned area
D. Apply lanolin ointment to the area

81. The most important reason to closely assess circumferential burns at least every hour is that they may result in:

A. Hypovolemia
B. Renal damage
C. Ventricular arrhythmias
D. Loss of peripheral pulses

82. During burn therapy, morphine is primarily administered IV for pain management because this route:

A. Delays absorption to provide continuous pain relief
B. Facilitates absorption because absorption from muscles is not dependable
C. Allows for discontinuance of the medication if respiratory depression develops
D. Avoids causing additional pain from IM injections

83. The medication that *best* penetrates eschar is:

A. Mafenide acetate (Sulfamylon)
B. Silver sulfadiazine (Silvadene)
C. Neomycin sulfate (Neosporin)
D. Povidone-iodine (Betadine)

84. When the nurse is evaluating lab data for a client 18–24 hours after a major thermal burn, the expected physiological changes would include which of the following?

A. Elevated serum sodium
B. Elevated serum calcium
C. Elevated serum protein
D. Elevated hematocrit

85. The nurse notes hyperventilation in a client with a thermal injury. She recognizes that this may be a reaction to which of the following medications if applied in large amounts?

A. Neosporin sulfate
B. Mafenide acetate
C. Silver sulfadiazine
D. Povidone-iodine

86. The primary reason for sending a burn client home with a pressure garment, such as a Jobst garment, is that the garment:

A. Decreases hypertrophic scar formation
B. Assists with ambulation
C. Covers burn scars and decreases the psychological impact during recovery
D. Increases venous return and cardiac output by normalizing fluid status

87. A client with emphysema is placed on diuretics. In order to avoid potassium depletion as a side effect of the drug therapy, which of the following foods should be included in his diet?

A. Celery
B. Potatoes
C. Tomatoes
D. Liver

88. Which of the following would the nurse expect to find following respiratory assessment of a client with advanced emphysema?

A. Distant breath sounds
B. Increased heart sounds
C. Decreased anteroposterior chest diameter
D. Collapsed neck veins

89. The nurse assists a client with advanced emphysema to the bathroom. The client becomes extremely short of breath while returning to bed. The nurse should:

A. Increase his nasal O_2 to 6 L/min
B. Place him in a lateral Sims' position
C. Encourage pursed-lip breathing
D. Have him breathe into a paper bag

90. Signs and symptoms of an allergy attack include which of the following?

A. Wheezing on inspiration
B. Increased respiratory rate
C. Circumoral cyanosis
D. Prolonged expiration

91. A 55-year-old man is admitted to the hospital with complaints of fatigue, jaundice, anorexia, and clay-colored stools. His admitting diagnosis is "rule out hepatitis." Laboratory studies reveal elevated liver enzymes and bilirubin. In obtaining his health history, the nurse should assess his potential for exposure to hepatitis.

Which of the following represents a high-risk group for contracting this disease?

A. Heterosexual males
B. Oncology nurses
C. American Indians
D. Jehovah's Witnesses

92. A diagnosis of hepatitis C is confirmed by a male client's physician. The nurse should be knowledgeable of the differences between hepatitis A, B, and C. Which of the following are characteristics of hepatitis C?

A. The potential for chronic liver disease is minimal.
B. The onset of symptoms is abrupt.
C. The incubation period is 2–26 weeks.
D. There is an effective vaccine for hepatitis B, but not for hepatitis C.

93. The nurse is aware that nutrition is an important aspect of care for a client with hepatitis. Which of the following diets would be *most* therapeutic?

A. High protein and low carbohydrate
B. Low calorie and low protein
C. High carbohydrate and high calorie
D. Low carbohydrate and high calorie

94. Which of the following nursing orders should be included in the plan of care for a client with hepatitis C?

A. The nurse should use universal precautions when obtaining blood samples.
B. Total bed rest should be maintained until the client is asymptomatic.
C. The client should be instructed to maintain a low semi-Fowler position when eating meals.
D. The nurse should administer an alcohol backrub at bedtime.

95. Which of the following should be included in discharge teaching for a client with hepatitis C?

A. He should take aspirin as needed for muscle and joint pain.
B. He may become a blood donor when his liver enzymes return to normal.
C. He should avoid alcoholic beverages during his recovery period.
D. He should use disposable dishes for eating and drinking.

96. A 27-year-old man was diagnosed with type I diabetes 3 months ago. Two weeks ago he complained of pain, redness, and tenderness in his right lower leg. He is admitted to the hospital with a slight elevation of temperature and vague complaints of "not feeling well." At 4:30 PM on the day of his admission, his blood glucose level is 50 mg; dinner will be served at 5:00 PM. The best nursing action would be to:

A. Give him 3 tbsp of sugar dissolved in 4 oz of grape juice to drink
B. Ask him to dissolve three pieces of hard candy in his mouth
C. Have him drink 4 oz of orange juice
D. Monitor him closely until dinner arrives

97. A male client receives 10 U of regular human insulin SC at 9:00 AM. The nurse would expect peak action from this injection to occur at:

A. 9:30 AM
B. 10:30 AM
C. 12 noon
D. 4:00 PM

98. A type I diabetic client is diagnosed with cellulitis in his right lower extremity. The nurse would expect which of the following to be present in relation to his blood sugar level?

A. A normal blood sugar level
B. A decreased blood sugar level
C. An increased blood sugar level
D. Fluctuating levels with a predawn increase

99. The physician has ordered that a daily exercise program be instituted by a client with type I diabetes following his discharge from the hospital. Discharge instructions about exercise should include which of the following?

A. Exercise should be performed 30 minutes before meals.
B. A snack may be needed before and/or during exercise.
C. Hyperglycemia may occur 2–4 hours after exercise.
D. The blood glucose level should be 100 mg or below before exercise is begun.

100. Dietary planning is an essential part of the diabetic client's regimen. The American Diabetes Association recommends which of the following caloric guidelines for daily meal planning?

A. 50% complex carbohydrate, 20%–25% protein, 20%–25% fat
B. 45% complex carbohydrate, 25%–30% protein, 30%–35% fat
C. 70% complex carbohydrate, 20%–30% protein, 10%–20% fat
D. 60% complex carbohydrate, 12%–15% protein, 20%–25% fat

1. **(C)** Client need: health promotion and maintenance; subcategory: growth and development through the life span; content area: maternity

   RATIONALE

   (A) March 27 is a miscalculation. (B) February 1 is a miscalculation. (C) February 27 is the correct answer. To calculate the estimated date of confinement using Nägele's rule, subtract 3 months from the date that the last menstrual cycle began and then add 7 days to the result. (D) January 3 is a miscalculation.

2. **(A)** Client need: health promotion and maintenance; subcategory: growth and development through the life span; content area: maternity

   RATIONALE

   (A) Nausea and vomiting are experienced by almost half of all pregnant women during the first 3 months of pregnancy as a result of elevated human chorionic gonadotropin levels and changed carbohydrate metabolism. (B) Quickening is the mother's perception of fetal movement and generally does not occur until 18–20 weeks after the last menstrual period in primigravidas, but it may occur as early as 16 weeks in multigravidas. (C) During the first trimester there should be only a modest weight gain of 2–4 lb. It is not uncommon for women to lose weight during the first trimester owing to nausea and/or vomiting. (D) Physical changes are not apparent until the second trimester, when the uterus rises out of the pelvis.

3. **(D)** Client need: health promotion and maintenance; subcategory: prevention and early detection of disease; content area: maternity

   RATIONALE

   (A, B, C) No amount of alcohol has been determined safe for pregnant women. Alcohol should be avoided owing to the risk of fetal alcohol syndrome. (D) The recommended safe dosage of alcohol consumption during pregnancy is none.

4. **(D)** Client need: physiological integrity; subcategory: reduction of risk potential; content area: maternity

   RATIONALE

   (A) Iron-deficiency anemia can occur throughout pregnancy and is not age related. (B) STDs can occur prior to or during pregnancy and are not age related. (C) Intrauterine growth retardation is an abnormal process where fetal development and maturation are delayed. It is not age related. (D) Physical risks for the pregnant client older than 35 include increased risk for PIH, cesarean delivery, fetal and neonatal mortality, and trisomy.

5. **(B)** Client need: health promotion and maintenance; subcategory: prevention and early detection of disease; content area: maternity

   RATIONALE

   (A) She is probably not compliant with her diet and exercise program. Recommended weight gain during second and third trimesters is approximately 12 lb. (B) Because of her excessive weight gain of 10 lb in 2 months, she needs re-evaluation of her eating habits and reinforcement of proper dietary habits for pregnancy. A 2200-calorie diet is recommended for most pregnant women with a weight gain of 27–30 lb over the 9-month period. With rapid and excessive weight gain, PIH should also be suspected. (C) She does not need to increase her caloric intake, but she does need to re-evaluate dietary habits. Ten pounds in 2 months is excessive weight gain during pregnancy, and health teaching is warranted. (D) Restrictive dieting is not recommended during pregnancy.

6. **(D)** Client need: physiological integrity; subcategory: physiological adaptation; content area: maternity

   RATIONALE

   (A) There is a rise in glomerular filtration rate in the kidneys in conjunction with decreased tubular glucose reabsorption, resulting in glycosuria. (B) Insulin is inhibited by increased levels of estrogen. (C) Insulin is inhibited by increased levels of progesterone. (D) Human placental lactogen levels increase later in pregnancy. This hormonal antagonist reduces insulin's effectiveness, stimulates lipolysis, and increases the circulation of free fatty acids.

7. **(A)** Client need: physiological integrity; subcategory: reduction of risk potential; content area: maternity

   RATIONALE

   (A) The recommended range is 70–120 mg/dL to reduce the risk of perinatal mortality. (B, C, D) These levels are not recommended. The higher the blood glucose, the worse the prognosis for the fetus. Hypoglycemia can also have detrimental effects on the fetus.

8. **(D)** Client need: health promotion and maintenance; subcategory: prevention and early detection of disease; content area: maternity

   RATIONALE

   (A) This is not a normal occurrence. Late decelerations need prompt intervention for immediate infant recovery. (B) To increase O_2 perfusion to the unborn infant, the mother should be placed on her left side. (C) IV fluids should be increased, not decreased. (D) Immediate action is warranted, such as reporting findings, turning mother on left side, administering O_2, discontinuing oxytocin (Pitocin), assessing maternal blood pressure and the labor process, preparing for immediate cesarean delivery, and explaining plan of action to client.

9. **(A)** Client need: physiological integrity; subcategory: pharmacological and parenteral therapies; content area: maternity

   RATIONALE

   (A) $MgSO_4$ is classified as an anticonvulsant drug. In preeclampsia management, $MgSO_4$ is used for prevention of seizures. (B) $MgSO_4$ has been used to inhibit hyperactive labor, but results are questionable. (C) Negative side effects such as respiratory depression should not be confused with generalized sedation. (D) $MgSO_4$ does not affect lung maturity. The infant should be assessed for neuromuscular and respiratory depression.

10. **(C)** Client need: physiological integrity; subcategory: reduction of risk potential; content area: maternity

    RATIONALE

    (A) Apgar scores are not related to the infant's care, but to the infant's physical condition. (B) Apgar scores assess the current physical condition of the infant and are not related to future environmental adaptation. (C) The purpose of the Apgar system is to evaluate the physical condition of the newborn at birth and to determine if there is an immediate need for resuscitation. (D) Congenital malformations are not one of the areas assessed with Apgar scores.

11. **(A)** Client need: physiological integrity; subcategory: reduction of risk potential; content area: maternity

    RATIONALE

    (A) Seven out of a possible perfect score of 10 is correct. Two points are given for heart rate above 100; 1 point is given for slow, irregular respiratory effort; 1 point is given for some flexion of extremities in assessing muscle tone; 2 points are given for vigorous cry in assessing reflex irritability; 1 point is assessed for color when the body is pink with blue extremities (acrocyanosis). (B) For a perfect Apgar score of 10, the infant would have a heart rate over 100 but would also have a good cry, active motion, and be completely pink. (C) For an Apgar score of 8 the respiratory rate, muscle tone, or color would need to fall into the 2-point rather than the 1-point category. (D) For this infant to receive an Apgar score of 9, four of the areas evaluated would need ratings of 2 points and one area, a rating of 1 point.

12. **(B)** Client need: health promotion and maintenance; subcategory: prevention and early detection of disease; content area: maternity

RATIONALE

(A) This choice would provide more unwanted fat and sugar than protein. (B) Skim milk would add protein. Eggs are good sources of protein while low in fat and calories. (C) The benefit of protein from ice cream would be outweighed by the fat content. Chocolate syrup has caffeine, which is contraindicated or limited in pregnancy. (D) Although most animal proteins are higher in protein than plant proteins, gelatin is not. It loses protein during the processing for food consumption.

13. **(B)** Client need: psychosocial integrity; subcategory: coping and adaptation; content area: maternity

RATIONALE

(A) This answer does not hold the client accountable for her own health. (B) The nurse should explore potential reasons for the client's anxiety: are there small children at home, is the husband out of town? The nurse should aid the client in seeking support or interventions to decrease the anxiety of hospitalization. (C) Repeating the physician's reason for recommending hospitalization may not aid the client in dealing with her reasons for anxiety. (D) The concern for self and welfare of baby may be secondary to a woman who is in a crisis situation. The nurse should explore the client's potential reasons for anxiety. For example, is there another child in the home who is ill, or is there a husband who is overseas and not able to return on short notice?

14. **(D)** Client need: physiological integrity; subcategory: physiological adaptation; content area: maternity

RATIONALE

(A) Frequently the mother experiences a shaking chill immediately after delivery, which is related to a nervous response or to vasomotor changes. If not followed by a fever, it is clinically innocuous. (B) The pulse rate during the immediate postpartal period may be low but presents no cause for alarm. The body attempts to adapt to the decreased pressures intra-abdominally as well as from the reduction of blood flow to the vascular bed. (C) Urinary output increases during the early postpartal period (12–24 hours) owing to diuresis. The kidneys must eliminate an estimated 2000–3000 mL of extracellular fluid associated with a normal pregnancy. (D) A temperature of 100.4°F (38°C) may occur after delivery as a result of exertion and dehydration of labor. However, any temperature greater than 100.4°F needs further investigation to identify any infectious process.

15. **(D)** Client need: health promotion and maintenance; subcategory: prevention and early detection of disease; content area: med/surg

RATIONALE

(A) Mammograms are less effective than breast self-examination for the diagnosis of abnormalities in younger women, who have denser breast tissue. They are more effective for women older than 40. (B) Up to 15% of early-stage breast cancers are detected by physical examination; however, 95% are detected by women doing breast self-examination. (C) Ultrasound is used primarily to determine the location of cysts and to distinguish cysts from solid masses. (D) Monthly breast self-examination has been shown to be the most effective method for early detection of breast cancer. Approximately 95% of lumps are detected by women themselves.

16. **(C)** Client needs: health promotion and maintenance; subcategories: prevention and early detection of disease; content area: med/surg

RATIONALE

(A) Women who begin menarche late (after 13 years old) have a lower risk of developing breast cancer than women who have begun earlier. Average age for menarche is 12.5 years. (B) Women who have never been pregnant have an increased risk for breast cancer, but a positive family history poses an even greater risk. (C) A positive family history puts a woman at an increased risk of developing breast cancer. It is recommended that mammography screening begin 5 years before the age at which an immediate female relative was diagnosed with breast cancer. (D) Early menopause decreases the risk of developing breast cancer.

17. **(D)** Client need: physiological integrity; subcategory: reduction of risk potential; content area: med/surg

RATIONALE

(A) Diaphanography, also known as transillumination, is a painless, noninvasive imaging technique that involves shining a light source through the breast tissue to visualize the interior. It must be used in conjunction with a mammogram and physical examination. (B) Mammography is a useful tool for screening but is not considered a means of diagnosing breast cancers. (C) Thermography is a pictorial representation of heat patterns on the surface of the breast. Breast cancers appear as a "hot spot" owing to their higher metabolic rate. (D) Biopsy either by needle aspiration or by surgical incision is the primary diagnostic technique for confirming the presence of cancer cells.

18. **(B)** Client need: physiological integrity; subcategory: physiological adaptation; content area: med/surg

RATIONALE

(A) Although tumor size is a factor in classification of cancer growth, it is not an indicator of lymph node spread. (B) Axillary node status is the most important indicator for predicting how far the cancer has spread. If the lymph nodes are positive for cancer cells, the prognosis is poorer. (C) The client's previous history of cancer puts her at an increased risk for breast cancer recurrence, especially if the cancer occurred in the other breast. It does not predict prognosis, however. (D) The estrogen-progesterone assay test is used to identify present tumors being fed from an estrogen site within the body. Some breast cancers grow rapidly as long as there is an estrogen supply such as from the ovaries. The estrogen-progesterone assay test does not indicate the prognosis.

19. **(A)** Client need: health promotion and maintenance; subcategory: prevention and early detection of disease; content area: med/surg

RATIONALE

(A) *Chlamydia trachomatis* infection is the most common STD in the United States. The Centers for Disease Control and Prevention recommend screening of all high-risk women, such as adolescents and women with multiple sex partners. (B) Herpes simplex genitalia is estimated to be found in 5–20 million people in the United States and is rising in occurrence yearly. (C) Syphilis is a chronic infection caused by *Treponema pallidum*. Over the last several years the number of people infected has begun to increase. (D) Gonorrhea is a bacterial infection caused by the organism *Neisseria gonorrhoeae*. Although gonorrhea is common, chlamydia is still the most common STD.

20. **(C)** Client need: psychosocial integrity; subcategory: psychosocial adaptation; content area: psychiatric

    RATIONALE

    (A) During the manic phase of bipolar disorder, clients have short attention spans and may be abusive toward authority figures. (B) Introspection requires focusing and concentration; clients with mania experience flight of ideas, which prevents concentration. (C) Grandiosity and an inflated sense of self-worth are characteristic of this disorder. (D) Feelings of helplessness and hopelessness are symptoms of the depressive stage of bipolar disorder.

21. **(B)** Client need: physiological integrity; subcategory: reduction of risk potential; content area: psychiatric

    RATIONALE

    (A) This range is too low to be therapeutic. (B) This is the therapeutic range for lithium. (C) This range is above the therapeutic level. (D) This range is toxic and may cause severe side effects.

22. **(C)** Client need: physiological integrity; subcategory: reduction of risk potential; content area: psychiatric

    RATIONALE

    (A) These symptoms are indicative of lithium toxicity. A stat dose of lithium could be fatal. (B) These are toxic effects of lithium therapy. (C) The client is exhibiting symptoms of lithium toxicity, which may be validated by lab studies. (D) There is no known lithium antidote.

23. **(C)** Client need: psychosocial integrity; subcategory: coping and adaptation; content area: psychiatric

    RATIONALE

    (A) This activity is too competitive, and the manic client might become abusive toward the other clients. (B) During mania, the client's attention span is too short to accomplish this task. (C) This activity uses gross motor skills, eases tension, and expands excess energy. A staff member is better equipped to interact therapeutically with clients. (D) This activity requires the use of fine motor skills and is very tedious.

24. **(A)** Client need: health promotion and maintenance; subcategory: prevention and early detection of disease; content area: psychiatric

    RATIONALE

    (A) The manic client is unable to sit still long enough to eat an adequate meal. Small, frequent feedings with finger foods allow him to eat during periods of activity. (B) This type of therapy should be implemented when other methods have been exhausted. (C) The manic client should not be in control of his treatment plan. This type of client may forget to eat. (D) The manic client is unable to sit down to eat full meals.

25. **(D)** Client need: psychosocial integrity; subcategory: coping and adaptation; content area: psychiatric

    RATIONALE

    (A) This response does not acknowledge the client's feelings. (B) This is a closed question and does not encourage communication. (C) This response negates the client's feelings and does not require a response from the client. (D) This acknowledges the client's implied thoughts and feelings and encourages a response.

26. **(A)** Client need: psychosocial integrity; subcategory: coping and adaptation; content area: psychiatric

    RATIONALE

    (A) This is a high-risk factor for potential suicide. (B) A previous suicide attempt is a definite risk factor for subsequent attempts. (C) Every threat of suicide should be taken seriously. (D) The client should be asked directly about his or her intent to do bodily harm. The client is never hurt by direct, respectful questions.

27. **(B)** Client need: physiological integrity; subcategory: reduction of risk potential; content area: psychiatric

    RATIONALE

    (A) Fluoxetine is not a tricyclic antidepressant. It is an atypical antidepressant. (B) This statement is true. (C) These foods are high in tyramine and should be avoided when the client is taking MAO inhibitors. Fluoxetine is not an MAO inhibitor. (D) Fatal reactions have been reported in clients receiving fluoxetine in combination with MAO inhibitors.

28. **(C)** Client need: psychosocial integrity; subcategory: coping and adaptation; content area: psychiatric

    RATIONALE

    (A) This response does not acknowledge the client's feelings and may increase his feelings of guilt. (B) This response denotes false reassurance. (C) This response acknowledges the client's feelings and invites a response. (D) This response changes the subject and does not allow the client to talk about his feelings.

29. **(B)** Client need: psychosocial integrity; subcategory: psychosocial adaptation; content area: psychiatric

    RATIONALE

    (A) This statement represents a short-term goal. (B) Long-term therapy should be directed toward assisting the client to cope effectively with stress. (C) Suicide contracts represent short-term interventions. (D) This statement represents an unrealistic goal. Stressful situations cannot be avoided in reality.

30. **(A)** Client need: psychosocial integrity; subcategory: psychosocial adaptation; content area: psychiatric

    RATIONALE

    (A) When the severely depressed client suddenly begins to feel better, it often indicates that the client has made the decision to kill himself or herself and has developed a plan to do so. (B) Improvement in behavior is not indicative of an exacerbation of depressive symptoms. (C) The depressed client has a tendency for self-violence, not violence toward others. (D) Depressive behavior is not always accompanied by psychotic behavior.

31. **(A)** Client need: psychosocial integrity; subcategory: psychosocial adaptation; content area: psychiatric

    RATIONALE

    (A) These clients are at high risk for seizures during the 1st week after cessation of alcohol intake. (B) Fluid intake should be increased to prevent dehydration. (C) Environmental stimuli should be decreased to prevent precipitation of seizures. (D) Application of restraints may cause the client to increase his or her physical activity and may eventually lead to exhaustion.

32. **(B)** Client need: psychosocial integrity; subcategory: psychosocial adaptation; content area: psychiatric

    RATIONALE

    (A) These delusions are related to the belief that an individual has an incurable illness. (B) These delusions are related to feelings of self-importance and uniqueness. (C) These delusions are related to feelings of being conspired against. (D) These delusions are related to denial of self-existence.

33. **(B)** Client need: psychosocial integrity; subcategory: psychosocial adaptation; content area: psychiatric

    RATIONALE

    (A) Auditory hallucinations involve sensory perceptions of hearing. (B) Gustatory hallucinations involve sensory perceptions of taste. (C) Olfactory hallucinations involve sensory perceptions of smell. (D) Visceral hallucinations involve sensory perceptions of sensation.

34. **(B)** Client need: psychosocial integrity; subcategory: coping and adaptation; content area: psychiatric

RATIONALE

(A) Displacement involves transferring feelings to a more acceptable object. (B) Projection involves attributing one's thoughts or feelings to another person. (C) Reaction formation involves transforming an unacceptable impulse into the opposite behavior. (D) Suppression involves the intentional exclusion of unpleasant thoughts or experiences.

35. **(B)** Client need: physiological integrity; subcategory: physiological adaptation; content area: pediatrics

RATIONALE

(A) The kidney can survive after 30 minutes of water submersion. (B) The cerebral neurons sustain irreversible damage after 4–6 minutes of water submersion. (C) The heart can survive up to 30 minutes of water submersion. (D) The lungs can survive up to 30 minutes of water submersion.

36. **(A)** Client need: physiological integrity; subcategory: physiological adaptation; content area: pediatrics

RATIONALE

(A) Waterhouse-Friderichsen syndrome is peripheral circulatory collapse, which may result in extensive and diffuse intravascular coagulation and thrombocytopenia resulting in death. (B) Syndrome of inappropriate antidiuretic hormone is a complication of meningitis, but it is not Waterhouse-Friderichsen syndrome. (C) Cerebral edema resulting in hydrocephalus is a complication of meningitis, but it is not Waterhouse-Friderichsen syndrome. (D) Auditory nerve damage resulting in permanent hearing loss is a complication of meningitis, but it is not Waterhouse-Friderichsen syndrome.

37. **(D)** Client need: physiological integrity; subcategory: physiological adaptation; content area: pediatrics

RATIONALE

(A) Urinary tract symptoms are not commonly associated with Lyme disease. (B) A fever of 103°F is not characteristic of Lyme disease. (C) The rash that is associated with Lyme disease does not appear on the palms of the hands and the soles of the feet. (D) Classic symptoms of Lyme disease include headache, malaise, fatigue, anorexia, stiff neck, generalized lymphadenopathy, splenomegaly, conjunctivitis, sore throat, abdominal pain, and cough.

38. **(C)** Client need: physiological integrity; subcategory: physiological adaptation; content area: pediatrics

RATIONALE

(A) Mites are not the common vector of Lyme disease. (B) Fleas are not the common vector of Lyme disease. (C) Ticks are the common vector of Lyme disease. (D) Mosquitoes are not the common vector of Lyme disease.

39. **(A)** Client need: physiological integrity; subcategory: reduction of risk potential; content area: pediatrics

RATIONALE

(A) Polymerase chain reaction is the laboratory technique specific for Lyme disease. (B) Heterophil antibody test is used to diagnose mononucleosis. (C) Lyme disease does not decrease the serum calcium level. (D) Lyme disease does not increase the serum potassium level.

40. **(B)** Client need: physiological integrity; subcategory: basic care and comfort; content area: pediatrics

RATIONALE

(A) The client is not placed on complete bed rest for 6 weeks. (B) Tetracycline is the treatment of choice for children with Lyme disease who are over the age of 9. (C) IV amphotericin B is the treatment for histoplasmosis. (D) The client is not restricted to a high-protein diet with limited fluids.

41. **(C)** Client need: physiological integrity; subcategory: reduction of risk potential; content area: pediatrics

RATIONALE

(A) Blood pressure can remain normotensive even in a state of hypovolemia. (B) Serum potassium is not reliable for determining adequacy of fluid resuscitation. (C) Urine output, alteration in sensorium, and capillary refill are the most reliable indicators for assessing adequacy of fluid resuscitation. (D) Pulse rate may vary for many reasons and is not a reliable indicator for assessing adequacy of fluid resuscitation.

42. **(A)** Client need: physiological integrity; subcategory: reduction of risk potential; content area: pediatrics

RATIONALE

(A) The child's weight supplies the countertraction for Bryant's traction; the buttocks are slightly elevated off the bed, and the hips are flexed at a 90-degree angle. Both legs are suspended by skin traction. (B) The child in Buck's extension traction maintains the legs extended and parallel to the bed. (C) The child in Russell traction maintains hip flexion of the affected leg at the prescribed angle with the leg extended. (D) The child in "90–90" traction maintains both hips and knees at a 90-degree flexion angle and the back is flat on the bed.

43. **(C)** Client need: physiological integrity; subcategory: physiological adaptation; content area: pediatrics

RATIONALE

(A) Bleeding, bruising, and hemorrhage may occur due to injury but are not classic signs of ischemia. (B) An increase in serum levels of creatinine, alkaline phosphatase, and aspartate transaminase is related to the disruption of muscle integrity. (C) Classic signs of ischemia related to vascular injury secondary to long bone fractures include the five "P's": pain, pallor, pulselessness, paresthesia, and paralysis. (D) Generalized swelling, pain, and diminished functional use with muscle rigidity and crepitus are common clinical manifestations of a fracture but not ischemia.

44. **(A)** Client need: physiological integrity; subcategory: reduction of risk potential; content area: pediatrics

RATIONALE

(A) Stephens-Johnson syndrome is a toxic effect of phenytoin. (B) Folate deficiency is a side effect of phenytoin, but not a toxic effect. (C) Leukopenic aplastic anemia is a toxic effect of carbamazepine (Tegretol). (D) Granulocytosis and nephrosis are toxic effects of trimethadione (Tridione).

45. **(C)** Client need: physiological integrity; subcategory: physiological adaptation; content area: pediatrics

RATIONALE

(A) The temperature elevation related to febrile seizures generally exceeds 101°F, and seizures occur during the temperature rise rather than after a prolonged elevation. (B) Febrile seizures may recur and are more likely to do so when the first seizure occurs in the 1st year of life. (C) There is little risk of neurological deficit, mental retardation, or altered behavior secondary to febrile seizures. (D) Febrile seizures are associated with disease of the central nervous system.

46. **(B)** Client need: physiological integrity; subcategory: physiological adaptation; content area: pediatrics

RATIONALE

(A) Anemia and vomiting are not cardinal signs of diabetes insipidus. (B) Polyuria and polydipsia are the cardinal signs of diabetes insipidus. (C) Irritability relieved by feeding water, not formula, is a common sign, but not the cardinal sign, of diabetes insipidus. (D) Hypothermia and azotemia are signs, but not cardinal signs, of diabetes insipidus.

47. **(D)** Client need: physiological integrity; subcategory: physiological adaptation; content area: pediatrics

    RATIONALE

    (A) Weight should be obtained daily. (B) Fluid is not restricted but is given according to urine output. (C) The medication does not have to be stored in a refrigerator. (D) Holding the vial under warm water for 10–15 minutes or rolling between your hands and shaking vigorously before drawing medication into the syringe activates the medication in the oil solution.

48. **(B)** Client need: physiological integrity; subcategory: physiological adaptation; content area: pediatrics

    RATIONALE

    (A) A rash with vesicular scabs in all stages (macule, papule, vesicle, and crusts). (B) A rash that appears profusely on the trunk and sparsely on the extremities. (C) A rash that first appears on the neck and spreads downward is characteristic of rubeola and rubella. (D) A rash, especially on the cheeks, that gives a "slapped-cheek" appearance is characteristic of roseola.

49. **(D)** Client need: physiological integrity; subcategory: basic care and comfort; content area: pediatrics

    RATIONALE

    (A) Maintaining a low-humidified environment. (B) Avoiding furry, soft stuffed animals for play, which may increase symptoms of allergy. (C) Avoiding showering, which irritates the dermatitis, and encouraging bathing 4 times a day in colloid bath for temporary relief. (D) Wrapping hands in soft cotton gloves to prevent skin damage during scratching.

50. **(A)** Client need: psychosocial integrity; subcategory: coping and adaptation; content area: pediatrics

    RATIONALE

    (A) The priority nursing goal when working with an autistic child is establishing a trusting relationship. (B) Maintaining a relationship with the family is important but having the trust of the child is a priority. (C) To promote involvement in school activities is inappropriate for a child who is autistic. (D) Maintaining nutritional requirements is not the primary problem of the autistic child.

51. **(B)** Client need: physiological integrity; subcategory: reduction of risk potential; content area: pediatrics

    RATIONALE

    (A) The IV line should not be discontinued because other IV medications will be needed. (B) Stop the medication and begin a normal saline infusion. The child is exhibiting signs of an allergic reaction and could go into shock if the medication is not stopped. The line should be kept opened for other medication. (C) Taking vital signs and reporting to the physician is not an adequate intervention because the IV medication continues to flow. (D) Assessing urinary output and, if it is 30 mL an hour, maintaining current treatment is an inappropriate intervention owing to the child's obvious allergic reaction.

52. **(C)** Client need: physiological integrity; subcategory: physiological adaptation; content area: pediatrics

    RATIONALE

    (A) An enlarged penis is not a sign of chlamydia. (B) Secondary lymphadenitis is a complication of lymphogranuloma venereum. (C) Untreated chlamydial infection can spread from the urethra, causing epididymitis, which presents as a tender, scrotal swelling. (D) Hepatomegaly is not a complication.

53. **(C)** Client need: physiological integrity; subcategory: reduction of risk potential; content area: pediatrics

    RATIONALE

    (A) Diluted fruit juices are not recommended for rehydration because they tend to aggravate the diarrhea. (B) Diluted soft drinks have a high-carbohydrate content, which aggravates the diarrhea. (C) Soy-based, lactose-free formula reduces stool output and duration of diarrhea in most infants. (D) Regular formulas contain lactose, which can increase diarrhea.

54. **(D)** Client need: physiological integrity; subcategory: physiological adaptation; content area: med/surg

    RATIONALE

    (A) Decreased stroke volume and blood pressure will occur secondary to decreased diastolic filling. (B) Tachycardia primarily decreases diastole; systolic time changes very little. (C) Contractility decreases owing to the decreased filling time and decreased time for fiber lengthening. (D) Decreased O_2 supply due to decreased time for filling of the coronary arteries increases ischemia and infarct size. Tachycardia primarily robs the heart of diastolic time, which is the primary time for coronary artery filling.

55. **(A)** Client need: physiological integrity; subcategory: physiological adaptation; content area: med/surg

    RATIONALE

    (A) Inotropic therapy will increase contractility, which will increase myocardial O_2 demand. (B) Decreased heart rate to the point of bradycardia will increase coronary artery filling time. This should be used cautiously because tachycardia may be a compensatory mechanism to increase cardiac output. (C) The goal in the care of the MI client with angina is to maintain a balance between myocardial O_2 supply and demand. (D) Decrease in systemic vascular resistance by drug therapy, such as IV nitroglycerin or nitroprusside, or intra-aortic balloon pump therapy, would decrease myocardial work and O_2 demand.

56. **(D)** Client need: physiological integrity; subcategory: reduction of risk potential; content area: med/surg

    RATIONALE

    (A) Norepinephrine's side effects are primarily related to safe, effective care environment and include decreased peripheral perfusion and bradycardia. (B) Dobutamine's side effects include increased heart rate and blood pressure, ventricular ectopy, nausea, and headache. (C) Propranolol's side effects include elevated blood urea nitrogen, serum transaminase, alkaline phosphatase, and lactic dehydrogenase. (D) Epinephrine increases serum glucose levels by increasing glycogenolysis and inhibiting insulin release. Prolonged use can elevate serum lactate levels, leading to metabolic acidosis, increased urinary catecholamines, false elevation of blood urea nitrogen, and decreased coagulation time.

57. **(D)** Client need: physiological integrity; subcategory: reduction of risk potential; content area: med/surg

    RATIONALE

    (A) Verapamil has the respiratory side effect of nasal or chest congestion, dyspnea, shortness of breath (SOB), and wheezing. (B) Amrinone has the effect of increased contractility and dilation of the vascular smooth muscle. It has no noted respiratory side effects. (C) Epinephrine has the effect of bronchodilation through β stimulation. (D) Propranolol, esmolol, and labetalol are all β-blocking agents, which can increase airway resistance and cause bronchospasms.

58. **(C)** Client need: physiological integrity; subcategory: reduction of risk potential; content area: med/surg

    RATIONALE

    (A) Hypokalemia can cause digoxin toxicity. Administration of KCl would prevent this. (B) Thyroid agents decrease digoxin levels. (C) Quinidine increases digoxin levels dramatically. (D) Theophylline is not noted to have an effect on digoxin levels.

59. **(A)** Client need: physiological integrity; subcategory: physiological adaptation; content area: med/surg

RATIONALE

(A) Sinus bradycardia and atrioventricular (AV) heart block are usually a result of right coronary artery occlusion. The right coronary artery perfuses the sinoatrial and AV nodes in most individuals. (B) Occlusion of the left main coronary artery causes bundle branch blocks and premature ventricular contractions. (C) Occlusion of the circumflex artery does not cause bradycardia. (D) Sinus tachycardia occurs primarily with left anterior descending coronary artery occlusion because this form of occlusion impairs left ventricular function.

60. **(C)** Client need: physiological integrity; subcategory: physiological adaptation; content area: med/surg

RATIONALE

(A) Pericarditis can cause dyspnea but primarily causes chest pain. (B) Anxiety can cause dyspnea resulting in SOB, yet it is not typically influenced by degree of head elevation. (C) The inability to oxygenate well without being upright is most indicative of congestive heart failure, due to alveolar drowning. (D) Angina causes primarily chest pain; any SOB associated with angina is not influenced by body position.

61. **(D)** Client need: physiological integrity; subcategory: physiological adaptation; content area: med/surg

RATIONALE

(A) The purpose of the study is not to provide a baseline for further tests. (B) The test causes an increase in O_2 demand beyond that required to perform usual daily activities. (C) Monitoring does occur, but the test is not for the purpose of cardiac toning and conditioning. (D) Exercise ECG, or stress testing, is designed to elevate the peripheral and myocardial needs for O_2 to evaluate the ability of the myocardium and coronary arteries to meet the additional demands.

62. **(D)** Client need: physiological integrity; subcategory: physiological adaptation; content area: med/surg

RATIONALE

(A) These signs are seen in pulmonic stenosis or in response to pulmonary congestion and edema and mitral stenosis. (B) These signs are seen primarily in mitral stenosis or as a late sign in aortic stenosis after left ventricular failure. (C) These signs are seen primarily in right-sided heart valve dysfunction. (D) Left ventricular hypertrophy occurs to increase muscle mass and overcome the stenosis; left ventricular pressures increase as left ventricular volume increases owing to insufficient emptying.

63. **(B)** Client need: physiological integrity; subcategory: physiological adaptation; content area: med/surg

RATIONALE

(A) Side effects of digoxin include headache, hypotension, AV block, blurred vision, and yellow-green halos. (B) Side effects of lidocaine include heart block, headache, dizziness, confusion, tremor, lethargy, and convulsions. (C) Side effects of quinidine include heart block, hepatotoxicity, thrombocytopenia, and respiratory depression. (D) Side effects of nitroglycerin include postural hypotension, headache, dizziness, and flushing.

64. **(C)** Client need: physiological integrity; subcategory: physiological adaptation; content area: med/surg

RATIONALE

(A) Hyperacute T waves occur with hyperkalemia. (B) Prolongation of the P R interval occurs with first-degree AV block. (C) Horizontal ST-segment depression of ≥ 1 mm during exercise is definitely a positive criterion on the exercise ECG test. (D) Pathological Q waves occur with MI.

65. **(C)** Client need: physiological integrity; subcategory: physiological adaptation; content area: med/surg

RATIONALE

(A) No S_3 or S_4 are noted with pericarditis. (B) No change in pulse pressure occurs. (C) The symptoms of pericarditis vary with the cause, but they usually include chest pain, dyspnea, tachycardia, rise in temperature, and friction rub caused by fibrin or other deposits. The pain seen with pericarditis typically worsens with deep inspiration. (D) Tamponade is not typically seen early on, and no change in pulse pressure occurs.

66. **(D)** Client need: physiological integrity; subcategory: physiological adaptation; content area: med/surg

RATIONALE

(A, B, C) Clinical manifestations of right-sided heart failure are weakness, peripheral edema, jugular venous distention, hepatomegaly, jaundice, and elevated central venous pressure. (D) Clinical manifestations of left-sided heart failure are left ventricular dysfunction, decreased cardiac output, hypotension, and the backward failure as a result of increased left atrium and pulmonary artery pressures, pulmonary edema, and rales.

67. **(A)** Client need: physiological integrity; subcategory: reduction of risk potential; content area: med/surg

RATIONALE

(A) Positive inotropic agents should not be administered owing to their action of increasing myocardial contractility. Increased ventricular contractility would increase outflow tract obstruction in the client with hypertrophic cardiomyopathy. (B) Vasodilators are not typically prescribed but are not contraindicated. (C) Diuretics are used with caution to avoid causing hypovolemia. (D) Antidysrhythmics are typically needed to treat both atrial and ventricular dysrhythmias.

68. **(A)** Client need: physiological integrity; subcategory: reduction of risk potential; content area: med/surg

RATIONALE

(A) Stinging or burning when nitroglycerin is placed under the tongue is to be expected. This effect indicates that the medication is potent and effective for use. Failure to have this response means that the client needs to get a new bottle of nitroglycerin. (B, C, D) The other responses are not expected in this situation and are not even side effects.

69. **(A)** Client need: physiological integrity; subcategory: pharmacological and parenteral therapies; content area: med/surg

RATIONALE

(A) Phentolamine is given to counteract the α-adrenergic effects that cause ischemia and necrosis of local tissue. (B) Epinephrine is an endogenous catecholamine that produces vasoconstriction and increases heart rate and contractility. (C) Phenylephrine causes constriction of arterioles of skin, mucous membranes, and viscera, which in turn can cause ischemia and necrosis. (D) Sodium bicarbonate is an alkalinizing agent that is incompatible with dopamine.

70. **(C)** Client need: physiological integrity; subcategory: physiological adaptation; content area: med/surg

RATIONALE

(A) Increased CO_2 will occur in both acute and chronic respiratory acidosis. (B) Hypoxia does not determine acid-base status. (C) Elevation of HCO_3 is a compensatory mechanism in acidosis that occurs almost immediately, but it takes hours to show any effect and days to reach maximum compensation. Renal disease and diuretic therapy may impair the ability of the kidneys to compensate. (D) Base excess is a nonrespiratory contributor to acid-base balance. It would increase to compensate for acidosis.

71. **(C)** Client need: physiological integrity; subcategory: physiological adaptation; content area: med/surg

RATIONALE

(A, B, D) These occur in both tension pneumothorax and open pneumothorax. (C) The tension pneumothorax acts like a one-way valve so that the pneumothorax increases with each breath. Eventually, it occupies enough space to shift mediastinal tissue toward the unaffected side away from the midline. Tracheal deviation, movement of point of maximum impulse, and decreased cardiac output will occur. The other three options will occur in both types of pneumothorax.

72. **(A)** Client need: physiological integrity; subcategory: physiological adaptation; content area: med/surg

    RATIONALE

    (A) Basilar skull fractures are fractures of the base of the skull. Blood behind the eardrum or blood or cerebrospinal fluid (CSF) leaking from the ear are indicative of a dural laceration. Basilar skull fractures are the only type with these symptoms. (B, C, D) These do not typically cause dural lacerations and CSF leakage.

73. **(B)** Client need: physiological integrity; subcategory: physiological adaptation; content area: med/surg

    RATIONALE

    (A) If cervical spine injury is suspected, the airway should be maintained using the jaw thrust method that also protects the cervical spine. (B) Primary intervention is protection of the airway and adequate ventilation. (C, D) All other interventions are secondary to adequate ventilation.

74. **(C)** Client need: physiological integrity; subcategory: physiological adaptation; content area: med/surg

    RATIONALE

    (A) No change in the breath sounds occurs as a direct result of the mediastinal shift. (B) Crepitus can occur owing to the primary disorder, not to the mediastinal shift. (C) Mediastinal shift occurs primarily with tension pneumothorax, but it can occur with very large hemothorax or pneumothorax. Mediastinal shift causes trachial deviation and deviation of the heart's point of maximum impulse. (D) No change in the heart sounds occurs as a result of the mediastinal shift.

75. **(A)** Client need: physiological integrity; subcategory: physiological adaptation; content area: med/surg

    RATIONALE

    (A) Priapism in the trauma client is due to the neurological dysfunction seen in spinal cord injury. Priapism is an abnormal erection of the penis; it may be accompanied by pain and tenderness. This may disappear as spinal cord edema is relieved. (B) Priapism is not associated with death. (C) Urinary retention, rather than incontinence, may occur. (D) Reproductive dysfunction may be a secondary problem.

76. **(A)** Client need: physiological integrity; subcategory: physiological adaptation; content area: med/surg

    RATIONALE

    (A) Neurogenic shock is caused by injury to the cervical region, which leads to loss of sympathetic control. This loss leads to vasodilation of the vascular beds, bradycardia resulting from the lack of sympathetic balance to parasympathetic stimuli from the vagus nerve, and the loss of the ability to sweat below the level of injury. In neurogenic shock, the client is hypotensive but bradycardic with warm, dry skin. (B) In hypovolemic shock, the client is hypotensive and tachycardic with cool skin. (C) In hypovolemic shock, the capillary refill would be ≥ 5 seconds. (D) In neurogenic shock, there is no capillary delay, the vascular beds are dilated, and peripheral flow is good.

77. **(D)** Client need: physiological integrity; subcategory: physiological adaptation; content area: med/surg

    RATIONALE

    (A) An increase in core body temperature increases metabolism and results in an increase in ICP. (B) Decreased serum osmolality indicates a fluid overload and may result in an increase in ICP.

(C) Hypo-osmolar fluids are generally voided in the neurologically compromised. Using IV fluids such as D_5W results in the dextrose being metabolized, releasing free water that is absorbed by the brain cells, leading to cerebral edema. (D) Hypercapnia and hypoventilation, which cause retention of CO_2 and lead to respiratory acidosis, both increase ICP. CO_2 is the most potent vasodilator known.

78. **(D)** Client need: physiological integrity; subcategory: physiological adaptation; content area: med/surg

    RATIONALE

    (A) Basilar skull fracture may cause dural lacerations, which result in CSF leaking from the ears or nose. Insertion of a tube could lead to CSF going into the brain tissue or sinuses. (B) Tamponading flow could worsen the problem and increase ICP. (C) Suction could increase brain damage and dislocate tissue. (D) Testing the fluid from the nares would determine the presence of CSF. Elevation of the head, notification of the medical staff, and prophylactic antibiotics are appropriate therapy.

79. **(C)** Client need: physiological integrity; subcategory: physiological adaptation; content area: med/surg

    RATIONALE

    (A) Tachypnea is not a symptom. (B) Circumoral pallor is not a symptom. (C) Autonomic dysreflexia is an uninhibited and exaggerated reflex of the autonomic nervous system to stimulation, which results in vasoconstriction and elevated blood pressure. (D) Pallor and itching are not symptoms.

80. **(B)** Client need: physiological integrity; subcategory: physiological adaptation; content area: med/surg

    RATIONALE

    (A) In the past, neutralizing solutions were recommended, but presently there is concern that these solutions extend the depth of burn area. (B) The use of large amounts of water to flush the area is recommended for chemical burns. (C) Calcium chloride is not recommended therapy and would likely worsen the problem. (D) Lanolin is of no benefit in the initial treatment of a chemical injury and may actually extend a thermal injury.

81. **(D)** Client need: physiological integrity; subcategory: physiological adaptation; content area: med/surg

    RATIONALE

    (A) Hypovolemia could be a result of fluid loss from thermal injury, but not as a result of the circumferential injury. (B) Renal damage is typically seen because of prolonged hypovolemia or myoglobinuria. (C) Electrical injuries and electrolyte changes typically cause arrhythmias in the burn client. (D) Full-thickness circumferential burns are nonelastic and result in an internal tourniquet effect that compromises distal blood flow when the area involved is an extremity. Circumferential full-thickness torso burns compromise respiratory motion and, when extreme, cardiac return.

82. **(B)** Client need: physiological integrity; subcategory: pharmacological and parenteral therapies; content area: med/surg

    RATIONALE

    (A) Absorption would be increased, not decreased. (B) IM injections should not be used until the client is hemodynamically stable and has adequate tissue perfusion. Medications will remain in the subcutaneous tissue with the fluid that is present in the interstitial spaces in the acute phase of the thermal injury. The client will have a poor response to the medication administered, and a "dumping" of the medication can occur when the medication and fluid are shifted back into the intravascular spaces in the next phase of healing. (C) IV administration of the medication would hasten respiratory compromise, if present. (D) The desire to avoid causing the client additional pain is not a primary reason for this route of administration.

83. **(A)** Client need: physiological integrity; subcategory: physiological adaptation; content area: med/surg

    RATIONALE

    (A) Mafenide acetate is bacteriostatic against gram-positive and gram-negative organisms and is the agent that best penetrates eschar. (B) Silver sulfadiazine poorly penetrates eschar. (C) Neomycin sulfate does not penetrate eschar. (D) Povidone-iodine does not penetrate eschar.

84. **(D)** Client need: physiological integrity; subcategory: physiological adaptation; content area: med/surg

    RATIONALE

    (A) Sodium enters the edema fluid in the burned area, lowering the sodium content of the vascular fluid. Hyponatremia may continue for days to several weeks because of sodium loss to edema, sodium shifting into the cells, and later, diuresis. (B) Hypocalcemia occurs because of calcium loss to edema fluid at the burned site (third space fluid). (C) Protein loss occurs at the burn site owing to increased capillary permeability. Serum protein levels remain low until healing occurs. (D) Hematocrit level is elevated owing to hemoconcentration from hypovolemia. Anemia is present in the postburn stage owing to blood loss and hemolysis, but it cannot be assessed until the client is adequately hydrated.

85. **(B)** Client need: physiological integrity; subcategory: physiological adaptation; content area: med/surg

    RATIONALE

    (A) The side effects of neomycin sulfate include rash, urticaria, nephrotoxicity, and ototoxicity. (B) The side effects of mafenide acetate include bone marrow suppression, hemolytic anemia, eosinophilia, and metabolic acidosis. The hyperventilation is a compensatory response to the metabolic acidosis. (C) The side effects of silver sulfadiazine include rash, itching, leukopenia, and decreased renal function. (D) The primary side effect of povidone-iodine is decreased renal function.

86. **(A)** Client need: physiological integrity; subcategory: reduction of risk potential; content area: med/surg

    RATIONALE

    (A) Tubular support, such as that received with a Jobst garment, applies tension of 10–20 mm Hg. This amount of uniform pressure is necessary to prevent or reduce hypertrophic scarring. Clients typically wear a pressure garment for 6–12 months during the recovery phase of their care. (B) Pressure garments have no ambulatory assistive properties. (C) Pressure garments can worsen the psychological impact of burn injury, especially if worn on the face. (D) Pressure garments do not normalize fluid status.

87. **(B)** Client need: physiological integrity; subcategory: physiological adaptation; content area: med/surg

    RATIONALE

    (A) Celery is high in sodium. (B) Potatoes are high in potassium. (C) Tomatoes are high in sodium. (D) Liver is high in iron.

88. **(A)** Client need: physiological integrity; subcategory: physiological adaptation; content area: med/surg

    RATIONALE

    (A) Distant breath sounds are found in clients with emphysema owing to increased anteroposterior chest diameter, overdistention, and air trapping. (B) Deceased heart sounds are present because of the increased anteroposterior chest diameter. (C) A barrel-shaped chest is characteristic of emphysema. (D) Increased distention of neck veins is found owing to right-sided heart failure, which may be present in advanced emphysema.

89. **(C)** Client need: physiological integrity; subcategory: physiological adaptation; content area: med/surg

    RATIONALE

    (A) Giving too high a concentration of O_2 to a client with emphysema may remove his stimulus to breathe. (B) The client should sit forward with his hands on his knees or an overbed table and with shoulders elevated. (C) Pursed-lip breathing helps the client to blow off CO_2 and to keep air passages open. (D) Covering the face of a client extremely short of breath may cause anxiety and further increase dyspnea.

90. **(D)** Client need: physiological integrity; subcategory: physiological adaptation; content area: med/surg

    RATIONALE

    (A) Wheezing occurs during expiration when air movement is impaired because of constricted edematous bronchial lumina. (B) Respirations are difficult, but the rate is frequently normal. (C) The circumoral area is usually pale. Cyanosis is not an early sign of hypoxia. (D) Expiration is prolonged because the alveoli are greatly distended and air trapping occurs.

91. **(B)** Client need: health promotion and maintenance; subcategory: prevention and early detection of disease; content area: med/surg

    RATIONALE

    (A) Homosexual males, not heterosexual males, are at high risk for contracting hepatitis. (B) Oncology nurses are employed in high-risk areas and perform invasive procedures that expose them to potential sources of infection. (C) The literature does not support the idea that any ethnic groups are at higher risk. (D) There is no evidence that any religious groups are at higher risk.

92. **(C)** Client need: physiological integrity; subcategory: physiological adaptation; content area: med/surg

    RATIONALE

    (A) Hepatitis C and B may result in chronic liver disease. Hepatitis A has a low potential for chronic liver disease. (B) Hepatitis C and B have insidious onsets. Hepatitis A has an abrupt onset. (C) Incubation periods are as follows: hepatitis C is 2–26 weeks, hepatitis B is 6–20 weeks, and hepatitis A is 2–6 weeks. (D) Only hepatitis B has an effective vaccine.

93. **(C)** Client need: physiological integrity; subcategory: basic care and comfort; content area: med/surg

    RATIONALE

    (A) Protein increases the workload of the liver. Increased carbohydrates provide needed calories and promote palatability. (B) Dietary intake should be adequate to ensure wound healing. (C) Increased carbohydrates provide needed calories. (D) A high-calorie diet is best obtained from carbohydrates because of their palatability. Fats increase the workload of the liver.

94. **(A)** Client need: physiological integrity; subcategory: physiological adaptation; content area: med/surg

    RATIONALE

    (A) The source of infection with hepatitis C is contaminated blood products. (B) Modified bed rest should be maintained while the client is symptomatic. Routine activities can be slowly resumed once the client is asymptomatic. (C) Nausea and vomiting occur frequently with hepatitis C. A high Fowler position may decrease the tendency to vomit. (D) The buildup of bilirubin in the client's skin may cause pruritus. Alcohol is a drying agent.

95. **(C)** Client need: physiological integrity; subcategory: reduction of risk potential; content area: med/surg

    RATIONALE

    (A) Aspirin is hepatotoxic, may increase bleeding, and should be avoided. (B) Blood should not be donated by a client who has had hepatitis C because of the possibility of transmission of disease. (C) Alcohol is detoxified in the liver. (D) Hepatitis C is not spread through the oral route.

96. **(C)** Client need: physiological integrity; subcategory: physiological adaptation; content area: med/surg

RATIONALE

(A) The combination of sugar and juice will increase the blood sugar beyond the normal range. (B) Concentrated sweets are not absorbed as fast as juice; consequently, they elevate the blood sugar beyond the normal limit. (C) Four ounces of orange juice will act immediately to raise the blood sugar to a normal level and sustain it for 30 minutes until supper is served. (D) There is an increased potential for the client's blood sugar to decrease even further, resulting in diabetic coma.

97. **(C)** Client need: physiological integrity; subcategory: physiological adaptation; content area: med/surg

RATIONALE

(A) This is too early for peak action to occur. (B) This is too early for peak action to occur. (C) Regular insulin peak action occurs 2–4 hours after administration. (D) This is too late for peak action to occur.

98. **(C)** Client need: physiological integrity; subcategory: physiological adaptation; content area: med/surg

RATIONALE

(A) Blood sugar levels increase when the body responds to stress and illness. (B) Blood sugar levels increase when the body responds to stress and illness. (C) Hyperglycemia occurs because glucose is produced as the body responds to the stress and illness of cellulitis. (D) Blood sugar levels remain elevated as long as the body responds to stress and illness.

99. **(B)** Client need: physiological integrity; subcategory: reduction of risk potential; content area: med/surg

RATIONALE

(A) Exercise should not be performed before meals because the blood sugar is usually lower just prior to eating; therefore, there is an increased risk for hypoglycemia. (B) Exercise lowers blood sugar levels; therefore, a snack may be needed to maintain the appropriate glucose level. (C) Exercise lowers blood sugar levels. (D) Exercise lowers blood sugar levels. If the blood glucose level is 100 mg or below at the start of exercise, the potential for hypoglycemia is greater.

100. **(D)** Client need: physiological integrity; subcategory: reduction of risk potential; content area: med/surg

RATIONALE

(A) The percentage of carbohydrates is too low to maintain blood sugar levels. The percent range of protein is too high and may cause extra workload on the kidney as it is metabolized. (B) The percentage of carbohydrates is too low to maintain blood sugar levels. The percent range of protein is too high and may cause extra workload on the kidney. (C) The percentage of carbohydrates is too high; the percent range of protein is too high, and of fat, too low. (D) This combination provides enough carbohydrates to maintain blood glucose levels, enough protein to maintain body repair, and enough fat to ensure palatability.

TEST 2

Joliet Junior College-Nursing Education Test

MOCK NCLEX-RN BOARD REVIEW TEST QUESTIONS

1. A 74-year-old female client is 3 days postoperative. She has an indwelling catheter and has been progressing well. While the nurse is in the room, the client states, "Oh dear, I feel like I have to urinate again!" Which of the following is the most appropriate initial nursing response?

   A. Assure her that this is most likely the result of bladder spasms.
   B. Check the collection bag and tubing to verify that the catheter is draining properly.
   C. Instruct her to do Kegel exercises to diminish the urge to void.
   D. Ask her if she has felt this way before.

2. In cleansing the perineal area around the site of catheter insertion, the nurse would:

   A. Wipe the catheter toward the urinary meatus
   B. Wipe the catheter away from the urinary meatus
   C. Apply a small amount of talcum powder after drying the perineal area
   D. Gently insert the catheter another ½ inch after cleansing to prevent irritation from the balloon

3. Nursing interventions designed to decrease the risk of infection in a client with an indwelling catheter include:

   A. Cleanse area around the meatus twice a day
   B. Empty the catheter drainage bag at least daily
   C. Change the catheter tubing and bag every 48 hours
   D. Maintain fluid intake of 1200–1500 mL every day

4. A client tells the nurse that she has had a history of urinary tract infections. The nurse would do further health teaching if she verbalizes she will:

   A. Drink at least 8 oz of cranberry juice daily
   B. Maintain a fluid intake of at least 2000 mL daily
   C. Wash her hands before and after voiding
   D. Limit her fluid intake after 6 PM so that there is not a great deal of urine in her bladder while she sleeps

5. An 83-year-old client has been hospitalized following a fall in his home. He has developed a possible fecal impaction. Which of the following assessment findings would be most indicative of a fecal impaction?

   A. Boardlike, rigid abdomen
   B. Loss of the urge to defecate
   C. Liquid stool
   D. Abdominal pain

6. The nurse provides a male client with diet teaching so that he can help prevent constipation in the future. Which food choices indicate that this teaching has been understood?

   A. Omelette and hash browns
   B. Pancakes and syrup
   C. Bagel with cream cheese
   D. Cooked oatmeal and grapefruit half

7. One of the medications that is prescribed for a male client is furosemide (Lasix) 80 mg bid. To reduce his risk of falls, the nurse would teach him to take this medication:

   A. On arising and no later than 6 PM
   B. At evenly spaced intervals, such as 8 AM and 8 PM
   C. With at least one glass of water per pill
   D. With breakfast and at bedtime

8. The nurse teaches a male client ways to reduce the risks associated with furosemide therapy. Which of the following indicates that he understands this teaching?

   A. "I'll be sure to rise slowly and sit for a few minutes after lying down."
   B. "I'll be sure to walk at least 2–3 blocks every day."
   C. "I'll be sure to restrict my fluid intake to four or five glasses a day."

D. "I'll be sure not to take any more aspirin while I am on this drug."

9. A client is taught to eat foods high in potassium. Which food choices would indicate that this teaching has been successful?

   A. Pork chop, baked acorn squash, brussel sprouts
   B. Chicken breast, rice, and green beans
   C. Roast beef, baked potato, and diced carrots
   D. Tuna casserole, noodles, and spinach

10. The nurse would be sure to instruct a client on the signs and symptoms of an eye infection and hemorrhage. These signs and symptoms would include:

    A. Blurred vision and dizziness
    B. Eye pain and itching
    C. Feeling of eye pressure and headache
    D. Eye discharge and hemoptysis

11. The nurse would teach a male client ways to minimize the risk of infection after eye surgery. Which of the following indicates the client needs further teaching?

    A. "I will wash my hands before instilling eye medications."
    B. "I will wear sunglasses when going outside."
    C. "I will wear an eye patch for the first 3 postoperative days."
    D. "I will maintain the sterility of the eye medications."

12. With a geriatric client, the nurse should also assess whether he has been obtaining a yearly vaccination against influenza. Why is this assessment important?

    A. Influenza is growing in our society.
    B. Older clients generally are sicker than others when stricken with flu.
    C. Older clients have less effective immune systems.
    D. Older clients have more exposure to the causative agents.

13. In evaluating the laboratory results of a client with severe pressure ulcers, the nurse finds that her albumin level is low. A decrease in serum albumin would contribute to the formation of pressure ulcers because:

    A. The proteins needed for tissue repair are diminished.
    B. The iron stores needed for tissue repair are inadequate.
    C. A decreased serum albumin level indicates kidney disease.
    D. A decreased serum albumin causes fluid movement into the blood vessels, causing dehydration.

14. Which of the following menu choices would indicate that a client with pressure ulcers understands the role diet plays in restoring her albumin levels?

    A. Broiled fish with rice
    B. Bran flakes with fresh peaches
    C. Lasagna with garlic bread
    D. Cauliflower and lettuce salad

15. The nurse observes that a client has difficulty chewing and swallowing her food. A nursing response designed to reduce this problem would include:

    A. Ordering a full liquid diet for her
    B. Ordering five small meals for her
    C. Ordering a mechanical soft diet for her
    D. Ordering a puréed diet for her

16. When a client with pancreatitis is discharged, the nurse needs to teach him how to prevent another occurrence of acute pancreatitis. Which of the following statements would indicate he has an understanding of his disease?

    A. "I will not eat any raw or uncooked vegetables."
    B. "I will limit my alcohol to one cocktail per day."
    C. "I will look into attending Alcoholics Anonymous meetings."
    D. "I will report any changes in bowel movements to my doctor."

17. A 54-year-old client is admitted to the hospital with a possible gastric ulcer. He is a heavy smoker. When discussing his smoking habits with him, the nurse should advise him to:

    A. Smoke low-tar, filtered cigarettes
    B. Smoke cigars instead
    C. Smoke only right after meals
    D. Chew gum instead

18. Iron dextran (Imferon) is a parenteral iron preparation. The nurse should know that it:

    A. Is also called intrinsic factor
    B. Must be given in the abdomen
    C. Requires use of the Z-track method
    D. Should be given SC

19. A nasogastric (NG) tube inserted preoperatively is attached to low, intermittent suctions. A client with an NG tube exhibits these symptoms: He is restless; serum electrolytes are Na 138, K 4.0, blood pH 7.53. This client is most likely experiencing:

    A. Hyperkalemia
    B. Hyponatremia
    C. Metabolic acidosis
    D. Metabolic alkalosis

20. A client is experiencing muscle weakness and lethargy. His serum K+ is 3.2. What other symptoms might he exhibit?

    A. Tetany
    B. Dysrhythmias
    C. Numbness of extremities
    D. Headache

21. Following a gastric resection, which of the following actions would the nurse reinforce with the client in order to alleviate the distress from dumping syndrome?

    A. Eating three large meals a day
    B. Drinking small amounts of liquids with meals
    C. Taking a long walk after meals
    D. Eating a low-carbohydrate diet

22. Azulfidine (Sulfasalazine) may be ordered for a client who has ulcerative colitis. Which of the following is a nursing implication for this drug?

    A. Limit fluids to 500 mL/day.
    B. Administer 2 hours before meals.

C. Observe for skin rash and diarrhea.

D. Monitor blood pressure, pulse.

23. Other drugs may be ordered to manage a client's ulcerative colitis. Which of the following medications, if ordered, would the nurse question?

    A. Methylprednisolone sodium succinate (Solu-Medrol)
    B. Loperamide (Imodium)
    C. Psyllium
    D. 6-Mercaptopurine

24. A male client is scheduled for a liver biopsy. In preparing him for this test, the nurse should:

    A. Explain that he will be kept NPO for 24 hours before the exam
    B. Practice with him so he will be able to hold his breath for 1 minute
    C. Explain that he will be receiving a laxative to prevent a distended bowel from applying pressure on the liver
    D. Explain that his vital signs will be checked frequently after the test

25. After a liver biopsy, the best position for the client is:

    A. High Fowler
    B. Prone
    C. Supine
    D. Right lateral

26. A complication for which the nurse should be alert following a liver biopsy is:

    A. Hepatic coma
    B. Jaundice
    C. Ascites
    D. Shock

27. Which nursing implication is appropriate for a client undergoing a paracentesis?

    A. Have the client void before the procedure.
    B. Keep the client NPO.
    C. Observe the client for hypertension following the procedure.
    D. Place the client on the right side following the procedure.

28. The nurse would assess the client's correct understanding of the fertility awareness methods that enhance conception, if the client stated that:

    A. "My sexual partner and I should have intercourse when my cervical mucosa is thick and cloudy."
    B. "At ovulation, my basal body temperature should rise about 0.5°F."
    C. "I should douche immediately after intercourse."
    D. "My sexual partner and I should have sexual intercourse on day 14 of my cycle regardless of the length of the cycle."

29. A couple is planning the conception of their first child. The wife, whose normal menstrual cycle is 34 days in length, correctly identifies the time that she is *most* likely to ovulate if she states that ovulation should occur on day:

    A. 14 ± 2 days
    B. 16 ± 2 days

C. 20 ± 2 days

D. 22 ± 2 days

30. A client is pregnant with her second child. Her last menstrual period began on January 15. Her expected date of delivery would be:

    A. October 8
    B. October 15
    C. October 22
    D. October 29

31. The nurse instructs a pregnant client (G_2P_1) to rest in a side-lying position and avoid lying flat on her back. The nurse explains that this is to avoid "vena caval syndrome," a condition which:

    A. Occurs when blood pressure increases sharply with changes in position
    B. Results when blood flow from the extremities is blocked or slowed
    C. Is seen mainly in first pregnancies
    D. May require medication if positioning does not help

32. A pregnant client comes to the office for her first prenatal examination at 10 weeks. She has been pregnant twice before; the first delivery produced a viable baby girl at 39 weeks 3 years ago; the second pregnancy produced a viable baby boy at 36 weeks 2 years ago. Both children are living and well. Using the GTPAL system to record her obstetrical history, the nurse should record:

    A. 3-2-0-0-2
    B. 2-2-0-2-2
    C. 3-1-1-0-2
    D. 2-1-1-0-2

33. A pregnant client comes to the office for her first prenatal examination at 10 weeks. She has been pregnant twice before; the first delivery produced a viable baby girl at 39 weeks 3 years ago; the second pregnancy produced a viable baby boy at 36 weeks 2 years ago. Both children are living and well. Using the gravida and para system to record the client's obstetrical history, the nurse should record:

    A. Gravida 3 para 1
    B. Gravida 3 para 2
    C. Gravida 2 para 1
    D. Gravida 2 para 2

34. A gravida 2 para 1 client is hospitalized with severe preeclampsia. While she receives magnesium sulfate ($MgSO_4$) therapy, the nurse knows it is safe to repeat the dosage if:

    A. Deep tendon reflexes are absent
    B. Urine output is 20 mL/hr
    C. $MgSO_4$ serum levels are ≥15 mg/dL
    D. Respirations are ≥16 breaths/min

35. Prenatal clients are routinely monitored for early signs of pregnancy-induced hypertension (PIH). For the prenatal client, which of the following blood pressure changes from baseline would be *most* significant for the nurse to report as indicative of PIH?

    A. 136/88 to 144/93
    B. 132/78 to 124/76

C. 114/70 to 140/88
D. 140/90 to 148/98

36. In assisting preconceptual clients, the nurse should teach that the corpus luteum secretes progesterone, which thickens the endometrial lining in which of the phases of the menstrual cycle?

A. Menstrual phase
B. Proliferative phase
C. Secretory phase
D. Ischemic phase

37. A client decided early in her pregnancy to breast-feed her first baby. She gave birth to a normal, full-term girl and is now progressing toward the establishment of successful lactation. To remove the baby from her breast, she should be instructed to:

A. Gently pull the infant away
B. Withdraw the breast from the infant's mouth
C. Compress the areolar tissue until the infant drops the nipple from her mouth
D. Insert a clean finger into the baby's mouth beside the nipple

38. A gravida 2 para 1 client delivered a full-term newborn 12 hours ago. The nurse finds her uterus to be boggy, high, and deviated to the right. The *most* appropriate nursing action is to:

A. Notify the physician
B. Place the client on a pad count
C. Massage the uterus and re-evaluate in 30 minutes
D. Have the client void and then re-evaluate the fundus

39. A client delivered her first-born son 4 hours ago. She asks the nurse what the white cheeselike substance is under the baby's arms. The nurse should respond:

A. "This is a normal skin variation in newborns. It will go away in a few days."
B. "Let me have a closer look at it. The baby may have an infection."
C. "This material, called vernix, covered the baby before it was born. It will disappear in a few days."
D. "Babies sometimes have sebaceous glands that get plugged at birth. This substance is an example of that condition."

40. A client is in early labor. Her fetus is in a left occipitoanterior (LOA) position; fetal heart sounds are *best* auscultated just:

A. Below the umbilicus toward left side of mother's abdomen
B. Below the umbilicus toward right side of mother's abdomen
C. At the umbilicus
D. Above the umbilicus to the left side of mother's abdomen

41. In performing the initial nursing assessment on a client at the prenatal clinic, the nurse will know that which of the following alterations is abnormal during pregnancy?

A. Striae gravidarum
B. Chloasma

C. Dysuria
D. Colostrum

42. A 35-weeks-pregnant client is undergoing a nonstress test (NST). During the 20-minute examination, the nurse notes three fetal movements accompanied by accelerations of the fetal heart rate, each $\geq$15 bpm, lasting 15 seconds. The nurse interprets this test to be:

A. Nonreactive
B. Reactive
C. Positive
D. Negative

43. The nurse is caring for a laboring client. Assessment data include cervical dilation 9 cm; contractions every 1–2 minutes; strong, large amount of "bloody show." The most appropriate nursing goal for this client would be:

A. Maintain client's privacy.
B. Assist with assessment procedures.
C. Provide strategies to maintain client control.
D. Enlist additional caregiver support to ensure client's safety.

44. A client is admitted to the labor unit. On vaginal examination, the presenting part in a cephalic presentation was at station plus two. Station 12 means that the:

A. Presenting part is 2 cm above the level of the ischial spines
B. Biparietal diameter is at the level of the ischial spines
C. Presenting part is 2 cm below the level of the ischial spines
D. Biparietal diameter is 5 cm above the ischial spines

45. A pregnant client is at the clinic for a third trimester prenatal visit. During this examination, it has been determined that her fetus is in a vertex presentation with the occiput located in her right anterior quadrant. On her chart this would be noted as:

A. Right occipitoposterior
B. Right occipitoanterior
C. Right sacroanterior
D. LOA

46. Assessment of parturient reveals the following: cervical dilation 6 cm and station 22; no progress in the last 4 hours. Uterine contractions decreasing in frequency and intensity. Marked molding of the presenting fetal head is described. The physician orders, "Begin oxytocin induction at 1 mU/min." The nurse should:

A. Begin the oxytocin induction as ordered
B. Increase the dosage by 2 mU/min increments at 15-minute intervals
C. Maintain the dosage when duration of contractions is 40–60 seconds and frequency is at 2½–4 minute intervals
D. Question the order

47. A client in active labor asks the nurse for coaching with her breathing during contractions. The client has attended Lamaze birth preparation classes. Which of the following is the *best* response by the nurse?

A. "Keep breathing with your abdominal muscles as long as you can."

B. "Make sure you take a deep cleansing breath as the contractions start, focus on an object, and breathe about 16–20 times a minute with shallow chest breaths."

C. "Find a comfortable position before you start a contraction. Once the contraction has started, take slow breaths using your abdominal muscles."

D. "If a woman in labor listens to her body and takes rapid, deep breaths, she will be able to deal with her contractions quite well."

48. A client is being discharged and will continue enteral feedings at home. Which of the following statements by a family member indicates the need for further teaching?

A. "If he develops diarrhea lasting for more than 2–3 days, I will contact the doctor or nurse."

B. "I should anticipate that he will gain about 1 lb/day now that he is on continuous feedings."

C. "It is important to keep the head of his bed elevated or sit him in the chair during feedings."

D. "I should use prepared or open formula within 24 hours and store unused portions in the refrigerator."

49. A 74-year-old obese man who has undergone open reduction and internal fixation of the right hip is 8 days postoperative. He has a history of arthritis and atrial fibrillation. He admits to right lower leg pain, described as "a cramp in my leg." An appropriate nursing action is to:

A. Assess for pain with plantiflexion

B. Assess for edema and heat of the right leg

C. Instruct him to rub the cramp out of his leg

D. Elevate right lower extremity with pillows propped under the knee

50. A male client is started on IV anticoagulant therapy with heparin. Which of the following laboratory studies will be ordered to monitor the therapeutic effects of heparin?

A. Partial thromboplastin time

B. Hemoglobin

C. Red blood cell (RBC) count

D. Prothrombin time

51. A client is being discharged on warfarin (Coumadin), an oral anticoagulant. The nurse instructs him about using this drug. Which following response by the client indicates the need for further teaching?

A. "I should shave with my electric razor while on Coumadin."

B. "I will inform my dentist that I am on anticoagulant therapy before receiving dental work."

C. "I will continue with my usual dosage of aspirin for my arthritis when I return home."

D. "I will wear an ID bracelet stating that I am on anticoagulants."

52. A 68-year-old woman is admitted to the hospital with chronic obstructive pulmonary disease (COPD). She is started on an aminophylline infusion. Three days later she is breathing easier. A serum theophylline level is drawn. Which of the following values represents a therapeutic level?

A. 14 μg/mL

B. 25 μg/mL

C. 4 μg/mL

D. 30 μg/mL

53. A client is being discharged with albuterol (Proventil) and beclomethasone dipropionate (Vanceril) to be administered via inhalation three times a day and at bedtime. Client teaching regarding the sequential order in which the drugs should be administered includes:

A. Glucocorticoid followed by the bronchodilator

B. Bronchodilator followed by the glucocorticoid

C. Alternate successive administrations

D. According to the client's preference

54. To prevent fungal infections of the mouth and throat, the nurse should teach clients on inhaled steroids to:

A. Rinse the plastic holder that aerosolizes the drug with hydrogen peroxide every other day

B. Rinse the mouth and gargle with warm water after each use of the inhaler

C. Take antacids immediately before inhalation to neutralize mucous membranes and prevent infection

D. Rinse the mouth before each use to eliminate colonization of bacteria

55. Which of the following would indicate the need for further teaching for the client with COPD? The client verbalizes the need to:

A. Eat high-calorie, high-protein foods

B. Take vitamin supplementation

C. Eliminate intake of milk and milk products

D. Eat small, frequent meals

56. A dose of theophylline may need to be altered if a client with COPD:

A. Is allergic to morphine

B. Has a history of arthritis

C. Operates machinery

D. Is concurrently on cimetidine for ulcers

57. The nurse working in a prenatal clinic needs to be alert to the cardinal signs and symptoms of PIH because:

A. Immediate treatment of mild PIH includes the administration of a variety of medications

B. Psychological counseling is indicated to reduce the emotional stress causing the blood pressure elevation

C. Self-discipline is required to control caloric intake throughout the pregnancy

D. The client may not recognize the early symptoms of PIH

58. Which of the following changes in blood pressure readings should be of greatest concern to the nurse when assessing a prenatal client?

A. 130/88 to 144/92

B. 136/90 to 148/100

C. 150/96 to 160/104

D. 118/70 to 130/88

59. A 16-year-old client comes to the prenatal clinic for her monthly appointment. She has gained 14 lb from her 7th to 8th month; her face and hands indicate edema. She is diagnosed as having PIH and referred to the high-risk prenatal clinic. The client's weight increase is most likely due to:

A. Overeating and subsequent obesity
B. Obesity prior to conception
C. Hypertension due to kidney lesions
D. Fluid retention

60. MgSO$_4$ is ordered IV following the established protocol for a client with severe PIH. The anticipated effects of this therapy are anticonvulsant and:

A. Vasoconstrictive
B. Vasodilative
C. Hypertensive
D. Antiemetic

61. A nurse should carefully monitor a client for the following side effect of MgSO$_4$:

A. Visual blurring
B. Tachypnea
C. Epigastric pain
D. Respiratory depression

62. MgSO$_4$ blood levels are monitored and the nurse would be prepared to administer the following antidote for MgSO$_4$ side effects or toxicity:

A. Magnesium oxide
B. Calcium hydroxide
C. Calcium gluconate
D. Naloxone (Narcan)

63. A client with severe PIH receiving MgSO$_4$ is placed in a quiet, darkened room. The nurse bases this action on the following understanding:

A. The client is restless.
B. The elevated blood pressure causes photophobia.
C. Noise or bright lights may precipitate a convulsion.
D. External stimuli are annoying to the client with PIH.

64. A 26-year-old client is admitted to the labor, delivery, recovery, postpartum unit. The nurse completes her assessment and determines the client is in the first stage of labor. The nurse should instruct her:

A. To hold her breath during contractions
B. To be flat on her back
C. Not to push with her contractions
D. To push before becoming fully dilated

65. In addition to changing the mother's position to relieve cord pressure, the nurse may employ the following measure(s) in the event that she observes the cord out of the vagina:

A. Immediately pour sterile saline on the cord, and repeat this every 15 minutes to prevent drying.
B. Cover the cord with a wet sponge.
C. Apply a cord clamp to the exposed cord, and cover with a sterile towel.
D. Keep the cord warm and moist by continuous applications of warm, sterile saline compresses.

66. Which of the following signs might indicate a complication during the labor process with vertex presentation?

A. Fetal tachycardia to 170 bpm during a contraction
B. Nausea and vomiting at 8–10 cm dilation
C. Contraction lasting 60 seconds
D. Appearance of dark-colored amniotic fluid

67. A client is admitted to the hospital for an induction of labor owing to a gestation of 42 weeks confirmed by dates and ultrasound. When she is dilated 3 cm, she has a contraction of 70 seconds. She is receiving oxytocin. The nurse's first intervention should be to:

A. Check FHT
B. Notify the attending physician
C. Turn off the IV oxytocin
D. Prepare for the delivery because the client is probably in transition

68. During a client's first postpartum day, the nurse assessed that the fundus was located laterally to the umbilicus. This may be due to:

A. Endometritis
B. Fibroid tumor on the uterus
C. Displacement due to bowel distention
D. Urine retention or a distended bladder

69. The nurse would be concerned if a client exhibited which of the following symptoms during her postpartum stay?

A. Pulse rate of 50–70 bpm by her third postpartum day
B. Diuresis by her second or third postpartum day
C. Vaginal discharge or rubra, serosa, then rubra
D. Diaphoresis by her third postpartum day

70. A postpartum client complains of rectal pressure and severe pain in her perineum; this may be indicative of:

A. Afterbirth pains
B. Constipation
C. Cystitis
D. A hematoma of the vagina or vulva

1. **(B)** Client need: physiological integrity; subcategory: basic care and comfort; content area: med/surg

   RATIONALE

   (A) Although this may be an appropriate response, the initial response would be to assure the patency of the catheter. (B) The most frequent reason for an urge to void with an indwelling catheter is blocked tubing. This response would be the best initial response. (C) Kegel exercises while a retention catheter is in place would not help to prevent a voiding urge and could irritate the urethral sphincter. (D) Though the nurse would want to ascertain whether the client has felt the same urge to void before, the initial response should be to assure the patency of the catheter.

2. **(B)** Client need: physiological integrity; subcategory: reduction of risk potential; content area: med/surg

   RATIONALE

   (A) Wiping toward the urinary meatus would transport microorganisms from the external tubing to the urethra, thereby increasing the risk of bladder infection. (B) Wiping away from the urinary meatus would remove microorganisms from the point of insertion of the catheter, thereby decreasing the risk of bladder infection. (C) Talcum powder should not be applied following catheter care, because powders contribute to moisture retention and infection likelihood. (D) The catheter should never be inserted further into the urethra, because this would serve no useful purpose and would increase the risk of infection.

3. **(A)** Client need: physiological integrity; subcategory: reduction of risk potential; content area: med/surg

   RATIONALE

   (A) Catheter site care is to be done at least twice daily to prevent pathogen growth at the catheter insertion site. (B) Catheter drainage bags are usually emptied every 8 hours to prevent urine stasis and pathogen growth. (C) Tubing and collection bags are not changed this often, because research studies have not demonstrated the efficacy of this practice. (D) Fluid intake needs to be in the 2000–2500 mL range if possible to help irrigate the bladder and prevent infection.

4. **(D)** Client need: health promotion and maintenance; subcategory: prevention and early detection of disease; content area: med/surg

   RATIONALE

   (A) Cranberry juice helps to maintain urine acidity, thereby retarding bacterial growth. (B) A generous fluid intake will help to irrigate the bladder and to prevent bacterial growth within the bladder. (C) Hand washing is an effective means of preventing pathogen transmission. (D) Restricting fluid intake would contribute to urinary stasis, which in turn would contribute to bacterial growth.

5. **(C)** Client need: physiological integrity; subcategory: physiological adaptation; content area: med/surg

   RATIONALE

   (A) A boardlike, rigid abdomen would point to a perforated bowel, not a fecal impaction. (B) When a client is fecally impacted, a common symptom is the urge to defecate but the inability to do so. (C) When an impaction is present, only liquid stool will be able to pass around the impacted site. (D) Abdominal pain without distention is not a sign of a fecal impaction.

6. **(D)** Client need: physiological integrity; subcategory: basic care and comfort; content area: med/surg

   RATIONALE

   (A) Eggs and hash browns do not provide much fiber and bulk, so they do not effectively prevent constipation. (B) Pancakes and syrup also have little fiber and bulk, so they do not effectively prevent constipation. (C) Bagel and cream cheese do not provide intestinal bulk. (D) A combination of oatmeal and fresh fruit will provide fiber and intestinal bulk.

7. **(A)** Client need: physiological integrity; subcategory: reduction of risk potential; content area: med/surg

   RATIONALE

   (A) This option provides adequate spacing of the medication and will limit the client's need to get up to go to the bathroom during the night hours, when he is especially at high risk for falls. (B) This option would result in the need to get up during the night to urinate and would thus increase the risk of falls. This option also does not take into consideration the client's usual daily routine. (C) Taking this medication with at least one glass of water would not have an impact on the risk of falls. (D) This option would result in the need to get up during the night to urinate and would thus increase the risk of falls.

8. **(A)** Client need: physiological integrity; subcategory: reduction of risk potential; content area: med/surg

   RATIONALE

   (A) This response will help to prevent the occurrence of postural hypotension, a common side effect of this drug and a common reason for falls. (B) Although walking is an excellent exercise, it is not specific to the reduction of risks associated with diuretic therapy. (C) Clients on diuretic therapy are generally taught to ensure that their fluid intake is at least 2000–3000 mL daily, unless contraindicated. (D) Aspirin is a safe drug to take along with furosemide.

9. **(A)** Client need: physiological integrity; subcategory: basic care and comfort; content area: med/surg

   RATIONALE

   (A) Both acorn squash and brussels sprouts are potassium-rich foods. (B) None of these foods is considered potassium rich. (C) Only the baked potato is a potassium-rich food. (D) Spinach is the only potassium-rich food in this option.

10. **(B)** Client need: physiological integrity; subcategory: physiological adaptation; content area: med/surg

    RATIONALE

    (A) Although blurred vision may occur, dizziness would not be associated with an infection or hemorrhage. (B) Eye pain is a symptom of hemorrhage within the eye, and itching is associated with infection. (C) Nausea and headache would not be usual symptoms of eye hemorrhage or infection. (D) Some eye discharge might be anticipated if an infection is present; hemoptysis would not.

11. **(C)** Client need: physiological integrity; subcategory: reduction of risk potential; content area: med/surg

    RATIONALE

    (A) Hand washing would be an important action designed to prevent transmission of pathogens from the hands to the eye. (B) Wearing sunglasses when going outside will prevent airborne pathogens from entering the eye. (C) Eye patches are most frequently ordered to be worn while the client sleeps or naps, not constantly for this length of time. (D) Eye medications are sterile; clients need to be taught how to maintain this sterility.

12. **(C)** Client need: health promotion and maintenance; subcategory: prevention and early detection of disease; content area: med/surg

RATIONALE

(A) Although influenza is common, the elderly are more at risk because of decreased effectiveness of their immune system, not because the incidence is increasing. (B) Older clients have the same degree of illness when stricken as other populations. (C) As people age, their immune system becomes less effective, increasing their risk for influenza. (D) Older clients have no more exposure to the causative agents than do school-age children, for example.

13. **(A)** Client need: physiological integrity; subcategory: reduction of risk potential; content area: med/surg

RATIONALE

(A) Serum albumin levels indicate the adequacy of protein stores available for tissue repair. (B) Serum albumin does not measure iron stores. (C) Serum albumin levels do not measure kidney function. (D) A decreased serum albumin level would cause fluid movement out of blood vessels, not into them.

14. **(A)** Client need: physiological integrity; subcategory: basic care and comfort; content area: med/surg

RATIONALE

(A) Broiled fish and rice are both excellent sources of protein. (B) Fresh fruits are not a good source of protein. (C) Foods in the bread group are not high in protein. (D) Most vegetables are not high in protein; peas and beans are the major vegetables higher in protein.

15. **(C)** Client need: physiological integrity; subcategory: basic care and comfort; content area: med/surg

RATIONALE

(A) Full liquids would be difficult to swallow if the muscle control of the swallowing act is affected; this is a probable reason for her difficulties, given her medical diagnosis of multiple sclerosis. (B) Five small meals would do little if anything to decrease her swallowing difficulties, other than assure that she tires less easily. (C) A mechanical soft diet should be easier to chew and swallow, because foods would be more evenly consistent. (D) A pureed diet would cause her to regress more than might be needed; the mechanical soft diet should be tried first.

16. **(C)** Client need: physiological integrity; subcategory: basic care and comfort; content area: med/surg

RATIONALE

(A) Raw or uncooked vegetables are all right to eat postdischarge. (B) This client must avoid any alcohol intake. (C) The client displays awareness of the need to avoid alcohol. (D) This action would be pertinent only if fatty stools associated with chronic hepatitis were the problem.

17. **(C)** Client need: physiological integrity; subcategory: reduction of risk potential; content area: med/surg

RATIONALE

(A, B, D) Cigarettes, cigars, and chewing gum would stimulate gastric acid secretion. (C) Smoking on a full stomach minimizes effect of nicotine on gastric acid.

18. **(C)** Client need: physiological integrity; subcategory: pharmacological and parenteral therapies; content area: med/surg

RATIONALE

(A) Intrinsic factor is needed to absorb vitamin B_{12}. (B) Iron dextran is given parenterally, but Z-track in a large muscle. (C) A Z-track method of injection is required to prevent staining and irritation of the tissue. (D) An SC injection is not deep enough and may cause subcutaneous fat abscess formation.

19. **(D)** Client need: physiological integrity; subcategory: physiological adaptation; content area: med/surg

RATIONALE

(A) Sodium level is within normal limits. (B) Sodium level is within normal limits. (C) pH level is consistent with alkalosis.

(D) With an NG tube attached to low, intermittent suction, acids are removed and a client will develop metabolic alkalosis.

20. **(B)** Client need: physiological integrity; subcategory: physiological adaptation; content area: med/surg

RATIONALE

(A) Tetany is seen with low calcium. (B) Low potassium causes dysrhythmias because potassium is responsible for cardiac muscle activity. (C) Numbness of extremities is seen with high potassium. (D) Headache is not associated with potassium excess or deficiency.

21. **(D)** Client need: physiological integrity; subcategory: reduction of risk potential; content area: med/surg

RATIONALE

(A) Six small meals are recommended. (B) Liquids after meals increase the time food empties from the stomach. (C) Lying down after meals is recommended to prevent gravity from producing dumping. (D) A low-carbohydrate diet will prevent a hypertonic bolus, which causes dumping.

22. **(C)** Client need: physiological integrity; subcategory: reduction of risk potential; content area: med/surg

RATIONALE

(A) Fluids up to 2500–3000 mL/day are needed to prevent kidney stones. (B) The client should be instructed to take oral preparations with meals or snacks to lessen gastric irritation. (C) Sulfasalazine causes skin rash and diarrhea. (D) Blood pressure and pulse are not altered by sulfasalazine.

23. **(D)** Client need: physiological integrity; subcategory: physiological adaptation; content area: med/surg

RATIONALE

(A) Methylprednisolone sodium succinate is used for its anti-inflammatory effects. (B) Loperamide would be used to control diarrhea. (C) Psyllium may improve consistency of stools by providing bulk. (D) An immunosuppressant such as 6-mercaptopurine is used for chronic unrelenting Crohn's disease.

24. **(D)** Client need: physiological integrity; subcategory: reduction of risk potential; content area: med/surg

RATIONALE

(A) There is no NPO restriction prior to a liver biopsy. (B) The client would need to hold his breath for 5–10 seconds. (C) There is no pretest laxative given. (D) Following the test, the client is watched for hemorrhage and shock.

25. **(D)** Client need: physiological integrity; subcategory: reduction of risk potential; content area: med/surg

RATIONALE

(A) This position does not help to prevent bleeding. (B) This position does not help to prevent bleeding. (C) This position does not help to prevent bleeding. (D) The right lateral position would allow pressure on the liver to prevent bleeding.

26. **(D)** Client need: physiological integrity; subcategory: physiological adaptation; content area: med/surg

RATIONALE

(A) Hepatic coma may occur in liver disease due to the increased NH_3 levels, not due to liver biopsy. (B) Jaundice may occur due to increased bilirubin levels, not due to liver biopsy. (C) Ascites would occur due to portal hypertension, not due to liver biopsy. (D) Hemorrhage and shock are the most likely complications after liver biopsy because of already existing bleeding tendencies in the vascular makeup of the liver.

27. **(A)** Client need: physiological integrity; subcategory: reduction of risk potential; content area: med/surg

RATIONALE

(A) A full bladder would impede withdrawal of ascitic fluid. (B) Keeping the client NPO is not necessary. (C) The client may exhibit signs and symptoms of shock and hypertension. (D) No position change is needed after the procedure.

28. **(B)** Client need: health promotion and maintenance; subcategory: growth and development through the life span; content area: maternity
RATIONALE
(A) At ovulation, the cervical mucus is increased, stretchable, and watery clear. (B) Under the influence of progesterone, the basal body temperature increases slightly after ovulation. (C) To enhance fertility, measures should be taken that promote retention of sperm rather than removal. (D) Ovulation, the optimal time for conception, occurs 14 ± 2 days before the next menses; therefore, the date of ovulation is directly related to the length of the menstrual cycle.

29. **(C)** Client need: health promotion and maintenance; subcategory: growth and development through the life span; content area: maternity
RATIONALE
(A) Ovulation is dependent on average length of menstrual cycle, not standard 14 days. (B) Ovulation occurs 14 ± 2 days before next menses (34 minus 14 does not equal 16). (C) Ovulation occurs 14 ± 2 days before next menses (34 minus 14 equals 20). (D) Ovulation occurs 14 ± 2 days before next menses (34 minus 14 does not equal 22).

30. **(C)** Client need: health promotion and maintenance; subcategory: growth and development through the life span; content area: maternity
RATIONALE
(A) Incorrect application of Nägele's rule: correctly subtracted 3 months but subtracted 7 days rather than added. (B) Incorrect application of Nägele's rule: correctly subtracted 3 months but did not add 7 days. (C) Correct application of Nägele's rule: correctly subtracted 3 months and added 7 days. (D) Incorrect application of Nägele's rule: correctly subtracted 3 months but added 14 days instead of 7 days.

31. **(B)** Client need: physiological integrity; subcategory: physiological adaptation; content area: maternity
RATIONALE
(A) Blood pressure changes are predominantly due to pressure of the gravid uterus. (B) Pressure of the gravid uterus on the inferior vena cava decreases blood return from lower extremities. (C) Inferior vena cava syndrome is experienced in the latter months of pregnancy regardless of parity. (D) There are no medications useful in the treatment of interior vena cava syndrome; alleviating pressure by position changes is effective.

32. **(C)** Client need: health promotion and maintenance; subcategory: growth and development through the life span; content area: maternity
RATIONALE
(A) This answer is an incorrect application of the GTPAL method. One prior pregnancy was a preterm birth at 36 weeks (T = 1, P = 1; not T = 2). (B) This answer is an incorrect application of the GTPAL method. The client is currently pregnant for the third time (G = 3, not 2), one prior pregnancy was preterm (T = 1, P = 1; not T = 2), and she has had no prior abortions (A = 0). (C) This answer is the correct application of GTPAL method. The client is currently pregnant for the third time (G = 3), her first pregnancy ended at term (>37 weeks) (T = 1), her second pregnancy ended preterm 20–33 weeks) (P = 1), she has no history of abortion (A = 0), and she has two living children (L = 2). (D) This answer is an incorrect application of the GTPAL method. The client is currently pregnant for the third time (G = 3, not 2).

33. **(B)** Client need: health promotion and maintenance; subcategory: growth and development through the life span; content area: maternity

RATIONALE
(A) This answer is an incorrect application of gravida and para. The client has had two prior deliveries of more than 20 weeks' gestation; therefore, para equals 2, not 1. (B) This answer is the correct application of gravida and para. The client is currently pregnant for the third time (G = 3), regardless of the length of the pregnancy, and has had two prior pregnancies with birth after the 20th week (P = 2), whether infant was alive or dead. (C) This answer is an incorrect application of gravida and para. The client is currently pregnant for the third time (G = 3, not 2); prior pregnancies lasted longer than 20 weeks (therefore, P = 2, not 1). (D) This is an incorrect application of gravida and para. Client is currently pregnant for third time (G = 3, not 2).

34. **(D)** Client need: physiological integrity; subcategory: physiological adaptation; content area: maternity
RATIONALE
(A) MgSO₄ is a central nervous system depressant. Loss of reflexes is often the first sign of developing toxicity. (B) Urinary output at <25 mL/hr or 100 mL in 4 hours may result in the accumulation of toxic levels of magnesium. (C) The therapeutic serum range for MgSO₄ is 6–8 mg/dL. Higher levels indicate toxicity. (D) Respirations of ≥16 breaths/min indicate that toxic levels of magnesium have not been reached. Medication administration would be safe.

35. **(C)** Client need: physiological integrity; subcategory: physiological adaptation; content area: maternity
RATIONALE
(A) These blood pressure changes reflect only an 8 mm Hg systolic and a 5 mm Hg diastolic increase, which is insufficient for blood pressure changes indicating PIH. (B) These blood pressure changes reflect a decrease in systolic pressure of 8 mm Hg and diastolic pressure of 2 mm Hg; these values are not indicative of blood pressure increases reflecting PIH. (C) The definition of PIH is an increase in systolic blood pressure of 30 mm Hg and/or diastolic blood pressure of 15 mm Hg. These blood pressures reflect a change of 26 mm Hg systolically and 18 mm Hg diastolically. (D) These blood pressures reflect a change of only 8 mm Hg systolically and 8 mm Hg diastolically, which is insufficient for blood pressure changes indicating PIH.

36. **(C)** Client need: health promotion and maintenance; subcategory: growth and development through the life span; content area: maternity
RATIONALE
(A) Menses occurs during the menstrual phase, during which levels of both estrogen and progesterone are decreased. (B) The ovarian hormone responsible for the proliferative phase, during which the uterine endometrium enlarges, is estrogen. (C) The ovarian hormone responsible for the secretory phase is progesterone, which is secreted by the corpus luteum and causes marked swelling in the uterine endometrium. (D) The corpus luteum begins to degenerate in the ischemic phase, causing a fall in both estrogen and progesterone.

37. **(D)** Client need: health promotion and maintenance; subcategory: growth and development through the life span; content area: maternity
RATIONALE
(A) In pulling the infant away from the breast without breaking suction, nipple trauma is likely to occur. (B) In pulling the breast away from the infant without breaking suction, nipple trauma is likely to occur. (C) Compressing the maternal tissue does not break the suction of the infant on the breast and can cause nipple trauma. (D) By inserting a finger into the infant's mouth beside the nipple, the lactating mother can break the suction and the nipple can be removed without trauma.

38. **(D)** Client need: physiological integrity; subcategory: physiological adaptation; content area: maternity

RATIONALE

(A) The nurse should initiate actions to remove the most frequent cause of uterine displacement, which involves emptying the bladder. Notifying the physician is an inappropriate nursing action. (B) The pad count gives an estimate of blood loss, which is likely to increase with a boggy uterus; but this action does not remove the most frequent cause of uterine displacement, which is a full bladder. (C) Massage may firm the uterus temporarily, but if a full bladder is not emptied, the uterus will remain displaced and is likely to relax again. (D) The most common cause of uterine displacement is a full bladder.

39. **(C)** Client need: health promotion and maintenance; subcategory: growth and development through the life span; content area: maternity

RATIONALE

(A) This response identifies the fact that vernix is a normal neonatal variation, but it does not teach the client medical terms that may be useful in understanding other healthcare personnel. (B) This response may raise maternal anxiety and incorrectly identifies a normal neonatal variation. (C) This response correctly identifies this neonatal variation and helps the client to understand medical terms as well as the characteristics of her newborn. (D) Blocked sebaceous glands produce milia, particularly present on the nose.

40. **(A)** Client need: health promotion and maintenance; subcategory: growth and development through the life span; content area: maternity

RATIONALE

(A) LOA identifies a fetus whose back is on its mother's left side, whose head is the presenting part, and whose back is toward its mother's anterior. It is easiest to auscultate fetal heart tones (FHTs) through the fetus's back. (B) The identified fetus's back is on its mother's left side, not right side. It is easiest to auscultate FHTs through the fetus's back. (C) In an LOA position, the fetus's head is presenting with the back to the left anterior side of the mother. The umbilicus is too high of a landmark for auscultating the fetus's heart rate through its back. (D) This is the correct auscultation point for a fetus in the left sacroanterior position, where the sacrum is presenting, not LOA.

41. **(C)** Client need: health promotion and maintenance; subcategory: growth and development through the life span; content area: maternity

RATIONALE

(A) Striae gravidarum are the normal stretch marks that frequently occur on the breasts, abdomen, and thighs as pregnancy progresses. (B) Chloasma is the "mask of pregnancy" that normally occurs in many pregnant women. (C) Dysuria is an abnormal danger sign during pregnancy and may indicate a urinary tract infection. (D) Colostrum is a yellow breast secretion that is normally present during the last trimester of pregnancy.

42. **(B)** Client need: health promotion and maintenance; subcategory: growth and development through the life span; content area: maternity

RATIONALE

(A) In a nonreactive NST, the criteria for reactivity are not met. (B) A reactive NST shows at least two accelerations of FHR with fetal movements, each 15 bpm, lasting 15 seconds or more, over 20 minutes. (C, D) This term is used to interpret a contraction stress test (CST), or oxytocin challenge test, not an NST.

43. **(C)** Client need: health promotion and maintenance; subcategory: growth and development through the life span; content area: maternity

RATIONALE

(A) Privacy may help the laboring client feel safer, but measures that enhance coping take priority. (B) The frequency of assessments do increase in transition, but helping the client to maintain control and cope with this phase of labor takes on importance. (C) This laboring client is in transition, the most difficult part of the first stage of labor because of decreased frequency, increased duration and intensity, and decreased resting phase of the uterine contraction. The client's ability to cope is most threatened during this phase of labor, and nursing actions are directed toward helping the client to maintain control. (D) Safety is a concern throughout labor, but helping the client to cope takes on importance in transition.

44. **(C)** Client need: health promotion and maintenance; subcategory: growth and development through the life span; content area: maternity

RATIONALE

(A) Station is the relationship of the presenting part to an imaginary line drawn between the ischial spines. If the presenting part is above the ischial spines, the station is negative. (B) When the biparietal diameter is at the level of the ischial spines, the presenting part is generally at a $+4$ or $+5$ station. (C) Station is the relationship of the presenting part to an imaginary line drawn between the ischial spines. If the presenting part is below the ischial spines, the station is positive. Thus, 2 cm below the ischial spines is the station $+2$. (D) When the biparietal diameter is above the ischial spines by 5 cm, the presenting part is usually engaged or at station 0.

45. **(B)** Client need: health promotion and maintenance; subcategory: growth and development through the life span; content area: maternity

RATIONALE

(A) The fetus in the right occipitoposterior position would be presenting with the occiput in the maternal right posterior quadrant. (B) Fetal position is defined by the location of the fetal presenting part in the four quadrants of the maternal pelvis. The right occipitoanterior is a fetus presenting with the occiput in mother's right anterior quadrant. (C) The fetus in right sacroanterior position would be presenting a sacrum, not an occiput. (D) The fetus in left occipitoanterior position would be presenting with the occiput in the mother's left anterior quadrant.

46. **(D)** Client need: physiological integrity; subcategory: pharmacological and parenteral therapies; content area: maternity

RATIONALE

(A) Oxytocin stimulates labor but should not be used until CPD (cephalopelvic disproportion) is ruled out in a dysfunctional labor. (B) This answer is the correct protocol for oxytocin administration, but the medication should not be used until CPD is ruled out. (C) This answer is the correct manner to interpret effective stimulation, but oxytocin should not be used until CPD is ruled out. (D) This answer is the appropriate nursing action because the scenario presents a dysfunctional labor pattern that may be caused by CPD. Oxytocin administration is contraindicated in CPD.

47. **(B)** Client need: health promotion and maintenance; subcategory: growth and development through the life span; content area: maternity

RATIONALE

(A) Lamaze childbirth preparation teaches the use of chest, not abdominal, breathing. (B) In Lamaze preparation, every patterned breath is preceded by a cleansing breath; as labor progresses, shallow, paced breathing is found to be effective. (C) It is important to assume a comfortable position in labor, but the Lamaze-prepared laboring woman is taught to breathe with her chest, not abdominal, muscles. (D) When deep chest breathing patterns are used in Lamaze preparation, they are slowly paced at a rate of 6–9 breaths/min.

48. **(B)** Client need: physiological integrity; subcategory: reduction of risk potential; content area: med/surg

    RATIONALE

    (A) Diarrhea is a complication of tube feedings that can lead to dehydration. Diarrhea may be the result of hypertonic formulas that can draw fluid into the bowel. Other causes of diarrhea may be bacterial contamination, fecal impaction, medications, and low albumin. (B) A consistent weight gain of more than 0.22 kg/day (½ lb/day) over several days should be reported promptly. The client should be evaluated for fluid volume excess. (C) Elevating the client's head prevents reflux and thus formula from entering the airway. (D) Bacteria proliferate rapidly in enteral formulas and can cause gastroenteritis and even sepsis.

49. **(B)** Client need: physiological integrity; subcategory: physiological adaptation; content area: med/surg

    RATIONALE

    (A) Calf pain with dorsiflexion of the foot (Homans' sign) can be a sign of a deep venous thrombosis; however, it is not diagnostic of the condition. (B) Swelling and warmth along the affected vein are commonly observed clinical manifestations of a deep venous thrombosis as a result of inflammation of the vessel wall. (C) Rubbing or massaging of the affected leg is contraindicated because of the risk of the clot breaking loose and becoming an embolus. (D) A pillow behind the knee can be constricting and further impair blood flow.

50. **(A)** Client need: physiological integrity; subcategory: reduction of risk potential; content area: med/surg

    RATIONALE

    (A) Partial thromboplastin time is used to monitor the effects of heparin, and dosage is adjusted depending on test results. It is a screening test used to detect deficiencies in all plasma clotting factors except factors VII and XIII and platelets. (B) Hemoglobin is the main component of RBCs. Its main function is to carry O_2 from the lungs to the body tissues and to transport CO_2 back to the lungs. (C) RBC count is the determination of the number of RBCs found in each cubic millimeter of whole blood. (D) PT is used to monitor the effects of oral anticoagulants, e.g., coumarin-type anticoagulants.

51. **(C)** Client need: physiological integrity; subcategory: reduction of risk potential; content area: med/surg

    RATIONALE

    (A) Using an electric razor prevents the risk of cuts while shaving. (B) Any physician or dentist should be informed of anticoagulant therapy because of the risk of bleeding due to a prolonged PT. (C) The client should be instructed to consult his physician. Aspirin is avoided because it potentiates the affects of oral anticoagulants by interfering with platelet aggregation. (D) Identification bracelets are necessary to direct treatment, especially in an emergency situation.

52. **(A)** Client need: physiological integrity; subcategory: pharmacological and parenteral therapies; content area: med/surg

    RATIONALE

    (A) The therapeutic blood level range of theophylline is 10–20 mg/mL. Therapeutic drug monitoring determines effective drug dosages and prevents toxicity. (B, D) This value is a toxic level of the drug. (C) This value is a nontherapeutic level of the drug.

53. **(B)** Client need: physiological integrity; subcategory: physiological adaptation; content area: med/surg

    RATIONALE

    (A) The client would not receive therapeutic effects of the glucocorticoid when it is inhaled through constricted airways. (B) Bronchodilating the airways *first* allows for the glucocorticoid to be inhaled through open airways and increases the penetration of the steroid for maximum effectiveness of the drug. (C) Inac-

curate use of the inhalers will lead to decreased effectiveness of the treatment. (D) Client teaching regarding the use and effects of inhalers will promote client understanding and compliance.

54. **(B)** Client need: health promotion and maintenance; subcategory: prevention and early detection of disease; content area: med/surg

    RATIONALE

    (A) It is sufficient to rinse the plastic holders with warm water at least once per day. (B) It is important to rinse the mouth after each use to minimize the risk of fungal infections by reducing the droplets of the glucocorticoid left in the oral cavity. (C) Antacids act by neutralizing or reducing gastric acid, thus decreasing the pH of the stomach. "Neutralizing" the oral mucosa prior to inhalation of a steroid inhaler does not minimize the risk of fungal infections. (D) Rinsing prior to the use of the glucocorticoid will not eliminate the droplets left on the oral mucous membranes following the use of the inhaler.

55. **(C)** Client need: physiological integrity; subcategory: basic care and comfort; content area: med/surg

    RATIONALE

    (A) Protein is vital for the maintenance of muscle to aid in breathing. A high-calorie diet using higher fat than carbohydrate content is given because clients are unable to breathe off the excess CO_2 that is an end product of carbohydrate metabolism. (B) Inadequate nutritional status, in particular, deficiencies in vitamins A and C, decreases resistance to infection. (C) Milk does not make mucus thicker. It may coat the back of the throat and make it feel thicker. Rinsing the mouth with water after drinking milk will prevent this problem. (D) Small, frequent meals minimize a fullness sensation and reduce pressure on the diaphragm. The work of breathing and SOB are also reduced.

56. **(D)** Client need: physiological integrity; subcategory: reduction of risk potential; content area: med/surg

    RATIONALE

    (A) The effects of morphine or an allergic response to the drug will not affect theophylline clearance. (B) Xanthines are used cautiously in clients with severe cardiac disease, liver disease, cor pulmonale, hypertension, or hyperthyroidism. Arthritis does not influence the dosage of theophylline. (C) Theophylline does not cause sedation or drowsiness. Conversely, its side effects may be exhibited by central nervous system stimulation. (D) Cimetidine decreases theophylline clearance from the system and increases theophylline levels in the blood, thus increasing the risk of toxicity.

57. **(D)** Client need: health promotion and maintenance; subcategory: prevention and early detection of disease; content area: maternity

    RATIONALE

    (A) Mild PIH is not treated with medications. (B) Emotional stress is not the cause of blood pressure elevation in PIH. (C) Excessive caloric intake is not the cause of weight gain in PIH. (D) The client most frequently is not aware of the signs and symptoms in mild PIH.

58. **(D)** Client need: health promotion and maintenance; subcategory: prevention and early detection of disease; content area: maternity

    RATIONALE

    (A, B, C) The individual's systolic and diastolic changes are more significant than the relatively high initial blood pressure readings. (D) The systolic pressure went up 12 mm Hg and the diastolic pressure 18 mm Hg. This is a more significant rise than the increases in A–C choices, and client should receive more frequent evaluations and care.

59. **(D)** Client need: physiological integrity; subcategory: physiological adaptation; content area: maternity

RATIONALE

(A) Overeating can lead to obesity, but not to edema. (B) There is no indication of obesity prior to pregnancy. PIH is more prevalent in the underweight than in the obese in this age group. (C) Hypertension can be due to kidney lesions, but it would have been apparent earlier in the pregnancy. (D) The weight gain in PIH is due to the retention of sodium ions and fluid and is one of the three cardinal symptoms of PIH.

60. **(B)** Client need: physiological integrity; subcategory: pharmacological and parenteral therapies; content area: maternity

RATIONALE

(A) An anticonvulsant effect is the goal of drug therapy for PIH. However, we would not want to increase the vasoconstriction that is already present. This would make the symptoms more severe. (B) An anticonvulsant effect and vasodilation are the desired outcomes when administering this drug. (C) An anticonvulsant effect is the goal of drug therapy for PIH; however, hypertensive drugs would increase the blood pressure even more. (D) An anticonvulsant effect is the goal of drug therapy for PIH. $MgSO_4$ is not classified as an antiemetic. Antiemetics are not indicated for PIH treatment.

61. **(D)** Client need: physiological integrity; subcategory: pharmacological and parenteral therapies; content area: maternity

RATIONALE

(A, C) The nurse should provide good distractors because these symptoms indicate that PIH has become more severe and may precede the convulsive or eclamptic phase. (B) This is the opposite side effect of this medication. (D) This is a common side effect of this medication and needs to be monitored and recorded frequently.

62. **(C)** Client need: physiological integrity; subcategory: pharmacological and parenteral therapies; content area: maternity

RATIONALE

(A, B) These drugs are not antidotes for $MgSO_4$. (C) This drug is the standard antidote and should always be readily available when $MgSO_4$ is being administered. (D) This drug is an antidote for narcotics, not $MgSO_4$.

63. **(C)** Client need: physiological integrity; subcategory: pharmacological and parenteral therapies; content area: maternity

RATIONALE

(A) The client may be anxious and hyperresponsive to stimuli but not necessarily restless. (B) This is not a physiological response to an elevated blood pressure in PIH. (C) The nurse must know the nursing measures that decrease the potential for convulsions. A quiet, darkened room decreases stimuli and promotes rest. (D) External stimuli might induce a convulsion but are not annoying to the client with PIH.

64. **(C)** Client need: health promotion and maintenance; subcategory: growth and development through the life span; content area: maternity

RATIONALE

(A) This nursing action may cause hyperventilation. (B) This nursing action could cause inferior vena cava syndrome. (C) The client is allowed to push only after complete dilation during the second stage of labor. The nurse needs to know the stages of labor. (D) If the client pushes before dilation, it could cause cervical edema and/or edema to the fetal scalp; both of these could contribute to increased risk of complications.

65. **(D)** Client need: physiological integrity; subcategory: physiological adaptation; content area: maternity

RATIONALE

(A) Saline should be warmed; waiting 15 minutes may not keep the cord moist. (B) This choice does not specify what the sponge was "wet" with. (C) This measure would stop circulation to the fetus. (D) The cord should be kept warm and moist to maintain fetal circulation. This measure is an accepted nursing action.

66. **(D)** Client need: physiological integrity; subcategory: physiological adaptation; content area: maternity

RATIONALE

(A) Fetal tachycardia may indicate fetal hypoxia; however, 170 bpm is only mild tachycardia. (B) Nausea and vomiting occur frequently during transition and are not a complication. (C) Contractions frequently last 60–90 seconds during the transitional phase of labor and are not considered a complication as long as the uterus relaxes completely between contractions. (D) Passage of meconium in a vertex presentation is a sign of fetal distress; this may be normal in a breech presentation owing to pressure on the presenting part.

67. **(C)** Client need: health promotion and maintenance; subcategory: growth and development through the life span; content area: maternity

RATIONALE

(A) FHT should be monitored continuously with an induction of labor; this is an accepted standard of care. (B) The physician should be notified, but this is not the first intervention the nurse should do. (C) The standard of care for an induction according to the Association of Women's Health, Obstetric, and Neonatal Nurses and American College of Obstetrics and Gynecology is that contractions should not exceed 60 seconds in an induction. Inductions should simulate normal labor; 70-second contractions during the latent phase (3 cm) are not the norm. The next contractions can be longer and increase risks to the mother and fetus. (D) Contractions lasting 60–90 seconds during transition are typical; this provides a good distractor. The nurse needs to be knowledgeable of the phases and stages of labor.

68. **(D)** Client need: health promotion and maintenance; subcategory: growth and development through the life span; content area: maternity

RATIONALE

(A, B) Endometritis, urine retention, or bladder distention provide good distractors because they may delay involution but do not usually cause the uterus to be lateral. (C) Bowel distention and constipation are common in the postpartum period but do not displace the uterus laterally. (D) Urine retention or bladder distention commonly displaces the uterus to the right and may delay involution.

69. **(C)** Client need: physiological integrity; subcategory: physiological adaptation; content area: maternity

RATIONALE

(A) Bradycardia is an expected assessment during the postpartum period. (B) Diuresis can occur during labor and the postpartum period and is an expected physiological adaptation. (C) A return of rubra after the serosa period may indicate a postpartal complication. (D) Diaphoresis, especially at night, is an expected physiological change and does not indicate an infectious process. Bradycardia, diuresis, and diaphoresis are normal postpartum physiological responses to adjust the cardiac output and blood volume to the nonpregnant state.

70. **(D)** Client need: physiological integrity; subcategory: physiological adaptation; content area: maternity

RATIONALE

(A) Afterbirth pains are a common complaint in the postpartum client, but they are located in the uterus. (B) Constipation may cause rectal pressure but is not usually associated with "severe pain." (C) Cystitis may cause pain, but the location is different. (D) Hematomas are frequently associated with severe pain and pressure. Further assessments are indicated for this client.

TEST 3

McNeese State University College of Nursing Test

MOCK NCLEX-RN BOARD REVIEW TEST QUESTIONS

1. After a 10-year-old child with insulin-dependent diabetes mellitus receives her dinner tray, she tells the nurse that she hates broccoli and wants some corn on the cob. The nurse's appropriate response is:

   A. "No vegetable exchanges are allowed."
   B. "Corn and other starchy vegetables are considered to be bread exchanges."
   C. "Yes, you may exchange any vegetable for any other vegetable."
   D. "Yes, but only one-half ear is allowed."

2. The nurse is teaching a 10-year-old insulin-dependent diabetic how to administer insulin. Which one of the following steps must be taught for insulin administration?

   A. Never use abdominal site for a rotation site.
   B. Pinch the skin up to form a subcutaneous pocket.
   C. Avoid applying pressure after injection.
   D. Change needles after injection.

3. In assessing the nature of the stool of a client who has cystic fibrosis, what would the nurse expect to see?

   A. Clay-colored stools
   B. Steatorrhea stools
   C. Dark brown stools
   D. Blood-tinged stools

4. A group of nursing students at a local preschool day care center are going to screen each child's fine and gross motor, language, and social skills. The students will use which one of the most widely used screening tests?

   A. Revised Prescreening Developmental Questionnaire
   B. Goodenough Draw-a-Person Screening Test
   C. Denver Development Screening Test
   D. Caldwell Home Inventory

5. A mother came to the pediatric clinic with her 17-month-old child. The mother would like to begin toilet training. What should the nurse teach her about implementing toilet training?

   A. Take two or three favorite toys with the child.
   B. Have a child-sized toilet seat or training potty on hand.
   C. Explain to the child she is going to "void" and "defecate."
   D. Show disapproval if she does not void or defecate.

6. A mother is unsure about the type of toys for her 17-month-old child. Based on knowledge of growth and development, what toy would the nurse suggest?

   A. A pull toy to encourage locomotion
   B. A mobile to improve hand-eye coordination
   C. A large toy with movable parts to improve pincer grasp
   D. Various large colored blocks to teach visual discrimination

7. A 16-year-old student has a long history of bronchial asthma and has experienced several severe asthmatic attacks during the school year. The school nurse is required to administer 0.2 mL of 1/1000 solution of epinephrine SC during an asthma attack. How does the school nurse evaluate the effectiveness of this intervention?

   A. Increased pulse rate
   B. Increased expectorate of secretions
   C. Decreased inspiratory difficulty
   D. Increased respiratory rate

8. Respiratory function is altered in a 16-year-old asthmatic. Which of the following is the cause of this alteration?

   A. Altered surfactant production
   B. Paradoxical movements of the chest wall
   C. Increased airway resistance
   D. Continuous changes in respiratory rate and depth

9. A mother frantically calls the emergency room (ER) asking what to do about her 3-year-old girl who was found eating pills out of a bottle in the medicine cabinet. The ER nurse tells the mother to:

   A. Give the child 15 mL of syrup of ipecac.
   B. Give the child 10 mL of syrup of ipecac with a sip of water.
   C. Give the child 1 cup of water to induce vomiting.
   D. Bring the child to the ER immediately.

10. A mother brings her 3-year-old child who is unconscious but breathing to the ER with an apparent drug overdose. The mother found an empty bottle of aspirin next to her child in the bathroom. Which nursing action is the most appropriate?

    A. Put in a nasogastric tube and lavage the child's stomach.
    B. Monitor muscular status.
    C. Teach mother poison prevention techniques.
    D. Place child on respiratory assistance.

11. A parent told the public health nurse that her 6-year-old son has been taking tetracycline for a chronic skin condition. The parent asked if this could cause any problems for the child. What should the nurse explain to the parent?

    A. Giving tetracycline to a child younger than 8 years may cause permanent staining of his teeth.
    B. If you give tetracycline with milk, it may be absorbed readily.
    C. The medication should be given to adults, not children.
    D. Secondary infections of chronic skin disorders do not respond to antibiotics.

12. A 6-month-old infant has developmental delays. His weight falls below the 5th percentile when plotted on a growth chart. A diagnosis of failure to thrive is made. What behaviors might indicate the possibility of maternal deprivation?

    A. Responsive to touch, wants to be held
    B. Uncomforted by touch, refuses bottle
    C. Maintains eye-to-eye contact
    D. Finicky eater, easily pacified, cuddly

13. A mother continues to breast-feed her 3-month-old infant. She tells the nurse that over the past 3 days she has not been producing enough milk to satisfy the infant. The nurse advises the mother to do which of the following?

    A. "Start the child on solid food."
    B. "Nurse the child more frequently during this growth spurt."
    C. "Provide supplements for the child between breast-feeding so you will have enough milk."
    D. "Wait 4 hours between feedings so that your breasts will fill up."

14. An 8-week-old infant has been diagnosed with gastro-esophageal reflux. The nurse is teaching the infant's mother to care for the infant at home. Which one of the following statements by the nurse is appropriate regarding the infant's home care?

    A. "Lay the infant flat on her left side after feeding."
    B. "Feed the infant every 4 hours with half-strength formula."
    C. "Antacids need to be given an hour before feeding."
    D. "Play activities should be carried out before instead of after feedings."

15. The nurse is preparing a 6-year-old child for an IV insertion. Which one of the following statements by the nurse is appropriate when preparing a child for a potentially painful procedure?

    A. "Some say this feels like a pinch or a bug bite. You tell me what it feels like."
    B. "This is going to hurt a lot; close your eyes and hold my hand."
    C. "This is a terrible procedure, so don't look."
    D. "This will hurt only a little; try to be a big boy."

16. The nurse enters the playroom and finds an 8-year-old child having a grand mal seizure. Which one of the following actions should the nurse take?

    A. Place a tongue blade in the child's mouth.
    B. Restrain the child so he will not injure himself.
    C. Go to the nurses station and call the physician.
    D. Move furniture out of the way and place a blanket under his head.

17. A six-month-old infant is receiving ribavirin for the treatment of respiratory syncytial virus. Ribavirin is administered via which one of the following routes?

    A. Oral
    B. IM
    C. IV
    D. Aerosol

18. A 5-year-old child has suffered second-degree thermal burns over 30% of her body. Forty-eight hours after the burn injury, the nurse must begin to monitor the child for which one of the following complications?

    A. Fluid volume deficit
    B. Fluid volume excess
    C. Decreased cardiac output
    D. Severe hypotension

19. Which one of the following is considered a reliable indicator for assessing the adequacy of fluid resuscitation in a 3-year-old child who suffered partial- and full-thickness burns to 25% of her body?

    A. Urine output
    B. Edema
    C. Hypertension
    D. Bulging fontanelle

20. A 4-year-old child is being discharged from the hospital after being treated for severe croup. Which one of the following instructions should the nurse give to the child's mother for the home treatment of croup?

    A. Take him in the bathroom, turn on the hot water, and close the door.
    B. Give him a dose of antihistamine.
    C. Give large amounts of clear liquids if drooling occurs.
    D. Place him near a cool mist vaporizer and encourage crying.

21. A 7-year-old child is brought to the ER at midnight by his mother after symptoms appeared abruptly. The nurse's initial assessment reveals a temperature of 104.5°F (40.3°C), difficulty swallowing, drooling, absence of a spontaneous cough, and agitation. These symptoms are indicative of which one of the following?

    A. Acute tracheitis
    B. Acute spasmodic croup
    C. Acute epiglottis
    D. Acute laryngotracheobronchitis

22. The nurse is teaching a mother care of her child's spica cast. The mother states that he complains of itching under the edge of the cast. One nonpharmacological technique the nurse might suggest would be:

    A. "Blowing air under the cast using a hair dryer on cool setting often relieves itching."
    B. "Slide a ruler under the cast and scratch the area."
    C. "Guide a towel under and through the cast and move it back and forth to relieve the itch."
    D. "Gently thump on cast to dislodge dried skin that causes the itching."

23. A 30-year-old client has just been treated in the ER for bruises and abrasions to her face and a broken arm from domestic violence, which has been increasing in frequency and intensity over the last few months. The nurse assesses her as being very anxious, fearful, bewildered, and feeling helpless as she states, "I don't know what to do, I'm afraid to go home." The best response by the nurse to the client would be:

    A. "I wouldn't want to go home either; call a friend who could help you."
    B. "Did you do something that could have made him so angry?"
    C. "Let's talk about people and resources available to you so that you don't have to go home."
    D. "I'll call the police and they will take care of him, and you can go home and get some rest."

24. A 26-year-old client is in a treatment center for aprazolam (Xanax) abuse and continues to manifest moderate levels of anxiety 3 weeks into the rehabilitation program, often requesting medication for "his nerves." Included in the client's plan of care is to identify alternate methods of coping with stress and anxiety other than use of medication. After intervening with assistance in stress reduction techniques, identifying feelings and past coping, the nurse evaluates the outcome as being met if:

    A. Client promises that he will not abuse aprazolam after discharge
    B. Client demonstrates use of exercise or physical activity to handle nervous energy following conflicts of everyday life
    C. Client is able to verbalize effects of substance abuse on the body
    D. Client has remained substance free during hospitalization and is discharged

25. A 23-year-old borderline client is admitted to an inpatient psychiatric unit following an impulsive act of self-mutilation. A few hours after admission, she requests special privileges, and when these are not granted, she stands up and angrily shouts that the people on the unit do not care, and she storms across the room. The nurse should respond to this behavior by:

    A. Placing her in seclusion until the behavior is under control
    B. Walking up to the client and touching her on the arm to get her attention
    C. Communicating a desire to assist the client to regain control, offering a one-to-one session in a quiet area
    D. Confronting the client, letting her know the consequences for getting angry and disrupting the unit

26. A 56-year-old client is admitted to the psychiatric unit in a state of total despair. She feels hopeless and worthless, has a flat affect and very sad appearance, and is unable to feel pleasure from anything. Her husband has been assisting her at home with the housework and cooking; however, she has not been eating much, lies around or sits in a chair most of the day, and is becoming confused and thinks her family does not want her around anymore. In assessing the client, the nurse determines that her behavior is consistent with:

    A. Transient depression
    B. Mild depression
    C. Moderate depression
    D. Severe depression

27. A 56-year-old psychiatric inpatient has had recurring episodes of depression and chronic low self-esteem. She feels that her family does not want her around, experiences a sense of helplessness, and has a negative view of herself. To assist the client in focusing on her strengths and positive traits, a strategy used by the nurse would be to:

    A. Tell the client to attend all structured activities on the unit
    B. Encourage or direct client to attend activities that offer simple methods to attain success
    C. Increase the client's self-esteem by asking that she make all decisions regarding attendance in group activities
    D. Not allow any dependent behaviors by the client because she must learn independence and will have to ask for any assistance from staff

28. A 42-year-old client on an inpatient psychiatric unit comments that he was brought to the hospital by his wife because he had taken too many pills and states, "I just couldn't take it anymore." The nurse's best response to this disclosure would be:

    A. "You shouldn't do things like that, just tell someone you feel bad."
    B. "Tell me more about what you couldn't take anymore."
    C. "I'm sure you probably didn't mean to kill yourself."
    D. "How long have you been in the hospital."

29. A 42-year-old client with bipolar disorder has been hospitalized on the inpatient psychiatric unit. She is dancing around, talking incessantly, and singing. Much of

the time the client is anorexic and eats very little from her tray before she is up and about again. The nurse's intervention would be to:

A. Confront the client with the fact that she will have to eat more from her tray to sustain her
B. Try to get the client to focus on her eating by offering a detailed discussion on the importance of nutrition
C. Let her have snacks and drinks anytime that she wants them because she will not eat at regular meal times
D. Not expect the client to sit down for complete meals; monitor intake, offering snacks and juice frequently

30. Assessment of severe depression in a client reveals feelings of hopelessness, worthlessness; inability to feel pleasure; sleep, psychomotor, and nutritional alterations; delusional thinking; negative view of self; and feelings of abandonment. These clinical features of the client's depression alert the nurse to prioritize problems and care by addressing which of the following problems first:

A. Nutritional status
B. Impaired thinking
C. Possible harm to self
D. Rest and activity impairment

31. The nurse is assessing and getting a history from a client treated for depression with a monoamine oxidase (MAO) antidepressant. The *most* serious side effect associated with this antidepressant and the ingestion of tyramine in aged foods may be:

A. Hypertensive crisis
B. Severe rash
C. Severe hypotension
D. Severe diarrhea

32. A cardinal symptom of the schizophrenic client is hallucinations. A nurse identifies this as a problem in the category of:

A. Impaired communication
B. Sensory-perceptual alterations
C. Altered thought processes
D. Impaired social interaction

33. A schizophrenic client who is experiencing thoughts of having special powers states that "I am a messenger from another planet and can rule the earth." The nurse assesses this behavior as:

A. Ideas of reference
B. Delusions of persecution
C. Thought broadcasting
D. Delusions of grandeur

34. A client experiencing delusions states, "I came here because there were people surrounding my house that wanted to take me away and use my body for science." The best response by the nurse would be:

A. "Describe the people surrounding your house that want to take you away."
B. "I need more information on why you think others want to use your body for science."
C. "There were no people surrounding your house, your relatives brought you here, and no one really wants your body for science."
D. "I know that must be frightening for you; let the staff know when you are having thoughts that trouble you."

35. A 16-year-old client with anorexia nervosa is on an inpatient psychiatric unit. She has a fear of gaining weight and is refusing to eat sufficient amounts to maintain body weight for her age, height, and stature. To assist with the problem of powerlessness and plan for the client to no longer need to withhold food to feel in control, the nurse uses the following strategy:

A. Establish a structured environment with routine tasks and activities. Also, serve meals at the same time each day.
B. Distract the client during meals to get her to eat because she must take in sufficient amounts to keep from starving.
C. Do frequent room checks to be sure that the client is not hiding food or throwing it away.
D. Listen attentively and participate in in-depth discussions about food, because these actions may encourage her to eat.

36. A 45-year-old male client was admitted to a chemical dependency treatment center following legal problems related to alcohol abuse. He states, "I know that alcohol is a problem for some people, but I can stop whenever I want to. I'm never sick or miss work, and no one can complain about me." During the initial assessment, the best response by the nurse would be:

A. "The fact is you are an alcoholic or you wouldn't be here."
B. "I understand it took strength to admit yourself to the unit, and I will do my part to help you to stay alcohol-free."
C. "If you can stop drinking when you want to, why don't you stop?"
D. "It's good that you can stop drinking when you want to."

37. A 79-year-old client with Alzheimer's disease is exhibiting significant memory impairment, cognitive impairment, extremely impaired judgment in social situations, and agitation when placed in a new situation or around unfamiliar people. The nurse should include the following strategy in the client's care:

A. Maintain routines and usual structure and adhere to schedules.
B. Encourage the client to attend all structured activities on the unit, whether she wants to or not.
C. Ask the client to go to an activity once. If she gives no response right away, change the question around, asking the same thing.
D. Give the client two or three choices to decide what she wants to do.

38. The nurse working with a client who is out of control should follow a model of intervention that includes which of the following?

A. Approach the client on a continuum of least restrictive care.

B. Challenge client's behavior immediately with steps to prevent injury to self or others.

C. Leave the aggressive client to himself or herself, and take other clients away.

D. To ensure safety of other clients, place client in seclusion immediately when he or she begins shouting.

39. When planning care for the passive-aggressive client, the nurse includes the following goal:

A. Allow the client to use humor, because this may be the only way this client can express self.

B. Allow the client to express anger by using "I" messages, such as "I was angry when . . .," etc.

C. Allow the client to have time away from therapeutic responsibilities.

D. Allow the client to give excuses if he forgets to give staff information.

40. A client calls the prenatal clinic to schedule an appointment. She states she has missed three menstrual periods and thinks she might be pregnant. During her first visit to the prenatal clinic, it is confirmed that she is pregnant. The registered nurse (RN) learns that her last menstrual period began on June 10. According to Nägele's rule, the estimated date of confinement is:

A. March 17
B. June 3
C. August 30
D. January 10

41. At 16 weeks' gestation, a pregnant client is admitted to the maternity unit to have a McDonald procedure (cerclage) done. She tells the RN who is admitting her to the unit that her physician had explained what this procedure was, but that she did not understand. The RN explains to the client that the purpose for this procedure is to:

A. Reinforce an incompetent cervix
B. Repair the amniotic sac
C. Evaluate cephalopelvic disproportion
D. Dilate the cervix

42. A pregnant client continues to visit the clinic regularly during her pregnancy. During one of her visits while lying supine on the examining table, she tells the RN that she is becoming light-headed. The RN notices that the client has pallor in her face and is perspiring profusely. The first intervention the RN should initiate is to:

A. Place the examining table in the Trendelenburg position
B. Assess the client to see if she is having vaginal bleeding
C. Obtain the client's vital signs immediately
D. Help the client to a sitting position

43. At 30 weeks' gestation, a client is admitted to the unit in premature labor. Her contractions are every 5 minutes and last 60 seconds, her cervix is closed, and the suture placed around her cervix during her 16th week of gestation, when she had the MacDonald procedure, can still be felt by the physician. The amniotic sac is still intact. She is very concerned about delivering prematurely. She asks the RN, "What is the greatest risk to my baby if it is born prematurely?" The RN's answer should be:

A. Hyperglycemia
B. Hypoglycemia

C. Lack of development of the intestines
D. Lack of development of the lungs

44. At 30 weeks' gestation, a client is admitted to the unit in premature labor. Her physician orders that an IV be started with 500 mL D_5W mixed with 150 mg of ritodrine stat. The RN prepares the IV solution with the medication. The RN knows that clients receiving the medication ritodrine IV should be observed closely for which one of the following side effects:

A. Hypoglycemia
B. Hyperkalemia
C. Tachycardia
D. Increase in hematocrit and hemoglobin

45. At 32 weeks' gestation, a client is scheduled for a fetal activity test (nonstress test). She calls the clinic and asks the RN, "How do I prepare for the test I am scheduled for?" The RN will most likely inform her of the following instructions to help prepare her for the test:

A. "You need to know that an IV is always started before the test."

B. "You will need to drink 6 to 8 glasses of water to fill your bladder."

C. "Do not eat any food or drink any liquids before the test is started."

D. "You will have to remain as still as you possibly can."

46. After the fetal activity test (nonstress test) is completed, the RN is looking at the test results on the monitor strip. The RN observes that the fetal heart accelerated 5 beats/min with each fetal movement. The accelerations lasted ≥15 seconds and occurred 3 times during the 20-minute test. The RN knows that these test results will be interpreted as:

A. A reactive test
B. A nonreactive test
C. An unsatisfactory test
D. A negative test

47. At 38 weeks' gestation, a client is in active labor. She is using her Lamaze breathing techniques. The RN is coaching her breathing and encouraging her to relax and work with her contractions. Which one of the following complaints by the client will alert the RN that she is beginning to hyperventilate with her breathing?

A. "I am cold."
B. "I have a backache."
C. "I feel dizzy."
D. "I am nauseous."

48. After performing a sterile vaginal exam on a client who has just been admitted to the unit in active labor and placed on an electronic fetal monitor, the RN assesses that the fetal head is at 21 station. She documents this on the monitor strip. Fetal head at 21 station means that the fetal head is located where in the pelvis?

A. One centimeter below the ischial spines
B. One centimeter above the ischial spines
C. Has not entered the pelvic inlet yet
D. Located in the pelvic outlet

49. A client has been admitted to the labor and delivery unit in active labor. After assessing her, the RN notes that the client's fetus position is left occipital posterior. Which of the following statements best describes what this means to the labor process:

    A. Decreases the overall time of the labor process
    B. Prolongs the client's first stage of labor
    C. Decreases the time of the client's first stage of labor
    D. Prolongs the client's third stage of labor

50. A client is in active labor and has been admitted to the labor and delivery unit. The RN has just done a sterile vaginal exam and determines that the client is dilated 5 cm, effaced 85%, and the fetus's head is at 0 station. She asks if she could have a lumbar epidural now. The epidural is started, and the anesthetic agent used is bupivacaine (Marcaine). After the client has received her lumbar epidural, it is important for the RN to monitor her for which of the following side effects:

    A. Hypertension
    B. Hypotension
    C. Hypoglycemia
    D. Hyperglycemia

51. A client has been in labor for 10 hours. Her contractions have become hypoactive and slowed in duration. The fetus is at 0 station, cervix is dilated 8 cm and effaced 90%. The physician orders an oxytocin (Pitocin) infusion to be started at once. The RN begins the oxytocin infusion. It is important that the RN discontinue the infusion if which one of the following occur?

    A. The client's contractions are <2 minutes apart.
    B. Duration of the contractions are 60 seconds.
    C. The uterus relaxes between contractions.
    D. The client complains that she is tired.

52. The client has been in active labor for the last 12 hours. During the last 3 hours, labor has been augmented with oxytocin because of hypoactive uterine contractions. Her physician assesses her cervix as 95% effaced, 8 cm dilated, and the fetus is at 0 station. Her oral temperature is 100.2°F at this time. The physician orders that she be prepared for a cesarean delivery. In preparing the client for the cesarean delivery, which one of the following physician's orders should the RN question?

    A. Administer meperidine (Demerol) 100 mg IM 1 hour prior to the delivery.
    B. Discontinue the oxytocin infusion.
    C. Insert an indwelling Foley catheter prior to delivery.
    D. Prepare abdominal area from below the nipples to below the symphysis pubis area.

53. After an infant is delivered by cesarean delivery and placed on the warmer, the RN dries and assesses the infant. At 1 and 5 minutes after birth, the RN does the Apgar scoring of the infant. The RN knows that because this infant was delivered by cesarean section, he is at increased risk for having which one of the following?

    A. Cold stress
    B. Cyanosis
    C. Respiratory distress syndrome
    D. Seizures

54. After the RN is finished the initial assessment of a newborn baby and after the initial bonding between the newborn and the mother has taken place in the delivery room, the RN will bring the newborn to the well-baby nursery. Before the newborn is taken from the delivery room and brought to the well-baby nursery, the RN makes sure that which of the following interventions was completed?

    A. The physician verifies the exact time of birth.
    B. The nurse counts the instruments and sponges with the scrub nurse.
    C. The nurse instills prophylactic ointment in the conjunctival sacs of the newborn's eyes.
    D. The nurse makes sure the mother and her newborn have been tagged with identical bands.

55. On a mother's 2nd postpartum day after having a vaginal delivery, the RN is preparing to assess her perineum and anus as part of her daily assessment. The *best* position for the client to be placed in for this assessment is:

    A. Sims'
    B. Fowler's
    C. Prone
    D. Any position that the RN chooses

56. While the RN is assessing a mother's perineum on her 2nd postpartum day after having a vaginal delivery, the RN notes a large ecchymotic area located to the left of the mother's perineum. Which one of the following interventions should the RN initiate at this time?

    A. Have the client expose the area to air.
    B. Apply ice to the perineum.
    C. Encourage the client to take warm sitz baths.
    D. Inform the physician.

57. A mother who is breast-feeding her newborn asks the RN, "How can I express milk from my breasts manually?" The RN tells her that the correct method for manual milk expression includes using the thumb and the index finger to:

    A. Alternately compress and release each nipple
    B. Roll the nipple and gently pull the nipple forward
    C. Slide the thumb and index finger forward from the outer border of the areola toward the end of the nipple
    D. Compress and release each breast at the outer border of the areola

58. A client had a vaginal delivery 3 days ago and is discharged from the hospital on the 2nd day postpartum. She told the RN, "I need to start exercising so that I can get back into shape. Could you suggest an exercise I could begin with?" The RN could suggest which one of the following?

    A. Push-ups
    B. Jumping jacks
    C. Leg lifts
    D. Kegel exercises

59. A 60-year-old male client was hospitalized 3 days ago with the diagnosis of acute anterior wall myocardial infarction. Today he has been complaining of increasing weakness and shortness of breath. Crackles in both lung bases are audible on auscultation. He is developing:

A. An extension of his myocardial infarction
B. Pneumonia
C. Pulmonary edema
D. Pulmonary emboli

60. On admission, the client has signs and symptoms of pulmonary edema. The nurse places the client in the *most* appropriate position for a client in pulmonary edema, which is:

    A. High Fowler
    B. Lying on the left side
    C. Sitting in a chair
    D. Supine with feet elevated

61. A male client has been hospitalized with congestive heart failure. Medical management of heart failure focuses on improving myocardial contractility. This can be achieved by administering:

    A. Digoxin (Lanoxin) 0.25 mg po every day
    B. Furosemide (Lasix) 40 mg po every morning
    C. O_2 2 L/min via nasal cannula
    D. Nitroglycerin (Nitrol) 1 inch topically every 4 hours

62. A client's congestive heart failure has been treated, and he will soon be discharged. Discharge teaching should include instruction to call the physician if he notices a 2-lb weight gain in a 24-hour period. Increased weight gain may indicate:

    A. A diet too high in calories and saturated fat
    B. Decreasing cardiac output
    C. Decreasing renal function
    D. Development of diabetes insipidus

63. A client was not using his seat belt when involved in a car accident. He fractured ribs 5, 6, and 7 on the left and developed a left pneumothorax. Assessment findings include:

    A. Crackles and paradoxical chest wall movement
    B. Decreased breath sounds on the left and chest pain with movement
    C. Rhonchi and frothy sputum
    D. Wheezing and dry cough

64. A client has a chest tube placed in his left pleural space to re-expand his collapsed lung. In a closed-chest drainage system, the purpose of the water seal is to:

    A. Prevent air from entering the pleural space
    B. Prevent fluid from entering the pleural space
    C. Provide a means to measure chest drainage
    D. Provide an indicator of respiratory effort

65. A client was admitted with rib fractures and a pneumothorax, which were sustained as a result of a motor vehicle accident. A chest tube was placed on the left side to reinflate his lung, and he was transferred to a client unit. Twenty-four hours after admission he continues to have bloody sputum, develops increasing hypoxemia, and his chest x-ray shows patchy infiltrates. The nurse analyzes these symptoms as being consistent with:

    A. Pneumonia
    B. Pulmonary contusions
    C. Pulmonary edema
    D. Tension pneumothorax

66. A 66-year-old female client has smoked 2 packs of cigarettes per day for 20 years. Her arterial blood gases on room air are as follows: pH 7.35; PO_2 70 mm Hg; PCO_2 55 mm Hg; HCO_3 32 mEq/L. These blood gases reflect:

    A. Compensated metabolic acidosis
    B. Compensated respiratory acidosis
    C. Compensated respiratory alkalosis
    D. Uncompensated respiratory acidosis

67. A female client who has chronic obstructive pulmonary disease (COPD) has presented in the emergency department with cough productive of yellow sputum and increasing shortness of breath. On room air, her blood gases are as follows: pH 7.30 mm Hg, PCO_2 60 mm Hg, PO_2 55 mm Hg, HCO_3 32 mEq/L. These arterial blood gases reflect:

    A. Compensated respiratory acidosis
    B. Normal blood gases
    C. Uncompensated metabolic acidosis
    D. Uncompensated respiratory acidosis

68. A 19-year-old client has sustained a C-7 fracture, which resulted in his spinal cord being partially transected. By 2 weeks' postinjury, his neck has been surgically stabilized, and he has been transferred from the intensive care unit. A potential life-threatening complication the nurse monitors the client for is:

    A. Autonomic dysreflexia
    B. Bradycardia
    C. Central cord syndrome
    D. Spinal shock

69. A 17-year-old client has a T-4 spinal cord injury. At present, he is learning to catheterize himself. When he says, "This is too much trouble. I would rather just have a Foley." An appropriate response for the RN teaching him would be:

    A. "I know. It is a lot to learn. In the long run, though, you will be able to reduce infections if you do an intermittent catheterization program."
    B. "It is not too much trouble. This is the best way to manage urination."
    C. "OK. I'll ask your physician if we can replace the Foley."
    D. "You need to learn this because your doctor ordered it."

70. A client's physician has prescribed theophylline (Theo-Dur) to help control the bronchospasm associated with the client's COPD. Instructions that should be given to the client include:

    A. "Call your physician if you develop palpitations, dizziness, or restlessness."
    B. "Cigarette smoking may significantly increase the risk for theophylline toxicity."
    C. "Take this medication on an empty stomach."
    D. "Do not take your medicine if your pulse is less than 60 beats per minute."

71. A 19-year-old client fell off a ladder approximately 3 ft to the ground. He did not lose consciousness but was taken to the emergency department by a friend to have a scalp laceration sutured. The nurse instructs the client to:

A. Clean the sutured laceration twice a day with povidone-iodine (Betadine)
B. Remove his scalp sutures after 5 days
C. Return to the hospital immediately if he develops confusion, nausea, or vomiting
D. Take meperidine 50 mg po q4–6h prn for headache

72. A male client has asthma and his physician has prescribed beclomethasone (Vanceril) 3 puffs tid in addition to his other medications. After taking his beclomethasone, the client should be instructed to:

A. Clean his inhaler with warm water and soak it in a 10% bleach solution
B. Drink a glass of water
C. Sit and rest
D. Use his bronchodilator inhaler

73. A 70-year-old client has pneumonia and has just had a respiratory arrest. He has just been intubated with an 8-mm endotracheal tube. During auscultation of his chest, breath sounds were found to be absent on the left side. The nurse identifies the *most* likely cause of this as:

A. Inappropriate endotracheal tube size
B. Left-sided pneumothorax
C. Right mainstem bronchus intubation
D. Pneumonia

74. A 55-year-old client is unconscious, and his physician has decided to begin tube feeding him using a small-bore silicone feeding tube (Keofeed, Duo-Tube). After the tube is inserted, the nurse identifies the *most* reliable way to confirm appropriate placement is to:

A. Aspirate gastric contents
B. Auscultate air insufflated through the tube
C. Obtain a chest x-ray
D. Place the tip of the tube under water and observe for air bubbles

75. A 70-year-old client is almost finished receiving her second unit of packed red blood cells. The client, who weighs 80 lb, has started complaining of being short of breath and now has crackles in the bases of her lungs. After slowing or stopping the transfusion, the *most* appropriate initial nursing action would be to:

A. Raise the client's head and place her feet in a dependent position
B. Notify the physician
C. Place the client on 2 liters of O_2 via nasal cannula
D. Administer furosemide (Lasix) 20 mg IV push

76. A 52-year-old client's abdominal aortic aneurysm ruptured. She received rapid massive blood transfusions for

bleeding. One potential complication of blood administration for which she is especially at risk is:

A. Air embolus
B. Circulatory overload
C. Hypocalcemia
D. Hypokalemia

77. A 67-year-old client will be undergoing a coronary arteriography in the morning. Client teaching about post-procedure nursing care should include that:

A. Bed rest with bathroom privileges will be ordered
B. He will be kept NPO for 8–12 hours
C. Some oozing of blood at the arterial puncture site is normal
D. The leg used for arterial puncture should be kept straight for 8–12 hours

78. A client had a myocardial infarction 5 days ago. His physician has ordered an echocardiogram to determine how his myocardial infarction has affected his ventricular wall motion. When the client asks if this test is painful, an appropriate response is:

A. "No, but you must be able to ride on a stationary bicycle while the test is being performed."
B. "No, but you will have to lie still and the gel that is used may be cool."
C. "Yes, but your physician will be there and will order pain medicine for you."
D. "Your physician has ordered medicine, which you will be given before you go for the test, which will make you sleepy."

79. A 55-year-old man has recently been diagnosed with hypertension. His physician orders a low-sodium diet for him. When he asks, "What does salt have to do with high blood pressure?" the nurse's initial response would be:

A. "The reason is not known why hypertension is associated with a high-salt diet."
B. "Large amounts of salt in your diet can cause you to retain fluid, which increases your blood pressure."
C. "Salt affects your blood vessels and causes your blood pressure to be high."
D. "Salt is needed to maintain blood pressure, but too much causes hypertension."

80. A client has consented to have a central venous catheter placed. The *best* position in which to place the client is the Trendelenburg position. The reason is that the Trendelenburg position:

A. Allows the physician to visualize the subclavian vein
B. Reduces the possibility of air embolism
C. Reduces the possibility of hematoma formation
D. Makes the procedure more comfortable for the client

1. **(B)** Client need: health promotion and maintenance; subcategory: prevention and early detection of disease; content area: pediatrics

   RATIONALE

   (A) Vegetable exchanges are parts of the exchange program in a diabetic diet, but vegetables cannot be exchanged for breads. (B) Corn is considered a bread exchange, not a vegetable exchange. (C) Vegetables can be exchanged for vegetables. Corn is considered a bread exchange. (D) One-half ear of corn is considered one bread exchange, not a vegetable exchange.

2. **(B)** Client need: safe, effective care environment; subcategory: safety and infection control; content area: pediatrics

   RATIONALE

   (A) Sites for injection need to be rotated, including abdominal sites, to enhance insulin absorption. (B) The pinch technique is the most effective method for obtaining skin tightness to allow easy entrance of the needle to subcutaneous tissues. (C) Massaging the site of injection facilitates absorption of the insulin. (D) Changing the needle will break the sterility of the system. It has become acceptable practice to reuse disposable needles and syringes for 3–7 days.

3. **(B)** Client need: physiological integrity; subcategory: physiological adaptation; content area: pediatrics

   RATIONALE

   (A) Clay-colored stools indicate dysfunction of the liver or biliary tract. (B) In the early stages of cystic fibrosis, fat absorption is primarily affected resulting in fat, foul, frothy, bulky stools. (C) Dark brown stools indicate normal passage through the colon. (D) Blood-tinged stools indicate dysfunction of the gastrointestinal (GI) tract.

4. **(C)** Client need: health promotion and maintenance; subcategory: prevention and early detection of disease; content area: pediatrics

   RATIONALE

   (A) The Revised Prescreening Developmental Questionnaire is more age appropriate and offers simplified parent scoring and easier comparison. It is used by parents instead of professionals. (B) The Goodenough Draw-a-Person test is used to assess intellectual development. (C) The Denver Developmental Screening Test is one of the most widely used screening tests. It offers a concise, easy-to-administer, systematic approach to assessing the preschool child. It is widely used because of its reliability and validity. (D) The Caldwell Home Inventory is used to assess the home environment in areas of social, emotional, and cognitive supports.

5. **(B)** Client need: health promotion and maintenance; subcategory: growth and development through the life span; content area: pediatrics

   RATIONALE

   (A) Giving her toys will distract her and interfere with toilet training because of inappropriate reinforcement. (B) A child-sized toilet seat or training potty gives a child a feeling of security. (C) She should use words that are age appropriate for the child. (D) Children should be praised for cooperative behavior and/or successful evacuation.

6. **(A)** Client need: health promotion and maintenance; subcategory: growth and development through the life span; content area: pediatrics

   RATIONALE

   (A) Increased locomotive skills make push-pull toys appropriate for the energetic toddler. (B) Infants progress from reflex activity through simple repetitive behaviors to imitative behavior. Hand-eye coordination forms the foundation of other movements. (C) At age 8 months, infants begin to have pincer grasp. Toys that help infants develop the pincer grasp are recommended for this age group. (D) Various large colored blocks are suggested toys for infants 6–12 months of age to help visual stimulation.

7. **(C)** Client need: physiological integrity; subcategory: pharmacological and parenteral therapies; content area: pediatrics

   RATIONALE

   (A) A side effect of epinephrine is fatal ventricular fibrillation owing to its effects on cardiac stimulation. (B) Medications used to treat asthma are designed to decrease bronchospasm, not to increase expectorate of secretions. (C) Epinephrine decreased inspiratory difficulty by stimulating α-, β_1-, and β_2-receptors causing sympathomimetic stimulation (e.g., bronchodilation). (D) The person with asthma fights to inspire sufficient air thus increasing respiratory rate.

8. **(C)** Client need: physiological integrity; subcategory: physiological adaptation; content area: pediatrics

   RATIONALE

   (A) Altered surfactant production is found in sudden infant death syndrome. (B) Paradoxical breathing occurs when a negative intrathoracic pressure is transmitted to the abdomen by a weakened, poorly functioning diaphragm. (C) Asthma is characterized by spasm and constriction of the airways resulting in increased resistance to airflow. (D) If the pulmonary tree is obstructed for any reason, inspired air has difficulty overcoming the resistance and getting out. The rate of respiration increases in order to compensate, thus increasing air exchange.

9. **(D)** Client need: physiological integrity; subcategory: reduction of risk potential; content area: pediatrics

   RATIONALE

   (A) Before giving any emetic, the substance ingested must be known. (B) At least 8 oz of water should be administered along with ipecac syrup to increase volume in the stomach and facilitate vomiting. (C) Water alone will not induce vomiting. An emetic is necessary to facilitate vomiting. (D) Vomiting should never be induced in an unconscious client because of the risk of aspiration.

10. **(A)** Client need: physiological integrity; subcategory: physiological adaptation; content area: pediatrics

    RATIONALE

    (A) The immediate treatment for drug overdose is removal of the drug from the stomach by either forced emesis or gastric lavage. The child's unconscious state prohibits forced emesis. (B) Toxic amounts of salicylates directly affect the respiratory system, which could lead to respiratory failure. (C) The mother's anxiety is probably so high that preventive guidance will be ineffective. (D) Respiratory assistance is not needed if the child's respiratory function is unaltered.

11. **(A)** Client need: physiological integrity; subcategory: pharmacological and parenteral therapies; content area: pediatrics

    RATIONALE

    (A) Tetracycline should be avoided during tooth development because it interferes with enamel formation and dental pigmentation. (B) Milk interferes with the absorption of tetracyclines. (C) Children older than 9 years or past the tooth development stage may be given tetracycline. (D) Secondary infections of chronic skin disorders may respond to antibiotics such as penicillin or tetracyclines.

12. **(B)** Client need: psychosocial integrity; subcategory: coping and adaptation; content area: pediatrics

RATIONALE

(A) Normal infant attachment behaviors include responding to touch and wanting to be held. (B) Maternal deprivation behaviors include poor feeding, stiffening and refusal to eat, and inconsistencies in responsiveness. (C) Attachment behavior includes maintaining eye contact. (D) Maternal deprivation behaviors include displeasure with touch and physical contact.

13. **(B)** Client need: health promotion and maintenance; subcategory: growth and development through the life span; content area: maternity

RATIONALE

(A) Solid foods introduced before 4–6 months of age are not compatible with the abilities of the GI tract and the nutritional needs of the infant. (B) Production of milk is supply and demand. A common growth spurt occurs at 3 months of age, and more frequent nursing will increase the milk supply to satisfy the infant. (C) Supplementation will decrease the infant's appetite and in turn decrease the milk supply. When the infant nurses less often or with less vigor, the amount of milk produced decreases. (D) Rigid feeding schedules lead to a decreased milk supply, whereas frequent nursing signals the mother's body to produce a correspondingly increased amount of milk.

14. **(D)** Client need: physiological integrity; subcategory: reduction of risk potential; content area: pediatrics

RATIONALE

(A) Elevating the child's head to a 30-degree angle is the recommended position for gastroesophageal reflux. The supine position predisposes the child to aspiration. (B) Small, frequent feedings with thickened formula are recommended to minimize vomiting. (C) Antacids should be given at the same time as the feeding to improve their buffering action. (D) The infant should be kept still after feedings to reduce the risk of vomiting and aspiration. Vigorous activities should be carried out before feedings.

15. **(A)** Client need: psychosocial integrity; subcategory: coping and adaptation; content area: pediatrics

RATIONALE

(A) Educating the child about the pain may lessen anxiety. The child should be prepared for a potentially painful procedure but avoid suggesting pain. The nurse should allow the child his own sensory perception and evaluation of the procedure. (B) The nurse should avoid absolute descriptive statements and allow the child his own perception of the procedure. (C) The nurse should avoid evaluative statements or descriptions and give the child control in describing his reactions. (D) False statements regarding a painful procedure will cause a loss of trust between the child and the nurse.

16. **(D)** Client need: physiological integrity; subcategory: physiological adaptation; content area: pediatrics

RATIONALE

(A) The nurse should not put anything in the child's mouth during a seizure; this action could obstruct the airway. (B) Restraining the child's movements could cause constrictive injury. (C) Staying with the child during a seizure provides protection and allows the nurse to observe the seizure activity. (D) The nurse should provide safety for the child by moving objects and protecting the head.

17. **(D)** Client need: physiological integrity; subcategory: pharmacological and parenteral therapies; content area: pediatrics

RATIONALE

(A) Ribavirin is not supplied in an oral form. (B) Ribavirin is administered by aerosol in order to decrease the duration of viral shedding within the infected tissue. (C) Ribavirin is not approved for IV use to treat respiratory syncytial virus. (D) Ribavirin is a synthetic antiviral agent supplied as a crystalline powder that is reconstituted with sterile water. A Small Aerosol Particle Generator unit aerosolizes the medication for delivery by oxygen hood, croup tent, or aerosol mask.

18. **(B)** Client need: physiological integrity; subcategory: physiological adaptation; content area: pediatrics

RATIONALE

(A) Fluid volume deficit resulting from fluid shifts to the interstitial spaces occurs in the first 48 hours. (B) Forty-eight hours to 72 hours after the burn injury and fluid resuscitation, capillary permeability is restored and fluid requirements decrease. Interstitial fluid returns rapidly to the vascular compartment, and the nurse must monitor the child for signs and symptoms of hypervolemia. (C) Increased cardiac output results as fluids shift back to the vascular compartment. (D) Hypertension is the result of hypervolemia.

19. **(A)** Client need: physiological integrity; subcategory: physiological adaptation; content area: pediatrics

RATIONALE

(A) Urinary output is a reliable indicator of renal perfusion, which in turn indicates that fluid resuscitation is adequate. IV fluids are adjusted based on the urinary output of the child during fluid resuscitation. (B) Edema is an indication of increased capillary permeability following a burn injury. (C) Hypertension is an indicator of fluid volume excess. (D) Fontanelles close by 18 months of age.

20. **(A)** Client need: physiological integrity; subcategory: physiological adaptation; content area: pediatrics

RATIONALE

(A) Initial home treatment of croup includes placing the child in an environment of high humidity to liquefy and mobilize secretions. (B) Antihistamines should be avoided because they can cause thickening of secretions. (C) Drooling is a characteristic sign of airway obstruction and the child should be taken directly to the emergency room. (D) Crying increases respiratory distress and hypoxia in the child with croup. The nurse should promote methods that will calm the child.

21. **(C)** Client need: physiological integrity; subcategory: physiological adaptation; content area: pediatrics

RATIONALE

(A) Clinical manifestations of acute tracheitis include a 2–3 day history of URI, croupy cough, stridor, purulent secretions, high fever. (B) Clinical manifestations of spasmodic croup include a history of URI, croupy cough, stridor, dyspnea, low-grade fever, and a slow progression. The age group most affected is 3 months to 3 years. (C) Three clinical observations have been found to be predictive of epiglottitis: the presence of drooling, absence of spontaneous cough, and agitation. Epiglottitis has a rapid onset that is accompanied by high fever and dysphagia. (D) Clinical manifestations of acute laryngotracheobronchitis (LTB) include slow onset with a history of URI, low-grade fever, stridor, brassy cough, and irritability.

22. **(A)** Client need: physiological integrity; subcategory: basic care and comfort; content area: pediatrics

RATIONALE

(A) Cool air will often relieve pruritus without damaging the cast or irritating the skin. (B) The nurse should never force anything under the cast, because the cast may become damaged and skin breakdown may occur. (C) Forcing an object under the cast could lead to cast damage and skin breakdown. The object may become lodged under the cast necessitating cast removal. (D) This technique does not dislodge skin cells. It could damage the cast and cause skin breakdown.

23. **(C)** Client need: psychosocial integrity; subcategory: psychosocial adaptation; content area: med/surg

RATIONALE

(A) A person in crisis needs support, assistance, and direction from a caregiver rather than just an instruction. (B) A battered person may feel guilt and think that they cause the abuser's behavior; however, the abuser has the problem and goes through phases of violence. (C) The nurse should provide support and guidance to the client in crisis by offering alternatives and assist in referrals. (D) Focusing on help from law enforcement may be a very temporary solution, because the victim may be fearful of pressing charges. This answer does not address the crisis of going home.

24. **(B)** Client need: psychosocial integrity; subcategory: psychosocial adaptation; content area: psychiatric

RATIONALE

(A) This client response does not address stress reduction techniques. Verbal response focuses only on the problem. (B) Exercise or physical activity is a common strategy or coping technique used to reduce stress and anxiety. (C) Verbalizing effects of substance abuse on the body may help with insight and break through denial, but it is not a strategy to reduce anxiety. (D) Remaining substance-free does indicate motivation to change lifestyle of substance abuse or dependence, and it is not a stress reduction strategy in itself.

25. **(C)** Client need: psychosocial integrity; subcategory: psychosocial adaptation; content area: psychiatric

RATIONALE

(A) Threatening a client with punitive action is violating a client's rights and could escalate the client's anger. (B) Angry clients need respect for personal space, and physical contact may be perceived as a threatening gesture escalating anger. (C) Client lacks sufficient self-control to limit own maladaptive behavior; she may need assistance from staff. (D) Confronting an angry client may escalate her anger to further acting out, and consequences are for acting out anger aggressively, not for getting angry or feeling angry.

26. **(D)** Client need: psychosocial integrity; subcategory: coping and adaptation; content area: psychiatric

RATIONALE

(A) Transient depression manifests as sadness or the "blues" as seen with everyday disappointments and is not necessarily dysfunctional. (B) Mild depression manifests as symptoms seen with grief response, such as denial, sadness, withdrawal, somatic symptoms, and frequent or continuous thoughts of the loss. (C) Moderate depression manifests as feelings of sadness, negativism; low self-esteem; rumination about life's failures; decreased interest in grooming and eating; and possibly sleep disturbances. These symptoms are consistent with dysthymia. (D) Severe depression manifests as feelings of total despair, hopelessness, emptiness, inability to feel pleasure; possibly extreme psychomotor retardation; inattention to hygiene; delusional thinking; confusion; self-blame; and suicidal thoughts. These symptoms are consistent with major depression.

27. **(B)** Client need: psychosocial integrity; subcategory: coping and adaptation; content area: psychiatric

RATIONALE

(A) The nurse should encourage activities gradually, as client's energy level and tolerance for shared activities improve. (B) Activities that focus on strengths and accomplishments, with uncomplicated tasks, minimize failure and increase self-worth. (C)

Asking a client to set a goal to make all decisions about attending group activities is unrealistic, and such decisions are not always under the client's control; this sets up the client for further failure and possibly decreased self-worth. (D) Encouragement toward independence does promote increased feelings of self-worth; however, clients may need assistance with decision making and problem solving for various situations and on an individual basis.

28. **(B)** Client need: psychosocial integrity; subcategory: coping and adaptation; content area: psychiatric

RATIONALE

(A) Disapproving gives the impression that the nurse has a right to pass judgment on the client's thoughts, actions, or ideas. (B) Giving a broad opening gives the client encouragement to continue with verbalization. (C) Failing to acknowledge the client's feelings conveys a lack of understanding and empathy. (D) Changing the subject takes the conversation away from the client and is indicative of the nurse's anxiety or insensitivity.

29. **(D)** Client need: psychosocial integrity; subcategory: psychosocial adaptation; content area: psychiatric

RATIONALE

(A) The manic client's mood may easily change from euphoric to irritable. The nurse should avoid confrontation and let the client know what she can do, rather than what she cannot. (B) Although helpful to refocus or redirect the manic client to discuss only one topic at a time, distractibility is very high and it's best to avoid long discussions. (C) Manic clients have a tendency to manipulate persons in their environment. Staff should monitor intake, including at mealtime and snacks, and be consistent in their approach to meeting nutritional needs. (D) Manic clients may not sit and eat complete meals, but they can carry foods and liquids from regular meals with them. Staff can monitor and give high-caloric and high-energy snacks and liquids.

30. **(C)** Client need: psychosocial integrity; subcategory: psychosocial adaptation; content area: psychiatric

RATIONALE

(A) Anorexia and weight loss are problems that need attention in severe depression, but they can be addressed secondary to immediate concerns. (B) Impaired thinking and confusion are problems in severe depression that are addressed with administration of medication, through group and individual psychotherapy, and through activity therapy as motivation and interest increase. (C) Possible harm to self as with suicidal ideation; a suicide plan, means to execute plan; and/or overt gestures or an attempt must be addressed as an immediate concern and safety measures implemented appropriate to the risk of suicide. (D) Rest and activity impairment may take time and further assessment to determine client's sleep pattern and amount of psychomotor retardation with the more immediate concern for safety present.

31. **(A)** Client needs: physiological integrity; subcategory: pharmacological and parenteral therapies; content area: psychiatric

RATIONALE

(A) The most serious adverse reactions of MAO inhibitors involve blood pressure and ingestion of tyramine-containing foods, which may provoke a hypertensive crisis. (B) MAO inhibitors cause adverse reactions affecting the central nervous system and serious adverse reactions involving blood pressure. (C) MAO inhibits false neurotransmitters (phenylalanines) and may produce hypotensive reactions from gradual accumulation of these neurotransmitters. (D) The most serious adverse reactions of MAO inhibitors involve blood pressure.

32. **(B)** Client need: psychosocial integrity; subcategory: psychosocial adaptation; content area: psychiatric

RATIONALE

(A) Impaired communication refers to decreased ability or inability to use or understand language in an interaction. (B) In sensory-perceptual alterations an individual has distorted, impaired, or exaggerated responses to incoming stimuli (i.e., a hallucination, which is a false sensory perception that is not associated with real external stimuli). (C) An altered thought processes problem statement is used when an individual experiences a disruption in cognitive operations and activities (i.e., delusions, loose associations, ideas of reference). (D) In impaired social interaction, the individual participates too little or too much in social interactions.

33. **(D)** Client need: psychosocial integrity; subcategory: psychosocial adaptation; content area: psychiatric

RATIONALE

(A) Clients experiencing ideas of reference believe that information from the environment (e.g., the television) is referring to them. (B) Clients experiencing delusions of persecution believe that others in the environment are plotting against them. (C) Clients experiencing thought broadcasting perceive that others can hear their thoughts. (D) Clients experiencing delusions of grandeur think that they are omnipotent and have superhuman powers.

34. **(D)** Client need: psychosocial integrity; subcategory: psychosocial adaptation; content area: psychiatric

RATIONALE

(A) Focusing on the delusional content does not reinforce reality. (B) Pursuing details or more information on the delusion reinforces the false belief and further distances the client from reality. (C) Challenging the client's delusional system may force the client to defend it, and you cannot change the delusion through logic. (D) Focusing on the feeling can reinforce reality and discourage the false belief. Seeking out staff when thoughts are troublesome can help to decrease anxiety.

35. **(A)** Client need: psychosocial integrity; subcategory: psychosocial adaptation; content area: psychiatric

RATIONALE

(A) Anorexia nervosa clients feel out of control. Providing a structured environment offers safety and comfort and can help them to develop internal control, thus reducing their need to control by self-starvation. (B) Distraction does not focus on the client's need for control. (C) Doing frequent room checks reinforces feelings of powerlessness and the need to continue with the dysfunctional behavior. (D) Participating in long discussions about food does not make the client want to eat, but rather this strategy allows her to indulge in her preoccupation and to continue with the dysfunctional behavior.

36. **(B)** Client need: psychosocial integrity; subcategory: psychosocial adaptation; content area: psychiatric

RATIONALE

(A) Direct confrontation initially is nontherapeutic and may result in the client becoming frustrated and wanting to leave. (B) A positive, supportive attitude builds trust, and identifying positive strength raises self-esteem. Offering help allows the client to feel that he is not alone in dealing with problems. (C) Asking the client why or to give an explanation for his behavior puts him in a position of having to justify his behavior to the nurse. (D) Giving approval or placing a value on feelings or a behavior may limit the client's freedom to behave in a way that may displease another. This response may lead to seeking praise instead of progress.

37. **(A)** Client need: psychosocial integrity; subcategory: coping and adaptation; content area: psychiatric

RATIONALE

(A) Alzheimer's clients cope poorly with changes in routine because of memory deficits. Schedule changes cause confusion and frustration, whereas adhering to schedules is helpful and supports orientation. (B) Insisting that the client go to all unit activities may antagonize her and increase her agitation because of cognitive impairments. It may be better to allow the client time for calming down or distraction rather than to insist that she attend every activity. (C) When repeating a question, allow time first for a response; then use the same words the second time to avoid further confusion. (D) The nurse should avoid giving several choices at once. Cognitively impaired clients will become more frustrated with making decisions.

38. **(A)** Client needs: psychosocial integrity; subcategory: coping and adaptation; content area: psychiatric

RATIONALE

(A) Approaching a client's aggressive behavior on a continuum of least restrictive care is in agreement with his or her rights (i.e., verbal methods to help maintain control, medication, seclusion, and restraints, as necessary). (B) Approaching a client in a challenging manner is threatening and inappropriate. A nonchallenging and calm approach reflects staff in control and may increase client's internal control. (C) It is inappropriate to leave an aggressive client who is acting out alone. The nurse should acquire qualified help to prevent client from harm or injury to self or others. (D) Moving a client to seclusion immediately for shouting is inappropriate. The nurse should offer the client an opportunity to control self with limit setting. The client should understand that the staff will assist with control if necessary (i.e., quietly accompany out of environment to decrease stimulation and allow for verbalization) employing the least restrictive care model of intervention.

39. **(B)** Client need: psychosocial integrity; subcategory: coping and adaptation; content area: psychiatric

RATIONALE

(A) Ceasing to use humor and sarcasm is a more appropriate goal, because this client uses these behaviors covertly to express aggression instead of being open with anger. (B) Use of "I" messages demonstrates proper use of assertive behavior to express anger instead of passive-aggressive behavior. (C) Client is expected to complete share of work in therapeutic community because he has often obstructed other's efforts by failing to do his share. (D) Client has used conveniently forgetting or withholding information as a passive-aggressive behavior, which is not acceptable.

40. **(A)** Client need: health promotion and maintenance; subcategory: growth and development through the life span; content area: maternity

RATIONALE

(A) Using Nägele's rule, count back 3 calendar months from the first day of the last menstrual period. The answer is March 10. Then add 7 days and 1 year, which would be March 17 of the following year. (B, C, D) This date is incorrect.

41. **(A)** Client need: physiological integrity; subcategory: reduction of risk potential; content area: maternity

RATIONALE

(A) The treatment most commonly uses the Shirodkar-Barter procedure (McDonald procedure) or cerclage to enforce the weakened cervix by encircling it with a suture at the level of the internal os. (B) There is no known procedure that is used to repair the amniotic sac. (C) Cephalopelvic disproportion is evaluated later in pregnancy. It is not related to this procedure. (D) No procedure is done to dilate the cervix at 16 weeks' gestation unless the pregnancy is to be terminated.

42. **(D)** Client need: physiological integrity; subcategory: physiological adaptation; content area: maternity

RATIONALE

(A) This position would cause the gravid uterus to bear the increased pressure of the vena cava, which could lead to maternal hypotension, in turn causing the client to continue to have pallor and to feel light-headed. (B) This would not be the first intervention the RN should initiate. The RN should understand the supine position and its effect on the gravid uterus and vena cava. (C) The RN's first intervention should be one that helps to alleviate the client's symptoms. Obtaining her vital signs will not alleviate her symptoms. (D) This would move the gravid uterus off of the client's vena cava, which would alleviate the maternal hypotension that is the cause of her symptoms.

43. **(D)** Client need: psychosocial integrity; subcategory: coping and adaptation; content area: maternity

RATIONALE

(A) Any infant would be at risk for hyperglycemia because the infant's liver is missing the islets of Langerhans, which secrete insulin to break down glucose for cellular use. Prematurity is not an added risk for hyperglycemia. (B) Both premature and mature infants can be at risk for hypoglycemia if their mother had gestational diabetes during pregnancy or entered the pregnancy with diabetes mellitus. These infants are exposed to high levels of maternal glucose while in utero, which causes the islets of Langerhans in the infant's liver to produce insulin. After birth when the umbilical cord is severed, the generous amount of maternal blood glucose is eliminated; however, there is continued islet cell hyperactivity in the infant's liver, which can lead to excessive insulin levels and depleted blood glucose. (C) Mature infants are born with an immature GI system. The nervous control of the stomach is incomplete at birth, salivary glands are immature at birth, and the intestinal tract is sterile. This is not the greatest risk to the premature infant. (D) Infants born before 37 weeks' gestation are at greatest risk for an insufficient amount of surfactant in the alveoli system of the lungs. Surfactant helps to prevent lung collapse and ensures stability of the respiratory system so that the infant can maintain his own respirations once the umbilical cord is severed at birth.

44. **(C)** Client need: physiological integrity; subcategory: pharmacological and parenteral therapies; content area: maternity

RATIONALE

(A) Ritodrine is a sympathomimetic α_2-adrenergic agonist that can cause an elevation of blood glucose and plasma insulin in pregnant women. Hyperglycemia can occur in women with abnormal carbohydrate metabolism because of their inability to release more insulin. (B) Hypokalemia can occur resulting from the action of the β-mimetics. It results from a displacement of the extracellular potassium into the intracellular space. (C) Ritodrine causes vasodilation of vessel walls, which can lead to hypotension. The body compensates by increasing heart rate and pulse pressure. (D) There is a lowering of serum iron resulting from the action of β-mimetics to activate hematopoiesis.

45. **(D)** Client need: psychosocial integrity; subcategory: coping and adaptation; content area: maternity

RATIONALE

(A) An IV line is not started in a nonstress test, because this test is used as an indicator of fetal well-being. This test measures fetal activity and heart rate acceleration. (B) The bladder does not have to be full prior to this test. It is not a sonogram test where a full bladder enables other structures to be scanned. (C) It has been proved that eating or drinking liquids prior to the test can assist in increasing fetal activity. (D) Any maternal activity will interfere with the results of the test.

46. **(A)** Client need: physiological integrity; subcategory: reduction of risk potential; content area: maternity

RATIONALE

(A) A nonstress test that shows at least two accelerations of the fetal heart rate of 15 bpm with fetal activity, lasting ≥15 seconds over a 20-minute period. (B) Reactive criteria are not met. The accelerations of the fetal heart rate are not at least 15 bpm and do not last 15 seconds. This could mean fetal well-being is compromised. Usually a contraction stress test is ordered if the nonstress test results are negative. (C) An unsatisfactory test means the data cannot be interpreted, or there was inadequate fetal activity. If this happens, usually the test is ordered to be done at a later date. (D) A negative test is a term used to describe the results of a contraction stress test.

47. **(C)** Client need: physiological integrity; subcategory: physiological adaptation; content area: maternity

RATIONALE

(A) Cold is not a symptom of hyperventilation. This could be due to the temperature of the room. (B) Backache is not a symptom of hyperventilation. This is probably due to the gravid uterus and its effect on the back muscles, or it may be due to the client's position in bed. (C) Dizziness is the first symptom of hyperventilation. It occurs because the body is eliminating too much CO_2. (D) Nausea is not a symptom of hyperventilation. It could be a symptom of pain.

48. **(B)** Client need: health promotion and maintenance; subcategory: growth and development through the life span; content area: maternity

RATIONALE

(A) The ischial spines are located on both sides of the midpelvis. These spines mark the diameter of the narrowest part of the pelvis that the fetus will encounter. They are not sharp protrusions that will harm the fetus. Station refers to the relationship between the ischial spines in the pelvis and the fetus. The ischial spines are designated at 0 station. If the presenting part of the fetus is located above the ischial spines, a negative number is assigned, noting the number of centimeters above the ischial spines. Therefore, 1 centimeter below the ischial spines is designated as +1 station. (B) See explanation in A. One centimeter above the ischial spines is designated as +1 station. (C) The pelvic inlet is the first part of the pelvis that the fetus enters in routine delivery. The midpelvis is the second part of the pelvis to be entered by the fetus. The ischial spines are located on both sides of the midpelvis. (D) The pelvic outlet is the last part of the pelvis that the fetus will enter. When the fetus reaches this part of the pelvis, birth is near.

49. **(B)** Client need: health promotion and maintenance; subcategory: growth and development through the life span; content area: maternity

RATIONALE

(A) Posterior position causes a larger diameter of the fetal head to enter the pelvis than an anterior position. Pressure on the sacral nerves is increased, and it takes the fetus a longer time to enter the pelvic inlet. (B) This position will prolong the first stage of labor. When the larger diameter of the fetal head enters the pelvis first, it will have a more difficult time accommodating to the pelvis; therefore, it will take a longer time for the fetus to move through the pelvis. (C) It will increase the time of labor because the larger diameter of the fetal head will have a more difficult time accommodating to the pelvic inlet and thus will move through the pelvis slower. (D) In the third stage of labor the placenta is delivered; therefore, the infant has been delivered.

50. **(B)** Client need: health promotion and maintenance; subcategory: growth and development through the life span; content area: maternity

RATIONALE

(A) The medication bupivacaine will cause vasodilation in the vascular system, and this does not result in elevation of the maternal blood pressure. (B) The medication bupivacaine will cause vasodilation in the vascular system, and this will result in lowering the maternal blood pressure. (C) Bupivacaine does not interfere with the functioning of the endocrine system. (D) Bupivacaine does not interfere with the functioning of the endocrine system.

51. **(A)** Client need: physiological integrity; subcategory: pharmacological and parenteral therapies; content area: maternity

    RATIONALE

    (A) It is very important that there is a resting phase or relaxation period between the contractions. During this period, the uterus, placenta, and umbilical vessels re-establish blood flow. No resting phase between contractions can lead to fetal bradycardia, fetal hypoxia, and acidosis. It can also result in a tetanic contraction, which can cause uterine rupture. (B) The goal of the oxytocin infusion is to help establish a contraction pattern lasting 45–60 seconds occurring every 2 minutes and a uterine tonus of 60–70 mm Hg. (C) This choice is correct. The uterus has time to recover from the contraction. (D) The client's tiring is no indication to stop the infusion. She will be tired even without the infusion.

52. **(A)** Client need: physiological integrity; subcategory: reduction of risk potential; content area: maternity

    RATIONALE

    (A) Meperidine is a narcotic analgesic medication that crosses the placental barrier and reaches the fetus, causing respiratory depression in the fetus. A narcotic medication should never be included in the preoperative order for a cesarean delivery. (B) Oxytocin infusion would be discontinued if client is being prepared for a cesarean delivery because the medication would not be needed. (C) The bladder is always emptied prior to and during the surgical intervention to prevent the urinary bladder from accidentally being incised while the uterine incision is made. (D) The abdominal area is always prepared to rid the area of hair before the abdominal incision is made. Abdominal hair cannot be sterilized and could become a source for postoperative incisional infection.

53. **(C)** Client need: physiological integrity; subcategory: reduction of risk potential; content area: maternity

    RATIONALE

    (A) The infant is placed on the warmer and dried after birth. Cold stress occurs when the infant is not dried and kept warm. (B) The fact that this infant was born by cesarean delivery does not place him at a greater risk for cyanosis than an infant delivered vaginally. Cyanosis occurs when infants cannot oxygenate their blood after the umbilical cord is severed. (C) Infants born by cesarean delivery are at a higher risk for developing respiratory distress syndrome because these infants do not pass through the pelvis, where the chest is compressed and fluid is able to escape from the lungs. (D) Cesarean-delivered infants are not at greater risk for seizures than infants delivered vaginally.

54. **(D)** Client need: safe, effective care environment; subcategory: safety and infection control; content area: maternity

    RATIONALE

    (A) The delivery room personnel are responsible for verifying time of birth. (B) The scrub and circulating nurses count sponges and instruments. (C) This intervention is done in the nursery. (D) Tagging the mother and infant with identical bands is of utmost importance. The mother wears one band, and the newborn wears two. Identical numbers on the three bands provide identification for the newborn and the birth mother. Every time the newborn is brought to the mother after delivery, those bands are checked to be sure that the numbers are identical.

55. **(A)** Client need: health promotion and maintenance; subcategory: prevention and early detection of disease; content area: maternity

    RATIONALE

    (A) The Sims' position is the best position for assessment of the perineum and anus. The top leg is placed over the bottom leg, and the RN raises the upper buttocks to fully expose the perineum and anus. (B) Fowler's position is a sitting position, and the perineum and anus would not be exposed. (C) The prone position would have the mother on her back, and her perineum and anus would not be exposed. (D) The position of choice should always be the Sims'.

56. **(C)** Client need: physiological integrity; subcategory: physiological adaptation; content area: maternity

    RATIONALE

    (A) The area is bruised and painful. This action would do nothing to help with the healing process of the perineum or to provide comfort. (B) Ice is effective immediately after birth to reduce edema and discomfort, but not on the 2nd postpartum day. (C) Sitz baths are useful if the perineum has been traumatized, because the moist heat increases circulation to the area to promote healing, relaxes tissue, and decreases edema. (D) The physician is not notified of bruising, but if a hematoma is present, then the physician is notified.

57. **(D)** Client need: health promotion and maintenance; subcategory: growth and development through the life span; content area: maternity

    RATIONALE

    (A) Manipulation of nipples will cause soreness and trauma. (B) Pulling the nipples will cause discomfort and soreness. (C) Sliding the thumb and index finger forward over the nipple will cause soreness. (D) The best method to express milk from the breast is to position the thumb and index finger at the outer border of the areola and compress. This is the location of the milk sinuses.

58. **(D)** Client need: health promotion and maintenance; subcategory: growth and development through the life span; content area: maternity

    RATIONALE

    (A, B, C) This exercise is too strenuous at this time. (D) This exercise is recommended for the first few days after delivery. It helps to stimulate muscle tonus in the area of the perineum and the area around the urinary meatus and vagina.

59. **(C)** Client need: physiological integrity; subcategory: physiological adaptation; content area: med/surg

    RATIONALE

    (A) Extensions of his myocardial infarction would be chest pain unrelieved with nitroglycerin, cardiac enzyme elevations, and electrocardiographic changes. (B) Persons with pneumonia may complain of weakness and shortness of breath and have crackles in their lung bases. However, they would also have sputum production and leukocytosis. (C) Persons who have had myocardial infarctions (especially anterior wall) are at risk of developing left ventricular heart failure, which is a major cause of pulmonary edema. Pulmonary edema is manifest by shortness of breath, weakness, and crackles on auscultation of the lung fields. (D) Pulmonary emboli may be accompanied by shortness of breath, weakness, and crackles. However, the pulmonary hypertension that accompanies pulmonary emboli results in signs of increased systemic venous pressure as well.

60. **(A)** Client need: physiological integrity; subcategory: reduction of risk potential; content area: med/surg

RATIONALE

(A) High Fowler position decreases venous return to the heart and permits greater lung expansion so that oxygenation is maximized. (B) Lying on the left side may improve perfusion to the left lung but does not promote lung expansion. (C) Sitting in a chair will decrease venous return and promote maximal lung expansion. However, clients with pulmonary edema can deteriorate quickly and require intubation and mechanical ventilation. If a client is sitting in a chair when this deterioration happens, it will be difficult to intervene quickly. (D) The supine with feet elevated position increases venous return and will worsen pulmonary edema.

61. **(A)** Client need: physiological integrity; subcategory: pharmacological and parenteral therapies; content area: med/surg

RATIONALE

(A) Digoxin is a cardiac glycoside given to clients in heart failure to improve their myocardial contractility. (B) Furosemide is a loop diuretic given to clients in heart failure to promote diuresis. (C) O_2 is given to clients in heart failure to increase oxygenation and to prevent or treat hypoxemia. (D) Nitroglycerin is a nitrate given to clients in heart failure to increase their cardiac output by decreasing the peripheral resistance that the left ventricle must pump against.

62. **(B)** Client need: health promotion and maintenance; subcategory: prevention and early detection of disease; content area: med/surg

RATIONALE

(A) Increased calories may result in weight gain, but there is no indication in this question that this man's diet has changed in a way that would result in increased calories. (B) Decreasing cardiac output stimulates the renin-angiotensin-aldosterone cycle and results in fluid retention, which is reflected by weight gain. (C) Decreasing renal function may result in fluid retention, but this question gives no indication that this man has any renal problems. (D) Profound diuresis occurs with diabetes insipidus, which results in weight loss.

63. **(B)** Client need: physiological integrity; subcategory: physiological adaptation; content area: med/surg

RATIONALE

(A) Crackles are caused by air moving through moisture in the small airways and occur with pulmonary edema. Paradoxical chest wall movement occurs with flail chest when a segment of the thorax moves outward on inspiration and inward on expiration. (B) Decreased breath sounds occur when a lung is collapsed or partially collapsed. Chest pain with movement occurs with rib fractures. (C) Rhonchi are caused by air moving through large fluid-filled airways. Frothy sputum may occur with pulmonary edema. (D) Wheezing is caused by fluid in large airways already narrowed by mucus or bronchospasm. Dry cough could indicate a cardiac problem.

64. **(A)** Client need: physiological integrity; subcategory: reduction of risk potential; content area: med/surg

RATIONALE

(A) A chest tube extends from the pleural space to a collection device. The tube is placed below the surface of the saline so that air cannot enter the pleural space. (B) Fluid may enter the pleural space as a result of injury or disease. A chest tube may drain fluid from the pleural space, but the water seal is not involved in this. (C) Chest drainage should be measured, but the water seal is not involved in this. (D) Fluctuations in the tube in the water-sealed bottle will give an indication of respiratory effort, but that is not the purpose of the water seal.

65. **(B)** Client need: physiological integrity; subcategory: physiological adaptation; content area: med/surg

RATIONALE

(A) Pneumonia may be reflected by patchy infiltrates. In addition, fever, an increasing white blood cell count, and copious sputum production would be present. (B) Blunt chest trauma causes a bruising process in which interstitial and alveolar edema and hemorrhage occur. This is manifest by gradual deterioration over 24 hours of arterial blood gases and the continued production of bloody sputum. Patchy infiltrates are evident on chest x-ray 24 hours postinjury. (C) Pulmonary edema usually results from left heart failure. It is manifest by pink, frothy sputum; increasing dyspnea; tachycardia; and crackles on auscultation. (D) Tension pneumothorax is a potential complication for someone with rib fractures and a chest tube. It is manifest by diminished breath sounds on the affected side, rapidly deteriorating arterial blood gases in the presence of an open airway, and shock that is unexplained by other injuries.

66. **(B)** Client need: physiological integrity; subcategory: physiological adaptation; content area: med/surg

RATIONALE

(A) In compensated metabolic acidosis, the pH level is normal, the PCO_2 level is decreased, and the HCO_3 level is decreased. The client's primary alteration is an inability to remove excess acid via the kidneys. The lungs compensate by hyperventilating and decreasing PCO_2. (B) In compensated respiratory acidosis, the pH level is normal, the PCO_2 level is elevated, and the HCO_3 level is elevated. The client's primary alteration is an inability to remove CO_2 from the lungs, so over time, the kidneys increase reabsorption of HCO_3 to buffer the CO_2. (C) In compensated respiratory alkalosis, the pH level is normal, the PCO_2 level is decreased, and the HCO_3 level is decreased. The client's primary alteration is hyperventilation, which decreases PCO_2. The client compensates by increasing the excretion of HCO_3 from the body. (D) In uncompensated respiratory acidosis, the pH level is decreased, the PCO_2 level is increased, and the HCO_3 level is normal. The client's primary alteration is an inability to remove CO_2 from the lungs. The kidneys have not compensated by increasing HCO_3 reabsorption.

67. **(D)** Client need: physiological integrity; subcategory: physiological adaptation; content area: med/surg

RATIONALE

(A) In compensated respiratory acidosis, the pH level is normal, the PCO_2 level is elevated, and the HCO_3 level is elevated. The client's primary alteration is an inability to remove CO_2 from the lungs, so over time, the kidneys increase reabsorption of HCO_3 to buffer the CO_2. (B) Normal ranges for arterial blood gases for adults and children are as follows: pH 7.35–7.45, PO_2 80–100 mm Hg, PCO_2 35–45 mm Hg, HCO_3 21–28 mEq/L. (C) In uncompensated metabolic acidosis the pH level is decreased, the PCO_2 level is normal, and the HCO_3 level is decreased. The client's primary alteration is an inability to remove excess acid via the kidneys. The lungs are unable to clear the increased acid. (D) In uncompensated respiratory acidosis, the pH level is decreased, the PCO_2 level is increased, and the HCO_3 level is normal. In a person with long-standing COPD, the HCO_3 level will rise gradually over time to compensate for the gradually increasing PCO_2, and the person's pH level will be normal. When a person with COPD becomes acutely ill, the kidneys do not have time to increase the reabsorption of HCO_3, so the person's pH level will reflect acidosis even though the HCO_3 is elevated.

68. **(A)** Client need: physiological integrity; subcategory: reduction of risk potential; content area: med/surg

RATIONALE

(A) Autonomic dysreflexia is the exaggerated sympathetic nervous system response to various stimuli in the anesthetized area. Sympathetic stimulation results in severe, uncontrolled hypertension, which may result in myocardial infarction or cerebral hemorrhage. (B) Bradycardia occurs as a result of sympathetic blockade in the immediate postinjury period. After spinal shock recedes, cardiovascular stability returns, but the client will be bradycardiac for life. (C) Central cord syndrome is a specific type of spinal cord injury that occurs as a result of either hyperextension injuries or disrupted blood flow to the spinal cord. (D) Spinal shock occurs in the immediate postinjury phase and usually resolves in approximately 72 hours.

69. **(A)** Client need: health promotion and maintenance; subcategory: prevention and early detection of disease; content area: med/surg

RATIONALE

(A) This response acknowledges the client's feelings, gives him factual information, and acknowledges that the final decision is his. (B) This response is judgmental and discourages the client from expressing his feelings about the procedure. (C) Catheterization is a procedure that takes time to learn, but which, for the spinal cord–injured client, can significantly reduce the incidence of urinary tract infections. A young client with a T-4 injury has the hand function to learn this procedure fairly easily. (D) The final decision about bladder elimination management ultimately rests with the client and not the physician.

70. **(A)** Client need: physiological integrity; subcategory: pharmacological and parenteral therapies; content area: med/surg

RATIONALE

(A) Indications of theophylline toxicity include palpitations, dizziness, restlessness, nausea, vomiting, shakiness, and anorexia. (B) Cigarette smoking significantly lowers theophylline plasma levels. (C) Theophylline should be taken with food to decrease stomach upset. (D) These instructions are appropriate for someone taking digoxin.

71. **(C)** Client need: health promotion and maintenance; subcategory: prevention and early detection of disease; content area: med/surg

RATIONALE

(A) Povidone-iodine is very irritating to skin and should not be routinely used. (B) Sutures should not be removed by the client. (C) Confusion, nausea, vomiting, and behavioral changes may indicate increasing intracranial pressure as a result of intracerebral bleeding. (D) Use of a narcotic opiate such as meperidine is not recommended in clients with a possible head injury because it may produce sedation, pupil changes, euphoria, and respiratory depression, which may mask the signs of increasing intracranial pressure.

72. **(B)** Client need: physiological integrity; subcategory: pharmacological and parenteral therapies; content area: med/surg

RATIONALE

(A) Inhalers should be cleaned once a day. They should be taken apart, washed in warm water, and dried according to manufacturer's instructions. Soaking in bleach is inappropriate. (B) A common side effect of inhaled steroid preparations is oral candidal infection. This can be prevented by drinking a glass of water or gargling after using a steroid inhaler. (C) There is nothing wrong with sitting and resting after using a steroid inhaler, but it is not necessary. (D) If a person is using a steroid inhaler as well as a bronchodilator inhaler, the bronchodilator should always be used first. The reason for this is that the bronchodilator opens up the person's airways so that when the steroid inhaler is used next, there will be better distribution of medication.

73. **(C)** Client need: physiological integrity; subcategory: physiological adaptation; content area: med/surg

RATIONALE

(A) Appropriate endotracheal tube sizes for adults range from 7.0–8.5 mm. (B) Pneumothorax could be indicated by an ab-

sence of breath sounds on the affected side. However, in a recently intubated client, the first priority would be to consider tube malposition. (C) During intubation, the right mainstem bronchus can be inadvertently entered if the endotracheal tube is inserted too far. Left mainstem bronchus intubation almost never occurs because of the angle of the left mainstem bronchus. (D) Breath sounds for someone with pneumonia may be decreased over the areas of consolidation. However, in a recently intubated client, the first priority would be to consider tube malposition.

74. **(C)** Client need: physiological integrity; subcategory: reduction of risk potential; content area: med/surg

RATIONALE

(A) Aspiration of gastric contents is usually a reliable way to verify tube placement. However, if the client has dark respiratory secretions from bleeding, tube feedings could be mistaken for respiratory secretions; in other words, aspirating an empty stomach is less reliable in this instance. In addition, it is common for small-bore feeding tubes to collapse when suction pressure is applied. (B) Insufflation of air into large-bore nasogastric tubes can usually be clearly heard. In small-bore tubes, it is more difficult to hear air, and it is difficult to distinguish between air in the stomach and air in the esophagus. (C) A chest x-ray is the most reliable means to determine placement of small-bore nasogastric tubes. (D) Observing for air bubbles when the tip is held under water is an unreliable means to determine correct tube placement for all types of nasogastric tubes. Air may come from both the respiratory tract and the stomach, and the client who is breathing shallowly may not force air out of the tube into the water.

75. **(A)** Client need: physiological integrity; subcategory: reduction of risk potential; content area: med/surg

RATIONALE

(A) Raising the client's head and placing her feet in a dependent position is an independent nursing action that can be taken to decrease venous return and to reduce pulmonary congestion. (B) Notifying the physician is an appropriate action that should be taken after the client is positioned to maximize her respiratory status. (C) Placing the client on O_2 may be done with a physician's order or according to an institution's standing orders; however, other actions should be taken first. (D) Furosemide 20 mg IV push is an appropriate medication for the client, but it must be ordered by her physician.

76. **(C)** Client need: physiological integrity; subcategory: pharmacological and parenteral therapies; content area: med/surg

RATIONALE

(A) Air embolism is a potential complication of blood administration, but it is fairly rare and can be prevented by using good IV technique. (B) Circulatory overload is a potential complication of blood administration, but because this client is actively bleeding, she is not at high risk for overload. (C) Hypocalcemia is a potential complication of blood administration that occurs in situations where massive transfusion has occurred over a short period of time. It occurs because the citrate in stored blood binds with the client's calcium. Another potential complication for which this client is especially at risk is hypothermia, which can be prevented by using a blood warmer to administer the blood. (D) Hypokalemia is not a complication of blood administration.

77. **(D)** Client need: physiological integrity; subcategory: reduction of risk potential; content area: med/surg

RATIONALE

(A) Bed rest will be ordered for 8–12 hours postprocedure. Flexing of the leg at the arterial puncture site will occur if the client gets out of bed, and this is contraindicated after arteriography. (B) The client will be able to eat as soon as he is alert enough to swallow safely and that will depend on what medications are used for sedation during the procedure. (C) Oozing at the arterial puncture site is not normal and should be closely evaluated. (D) The leg where the arterial puncture occurred must be kept straight for 8–12 hours to minimize the risk of bleeding.

78. **(B)** Client need: physiological integrity; subcategory: reduction of risk potential; content area: med/surg

    RATIONALE
    (A) Riding a stationary bicycle or walking on a treadmill is done during a stress test. (B) During an echocardiogram, the client must lie supine while a technician performs the test. To perform the test, the technician uses a conductive gel and a transducer to obtain ultrasound tracings of the heart. (C) A physician need not be present during an echocardiogram, and it is neither invasive nor painful. (D) There is no premedication required for an echocardiogram.

79. **(B)** Client need: health promotion and maintenance; subcategory: prevention and early detection of disease; content area: med/surg

RATIONALE
(A) This response is untrue. (B) Decreasing salt intake reduces fluid retention and decreases blood pressure. (C) Salt does not have an effect on the blood vessels themselves, but on fluid retention, which accompanies salt intake. (D) This response is untrue.

80. **(B)** Client need: physiological integrity: subcategory: reduction of risk potential; content area: med/surg

    RATIONALE
    (A) The subclavian vein is not visible during central line insertion regardless of the client's position. (B) The Trendelenburg position reduces the possibility of air embolism because it places slight positive pressure on the central veins. It also distends the veins, and distention facilitates insertion. (C) This response is untrue; it has no effect on hematoma formation. (D) This position is not necessarily more comfortable for the client, and many clients, especially those who may be short of breath, may find the position uncomfortable and difficult to maintain.

TEST 4

Nicholls State University Test

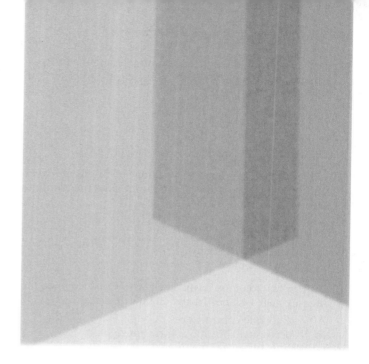

MOCK NCLEX-RN BOARD REVIEW TEST QUESTIONS

1. A newborn infant is exhibiting signs of respiratory distress. Which of the following would the nurse recognize as the earliest clinical sign of respiratory distress?

   A. Cyanosis
   B. Increased respirations
   C. Sternal and subcostal retractions
   D. Decreased respirations

2. A nurse is performing a vaginal exam on a client in active labor. An important landmark to assess during labor and delivery are the ischial spines because:

   A. Ischial spines are the narrowest diameter of the pelvis
   B. Ischial spines are the widest diameter of the pelvis
   C. They represent the inlet of birth canal
   D. They measure pelvic floor

3. The nurse instructs a client on the difference between true labor and false labor. The nurse explains, "In true labor:

   A. Uterine contractions will weaken with walking."
   B. Uterine contractions will strengthen with walking."
   C. The cervix does not dilate."
   D. The fetus does not descend."

4. A first-trimester primigravida is diagnosed with anemia. The nurse should suspect that this anemia is a result of:

   A. Mother's increased blood volume
   B. Mother's decreased blood volume
   C. Fetal blood volume increase
   D. Increase in iron absorption

5. In client teaching, the nurse should emphasize that fetal damage occurs more frequently with ingestion of drugs during:

   A. First trimester
   B. Second trimester
   C. Third trimester
   D. Every trimester

6. A laboring client presents with a prolapsed cord. The nurse should immediately place the client in what position?

   A. Reverse Trendelenburg
   B. Fowler's
   C. Trendelenburg
   D. Sims'

7. A client suspects that she is pregnant. She reports two missed menstrual periods. The first day of her last menstrual period was August 3. Her estimated date of confinement would be:

   A. November 7
   B. November 10
   C. May 7
   D. May 10

8. An elective saline abortion has been performed on a 3-week primigravida. Following the procedure, the nurse should be alert for which early side effect?

   A. Water satiety
   B. Thirst
   C. Edema
   D. Diabetes insipidus

9. Assessment of a newborn for Apgar scoring includes observation for:

   A. Pupil response
   B. Respiratory rate
   C. Heart rate
   D. Babinski's reflex

10. Painless vaginal bleeding in the last trimester may be caused by:

    A. Menstruation
    B. Abruptio placentae
    C. Placenta previa
    D. Polyhydramnios

11. The nurse should facilitate bonding during the postpartum period. What should the nurse expect to observe in the taking-hold phase?

    A. Mother is concerned about her recovery.
    B. Mother calls infant by name.
    C. Mother lightly touches infant.
    D. Mother is concerned about her weight gain.

12. The physician is preparing to induce labor on a 40-week multigravida. The nurse should anticipate the administration of:

    A. Oxytocin (Pitocin)
    B. Progesterone
    C. Vasopressin (Pitressin)
    D. Ergonovine maleate

13. A primigravida is at term. The nurse can recognize the second stage of labor by the client's desire to:

    A. Push during contractions
    B. Hyperventilate during contractions
    C. Walk between contractions
    D. Relax during contractions

14. A pregnant client during labor is irritable and feels the urge to vomit. The nurse should recognize this as the:

    A. Fourth stage of labor
    B. Third stage of labor
    C. Transition stage of labor
    D. Second stage of labor

15. A pregnant client experiences spontaneous rupture of membranes. The first nursing action is to:

    A. Assess the client's respirations
    B. Notify the physician
    C. Auscultate fetal heart rate
    D. Transfer to delivery suite

16. A pregnant client experiences a precipitous delivery. The nursing action during a precipitous delivery is to:

    A. Control the delivery by guiding expulsion of fetus
    B. Leave the room to call the physician
    C. Push against the perineum to stop delivery
    D. Cross client's legs tightly

17. Following a vaginal delivery, the postpartum nurse should observe for:

    A. Dystocia, kraurosis
    B. Chadwick's sign
    C. Fatigue, hemorrhoids
    D. Hemorrhage and infection

18. A client who is 7 months pregnant is diagnosed with pyelonephritis. The nurse anticipates the physician ordering:

    A. Oxytocin
    B. Magnesium sulfate (MgSO$_4$)
    C. Ampicillin
    D. Tetracycline

19. A newborn is admitted to the newborn nursery with tremors, apnea periods, and poor sucking reflex. The nurse should suspect:

    A. Central nervous system damage
    B. Hypoglycemia

    C. Hyperglycemia
    D. These are normal newborn responses to extrauterine life

20. A premature infant needs supplemental O$_2$ therapy. A nursing intervention that reduces the risk of retrolental fibroplasia is to:

    A. Maintain O$_2$ at <40%
    B. Maintain O$_2$ at ≥40%
    C. Give moist O$_2$ at ≥40%
    D. Maintain on 100% O$_2$

21. A client presents to the psychiatric unit crying hysterically. She is diagnosed with severe anxiety disorder. The first nursing action is to:

    A. Demand that she relax
    B. Ask what is the problem
    C. Stand or sit next to her
    D. Give her something to do

22. A schizophrenic is admitted to the psychiatric unit. What affect would the nurse expect to observe?

    A. Anger
    B. Apathy and flatness
    C. Smiling
    D. Hostility

23. A 16-year-old client reports a weight loss of 20% of her previous weight. She has a history of food binges followed by self-induced vomiting (purging). The nurse should suspect a diagnosis of:

    A. Anorexia nervosa
    B. Anorexia hysteria
    C. Bulimia
    D. Conversion reaction

24. A 24-year-old client presents to the emergency department protesting "I am God." The nurse identifies this as a:

    A. Delusion
    B. Illusion
    C. Hallucination
    D. Conversion

25. A 30-year-old client has a history of several recent traumatic experiences. She presents at the physician's office with a complaint of blindness. Physical exam and diagnostic testing reveal no organic cause. The nurse recognizes this as:

    A. Delusion
    B. Illusion
    C. Hallucination
    D. Conversion

26. A 40-year-old client is admitted to the hospital for tests to diagnose cancer. Since his admission, he has become dependent and demanding to the nursing staff. The nurse identifies this behavior as which defense mechanism?

    A. Denial
    B. Displacement
    C. Regression
    D. Projection

27. A young boy tells the nurse, "I don't like my Dad to kiss or hug my Mom. I love my Mom and want to marry her."

The nurse recognizes this stage of growth and development as:

A. Electra complex
B. Oedipus complex
C. Superego
D. Ego

28. A client was prescribed a major tranquilizer 2 months ago. One month ago she was placed on benztropine (Cogentin). What would indicate that benztropine therapy is effective?

A. Smooth, coordinated voluntary movement
B. Tremors
C. Rigidity
D. Muscle weakness

29. A client is diagnosed with organic brain disorder. The nursing care should include:

A. Organized, safe environment
B. Long, extended family visits
C. Detailed explanations of procedures
D. Challenging educational programs

30. A 4-year-old child has Down syndrome. The community health nurse has coordinated a special preschool program. The nurse's primary goal is to:

A. Provide respite care for the mother
B. Facilitate optimal development
C. Provide a demanding and challenging educational program
D. Prepare child to enter mainstream education

31. A 13-year-old hemophiliac is hospitalized for hemarthrosis of his right knee. To relieve the pain, the nurse should:

A. Place on bed rest; elevate and splint the right knee
B. Apply moist heat to the right knee
C. Administer aspirin for pain
D. Encourage active range of motion to right knee

32. A 3-month-old infant has had a unilateral cleft lip repair. He has resumed feedings of oral formula. The nurse should feed the infant with:

A. Gavage tube
B. Nipple and bottle
C. A straw and cup
D. Syringe

33. A 3-year-old child is admitted with a diagnosis of possible noncommunicating hydrocephalus. What is the first symptom that indicates increased intracranial pressure?

A. Bulging fontanelles
B. Seizure
C. Headache
D. Ataxia

34. What is the appropriate nursing action for a child with increased intracranial pressure?

A. Head of bed elevated 45 degrees with child's head maintained in a neutral position
B. Child lying flat
C. Head turned to side
D. Frequent visitation for stimulation

35. A client is 2 hours post ventriculoperitoneal shunt placement. How should the nurse position the client?

A. Head of bed elevated 30 degrees on nonoperative side
B. Head of bed elevated 30 degrees on operative side
C. Bed flat on operative side
D. Bed flat on nonoperative side

36. A type I diabetic client delivers a male newborn. The newborn is 45 minutes old. What is the primary nursing goal in the nursery during the first hours for this newborn?

A. Bonding
B. Maintain normal blood sugar
C. Maintain normal nutrition
D. Monitor intake and output

37. A 16-month-old infant is being prepared for tetralogy of Fallot repair. In the nursing assessment, which lab value should elicit further assessment and requires notification of physician?

A. pH 7.39
B. White blood cell (WBC) count 10,000 WBCs/mm³
C. Hematocrit 60%
D. Bleeding time of 4 minutes

38. A 2-month-old infant is receiving IV fluids with a volume control set. The nurse uses this type of tubing because it:

A. Prevents administration of other drugs
B. Prevents entry of air into tubing
C. Prevents inadvertent administration of a large amount of fluids
D. Prevents phlebitis

39. Which type of insulin can be administered by a continuous IV drip?

A. Humulin N
B. NPH insulin
C. Regular insulin
D. Lente insulin

40. A physician's order reads: Administer furosemide oral solution 0.5 mL stat. The furosemide bottle dosage is 10 mg/mL. What dosage of furosemide should the nurse give to this infant?

A. 5 mg
B. 0.5 mg
C. 0.05 mg
D. 20 mg

41. A physician's order reads: Administer KCl 10% oral solution 1.5 mL. The KCl bottle reads 20 mEq/15 mL. What dosage should the nurse administer to the infant?

A. 1 mEq
B. 1.13 mEq
C. 2 mEq
D. Not enough information to calculate

42. A 1000-mL dose of lactated Ringer's solution is to be infused in 8 hours. The drop factor for the tubing is 10 gtt/mL. How many drops per minute should the nurse administer?

A. 125 gtt/min
B. 48 gtt/min
C. 20 gtt/min
D. 21 gtt/min

43. A 1000-mL dose of D₅W ½ normal saline is to be infused in 8 hours. The drop factor for the tubing is 60 gtt/min. How many drops per minute should the nurse administer?

A. 75 gtt/min
B. 100 gtt/min
C. 125 gtt/min
D. 150 gtt/min

44. A physician's order reads: 0.25 normal saline at 50 mL/hr until discontinued. The nurse is using a micro-drip tubing set. How many drops per minute should the nurse administer?

A. 1 gtt/min
B. 5 gtt/min
C. 50 gtt/min
D. 100 gtt/min

45. A 6-year-old child is attending a pediatric clinic for a routine examination. What should the nurse assess for while conducting a vision screening?

A. Hearing test
B. Gait
C. Strabismus
D. Papilledema

46. An 11-year-old boy has received a partial-thickness burn to both legs. He presents to the emergency room approximately 15 minutes after the accident in excruciating pain with charred clothing to both legs. What is the first nursing action?

A. Apply ice packs to both legs.
B. Begin débridement by removing all charred clothing from wound.
C. Apply Silvadene cream (silver sulfadiazine).
D. Immerse both legs in cool water.

47. A burn victim's immunization history is assessed by the nurse. Which immunization is of priority concern?

A. Oral poliovirus vaccine
B. Inactivated poliovirus vaccine
C. Tetanus toxoid
D. Hepatitis B vaccine

48. A newborn has been delivered with a meningo-myelocele. The nursery nurse should position the newborn:

A. Prone
B. Supine
C. Side lying
D. Semi-Fowler

49. Nursing care of the infant prior to surgical closure of a meningomyelocele would include:

A. Cover sac with dry sterile dressing
B. Cover sac with saline-soaked sterile dressing
C. Do not apply dressing; keep sac open to air
D. Aspirate any fluid from sac

50. A 35-year-old client is admitted to the hospital with diabetic ketoacidosis. Results of arterial blood gases are pH 7.2, PaO₂ 90, PaCO₂ 45, and HCO₃ 16. The nursing assessment of arterial blood gases indicate the presence of:

A. Respiratory alkalosis
B. Respiratory acidosis
C. Metabolic alkalosis
D. Metabolic acidosis

51. A client presents to the emergency room with cyanosis, coughing, tachypnea, and tachycardia. She has a history of asthma. Arterial blood gas values are pH 7.28, PaO₂ 54, PaCO₂ 60, and HCO₃ 24. The nursing assessment of arterial blood gases indicate the presence of:

A. Respiratory alkalosis
B. Respiratory acidosis
C. Metabolic alkalosis
D. Metabolic acidosis

52. A 40-year-old client is admitted to the coronary care unit with chest pain and shortness of breath. The physician diagnosed an anterior wall myocardial infarction. What tests should the nurse anticipate?

A. Reticulocyte count, creatinine phosphokinase (CPK)
B. Aspartate transaminase, alanine transaminase
C. Sedimentation rate, WBC count
D. Lactic dehydrogenase, CPK

53. The nurse needs to be aware that the *most* common early complication of a myocardial infarction is:

A. Diabetes mellitus
B. Anaphylactic shock
C. Cardiac hypertrophy
D. Cardiac dysrhythmia

54. A client is being treated for congestive heart failure. His medical regimen consists of digoxin (Lanoxin) 0.25 mg po daily and furosemide 20 mg po bid. Which laboratory test should the nurse monitor?

A. Intake and output
B. Calcium
C. Potassium
D. Magnesium

55. In the coronary care unit, a client has developed multi-focal premature ventricular contractions. The nurse should anticipate the administration of:

A. Furosemide
B. Nitroglycerin
C. Lidocaine
D. Digoxin

56. A client has received digoxin 0.25 mg po daily for 2 weeks. Which of the following digoxin levels indicates toxicity?

A. 0.5 ng/mL
B. 1.0 ng/mL
C. 2.0 ng/mL
D. 3.0 ng/mL

57. A client has developed congestive heart failure secondary to his myocardial infarction. Discharge diet instructions should emphasize the reduction or avoidance of:

    A. Fresh vegetables and fruit
    B. Canned vegetables and fruit
    C. Breads, cereals, and rice
    D. Fish

58. A client takes warfarin (Coumadin) 15 mg po daily. To evaluate the medication's effectiveness, the nurse should monitor the:

    A. prothrombin time (PT)
    B. partial thromboplastin time (PTT)
    C. PTT-C
    D. Fibrin split products

59. Prior to administering digoxin to a client with congestive heart failure, the nurse needs to assess:

    A. Respiratory rate for 1 minute
    B. Radial pulse for 1 minute
    C. Radial pulse for 2 minutes
    D. Apical pulse for 1 minute

60. A client is diagnosed with *Mycobacterium* tuberculosis. He is placed in respiratory isolation, intubated, and receives mechanical ventilation. When performing suctioning, the nurse should:

    A. Suction for a maximum of 20 seconds
    B. Hyperoxygenate before and after suctioning
    C. Suction for a maximum of 30 seconds
    D. Maintain clean technique during suctioning

61. The physician prescribes a medical regimen of isoniazid, rifampin, and vitamin B_6 for a tuberculosis client. The nurse instructs the client that B_6 is given because it:

    A. Increases activity of isoniazid
    B. Increases activity of rifampin
    C. Improves nutritional status
    D. Reduces peripheral neuropathy

62. Which of the following nursing actions is essential to prevent drug-resistant tuberculosis?

    A. Monitor liver function.
    B. Monitor renal function.
    C. Assess knowledge of respiratory isolation.
    D. Monitor compliance with drug therapy.

63. To facilitate maximum air exchange, the nurse should position the client in:

    A. High Fowler
    B. Orthopneic
    C. Prone
    D. Flat-supine

64. A client has been diagnosed with congestive heart failure. His fluid intake and output are strictly regulated. For lunch, he drank 8 oz of milk, 4 oz of tea, and 6 oz of coffee. His intake would be recorded as:

    A. 500 mL
    B. 540 mL
    C. 600 mL
    D. 655 mL

65. The client tells the nurse, "I have pain in my left shoulder." This is considered:

    A. Evaluation process
    B. Objective information
    C. Subjective information
    D. Complaining

66. Before completing a nursing diagnosis, the nurse must first:

    A. Write goals and objectives
    B. Perform an assessment
    C. Plan interventions
    D. Perform evaluation

67. A 70-year-old homeless woman is admitted with pneumonia. She is weak, emaciated, and febrile. The physician orders enteral feedings intermittently by nasogastric tube. When inserting the nasogastric tube, once the tube passes through the oropharynx, the nurse will instruct the client to:

    A. Tilt her head backwards
    B. Swallow as tube passes
    C. Hold breath as tube passes
    D. Cough as tube passes

68. When assessing residual volume in tube feeding, the feeding should be delayed if the amount of gastric contents (residual) exceeds:

    A. 20 mL
    B. 25 mL
    C. 30 mL
    D. 50 mL

69. A client has a history of alcoholism. He is currently diagnosed with cirrhosis of the liver. The nurse would expect him to be on which type of diet?

    A. High protein and high calorie
    B. High calorie and high carbohydrate
    C. Low-fat 2-g sodium diet
    D. High protein and high fat

70. A client has ascites, which is caused by:

    A. Decreased plasma proteins
    B. Electrolyte imbalance
    C. Decreased renal function
    D. Portal hypertension

71. A common complication of cirrhosis of the liver is prolonged bleeding. The nurse should be prepared to administer?

    A. Vitamin C
    B. Vitamin K
    C. Vitamin E
    D. Vitamin A

72. A 45-year-old client has a permanent colostomy. Which of the following foods should he avoid?

    A. Peanut butter and jelly sandwich and milk
    B. Corn beef and cabbage and boiled potatoes
    C. Oatmeal, whole-wheat toast, and milk
    D. Tuna on whole-wheat bread and iced tea

73. On an assessment of a client's mouth, the nurse notices white patches on the buccal mucosa. The nurse tries to obtain a sample for a culture, but the lesion cannot be rubbed off. The nurse would suspect that this lesion is:
    A. Xerosteromia
    B. Candidiasis
    C. Leukoplakia
    D. Stomatitis

74. A client on the infectious disease unit is discussing transmission of human immunodeficiency virus (HIV). The nurse would need to provide more client education based on which client statement?
    A. "HIV is a virus transmitted by sexual contact."
    B. "Condoms reduce the transmission of HIV."
    C. "HIV is a virus that is easily transmitted by casual contact."
    D. "HIV can be transmitted to an unborn infant."

75. A 26-year-old client is diagnosed with an astrocytoma, a benign brain tumor. From the nurse's knowledge of the central nervous system, the nurse knows that benign tumors:
    A. Can be just as dangerous as malignant tumors
    B. Grow more rapidly than malignant tumors
    C. Do not warrant concern because they do not become malignant tumors
    D. Can be removed surgically

76. A 55-year-old client is admitted with a diagnosis of renal calculi. He presented with severe right flank pain, nausea, and vomiting. The *most* important nursing action for him at this time is:
    A. Intake and output measurement
    B. Daily weights
    C. Straining of all urine
    D. Administration of O_2 therapy

77. A client's renal calculi are identified as consisting of calcium phosphate. Which of the following diets would be appropriate?
    A. High calcium, low phosphorus
    B. Low calcium, high phosphorus
    C. Two-gram sodium diet
    D. Low calcium and phosphorus, acid ash

78. A client is admitted to the hospital with diabetic ketoacidosis. The emergency room nurse should anticipate the administration of:
    A. Humulin N
    B. Humulin R
    C. Humulin U
    D. Humulin L

79. A client is diagnosed with diabetic ketoacidosis. The nurse should be prepared to administer which of the following IV solutions?
    A. D_5 in normal saline
    B. D_5W
    C. 0.9 normal saline
    D. D_5 in lactated Ringer's

MOCK NCLEX-RN BOARD REVIEW TEST ANSWERS

1. **(C)** Client need: physiological integrity; subcategory: physiological adaptation; content area: maternity

   RATIONALE

   (A) Cyanosis is a late clinical sign of respiratory distress. (B) Rapid respirations are normal in a newborn. (C) The newborn has to exert an extra effort for ventilation, which is accomplished by using the accessory muscles of ventilation. The diaphragm and abdominal muscles are immature and weak in the newborn. (D) Decreased respirations are a late clinical sign. In the newborn, decreased respirations precede respiratory failure.

2. **(A)** Client need: health promotion and maintenance; subcategory: growth and development through the life span; content area: maternity

   RATIONALE

   (A) The fetal descent, or station, is determined by the relationship of the presenting part to the spine. (B) Ischial spines are the narrowest measurement. (C) Ischial spines measure the pelvic outlet. (D) Pelvic floor measurement is not related to fetal descent.

3. **(B)** Client need: health promotion and maintenance; subcategory: growth and development through the life span; content area: maternity

   RATIONALE

   (A) Uterine contractions increase with activity. (B) Walking will increase the strength and regularity of uterine contractions in true labor. (C) Uterine contractions that are strong and regular facilitate cervical dilation. (D) Regular, strong uterine contractions, as in true labor, result in fetal descent.

4. **(A)** Client need: physiological integrity; subcategory: physiological adaptation; content area: maternity

   RATIONALE

   (A) Maternal blood volume increases at the end of the first trimester leading to a dilutional anemia. (B) Maternal blood volume increases. (C) Fetal blood volume is minimal in the first trimester. (D) Increased iron absorption would facilitate the manufacturing of erythrocytes and decrease anemia.

5. **(A)** Client need: health promotion and maintenance; subcategory: prevention and early detection of disease; content area: maternity

   RATIONALE

   (A) Organogenesis occurs in the first trimester. Fetus is most susceptible to malformation during this period. (B) Organogenesis has occurred by the second trimester. (C) Fetal development is complete by this time. (D) The dangerous period for fetal damage is the first trimester, not the entire pregnancy.

6. **(C)** Client need: physiological integrity; subcategory: reduction of risk potential; content area: maternity

   RATIONALE

   (A) Reverse Trendelenburg position increases pressure on the perineum. This position will not relieve cord pressure. (B) Fowler's position increases perineal pressure. Cord pressure would not be relieved. (C) Trendelenburg position will decrease perineal pressure. Cord compression will be decreased and increase in fetal blood flow occurs. (D) Sims' position does not relieve pressure on cord or perineum.

7. **(D)** Client need: health promotion and maintenance; subcategory: growth and development through the life span; content area: maternity

   RATIONALE

   (A) Wrong calculation (B) Wrong calculation (C) Wrong calculation (D) Nägele's rule is: Expected Date of Confinement = Last Menstrual Period − 3 months + 7 days + 1 year

8. **(B)** Client need: physiological integrity; subcategory: reduction of risk potential; content area: maternity

   RATIONALE

   (A) If the client is experiencing water satiety, there is no more desire for water. (B) Absorption of saline into circulation rather than into amniotic sac increases serum sodium and desire for water. (C) Edema can be a late side effect caused by water intoxication. (D) Diabetes insipidus occurs as a result of deficient antidiuretic hormone.

9. **(C)** Client need: health promotion and maintenance; subcategory: growth and development through the life span; content area: maternity

   RATIONALE

   (A) Pupil response should be assessed but is not part of Apgar scoring. (B) Respiratory effort is an essential part of Apgar scoring, not respiratory rate. (C) Heart rate is the most critical component of Apgar scoring. (D) Assessment of Babinski's reflex is not a component of Apgar scoring.

10. **(C)** Client need: physiological integrity; subcategory: physiological adaptation; content area: maternity

    RATIONALE

    (A) Menstruation should not occur during pregnancy. (B) Abruptio placentae is marked by painful vaginal bleeding following a premature placental detachment after 20th week of gestation. (C) A low-lying placenta separates from the uterine wall as the uterus contracts and cervix dilates. This separation causes painless bleeding in the 7th-8th month. (D) Polyhydramnios is excessive amniotic fluid.

11. **(B)** Client need: psychosocial integrity; subcategory: coping and adaptation; content area: maternity

    RATIONALE

    (A) This observation can be made during the taking-in phase when the mother's needs are more important. (B) This observation can be made during the taking-hold phase when the mother is actively involved with herself and the infant. (C, D) This observation can be made during the taking-in phase.

12. **(A)** Client need: physiological integrity; subcategory: pharmacological and parenteral therapies; content area: maternity

    RATIONALE

    (A) Oxytocin is a hormone secreted by the neurohypophysis during suckling and parturition that produces strong uterine contractions. (B) Progesterone has a quiescence effect on the uterus. (C) Vasopressin is an antidiuretic hormone that promotes water reabsorption by the renal tubules. (D) Ergonovine produces dystocia as a result of sustained uterine contractions.

13. **(A)** Client need: health promotion and maintenance; subcategory: growth and development through the life span; content area: maternity

    RATIONALE

    (A) The second stage of labor is characterized by uterine contractions, which cause the client to bear down. (B) Slow, deep, rhythmic breathing facilitates the laboring process. Hyperventilation is abnormal breathing resulting from loss of pain control. (C) The client should remain on bed rest during labor. (D) Contractions result in discomfort.

14. **(C)** Client need: health promotion and maintenance; subcategory: growth and development through the life span; content area: maternity

    RATIONALE

    (A) The fourth stage begins after expulsion of the placenta. Client symptoms are: fatigue; chills; scant, bloody vaginal discharge; and nausea. (B) The third stage is from birth to expulsion of placenta. Client symptoms are uterine contractions, gush of blood, and perineal pain. (C) The transition stage is characterized by strong uterine contractions and cervical dilation. Client symptoms are irritability, restlessness, belching, muscle tremors, nausea, and vomiting. (D) The second stage is characterized by full dilation of cervix. Client symptoms are perineal bulge, pushing with contractions, great irritability, and leg cramps.

15. **(C)** Client need: health promotion and maintenance; subcategory: growth and development through the life span; content area: maternity

    RATIONALE

    (A) Immediately following membrane rupture, the fetus is at risk for complications, not necessarily the mother. (B) The physician is notified after the nurse completes an assessment of the mother's and fetus's conditions. (C) Rupture of membranes facilitates fetal descent. A potential complication is cord prolapse, which is assessed by auscultating fetal heart rate. (D) Rupture of membranes does not necessarily indicate readiness to deliver.

16. **(A)** Client need: physiological integrity; subcategory: physiological adaptation; content area: maternity

    RATIONALE

    (A) Controlling the rapid delivery will reduce the risk of fetal injury and perineal lacerations. (B) The nurse should always remain with a client experiencing a precipitous delivery. (C) Pushing against the perineum may cause fetal distress. (D) Crossing of legs may cause fetal distress and does not stop the delivery process.

17. **(D)** Client need: physiological integrity; subcategory: physiological adaptation; content area: maternity

    RATIONALE

    (A) Dystocia is difficult labor. The delivery has occurred. Kraurosis is atrophy and dryness of skin and any mucous membrane (vulva). (B) Chadwick's sign is a bluish color of vaginal mucosa suggestive of pregnancy. (C) Fatigue is a common symptom in the postpartal period. Hemorrhoids may occur with pregnancy. (D) Hemorrhage and infection are potential complications of vaginal delivery. Hemorrhage may result from retained placental fragments or soft uterus. Infection may occur from the introduction of organisms into the uterus during the delivery.

18. **(C)** Client need: physiological integrity; subcategory: pharmacological and parenteral therapies; content area: maternity

    RATIONALE

    (A) Oxytocin is prescribed to stimulate uterine contractions. (B) $MgSO_4$ is a central nervous system depressant prescribed to prevent and control convulsions related to preeclampsia. (C) Ampicillin is a penicillin derivative with no known teratogenic effects. This is the safest antibiotic during pregnancy. (D) Tetracycline stains teeth yellow and is not as safe as ampicillin during pregnancy.

19. **(B)** Client need: physiological integrity; subcategory: physiological adaptation; content area: maternity

    RATIONALE

    (A) Central nervous system damage presents as seizures, decreased arousal, and absence of newborn reflexes. (B) In a diabetic mother, the infant is exposed to high serum glucose. The fetal pancreas produces large amounts of insulin, which causes hypoglycemia after birth. (C) Hypoglycemia is a common newborn problem. Increased insulin production causes hypoglycemia, not hyperglycemia. (D) These are not normal adaptive behaviors to extrauterine life.

20. **(A)** Client need: physiological integrity; subcategory: reduction of risk potential; content area: maternity

    RATIONALE

    (A) Retrolental fibroplasia is the result of prolonged exposure to high levels of O_2 in premature infants. Complications are hemorrhage and retinal detachment. (B, C, D) O_2 concentration is too high.

21. **(C)** Client need: psychosocial integrity; subcategory: coping and adaptation; content area: psychiatric

    RATIONALE

    (A) This nursing action is too controlling and authoritative. It could increase the client's anxiety level. (B) In her anxiety state, the client cannot rationally identify a problem. (C) This nursing action conveys a message of caring and security. (D) Giving the client a task would increase her anxiety. This would be a late nursing action.

22. **(B)** Client need: psychosocial integrity; subcategory: psychosocial adaptation; content area: psychiatric

    RATIONALE

    (A) Anger is an emotion that is not necessarily present in schizophrenia. (B) Lack of response to or involvement with environment and distancing are characteristic of schizophrenia. (C) Euphoria is more characteristic of manic-depressive disorder (bipolar disorder). (D) Hostility is an emotion that is not necessarily present in schizophrenia.

23. **(C)** Client need: psychosocial integrity; subcategory: psychosocial adaptation; content area: psychiatric

    RATIONALE

    (A) Anorexia nervosa is characterized by self-starvation. (B) Anorexia hysteria is not a known disease or disorder. (C) Bulimia is characterized by food binges and self-induced vomiting. (D) Conversion reaction is a defense mechanism.

24. **(A)** Client need: psychosocial integrity; subcategory: psychosocial adaptation; content area: psychiatric

    RATIONALE

    (A) Delusion is a false belief. (B) Illusion is the misrepresentation of a real, external sensory experience. (C) Hallucination is a false sensory perception involving any of the senses. (D) Conversion is the expression of intrapsychic conflict through sensory or motor manifestations.

25. **(D)** Client need: psychosocial integrity; subcategory: coping and adaptation; content area: psychiatric

    RATIONALE

    (A) The client's blindness is real. Delusion is a false belief. (B) Illusion is the misrepresentation of a real, external sensory experience. (C) Hallucination is a false sensory perception involving any of the senses. (D) Conversion is the expression of intrapsychic conflict through sensory or motor manifestations.

26. **(C)** Client need: psychosocial integrity; subcategory: coping and adaptation; content area: psychiatric

    RATIONALE

    (A) Denial is the disowning of consciously intolerable thoughts. (B) Displacement is the referring of a feeling or emotion from one person, object, or idea to another. (C) Regression is returning to an earlier stage of development. (D) Projection is attributing one's own thoughts, feelings, or impulses to another person.

27. **(B)** Client need: psychosocial integrity; subcategory: coping and adaptation; content area: pediatrics

RATIONALE

(A) The Electra complex is the erotic attachment of the female child to the father. (B) The Oedipus complex is characterized by jealousy toward the parent of the same sex and erotic attachment to the parent of the opposite sex. (C) The superego as described by Freud is the part of personality that is associated with internalized parental and societal control. (D) The ego as described by Freud is the part of personality that is associated with reality assessment.

28. **(A)** Client need: physiological integrity; subcategory: pharmacological and parenteral therapies; content area: psychiatric

RATIONALE

(A) Benztropine is prescribed to decrease or alleviate extrapyramidal side effects of major tranquilizers. Smooth, coordinated voluntary movement indicates minimal extrapyramidal side effects. (B) Tremors are an extrapyramidal side effect. (C) Rigidity is an extrapyramidal side effect. (D) Muscle weakness is an extrapyramidal side effect.

29. **(A)** Client need: physiological integrity; subcategory: basic care and comfort; content area: psychiatric

RATIONALE

(A) A priority nursing goal is attending to the client's safety and well-being. Reorient frequently, remove dangerous objects, and maintain consistent environment. (B) Short, frequent visits are recommended to avoid overstimulation and fatigue. (C) Short, concise, simple explanations are easier to understand. (D) Mental capability and attention span deficits make learning difficult and frustrating.

30. **(B)** Client need: psychosocial integrity; subcategory: coping and adaptation; content area: pediatrics

RATIONALE

(A) Respite care for the family may be needed, but it is not the primary goal of a preschool program. (B) Facilitation of optimal growth and development is essential for every child. (C) A demanding and challenging educational program may predispose the child to failure. Children with retardation should begin with simple and challenging educational programs. (D) Mental retardation associated with Down syndrome may not permit mainstream education. A preschool program's primary goal is not preparation for mainstream education but continuation of optimal development.

31. **(A)** Client need: physiological integrity; subcategory: basic care and comfort; content area: pediatrics

RATIONALE

(A) Immobilization, splinting, and bed rest will reduce the bleeding. Once bleeding is reduced or stopped, the pain will subside. (B) Moist heat causes vasodilation and bleeding. Ice or cold compresses should be applied. (C) Aspirin decreases platelet aggregation, which causes bleeding. (D) Active range of motion aggravates bleeding and damages the synovial sac during bleeding episodes.

32. **(D)** Client need: physiological integrity; subcategory: basic care and comfort; content area: pediatrics

RATIONALE

(A) A gavage tube may damage suture line. It is the most invasive and should be the last measure. (B) A nipple and bottle require sucking, which may damage sutures. (C) A 3-month-old infant is not able to drink from a straw. (D) A syringe allows for the formula to be placed to the side and back of the mouth. This minimizes the amount of sucking needed.

33. **(C)** Client need: health promotion and maintenance; subcategory: prevention and early detection of disease; content area: pediatrics

RATIONALE

(A) Bulging fontanelles are a symptom of increased intracranial pressure in infants. (B) Seizure is a late sign of increased intracranial pressure. (C) Headache is a very early symptom of increased intracranial pressure in the child. (D) Ataxia is a late sign of increased intracranial pressure.

34. **(A)** Client need: physiological integrity; subcategory: reduction of risk potential; content area: pediatrics

RATIONALE

(A) Elevation of head of bed and neutral head position promote drainage of cerebrospinal fluid. (B) Flat position increases intracranial pressure and impedes cerebrospinal fluid drainage. (C) Head turned to either side impedes cerebrospinal fluid drainage. (D) Child should be in a calm, quiet environment with minimal stimulation.

35. **(D)** Client need: physiological integrity; subcategory: reduction of risk potential; content area: pediatrics

RATIONALE

(A) Elevation of head on nonoperative side would be the position for the late postoperative period. (B) Positioning on operative side puts pressure on the suture lines and on the shunt valve. Elevation of head in immediate postoperative period may cause rapid reduction of cerebrospinal fluid. (C) Placement on operative side puts pressure on the suture lines and shunt valve. (D) Flat position on nonoperative side in the immediate postoperative period prevents pressure on shunt valve and rapid reduction in cerebrospinal fluid.

36. **(B)** Client need: physiological integrity; subcategory: reduction of risk potential; content area: maternity

RATIONALE

(A) Bonding is necessary but would not be the priority with this newborn in the nursery. (B) The infant will be at risk for hypoglycemia because of excess insulin production. (C) Normal nutrition is a goal for all newborns. (D) Monitoring intake and output is necessary but is not the most critical nursing goal.

37. **(C)** Client need: physiological integrity; subcategory: reduction of risk potential; content area: pediatrics

RATIONALE

(A) Normal pH of arterial blood gases for an infant is 7.35–7.45. (B) Normal white blood cell count in an infant is 6,000–17,500 WBCs/mm^3. (C) Normal hematocrit in infant is 28%–42%. A 60% hematocrit may indicate polycythemia, a common complication of cyanotic heart disease. (D) Normal bleeding time is 2–7 minutes.

38. **(C)** Client need: physiological integrity; subcategory: pharmacological and parenteral therapies; content area: pediatrics

RATIONALE

(A) A volume control set has a chamber that permits the administration of compatible drugs. (B) Air may enter a volume control set when tubing is not adequately purged. (C) A volume control set allows the nurse to control the amount of fluid administered over a set period. (D) Contamination of volume control set may cause phlebitis.

39. **(C)** Client need: physiological integrity; subcategory: pharmacological and parenteral therapies; content area: med/surg

RATIONALE

(A) Humulin N cannot be administered IV. (B) NPH insulin cannot be administered IV. (C) Regular insulin is the only insulin that can be administered IV. (D) Lente insulin cannot be administered IV.

40. **(A)** Client need: physiological integrity; subcategory: pharmacological and parenteral therapies; content area: pharmacology

RATIONALE

(A) 1 mg = 0.1 mL, then $0.5 \text{ mL} \times \dfrac{1.0 \text{ mg}}{0.1 \text{ mL}} = 55 \text{ mg}$. (B) This answer is a miscalculation. (C) This answer is a miscalculation. (D) This answer is a miscalculation.

41. **(C)** Client need: physiological integrity; subcategory: pharmacological and parenteral therapies; content area: pharmacology

RATIONALE

(A) This answer is a miscalculation. (B) This answer is a miscalculation. (C) 1.33 mEq = 1 mL, then $1.5 \text{ mL} \times \dfrac{1.33 \text{ mEq}}{1 \text{ mL}} =$ 1.99, or 2 mEq. (D) Information is adequate for calculation.

42. **(D)** Client need: physiological integrity; subcategory: pharmacological and parenteral therapies; content area: pharmacology

RATIONALE

(A) This answer is a miscalculation. (B) This answer is a miscalculation. (C) This answer has not been rounded off to an even number. (D) $\dfrac{1{,}000 \text{ mL} \times 10 \text{ gtt/mL}}{8 \text{ hr} \times 60 \text{ min/hr}} = \dfrac{10{,}000}{480} = 20.8$, or 21 gtt/min.

43. **(C)** Client need: physiological integrity; subcategory: pharmacological and parenteral therapies; content area: pharmacology

RATIONALE

(A) This answer is a miscalculation. (B) This answer is a miscalculation. (C) $\dfrac{1{,}000 \text{ mL} \times 60 \text{ gtt/mL}}{8 \text{ hr} \times 60 \text{ min/hr}} = \dfrac{60{,}000}{480} = 125 \text{ gtt/min}$. (D) This answer is a miscalculation.

44. **(C)** Client need: physiological integrity; subcategory: pharmacological and parenteral therapies; content area: pharmacology

RATIONALE

(A) This answer is a miscalculation. (B) This answer is a miscalculation. (C) $\dfrac{50 \text{ mL} \times 60 \text{ gtt/mL}}{60 \text{ min}} = \dfrac{3{,}000}{60} = 50 \text{ gtt/min}$. (D) This answer is a miscalculation.

45. **(C)** Client need: health promotion and maintenance; subcategory: prevention and early detection of disease; content area: pediatrics

RATIONALE

(A) Hearing should be assessed separately. (B) Gait should be assessed separately. Client usually remains in one place for vision screening. Gait is part of neurological assessment. (C) Strabismus is crossing of eyes or outward deviation, which may cause diplopia or ambylopia. It is easily assessed during vision screening. (D) Papilledema is assessed by an ophthalmoscopic examination, which follows vision screening. It is part of neurological assessment.

46. **(D)** Client need: physiological integrity; subcategory: physiological adaptation; content area: pediatrics

RATIONALE

(A) Ice creates a dramatic temperature change in the tissue, which can cause further thermal injury. (B) Charred clothing should not be removed from wound first. This creates further tissue damage. Débridement is not the first nursing action. (C) Applying silver sulfadiazine cream first insulates heat in injured tissue and increases potential for infection. (D) Emergency care of a thermal burn is immersing both legs in cool water. Cool water permits gradual temperature change and prevents further thermal damage.

47. **(C)** Client need: health promotion and maintenance; subcategory: prevention and early detection of disease; content area: pediatrics

RATIONALE

(A) Oral poliovirus vaccine is given to prevent polio. Polio is transmitted by direct contact with an infected person. (B) Inactivated poliovirus vaccine is given to adults and immunosuppressed individuals. Polio is transmitted by direct contact with an infected person. (C) Tetanus toxoid prevents tetanus. Tetanus is transmitted through contaminated wounds. (D) Hepatitis B vaccine prevents hepatitis B infection. Hepatitis B is transmitted through contact with infected blood or body fluids.

48. **(A)** Client need: physiological integrity; subcategory: basic care and comfort; content area: maternity

RATIONALE

(A) The prone position reduces pressure and tension on the sac. Primary nursing goals are to prevent trauma and infection of the sac. (B) The supine position exerts pressure on the sac. (C) Newborns usually cannot maintain side-lying position. (D) The semi-Fowler position exerts pressure on the sac.

49. **(B)** Client need: physiological integrity; subcategory: reduction of risk potential; content area: pediatrics

RATIONALE

(A) A dry, sterile dressing would adhere to the sac, causing tissue damage. (B) A saline-soaked sterile dressing protects the sac from contamination by air and prevents drying. (C) A sac open to air causes drying and potential for contamination. (D) This intervention is not an independent nursing action.

50. **(D)** Client need: physiological integrity; subcategory: physiological adaptation; content area: med/surg

RATIONALE

(A) Respiratory alkalosis is determined by elevated pH and low $PaCO_2$. (B) Respiratory acidosis is determined by low pH and elevated $PaCO_2$. (C) Metabolic alkalosis is determined by elevated pH and HCO_3. (D) Metabolic acidosis is determined by low pH and HCO_3.

51. **(B)** Client need: physiological integrity; subcategory: physiological adaptation; content area: med/surg

RATIONALE

(A) Respiratory alkalosis is determined by elevated pH and low $PaCO_2$. (B) Respiratory acidosis is determined by low pH and elevated $PaCO_2$. (C) Metabolic alkalosis is determined by elevated pH and HCO_3. (D) Metabolic acidosis is determined by low pH and HCO_3.

52. **(D)** Client need: physiological integrity; subcategory: reduction of risk potential; content area: med/surg

RATIONALE

(A) Reticulocyte count measures the number of immature erythrocytes. CPK is an enzyme released from injured myocardial tissue. (B) Aspartate transaminase is an enzyme released from injured myocardial tissue. Alanine transaminase is an enzyme released for general tissue destruction, which is specific for liver injury. (C) Sedimentation rate is a nonspecific test for inflammation. (D) Lactic dehydrogenase and CPK are enzymes released from injured myocardial tissue.

53. **(D)** Client need: physiological integrity; subcategory: physiological adaptation; content area: med/surg

RATIONALE

(A) Diabetes mellitus is not a common complication of myocardial infarction. (B) Anaphylactic shock is an allergic reaction. (C) Cardiac hypertrophy is a late potential complication. It is a common complication of congestive heart failure. (D) Myocardial infarction causes tissue damage, which may interrupt electrical impulses. Myocardial irritability results from lack of oxygenated tissue.

54. **(C)** Client need: physiological integrity; subcategory: reduction of risk potential; content area: med/surg

    RATIONALE

    (A) Intake and output are not laboratory tests. (B) Serum calcium levels are not affected by digoxin or furosemide. (C) Furosemide is a non–potassium-sparing loop diuretic. Hypokalemia is a common side effect of furosemide and may enhance digoxin toxicity. (D) Serum magnesium levels are not affected by digoxin or furosemide.

55. **(C)** Client need: physiological integrity; subcategory: pharmacological and parenteral therapies; content area: med/surg

    RATIONALE

    (A) Furosemide is a loop diuretic. (B) Nitroglycerin is a vasodilator. (C) Lidocaine is the drug of choice to treat ectopic ventricular beats. (D) Digoxin slows down the electrical impulses and increases ventricular contractions, but it does not rapidly correct ventricular ectopy.

56. **(D)** Client need: physiological integrity; subcategory: pharmacological and parenteral therapies; content area: med/surg

    RATIONALE

    (A) 0.5 ng/mL of digoxin is a subtherapeutic level, not a toxic one. (B) 1.0 ng/mL is a therapeutic level. (C) 2.0 ng/mL is a therapeutic level. (D) Digoxin's therapeutic level is 0.8–2.0 ng/mL. Digoxin's toxic level is >2.0 ng/mL.

57. **(B)** Client need: health promotion and maintenance; subcategory: prevention and early detection of disease; content area: med/surg

    RATIONALE

    (A) Fresh vegetables and fruits are excellent sources of essential vitamins. (B) Canned and frozen foods have a high sodium content. Labels of all canned foods should be read to determine if sodium is used in any form. (C) Bread, cereal, and rice are excellent sources of carbohydrates. (D) Fish is an excellent source of protein.

58. **(A)** Client need: physiological integrity; subcategory: reduction of risk potential; content area: med/surg

    RATIONALE

    (A) PT evaluates adequacy of extrinsic clotting pathway. Adequacy of warfarin therapy is monitored by PT. (B) PTT evaluates adequacy of intrinsic clotting pathway. Adequacy of heparin therapy is monitored by PTT. (C) There is no such laboratory test. (D) Fibrin split products indicate fibrinolysis. This is a screening test for disseminated intravascular coagulation. Heparin therapy may increase fibrin split products.

59. **(D)** Client need: physiological integrity; subcategory: reduction of risk potential; content area: med/surg

    RATIONALE

    (A) Respiratory rate is not directly affected by digoxin therapy. (B) A radial pulse is not as accurate as an apical pulse. Dysrhythmias may not be detected. (C) A radial pulse is not as accurate as an apical pulse, regardless of assessment time. (D) Apical pulse should be measured for 1-minute prior to digoxin administration. Digoxin decreases the heart rate. Digoxin should be withheld if apical rates are <60 bpm or >120 bpm.

60. **(B)** Client need: physiological integrity; subcategory: physiological adaptation; content area: med/surg

    RATIONALE

    (A) The maximum time for suctioning is 10–15 seconds. (B) Supplemental O_2 should be administered before and after suctioning to reduce hypoxia. (C) The maximum time for suctioning is 10–15 seconds. (D) Strict sterile technique should be used during suctioning.

61. **(D)** Client need: physiological integrity; subcategory: pharmacological and parenteral therapies; content area: med/surg

    RATIONALE

    (A) Vitamin B_6 does not enhance the activity of isoniazid. (B) Vitamin B_6 does not enhance the activity of rifampin. (C) A vitamin alone does not improve nutritional status. (D) Isoniazid leads to Vitamin B_6 deficiency, which is manifested as peripheral neuropathy.

62. **(D)** Client need: health promotion and maintenance; subcategory: prevention and early detection of disease; content area: med/surg

    RATIONALE

    (A) Monitoring liver function will not prevent the development of drug-resistant organisms. (B) Monitoring renal function will not prevent the development of drug-resistant organisms. (C) Knowledge of respiratory isolation will reduce transmission of tuberculosis but will not prevent development of drug-resistant organisms. (D) Noncompliance with prescribed antituberculosis drug regimen is the primary cause of drug-resistant organisms. Noncompliance permits the mutation of organisms.

63. **(B)** Client need: physiological integrity; subcategory: basic care and comfort; content area: med/surg

    RATIONALE

    (A) The high Fowler position does increase air exchange, but not to the extent of orthopneic position. (B) The orthopneic position is a sitting position that allows maximum lung expansion. (C) The prone position places pressure on diaphragm and does not promote maximum air exchange. (D) The flat-supine position places pressure on diaphragm by abdominal organs and does not promote maximum air exchange.

64. **(B)** Client need: physiological integrity; subcategory: basic care and comfort; content area: med/surg

    RATIONALE

    (A, C, D) This answer is a miscalculation. (B) 1 oz = 30 mL; therefore, $18 \text{ oz} \times \dfrac{30 \text{ mL}}{1 \text{ oz}} = 540 \text{ mL}$.

65. **(C)** Client need: physiological integrity; subcategory: physiological adaptation; content area: med/surg

    RATIONALE

    (A) Evaluation process follows a nursing intervention. (B) Objective information can be measured. (C) Subjective information is provided by a person. (D) Client is reporting a symptom that needs to be assessed.

66. **(B)** Client need: safe, effective care environment; subcategory: management of care; content area: med/surg

    RATIONALE

    (A) Goals and objectives are based on a nursing assessment and diagnosis. (B) Assessment is the first step of nursing process. (C) Interventions are nursing actions to meet goals and objectives. (D) Evaluation process follows nursing interventions.

67. **(B)** Client need: physiological integrity; subcategory: reduction of risk potential; content area: med/surg

    RATIONALE

    (A) Head should be tilted slightly forward to facilitate insertion. (B) Swallowing assists with insertion of tube and closes off airway. (C) Client should be swallowing as tube passes; holding the breath facilitates nothing. (D) Coughing may expel tube.

68. **(D)** Client need: physiological integrity; subcategory: reduction of risk potential; content area: med/surg

    RATIONALE

    (A) A residual volume of 20 mL is not excessive. (B) A residual volume of 25 mL is not excessive. (C) A residual volume of 30 mL is not excessive. (D) Tube feedings should be withheld and physician notified for residual volumes of 50–100 mL.

69. **(B)** Client need: physiological integrity; subcategory: basic care and comfort; content area: med/surg

    RATIONALE

    (A) A high-protein diet is contraindicated in hepatic disease. (B) High carbohydrates provide high-caloric content to prevent tissue catabolism. (C) A low-fat 2-g sodium diet is a cardiac diet; however, a low-fat diet would be beneficial. (D) A high-protein and high-fat diet is contraindicated in hepatic disease.

70. **(A)** Client need: physiological integrity; subcategory: physiological adaptation; content area: med/surg

    RATIONALE

    (A) A decrease in plasma proteins causes a decrease in intravascular osmotic pressure resulting in leakage of fluid into peritoneal cavity. (B) Fluid and electrolyte imbalance may occur as a result of the ascites. (C) Ascites is a result of hepatic malfunction, not renal malfunction. (D) Portal hypertension causes esophageal varices, not ascites.

71. **(B)** Client need: physiological integrity; subcategory: reduction of risk potential; content area: med/surg

    RATIONALE

    (A) Vitamin C does not directly affect clotting. (B) Vitamin K is a fat-soluble vitamin that depends on liver function for absorption. Vitamin K is essential for clotting. (C) Vitamin E does not directly affect clotting. (D) Vitamin A does not directly affect clotting.

72. **(B)** Client need: physiological integrity; subcategory: basic care and comfort; content area: med/surg

    RATIONALE

    (A, C, D) These foods are allowed with a colostomy. (B) Gas-forming foods such as cabbage should be avoided.

73. **(C)** Client need: physiological integrity; subcategory: physiological adaptation; content area: med/surg

    RATIONALE

    (A) Xerostomia is dry mouth. (B) Candidiasis can be rubbed off, but it will bleed. (C) Leukoplakia cannot be rubbed off. (D) Stomatitis is caused by candidiasis and gram-negative bacteria.

74. **(C)** Client need: health promotion and maintenance; subcategory: prevention and early detection of disease; content area: med/surg

    RATIONALE

    (A) HIV is transmitted through unprotected sexual contact. (B) Condoms are an effective barrier to prevent HIV transmission. (C) HIV is not easily transmitted by casual contact. (D) HIV can be transmitted intrauterinely at the time of delivery, and by breast-feeding.

75. **(A)** Client need: physiological integrity; subcategory: physiological adaptation; content area: med/surg

    RATIONALE

    (A) Both a benign and a malignant tumor can displace or destroy nearby structures or increase intracranial pressure. (B) Benign or malignant brain tumors grow at different rates depending on the type of tumor. (C) Some benign tumors do become malignant tumors. (D) Whether or not a tumor is operable depends on its location and the amount of damage its removal will cause.

76. **(C)** Client need: physiological integrity; subcategory: reduction of risk potential; content area: med/surg

    RATIONALE

    (A) Intake and output measurements are important but must be accompanied by straining urine. (B) Daily weights would not provide for identification of calculi. (C) Straining urine provides for assessment of calculi and evaluation of calculi descent through ureters and urethra. (D) O_2 therapy should not be necessary for renal calculi.

77. **(D)** Client need: physiological integrity; subcategory: physiological adaptation; content area: med/surg

    RATIONALE

    (A) The stones consist of calcium and phosphorus; therefore, these minerals should be avoided. A high-calcium diet is contraindicated. (B) A high-phosphorus diet is contraindicated. (C) A 2-g sodium diet is a cardiac diet. (D) A low-calcium and phosphorus diet will reduce further calculi formation.

78. **(B)** Client need: physiological integrity; subcategory: pharmacological and parenteral therapies; content area: med/surg

    RATIONALE

    (A) Intermediate-acting insulin is not indicated in an emergency. (B) Regular insulin is rapid acting and indicated in an emergency situation. (C) Long-acting insulin is not indicated in an emergency situation. (D) Intermediate-acting insulin is not indicated in an emergency situation.

79. **(C)** Client need: physiological integrity; subcategory: pharmacological and parenteral therapies; content area: med/surg

    RATIONALE

    (A) D_5 in normal saline would increase serum glucose. (B) D_5W would increase serum glucose. (C) A concentration of 0.9 NS is used to correct extracellular fluid depletion. (D) D_5 in Ringer's lactate would increase serum glucose.

TEST 5

University of Arkansas for Medical Sciences Test

MOCK NCLEX-RN BOARD REVIEW TEST QUESTIONS

1. The nurse is caring for a client who has diabetes insipidus. The nurse would describe this client's urine output pattern as:

    A. Anuria
    B. Oliguria
    C. Dysuria
    D. Polyuria

2. A male client was involved in a motor vehicle accident earlier in the day. The nurse caring for him on evenings notices that on admission to the hospital, he lost a lot of blood and required multiple blood transfusions. The nurse would anticipate which blood product would be ordered when a large blood loss has occurred?

    A. Whole blood
    B. Platelets
    C. Fresh frozen plasma
    D. Packed red blood cells

3. An expected response to sodium polystyrene sulfonate (Kayexalate) is:

    A. Increase in serum magnesium
    B. Increase in serum HCO_3
    C. Decrease in serum potassium
    D. Decrease in serum calcium

4. Cheyne-Stokes respiratory pattern can be associated with which of the following conditions?

    A. Diabetic ketoacidosis
    B. Fever
    C. Increased intracranial pressure
    D. Spinal meningitis

5. When providing dietary teaching to an individual who has diabetes mellitus, type II, the nurse discusses the importance of consuming the recommended daily allowance of which of the following electrolytes?

    A. Potassium
    B. Magnesium
    C. Sodium
    D. HCO_3

6. A physician tells the nurse that he wants to orally intubate a client with a No. 8 endotracheal tube. The finding of normal breath sounds on the right side of the chest and diminished, distant breath sounds on the left side of the chest of a newly intubated client is probably due to:

    A. A left hemothorax
    B. A right hemothorax
    C. Intubation of the right mainstem bronchus
    D. An inadequate mechanical ventilator

7. Which of the following blood gas parameters primarily reflects respiratory function?

    A. P_{CO_2}
    B. CO_2 content of the blood
    C. HCO_3
    D. Base excess

8. Endotracheal tube cuff pressure should never exceed:

    A. 10 mm Hg
    B. 20 mm Hg
    C. 45 mm Hg
    D. 60 mm Hg

9. The physician prescribes phenytoin (Dilantin) for a client with seizure disorders. Phenytoin can only be mixed with which of the following solutions?

    A. Ringer's lactate
    B. D_5 in water
    C. D_5 with Ringer's lactate
    D. Normal saline

10. A client sustained second- and third-degree burns to his face, neck, and upper chest. Which of the following

nursing diagnoses would be given the highest priority in the first 8 hours' postburn?

A. Fluid volume deficit secondary to alteration in skin integrity
B. Alteration in comfort secondary to alteration in skin integrity
C. Alteration in sensation secondary to third-degree burn
D. Alteration in airway integrity secondary to edema of neck and face, which in turn is secondary to alteration in skin integrity

11. A post-lung surgery client is placed on a chest tube drainage system. When explaining to the family how the system works, the nurse states that the water-seal bottle of a three-bottle chest drainage system serves which of the following purposes?

A. Collection bottle for drainage
B. Pressure regulator
C. Preventing accumulation of blood around the heart
D. Preventing air from entering the chest upon inspiration

12. Which of the following serum laboratory values would the nurse monitor during gentamicin therapy?

A. Creatinine
B. Sodium
C. Calcium
D. Potassium

13. While changing the dressing on a client's central line, the nurse notices redness and warmth at the needle insertion site. Which of the following actions would be appropriate to implement based on this finding?

A. Discontinue the central line.
B. Begin a peripheral IV.
C. Document in the nurse's notes and notify the physician after redressing the site.
D. Clean the site well and redress.

14. The nurse is caring for a client who has had a tracheostomy for 7 years. The client is started on a full-strength tube feeding at 75 mL/hr. Prior to starting the tube feeding, the nurse confirms placement of the tube in the stomach. The hospital policy states that all tube feeding must be dyed blue. On suctioning, the nurse notices the sputum to be a blue color. This is indicative of which of the following?

A. The client aspirated tube feeding.
B. The nurse has placed the suction catheter in the esophagus.
C. This is a normal finding.
D. The feeding is infusing into the trachea.

15. The nurse is caring for a client with pancreatitis. Which of the following IV medications would the nurse expect the physician to prescribe for control of pain in this client?

A. Morphine sulfate
B. Kerolac tromethamine (Toradol)
C. Promethazine (Phenergan)
D. Meperidine (Demerol)

16. The nurse begins morning assessment on a male client and notices that she is unable to palpate either of his dorsalis pedis pulses in his feet. What is the first nursing action after assessing this finding?

A. Palpate these pulses again in 15 minutes.
B. Use a Doppler to determine presence and strength of these pulses.
C. Document the finding that the pulses are not palpable.
D. Call the physician and notify the physician of this finding.

17. The physician has prescribed metoclopramide (Reglan). When assessing the client, the nurse would expect to find which of the following responses?

A. Increase in gastric secretions
B. Increase in peristalsis
C. Disorientation
D. Drowsiness

18. A 33-year-old client was brought into the emergency room unconscious, and it is determined that surgery is needed. Informed consent must be obtained from his next of kin. The sequence in which the next of kin would be asked for the consent would be:

A. Parent, spouse, adult child, sibling
B. Spouse, adult child, parent, sibling
C. Spouse, parent, sibling, adult child
D. Parent, spouse, sibling, adult child

19. A client had abdominal surgery this morning. The nurse notices that there is a small amount of bloody drainage on his surgical dressing. The nurse would document this as what type of drainage?

A. Serosanguinous
B. Purulent
C. Sanguinous
D. Catarrhal

20. A client had a hemicolectomy performed 2 days ago. Today, when the nurse assesses the incision, a small part of the abdominal viscera is seen protruding through the incision. This complication of wound healing is known as:

A. Excoriation
B. Dehiscence
C. Decortication
D. Evisceration

21. The nurse documents a client's surgical incision as having red granulated tissue. This indicates that the wound is:

A. Infected
B. Not healing
C. Necrotic
D. Healing

22. A client has returned to the unit following a left femoral popliteal bypass graft. Six hours later, his dorsalis pedis pulse cannot be palpated, and his foot is cool and dusky. The nurse should:

A. Continue to monitor the foot
B. Notify the physician immediately
C. Reposition and reassess the foot
D. Assure the client that his foot is fine

23. A client is to have a coronary artery bypass graft performed in the morning using a saphenous vein. He wants to know why the physician does not use the internal mammary artery for his bypass graft because his friend's physician uses this artery. The nurse tells the client that the internal mammary artery:

    A. Takes more time to remove
    B. Has a greater risk of becoming reoccluded
    C. Is smaller in diameter
    D. Has too many valves

24. A client returns to the cardiovascular intensive care unit following his coronary artery bypass graft. In planning his care, the most important electrolyte the nurse needs to monitor will be:

    A. Chloride
    B. HCO_3
    C. Potassium
    D. Sodium

25. A client is being discharged from the hospital today. The discharge teaching for care of her colostomy included which of the following basic principles for protecting the skin around her stoma:

    A. Taping a pouch that is leaking
    B. Cutting the skin barrier 1½ inches larger than the stoma
    C. Changing the pouch only when leakage occurs
    D. Using a skin sealant under pouch adhesives

26. A client is being discharged from the hospital tomorrow following a colon resection with a left colostomy. The nurse knows that the client understands the discharge teaching about care of her colostomy when she says:

    A. "I know that I am not supposed to irrigate my colostomy."
    B. "My stool will be soft like paste."
    C. "My stoma should be red and slightly raised."
    D. "The skin around my stoma may become irritated from the enzymes in my stool."

27. A client had a right below-the-knee amputation 4 days ago. He is complaining of pain in his right lower leg. The nurse should:

    A. Remind the client that he no longer has that part of his leg and assure him he will be OK
    B. Call the physician to request a psychological consultation for the client
    C. Turn on the television to distract the client's attention from his amputated leg
    D. Give the client his order of Demerol 50 mg IM prn

28. A client has returned to the unit from the recovery room after having a thyroidectomy. The nurse knows that a major complication after a thyroidectomy is:

    A. Respiratory obstruction
    B. Hypercalcemia
    C. Fistula formation
    D. Myxedema

29. A client had a transurethral resection of the prostate yesterday. He is concerned about the small amount of blood that is still in his urine. The nurse explains that the blood in his urine:

    A. Should not be there on the second day
    B. Will stop when the Foley catheter is removed
    C. Is normal and he need not be concerned about it
    D. Can be removed by irrigating the bladder

30. A 72-year-old male client had the Foley catheter that was inserted during the transurethral resection of his prostate removed today. He is concerned about the urinary incontinence he is having since removal of the Foley catheter. The nurse explains that:

    A. He should not be concerned about it because it will resolve quickly
    B. This is usually temporary
    C. The nurse will keep him dry, and he should notify the nurse when this happens
    D. This is related to the bladder spasms and will soon stop

31. A 48-year-old female client is going to have a cholecystectomy in the morning. In planning for her postoperative care, the nurse is aware that a priority nursing diagnosis for her will be high risk for:

    A. Knowledge deficit
    B. Urinary retention
    C. Impaired physical mobility
    D. Ineffective breathing pattern

32. A client is having a pneumonectomy done today, and the nurse is planning her postoperative care. Nursing interventions for a postoperative left pneumonectomy would include:

    A. Monitoring the chest tubes
    B. Positioning the client on the right side
    C. Positioning the client in semi-Fowler position with a pillow under the shoulder and back
    D. Monitoring the right lung for an increase in rales

33. A client returned to the unit following a pneumonectomy. As the nurse is assessing her incision, she notices fresh blood on the dressing. The nurse should first:

    A. Reinforce the dressing.
    B. Continue to monitor the dressing.
    C. Notify the physician.
    D. Note the time and amount of blood.

34. A client had a renal transplant 3 months ago. He has suddenly developed graft tenderness, an increased white blood cell count, and malaise. The client is experiencing which type of rejection?

    A. Acute
    B. Chronic
    C. Hyperacute
    D. Hyperchronic

35. A client has received preoperative teaching for the vertical partial laryngectomy that he is scheduled to have in the morning. The nurse determines that the teaching has been effective when the client states:

    A. "I know I will need special swallowing training after my surgery."

B. "The quality of my voice will be excellent after surgery."

C. "I will have very little difficulty swallowing after surgery."

D. "I may also have to have a radical neck dissection done."

36. A client is having a vertical partial laryngectomy, and the nurse is planning his postoperative care. A priority postoperative nursing diagnosis for a client having a vertical partial laryngectomy would be:

A. Activity intolerance
B. Ineffective airway clearance
C. High risk for infection
D. Altered oral mucous membrane

37. A client is going to have a pneumonectomy in the morning. She had a previous negative surgical experience, is talking rapidly, and has an increased pulse and respiratory rate. Nursing interventions for this client should include:

A. Providing opportunities to ask questions and talk about concerns
B. Providing distractors such as reading or watching television
C. Telling her that she should not be so nervous and assuring her that everything will be OK
D. Reminding her that this surgery is not as extensive as her past surgery was

38. On admission to the inpatient unit, a 34-year-old client is able to follow simple directions, but with great difficulty. He is worried about how he can keep clean in such a public place and repeatedly dusts his bureau, straightens his bed, and adjusts the clothes in his closet. The client is experiencing a severe level of anxiety. Which response by the nurse would be *most* therapeutic in initially attempting to reduce his anxiety?

A. "You will not be allowed to remain in your room if you continue to bother things."
B. "I can see how uncomfortable you are, but I would like you to walk with me so I can show you around the unit."
C. "Tell me why your room needs to be so clean."
D. "I've inspected this room and it is perfectly clean."

39. The physician prescribes amitriptyline (Elavil) for a client. What does the patient need to know about this medication?

A. Prolonged use of this medication will result in extrapyramidal side effects.
B. When the medication is effective, he will experience no anxiety.
C. The medication should relieve his symptoms of depression.
D. Blood must be drawn weekly to test for toxicity.

40. The health team needs to realize that the compulsive concern with cleanliness that a client with severe anxiety exhibits is most likely an attempt to:

A. Reduce his anxiety
B. Avoid going to psychotherapy

C. Manipulate the health team members
D. Increase his self-image by showing higher standards than the fellow clients

41. A successful executive left her job and became a housewife after her marriage to a plastic surgeon. She started doing volunteer work for a charity organization. She developed pain in her legs that advanced to the point of paralysis. Her physicians can find no organic basis for the paralysis. The client's behavior can be described as:

A. Housework phobia
B. Malingering
C. Conversion reaction
D. Agoraphobia

42. A 28-year-old client performs a long, involved ritual in getting up and preparing for the day. He became unable to get to his job before noon. His family, in desperation, has admitted him to the hospital's psychiatric unit. On the unit, he is always late for breakfast, which is served at 8 am. The nurse identifies that the *best* approach to this problem is to:

A. Allow him to eat late
B. Suggest that he do the rituals after breakfast
C. Get him up early so that he can complete the ritual before breakfast
D. Ask him to get all the other clients up so that he will forget about his ritual

43. A 25-year-old lawyer who is married with three young children works long hours in an effort to become a partner in the law firm. Following a recent hospitalization for a bleeding ulcer, he was referred for therapy to treat this psychophysiological disorder. On meeting with the therapist, he informed him or her that he was a busy man and did not have much time for this "psych stuff." When guiding the client to ventilate his feelings, the therapist can expect him to express feelings of:

A. Guilt
B. Shame
C. Despair
D. Anger

44. Plans for the care of a client with an ulcer caused by emotional problems need to take into consideration that:

A. His priority needs are limited to medical management
B. There is no real psychological basis for his illness
C. The disorder is a threat to his physical well-being
D. He is unable to participate in planning his care

45. A client has been uncomfortable in crowds all her life. After the birth of her child, she has been housebound unless her husband can accompany her to the grocery store and for medical appointments. His schedule will not allow for this, and he has insisted that she must be more independent. Her anxiety has increased to the point of panic. The client has been diagnosed with agoraphobia. Which statement is true about this disorder?

A. The behavior is not considered disabling.
B. More men suffer from agoraphobia than women.
C. The fears are persistent, and avoidance is used as the coping mechanism.

D. Agoraphobia moves into remission when treated with chlorpromazine.

46. A 22-year-old single woman was admitted to the psychiatric hospital by her mother, who reported bizarre behavior. Except for going to work, she spends all her time in her room and expresses concern over neighbors spying on her. She has fears of the telephone being "bugged." Her diagnosis is schizophrenia. One nurse per shift is assigned to work with the client. The primary reason for this plan would be to:

A. Protect her from suicide
B. Enable her to develop trust
C. Supervise her medication regimen
D. Involve her in groups for social interaction

47. The 4th of July holiday comes while a client is in the hospital being treated for schizophrenia. She is taking chlorpromazine and has improved to the point of being allowed to go with a group to the park for a picnic. The side effect of chlorpromazine that the nurse needs to keep in mind during this outing is:

A. Hypotension
B. Photosensitivity
C. Excessive appetite
D. Dryness of the mouth

48. Except for initial explosiveness on admission, a client diagnosed with schizophrenia stays in her room. She continues to believe other people are out to get her. A nursing intervention basic to improving withdrawn behavior is:

A. Assigning her to occupational therapy
B. Having her sit with the nurses while they chart
C. Helping her to make friends
D. Facilitating communication

49. A 32-year-old mother of two was brought to the hospital by her husband. He reported that his wife could no longer manage the house and children. She does not sleep and talks day and night. She has purchased some very expensive clothes. The nurse noted that the client speaks rapidly and changes the subject irrationally. This is an example of:

A. Flight of ideas
B. Delusions
C. Hallucinations
D. Echolalia

50. A client is placed on lithium therapy for her manic-depressive illness. When monitoring the client, the nurse assesses the laboratory blood values. Toxicity may occur with lithium therapy when the blood level is above:

A. 1.0 mEq/L
B. 2.2 mEq/L
C. 0.03 mEq/L
D. 1.5 mEq/L

51. A client's behavior is annoying other clients on the unit. He is meddling with their belongings and dominating the group. The best approach by the nurse is to:

A. Seclude him in his room.
B. Set limits on his behavior.

C. Have his medication increased.
D. Ignore him and tell the other clients that these behaviors are due to his illness and that they should understand.

52. A client is hyperactive and not sleeping. She will not remain at the table during mealtime. She is getting very limited calories and is using a lot of energy in her hyperactive state. The most therapeutic nursing action is to:

A. Insist that she remain at the table and eat a balanced diet.
B. Order a high-calorie diet with supplements.
C. Provide nutritious finger foods several times a day.
D. Offer to go to the dining room with her and allow her to open the food and inspect what she eats.

53. A hyperactive client is experiencing flight of ideas. The *most* therapeutic activity for him would be:

A. Doing crafts in occupational therapy
B. Working a 1000-piece puzzle
C. Playing bridge with three other clients
D. Playing basketball in the gym

54. A client is a depressed, 48-year-old salesman. A serious concern for the nurse working with depressed clients is the potential of suicide. The time that suicide is *most* likely to occur is:

A. In the acutely depressed state
B. When the depression starts to lift
C. In the denial phase
D. During a manic episode

55. Succinylcholine chloride (Anectine) is ordered prior to electroconvulsive therapy treatment for depressed clients. The nurse explains that the purpose of the drug is to:

A. Relax muscles
B. Relieve anxiety
C. Reduce secretions
D. Act as an anesthetic

56. The nurse teaches a pregnant client that a high-risk symptom occurring at any time during pregnancy that needs to be reported immediately to a healthcare provider is:

A. Constipation
B. Urinary frequency
C. Breast tenderness
D. Abdominal pain

57. At her first prenatal visit, a 21-year-old woman who is gravida 2, para 0, ab 1, is currently at 32 weeks' gestation and has a history of drug abuse, smoking, and occasional ethyl alcohol use. Fetal ultrasound tests indicate poor fetal growth. The *most* likely reason for the infant's intrauterine growth retardation is:

A. The client's young age
B. The client's previous abortion
C. The client's history of drug, ethyl alcohol, and tobacco use
D. The client's late prenatal care

58. When teaching a class of nursing students, the nurse asks why the embryonic period (weeks 4–8) of pregnancy is so critical.

    A. Duplication of genetic information takes place.
    B. Organogenesis occurs.
    C. Subcutaneous fat builds up steadily.
    D. Kidneys begin to secrete urine.

59. What specific hormone must be present in serum or urine laboratory tests used to diagnose pregnancy?

    A. Human chorionic gonadotropin
    B. Estrogen
    C. α-fetoprotein
    D. Sphingomyelin

60. A nurse is taking a maternal history for a client at her first prenatal visit. Her pregnancy test was positive, she has two living children, she had one spontaneous abortion, and one infant died at the age of 3 months. Which of the following best describes the client at the present?

    A. Gravida 4, para 2, ab 1
    B. Gravida 5, para 3, ab 1
    C. Gravida 5, para 4, ab 0
    D. Gravida 4, para 3, ab 0

61. A client is now pregnant for the second time. Her first child weighed 4536 g at delivery. The client's glucose tolerance test shows elevated blood sugar levels. Because she only shows signs of diabetes when she is pregnant, she is classified as having:

    A. Insulin-dependent diabetes
    B. Type II diabetes mellitus
    C. Type I diabetes mellitus
    D. Gestational diabetes mellitus

62. Prior to an amniocentesis, a fetal ultrasound is done in order to:

    A. Evaluate fetal lung maturity
    B. Evaluate the amount of amniotic fluid
    C. Locate the position of the placenta and fetus
    D. Ensure that the fetus is mature enough to perform the amniocentesis

63. A 17-year-old pregnant client who is gravida 1, para 0, is at 36 weeks' gestation. Based on the nurse's knowledge of the maternal physiological changes in pregnancy, which of these findings would be of concern?

    A. Complaints of dyspnea
    B. Edema of face and hands
    C. Pulse of 65 bpm at 8 weeks, 73 bpm at 36 weeks
    D. Hematocrit 39%

64. Based on your knowledge of genetic inheritance, which of these statements is true for autosomal recessive genetic disorders?

    A. Heterozygotes are affected.
    B. The disorder is always carried on the X chromosome.
    C. Only females are affected.
    D. Two affected parents always have affected children.

65. Chorioamnionitis is a maternal infection that is usually associated with:

    A. Prolonged rupture of membranes
    B. Postterm deliveries
    C. Maternal pyelonephritis
    D. Maternal dehydration

66. A client has been diagnosed with thrombophlebitis. She asks, "What is the most likely cause of thrombophlebitis during my pregnancy?" The nurse explains:

    A. Increased levels of the coagulation factors and a decrease in fibrinolysis
    B. An inadequate production of platelets
    C. An inadequate intake of folic acid during pregnancy
    D. An increase in fibrinolysis and a decrease in coagulation factors

67. Following the delivery of a healthy newborn, a client has developed thrombophlebitis and is receiving heparin IV. What are the signs and symptoms of a heparin overdose for which the nurse would need to observe during postpartum care of the client?

    A. Dysuria
    B. Epistaxis, hematuria, dysuria
    C. Vertigo, hematuria, ecchymosis
    D. Hematuria, ecchymosis, and epistaxis

68. A client who is a breast-feeding mother develops mastitis. The clinical signs and symptoms of mastitis include:

    A. Marked engorgement, elevated temperature, chills, and breast pain with an area that is red and hardened
    B. Marked engorgement and breast pain
    C. Elevated temperature and general malaise
    D. Cracked nipple with complaints of soreness

69. A 34-year-old client who is gravida 1, para 0 has a history of infertility and conceived this pregnancy while taking fertility drugs. She is at 32 weeks' gestation and is carrying triplets. She is complaining of low back pain and a feeling of pelvic pressure. Her cervical exam reveals a long, closed cervix. The nurse notes that the client is experiencing mild uterine contractions every 7–8 minutes after the nurse has placed her on the fetal monitor. Her condition should indicate that:

    A. Her cervix shows she will likely deliver soon
    B. The nurse should not be alarmed because mild uterine activity is common at 32 weeks' gestation
    C. She may be in preterm labor because this is more common with multiple pregnancies
    D. She most likely has a urinary tract infection (UTI) because this is common with pregnancy

70. The *most* frequent cause of early postpartum hemorrhage is:

    A. Hematoma
    B. Coagulation disorders
    C. Uterine atony
    D. Retained placental fragments

71. A client has just been transferred to the floor from the labor and delivery unit following delivery of a stillborn term infant. She is very despondent. When the nurse attempts to take her vital signs, she responds in anger, stating, "You leave me alone. You don't care anything

about me. It's people like you who let my baby die." The nurse's best course of action is to:

A. Quietly leave her room, allowing her more private time to deal with her loss.

B. Tell her that what happened was for the best and that she is still young and can have other children.

C. Tell her how sorry you are, and let her know that her child is now a little angel in heaven.

D. Tell her how sorry you are about the loss of her baby, and acknowledge her anger as being a normal stage of grief. Assure her that you are there to help her in any way you can.

72. When a client arrives on the labor and delivery unit, she informs the nurse that she has been having contractions for the last 5 hours. Now the pain is constant and not cyclical as it was earlier. The nurse considers the possibility of uterine rupture. Which of the following symptoms would be consistent with a uterine rupture?

A. A large gush of clear fluid from the vagina

B. Systolic hypertension

C. Abdominal rigidity

D. Increased fetal movements

73. A mother called the physician's office to ask if it would help relieve her small daughter's abdominal pain if she gave an enema and placed a heating pad on the abdomen. Her daughter has a fever and has vomited twice. The nurse's response is based on the knowledge that:

A. The symptoms could easily have been caused by constipation, which an enema would relieve

B. Heat would help to relax the abdominal muscles and relieve her pain

C. Both heat and enemas stimulate intestinal motility and could increase the risk of perforation

D. Complaints of stomach ache are common in young children and are generally best ignored

74. An 8-year-old child is admitted to the hospital for surgery. She has had no previous hospitalizations, and both she and her family appear anxious and fearful. It will be most helpful for the nurse to:

A. Take the child to her room and calmly and matter-of-factly begin to get her ready to go to the operating room

B. Take time to orient the child and her family to the hospital and the forthcoming events

C. Explain that as soon as the child goes to the operating room she will have time to answer any questions the family has

D. Tell the child and her family that there is nothing to worry about, that the operation will not take long, and she will soon be as "good as new"

75. Following a bicycle accident, a 12-year-old client sustained a complete fracture of the left femur. He was placed in 90°–90° skeletal traction with a pin in the distal end of the femur to achieve realignment and immobilization of the left femur. When providing nursing care, it is important for the nurse to remember that:

A. The nurse may lift only the weights that are applying traction in order to reposition him in bed

B. The client will need special skin care at the pin site according to hospital policy or the physician's preference

C. The traction pull should result in an immediate increase in comfort and reduce the need for pain medication

D. The client should be discouraged from participating in self-care activities to avoid the risk of disrupting the traction

76. A 10-year-old client with a pin in the right femur is immobilized in traction. He is exhibiting behavioral changes including restlessness, difficulty with problem solving, inability to concentrate on activities, and monotony. Which of the following nursing implementations would be most effective in helping him cope with immobility?

A. Providing him with books, challenging puzzles, and games as diversionary activities

B. Allowing him to do as much for himself as he is able, including learning to do pin-site care under supervision

C. Having a volunteer come in to sit with the client and to read him stories

D. Stimulating rest and relaxation by gentle rubbing with lotion and changing the client's position frequently

77. Following a fracture of the left femur, a client develops symptoms of osteomyelitis. During the acute phase of osteomyelitis, nursing care is directed toward:

A. Moving or turning the client's left leg carefully to minimize pain and discomfort

B. Allowing the client out of bed only in a wheelchair or gurney to minimize weight bearing on the left leg

C. Providing the client with a high-protein, high-fiber diet to promote healing

D. Instituting physical therapy to ensure restoration of optimal functioning of the leg

78. Several months after antibiotic therapy, a child is readmitted to the hospital with an exacerbation of osteomyelitis, which is now in the chronic stage. The mother appears anxious and asks what she could have done to prevent the exacerbation. The nurse's response is based on the knowledge that chronic osteomyelitis:

A. Is caused by poor physical conditions or poor nutrition

B. Often results from unhygienic conditions or an unclean environment

C. Is directly related to sluggish circulation in the affected limb

D. May develop from sinuses in the involved bone that retain infectious material

79. A 5-year-old child was recently diagnosed as having acute lymphoid leukemia. She is hospitalized for additional tests and to begin a course of chemotherapy designed to induce a remission. She is scheduled to have a bone marrow aspiration tomorrow. She has had a bone marrow test previously and is apprehensive about having another. Which of the following interventions will be most effective in relieving her anxiety?

A. Explain what will take place and what she will see, feel, and hear.

B. Remind her that she has had this procedure before and that it is nothing to be afraid of.

C. Tell her not to worry about it, that it will be over soon and she can join her friends in the playroom.

D. Give her a big hug and tell her that she is a big girl now and that she will do just fine.

80. Parents of children receiving chemotherapy should be warned that alopecia is a side effect and that:

A. Children seldom show concern about losing their hair

B. The hair will come out gradually, and the loss will not be noticeable for some time

C. It is best for girls to choose a wig similar to their hair style and color before the hair falls out

D. The parents will soon get used to seeing their children without hair, and it will no longer bother them

81. A child receiving chemotherapeutic drugs experiences a loss of appetite directly related to the therapy. Which of the following strategies should be most effective in encouraging the child to eat?

A. Provide a well-balanced diet at usual times, and restrict dessert if the child fails to eat well.

B. Schedule procedures immediately after eating so that the child will not be tired or in pain at mealtime.

C. Offer the child a diet with a wider variety of foods and with more seasoning than her usual diet.

D. Offer the child smaller meals more frequently than usual, and include as many of her favorite foods as possible.

82. A child becomes neutropenic and is placed on protective isolation. The purpose of protective isolation is to:

A. Protect the child from infection

B. Provide the child with privacy

C. Protect the family from curious visitors

D. Isolate the child from other clients and the nursing staff

83. A client is experiencing mucosal cell damage secondary to chemotherapy. Because of mucosal ulcers, eating has become increasingly uncomfortable for her. Which of the following interventions would be most effective in getting her to eat?

A. Local anesthetics or mouth washes applied to ulcers 30 minutes prior to meals

B. A bland, moist, soft diet

C. Staying with the client and providing distraction during meals

D. Cleaning the mouth carefully with lemon glycerin swabs and milk of magnesia before meals

84. A 15-year-old client was diagnosed as having cystic fibrosis at 8 months of age. He is in the hospital for a course of IV antibiotic therapy and vigorous chest physiotherapy. He has a poor appetite. The nurse can *best* help him to meet the desired outcome of consuming a prescribed number of calories by:

A. Including the client in planning sessions to select the type of meal plan and foods for his diet

B. Working with the nutritionist to devise a diet with significantly increased calories

C. Selecting foods for the client's diet that are high in calories and instituting a strict calorie count

D. Constantly providing him with chips, dips, and candies, because the number of calories consumed is more important than the quality of foods

85. The *most* appropriate method of evaluating whether the diet of a child with cystic fibrosis is meeting his caloric needs is:

A. Careful monitoring of weight loss or gain

B. Carefully recording amounts and types of foods ingested

C. Keeping a strict account of the number of calories ingested

D. Keeping a careful account of the amount of pancreatic enzymes ingested

86. A client with cystic fibrosis exhibits activity intolerance related to the pulmonary problems associated with his disease. However, he needs to be encouraged to participate in daily physical exercise. The ultimate aim of exercise is to:

A. Create a sense of well-being and self-worth

B. Help him overcome respiratory infections

C. Establish an effective, habitual breathing pattern

D. Promote normal growth and development

87. As a nurse works with an adolescent with cystic fibrosis, the nurse begins to notice that he appears depressed and talks about suicide and feelings of worthlessness. This is an important factor to consider in planning for his care because:

A. It may be a bid for attention and an indication that more diversionary activity should be planned for him

B. No threat of suicide should be ignored or challenged in any way

C. He needs to be observed carefully for signs that his depression has been relieved

D. He needs to be confronted with his feelings and forced to work through them

88. A 9-month-old infant is being examined in the general pediatric clinic for a routine well-child checkup. His immunizations are up to date, and his mother reports that he has had no significant illnesses or injuries. Which of the following signs would lead the nurse to believe that he has had a cerebral injury?

A. Hyperextension of the neck with evidence of pain on flexion

B. Holding the head to one side and pointing the chin toward the other side

C. Holding the head erect and in the midline when in a vertical position

D. Significant head lag when raised to a sitting position

89. During an examination, the nurse notes that an infant has diaper rash on the convex surfaces of his buttocks, inner thighs, and scrotum. Which of the following nursing interventions will be most effective in resolving the condition?

A. Coating the inflamed areas with zinc oxide

B. Using talcum powder on the inflamed areas to promote drying
C. Removing the diaper entirely for extended periods of time
D. Cleaning the inflamed area thoroughly with disposable wet "wipes" at each diaper change

90. A 10-month-old infant's mother says that he takes fresh whole milk eagerly, but that when she offered him baby foods at 6 months of age, he pushed them out of his mouth. Because he has gained weight appropriately, she has quit trying to get him to eat other foods. The nurse's response is based on the knowledge that:

A. Milk intake should be limited to no more than four 8-oz bottles per day and should be followed by iron-enriched cereal or other solid foods or juices
B. Milk is an excellent food and will meet his nutritional needs adequately until he is ready to eat solid foods
C. It is acceptable to continue to give him whole milk and to delay giving solid foods as long as he takes a vitamin supplement daily
D. He should be started on iron-enriched cereal, meat, vegetables, fruits, and juices prior to bottle feeds. Milk intake should be limited to 1 qt/day

1. **(D)** Client need: physiological integrity; subcategory: physiological adaptation; content area: med/surg

   RATIONALE

   (A) *Anuria* is defined as absence of urine output, which is not indicative of the urinary pattern of diabetes insipidus. (B) *Oliguria* is defined as <500 mL of urine per day, which is not a urinary output pattern associated with diabetes insipidus. (C) *Dysuria* is defined as difficult urination. Clients with diabetes insipidus do not have dysuria as a symptom of their disease. (D) Polyuria is a primary symptom of diabetes insipidus. These clients have decreased or absent vasopressin secretion, which causes water loss in the urine and sodium increases.

2. **(A)** Client need: health promotion and maintenance; subcategory: prevention and early detection of disease; content area: med/surg

   RATIONALE

   (A) Whole blood is the transfusion component of choice when large volumes of blood need to be replaced. Whole blood contains all blood components that are lost during active bleeding. (B) Platelet therapy is indicated for thrombocytopenia if the client's platelet count is below 15,000/mm^3. (C) Infusion of fresh frozen plasma is required when the prothrombin time and partial thromboplastic time are prolonged. (D) Packed red blood cells are transfused in instances of anemia with decreases in hematocrit and hemoglobin.

3. **(C)** Client need: physiological integrity; subcategory: pharmacological and parenteral therapies; content area: med/surg

   RATIONALE

   (A) Sodium polystyrene sulfonate administration will not increase serum magnesium. Hypermagnesemia is virtually unknown except for clients in renal failure. (B) Sodium polystyrene sulfonate administration is not known to increase serum bicarbonate. (C) Decrease in serum potassium, the expected response of sodium polystyrene sulfonate, is secondary to the binding of this drug and potassium in the colon, and potassium is removed through the feces. (D) Serum calcium may actually increase with sodium polystyrene sulfonate administration, especially if calcium chloride is administered concurrently with this drug.

4. **(C)** Client need: physiological integrity; subcategory: physiological adaptation; content area: med/surg

   RATIONALE

   (A) Kussmaul's respirations are associated with diabetic ketoacidosis, severe hemorrhage, peritonitis, renal failure, and uremia. (B) Tachypnea (respiratory rate >25 breaths/min) is often associated with fever. (C) Cheyne-Stokes respiratory pattern is most often associated with increased intracranial pressure secondary to changes in pressure in the cerebral and cerebellar areas. (D) Biot's breathing is most frequently associated with spinal meningitis.

5. **(B)** Client need: physiological integrity; subcategory: physiological adaptation; content area: med/surg

   RATIONALE

   (A) Potassium intake that meets the recommended daily allowance is important, especially in clients who have a history of cardiac disease. (B) Low levels of magnesium can cause an increase in resistance to insulin and can lead to carbohydrate intolerance. (C) Sodium is an important electrolyte for all clients but has no direct effect on diabetes mellitus. (D) Bicarbonate plays an important role in acid-base balance. It is equally necessary for maintenance of all body functions.

6. **(C)** Client need: physiological integrity; subcategory: physiological adaptation; content area: med/surg

   RATIONALE

   (A) Although a left hemothorax could cause diminished and distant breath sounds, it is irrelevant to this situation. (B) A right hemothorax will not cause diminished and distant breath sounds on the left side of the chest. (C) The right mainstem bronchus is most frequently intubated in error because the angle of the right mainstem bronchus is very small as compared with that of the left mainstem bronchus. Because ventilation is only occurring on the right side, the nurse would auscultate diminished and distant breath sounds on the left. (D) An inadequate mechanical ventilator has no relationship to this situation.

7. **(A)** Client need: physiological integrity; subcategory: physiological adaptation; content area: med/surg

   RATIONALE

   (A) The lungs are responsible for regulation of CO_2, and this parameter primarily reflects respiratory function. (B) CO_2 content of the blood is an indirect measure of respiratory function. (C) HCO_3 is a measure of kidney function only and is important in acid-base balance. (D) Base excess represents the excess of HCO_3 and is not reflective of respiratory function.

8. **(B)** Client need: physiological integrity; subcategory: reduction of risk potential; content area: med/surg

   RATIONALE

   (A) Pressure ≤10 mm Hg places the client at risk for aspiration. (B) Pressure in the endotracheal tube cuff should never exceed 20 mm Hg, because higher pressure places the client at risk for tracheal erosion. (C) A pressure of 45 mm Hg is an extremely high pressure in the endotracheal tube cuff. This places the client at great risk for tracheal erosion. (D) A pressure of 60 mm Hg is an extremely high pressure in the endotracheal tube cuff. This places the client at great risk for tracheal erosion.

9. **(D)** Client need: physiological integrity; subcategory: pharmacological and parenteral therapies; content area: med/surg

   RATIONALE

   (A) Phenytoin will precipitate if mixed with Ringer's lactate and should not be administered. (B, C) Phenytoin will precipitate if mixed with D_5 in Ringer's lactate and should not be administered. (D) Phenytoin is compatible only with normal saline and should be mixed only with normal saline for administration.

10. **(D)** Client need: physiological integrity; subcategory: physiological adaptation; content area: med/surg

    RATIONALE

    (A) Fluid deficit is a high priority not only during the first 8 hours postburn, but also during the first 36 hours postburn. (B) Alteration in comfort is a high priority during the entire length of the client's hospitalization and on discharge. (C) Alteration in sensation is a high priority during the first 48–72 hours postburn. Lack of sensation may be indicative of lack of circulation. (D) Alteration in airway integrity is the highest priority for this client in the first 8 hours postburn. Failure to continually assess this client's airway status could result in poor ventilation and oxygenation, in addition to an inability to intubate the client secondary to excessive edema formation in the neck.

11. **(D)** Client need: physiological integrity; subcategory: reduction of risk potential; content area: med/surg

    RATIONALE

    (A) There is a separate collection bottle for drainage as part of a chest drainage system. (B) In a three-bottle chest drainage system, one bottle serves only as a pressure regulator. (C) Mediastinal chest tubes prevent accumulation of blood around the heart immediately following heart surgery. (D) The purpose of the water-seal bottle in any chest drainage setup is to allow air out of the chest, but not back in. This negative pressure promotes lung expansion.

12. **(A)** Client need: physiological integrity; subcategory: reduction of risk potential; content area: med/surg

RATIONALE

(A) A common side effect of gentamicin is nephrotoxicity. The serum laboratory test that best reflects kidney function is serum creatinine. (B) Serum sodium has no relationship to gentamicin. (C) Serum calcium has no relationship to gentamicin. (D) Serum potassium has no relationship to gentamicin. If a client has impaired renal function secondary to gentamicin administration, he or she may also have hyperkalemia as a secondary disorder.

13. **(C)** Client need: physiological integrity; subcategory: reduction of risk potential; content area: med/surg

RATIONALE

(A) The nurse may never discontinue a central line without a physician's order. (B) The nurse may never initiate a peripheral IV without a physician's order except in an emergency situation. (C) The nurse should always document findings and alert the physician to the findings as well. The physician may then initiate a new central line and order the current central line to be discontinued. (D) Besides cleaning and redressing, the nurse should always document the findings.

14. **(A)** Client need: safe, effective care environment; subcategory: safety and infection control; content area: med/surg

RATIONALE

(A) Once the feeding tube placement is confirmed in the stomach, aspiration can occur if the client's stomach becomes too full. When suctioning the trachea, if secretions resemble tube feeding, the client has aspirated the feeding. (B) Because the trachea provides direct access to a client's airway, it would not be possible to place the catheter in the esophagus. (C) Blue-colored sputum is never considered a normal finding and should be reported and documented. (D) The nurse confirmed placement of the feeding tube in the stomach prior to initiating the tube feeding; therefore, it is highly unlikely that the feeding tube would be located in the trachea.

15. **(D)** Client need: physiological integrity; subcategory: pharmacological and parenteral therapies; content area: med/surg

RATIONALE

(A) Morphine sulfate is contraindicated in clients with pancreatitis because it may cause spasms of the sphincter of Oddi and increase pancreatic pain. (B) Ketorolac tromethamine is currently not approved by the Food and Drug Administration for IV use. (C) Promethazine is a medication that has no analgesic properties. (D) Meperidine is the drug of choice for clients with pancreatitis. It will not cause spasms at the sphincter of Oddi, which can lead to increased pancreatic pain.

16. **(B)** Client need: physiological integrity; subcategory: reduction of risk potential; content area: med/surg

RATIONALE

(A) Palpating these pulses again in 15 minutes may only result in the same findings. (B) Any time during an assessment that the nurse is unable to palpate pulses, the nurse should then obtain a Doppler and assess for presence or absence of the pulse and pulse strength, if a pulse is present. (C) Pulses may be present and assessed through use of a Doppler. Absence of palpable pulses does not indicate absence of blood flow unless pulses cannot be located with a Doppler. (D) The nurse would only call the physician after determining that the pulses are absent by both palpation and Doppler.

17. **(B)** Client need: physiological integrity; subcategory: pharmacological and parenteral therapies; content area: med/surg

RATIONALE

(A) Metoclopramide does not stimulate gastric secretions. (B) This response is expected with metoclopramide, in addition to increasing gastric emptying. (C) Disorientation is a symptom of metoclopramide overdose. The drug should be discontinued. (D) Drowsiness is a symptom of metoclopramide overdose and the drug should be discontinued.

18. **(B)** Client need: safe, effective care environment; subcategory: management of care; content area: med/surg

RATIONALE

(A) Spouse and adult child would be asked before a parent. (B) The order of kin relationship for an adult, as determined from legal intestate succession, is usually spouse, adult child, parent, sibling. (C) Parent and sibling would be asked after adult child. (D) Spouse and adult child would be asked before parent. Sibling would be asked last.

19. **(C)** Client need: physiological integrity; subcategory: physiological adaptation; content area: med/surg

RATIONALE

(A) Drainage from a surgical incision usually proceeds from sanguinous to serosanguinous. (B) Purulent drainage usually indicates infection and should not be seen initially from a surgical incision. (C) Drainage from a surgical incision is initially sanguinous, proceeding to serosanguinous, and then to serous. (D) Catarrhal is a type of exudate seen in upper respiratory infections, not in surgical incisions.

20. **(D)** Client need: physiological integrity; subcategory: physiological adaptation; content area: med/surg

RATIONALE

(A) Excoriation is abrasion of the epidermis or of the coating of any organ of the body by trauma, chemicals, burns, or other causes. (B) Dehiscence is a partial or complete separation of the wound edges with no protrusion of abdominal tissue. (C) Decortication is removal of the surface layer of an organ or structure. It is a type of surgery, such as removing the fibrinous peel from the visceral pleura in thoracic surgery. (D) Evisceration occurs when the incision separates and the contents of the cavity spill out.

21. **(D)** Client need: physiological integrity; subcategory: physiological adaptation; content area: med/surg

RATIONALE

(A) The wound is not infected. An infected wound would contain pus, debris, and exudate. (B) The wound is healing properly. (C) A necrotic wound would appear black or brown. (D) The wound is healing properly and is filled with red granulated tissue and fragile capillaries.

22. **(B)** Client need: physiological integrity; subcategory: reduction of risk potential; content area: med/surg

RATIONALE

(A) The client is losing blood supply to his left foot. Continuing to monitor the foot will not help restore the blood supply to the foot. (B) The physician should be notified immediately because the client is losing blood supply to his left foot and is in danger of losing the foot and/or leg. (C) The presenting symptoms are of an emergency nature and require immediate intervention. (D) This action would be giving the client false assurance.

23. **(A)** Client need: physiological integrity; subcategory: reduction of risk potential; content area: med/surg

RATIONALE

(A) It does take more time to remove the internal mammary artery, and this is one reason why some physicians do not use it.

(B) There is not a greater risk of reocclusion. In fact, it may actually stay patent longer. (C) The internal mammary artery is actually larger in diameter than the saphenous vein. (D) The internal mammary artery does not have too many valves.

24. **(C)** Client need: physiological integrity; subcategory: reduction of risk potential; content area: med/surg

    RATIONALE

    (A) Chloride, HCO_3, and sodium will need to be monitored, but monitoring these electrolytes is not as important as potassium monitoring. (B) Chloride, HCO_3, and sodium will need to be monitored, but monitoring these electrolytes is not as important as potassium monitoring. (C) Potassium will need to be closely monitored because of its effects on the heart. Hypokalemia could result in supraventricular tachyarrhythmias. (D) Chloride, HCO_3, and sodium will need to be monitored, but monitoring these electrolytes is not as important as potassium monitoring.

25. **(D)** Client need: health promotion and maintenance; subcategory: prevention and early detection of disease; content area: med/surg

    RATIONALE

    (A) When a pouch seal leaks, the pouch should be immediately changed, not taped. Stool held against the skin can quickly result in severe irritation. (B) The skin barrier should be cut only slightly larger than the stoma (one-half inch). (C) The client should be taught to change pouches whenever possible before leakage occurs. (D) When skin sealant is used under the tape, the outermost layer of the epidermis remains intact. When no skin sealant is used, this layer is removed when the tape is removed.

26. **(C)** Client need: health promotion and maintenance; subcategory: prevention and early detection of disease; content area: med/surg

    RATIONALE

    (A) A left colostomy indicates an ascending colon resection. This type of colostomy can be irrigated. (B) The stool from an ascending colon resection should be formed. (C) The healthy stoma should be red and slightly raised. If it begins to turn dark or blue, the client should see the physician immediately. (D) The stool in the ascending colon does not usually have many enzymes in it. Stool from an ileostomy has more enzymes and is more irritating to the skin.

27. **(D)** Client need: physiological integrity; subcategory: physiological adaptation; content area: med/surg

    RATIONALE

    (A) The nurse is ignoring the client's pain. Telling the client that he will be OK will not relieve his phantom pain. (B) The client does not need a psychological consultation. Phantom pain is a normal sensation experienced by clients with amputations. (C) Using the television as a distractor will not relieve the client's phantom pain. (D) Phantom pain is a normal, very real experience for an amputee and should be treated with pain medication.

28. **(A)** Client need: physiological integrity; subcategory: reduction of risk potential; content area: med/surg

    RATIONALE

    (A) Respiratory obstruction due to edema of the glottis, bilateral laryngeal nerve damage, or tracheal compression from hemorrhage is a major complication after a thyroidectomy. (B) Hypocalcemia accompanied by tetany from accidental removal of one or more parathyroid glands is a major complication, not hypercalcemia. (C) Fistula formation is not a major complication associated with a thyroidectomy. It is a major complication with a laryngectomy. (D) Myxedema is hypothyroidism that occurs in adults and is not a complication of a thyroidectomy. A thyroidectomy client tends to develop thyroid storm, which is excess production of thyroid hormone.

29. **(C)** Client need: physiological integrity; subcategory: physiological adaptation; content area: med/surg

    RATIONALE

    (A) Some hematuria is usual for several days after surgery. (B) The client will continue to have a small amount of hematuria even after the Foley catheter is removed. (C) Some hematuria is usual for several days after surgery. The client should not be concerned about it unless it increases. (D) Irrigating the bladder will not remove the hematuria. Irrigation is done to remove blood clots and facilitate urinary drainage.

30. **(B)** Client need: psychosocial integrity; subcategory: coping and adaptation; content area: med/surg

    RATIONALE

    (A) This problem is temporary, but it may take some time to resolve, especially in an older man. (B) This problem is usually temporary, but it may take some time to resolve. (C) Keeping the client dry will not relieve his anxiety about his incontinence. (D) The bladder spasms are not the cause of the client's incontinence.

31. **(D)** Client need: physiological integrity; subcategory: reduction of risk potential; content area: med/surg

    RATIONALE

    (A) The client may have a knowledge deficit, but reducing the risk for knowledge deficit is not a priority nursing diagnosis postoperatively. (B) The client will have a Foley catheter for a day or two after surgery. Urinary retention is usually not a problem once the Foley catheter is removed. (C) A client having a cholecystectomy should not be physically impaired. In fact, the client is encouraged to begin ambulating soon after surgery. (D) Because of the location of the incision, the client having a cholecystectomy is reluctant to breathe deeply and is at risk for developing pneumonia. These clients have to be reminded and encouraged to take deep breaths.

32. **(D)** Client need: physiological integrity; subcategory: reduction of risk potential; content area: med/surg

    RATIONALE

    (A) Chest tubes are usually not necessary in a pneumonectomy because there is no lung to re-expand on the operative side. (B) The pneumonectomy client should be positioned on the back or operated side because the sutured bronchial stump may open, allowing fluid to drain into the unoperated side and drown the client. (C) The client should not have a pillow under the shoulder and back because of the subscapular incision. (D) Rales are commonly heard over the base of the remaining lung, but an increase could indicate circulatory overload and therefore should be closely monitored.

33. **(C)** Client need: physiological integrity; subcategory: physiological adaptation; content area: med/surg

    RATIONALE

    (A) The dressing should not be reinforced without first notifying the physician. The decision may be made by the physician to reinforce the dressing after assessing the amount of bleeding. (B) Blood on the dressing is unusual and should make the nurse aware that something more than continuing to monitor the dressing should be done. (C) The physician should be notified immediately, because if the bleeding persists, the client may have to be taken back to surgery. (D) The time and amount of blood do need to be recorded after the physician is notified.

34. **(A)** Client need: physiological integrity; subcategory: physiological adaptation; content area: med/surg

    RATIONALE

    (A) The sudden development of fever, graft tenderness, increased white blood count, and malaise are signs and symptoms of an acute rejection that commonly occurs at 3 months. (B) Chronic rejection occurs slowly over a period of months to years and mimics chronic renal failure. (C) Hyperacute rejection occurs immediately after surgery up to 48 hours postoperatively. (D) Hyperchronic rejection is not a type of rejection.

35. **(C)** Client need: physiological integrity; subcategory: reduction of risk potential; content area: med/surg

RATIONALE

(A) A client with a supraglottic (horizontal partial) laryngectomy would require special swallowing training, not a vertical partial laryngectomy. (B) The quality of the client's voice will be altered but adequate for communication. (C) The client will have minimal difficulty swallowing. (D) A radical neck dissection may be done with a total laryngectomy, but not with a partial laryngectomy.

36. **(B)** Client need: physiological integrity; subcategory: reduction of risk potential; content area: med/surg

RATIONALE

(A) The laryngectomy client should be able to gradually increase activities without difficulty. (B) The laryngectomy client may have copious amounts of secretions and require suctioning for the first 24–48 hours. The cannula will require cleaning even after the first 24 hours because mucus collects in it. (C) The client does have a potential for infection, but it is not a more important nursing priority than the ineffective airway clearance. (D) This problem is not a more important nursing priority than ineffective airway clearance. The client's mouth may become dry, but good oral care should take care of the dryness.

37. **(A)** Client need: psychosocial integrity; subcategory: coping and adaptation; content area: med/surg

RATIONALE

(A) This intervention will help to clarify any misunderstandings about the surgery and give the client an opportunity to verbalize concerns about the surgery. (B) Distractors will not alleviate the preoperative anxiety that the client is experiencing. This response actually denies the client's anxiety. (C) This intervention is false assurance and denies that anxiety is a normal response to the threat of surgery. (D) Psychological responses are not directly related to the extent of the surgery, because they are influenced by the client's past experiences.

38. **(B)** Client need: psychosocial integrity; subcategory: coping and adaptation; content area: psychiatric

RATIONALE

(A) This statement is punitive. (B) Acknowledging the anxiety and channeling it into some positive activity is therapeutic. (C) The client cannot say "why"; this statement puts the client on the defensive. (D) A rational approach, especially a judgmental one, is nontherapeutic.

39. **(C)** Client need: physiological integrity; subcategory: pharmacological and parenteral therapies; content area: psychiatric

RATIONALE

(A) Phenothiazines cause extrapyramidal symptoms. (B) No amount of medication can relieve all anxiety in all cases. (C) The purpose of amitriptyline is to relieve the symptoms of depression because it is an antidepressant. It increases the action of norepinephrine and serotonin on nerve cells. (D) Periodic blood tests are done when lithium is prescribed.

40. **(A)** Client need: psychosocial integrity; subcategory: coping and adaptation; content area: psychiatric

RATIONALE

(A) These behaviors are attempts to relieve anxiety. (B) Avoidance is not a pattern in the obsessive client. (C) Although these behaviors may seem to manipulate others, that is not the purpose behind the activity. (D) Inflated self-esteem is not a characteristic of the severely anxious client.

41. **(C)** Client need: psychosocial integrity; subcategory: coping and adaptation; content area: psychiatric

RATIONALE

(A) A typical phobia does not result in physical symptoms (i.e., paralysis). (B) Malingering is pretending to be ill. This person has a true paralysis. (C) A conversion reaction is a physical expression of an emotional conflict. It has no organic basis. (D) Agoraphobia is fear of public places.

42. **(C)** Client need: psychosocial integrity; subcategory: psychosocial adaptation; content area: psychiatric

RATIONALE

(A) Allowing him to eat late is not a solution to the problem because the ritual affects more than just this meal. (B) He is helpless to change this behavior because the rituals occur as a result of an irrational effort to control his anxiety. (C) To interfere with the ritual will increase anxiety. Until the basic problem is resolved, and in turn his need for the ritual relieved, arrange the schedule so that essential activities may be included (such as meals with the group). (D) This approach would be very disruptive to the other clients and would not serve to relieve the anxiety of the client.

43. **(D)** Client need: psychosocial integrity; subcategory: coping and adaptation; content area: psychiatric

RATIONALE

(A) Guilt relates to depression. (B) Shame is not associated with psychophysiological disorders. (C) Despair relates to depression. (D) Repressed anger is associated with psychophysiological disorders.

44. **(C)** Client need: physiological integrity; subcategory: physiological adaptation; content area: psychiatric

RATIONALE

(A) There may be a medical emergency that takes top priority; however, the basis of the problem is emotional. (B) The problem is a physical manifestation of an emotional conflict. (C) The bleeding ulcer can be life threatening. (D) For lifestyle change to occur, the client must participate in the planning of his care so that he is committed to changes that will have positive results.

45. **(C)** Client need: psychosocial integrity; subcategory: psychosocial adaptation; content area: psychiatric

RATIONALE

(A) Agoraphobia is the most pervasive and serious phobic disorder. (B) Women compose 70%–85% of agoraphobia sufferers. (C) Agoraphobia is an acute disorder that immobilizes the sufferer with extreme anxiety. (D) Chlorpromazine is not a drug used to treat phobias.

46. **(B)** Client need: psychosocial integrity; subcategory: psychosocial adaptation; content area: psychiatric

RATIONALE

(A) Suicide is a greater risk in depression than in schizophrenia. (B) The client is suspicious and needs help to develop trust, which is basic to her improvement. (C) Although she will be taking medication, drug therapy would not necessitate consistency in the nurses assigned. (D) A suspicious client should have limited exposure to groups, because group participation increases discomfort.

47. **(B)** Client need: physiological integrity; subcategory: pharmacological and parenteral therapies; content area: psychiatric

RATIONALE

(A) A decrease in blood pressure sometimes occurs with chlorpromazine. It would not be a factor influenced by a picnic in the park. (B) Protection from the sun is important in clients taking phenothiazines because they burn easily and severely. (C) An appetite increase sometimes occurs with chlorpromazine. It would not be affected by a picnic. (D) Dryness of the mouth may occur at any time and is not affected by the picnic outing.

48. **(D)** Client need: psychosocial integrity; subcategory: psychosocial adaptation; content area: psychiatric

    RATIONALE

    (A) The nurse does not make this assignment. (B) One-to-one observation is not appropriate. It does not focus on the client or encourage communication. (C) The client is too suspicious to accomplish this goal. (D) The withdrawn individual must learn to communicate on a one-to-one level before moving on to more threatening situations.

49. **(A)** Client need: psychosocial integrity; subcategory: coping and adaptation; content area: psychiatric

    RATIONALE

    (A) Rapidly moving from one topic to another without following any logical sequence is called flight of ideas. (B) False beliefs are delusions. (C) False sensory perceptions are hallucinations ("hearing voices"). (D) Repeating words is called echolalia.

50. **(D)** Client need: physiological integrity; subcategory: reduction of risk potential; content area: psychiatric

    RATIONALE

    (A) This value is a low blood level. (B) This value is a toxic blood level. (C) This value is a low blood level. (D) This value is the level at which most clients are maintained, and toxicity may occur if the level increases. The client should be monitored closely for symptoms, because some clients become toxic even at this level.

51. **(B)** Client need: psychosocial integrity; subcategory: psychosocial adaptation; content area: psychiatric

    RATIONALE

    (A) This action by the nurse would be punitive. (B) Consistent limit setting will help the client to know what is acceptable behavior. (C) This action is not within the nurse's scope of practice. (D) This could be dangerous to the client and to others and violates other clients' rights.

52. **(C)** Client need: psychosocial integrity; subcategory: psychosocial adaptation; content area: psychiatric

    RATIONALE

    (A) The client is not able to sit for long periods. Forcing her to remain at the table will increase her anxiety and cause her to become hostile. (B) This action will not ensure that the client eats what is ordered. Dietary orders are not within the nurse's scope of practice. (C) Providing finger foods increases the likelihood of eating for hyperactive persons. They may be eating "on the run." (D) These clients are not suspicious of the food or insecure in moving about the unit alone.

53. **(D)** Client need: psychosocial integrity; subcategory: psychosocial adaptation; content area: psychiatric

    RATIONALE

    (A) This activity requires motor skills and therefore would be difficult for a hyperactive client. (B) This activity would take too long, and the client would have difficulty concentrating owing to a limited attention span. (C) This client would not be able to concentrate enough to play card games. He would respond to all the stimuli in the area, become distracted, and leave the table. (D) This activity would allow the client to channel his energy in a positive way.

54. **(B)** Client need: psychosocial integrity; subcategory: psychosocial adaptation; content area: psychiatric

    RATIONALE

    (A) The client may be too disorganized in the acute phase to make a workable plan. (B) When the depression starts to lift, the client is able to make a workable plan. (C) There usually is not a significant denial phase related to depression. Suicide occurs in a state of despair and hopelessness. (D) Suicide is uncommon in the manic state. In this state, clients do not feel hopeless, but euphoric and overly confident.

55. **(A)** Client need: physiological integrity; subcategory: pharmacological and parenteral therapies; content area: psychiatric

    RATIONALE

    (A) Succinylcholine chloride relaxes muscles and decreases the intensity of the seizure. (B) Succinylcholine chloride does not relieve anxiety. (C) Atropine is given to reduce secretions. (D) Thiamylal sodium (Surital) or other phenobarbital preparations are used as brief anesthetics.

56. **(D)** Client need: health promotion and maintenance; subcategory: prevention and early detection of disease; content area: maternity

    RATIONALE

    (A) Constipation is a result of decreased peristalsis due to smooth muscle relaxation related to changing progesterone levels that occur during pregnancy. (B) Urinary frequency is a common result of the increasing size of the uterus and the resulting pressure it places on the bladder. (C) With the increased vascularity and hypertrophy of the mammary alveoli due to estrogen and progesterone level changes, the breasts will increase in size and may become tender. (D) Abdominal pain may be an indication of early spontaneous abortion, preterm delivery, or a placental abruption.

57. **(C)** Client need: physiological integrity; subcategory: physiological adaptation; content area: maternity

    RATIONALE

    (A) Although adolescents frequently have a higher incidence of low-birth-weight infants, this client is 21 years old. (B) Uncomplicated induced abortions have not been proved to influence the growth of infants of subsequent pregnancies. (C) Compounds in cigarettes and some illicit drugs cause maternal vasoconstriction and a subsequent reduction in O_2 availability for the fetus owing to the resulting reduction in uteroplacental blood flow. As few as one or two drinks of alcohol per day will decrease birth weight. (D) Although early prenatal care has been shown to improve pregnancy outcomes, not seeking care until the second week of gestation does not, in and of itself, cause intrauterine growth retardation.

58. **(B)** Client need: health promotion and maintenance; subcategory: growth and development through the life span; content area: maternity

    RATIONALE

    (A) Duplication of genetic material occurs during the pre-embryonic period (weeks 1–3) following conception. The exact duplication of genetic material is essential for cell differentiation, growth, and biological maintenance of the organism. (B) Weeks 4–8, known as the embryonic period, are the time organogenesis occurs and pose the greatest potential for major congenital malformations. All major internal and external organs and systems are formed. (C) Subcutaneous fat does not develop until the latter weeks of gestation. (D) Kidneys begin to secrete urine during the 13th–16th week.

59. **(A)** Client need: health promotion and maintenance; subcategory: prevention and early detection of disease; content area: maternity

    RATIONALE

    (A) Human chorionic gonadotropin is the biochemical basis for pregnancy tests. It is produced by the placenta to help maintain the corpus luteum. Its levels climb rapidly following conception, peaking at about 8 weeks and then gradually decreasing to low levels after 16 weeks. (B) Estrogen does steadily rise throughout pregnancy, increasing to 30 times that of prepregnancy levels. Although estrogen levels do change during pregnancy, it is not used as the main hormone of evaluation in pregnancy tests. (C) α-Fetoprotein is the major protein in the serum of the embryo. It is initially produced by the yolk sac. (D) Lecithin and sphingomyelin are two phospholipids of which fetal lung surfactant is composed. Levels are evaluated to determine fetal lung maturity.

60. **(B)** Client need: health promotion and maintenance; subcategory: growth and development through the life span; content area: maternity

    RATIONALE

    (A) This individual has been pregnant four times, delivered two children, and had one abortion. (B) Your client has been pregnant five times, delivered three children, and had one abortion. (C) This individual has been pregnant five times, delivered four children, and has not had an abortion. (D) This individual has been pregnant four times, delivered three children, and has not had an abortion.

61. **(D)** Client need: physiological integrity; subcategory: physiological adaptation; content area: maternity

    RATIONALE

    (A) Insulin-dependent diabetes mellitus, also known as type I diabetes, usually appears before the age of 30 years with an abrupt onset of symptoms requiring insulin for management. It is not related to onset during pregnancy. (B) Non-insulin–dependent diabetes (type II diabetes) usually appears in older adults. It has a slow onset and progression of symptoms. (C) This type of diabetes is the same as insulin-dependent diabetes. (D) Gestational diabetes mellitus has its onset of symptoms during pregnancy and usually disappears after delivery. These symptoms are usually mild and not life threatening, although they are associated with increased fetal morbidity and other fetal complications.

62. **(C)** Client need: health promotion and maintenance; subcategory: prevention and early detection of disease; content area: maternity

    RATIONALE

    (A) Amniocentesis can be performed to assess for lung maturity. Fetal ultrasound can be used for gestational dating, although it does not separately determine lung maturity. (B) Ultrasound can evaluate amniotic fluid volume, which may be used to determine congenital anomalies. (C) Amniocentesis involves removal of amniotic fluid for evaluation. The needle, inserted through the abdomen, is guided by ultrasound to avoid needle injuries, and the test evaluates the position of the placenta and the fetus. (D) Amniocentesis can be performed as early as the 15th–17th week of pregnancy.

63. **(B)** Client need: health promotion and maintenance; subcategory: growth and development through the life span; content area: maternity

    RATIONALE

    (A) Dyspnea is a common complaint during the third trimester owing to the increasing size of the uterus and the resulting pressure against the diaphragm. (B) Edema of the face, hands, or pitting edema after 12 hours of bed rest may be indicative of preeclampsia and would be of great concern to the healthcare provider. (C) An increase in heart rate of 10–15 bpm is a normal physiological change in pregnancy due to the multiple hemodynamic changes. (D) A hematocrit value of 39% is within the normal range. A value <35% would indicate anemia.

64. **(D)** Client need: physiological integrity; subcategory: physiological adaptation; content area: maternity

    RATIONALE

    (A) The term heterozygote refers to an individual with one normal and one mutant allele at a given locus on a pair of homolo-

gous chromosomes. An individual who is heterozygous for the abnormal gene does not manifest obvious symptoms. (B) Disorders carried on either the X or Y sex chromosome are referred to as sex-linked recessive. (C) Either sex may be affected by autosomal recessive genetic disorders because the responsible allele can be on any one of the 46 chromosomes. (D) If both parents are affected by the disorder and are not just carriers, then all their children would manifest the same disorder.

65. **(A)** Client need: physiological integrity; subcategory: physiological adaptation; content area: maternity

    RATIONALE

    (A) Chorioamnionitis is an inflammation of the chorion and amnion that is generally associated with premature or prolonged rupture of membranes. (B) Postterm deliveries have not been shown to increase the risk of chorioamnionitis unless there has been prolonged rupture of membranes. (C) Pyelonephritis is a kidney infection that develops in 20%–40% of untreated maternal UTIs. (D) Maternal dehydration, though of great concern, is not related to chorioamnionitis.

66. **(A)** Client need: physiological integrity; subcategory: physiological adaptation; content area: maternity

    RATIONALE

    (A) During pregnancy, the potential for thromboses increases owing to the increased levels of coagulation factors and a decrease in the breakdown of fibrin. (B) An inadequate production of platelets would result in thrombocytopenia with resulting signs and symptoms of bleeding such as petechiae, hematuria, or hematemesis. (C) A deficiency of folic acid during pregnancy produces a megaloblastic anemia. It is usually found in combination with iron deficiency. (D) This combination would result in bleeding disorders because more fibrin would be broken down and fewer clotting factors would be available.

67. **(D)** Client need: physiological integrity; subcategory: pharmacological and parenteral therapies; content area: maternity

    RATIONALE

    (A) Dysuria is not a common symptom of heparin overdose. (B) Although epistaxis and hematuria are common symptoms of heparin overdose, dysuria is not. (C) Vertigo is not a common symptom of heparin overdose. (D) Hematuria, ecchymosis, and epistaxis are the most common signs and symptoms of a heparin overdose. Others are thrombocytopenia, elevated liver enzymes, and local injection site complications.

68. **(A)** Client need: physiological integrity; subcategory: physiological adaptation; content area: maternity

    RATIONALE

    (A) Mastitis is a bacterial inflammation of the breast tissue found primarily in breast-feeding mothers. The bacteria usually enter the breast through a cracked nipple, or the infection results from stasis of milk behind a blocked duct. (B) With breast engorgement during breast-feeding, there may be marked breast pain. This is not necessarily a sign of infection. (C) Women may become ill during breast-feeding with other bacterial or viral infections that are not related to mastitis. (D) Improper care of the nipples or improper positioning of the infant during breast-feeding may result in cracked or sore nipples.

69. **(C)** Client need: physiological integrity; subcategory: physiological adaptation; content area: maternity

    RATIONALE

    (A) Her cervical exam is normal. There are no cervical changes at this time. (B) Braxton Hicks contractions may be common throughout pregnancy, but they are not regular. (C) Rhythmical contractions in conjunction with low back pain and pelvic pressure at 32 weeks in a woman carrying triplets are of great concern. She may be in preterm labor. (D) UTIs are common in pregnancy due to the enlarging uterus compressing the ureters and the stasis of urine. The woman would be more likely to complain of urinary frequency and urgency, fever or chills, and malodorous urine with a UTI.

70. **(C)** Client need: physiological integrity; subcategory: physiological adaptation; content area: maternity

RATIONALE

(A) Hematomas, which are the result of damage to a vessel wall without laceration of the tissue, are a cause, though not the most frequent cause. (B) Coagulation disorders are among the causes of postpartal hemorrhage, but they are less common. (C) The most frequent causes of hemorrhage in the postpartal period are related to an interference with involution of the uterus. Uterine atony is the most frequent cause, occurring in the first 24 hours after delivery. (D) Retained placental fragments are also a cause, although these bleeds usually occur 7–14 days after delivery.

71. **(D)** Client need: psychosocial integrity; subcategory: coping and adaptation; content area: maternity

RATIONALE

(A) Parents do need their privacy following a loss, but the nurse still has a responsibility to provide postpartum physical care. (B) This is a negative statement, which is not therapeutic. The client is not concerned about future children but is in the first stages of grief, denial, and anger. (C) This is a negative statement, which is not therapeutic. The client does not want to hear about her baby in heaven. She cannot believe that God could love or want her child more than she could. (D) Acknowledging that anger is normal and beneficial will help the client to understand the normal stages of grief. Expressing sorrow over her loss and assuring her that the support is there to take care of her physical and emotional needs will help to promote a trusting relationship.

72. **(C)** Client need: physiological integrity; subcategory: physiological adaptation; content area: maternity

RATIONALE

(A) This symptom would indicate a rupture of the membranes, which would be expected during labor. There would be no cause for alarm if the fluid were clear. (B) With uterine rupture and the risk of maternal shock secondary to blood loss, the most likely sign would be hypotension indicating hypovolemic shock. (C) In the event of a uterine rupture, an abdominal examination would likely reveal rigidity or tenderness. (D) The most likely finding would be a decrease in fetal movement related to fetal distress due to impaired uteroplacental blood flow. Maintaining the client on her left side would help to maximize uterine blood flow.

73. **(C)** Client need: physiological integrity; subcategory: physiological adaptation; content area: pediatrics

RATIONALE

(A) Constipation does not cause fever or vomiting but may cause anorexia. Risk of perforation outweighs the possible benefits of an enema. (B) Heat will not relieve her symptoms but will increase intestinal motility and increase the risk of perforation. (C) Heat and enemas are contraindicated where severe abdominal pain is suspected because they increase intestinal motility and the risk of perforation. (D) Complaints accompanied by physical symptoms such as pain, anorexia, and fever should never be ignored.

74. **(B)** Client need: psychosocial integrity; subcategory: coping and adaptation; content area: pediatrics

RATIONALE

(A) This action does nothing to prepare the child and her family for what will happen or to relieve their anxiety and fear. (B) This action provides security by preparing the child and the family for what will happen and will help to relieve fear and anxiety. (C) This action does nothing to help prepare the child for what will happen and does not give the parents permission to ask ques-

tions until later. (D) This action provides possibly false reassurance and may prevent the child and/or the family from asking pressing questions.

75. **(B)** Client need: physiological integrity; subcategory: reduction of risk potential; content area: pediatrics

RATIONALE

(A) Skeletal traction, including the weights that are applying the traction, is never released by the nurse. (B) It is necessary to keep the pin site clean and free from infection. (C) When first placed in traction, the client may experience increased discomfort as a result of the traction pull fatiguing the muscle. (D) When the child in traction is allowed to participate in his care, it gives him a measure of control and helps him to cope with the situation.

76. **(B)** Client need: psychosocial integrity; subcategory: coping and adaptation; content area: pediatrics

RATIONALE

(A) These activities could be frustrating for the client if he is having difficulty with problem solving and concentration. (B) Self-care is usually well received by the child, and it is one of the most useful interventions to help the child cope with immobility. (C) This may be helpful to the client if he has no visitors, but it does little to help him develop coping skills. (D) This will help to prevent skin irritation or breakdown related to immobility but will not help to prevent behavioral changes related to immobility.

77. **(A)** Client need: physiological integrity; subcategory: reduction of risk potential; content area: pediatrics

RATIONALE

(A) Any movement of his affected limb will cause discomfort to the child. (B) No weight bearing will be allowed until healing is well underway to avoid pathological fractures. (C) The child will be anorexic and may experience vomiting. Diet should be simple and high caloric until appetite returns and symptoms subside. (D) Physical therapy is instituted only after infection subsides.

78. **(D)** Client need: physiological integrity; subcategory: physiological adaptation; content area: pediatrics

RATIONALE

(A) Poor nutrition and/or poor physical conditions are factors that predispose to the development of osteomyelitis but do not cause it. (B) An unclean or unhygienic environment may predispose to the development of chronic osteomyelitis, but it does not cause an exacerbation of the previous infection. (C) Sluggish circulation through the medullary cavity during acute osteomyelitis may delay healing, but it does not cause the disease to become chronic. (D) Areas of sequestrum may be surrounded by dense bone, become honeycombed with sinuses, and retain infectious organisms for a long time.

79. **(A)** Client need: psychosocial integrity; subcategory: coping and adaptation; content area: pediatrics

RATIONALE

(A) Even though the child has had the procedure before, she will probably need additional explanations and emotional support. (B) The fact that the child has had the procedure before and possibly found it painful or uncomfortable may increase, not relieve, her stress. (C) This intervention does nothing to reassure the child and may well prevent her from expressing her feelings. (D) This does not prepare the child for the test and burdens her with the expectation that she act bigger and braver than she is.

80. **(C)** Client need: physiological integrity; subcategory: pharmacological and parenteral therapies; content area: pediatrics

RATIONALE

(A) Children may become depressed with a changed appearance and not want to look at themselves or have others see them. (B) The hair will fall out in clumps, causing patchy baldness that is quite noticeable and traumatic to children and their families. (C) Having a wig that looks like a girl's own hair can be a psychological boost to children and is helpful in fostering later adjustments to hair loss. (D) Families may become accustomed to seeing their children without hair, but the loss is traumatic to them and will continue to bother them.

81. **(D)** Client need: physiological integrity; subcategory: basic care and comfort; content area: pediatrics

RATIONALE

(A) Because the child's appetite is capricious at best, regular servings may be overwhelming. Praise the child for what is eaten. (B) The child will soon learn that procedures follow meals and may play with food rather than eat it to avoid or delay the procedure. (C) Young children usually do not like highly seasoned foods and may need the security of usual foods. Such a change may actually increase anorexia. (D) Small servings appear more achievable to the child, and the inclusion of favorite foods can add a sense of security.

82. **(A)** Client need: health promotion and maintenance; subcategory: prevention and early detection of disease; content area: pediatrics

RATIONALE

(A) The child no longer has normal white blood cells and is extremely susceptible to infection. (B) There are more appropriate ways to provide privacy, and there is no need to protect the child from healthy visitors. (C) Visitors and visiting hours may be at the client's and/or family's request without regard to the isolation precaution. (D) The child may have strong positive relationships with other clients or staff. As long as proper precautions are observed, there is no reason to isolate her from them.

83. **(B)** Client need: physiological integrity; subcategory: basic care and comfort; content area: pediatrics

RATIONALE

(A) Local anesthetics do temporarily relieve the pain but leave an unpleasant taste and numb feeling that are not conductive to eating. (B) Such a diet is less irritating to the damaged mucosa and is easier for the child to tolerate. (C) This intervention is helpful if the child has only anorexia. It does not work if the type and texture of the food increase oral discomfort. (D) Lemon glycerin swabs and milk of magnesia dry the oral mucosa and should be avoided.

84. **(A)** Client need: physiological integrity; subcategory: basic care and comfort; content area: pediatrics

RATIONALE

(A) The adolescent knows what he likes and will be more likely to eat if he has some control over his diet. (B) The nurses and nutritionist can plan an excellent diet, but it will not help the adolescent unless he eats it. (C) Eating is already a chore for this client. Adding a strict calorie count could make it even more burdensome. (D) Fats are particularly difficult for the cystic fibrosis client to digest. He does need a healthful diet, not just more calories.

85. **(A)** Client need: physiological integrity; subcategory: basic care and comfort; content area: pediatrics

RATIONALE

(A) Consistent weight gain, even if it is slow, is an indication that the child is eating and digesting sufficient calories. (B) Recording how much the child eats is useful, but it is not an indicator of how well his body is using the foods consumed. (C) Counting calories will indicate how much he is eating, but it will not reflect whether or not the foods are properly digested. (D) Keeping track of the enzyme intake will indicate compliance with medication but not whether the child is getting sufficient calories.

86. **(C)** Client need: health promotion and maintenance; subcategory: prevention and early detection of disease; content area: pediatrics

RATIONALE

(A) Regular exercise does promote a sense of well-being and self-worth, but this is not the ultimate goal of exercise for this client. (B) Regular chest physiotherapy, not exercise per se, helps to prevent respiratory infections. (C) Physical exercise is an important adjunct to chest physiotherapy. It stimulates mucus secretion, promotes a feeling of well-being, and helps to establish a habitual breathing pattern. (D) Along with adequate nutrition and minimization of pulmonary complications, exercise does help promote normal growth and development. However, exercise is promoted primarily to help establish a habitual breathing pattern.

87. **(B)** Client need: psychosocial integrity; subcategory: coping and adaptation; content area: pediatrics

RATIONALE

(A) Threats of suicide should always be taken seriously. (B) This client has a life-threatening chronic illness. He may be concerned about dying or he may actually be contemplating suicide. (C) Sometimes clients who have made the decision to commit suicide appear to be less depressed. (D) Forcing him to look at his feelings may cause him to build a defense against the depression with behavioral or psychosomatic disturbances.

88. **(D)** Client need: health promotion and maintenance; subcategory: prevention and early detection of disease; content area: pediatrics

RATIONALE

(A) This position is indicative of a possible meningeal irritation or infection such as meningitis. (B) This position is seen most frequently in infants who have had an injury to the sternocleidomastoid muscle. (C) Most infants aged 4 months and older are able to maintain this position. (D) Infants older than 6 months of age should not have significant head lag. This is a sign of cerebral injury and should be referred for further evaluation.

89. **(C)** Client need: health promotion and maintenance; subcategory: prevention and early detection of disease; content area: pediatrics

RATIONALE

(A) Zinc oxide is not usually applied to inflamed areas because it contributes to sweat retention. (B) Talcum powder is of questionable benefit and poses a hazard of accidental inhalation. (C) Removing the diaper and exposing the area to air and light facilitate drying and healing. (D) Infants may be sensitive to one or more agents in the wet "wipes." It is better to simply clean with a wet cloth.

90. **(D)** Client need: health promotion and maintenance; subcategory: growth and development through the life span; content area: pediatrics

RATIONALE

(A) If the infant is given the bottle first, he will be less likely to be hungry enough to eat the solid foods. (B) Milk is deficient in iron, vitamin C, zinc, and fluoride. It does not provide an adequate diet. (C) The vitamin supplement will help, but the infant needs an iron supplement. (D) Giving the solid food when the infant is hungriest will increase the likelihood that he will eat. The more solid food he takes, the less milk he will desire.

T E S T 6

Southeastern Louisiana University Test

MOCK NCLEX-RN BOARD REVIEW TEST QUESTIONS

1. A 9-month-old infant was diagnosed with nonorganic failure to thrive. During her hospitalization, primary nurses were assigned to initiate all infant feedings. The infant's parents question why they cannot feed their own child. Which of the following responses would be most appropriate by the nurse?

   A. By assigning the same nurses to the child, the nurses can begin to learn the infant's cues and feeding behaviors.
   B. The same nurses will prevent parental fatigue and frustration.
   C. The same nurses will prevent infant fatigue and frustration.
   D. Primary nurses will ensure privacy.

2. The parents of a 2-year-old child are ready to begin toilet training activities with him. His parents feel he is ready to train because he is now 2 years old. What would the nurse identify as readiness in this child?

   A. Patience by the child when wearing soiled diapers
   B. Communicating the urge to defecate or urinate
   C. The child awakening wet from his naps
   D. The age at which the child's siblings were trained

3. A 5-year-old child is hospitalized for an acute illness. The nurse encourages the family to bring her favorite objects from home. What is the nurse's rationale?

   A. To reduce fear of the unknown
   B. To keep the child calm
   C. To establish a trusting relationship
   D. To prevent or minimize separation anxiety

4. A 3-year-old child was hospitalized for acute laryngotracheobronchitis. During her hospitalization, the child was placed under an oxygen mist tent. The nurse's frequent monitoring of the child's temperature frightened her parents. Which response by the nurse would be most appropriate?

   A. Monitoring the temperature prevents undue chilling.
   B. Rapid temperature elevations can occur in children.
   C. Checking the temperature will prevent febrile seizures.
   D. Taking the child's temperature can prevent airway obstruction.

5. A school-age child with asthma is ready for discharge from the hospital. His physician has written an order to continue the theophylline given in the hospital as an oral home medication. Immediately prior to discharge, he complains of nausea and becomes irritable. His vital signs were normal except for tachycardia. What first nursing actions would be essential in this situation?

   A. Hold the child's discharge for 1 hour.
   B. Notify the physician immediately.
   C. Discharge the child as the physician ordered.
   D. Administer an antiemetic as necessary.

6. A neonate was admitted to the hospital with projectile vomiting. According to the parents, the baby had experienced vomiting episodes after feeding for the last 2 days. A medical diagnosis of hypertrophic pyloric stenosis was made. On assessment, the infant had poor skin turgor, sunken eyeballs, dry skin, and weight loss. Identify the number-one priority nursing diagnosis.

   A. Fluid volume deficit
   B. Altered nutrition
   C. Altered bowel elimination
   D. Anxiety

7. A baby who was diagnosed with pyloric stenosis has continued to have projectile vomiting. With prolonged vomiting, the infant is prone to:

   A. Respiratory acidosis
   B. Respiratory alkalosis
   C. Metabolic acidosis
   D. Metabolic alkalosis

8. Parents of young children often need anticipatory guidance from the nurse. Parents may have little knowledge regarding growth and development. Which of the following toys and activities would the nurse suggest as appropriate for a toddler?

    A. Cutting, pasting, string beads, music, dolls
    B. Mobiles, rattle, squeeze toys
    C. Pull-toys, large ball, dolls, sand and water play, music
    D. Simple card games, puzzles, bicycle, television

9. A 5-year-old child cries continually in her bed. Her parents have been unsuccessful in assisting her in expressing her feelings. Which activity should the nurse provide the child to assist her in expressing her feelings?

    A. Books with colorful pictures
    B. Music
    C. Riding toys
    D. Puppets

10. During his hospitalization, a 3-year-old child has become unusually aggressive in his play activities. His parents report this change in behavior to the primary nurse. How could the nurse explain the child's change in behavior?

    A. Deep-seated feelings of hostility
    B. A lack of interest in socializing
    C. Usual behavior for this child
    D. A coping response

11. Following her surgery, a 5-year-old child will return to the pediatric unit with a long-arm cast. She experienced a supracondylar fracture of the humerus near the elbow. Which nursing action is most essential during the first 24 hours after surgery and cast application?

    A. Mobilization of the child
    B. Discharge teaching
    C. Pain management
    D. Assessment of neurovascular status

12. A 9-month-old infant visits her pediatrician for a routine visit. A developmental assessment was initiated by the nurse. Which skill would cause the nurse to be concerned about the infant's developmental progression?

    A. She sits briefly alone with assistance.
    B. She creeps and crawls.
    C. She pulls herself to her feet with help.
    D. She stands while holding onto furniture.

13. Children often experience visual impairments. Refractive errors affect the child's visual activity. The main refractive error seen in children is myopia. The nurse explains to the child's parents that myopia may also be described as:

    A. Cataracts
    B. Farsightedness
    C. Nearsightedness
    D. Lazy eye

14. A client is experiencing visual problems at school. She has complained of difficulty seeing the blackboard and squinting. She no longer likes to participate in physical activities such as softball. The client has displayed possible classic symptoms of which refractive error?

    A. Astigmatism
    B. Hyperopia
    C. Myopia
    D. Amblyopia

15. An 18-year-old client enters the emergency room complaining of coughing, chest tightness, dyspnea, and sputum production. On physical assessment, the nurse notes agitation, nasal flaring, tachypnea, and expiratory wheezing. These signs should alert the nurse to:

    A. A tension pneumothorax
    B. An asthma attack
    C. Pneumonia
    D. Pulmonary embolus

16. The nurse is assisting a 4th-day postoperative cholecystectomy client in planning her meals for tomorrow's menu. Which vitamin is the most essential in promoting tissue healing?

    A. Vitamin C
    B. Vitamin B_1
    C. Vitamin D
    D. Vitamin A

17. As a postoperative cholecystectomy client completes tomorrow's dinner menu, the nurse knows that one of the following meal choices will *best* provide the essential vitamin(s) necessary for proper tissue healing?

    A. Liver, white rice, spinach, tossed salad, custard pudding
    B. Fish fillet, carrots, mashed potatoes, butterscotch pudding
    C. Roast chicken, gelatin with sliced fruit
    D. Chicken breast fillet in tomato sauce, potatoes, mustard greens, orange and strawberry slices

18. A 71-year-old client fell and injured her left leg while cooking in the kitchen. Her husband calls the ambulance, and she is taken to the emergency department at a local hospital. X-ray reports confirm that she has an intertrochanteric fracture of the left femur. Her left leg will require skeletal traction initially and then surgery. The nurse knows that this type of traction will be used:

    A. By inserting pins to provide steady pull on the bone
    B. To suspend the leg in a sling without pull on the extremity
    C. Intermittently to place a pull over the pelvis and lower spine
    D. With weights at both ends of the bed to maintain pull on the upper extremity

19. Pin care is a part of the care plan for a client who is in skeletal traction. When assessing the site of pin insertion, which one of the following findings would the nurse know as an indicator of normal wound healing?

    A. Exudate
    B. Crust
    C. Edema
    D. Erythema

20. A 47-year-old client comes to the emergency department complaining of moderate flank, abdominal, and

testicular pain with nausea of 4 hours' duration. After physical examination and obtaining the client's history, the physician suspects urethral obstruction by calculi. The nurse realizes that the physician will order which one of the following diagnostic studies to *best* confirm the diagnosis?

A. Cystoscopy
B. Kidneys, ureter, bladder, x-ray of abdomen
C. Intravenous pyelogram with excretory urogram
D. Ureterolithotomy

21. An obstructing stone in the renal pelvis or upper ureter causes:

A. Radiating pain into the urethra with labia pain experienced in females or testicular pain in males
B. Urinary frequency and dysuria
C. Severe flank and abdominal pain with nausea, vomiting, diaphoresis, and pallor
D. Dull, aching, back pain

22. A client who has gout is most likely to form which type of renal calculi?

A. Struvite stones
B. Staghorn calculi
C. Uric acid stones
D. Calcium stones

23. A 75-year-old client is hospitalized with pneumonia caused by gram-positive bacteria. Which one of the following best describes a gram-positive bacterial pneumonia?

A. *Klebsiella* pneumonia
B. Pneumococcal pneumonia
C. *Legionella pneumophila* pneumonia
D. *Escherichia coli* pneumonia

24. The nurse caring for a client who has pneumonia, which is caused by a gram-positive bacteria, inspects her sputum. Because the client's pneumonia is caused by a gram-positive bacteria, the nurse experts to find the sputum to be:

A. Bright red with streaks
B. Rust colored
C. Green colored
D. Pink-tinged and frothy

25. The nurse who is caring for a client with pneumonia assesses that the client has become increasingly irritable and restless. The nurse realizes that this is a result of:

A. Prolonged bed rest
B. The client's maintaining a semi-Fowler position
C. Cerebral hypoxia
D. IV fluids of 2.5–3 liters in 24 hours

26. A 22-year-old client who is being seen in the clinic for a possible asthma attack stops wheezing suddenly as the nurse is doing a lung assessment. Which one of the following nursing interventions is most important?

A. Place the client in a supine position.
B. Draw a blood sample for arterial blood gases.
C. Start O_2 at 4 L/min.
D. Establish a patent airway.

27. A 49-year-old obese woman has been admitted to the general surgery unit with choledocholithiasis. As the nurse is admitting her to the unit, she states, "The doctor said I have stones that need to be removed; where are they?" The nurse knows that the best explanation for this is to tell her that:

A. There are stones present in her gallbladder
B. There are stones present in her kidneys
C. There are stones present in her common bile duct
D. There are no stones, but her gallbladder is irritated and caused her nausea, vomiting, and pain

28. A 48-year-old client is being seen in her physician's office for complaints of indigestion, heartburn, right upper quadrant pain, and nausea of 4 days' duration, especially after meals. The nurse realizes that these symptoms may be associated with cholecystitis and therefore would check for which specific sign during the abdominal assessment?

A. Cullen's sign
B. Rebound tenderness
C. Murphy's sign
D. Turner's sign

29. When caring for a postoperative cholecystectomy client, the nurse assesses patency and documents drainage of the T-tube. The nurse recognizes that the expected amount of drainage during the first 24 hours postoperatively is:

A. 50–100 mL
B. 200–300 mL
C. 300–500 mL
D. 1000–1200 mL

30. The nurse recognizes that a client with the diagnosis of cholecystitis and cholelithiasis would expect to have stools that are:

A. Clay or gray colored
B. Watery and loose
C. Bright-red streaked
D. Black

31. A 52-year-old client who underwent an exploratory laparotomy for a bowel obstruction begins to complain of hunger on the third postoperative day. His nasogastric (NG) tube was removed this morning, and he has an IV of D_5W with 0.45% normal saline running at 125 mL/hr. He asks when he can get rid of his IV and start eating. The nurse recognizes that he will be able to begin taking oral fluids and nourishment when:

A. It is determined that he has no signs of wound infection
B. He is able to eat a full meal without evidence of nausea or vomiting
C. The nurse can detect bowel sounds in all four quadrants
D. His blood pressure returns to its preoperative baseline level or greater

32. A 47-year-old client has been admitted to the general surgery unit for bowel obstruction. The doctor has ordered that an NG tube be inserted to aid in bowel de-

compression. When preparing to insert a NG tube, the nurse measures from the:

A. Lower lip to the shoulder to the upper sternum
B. Tip of the nose to the lower lip to the umbilicus
C. End of the tube to the first measurement line on the tube
D. Tip of the nose to the ear lobe to the xiphoid process or midepigastric area

33. A 65-year-old client who has a new colostomy is preparing for discharge from the hospital. As part of the instructions on colostomy care, the nurse explains to the client that to regulate the bowel, colostomy irrigation should be performed at the same time each day. The best time is:

A. After meals
B. Before meals
C. Every 2 hours
D. At bedtime

34. A 72-year-old client with a new colostomy is being evaluated at the clinic today for constipation. When discussing diet with the client, the nurse recognizes that which one of the following foods most likely caused this problem?

A. Fried chicken
B. Eggs
C. Tapioca
D. Cabbage

35. When giving discharge instructions to a 24-year-old client who had a short-arm cast applied for a fractured right ulna, the nurse recognizes the importance of telling him that the drying time for a plaster of Paris cast is approximately:

A. 30 minutes
B. 1–4 hours
C. 12–24 hours
D. 24–72 hours

36. A 58-year-old client on a general surgery unit is scheduled for transurethral resection of the prostate (TURP) in 2 hours. The nurse explains to the client that this procedure means:

A. Removal of the prostate tissue by way of a lower abdominal midline incision through the bladder and into the prostate gland
B. Removal of prostate tissue by a resectoscope that is inserted through the penile urethra
C. Removal of the prostate tissue by an open surgical approach through an incision between the ischial tuberosities, the scrotum, and the rectum
D. Removal of prostate tissue by an open surgical approach through a low horizontal incision, bypassing the bladder, to the prostate gland

37. A postoperative TURP client returns from the recovery room to the general surgery unit and is in stable condition. One hour later the nurse assesses him and finds him to be confused and disoriented. She recognizes that this is most likely caused by:

A. Hypovolemic shock
B. Hypokalemia

C. Hypernatremia
D. Hyponatremia

38. A postoperative TURP client is ordered continuous bladder irrigations. Later in the evening on the first postoperative day, he complains of increasing suprapubic pain. When assessing the client, the nurse notes diminished flow of bloody urine and several large blood clots in the drainage tubing. Which one of the following should be the initial nursing intervention?

A. Call the physician about the problem.
B. Irrigate the Foley catheter.
C. Change the Foley catheter.
D. Administer a prescribed narcotic analgesic.

39. A postoperative prostatectomy client is preparing for discharge from the hospital the next morning. The nurse realizes that additional instructions are necessary when he states:

A. "If I drink 10 to 12 glasses of fluids each day, that will help to prevent any clot formation in my urine."
B. "The isometric exercises will help to strengthen my perineal muscles and help me control my urine."
C. "If I feel as though I have developed a fever, I will take a rectal temperature, which is the most accurate."
D. "I do not plan to do any heavy lifting until I visit my doctor again."

40. A 67-year-old postoperative TURP client has hematuria. The nurse caring for him reviews his postoperative orders and recognizes that which one of the following prescribed medications would best relieve this problem?

A. Acetaminophen suppository 650 mg
B. Meperidine 50 mg IM
C. Promethazine 25 mg IM
D. Aminocaproic acid (Amicar) 6 g/24 hr

41. A 52-year-old client is scheduled for a small-bowel resection in the morning. In conjunction with other preoperative preparation, the nurse is teaching her diaphragmatic breathing exercises. She will teach the client to:

A. Inhale slowly and deeply through the nose until the lungs are fully expanded, hold the breath a couple of seconds, and then exhale slowly through the mouth. Repeat 2–3 more times to complete the series every 1–2 hours while awake
B. Purse the lips and take quick, short breaths approximately 18–20 times/min
C. Take a large gulp of air into the mouth, hold it for 10–15 seconds, and then expel it through the nose. Repeat 4–5 times to complete the series
D. Inhale as deeply as possible and then immediately exhale as deeply as possible at a rate of approximately 20–24 times/min

42. A 27-year-old healthy primigravida is brought to the labor and birthing room by her husband at 32 weeks' gestation. She experienced a sudden onset of painless vaginal bleeding. Following an ultrasound examination, the diagnosis of bleeding secondary to complete placenta

previa is made. Expected assessment findings concerning the abdomen would include:

A. A rigid, boardlike abdomen
B. Uterine atony
C. A soft relaxed abdomen
D. Hypertonicity of the uterus

43. A 27-year-old primigravida stated that she got up from the chair to fix dinner and bright red blood was running down her legs. She denies any pain previously or currently. The client is very concerned about whether her baby will be all right. Her vital signs include P 120 bpm, respirations 26 breaths/min, BP 104/58 mm Hg, temperature 98.2°F, and fetal heart rate 146 bpm. Laboratory findings revealed hemoglobin 9.0 g/dL, hematocrit 26%, and coagulation studies within normal range. On admission, the peripad she wore was noted to be half saturated with bright red blood. A medical diagnosis of placenta previa is made. The priority nursing diagnosis for this client would be:

A. Decreased cardiac output related to excessive bleeding
B. Potential for fluid volume excess related to fluid resuscitation
C. Anxiety related to threat to self
D. Alteration in parenting related to potential fetal injury

44. A 27-year-old primigravida at 32 weeks' gestation has been diagnosed with complete placenta previa. Conservative management including bed rest is the proper medical management. The goal for fetal survival is based on fetal lung maturity. The test used to determine fetal lung maturity is:

A. Dinitrophenylhydrazine
B. Metachromatic stain
C. Blood serum phenylalanine test
D. Lecithin-sphingomyelin ratio

45. The nurse is notified that a 27-year-old primigravida diagnosed with complete placenta previa is to be admitted to the hospital for a cesarean section. The client is now at 36 weeks' gestation and is presently having bright red bleeding of moderate amount. On admission, the nursing intervention that the nurse should give the highest priority to is:

A. Shave the client's abdomen and arrange her lab work
B. Determine the status of the fetus by fetal heart tones
C. Start an IV infusion in the client's arm
D. Insert an indwelling catheter into her bladder

46. A 29-year-old client delivered her fifth child by the Lamaze method and developed a postpartal hemorrhage in the recovery room. What are the initial symptoms of shock that she may experience?

A. Marked elevation in blood pressure, respirations, and pulse
B. Decreased systolic pressure, cold skin, and anuria
C. Rapid pulse; narrowed pulse pressure; cool, moist skin
D. No urinary output, tachycardia, and restlessness

47. The nurse has been assigned a client who delivered a 6-lb, 12-oz baby boy vaginally 40 minutes ago. The initial

assessment of *greatest* importance for this client would be:

A. Length of her labor
B. Type of episiotomy
C. Amount of IV fluid to be infused
D. Character of the fundus

48. On the first postpartal day, a client tells the nurse that she has been changing her perineal pads every ½ hour because they are saturated with bright red vaginal drainage. When palpating the uterus, the nurse assesses that it is somewhat soft, 1 fingerbreadth above the umbilicus, and midline. The nursing action to be taken is to:

A. Gently massage the uterus until firm, express any clots, and note the amount and character of lochia
B. Catheterize the client and reassess the uterus
C. Begin IV fluids and administer oxytocic medication
D. Administer analgesics as ordered to relieve discomfort

49. The nurse assesses a client on the second postpartum day and finds a dark red discharge on the peripad. The stain appears to be about 5 inches long. Which of the following correctly describes the character and amount of lochia?

A. Lochia alba, light
B. Lochia serosa, heavy
C. Lochia granulosa, heavy
D. Lochia rubra, moderate

50. A 2-day-old infant boy has been diagnosed with an atrial septal defect due to a persistent patent foramen ovale. When explaining the diagnosis to the mother, the nurse includes in the discussion the function of the foramen ovale. In fetal circulation, the foramen ovale allows a portion of the blood to bypass the:

A. Left ventricle
B. Pulmonary system
C. Liver
D. Superior vena cava

51. A client has been admitted to the nursing unit with the diagnosis of severe anemia. She is slightly short of breath, has episodes of dizziness, and complains her heart sometimes feels like it will "beat out of her chest." The physician has ordered her to receive 2 U of packed red blood cells. The most important nursing action to be taken is:

A. Starting an 18-gauge IV infusion
B. Having the consent form on the chart
C. Administering the correct blood product to the correct client
D. Transfusing the blood in a 2-hour time frame

52. A client diagnosed with severe anemia is to receive 2 U of packed red blood cells. Prior to starting the blood transfusion, the nurse must:

A. Take a baseline set of vital signs
B. Hang Ringer's lactate as the companion fluid
C. Use microdrip tubing for the blood administration
D. Have the registered nurse in charge assume responsibility for verifying the client and blood product information

53. A client's transfusion of packed red blood cells has been infusing for 2 hours. She is complaining of a raised, itchy rash and shortness of breath. She is wheezing, anxious, and very restless. The nurse knows these assessment findings are congruent with:
    A. Hemolytic transfusion reaction
    B. Febrile transfusion reaction
    C. Circulatory overload
    D. Allergic transfusion reaction

54. Diagnostic assessment findings for an infant with possible coarctation of the aorta would include:
    A. A third heart sound
    B. A diastolic murmur
    C. Pulse pressure difference between the upper extremities
    D. Diminished or absent femoral pulses

55. Decreased pulmonary blood flow, right-to-left shunting, and deoxygenated blood reaching the systemic circulation are characteristic of:
    A. Tetralogy of Fallot
    B. Ventricular septal defect
    C. Patent ductus arteriosus
    D. Transposition of the great arteries

56. A 2-year-old child will undergo a cardiac catheterization tomorrow to evaluate his ventricular septal defect. Based on his developmental stage, the nurse:
    A. Uses pictures to explain the procedure to the child and his parents that evening
    B. Explains the procedure using simple words and sentences just before the preoperative sedation
    C. Asks the parents to explain the procedure to the child after she explains it to them
    D. Asks the parents to leave the room while the preoperative medication and instructions are given

57. Home-care instructions for the child following a cardiac catheterization should include:
    A. Notify the physician if a slight bruise develops around the insertion site.
    B. Use sponge bathing until stitches are removed.
    C. Give aspirin if the child complains of pain at the insertion site.
    D. Keep a clean, dry dressing on the insertion site for 2 days.

58. Nursing care for the parents of a child with a congenital heart defect would include:
    A. Encouraging the parents not to tell the child about the seriousness of the congenital heart defect, so the child will function as normally as possible
    B. Acknowledging the fear and concern surrounding their child's health and assisting the parents through the grieving process as they mourn the loss of their fantasized healthy child
    C. Identifying anger and resentment as destructive emotions that serve no purpose
    D. Expressing to the parents after the corrective surgery has been completed successfully that all their grief feelings will resolve

59. An infant with a congenital heart defect is being discharged with an order for the administration of digoxin elixir every 12 hours. The parents need to be taught when administering digoxin to the infant that:
    A. If the infant vomits within 30 minutes of the digoxin administration, repeat the dose
    B. They need to mix it with formula so the infant swallows it easily
    C. If the infant vomits two or more consecutive doses or becomes listless or anorexic, notify the physician
    D. If a dose of digoxin is skipped for more than 6 hours, a new timetable for administration must be developed

60. A 4-year-old child with a history of sickle cell anemia is admitted to the nursing unit with dizziness, shortness of breath, and pallor. Nursing assessment findings reveal tenderness in the abdomen. The child is most likely experiencing a/an:
    A. Aplastic crisis
    B. Vaso-occlusive crisis
    C. Dactylitis crisis
    D. Sequestration crisis

61. The primary focus of nursing interventions for the child experiencing sickle cell crisis is aimed toward:
    A. Maintaining an adequate level of hydration
    B. Providing pain relief
    C. Preventing infection
    D. O_2 therapy

62. A 30-year-old client is exhibiting auditory hallucinations. In working with this client, the nurse would be *most* effective if the nurse:
    A. Encourages the client to discuss the voices
    B. Attempts to direct the client's attention to the here and now
    C. Exhibits sincere interest in the delusional voices
    D. Gives the medication as necessary for the acting-out behavior

63. One week ago, a 21-year-old client with a diagnosis of bipolar disorder was started on lithium 300 mg po qid. A lithium level is ordered. The client's level is 1.3 mEq/L. The nurse recognizes that this level is considered to be:
    A. Within therapeutic range
    B. Below therapeutic range
    C. Above therapeutic range
    D. At a level of toxic poisoning

64. A client was exhibiting signs of mania and was recently started on lithium carbonate. She has no known physical problems. A teaching plan for this client would include which of the following?
    A. Regular foods should be eaten, including those that contain salt, such as bacon, ham, V-8 juice, and tomato juice.
    B. Restrict fluids to 1000 mL/day.
    C. Restrict foods that contain salt or sodium.
    D. Discontinue the medication if nausea occurs.

65. A behavioral modification program is recommended by the multidisciplinary team working with a 15-year-old

client with anorexia nervosa. A nursing plan of care based on this modality would include:

A. Role playing the client's eating behaviors
B. Restriction to the unit until she has gained 2 lb
C. Encouraging her to verbalize her feelings concerning food and food intake
D. Provision for a high-calorie, high-protein snack between meals

66. A 22-year-old client presents with a diagnosis of antisocial personality disorder and a history of using drugs, writing numerous checks with insufficient funds, and stealing. He appears charming and intelligent, and the other clients are impressed and want to be liked by him. The greatest problem that may arise from this situation is that:

A. He will manipulate the other clients for his own benefit
B. He will cause the other clients to become psychotic
C. He will become delusional and hallucinate as a result of the excess attention given to him by peers
D. He may exhibit self-mutilative behavior

67. In admitting a client to the psychiatric unit, the nurse must explain the rules and regulations of the unit. A client with antisocial personality disorder makes the following remark, "Forget all those rules. I always get along well with the nurses." Which nursing response to him would be most effective?

A. "OK, don't listen to the rules. See where you end up."
B. "I'm pleased that you get along so well with the staff. You must still know and abide by the rules."
C. "It is irrelevant whether you get along with the nurses."
D. "I'm not the other nurses. You better read the rules yourself."

68. A client was admitted to the hospital after falling in her home. At the time of admission, her blood alcohol level was 0.27 mg%. Her family indicates that she has been drinking a fifth of vodka a day for the past 9 months. She had her last drink 30 minutes prior to admission. Alcohol withdrawal symptoms would most likely be exhibited by her:

A. Two to 4 hours after the last drink
B. Six to 8 hours after the last drink
C. Immediately on admission
D. Twenty-four hours after the last drink

69. A client has begun to exhibit signs of alcohol withdrawal. Her blood pressure has risen from 120/60 to 190/100, pulse is increased from 88 to 110 bpm, and she is irritable and agitated and has gross motor tremors of the hands. The nurse notifies the doctor. The nurse can anticipate that the doctor will order which of the following?

A. An opiate such as propoxyphene napsylate (Darvocet)
B. A benzodiazepine such as chlordiazepoxide (Librium)
C. A tricyclic antidepressant such as amitriptyline (Elavil)
D. A phenothiazine such as chlorpromazine (Thorazine)

70. A 60-year-old woman exhibits forgetfulness, emotional lability, confusion, and decreased concentration. She has been unable to perform activities of daily living without assistance. After a thorough medical evaluation, a diagnosis of Alzheimer's disease was made. An appropriate nursing intervention to decrease the anxiety of this client would include:

A. Allowing the client to perform activities of daily living as much as possible unassisted
B. Confronting confabulations
C. Reality testing
D. Providing a highly stimulating environment

71. A 74-year-old client seen in the emergency room is exhibiting signs of delirium. His family states that he has not slept, eaten, or taken fluids for the past 24 hours. The planning of nursing care for a delirious client is based on which of the following premises?

A. The delirious client is capable of returning to his previous level of functioning.
B. The delirious client is incapable of returning to his previous level of functioning.
C. Delirium entails progressive intellectual and behavioral deterioration.
D. Delirium is an insidious process.

72. A 48-year-old client presents with a long history of severe depression unrelieved by medication. He is admitted to the hospital for electroconvulsive therapy. Family members are very concerned about this therapy and are requesting information about aftereffects of the treatment. The nurse informs the family that he will:

A. Have transient memory loss, confusion, and headache
B. Be alert and oriented immediately after the treatment
C. Have insomnia for the first few days
D. Require no special care after the procedure

73. An 80-year-old widow is living with her son and daughter-in-law. The home health nurse has been making weekly visits to draw blood for a prothrombin time test. The client is taking 5 mg of coumadin per day. She appears more debilitated, and bruises are noted on her face. Elder abuse is suspected. Which of the following are signs of persons who are at risk for abusing an elderly person?

A. A family member who is having marital problems and is regularly abusing alcohol
B. A person with adequate communication and coping skills who is employed by the family
C. A friend of the family who wants to help but is minimally competent
D. A lifelong friend of the client who is often confused

74. A 16-year-old client with a diagnosis of oppositional defiant disorder is threatening violence toward another child. In managing a potentially violent client, the nurse:

A. Must use the least restrictive measure possible to control the behavior
B. Should put the client in seclusion until he promises to behave appropriately

C. Should apply full restraints until the behavior is under control

D. Should allow other clients to observe the acting out so that they can learn from the experience

75. The nurse is planning a reality orientation program for a group of clients with organic brain syndrome at the mental health center. Props that could be used for this program are:

A. Month-old magazines that are provided by volunteers
B. Large maps and posters depicting area of current residence
C. A litter of kittens for the clients to pet
D. A library of biographical books

76. In working with a manipulative client, which of the following nursing interventions would be most appropriate?

A. Bargaining with the client as a strategy to control the behavior
B. Redirecting the client
C. Providing a consistent set of guidelines and rules
D. Assigning the client to different staff persons each day

77. Primary nursing diagnoses for the antisocial client are:

A. Alteration in perception and altered self-concept
B. Impaired social interaction, ineffective individual coping, and altered self-concept
C. Altered communication processes and altered recreational patterns
D. Altered body image and altered thought processes

78. A 25-year-old outpatient presents with a diagnosis of compulsive personality disorder. His coworkers become annoyed with his rigid, perfectionistic manner and preoccupation with trivial details and schedules. A nursing intervention appropriate for this client would include:

A. Encouraging him to engage in recreational activities
B. Avoiding discussion of his annoying behavior
C. Encouraging the client to set a time schedule and deadlines for himself
D. Contracting with him for the amount of time he will spend on the compulsive behaviors

79. The serial sevens test is often used to determine delirium and dementia. This test aids in assessing which of the following?

A. Abstract thinking
B. Ability to focus and concentrate thoughts
C. Judgment
D. Memory

80. A 14-year-old client has a history of lying, stealing, and destruction of property. Personal items of peers have been found missing. After group therapy, a peer approaches the nurse to report that he has seen the 14-year-old with some of the missing items. The best response of the nurse is to:

A. Request that he explain to the group why he took personal items from peers
B. Approach him when he is alone to inquire about his involvement in the incident

C. Imply to him that you doubt his involvement in the incident and request his denial
D. Confront him openly in group and request an apology

81. A 15-year-old client is admitted to the adolescent unit. The nurse recognizes that encouraging a client to speak openly depends on how clearly questions are phrased. Which of the following statements is most desirable in eliciting information from an adolescent client?

A. "Do you get along well with your family?"
B. "Do you communicate with your parents?"
C. "You don't hate your family, do you?"
D. "What is it like between you and your family?"

82. A 37-year-old client has been taking antipsychotic medication for the past 10 days. The nurse observes her walking with a shuffling gait and postural rigidity and notes a masklike expression on her face. Which side effect is this client exhibiting?

A. Dystonia
B. Parkinsonism
C. Tardive dyskinesia
D. Akathesia

83. Clients receiving antipsychotic drug therapy will often exhibit extrapyramidal side effects that are reversible with which of the following agents ordered by the physician?

A. Phenothiazines
B. Anticholinergics
C. Anti-Parkinsonian drugs
D. Tricyclic agents

84. A client who was started on antipsychotic medication 2 weeks ago is preparing for discharge from the hospital. Compliance with the medication regimen is important despite the mild side effects encountered. In order to increase the likelihood of medication compliance, the nurse would:

A. Discuss the disease process and the importance of the medication in prevention of symptoms.
B. Inform the client that additional side effects are to be expected and need not be reported.
C. Discuss the importance of getting blood drawn weekly to determine medication therapeutics.
D. Inform the client to cease taking the medication when all psychotic symptoms have cleared.

85. A depressed client is seen at the mental health center for follow-up after an attempted suicide 1 week ago. She has taken phenelzine sulfate (Nardil), a monoamine oxidase (MAO) inhibitor, for 7 straight days. She states that she is not feeling any better. The nurse explains that the drug must accumulate to an effective level before symptoms are totally relieved. Symptom relief is expected to occur within:

A. 10 days
B. 2–4 weeks
C. 2 months
D. 3 months

86. Because a client is taking an MAO inhibitor, it is necessary to discuss the need for adherence to a low-tyramine

diet. Which of the following are foods that she should avoid?

A. Pickled, aged, smoked, and fermented foods
B. Fresh vegetables
C. Broiled fresh fish and fowl
D. Fresh fruit such as apples and oranges

87. In working with mental health clients who are prescribed medication that must be taken on a routine basis, it is important for education to begin when the drug therapy is initiated. One of the first steps in the teaching process is to:

A. Explain the side effects of the medication
B. Discuss the danger of overmedication
C. Distribute written material to supplement verbal instructions
D. Explore the client's perception regarding medication therapy

88. A 29-year-old client is diagnosed with borderline personality disorder. He has aroused the nurse's anger by using a condescending tone of voice with other clients and staff persons. Which of the following statements from the nurse would be most appropriate in acknowledging feelings regarding the client's behavior?

A. "I feel angry when I hear that tone of voice."
B. "You make me angry when you talk to me that way."
C. "Are you trying to get me angry?"
D. "Why do you treat me that way?"

89. The mother of a 7-year-old mental health center client reports that the client has refused to attend gymnastics for the past 2 weeks. Prior to that time, the child liked going to this class and was attending 3 times a week. In talking with the client, the nurse would:

A. Ask her why she doesn't like gymnastics anymore
B. Ask her to describe how things were at gymnastics before she started refusing to go
C. Tell her that it is OK to be afraid of this activity
D. Reassure her that things will get better once she begins the classes again

90. A 42-year-old client presents with a diagnosis of paranoid schizophrenia. She has become increasingly restless and verbally argumentative, and her speech has become pressured. She is exhibiting signs of:

A. Depression
B. Agitation
C. Psychotic ideation
D. Anhedonia

91. A 50-year-old depressed client has recently lost his job. He has been reluctant to leave his hospital room. Nursing care would include:

A. Forcing the client to attend all unit activities
B. Encouraging the client to discuss why he is so sad
C. Monitoring elimination patterns
D. Providing sensory stimulation

92. A client was admitted to the hospital for a TURP. Within 48 hours of admission and 12 hours postoperatively, both the blood pressure and pulse increased. He became agitated, thought snakes were crawling on his arms and legs, and generally became unmanageable. He pulled out his IV and urinary catheter in attempt to rid himself of the snakes. He was sweating profusely. The admission nurse's notes indicated that the client admitted to "having a few drinks now and then." He is probably experiencing which of the following?

A. Major psychotic depression
B. Delirium tremens
C. Generalized anxiety disorder
D. Adjustment disorder with mixed features

MOCK NCLEX-RN BOARD REVIEW TEST ANSWERS

1. **(A)** Client need: health promotion and maintenance; subcategory: prevention and early detection of disease; content area: pediatrics

RATIONALE

(A) Consistent primary care nurses can better interpret infant cues and note feeding behaviors. (B) In nonorganic failure to thrive the parent-infant dyad has already experienced difficulties in the relationship. These parents may already feel dissatisfied and frustrated. The primary nurse would be unable to prevent this. (C) Assigning a primary nurse does not ensure that infant fatigue and frustration will not occur or can be prevented. (D) Providing privacy does not ensure a change in feeding behavior.

2. **(B)** Client need: health promotion and maintenance; subcategory: growth and development through the life span; content area: pediatrics

RATIONALE

(A) Children experience impatience with soiled diapers when readiness for training is apparent. They often desire to be changed immediately. (B) A child must be able to use verbal or nonverbal skills to communicate needs. (C) A readiness indicator would be awaking dry from naps. (D) The age at which a sibling was toilet trained has no implications for training this child.

3. **(D)** Client need: psychosocial integrity; subcategory: coping and adaptation; content area: pediatrics

RATIONALE

(A) Objects from home do not reduce fear of the unknown. Children need explanations, reassurance, and preparation for the unknown. Also, parental presence can promote comfort and feelings of security. (B) A calm, relaxed, and reassuring manner will assist in calming the child. The child's objects from home will not assist in calming the child. (C) A trusting relationship is based on the quality of the nurse-client relationship. Objects from home have no impact. (D) Favorite objects from home assist in creating a familiar setting. Also, these objects may prevent or minimize separation from the child's usual routine and family support.

4. **(A)** Client need: health promotion and maintenance; subcategory: prevention and early detection of disease; content area: pediatrics

RATIONALE

(A) The refrigerated cool mist tent creates a cool, moist environment. The child as well as bedding and clothing may become dampened. Monitoring the temperature of the child will ensure warmth and prevent chilling. (B) Only a low-grade fever is expected in laryngotracheobronchitis. (C) Febrile seizures are not expected with the low-grade fever. (D) Inflammation of the mucosal lining in the respiratory tract can cause airway obstruction. However, monitoring the child's temperature would not prevent airway obstruction.

5. **(B)** Client need: physiological integrity; subcategory: pharmacological and parenteral therapies; content area: pediatrics

RATIONALE

(A) Holding the child's discharge alone does not address the client's problem. (B) Nausea, tachycardia, and irritability are all symptoms of theophylline toxicity. The physician should be notified immediately so that a serum theophylline level can be ordered. Theophylline dose should be withheld until the physician is notified. (C) The child must be evaluated for theophylline toxicity before any discharge. (D) Cause of the nausea should be investigated before the administration of an antiemetic.

6. **(A)** Client need: physiological integrity; subcategory: physiological adaptation; content area: pediatrics

RATIONALE

(A) Fluid volume deficit is the major problem. Symptoms of dehydration are evident. The effects of fluid and electrolyte balance may be life threatening. Rehydration can be accomplished effectively through IV fluids and electrolytes. (B) Vomiting may also signal a nutritional problem. However, the nutritional problem would be secondary to fluid and electrolyte disturbances. The infant may also be placed on NPO status. (C) With vomiting, a decrease in the size and number of stools is expected. (D) The infant cannot verbalize feelings of anxiety. Anxiety would not be an appropriate diagnosis.

7. **(D)** Client need: physiological integrity; subcategory: physiological adaptation; content area: pediatrics

RATIONALE

(A) Respiratory acidosis is the result of problematic ventilation. Plasma pH decreases, while plasma PCO_2 and plasma HCO_3 increase. (B) Respiratory alkalosis results from increased respiratory rate and depth. Plasma pH increases, while plasma PCO_2 and plasma HCO_3 decrease. (C) Metabolic acidosis occurs when there is strong acid gain in the body. Plasma pH, PCO_2, and HCO_3 decrease. (D) Increased risk for metabolic alkalosis is due to a loss of hydrogen ions; depletion of potassium, sodium, and chloride when vomiting occurs. Plasma pH and plasma PCO_2 increase; plasma HCO_3 may decrease and then increase to compensate.

8. **(C)** Client need: health promotion and maintenance; subcategory: growth and development through the life span; content area: pediatrics

RATIONALE

(A) These activities are suited for the preschool-age child (3–5 years old). The activities are not safe for a toddler. (B) Infants (0–1 year) like these toys. (C) These activities provide the toddler (1–3 years old) with a variety of physical activities for play. (D) The toddler lacks the physical and cognitive abilities for these activities. The tasks are far better suited for the school-age child.

9. **(D)** Client need: psychosocial integrity; subcategory: coping and adaptation; content area: pediatrics

RATIONALE

(A) Books increase cognition, assist with fine motor skills, and augment language development. (B) Music provides auditory stimulation and large-muscle activity. (C) Riding toys provide large-muscle activity. (D) Puppets allow expression of feelings and fears that otherwise could not be directly communicated.

10. **(D)** Client need: psychosocial integrity; subcategory: coping and adaptation; content area: pediatrics

RATIONALE

(A) Unusually aggressive behavior does not indicate a deep-seated problem. (B) A lack of social interest results in poor participation in play activities with peers. Aggression would not be an expected behavior. (C) The aggressive behavior was newly developed and not a routine behavior. (D) Play provides the child with opportunities for coping and adaptation. Aggression during the play activities would indicate a coping response.

11. **(D)** Client need: physiological integrity; subcategory: reduction of risk potential; content area: pediatrics

RATIONALE

(A) Mobilization is important but not absolutely essential. (B) Discharge teaching should be initiated prior to surgery as well as during the postoperative period. (C) Assessment and management of pain are necessary and high in priority. (D) Neurovascular status of the extremity is of primary importance. The risk of circulatory impairment exists with any cast application. This type of fracture is common in children. A high incidence of neurovascular complications exists with fractures near the elbow.

12. **(A)** Client need: health promotion and maintenance; subcategory: prevention and early detection of disease; content area: pediatrics

    RATIONALE

    (A) The 9-month-old infant can sit alone for long periods. By the age of 6 months, many infants can pull themselves to a sitting position. (B, C, D) This skill represents normal development.

13. **(C)** Client need: health promotion and maintenance; subcategory: prevention and early detection of disease; content area: pediatrics

    RATIONALE

    (A) Cataracts are not considered refractive errors. Cataracts can be described as opacity of the lens. (B) *Hyperopia* is the term for farsightedness. One can see objects at a distance more clearly than close objects. (C) *Myopia* is the term for nearsightedness. Objects that are close in distance are more clearly seen. (D) Lazy eye refers to strabismus or misalignment of the eyes.

14. **(C)** Client need: health promotion and maintenance; subcategory: prevention and early detection of disease; content area: pediatrics

    RATIONALE

    (A) Visual images are blurred and distorted. (B) Symptoms are headaches, burning eyes, fatigue, squinting, and difficulty reading. (C) These symptoms are classic for myopia. (D) Amblyopia is not a refractive error. It is a loss of vision in one or both eyes.

15. **(B)** Client need: physiological integrity; subcategory: physiological adaptation; content area: med/surg

    RATIONALE

    (A) A tension pneumothorax is an accumulation of air in the pleural space. Important physical assessment findings to confirm this condition include cyanosis, jugular vein distention, absent breath sounds on the affected side, distant heart sounds, and lowered blood pressure. (B) Asthma is a disorder in which there is an airflow obstruction in the bronchioles and smaller bronchi secondary to bronchospasm, swelling of mucous membranes, and increased mucus production. Physical assessment reveals some important findings: agitation, nasal flaring, tachypnea, and expiratory wheezing. (C) Pneumonia is an acute bacterial or viral infection that causes inflammation of the lung in the alveolar and interstitial tissue and results in consolidation. Specific assessment findings to confirm this condition include decreased chest expansion caused by pleuritic pain, dullness on percussion over consolidated areas, decreased breath sounds, and increased vocal fremitus. (D) A pulmonary embolus is the passage of a foreign substance (blood clot, fat, air, or amniotic fluid) into the pulmonary artery or its branches, with subsequent obstruction of blood supply to lung tissue. Specific assessment findings that confirm this condition include tachypnea, tachycardia, crackles (rales), transient friction rub, diaphoresis, edema, and cyanosis.

16. **(A)** Client need: health promotion and maintenance; subcategory: prevention and early detection of disease; content area: med/surg

    RATIONALE

    (A) Vitamin C (ascorbic acid) is essential in promoting wound healing and collagen formation. (B) Vitamin B_1 (thiamine) maintains normal gastrointestinal (GI) functioning, oxidizes carbohydrates, and is essential for normal functioning of nervous tissue. (C) Vitamin D regulates absorption of calcium and phosphorus

from the GI tract and helps prevent rickets. (D) Vitamin A is necessary for the formation and maintenance of skin and mucous membranes. It is also essential for normal growth and development of bones and teeth.

17. **(D)** Client need: health promotion and maintenance; subcategory: prevention and early detection of disease; content area: med/surg

    RATIONALE

    (A) This meal choice provides more of the vitamins A, D, and K than of vitamin C. (B) This meal choice provides more of the vitamins A, B_{12}, and D than of vitamin C. (C) This meal choice provides more of the vitamins A, B_1 (thiamine), niacin, and microminerals than of vitamin C. (D) This meal choice provides foods rich in vitamin C, which are essential in tissue healing.

18. **(A)** Client need: physiological integrity; subcategory: reduction of risk potential; content area: med/surg

    RATIONALE

    (A) Skeletal traction is the application of traction directly to bone with the use of pins and wires or tongs for the purpose of providing a strong, steady, continuous longitudinal pull on the bone. It is indicated for preoperative immobilization and positioning of hip and femur fractures. (B) A type of skeletal traction (balanced suspension with a Thomas splint and Pearson attachment) uses a sling to support the extremity, but it also uses weights to provide a strong, steady continuous pull on the extremity. A sling is used instead of pins. (C) Pelvic traction provides an intermittent pull over the pelvis and bone, whereas skeletal traction is continuous. Pelvic traction does not use pins. (D) Skeletal traction uses weights at the end of the bed to provide a continuous pull on long bones. Weights are not applied to both ends of the bed.

19. **(B)** Client need: physiological integrity; subcategory: physiological adaptation; content area: med/surg

    RATIONALE

    (A) Exudate (moist, active drainage) is a clinical sign of wound infection. (B) Crust (dry, scaly) is part of the normal stages of wound healing and should not be removed from around the pin site. It usually sloughs off after the underlying tissue has healed. (C) Edema (swelling) is a clinical sign of wound infection. (D) Erythema (redness) is a clinical sign of wound infection.

20. **(C)** Client need: health promotion and maintenance; subcategory: prevention and early detection of disease; content area: med/surg

    RATIONALE

    (A) Cystoscopy is an endoscopic procedure that uses an instrument (a cystoscope) to visualize the internal bladder and ureter structures and to capture and remove an obstructing stone. (B) Kidney, ureter, bladder x-ray is used to outline gross structural changes in the kidneys, ureter, and bladder and will determine the general location of a stone. (C) An intravenous pyelogram with excretory urogram is used to visualize the kidneys, kidney pelvis, ureters, and bladder. This procedure is used specifically to determine whether urethral obstruction is partial or complete; it shows the exact location of the stone and dilation of the ureter above the stone. (D) Ureterolithotomy is a surgical procedure in which the ureter is incised and the stone is manually removed because the stone is unable to pass through the ureter independently.

21. **(C)** Client need: physiological integrity; subcategory: physiological adaptation; content area: med/surg

    RATIONALE

    (A) Radiating pain in the urethra in both sexes, extending into the labia in females and into the testicle or penis in the male, indicates a stone in the middle or lower segment of the ureter. (B) Urinary frequency and dysuria are caused by a stone in the terminal segment of the ureter within the bladder wall. (C) An obstructing stone in the renal pelvis or upper ureter causes severe flank and abdominal pain with nausea, vomiting, diaphoresis, and pallor. (D) Dull and aching pain may indicate early stages of hydronephrosis. Also, a stone in the renal pelvis or upper ureter causes severe flank and abdominal pain.

22. **(C)** Client need: physiological integrity; subcategory: physiological adaptation; content area: med/surg

    RATIONALE

    (A) The presence of urinary tract infection is a factor in the formation of struvite stones. (B) Staghorn calculi is the other name for struvite stones associated with urinary tract infection. (C) Clients who have gout form uric acid stones. (D) Clients who have increased urinary excretion of calcium form calcium stones.

23. **(B)** Client need: physiological integrity; subcategory: physiological adaptation; content area: med/surg

    RATIONALE

    (A) *Klebsiella* pneumonia is caused by gram-negative bacteria. (B) Pneumococcal pneumonia is caused by gram-positive bacteria. (C) *Legionella pneumophila* pneumonia is a nonbacterial pneumonia. (D) *E. coli* pneumonia is caused by gram-negative bacteria.

24. **(B)** Client need: physiological integrity; subcategory: physiological adaptation; content area: med/surg

    RATIONALE

    (A) Bright red sputum with streaks is associated with pneumonia caused by gram-negative bacteria, such as *Klebsiella* pneumonia. (B) Pneumococcal pneumonia, caused by gram-positive bacteria, has a characteristic productive cough with green or rust-colored sputum. (C) Green-colored sputum is more characteristic of *Pseudomonas* than of gram-positive bacterial pneumonia. (D) Pink-tinged and frothy sputum is more characteristic of pulmonary edema than of gram-positive bacterial pneumonia.

25. **(C)** Client need: physiological integrity; subcategory: physiological adaptation; content area: med/surg

    RATIONALE

    (A) Maintaining bed rest helps to decrease the O_2 needs of the tissues, which decreases dyspnea and workload on the respiratory system. (B) The semi-Fowler or high-Fowler position is necessary to aid in lessening pressure on the diaphragm from the abdominal organs, which facilitates comfort and easier breathing patterns. (C) Cerebral hypoxia causes the client with pneumonia to be increasingly irritable and restless and results from the client not obtaining enough O_2 to meet metabolic needs. (D) Proper hydration facilitates liquefaction of mucus trapped in the bronchioles and alveoli and enhances expectoration. Unless contraindicated, a reasonable amount of IV fluids to be administered is at least 2.5–3 liters in a 24-hour period.

26. **(D)** Client need: physiological integrity; subcategory: physiological adaptation; content area: med/surg

    RATIONALE

    (A) During impending respiratory failure or asthmatic complications, the client is placed in the high-Fowler position to facilitate comfort and promote optimal gas exchange. (B) Arterial blood gases are monitored in the treatment of respiratory failure during an asthma attack, but it is not an initial intervention. (C) O_2 therapy is used during an asthma attack, but it is not the initial intervention. The usual prescribed amount is a cautiously low flow rate of 1–2 L/min. (D) Wheezing is a characteristic clinical finding during an asthma attack. If wheezing suddenly ceases, it usually indicates a complete airway obstruction and requires immediate treatment for respiratory failure or arrest.

27. **(C)** Client need: physiological integrity; subcategory: physiological adaptation; content area: med/surg

    RATIONALE

    (A) *Cholelithiasis* is the correct term used to describe the presence of stones in the gallbladder. (B) *Nephrolithiasis*, or *renal calculi*, is the correct term used to describe the presence of stones in the kidney. (C) *Choledocholithiasis* is the correct term used to describe the presence of stones in the common bile duct. (D) *Cholecystitis* is the correct term used to describe inflammation of the gallbladder and can be associated with cystic duct obstructions from impacted stones.

28. **(C)** Client need: health promotion and maintenance; subcategory: prevention and early detection of disease; content area: med/surg

    RATIONALE

    (A) This sign is a faint blue discoloration around the umbilicus found in clients who have hemorrhagic pancreatitis. (B) This sign indicates areas of inflammation within the peritoneum, such as with appendicitis. It is a deep palpation technique used on a nontender area of the abdomen, and when the palpating hand is removed suddenly, the client experiences a sharp, stabbing pain at an area of peritoneal inflammation. (C) This sign is considered positive with acute cholecystitis when the client is unable to take a deep breath while the right upper quadrant is being deeply palpated. The client will elicit a sudden, sharp gasp, which means the gallbladder is acutely inflamed. (D) This is a sign of acute hemorrhagic pancreatitis and manifests as a green or purple discoloration in the flanks.

29. **(C)** Client need: physiological integrity; subcategory: reduction of risk potential; content area: med/surg

    RATIONALE

    (A) During the first 24 hours after surgery, the drainage is normally 300–500 mL and then decreases to about 200 mL in 24 hours during the next 3–4 days. (B) This range is the amount of drainage after the first 24 hours postoperatively. During the first 24 hours, it is 300–500 mL. (C) During the first 24 hours after surgery, this range is the expected amount of drainage. (D) The expected amount of drainage during the first 24 hours is 300–500 mL. An output of >500 mL should be reported to the physician, because an occlusion of some type, caused by a retained gallstone or an inflammatory process within the biliary drainage system, is evident.

30. **(A)** Client need: physiological integrity; subcategory: physiological adaptation; content area: med/surg

    RATIONALE

    (A) Clients who have obstruction in the biliary tract so that bile is not released into the duodenum experience a change in stools from brown to gray or clay colored. (B) This type of stool can occur with other GI problems, such as bacterial or viral infections, and other disease problems, and is not a common finding with biliary obstructions such as cholecystitis and cholelithiasis. (C) This type of stool is usually associated with a GI or bowel problem, such as lower GI bleeding, rather than with biliary obstructions. (D) This type of stool is usually associated with a GI or bowel problem, such as upper GI bleeding, rather than with biliary obstructions.

31. **(C)** Client need: physiological integrity; subcategory: physiological adaptation; content area: med/surg

    RATIONALE

    (A) The absence of wound infection is related to his surgical wound and not to postoperative GI functioning and return of peristalsis. (B) Routine postoperative protocol involves detection of bowel sounds and return of peristalsis before introduction of clear liquids, followed by progression of full liquids and a regular diet versus a full regular meal first. (C) Routine postoperative protocol for bowel obstruction is to assess for the return of bowel sounds within 72 hours after major surgery, because that is when bowel sounds normally return. If unable to detect bowel sounds, the surgeon should be notified immediately and have the client remain NPO. (D) Routine postoperative protocol for bowel obstruction and other major surgeries involves frequent monitoring of vital signs in the immediate postoperative period (in recovery room) and then every 4 hours, or more frequently if the client is unstable, on the nursing unit. This includes assessing for signs of hypovolemic shock. Vital signs usually stabilize within the first 24 hours postoperatively.

32. **(D)** Client need: physiological integrity; subcategory: reduction of risk potential; content area: med/surg

    RATIONALE

    (A) This measurement is <50 cm (48–49 cm). Fifty centimeters is considered the length necessary for the distal end of the tube to be in place in the stomach. This measurement is too short. (B) This measurement is <50 cm (47–48 cm). Fifty centimeters is considered the length necessary for the distal end of the tube to be in place in the stomach. This measurement is too short. (C) This measurement gives an approximate indication of the length necessary for the distal end of the tube to be in place in the stomach, but it is not as accurate as actually measuring the client (nose-ear-xiphoid). (D) This is the correct measurement of 50 cm from the tip of the client's nose to the tip of the earlobe to the xiphoid process (called the NEX [nose-ear-xiphoid] measurement). It is approximately equal to the distance necessary for the distal end of the tube to be located in the correct position in the stomach.

33. **(A)** Client need: physiological integrity; subcategory: basic care and comfort; content area: med/surg

    RATIONALE

    (A) Bowel movements should be regulated at a specific time each day to prevent "accidents." Irrigating after meals takes advantage of the gastrocolic reflex and time of increased peristalsis, so better results may be produced. After meals is the normal time that peristalsis begins in most persons and evacuation of feces occurs. (B) Irrigating before meals may cause poor results because of decreased gastrocolic reflex and decreased peristalsis. (C) Irrigating a colostomy every 2 hours may produce hyperactivity of the bowel, leading to irritation and diarrhea. This would not aid in regulation of the bowel. (D) If irrigation of a colostomy were done at bedtime, there is greater chance of having an "accident" during sleep. This would not be an advantageous practice of bowel regulation.

34. **(C)** Client need: physiological integrity; subcategory: basic care and comfort; content area: med/surg

    RATIONALE

    (A) Fried, greasy food, such as fried chicken, will produce diarrhealike stools in individuals with all types of GI ostomies. (B) Eggs will cause odor-producing stools in individuals with all types of GI ostomies. (C) Tapioca and rice products will cause constipation in individuals with all types of GI ostomies. (D) Cabbage will cause odor-producing and flatus-producing stools in individuals with all types of GI ostomies.

35. **(D)** Client need: health promotion and maintenance; subcategory: prevention and early detection of disease; content area: med/surg

    RATIONALE

    (A) Synthetic cast materials harden in 3–15 minutes. Weight bearing is permitted in 15–30 minutes. Drying time for plaster of Paris is about 24–72 hours. (B, C) Plaster of Paris cast materials are heavier than synthetic materials and require a drying time of 24–72 hours. Synthetic materials dry within 30 minutes. (D) Plaster of Paris cast materials are heavier than synthetic materials and require a longer period to set and dry. Even though setting time (hardening) is only 3–15 minutes, the drying time for plaster of Paris is 24–72 hours. This depends on the size and thickness of the cast, exposure to air, and humidity in the air.

36. **(B)** Client need: physiological integrity; subcategory: physiological adaptation; content area: med/surg

    RATIONALE

    (A) This describes a suprapubic (transvesical) prostatectomy procedure. (B) This is the correct description of a TURP procedure. (C) This describes a perineal prostatectomy procedure. (D) This describes a retropubic (extravesical) prostatectomy procedure.

37. **(D)** Client need: physiological integrity; subcategory: physiological adaptation; content area: med/surg

    RATIONALE

    (A) Early signs of hypovolemic shock include hypotension, tachycardia, tachypnea, pallor, and diaphoresis. (B) Early signs of potassium depletion include muscular weakness or paralysis, tetany, postural hypotension, weak pulse, shallow respirations, apathy, weak voice, and electrocardiographic changes. (C) Early signs of an elevated sodium level include dry oral mucous membranes, marked thirst, hypertension, tachycardia, oliguria or anuria, anxiety, and agitation. (D) This answer is correct. Important early clinical findings of a decreased sodium concentration include confusion and disorientation. Hyponatremia can occur after a TURP because absorption during surgery through the prostate veins can increase circulating blood volume and decrease sodium concentration.

38. **(B)** Client need: physiological integrity; subcategory: reduction of risk potential; content area: med/surg

    RATIONALE

    (A) The physician should be notified as problems arise, but in this case, the nurse can attempt to irrigate the Foley catheter first and call the physician if irrigation is unsuccessful. Notifying the physician of problems is a subsequent nursing intervention. (B) This answer is correct. Assessing catheter patency and irrigating as prescribed are the initial priorities to maintain continuous bladder irrigation. Manual irrigation will dislodge blood clots that have blocked the catheter and prevent problems of bladder distention, pain, and possibly fresh bleeding. (C) The Foley catheter would not be changed as an initial nursing intervention, but irrigation of the catheter should be done as ordered to dislodge clots that interfere with patency. (D) Even though the client complains of increasing suprapubic pain, administration of a prescribed narcotic analgesic is not the initial priority. The effect of the medication may mask the symptoms of a distended bladder and lead to more serious complications.

39. **(C)** Client need: health promotion and maintenance; subcategory: prevention and early detection of disease; content area: med/surg

    RATIONALE

    (A) This is correct health teaching. Drinking 10–12 glasses of clear liquid will help increase urine volumes and prevent clot formation. (B) This is correct health teaching. These types of exercises are prescribed by physicians to assist postprostatectomy clients to strengthen their perineal muscles. (C) This action is not recommended post-TURP because of the close proximity of the prostate and rectum. (D) This is correct healthcare teaching. The client should limit walking long distances, lifting heavy objects, or driving a car until these activities are cleared by the physician at the first office visit.

40. **(D)** Client need: physiological integrity; subcategory: pharmacological and parenteral therapies; content area: med/surg

    RATIONALE

    (A) Acetaminophen (Tylenol) has analgesic and antipyretic actions approximately equivalent to those of aspirin. It produces analgesia possibly by action on the peripheral nervous system. It reduces fever by direct action on the hypothalamus heat-regulating center with consequent peripheral vasodilation. It is generally used for temporary relief of mild to moderate pain, such as a simple headache, minor joint and muscle pains, and control of fever. (B) Meperidine is a narcotic agonist analgesic with properties similar to morphine except that it has a shorter duration of action and produces less depression of urinary retention and smooth muscle spasm. It is used for moderate to severe pain, for a preoperative medication, for support of anesthesia, and for obstetrical analgesia. In a postoperative TURP client, it would be used in conjunction with other medications for relief of moderate to severe pain, but not specifically for bladder spasms associated with TURP surgery. (C) Promethazine hydrochloride is an antihistamine, antiemetic preparation. It exerts antiserotonin, anticholinergic, and local anesthetic actions. It is used for symptomatic relief of various allergic conditions, motion sickness, nausea, and vomiting. It is used for preoperative, postoperative, and obstetrical sedation and as an adjunct to analgesics for control of pain. (D) This answer is correct because aminocaproic acid is prescribed specifically for hematuria. Aminocaproic acid is excreted in the urine. The nurse should be alert for possible signs of thrombosis, particularly in the extremities.

41. **(A)** Client need: health promotion and maintenance; subcategory: prevention and early detection of disease; content area: med/surg

RATIONALE

(A) This is the correct method of teaching diaphragmatic breathing, which allows full lung expansion to increase oxygenation, prevent atelectasis, and move secretions up and out of the lungs to decrease risk of pneumonia. (B) Quick, short breaths do not allow for full lung expansion and movement of secretions up and out of the lungs. Quick, short breaths may lead to O_2 depletion, hyperventilation, and hypoxia. (C) Expelling breaths through the nose does not allow for full lung expansion and the use of diaphragmatic muscles to assist in moving secretions up and out of the lungs. (D) Inhaling and exhaling at a rate of 20–24 times/min does not allow time for full lung expansion to increase oxygenation. This would most likely lead to O_2 depletion and hypoxia.

42. **(C)** Client need: physiological integrity; subcategory: physiological adaptation; content area: maternity

RATIONALE

(A) A rigid, boardlike abdomen is an assessment finding indicative of placenta abruptio. (B) A cause of postbirth hemorrhage is uterine atony. With placenta previa, uterine tone is within normal range. (C) The placenta is located directly over the cervical os in complete previa. Blood will escape through the os, resulting in the uterus and abdomen remaining soft and relaxed. (D) In placenta abruptio, hypertonicity of the uterus is caused by the entrapment of blood between the placenta and uterine wall, a retroplacental bleed. This does not exist in placenta previa.

43. **(A)** Client need: physiological integrity; subcategory: physiological adaptation; content area: maternity

RATIONALE

(A) Based on the client's history, presence of bright red vaginal bleeding, and hemoglobin value on admission, the priority nursing diagnosis would be decreased cardiac output related to excessive bleeding. (B) This nursing diagnosis is a potential problem that does not exist at the present time, and therefore is not the priority problem. (C) The client's expressed anxiety is for her child. The fetus will remain physiologically safe if the decreased cardiac output is resolved. (D) Initial spontaneous bleeding with placenta previa is rarely life threatening to the mother or the fetus. Delivery of the fetus will be postponed until fetal maturity is achieved and survival is likely.

44. **(D)** Client need: health promotion and maintenance; subcategory: prevention and early detection of disease; content area: maternity

RATIONALE

(A) Dinitrophenylhydrazine is a laboratory test used to detect phenylketonuria, maple syrup urine disease, and Lowe's syn-

drome. (B) Metachromatic stain is a laboratory test that may be used to diagnose Tay-Sachs and other lipid diseases of the central nervous system. (C) The blood serum phenylalanine test is diagnostic of phenylketonuria and can be used for wide-scale screening. (D) A lecithin-sphingomyelin ratio of at least 2:1 is indicative of fetal lung maturity, and survival of the fetus is likely.

45. **(B)** Client need: physiological integrity; subcategory: physiological adaptation; content area: maternity

RATIONALE

(A) These nursing actions are necessary prior to the cesarean section, but not immediately necessary to maintain physiological equilibrium. (B) Determining the physiological status of the fetus would constitute the highest priority in evaluating and maintaining fetal life. (C) These nursing actions are necessary prior to the cesarean section, but not immediately necessary to maintain physiological equilibrium. (D) These nursing actions are necessary prior to the cesarean section, but not immediately necessary to maintain physiological equilibrium.

46. **(C)** Client need: physiological integrity; subcategory: physiological adaptation; content area: maternity

RATIONALE

(A) Early shock does not exhibit the symptom of marked elevation in blood pressure. A narrowing of the pulse pressure is indicative of early shock. (B) Anuria is a clinical finding in late shock. (C) All of these clinical findings are congruent with early shock. (D) Absence of urinary output is a clinical finding in the late phase of shock.

47. **(D)** Client need: health promotion and maintenance; subcategory: growth and development through the life span; content area: maternity

RATIONALE

The length of labor has little bearing on the fourth stage of labor. The type of labor and delivery is significant. (B) The type of episiotomy will affect the client's comfort level. However, the nurse's assessment and implementations center on prevention of hemorrhage during the fourth stage of labor. The amount of bleeding from the episiotomy or hematoma formation is of higher priority than the type of episiotomy. (C) The amount of IV fluid to be infused is a nursing function to be attended to; however, it is lower in priority than determining if hemorrhaging is occurring. (D) Character of the fundus would be the priority nursing assessment because changes in uterine tone may identify possible postpartum hemorrhage.

48. **(A)** Client need: health promotion and maintenance; subcategory: growth and development through the life span; content area: maternity

RATIONALE

(A) Gentle massage and expression of clots will let the fundus return to a state of firmness, allowing the uterus to function as the "living ligature." (B) A distended bladder may promote uterine atony; however, after determining the bladder is distended, the nurse would have the client void. Catheterization is only done if normal bladder function has not returned. (C) Oxytocic medications are ordered and administered if the uterus does not remain contracted after gentle massage and determining if the bladder is empty. (D) The client is not complaining of discomfort or pain; therefore, analgesics are not necessary.

49. **(D)** Client need: health promotion and maintenance; subcategory: growth and development through the life span; content area: maternity

RATIONALE

(A) Lochia alba occurs approximately 10 days after birth and is yellow to white. A discharge is classified as light when less than a 4-inch stain exists. (B) Lochia serosa is pink to brown and occurs 3–4 days after delivery. A stain is classified as heavy when a peripad is saturated in 1 hour. (C) Lochia granulosa is not a proper classification. (D) Lochia rubra is red, consisting mainly of blood, debris, and bacteria, and lasts from the time of delivery to 3–4 days afterward. A stain is classified as moderate when less than a 6-inch stain exists.

50. **(B)** Client need: health promotion and maintenance; subcategory: growth and development through the life span; content area: maternity

    RATIONALE

    (A) The foramen ovale permits a percentage of the blood to shunt from the right atrium to the left atrium. The blood then goes to the left ventricle, permitting systemic fetal circulation with blood containing a higher O_2 saturation. (B) As the blood shunts from the right atrium to the left atrium, the pulmonary system is bypassed. The fetus receives O_2 from the maternal circulation, thereby permitting the partial bypass of the pulmonary system. (C) The foramen ovale is located in the atrial septum of the heart and does not affect the liver. (D) The superior vena cava returns blood to the heart, bringing blood to the location of the foramen ovale.

51. **(C)** Client need: physiological integrity; subcategory: reduction of risk potential; content area: med/surg

    RATIONALE

    (A) An 18-gauge IV is an appropriate size for administering blood; however, client safety demands that the right blood product must be administered. (B) The consent form is legally necessary to be on the chart, but client safety is maintained by giving the correct blood component to the correct client. (C) Administering the correct blood product to the correct client will maintain physiological safety and minimize transfusion reactions. (D) The blood administration should take place over the ordered time frame designated by the physician.

52. **(A)** Client need: physiological integrity; subcategory: reduction of risk potential; content area: med/surg

    RATIONALE

    (A) A baseline set of vital signs is necessary to determine if any transfusion reactions occur as the blood product is being administered. (B) The only companion fluid to be used during a blood transfusion is normal saline. The calcium in Ringer's lactate can cause clotting. (C) Only a blood administration set should be used. A microdrip tube would cause lysis of the red blood cells. (D) Proper identification of the recipient and the blood product must be validated by at least two people.

53. **(D)** Client need: physiological integrity; subcategory: pharmacological and parenteral therapies; content area: med/surg

    RATIONALE

    (A) A hemolytic transfusion reaction would be characterized by fever, chills, chest pain, hypotension, and tachypnea. (B) Fever, chills, and headaches are indicative of a febrile transfusion reaction. (C) Circulatory overload is manifest by dyspnea, cough, and pulmonary crackles. (D) Urticaria, pruritus, wheezing, and anxiety are indicative of an allergic transfusion reaction.

54. **(D)** Client need: physiological integrity; subcategory: physiological adaptation; content area: maternity

    RATIONALE

    (A) S_1 and S_2 in an infant with coarctation of the aorta are usually normal. S_3 and S_4 do not exist with this diagnosis. (B) Either no murmur will be heard or a systolic murmur from an associated cardiac defect will be heard along the left upper sternal border. A diastolic murmur is not associated with coarctation of the aorta. (C) Pulse pressure differences of ≥ 20 mm Hg exist between the upper extremities and the lower extremities. It is important to evaluate the upper and lower extremities with the appropriate-sized cuffs. (D) Femoral and pedal pulses will be diminished or absent in infants with coarctation of the aorta.

55. **(A)** Client need: physiological integrity; subcategory: physiological adaptation; content area: pediatrics

    RATIONALE

    (A) Tetralogy of Fallot is the most common cyanotic heart defect, which includes a VSD, pulmonary stenosis, an overriding aorta, and ventricular hypertrophy. The blood flow is obstructed because the pulmonary stenosis decreases the pulmonary blood flow and shunts blood through the VSD, creating a right-to-left shunt that allows deoxygenated blood the reach the systemic circulation. (B) A VSD alone creates a left-to-right shunt. The pressure in the left ventricle is greater than that of the right; therefore, the blood will shunt from the left ventricle to the right ventricle, increasing the blood flow to the lungs. No deoxygenated blood will reach the systemic circulation. (C) In patent ductus arteriosus, the pressure in the aorta is greater than in the pulmonary artery, creating a left-to-right shunt. Oxygenated blood from the aorta flows into the unoxygenated blood of the pulmonary artery. (D) Transposition of the great arteries results in two separate and parallel circulatory systems. The only mixing or shunting of blood is based on the presence of associated lesions.

56. **(B)** Client need: health promotion and maintenance; subcategory: growth and development through the life span; content area: pediatrics

    RATIONALE

    (A) A toddler is not capable of conceptualizing about the inside of his body and is concerned about body intactness; therefore, diagrams would not be useful. Also, the previous evening is too far from the procedure for the toddler to remember the instructions. (B) A simple explanation the morning of the procedure is the best developmental strategy to use, because it focuses on the toddler's need for parental support, body intactness, and short attention span. (C) A relationship between the nurse and the child needs to develop. Also, misinformation may be given to the child if the parents explain the procedure to the child. (D) The parents are the child's support system and need to be there to strengthen the child.

57. **(B)** Client need: health promotion and maintenance; subcategory: prevention and early detection of disease; content area: pediatrics

    RATIONALE

    (A) A small bruise may develop around the insertion site and is not a reason for alarm. (B) It is best to keep the child out of the bathtub until the sutures are removed. (C) Acetaminophen, not aspirin, is the drug of choice if there is pain at the insertion site. (D) The insertion site should be kept clean and dry and open to air.

58. **(B)** Client need: psychosocial integrity; subcategory: coping and adaptation; content area: pediatrics

    RATIONALE

    (A) It is important to discuss with parents the need to treat the child as they would any other children, but they must be truthful and honest with the child about the heart defect. As the child grows older, explanations can go into greater depth. (B) Parents of children with congenital heart defects go through a grieving process over the loss of their "healthy" child. The nurse needs to recognize these feelings and give the parents a role in the child's care when they are ready. (C) Anger and resentment are normal feelings that must be dealt with appropriately. (D) Parents may go through a second grieving process after the repair of the cardiac defect. During this grieving period, they mourn the loss of the "defective" child who now may be essentially "normal."

59. **(C)** Client need: physiological integrity; subcategory: pharmacological and parenteral therapies; content area: pediatrics

    RATIONALE

    (A) Occasionally the child may vomit. They should not repeat the dose because the amount of digoxin that was absorbed is unknown, and serum levels of digoxin that are too high are more dangerous than those that are temporarily too low. (B) To ensure that the entire dose of digoxin is received, never mix it with food or formula. (C) Vomiting, anorexia, and listlessness are all signs of digoxin toxicity and should be reported to the physician immediately. (D) If a dose is forgotten for more than 6 hours, the nurse should advise the parents to skip that dose and to continue the next dose as scheduled.

60. **(D)** Client need: physiological integrity; subcategory: physiological adaptation; content area: pediatrics

RATIONALE

(A) Aplastic anemia is characterized by a lack of reticulocytes in the blood. Platelet and white blood cell counts are usually not depressed. It is usually self-limiting, lasting 5–10 days. (B) Vaso-occlusive crisis is the most common type of crisis in sickle cell anemia. Sickled cells become clogged, leading to distal tissue hypoxia and infarction. Joints and extremities are the most commonly affected areas. (C) Dactylitis crisis, or "hand-foot syndrome," causes symmetrical infarction of the bones in the hands and feet, resulting in painful swelling in the soft tissues of the hands and feet. (D) Sequestration crisis occurs as enormous volumes of blood pool within the spleen. The spleen enlarges, causing tenderness. Signs of shock including pallor, tachypnea, and faintness result, related to the deficient intravascular volume. This type of crisis is potentially fatal.

61. **(A)** Client need: physiological integrity; subcategory: physiological adaptation; content area: pediatrics

RATIONALE

(A) Maintaining the hydration level is the focus for nursing intervention because dehydration enhances the sickling process. Both oral and parenteral fluids are used. (B) The pain is a result of the sickling process. Analgesics or narcotics will be used for symptom relief, but the underlying cause of the pain will be resolved with hydration. (C) Serious bacterial infections may result owing to splenic dysfunction. This is true at all times, not just during the acute period of a crisis. (D) O_2 therapy is used for symptomatic relief of the hypoxia resulting from the sickling process. Hydration is the primary intervention to alleviate the dehydration that enhances the sickling process.

62. **(B)** Client need: psychosocial integrity; subcategory: psychosocial adaptation; content area: psychiatric

RATIONALE

(A) This answer is incorrect. Encouraging discussion of the voices will reinforce the delusion. (B) This answer is correct. The nurse should appropriately present reality. (C) This answer is incorrect. Showing interest would reinforce the delusional system. (D) This answer is incorrect. The statement only indicates that the client is hearing voices. It does not state that the client is acting out.

63. **(A)** Client need: physiological integrity; subcategory: pharmacological and parenteral therapies; content area: psychiatric

RATIONALE

(A) This answer is correct. The therapeutic range is 1.0–1.5 mEq/L in the acute phase. Maintenance control levels are 0.6–1.2 mEq/L. (B, C) This answer is incorrect. A level of 1.3 mEq/L is within therapeutic range. (D) This answer is incorrect. Toxic poisoning is usually at the 2.0 level or higher.

64. **(A)** Client need: physiological integrity; subcategory: pharmacological and parenteral therapies; content area: psychiatric

RATIONALE

(A) This answer is correct. A balanced diet with adequate salt intake is necessary. (B) This answer is incorrect. The client must drink six to eight full glasses of fluid per day (2000–3000 mL/day). (C) This answer is incorrect. The client should be instructed to avoid fluctuations of sodium intake. Diet should be balanced, with an adequate salt intake. (D) This answer is incorrect. Nausea is a frequent side effect that can be minimized with administration of drug with meals or after eating food.

65. **(B)** Client need: psychosocial integrity; subcategory: psychosocial adaptation; content area: psychiatric

RATIONALE

(A) This answer is incorrect. Role playing is based on learning but is not based on the behavioral modification model. (B) This answer is correct. The behavioral modification model is based on negative and positive reinforcers to change behavior. (C) This answer is incorrect. Verbal catharsis is not an intervention based on behavioral modification. (D) This answer is incorrect. Although an acceptable nursing intervention, it is not based on behavioral modification.

66. **(A)** Client need: psychosocial integrity; subcategory: psychosocial adaptation; content area: psychiatric

RATIONALE

(A) This answer is correct. Persons with antisocial personality disorder typically are very manipulative. (B) This answer is incorrect. The client's behavior cannot cause another person to become psychotic. (C) This answer is incorrect. Psychosis is not a symptom of antisocial personality. One of the criteria for diagnosis of this disorder is that no psychosis be present. In addition, the client would love the attention. (D) This answer is incorrect. Self-mutilative behavior is characteristic of the borderline personality disorder.

67. **(B)** Client need: psychosocial integrity; subcategory: psychosocial adaptation; content area: psychiatric

RATIONALE

(A) This answer is incorrect. A nurse should be an appropriate role model. Threats are not appropriate. No limit setting was stated. (B) This answer is correct. The nurse made a positive statement followed by a simple, clear, concise setting of limits. (C) This answer is incorrect. It appears to have a negative connotation. There was no limit setting. (D) This answer is incorrect. The nurse obviously responded in a negative manner. Learning takes place more readily when one is accepted, not rejected. No limits were set.

68. **(B)** Client need: physiological integrity; subcategory: physiological adaptation; content area: psychiatric

RATIONALE

(A) This answer is incorrect. Alcohol withdrawal usually begins approximately 6–8 hours after the last drink. (B) This answer is correct. It takes approximately 6–8 hours for metabolism of alcohol. (C) This answer is incorrect. The alcohol is still in the system, as indicated by the high blood alcohol level. (D) This answer is incorrect. Symptoms of alcohol withdrawal usually begin within 6–8 hours of the last drink.

69. **(B)** Client need: physiological integrity; subcategory: pharmacological and parenteral therapies; content area: psychiatric

RATIONALE

(A) This answer is incorrect. Benzodiazepines are drugs of choice for alcohol withdrawal. (B) This answer is correct. The drug has a sedative effect, is safe, and has an anticonvulsant effect. (C) This answer is incorrect. Amitriptyline is an antidepressant. (D) This answer is incorrect. Chlorpromazine is most effective in psychotic disorders.

70. **(A)** Client need: psychosocial integrity; subcategory: psychosocial adaptation; content area: psychiatric

RATIONALE

(A) This answer is correct. The more the client is able to control her daily routine, the less anxiety she will experience. (B) This answer is incorrect. Confrontation tends to increase anxiety. (C) This answer is incorrect. Reality testing is an assessment tool. It does not decrease anxiety. (D) This answer is incorrect. A highly stimulating environment increases distractibility and anxiety.

71. **(A)** Client need: psychosocial integrity; subcategory: psychosocial adaptation; content area: psychiatric

    RATIONALE

    (A) This answer is correct. If the cause is removed, the delirious client will recover completely. (B) This answer is incorrect. The demented client is incapable of returning to previous level of functioning. The delirious client is capable of returning to previous functioning. (C) This answer is incorrect. The demented client, not the delirious client, has progressive intellectual and behavioral deterioration. (D) This answer is incorrect. Delirium develops rapidly, whereas dementia is insidious.

72. **(A)** Client need: psychosocial integrity; subcategory: psychosocial adaptation; content area: psychiatric

    RATIONALE

    (A) This answer is correct. The client will be confused and have a memory loss, which is usually temporary, after electroconvulsive shock therapy. (B) This answer is incorrect. The client will experience transient memory loss, look bewildered, and be confused initially. (C) This answer is incorrect. The client will sleep immediately following the treatment. (D) This answer is incorrect. Vital signs are taken at least hourly after treatment. The client is monitored for hypotension, tachycardia, respiratory problems, and possible seizure activity.

73. **(A)** Client need: psychosocial; subcategory: psychosocial adaptation; content area: psychiatric

    RATIONALE

    (A) This answer is correct. Two risk factors are identified in this answer. (B) This answer is incorrect. Persons at risk tend to lack communication skills and effective coping patterns. (C) This answer is incorrect. Persons at risk are usually family members or those reluctant to provide care. (D) This answer is incorrect. This individual has a vested interest in providing care.

74. **(A)** Client need: psychosocial integrity; subcategory: psychosocial adaptation; content area: psychiatric

    RATIONALE

    (A) This answer is correct. Least restrictive measures should always be attempted before a client is placed in seclusion or restraints. The nurse should first try a calm verbal approach, suggest a quiet room, or request that the client take "time-out" before placing the client in seclusion, giving medication as necessary, or restraining. (B) This answer is incorrect. A calm verbal approach or requesting that a client go to his room should be attempted before restraining. (C) This answer is incorrect. Restraints should be applied only after all other measures fail to control the behavior. (D) This answer is incorrect. Other clients should be removed from the area. It is often very anxiety producing for other clients to see a peer out of control. It could also lead to mass acting-out behaviors.

75. **(B)** Client need: psychosocial integrity; subcategory: psychosocial adaptation; content area: psychiatric

    RATIONALE

    (A) This answer is incorrect. Current magazines would be appropriate. (B) This answer is correct. Maps of the state and town and posters that depict current events in the area are appropriate props. (C) This answer is incorrect. Kittens would be appropriate for pet therapy, not reality therapy. (D) This answer is incorrect. Biographies depict a past, not a present, orientation.

76. **(C)** Client need: psychosocial integrity; subcategory: psychosocial adaptation; content area: psychiatric

    RATIONALE

    (A) This answer is incorrect. Bargaining is a manipulative act, which the nurse could expect from the client. (B) This answer is incorrect. Confrontation is an effective nursing strategy with manipulative behavior. Redirection is appropriate for the client who is out of touch with reality. (C) This answer is correct. Manipulative clients must abide by consistent rules. (D) This answer is incorrect. Manipulation is kept at a minimum if the same staff person is assigned to the client. Often the client will attempt to play staff persons against each other.

77. **(B)** Client need: psychosocial integrity; subcategory: psychosocial adaptation; content area: psychiatric

    RATIONALE

    (A) This answer is incorrect. Perception is not altered because the client is not psychotic. (B) This answer is correct. The antisocial client lacks responsibility, accountability, and social commitment; has impaired problem-solving ability; tends to overuse defense mechanisms; lies and steals; and is often grandiose concerning self. (C) This answer is incorrect. Altered communication processes do not characterize this client. The antisocial person communicates well and tends to have a charming personality. (D) This answer is incorrect. Altered thought processes refer to delusional thinking, which is bizarre and fixed, and do not characterize this client.

78. **(D)** Client need: psychosocial integrity; subcategory: psychosocial adaptation; content area: psychiatric

    RATIONALE

    (A) This answer is incorrect. The client will work hard at the activity instead of enjoying it. (B) This answer is incorrect. The nurse should allow the client to discuss these thoughts, within limits, not to avoid discussing them. (C) This answer is incorrect. The compulsive client tends to control time to excess. It should not be encouraged. (D) This answer is correct. A contract with the client regarding the amount of time that will be spent discussing the compulsive activities is appropriate. Time allotted should be gradually decreased.

79. **(B)** Client need: health promotion and maintenance; subcategory: prevention and early detection of disease; content area: psychiatric

    RATIONALE

    (A) This answer is incorrect. The test measures the abilities to concentrate and calculate. The use of proverbs is the most common way to test abstraction. (B) This answer is correct. The serial sevens test is a common test of calculation ability. It is difficult for the demented or delirious client to perform. (C) This answer is incorrect. The test for judgment should predict whether the individual will behave in a socially accepted manner. (D) This answer is incorrect. In testing memory, the nurse would attempt to get the client either to recall recent events or to think about past events.

80. **(B)** Client need: psychosocial integrity; subcategory: psychosocial adaptation; content area: psychiatric

    RATIONALE

    (A) This answer is incorrect. There is no proof that he removed the missing items. (B) This answer is correct. Anxiety and defensiveness are lessened if the individual is approached in this manner. (C) This answer is incorrect. It is difficult for one to admit to wrongdoing with this approach. (D) This answer is incorrect. He has not yet been proved guilty. Confrontation will only increase defensiveness and anxiety.

81. **(D)** Client need: psychosocial integrity; subcategory: coping and adaptation; content area: psychiatric

    RATIONALE

    (A, B) This statement can be answered with a simple yes or no. (C) This statement is asked in a negative manner and therefore has a negative connotation. (D) This statement is open ended and positively stated.

82. **(B)** Client need: physiological integrity; subcategory: pharmacological and parenteral therapies; content area: psychiatric

    RATIONALE

    (A) This answer is incorrect. Dystonia refers to severe, painful muscle contractions. (B) This answer is correct. Parkinsonism commonly occurs approximately 1–2 weeks after initiation of antipsychotic drug therapy. Traditional signs are masklike facies, postural rigidity, shuffling gait, and resting tremor. (C) This answer is incorrect. Tardive dyskinesia is characterized by involuntary muscle movements of the face, jaw, and tongue. (D) This answer is incorrect. Akathesia is motor restlessness.

83. **(B)** Client need: physiological integrity; subcategory: pharmacological and parenteral therapies; content area: psychiatric

    RATIONALE

    (A) This answer is incorrect. Phenothiazines are antipsychotic drugs and produce the symptoms. (B) This answer is correct. Anticholinergic agents are often used prophylactically for extrapyramidal symptoms. They balance cholinergic activity in the basal ganglia of the brain. (C) This answer is incorrect. Anti-Parkinsonian drugs would increase the symptoms. (D) This answer is incorrect. Tricyclic agents are used for symptoms of depression.

84. **(A)** Client need: physiological integrity; subcategory: reduction of risk potential; content area: psychiatric

    RATIONALE

    (A) This answer is correct. If the client is well informed about what reactions to expect from her medication, she is more likely to follow the treatment regimen. (B) This answer is incorrect. There are many side effects that are reversible by medication, and these must be reported to the nurse or physician. There are also more severe side effects, such as neuroleptic malignant syndrome, characterized by fever, tachycardia, and diaphoresis, which can be life threatening. (C) This answer is incorrect. There is no need for weekly blood tests if the drug regimen has been followed properly. (D) This answer is incorrect. The client should continue the medication until the physician recommends any change in the drug regimen. Symptoms will usually reappear if medication is discontinued.

85. **(B)** Client need: physiological integrity; subcategory: pharmacological and parenteral therapies; content area: psychiatric

    RATIONALE

    (A) This answer is incorrect. It can take up to 1 month for therapeutic effect of the medication. (B) This answer is correct. Because MAO inhibitors are slow to act, it takes 2–4 weeks before improvement of symptoms is noted. (C) This answer is incorrect. It can take up to 1 month for therapeutic effect of the medication. (D) This answer is incorrect. Therapeutic effects of the medication are noted within 1 month of drug therapy.

86. **(A)** Client need: physiological integrity; subcategory: pharmacological and parenteral therapies; content area: psychiatric

    RATIONALE

    (A) These foods may produce elevation in blood pressure when consumed during MAO inhibition therapy. (B) These foods have not been pickled, fermented, smoked, or aged. They contain very little, if any, tyramine or tryptophan. (C) As long as the meat has not been aged or smoked, it is within the dietary regimen. (D) Fresh fruits can be consumed as desired. However, the consumption of bananas is limited.

87. **(D)** Client need: physiological integrity; subcategory: pharmacological and parenteral therapies; content area: psychiatric

    RATIONALE

    (A, B, C) The nurse must first obtain information regarding the client's perception of the medication regimen. (D) The first step in the teaching process is to determine the client's perception.

88. **(A)** Client need: psychosocial integrity; subcategory: psychosocial adaptation; content area: psychiatric

    RATIONALE

    The nurse appropriately states how he or she feels when the client speaks in a condescending manner. (B) This statement indicates that the client has control over the nurse. No one makes another person angry; each individual has a choice. (C) "Why" questions usually put a person on the defensive. In addition, the client cannot "make" the nurse angry. The client does not have that control. (D) Again, a "why" statement places the client on the defensive.

89. **(B)** Client need: psychosocial integrity; subcategory: coping and adaptation; content area: psychiatric

    RATIONALE

    (A) The child has not said that she dislikes gymnastics. (B) The nurse will be able to obtain information on what events occurred at gymnastics prior to her refusal to attend. The nurse will also gain information about the child's perception of the problem. (C) The child has not said she is afraid to go to gymnastics. (D) False reassurance is inappropriate.

90. **(B)** Client need: psychosocial integrity; subcategory: psychosocial adaptation; content area: psychiatric

    RATIONALE

    (A) Signs of depression would include withdrawal, sadness, morbid thoughts, insomnia, early awakening, etc. (B) These clinical features are classic signs of agitation. (C) Psychotic ideation includes delusional thoughts, bizarre behavior, disorganized thinking, etc. (D) Anhedonia is the inability to experience pleasure.

91. **(C)** Client need: psychosocial integrity; subcategory: coping and adaptation; content area: psychiatric

    RATIONALE

    (A) The client should be encouraged to attend the unit activities. The nurse and client should choose a few activities for the client to attend that will be positive experiences for him. (B) The nurse should encourage the client to discuss his feelings and to begin to deal with the depression. (C) Depressed persons often have little appetite and poor fluid intake. Constipation is common. (D) A calm, consistent level of stimuli is most effective. Sensory deprivation and overstimulation should be avoided.

92. **(B)** Client need: psychosocial integrity; subcategory: psychosocial adaptation; content area: psychiatric

    RATIONALE

    (A) Symptoms of psychotic depression must exist for at least 2 weeks, and the symptoms must represent a change from previous functioning. (B) Delirium tremens occur approximately on the second or third day following cessation or reduction of alcohol intake. Symptoms would be all those described in the situation. (C) Symptoms exhibited by this client are not exhibited in clients with anxiety disorders, who manifest excessive or unrealistic worry about life circumstances for at least 6 months. (D) Symptoms for adjustment disorders with mixed emotional features (e.g., depression and anxiety) are different from those exhibited by the client in this situation.

TEST 7

Delgado Community College Charity School of Nursing Test

MOCK NCLEX-RN BOARD REVIEW TEST QUESTIONS

1. A 68-year-old client developed acute respiratory distress syndrome while hospitalized for pneumonia. After a respiratory arrest, an endotracheal tube was inserted. Several days later, numerous attempts to wean him from mechanical ventilation were ineffective, and a tracheostomy was created. For the first 24 hours following tracheostomy, it is important to minimize bleeding around the insertion site. The nurse can accomplish this by:

   A. Deflating the cuff for 10 minutes every other hour instead of 5 minutes every hour
   B. Avoiding manipulation of the tracheostomy including cuff deflation
   C. Reporting any signs of crepitus immediately to the physician
   D. Changing tracheostomy dressing only as necessary using one-half strength hydrogen peroxide to cleanse the site

2. A 43-year-old client is admitted to the hospital with a diagnosis of peripheral vascular disorder. She arrives in her room via stretcher and requires assistance to move to her bed. The nurse notes that her left leg is cold to touch. She complains of having recently experienced muscle spasms in that leg. To determine if these muscle spasms are indicative of intermittent claudication, the nurse would begin her assessment with the following question:

   A. "Would you describe the intensity, duration, and symptoms associated with your pain?"
   B. "Do you experience swelling at the end of the day in the affected and unaffected leg?"
   C. "Have you had any lesions of the affected leg that have been difficult to heal?"
   D. "Do your muscle spasms occur following rest, walking, or exercising?"

3. A client had a ruptured abdominal aortic aneurysm that was repaired surgically. Her postoperative recovery progressed without complications, and she is ready for discharge. Client education in preparation for discharge began 7 days ago on her admission to the nursing unit. Evaluation of nursing care related to client education is based on evaluation of expected outcomes. Which statement made by the client would indicate that she is ready for discharge?

   A. "I will not drive but ride in the front seat of the car with a seat belt on for my first doctor's appointment."
   B. "When I bathe tomorrow morning, I will be very careful not to get soap on my incision."
   C. "I am allowed to exercise by walking for short periods."
   D. "Teach my husband about the diet. He'll be doing all the cooking now."

4. A 67-year-old man had a physical examination prior to beginning volunteer work at the hospital. A routine chest x-ray demonstrated left ventricular hypertrophy. His blood pressure was 180/110. He is 45 lb overweight. His diet is high in sodium and fat. He has a strong family history of hypertension. The client is placed on antihypertensive medication; a low-sodium, low-fat diet; and an exercise regimen. On his next visit, compliance would *best* be determined by:

   A. A blood pressure reading of 130/70 with a 5-lb weight loss
   B. No side effects from antihypertensive medication and an accurate pill count
   C. No evidence of increased left ventricular hypertrophy on chest x-ray
   D. Serum blood levels of the antihypertensive medication within therapeutic range

5. A 55-year-old woman entered the emergency room by ambulance. Her primary complaint is chest pain. She is receiving O_2 via nasal cannula at 2 L/min for dyspnea. Which of the following findings in the client's nursing assessment demand immediate nursing action?

   A. Associated symptoms of indigestion and nausea
   B. Restlessness and apprehensiveness

C. Inability to tolerate assessment session with the admitting nurse

D. History of hypertension treated with pharmacological therapy

6. A 48-year-old client is in the surgical intensive care unit after having had three-vessel coronary artery bypass surgery yesterday. She is extubated, awake, alert and talking. She is receiving digitalis for atrial arrhythmias. This morning serum electrolytes were drawn. Which abnormality would require immediate intervention by the nurse after contacting the physician?

A. Serum osmolality is elevated indicating hemoconcentration. The nurse should increase IV fluid rate.

B. Serum sodium is low. The nurse should change IV fluids to normal saline.

C. Blood urea nitrogen is subnormal. The nurse should increase the protein in the client's diet as soon as possible.

D. Serum potassium is low. The nurse should administer KCl as ordered.

7. A male client received a heart-lung transplant 1 month ago at a local transplant center. While visiting the nursing center to have his blood pressure taken, he complains of recent weakness and fatigue. He also tells the nurse that he is considering stopping his cyclosporine because it is expensive and is causing his face to become round. He fears he will catch viruses and be more susceptible to infections. The nurse responds to this last statement by explaining that cyclosporine:

A. Is given to prevent rejection and makes him less susceptible to infection than other oral corticosteroids

B. Is available at discount pharmacies for a reduced price

C. Is usually not necessary after the first year following transplantation

D. May initially cause weakness, dizziness, and fatigue, but these side effects will gradually resolve themselves

8. A 23-year-old college student seeks medical attention at the college infirmary for complaints of severe fatigue. Her skin is pale, and she reports exertional dyspnea. She is admitted to the hospital with possible aplastic anemia. Laboratory values reflect anemia, and the client is prepared for a bone marrow biopsy. She refuses to sign the biopsy consent and states, "Can't you just get the doctor to give me a transfusion and let me go. This weekend begins spring break, and I have plans to go to Florida." At this time the nurse's greatest concern is that:

A. The client may contract an infection as a result of being exposed to large crowds at spring break

B. The client does not grasp the full impact of her illness

C. The client may require transfusion before leaving for spring break

D. The causative agent be identified and treatment begun

9. A 68-year-old man was recently diagnosed with end-stage renal disease. He has not yet begun dialysis but is experiencing severe anemia with associated symptoms of dyspnea on exertion and chest pain. Which statement *best* describes the management of anemia in renal failure?

A. Hematocrit levels usually remain slightly below normal in clients with renal failure.

B. Transfusion is often begun as early as possible to prevent complications of anemia such as dyspnea and angina.

C. Anemia in renal failure is frequently caused by low serum iron and ferritin and corrected by oral iron and ferritin replacement therapy.

D. The renal secretion of erythropoiesis is decreased. The bone marrow requires erythropoietin to mature red blood cells.

10. A female client has married recently. A month ago she visited her physician with complaints of burning on urination. She was given a prescription for trimethoprim-sulfamethoxazole (Bactrim) DS bid for 10 days. She was admitted through the emergency room on Saturday evening complaining of flank pain. Her temperature was 104°F. A preliminary urinalysis revealed 31 bacteria along with red and white blood cells in the urine. A preliminary diagnosis of pyelonephritis was made. During a nursing admission assessment, which statement by the client demonstrates a possible cause for pyelonephritis?

A. "I have not been drinking six to eight glasses of water each day as the nurse had instructed."

B. "I'm afraid I may have something wrong with my bladder because I have been getting bladder infections frequently since I've been married."

C. "I took the Bactrim for 6 or 7 days. The burning stopped, so I saved the rest of the medication for the next time."

D. "I recently had the flu, which could be settling in my kidneys now."

11. A male client was diagnosed 6 months ago with amyotrophic lateral sclerosis (ALS). The progression of the disease has been aggressive. He is unable to maintain his personal hygiene without assistance. Ambulation is most difficult, requiring him to use a wheelchair and rely on assistance for mobility. He recently has become severely dysphasic. Nursing interventions for dysphasia would be aimed toward prevention of:

A. Loss of ability to speak and communicate effectively

B. Aspiration and weight loss

C. Secondary infection resulting from poor oral hygiene

D. Drooling

12. A 70-year-old female client is admitted to the medical intensive care unit with a diagnosis of cerebrovascular accident (CVA). She is semicomatose, responding to pain and change in position. She is unable to speak or cough. In planning her nursing care for the first 24 hours following a CVA, which nursing diagnosis should receive the *highest* priority?

A. Ineffective airway clearance related to immobility, ineffective cough, and decreased level of consciousness

B. Altered cerebral tissue perfusion related to pathophysiological changes that decrease blood flow

C. Potential for injury related to impaired mobility and seizures

D. Impaired verbal communication related to aphasia

13. A 32-year-old female client is being treated for Guillain-Barré syndrome. She complains of gradually increasing muscle weakness over the past several days. She has noticed an increased difficulty in ambulating and fell yesterday. When conducting a nursing assessment, which finding would indicate a need for immediate further evaluation?

    A. Complaints of a headache
    B. Loss of superficial and deep tendon reflexes
    C. Complaints of shortness of breath
    D. Facial paralysis

14. A 19-year-old male client arrived via ambulance to the emergency room following a motorcycle accident. He is comatose. His face has evidence of dried blood. On assessment, the nurse notes an obvious injury to his left eye. The preferred positioning for a client with an obvious eye injury is:

    A. Reclining to control bleeding
    B. Any position in which the client is comfortable
    C. Side-lying, either left or right
    D. Sitting with head support

15. A female client has been hospitalized for several months following major abdominal surgery for a ruptured colon. A colostomy was created, and the large abdominal wound was left open and allowed to heal through granulation. She is receiving gentamicin IV for treatment of wound infection. Knowing this drug is ototoxic, the nurse would implement which of the following measures?

    A. Instruct the client to report any signs of tinnitus, dizziness or difficulty hearing.
    B. Advise the client to discontinue the drug at the first sign of dizziness.
    C. Order audiometric testing in order to determine if hearing loss is caused by an ototoxic drug or other cause.
    D. Instruct the client in Valsalva's maneuver to equalize middle ear pressure and to prevent hearing loss.

16. A male client has experienced low back pain for several years. He is the primary support of his wife and six children. Although he would qualify for disability, he plans to continue his employment as long as possible. His back pain has increased recently, and he is unable to control it with non-steroidal anti-inflammatory agents. He refuses surgery and cannot take narcotics and remain alert enough to concentrate at work. His physician has suggested application of a transcutaneous electrical nerve stimulation (TENS) unit. Which of the following is an appropriate rationale for using a TENS unit for relief of pain?

    A. TENS units have an ultrasonic effect that relaxes muscles, decreases joint stiffness, and increases range of motion.
    B. TENS units produce endogenous opioids that affect the central nervous system with analgesic potency comparable to morphine.
    C. TENS units work on the gate-control theory of pain; biostimulation therapy of large fibers block painful stimuli.

    D. TENS units prevent muscle spasms, decrease the potential for further injury, and minimize pressure on joints.

17. A male client had a right below-the-knee amputation 4 days ago. His incision is healing well. He has gotten out of bed several times and sat at the side of the bed. Each time after returning to bed, he has experienced pain as if it were located in his right foot. Which nursing measure indicates the nurse has a thorough understanding of phantom pain and its management?

    A. Phantom pain is entirely in the client's mind. The client should be instructed that the pain is psychological and should not be treated.
    B. The basis for phantom pain may occur because the nerves still carry pain sensation to the brain even though the limb has been amputated. The pain is real, intense, and should be treated.
    C. The cause of phantom pain is unknown. The nurse should provide the client with support, promote sleep, and handle the injured limb smoothly and gently.
    D. Phantom pain is caused by trauma, spasms, and edema at the incisional site. It will decrease when postoperative edema decreases. It should be treated with nonnarcotic medication whenever possible.

18. A 28-year-old woman was admitted to the hospital for a thyroidectomy. Postoperatively she is taken to the postanesthesia care unit for several hours. In preparing for the client's return to her room, which nursing measure best demonstrates the nurse's thorough understanding of possible postthyroidectomy complications?

    A. Dressings are placed at the bedside for dressing changes, which are to be done every 2 hours to best detect postoperative bleeding.
    B. Narcotics are readily available and administered when the client returns to her room to prevent excruciating pain.
    C. A tracheostomy set, O_2, and suction are available at the bedside.
    D. The nurse should instruct the client as soon as possible on alternative means of communication.

19. A male client is diagnosed with hypoparathyroidism. He has been on dialysis for several years. He is experiencing symptoms such as numbness of the lips, muscle weakness, carpopedal spasms, and wheezing. Given the client's symptoms, nursing assessment would focus on:

    A. Detection of tetany
    B. Detection of hypocalcemia to prevent seizures
    C. Evidence of depression
    D. Detection of premature cataract formation

20. A male client has been an insulin-dependent diabetic for approximately 30 years. He frequently indulges in high-sugar foods and forgets to take his insulin. He has not experienced acute diabetic emergencies over the years but is now beginning to demonstrate symptoms of diabetic peripheral neuropathy. This distresses him because dancing is one of his favorite pastimes. He decides to question his wife's home health nurse about diabetic peripheral neuropathy. The nurse points out his noncompliance to

his diabetic diet and insulin regimen. The client answers the nurse, "It has been my experience that the diabetic diet is very difficult to follow. As far as the insulin, isn't a fellow allowed to forget now and then?" The client's actions and response best demonstrate:

A. Depression
B. Anger
C. Denial
D. Bargaining

21. A female client was recently diagnosed with gastric cancer. She entered the hospital and had a total gastrectomy with esophagojejunostomy. Her postoperative recovery was uneventful. On conducting discharge teaching, the nurse discusses changes in bodily function and lifestyle changes with the client. In order to prevent pernicious anemia, the nurse stresses that the client must:

A. Receive monthly blood transfusions
B. Increase the amount of iron in her diet
C. Eat small quantities several times daily until she is able to tolerate food in moderate portions
D. Understand the need for Vitamin B_{12} replacement therapy

22. A female client was employed as a client care technician in a hemodialysis unit. She recently began to experience extreme fatigue, being able to sleep for 16–20 hours at a time. She also noted that her urine was tea colored, which she rationalized was a result of the vitamins she began taking to alleviate fatigue. She was diagnosed with hepatitis B. After a brief hospital stay, she is discharged to her parent's home. Her mother asks the nurse if any precautions are necessary to prevent transmission to the client's family. The nurse explains necessary precautions, which include:

A. Isolation of the client from the remainder of the family
B. Separate bathroom facilities if possible; if not, then cleansing daily of the facilities with a chloride solution
C. No necessary precautions because she is beyond the contagious phase
D. Laundering clothes separately in cold water with a chloride solution

23. A male client is admitted to the medical-surgical unit from the emergency room with a diagnosis of acute pancreatitis. The nurse performs the admission nursing assessment. He is NPO with IV fluids infusing at 100 mL/hour. He is experiencing excruciating abdominal pain. Based on an analysis of these data, which nursing diagnosis would receive the highest priority?

A. Pain related to stimulation of nerve endings associated with obstruction of the pancreatic tract
B. Fluid volume deficit related to vomiting and nasogastric tube drainage
C. Knowledge deficit related to treatment regimen
D. Altered nutrition: less than body requirements, related to inadequate intake associated with current anorexia, nausea, vomiting, and digestive enzyme loss

24. A male client has burns over 90% of his body after an automobile accident resulting in a fire. He was trapped inside the auto and pulled out by a bystander. After several months in the hospital and over 20 surgeries, dis-

charge planning has begun. Throughout his hospitalization the nursing staff has been aware of psychological changes the client faces after burns over a large portion of his body resulting in disfigurement. The nursing staff can best foster the client's self-esteem by:

A. Adhering to a strict schedule of diet, exercise, and wound care
B. Allowing him to go to physical therapy for whirlpool treatment when other clients were not in physical therapy
C. Following a standardized plan of care for burn clients formulated by a world-renowned burn center
D. Allowing him to plan, assist in, and perform his own care whenever possible

25. A 20-year-old client presents to the obstetrics-gynecology clinic for the first time. She tells the nurse that she is pregnant and wants to start prenatal care. After collecting some initial assessment data, the nurse measures her fundal height to be at the level of the umbilicus. The nurse estimates the fetal gestational age to be approximately:

A. 10 weeks
B. 16 weeks
C. 20 weeks
D. 30 weeks

26. A female client presents to the obstetric-gynecology clinic for a pregnancy test, the result which turns out to be positive. Her last menstrual period began December 10, 1993. Using Nägele's rule, the nurse estimates her date of delivery to be:

A. September 17, 1994
B. September 10, 1994
C. September 3, 1994
D. August 17, 1994

27. A female client comes for her second prenatal visit. The nurse-midwife tells her, "Your blood tests reveal that you do not show immunity to the German measles." Which notation will the nurse include in her plan of care for the client? "Will need . . .

A. Rh-immune globulin at the next visit"
B. Rh-immune globulin within 3 days of delivery"
C. Rubella vaccine at the next visit"
D. Rubella vaccine after delivery on the day of discharge"

28. A female client at 37 weeks' gestation has just undergone a nonstress test. The results were two fetal movements with a corresponding increase in fetal heart rate (FHR) of 15 bpm lasting 15 seconds within a 20-minute period. Her results would be classified as:

A. Reactive; needs follow-up contraction stress test
B. Reactive; no contraction stress test required
C. Non-reactive; needs follow-up contraction stress test
D. Non-reactive; no contraction stress test required

29. A female client at 36 weeks' gestation has been treated successfully for premature labor for 4 weeks. She has begun having uterine contractions today and has been admitted to the labor and delivery suite. Her amniocentesis results reveal a lecithin/sphingomyelin (L/S) ratio of 2

and positive phosphatidylglycerol (PG). These lab values indicate:

A. Placental maturity
B. Suspected chronic asphyxia
C. Cord compression
D. Fetal lung maturity

30. A primigravida with a blood type A negative is at 28 weeks' gestation. Today her physician has ordered a RhoGAM injection. Which statement by the client demonstrates that more teaching is needed related to this therapy?

A. "I'm getting this shot so that my baby won't develop antibodies against my blood, right?"
B. "I understand that if my baby is Rh positive I'll be getting another one of these injections."
C. "This shot should help to protect me in future pregnancies if this baby is Rh positive, like my husband."
D. "This shot will prevent me from becoming sensitized to Rh-positive blood."

31. At her monthly prenatal visit, a client reports experiencing heartburn. Which nursing measure should be included in her plan of care to help alleviate it?

A. Restrict fluid intake.
B. Use Alka-Seltzer as necessary.
C. Eat small, frequent bland meals.
D. Lie down after eating.

32. A client is dilated 8 cm and entering the transition phase of labor. Common behaviors of the laboring woman during transition are:

A. Frustration, vague in communication
B. Seriousness, some difficulty following directions
C. Calmness, follows directions easily
D. Excitement, openness to instructions

33. The FHR pattern in a laboring client begins to show early decelerations. The nurse would best respond by:

A. Notifying the physician
B. Changing the client to the left lateral position
C. Continuing to monitor the FHR closely
D. Administering O_2 at 8 L/min via face mask

34. A female client is admitted to the emergency department complaining of severe right-sided abdominal pain and vaginal spotting. She states that her last menstrual period was about 2 months ago. A positive pregnancy test result and ultrasonography confirm an ectopic pregnancy. The nurse could best explain to the client that her condition is caused by:

A. Abnormal development of the embryo
B. A distended or ruptured fallopian tube
C. A congenital abnormality of the tube
D. A malfunctioning of the placenta

35. A female client at 10 weeks' gestation complains to her physician of slight vaginal bleeding and mild cramps. On examination, her physician determines that her cervix is closed. The client is exhibiting signs of:

A. An inevitable abortion
B. A threatened abortion

C. An incomplete abortion
D. A missed abortion

36. A female client at 36 weeks' gestation is experiencing preterm labor. Her physician has prescribed two doses of betamethasone 12 mg IM q24h. The nurse explains that she is receiving this drug to:

A. Treat fetal respiratory distress syndrome
B. Prevent uterine infection
C. Promote fetal lung maturation
D. Increase uteroplacental circulation

37. A female client at 30 weeks' gestation is brought into the emergency department after falling down a flight of stairs. On examination, the physician notes a rigid, boardlike abdomen; FHR in the 160s; and stable vital signs. Considering possible abdominal trauma, which obstetric emergency must be anticipated?

A. Abruptio placentae
B. Ectopic pregnancy
C. Massive uterine rupture
D. Placenta previa

38. A 4 days postpartum client who is gravida 3, para 3, is examined by the home health nurse during her first postpartum home visit. The nurse notes that she has a pink vaginal discharge with a serosanguineous consistency. The nurse would most accurately chart the client's lochia as:

A. Rubra
B. Rosa
C. Serosa
D. Alba

39. A primipara is assessed on arrival to the postpartum unit. The nurse finds her uterus to be boggy. The nurse's first action should be to:

A. Call the physician
B. Assess her vital signs
C. Give the prescribed oxytocic drug
D. Massage her fundus

40. A female client plans to bottle-feed her newborn. Her physician has ordered bromocriptine (Parlodel) to suppress lactation. Which of the following instructions about bromocriptine should be given by the nurse?

A. Bromocriptine stimulates the production of prolactin.
B. Hypertension is a primary side effect.
C. Bromocriptine is generally taken for 5 days.
D. Her blood pressure must be stable before starting bromocriptine.

41. The postpartum nurse should include which of the following instructions to breast-feeding mothers?

A. Limit feeding times for several days to avoid nipple soreness.
B. Wash the nipples with soap and water before and after each feeding.
C. Daily caloric intake should be increased by 500 cal.
D. Breast milk is totally digestible by the baby because it contains lactose.

42. At 12 hours postvaginal delivery, a female client is without complications. Which of the following assessment findings would warrant further nursing interventions?

    A. Apical pulse of 52 bpm
    B. Uterine fundus palpable left of midline
    C. No bowel movement since delivery
    D. Oral temperature of 100.4°F

43. The nurse observes a client crying quietly. She has just experienced a spontaneous abortion at nine weeks' gestation. An appropriate response by the nurse would be:

    A. "It must be God's will and probably is for the best."
    B. "This must be a difficult time for you. Would you like to talk about it?"
    C. "I'm sure your other children will be a comfort for you."
    D. "Don't worry, you're still young. If I were you I'd just try again."

44. A 48-hour-old male infant is ordered to have phototherapy. When his mother questions the nurse about its purpose, the nurse explains that phototherapy:

    A. Prevents the development of ophthalmia neonatorum
    B. Assists the baby's clotting mechanism
    C. Breaks down bilirubin in the skin into substances that can be excreted in stool or urine
    D. Increases levels of unconjugated bilirubin, thereby preventing kernicterus (brain damage)

45. After instructing a female client on circumcision care, the nursery nurse asks her to restate some of the key points covered. Which statement shows that the client will properly care for her son's circumcision?

    A. "I'll make sure I soak the gauze with warm water first, before I take it off each time."
    B. "I'll make sure that I report any drainage around where they operated."
    C. "I'll apply alcohol to the area daily to clean it and prevent any infection."
    D. "I'll keep a close watch on it for a day or two."

46. A male infant is to be discharged home this morning. Which instruction related to his cord care should be included in his mother's discharge teaching plan?

    A. Keep the umbilical area moist with Vaseline until the stump falls off.
    B. Keep the umbilical area covered at all times with the diaper.
    C. Clean the umbilical cord with alcohol at each diaper change.
    D. Clean the umbilical cord daily with soap and water during the bath.

47. Which behavior by a female client feeding her newborn demonstrates that she needs more teaching related to safety and infant feeding?

    A. She uses the bulb syringe to help clear her baby's nose when milk is regurgitated.
    B. She places her infant on her right side after feeding her.
    C. She props the bottle in the crib to feed her baby, which allows her to write birth announcements and feed her baby at the same time.
    D. She burps her baby by placing her in a sitting position, supporting her head and neck and gently massaging her back.

48. Newborns are routinely screened for phenylketonuria. The nursery nurse ensures that this screening test is performed:

    A. Immediately after birth, because the most accurate result is obtained at this time
    B. After 2–3 days of milk ingestion
    C. At 2–3 days of age regardless of amount of milk feedings
    D. At 1 month, because the biochemical buildup of phenylalanine takes 1 month to detect

49. A 3-year-old child has had symptoms of influenza including fever, productive cough, nausea, vomiting, and sore throat for the past several days. In caring for a young child with symptoms of influenza, the mother must be cautioned about:

    A. Giving aspirin and bismuth subsalicylate (Pepto-Bismol) to treat the symptoms
    B. Giving clear liquids too soon
    C. Allowing the child to come in contact with other children for 3 days
    D. The possibility of pneumonia as a complication

50. A 10-year-old boy has been diagnosed with Legg-Calvé Perthes disease. Which of the client's responses would indicate compliance during initial therapy?

    A. Drinking large amounts of milk
    B. Not bearing weight on affected extremity
    C. Walking short distances 3 times/day
    D. Putting self on weight reduction diet

51. A 7-year-old girl has been diagnosed with juvenile arthritis and has been placed on daily aspirin. Which statement made by the parent indicates a need for further teaching?

    A. "My daughter takes her aspirin with her meals."
    B. "Her gums have been bleeding frequently. Maybe she is brushing too hard."
    C. "I give her aspirin on a regular schedule every day."
    D. "One sign of aspirin toxicity can be ringing in the ears."

52. A young child has been placed in a spica cast. The chief concern of the nurse during the first few hours is:

    A. Prevention of neurovascular complications
    B. Prevention of loss of muscle tone
    C. Immobilization of the affected limb
    D. Using heated fans to dry the cast

53. The pediatrician has diagnosed tinea capitis in an 8-year-old girl and has placed her on oral griseofulvin. The nurse should emphasize which of these instructions to the mother and/or child?

    A. Administer oral griseofulvin on an empty stomach for best results.
    B. Discontinue drug therapy if food tastes funny.

    C. May discontinue medication when the child experiences symptomatic relief.

    D. Observe for headaches, dizziness, and anorexia.

54. A 12-year-old girl has been diagnosed with insulin-dependent diabetes mellitus. Which of these principles would best guide her nutritional management?

    A. Concentrated sweets are taken during increased activity.

    B. Food restriction is imposed to reduce weight.

    C. Caloric distribution should be calculated to fit activity patterns.

    D. Fat requirements are increased owing to the possibility of ketoacidosis.

55. A 5-year-old has just had a tonsillectomy and adenoidectomy. Which of these nursing measures should be included in the postoperative care?

    A. Encourage the child to cough up blood if present.

    B. Give warm clear liquids when fully alert.

    C. Have child gargle and do toothbrushing to remove old blood.

    D. Observe for evidence of bleeding.

56. A 4-week-old infant is admitted to the emergency room in respiratory distress. Which of the following statements indicates the nurse's knowledge of the anatomy of the respiratory system in pediatric clients?

    A. The diameter of the trachea is much smaller in children than in adults.

    B. The tongue is proportionally smaller in children than in adults.

    C. The pediatric airway is more rigid than that of the adults.

    D. The length of the pediatric airway is longer in children than in adults.

57. A 10-year-old has been diagnosed with acute poststreptococcal glomerulonephritis. The clinical findings were proteinuria, moderately elevated blood pressure, and periorbital edema. Which dietary plan is most appropriate for this client?

    A. Low-protein diet

    B. Low-sodium diet

    C. Increased fluid intake

    D. High-cholesterol diet

58. A 6-year-old girl has been diagnosed with a urinary tract infection secondary to vesicoureteral reflux. Which statement by her mother indicates a need for further teaching?

    A. "I have taught her to wipe from front to back after urinating."

    B. "I make sure she drinks plenty of fluids every day."

    C. "She enjoys wearing nylon panties, but I make her change them everyday."

    D. "She tries to empty her bladder completely after she urinates, like I told her."

59. A 1-year-old child is to receive an IM injection ordered by his pediatrician. He has fallen asleep in his mother's arms when the nurse approaches. Which approach is most appropriate at this time?

    A. Give the injection in the vastus lateralis site before the child awakens.

    B. Awaken the child first and give the injection in the ventrogluteal site.

    C. Awaken the child first and give the injection in the dorsogluteal site.

    D. Ask the mother to place the child on the examination table and leave the room, and then give the injection in an appropriate site.

60. The physician has ordered that ampicillin 250 mg IV be given over 30 minutes. The medication is diluted as recommended in 10 mL in the volume control chamber of a set that has a tubing of 12 mL. Which nursing measure is most accurate considering these facts?

    A. Infuse volume at 44 mL/hr.

    B. Infuse volume at 22 mL/hr.

    C. Infuse volume at 10 mL/hr.

    D. Infuse volume at 30 mL/hr.

61. An infant weighing 15 lb has just been treated for severe diarrhea in the hospital. Discharge instructions by the nurse will include maintenance fluid requirements for the pediatric client. Which of the following values *best* indicates the nurse's understanding of normal fluid requirements for this infant?

    A. 240 mL/day

    B. 680 mL/day

    C. 330 mL/day

    D. 960 mL/day

62. A normal 3-year-old child is suspected of having meningitis. The doctor has ordered a lumbar puncture. In light of this procedure and developmental characteristics of this age group, which nursing measure is *most* appropriate?

    A. Emphasize those aspects of the procedure that require cooperation.

    B. Tell the child not to cry or yell.

    C. Tell the child that he will get a "stick" in his back.

    D. Use medical terminology when explaining the procedure to the client.

63. A mother brings a 6-month-old infant and a 4-year-old child to the nursing clinic for routine examination and screening. Which of these plans by the nurse would be *most* successful?

    A. Examine the 4 year old first.

    B. Provide time for play and becoming acquainted.

    C. Have the mother leave the room with one child, and examine the other child privately.

    D. Examine painful areas first to get them "over with."

64. An 11-month-old infant is admitted with a possible diagnosis of pyloric stenosis. Which of the following *best* describes the characteristic clinical manifestations of pyloric stenosis?

    A. Pain, especially when eating

    B. Poor appetite and sucking reflex

    C. Increased frequency and quantity of stools

    D. Palpable olive-shaped mass in the epigastrium just right of the umbilical cord

65. As soon as a child has been diagnosed as "hearing impaired," special education should begin. Which of the following special education tasks is the most difficult for a severely hearing-impaired child?

    A. Auditory training
    B. Speech
    C. Lip reading
    D. Signing

66. A 15-year-old child is admitted to the pediatric unit with a diagnosis of thalassemia. Which of the following would be included in educating the mother and child as part of discharge planning?

    A. Give oral iron medication every day.
    B. Have the child's blood pressure monitored every week.
    C. Know the signs and symptoms of iron overload.
    D. Keep exercise at a minimum to reduce stress.

67. An 8-year-old boy has been diagnosed with hemophilia. Which of the following diagnostic blood studies is characteristically abnormal in this disorder?

    A. Partial thromboplastin time
    B. Platelet count
    C. Complete blood count
    D. Bleeding time

68. A murmur has been discovered during the routine physical examination of a 1-year-old child. The parent is extremely concerned about this diagnosis. Which of the following explanations by the nurse indicates understanding of this dysfunction?

    A. The blood shifts from the right to the left atrium.
    B. Surgical closure by suture or patch is recommended before school age.
    C. Most atrial septal defects close spontaneously.
    D. The child can be treated medically with antibiotics to prevent bacterial endocarditis.

69. An alcoholic client who is completing the inpatient segment of a substance abuse program was placed on disulfiram (Antabuse) drug therapy. What should the nurse include in the discharge instructions?

    A. If disulfiram is taken and alcohol ingested, the client experiences nausea, vomiting and elevated blood pressure.
    B. Disulfiram is most effective when prescribed as late as possible in a recovery program.
    C. Disulfiram works on the desensitization principle.
    D. The effects of disulfiram can be triggered by alcohol 5 days to 2 weeks after the drug is discontinued.

70. An 82-year-old former restaurant owner walks to the nursing station and states, "I have to go. The restaurant opens at 11 am." Which response by the nurse is the most appropriate?

    A. "Go back to your room. You do not own a restaurant."
    B. "You are in the hospital now. Calm down."
    C. "You once owned a restaurant. Tell me about it."
    D. "It is snowing outside. The restaurant is closed."

71. A 15-year-old female adolescent is frequently breaking the rules of the unit. She has left the unit and was found smoking in the bathroom and spending a large amount of time in the male ward. Which statement by the nurse would best explain to the teenager why she must follow the rules of the unit?

    A. "It is not easy, but the rules must be followed so that everyone can get a fair chance."
    B. "If you do not follow the rules, you will be transferred to the closed, locked unit."
    C. "You are not being fair to the other clients by getting them involved in your deviant behavior."
    D. "Break the rules, all you want, but don't get caught again!"

72. A 45-year-old male client experiences a sense of depression because he has not yet achieved his life's goals. His career has not been satisfying. He is still looking for the right job. His wife spends too much money, and his children seem to ignore him while being very selfish. He is tired of all of their attitudes and is considering buying a red Corvette convertible. While obtaining these data concerning the client's feelings about his life, the nurse is able to determine he is experiencing what psychological crisis according to Erikson's stages?

    A. Identity versus role confusion
    B. Integrity versus despair
    C. Intimacy versus isolation
    D. Generativity versus self-absorption

73. A female client is anticipating a visit with her parents over the Thanksgiving holidays. She has recently begun experiencing periods of extreme shortness of breath, which her physician has labeled as panic attacks. Which of the following statements by the nurse would enhance therapeutic communication?

    A. "Why do you feel this way?"
    B. "Tell me about your dislike for your parents."
    C. "Don't worry, everything will be all right on your visit with your parents."
    D. "Perhaps you and I can discover what produces your anxiety."

74. A female client has experienced varying degrees of depression throughout her life. Now that she is postmenopausal, her depression has increased. She is unable to motivate herself to clean her house or even to get out of bed and get dressed in the morning. The client was begun on fluoxetine (Prozac) therapy. When educating her about fluoxetine, what might the nurse caution her about?

    A. A daily dose of fluoxetine may be taken in the morning or evening.
    B. Fluoxetine is not sedating; therefore, restrictions on driving and other hazardous activities are not necessary.
    C. Rashes or pruritus usually occur early in the therapy and are treatable without discontinuing the medication.
    D. It is safe to take over-the-counter or other prescription medications with fluoxetine.

75. A male client seeks counseling after his wife of 19 years threatened to divorce him. For most of their marriage, he has physically and verbally abused her. When asked

about his behavior in the process of the nursing assessment, the client states, "I was mean to my wife because she insists on cooking meals and wearing clothes that I do not like." This defense mechanism is an example of:

A. Repression
B. Regression
C. Reaction formation
D. Rationalization

76. A male client is admitted to the psychiatric unit after experiencing severe depression. He states that he intends to kill himself, but he asks the nurse not to repeat his intentions to other staff members. Which response demonstrates understanding and appropriate action on the part of the nurse?

A. "I understand you're depressed, but killing yourself is not a reasonable option."
B. "We need to discuss this further, but right now let's complete these forms."
C. "Don't do that, you have so much to live for. You have a wonderful wife and children. The client in the next room has no one."
D. "This is very serious. I do not want any harm to come to you. I will have to report this to the rest of the staff."

77. During the admitting mental health assessment, a client demonstrates involuntary muscular activity. He has a marked facial tic around the mouth that is distracting to the nurse during the interview. The nurse recognizes the behavior and documents it as:

A. Dyskinesia
B. Akathisia
C. Echopraxia
D. Echolalia

78. A female client is seeking counseling for personal problems. She admits to being very unhappy lately at both home and work. During the nursing assessment, she uses many defense mechanisms. Which statement or action made by the client is an example of adaptive suppression?

A. "I did not get the raise because my boss does not like me."
B. "I felt a lump in my breast 2 weeks ago. I put off getting it checked until after my sister's wedding."
C. "My son died 3 years ago. I still cannot bring myself to clean out his room."
D. "My husband told me this morning that he wants a divorce. I am upset, but I cannot discuss the matter with him until after my company's board meeting today."

79. When interviewing parents who are suspected of child abuse, the nurse would use which of the following interview techniques?

A. Be direct, honest, and attentive.
B. Approach them in the emergency room as soon as you suspect abuse to "clear the air" right away.
C. Ask the parents what they could have done differently to prevent this from happening to the child.
D. After the interview, call child protective services.

80. In an interview for suspected child abuse, the child's mother openly discusses her feelings. She feels her husband is too aggressive in disciplining their child. The child's father states, "Being a school custodian, I see kids every day that are bad because they did not get enough discipline at home. That will not happen to our child." Based on this remark, the nurse would make the following nursing diagnosis:

A. Fear related to retaliation by the father
B. Actual injury related to poor impulse control by the father
C. Ineffective coping
D. Altered family process related to physical abuse

81. A 40-year-old client has lived for 8 years with an abusive spouse. She married her husband in her senior year of high school after becoming pregnant. Shortly after the baby was born, he began to physically abuse her. She has attempted to leave him several times, but she has always returned. She is unable to support herself financially, and her husband threatens to kill her if she leaves him. This time, her husband has beaten her so badly she cannot stop the bleeding from the gash above her eye. She admits her husband caused her injury. In assessing a person after experiencing spousal abuse, which need has the highest priority?

A. Assess the level of anxiety, coping responses, and support systems.
B. Assess the history of physical abuse.
C. Assess suicide potential.
D. Assess drug and alcohol use.

82. As a nurse in the emergency room, you receive an outside call from an elderly woman who states she has just been raped. She states, "I know I must come to the hospital, but what do I do next?" You advise her to call the police, then come to the hospital emergency room. What action by the nurse would indicate an understanding of the examination process once the victim enters the emergency room?

A. Inform the victim not to wash, change clothes, douche, brush teeth, or eat or drink anything.
B. Inform the victim to bring insurance information with her to the hospital so she can be properly cared for.
C. Phone a rape counselor to begin working with the victim as soon as she enters the hospital.
D. Do not leave the victim alone to collect her thoughts.

83. A 14-year-old teenager is demonstrating behavior indicative of an obsessive-compulsive disorder. She is obsessed with her appearance. She will not leave her room until her hair, clothes, and makeup are perfect. She always dresses immaculately. Recently, she expressed disgust over her appearance after she gained 5 lb. After observing a marked weight loss over a 2-week period, her mother suspects that she is experiencing bulimia. She eats everything on her plate, then runs to the bathroom. In interviewing the teenager, she discusses in great detail all of the events leading to her bulimia, but not her feelings. What defense mechanism is she using?

A. Dissociation
B. Intellectualization

C. Rationalization

D. Displacement

84. A male client is experiencing extreme distress. He begins to pace up and down the corridor. What nursing intervention is appropriate when communicating with the pacing client?

A. Ask him to sit down. Speak slowly and use short, simple sentences.

B. Help him to recognize his anxiety.

C. Walk with him as he paces.

D. Increase the level of his supervision.

85. A 24-year-old graduate student recognizes that he has a phobia. He suffers severe anxiety when he is in darkness. It has altered his lifestyle because he is unable to go to a movie theater, concert, and other events that may require absence of light. The client is seeking assistance because he is no longer able to socialize with friends due to his phobia. The psychologist working with him is using desensitization. He has asked the nursing staff to assist the client in muscle relaxation techniques. What result would indicate client education has been successful?

A. He enters a movie theater, sits in his chair, and replaces anxiety with relaxation as the theater darkens.

B. He enters a concert, but as the lights dim, he does not experience anxiety.

C. He states that he no longer fears dark places.

D. He takes a part-time job as a photographic assistant. His job necessitates his working in a darkroom.

86. A female client has just died. Her family is requesting that all nursing staff leave the room. The family's religious leader has arrived and is ready to conduct a ceremony for the deceased in the room, requesting that only family members be present. The nurse assigned to the client should perform the appropriate nursing action, which might include:

A. Inform the family that it is the hospital's policy not to conduct religious ceremonies in client rooms.

B. Refuse to leave the room because the client's body is entrusted in the nurse's care until it can be brought to the morgue.

C. Tell the family that they may conduct their ceremony in the client's room; however, the nurse must attend.

D. Respect the client's family's wishes.

87. A female client has been recently diagnosed as bipolar. She has taken lithium for the past several weeks to control mania. What must be included in client education regarding lithium toxicity?

A. Maintain a normal diet; however, limit salt intake to no more than 3 g/day.

B. Take lithium between meals to increase absorption.

C. Withhold lithium if experiencing diarrhea, vomiting, or diaphoresis.

D. For pain or fever, avoid aspirin or acetaminophen (Tylenol). Nonsteroidal anti-inflammatory drugs are preferred.

88. For the past several months, an elderly female client with Alzheimer's disease has experienced paranoia; hallucinations; and aggressive, disruptive behavior. The family is utilizing haloperidol as needed to control her behavior. On nursing assessment, you note that the client demonstrates involuntary movements of the tongue and fingers. This may most likely indicate:

A. Tardive dyskinesia, which may be a side effect of antipsychotic medication

B. Early symptoms of Parkinson's disease

C. A more advanced stage of Alzheimer's disease than previously experienced by the client

D. The need to change her medication from haloperidol to another antipsychotic drug to lessen symptoms

89. A 32-year-old male client is a marketing representative. His job requires him to have a tremendous amount of energy during the day. He frequently uses cocaine to sustain his energy level. Lately he has increased his use of cocaine and even experimented with crack cocaine. Realizing he can no longer continue this destructive behavior, he is seeking treatment for cocaine addiction. In planning nursing care for the client's inpatient stay, which expected outcome is most appropriate?

A. He will attend four consecutive group educational sessions on substance abuse.

B. He will name activities that he would most likely be involved in posttreatment.

C. He will meet with his family in counseling sessions and discuss his feelings.

D. He will be able to deal with his feelings through participation in group therapy sessions.

1. **(B)** Client need: physiological integrity; subcategory: reduction of risk potential; content area: med/surg

RATIONALE
(A) The tracheal cuff should not be deflated within the first 24 hours following surgery. (B) To minimize bleeding, any manipulation, including cuff deflation, should be avoided. (C) Small amounts of crepitus are expected to occur; however, large amounts or expansion of the area of crepitus should be reported to the physician. (D) The tracheostomy site may be changed as often as necessary, but site care should be done with normal saline.

2. **(D)** Client need: physiological integrity; subcategory: physiological adaptation; content area: med/surg

RATIONALE
(A) Describing pain is an important aspect of the assessment; however, assessing activity preceding muscle spasms is equally important. (B) Edema may occur with peripheral vascular disease, but it is not of particular importance in assessing intermittent claudication. (C) Lesions may be present with peripheral vascular disease, but they are not an indication of intermittent claudication. (D) With intermittent claudication, muscle spasms occur intermittently, mainly with walking and after exercising. Rest may relieve muscle spasms.

3. **(C)** Client need: health promotion and maintenance; subcategory: prevention and early detection of disease; content area: med/surg

RATIONALE
(A) Postoperatively, clients with major abdominal surgery are instructed to avoid driving, riding in the front seat, and wearing seat belts because any sudden impact may injure a fresh incision. She should ride in back seat without a seat belt. (B) Clients should not sit in the tub and allow the incision to soak in water because this may predispose the client to infection. A short, cool shower would be preferable. Allowing soap to come in contact with the incision would not harm it and is frequently used as postoperative wound care at home on discharge from the hospital. (C) Activity instructions include: avoid sitting for long periods and get exercise by walking. Lifting more than 5 lb of weight is also prohibited. (D) The client must also learn her diet. Her husband cooking is probably a temporary measure unless he did the cooking prior to her hospitalization. A statement such as this may indicate the need for further exploration of feelings regarding her illness, dependence, and self-care expectations.

4. **(A)** Client need: health promotion and maintenance; subcategory: prevention and early detection of disease; content area: med/surg

RATIONALE
(A) A blood pressure within acceptable range best demonstrates compliance, but weight loss cannot be accomplished without adherence to medication, diet, and exercise. (B) Absence of side effects does not indicate compliance with medication. Pill counts can be misleading because the client can alter pill counts prior to visit. (C) Left ventricular hypertrophy is not an accurate measure of compliance because hypertrophy frequently does not decrease even with pharmacological management. (D) Therapeutic blood levels measure the drug level at the time of the test. There is no indication of compliance several days before testing.

5. **(B)** Client need: physiological integrity; subcategory: physiological adaptation; content area: med/surg

RATIONALE
(A) Indigestion or nausea may accompany angina or myocardial infarction, but they do not indicate imminent danger for the client. (B) Restlessness and apprehensiveness require immediate nursing action because they are indicative of very low oxygenation of body tissues and are frequently the first indication of impending cardiac or respiratory arrest. (C) It is common for the cardiac client to experience fatigue and inability to physically tolerate long assessment sessions. (D) A history of hypertension requires no immediate nursing intervention. In the situation described, the blood pressure is not given and therefore cannot be assumed to be elevated.

6. **(D)** Client need: physiological integrity; subcategory: reduction of risk potential; content area: med/surg

RATIONALE
(A) An elevated serum osmolality poses no immediate danger and is not corrected rapidly. (B) A low serum sodium alone does not warrant changing IV fluids to normal saline. Other assessment parameters, such as hydration status, must be considered. (C) A low serum blood urea nitrogen is not necessarily indicative of protein deprivation. It may also be the result of overhydration. (D) A low serum potassium potentiates the effects of digitalis, predisposing the client to dangerous arrhythmias. It must be corrected immediately.

7. **(A)** Client need: physiological integrity; subcategory: pharmacological and parenteral therapies; content area: med/surg

RATIONALE
(A) Cyclosporine is the immunosuppressive drug of choice. It provides immunosuppression but does not lower the white blood cell count; therefore, the client is less susceptible to infection. (B) Cyclosporine is available at discount pharmacies. The cost may be absorbed by health insurance, or Medicare, if the client is eligible. However, this statement does not address the entire problem verbalized by the client. (C) Immunosuppressive agents will be taken for the client's entire life because rejection can occur at any time. (D) These side effects do not necessarily resolve in time; however, the client may adapt.

8. **(B)** Client need: psychosocial integrity; subcategory: coping and adaptation; content area: med/surg

RATIONALE
(A) The client could contract an infection, but at this point it is not the most pertinent issue. (B) The client's statement indicates that she does not grasp the full impact of her illness. Further client education must be given, along with allowing her to express her feelings regarding her illness. (C) The client may require a transfusion, but this is a temporary measure because the causative agent has not been identified. Her feelings regarding her illness must be addressed in order for care to continue. (D) A bone marrow is done first to make a definitive diagnosis; then treatment may begin.

9. **(D)** Client need: physiological integrity; subcategory: physiological adaptation; content area: med/surg

RATIONALE
(A) Clients in renal failure typically have very low hematocrits, often in the range of 16–22%. (B) Transfusion is avoided unless the client exhibits acute symptoms such as dyspnea, chest pain, tachycardia, and extreme fatigue. When the client is given a transfusion, the bone marrow adjusts by producing less red blood cells. (C) Anemia in renal failure is caused primarily by decreased erythropoietin. Low serum iron and ferritin may aggravate the anemia and require treatment. (D) Decreased secretion of erythropoietin by the kidney is the primary cause of anemia. The bone marrow requires this hormone to mature red blood cells. Treatment is with replacement therapy.

10. **(C)** Client need: health promotion and maintenance; subcategory: prevention and early detection of disease; content area: med/surg

    RATIONALE

    (A) Although it is important that the client drink adequate fluids while treating a bladder infection with trimethoprim-sulfamethoxazole, the failure to do so will not cause pyelonephritis. (B) A stricture or abnormality may cause the progression of bladder infection to urinary tract infection, but this is rare. There is no indication in this situation that this has occurred. (C) The most common cause of pyelonephritis is improper treatment of bladder infections. The client typically feels better after several days, discontinues the medication, and saves the remainder for the next occurrence of a bladder infection. For this reason, it is imperative to provide client education related to completion of the prescribed medication. (D) There is no evidence that infection in another body system could cause pyelonephritis.

11. **(B)** Client need: health maintenance and prevention; subcategory: prevention and early detection of disease; content area: med/surg

    RATIONALE

    (A) Loss of ability to speak is not dysphasia. Although the client may have difficulty communicating, alternative measures can be developed to enhance communication. This goal, while important, is of a lesser priority. (B) Dysphasia is difficulty swallowing, which could result in aspiration of food and inability to eat, causing weight loss. (C) A secondary infection could result from poor oral hygiene, which could enhance the client's inability to eat, but this goal is of a lesser priority. (D) Drooling normally occurs in clients with amyotrophic lateral sclerosis and may require suctioning. Drooling, while aggravating for the client, does not pose an immediate danger.

12. **(A)** Client need: physiological integrity; subcategory: physiological adaptation; content area: med/surg

    RATIONALE

    (A) An effective airway is necessary to prevent hypoxia and subsequent cardiac arrest. (B) Cerebral tissue perfusion is necessary to preserve remaining cerebral tissue, but this goal is secondary to maintenance of an effective airway. (C) While prevention of injury is important, it is secondary to maintaining an effective airway and cerebral tissue perfusion. (D) Impaired verbal communication is not life threatening in the acute phase of recovery. It is the lowest priority of the nursing diagnoses listed.

13. **(C)** Client need: physiological integrity; subcategory: physiological adaptation; content area: med/surg

    RATIONALE

    (A) Headaches are not associated with Guillain-Barré syndrome. (B) Loss of superficial and deep tendon reflexes is expected with this diagnosis. (C) Complaints of shortness of breath must be further evaluated. Forty percent of all clients have some detectable respiratory weakness and should be prepared for a possible tracheostomy. Pneumonia is also a common complication of this syndrome. (D) Facial paralysis is expected and is not considered abnormal.

14. **(D)** Client need: physiological integrity; subcategory: physiological adaptation; content area: med/surg

    RATIONALE

    (A) A reclining position can cause a penetrating object to advance further into the eye. (B) Prevention of further injury is the priority, not comfort. (C) A side-lying position may increase intraocular and intracranial pressure if an accompanying head injury is suspected. (D) A sitting position with the head supported will prevent further injury while allowing injury care to take place.

15. **(A)** Client need: physiological integrity; subcategory: pharmacological and parenteral therapies; content area: med/surg

    RATIONALE

    (A) The first nursing measure is to instruct the client in which drug side effects to report. (B) Discontinuing the drug is not an independent nursing intervention and may compromise client care. (C) Audiometric testing will detect hearing loss, but it does not indicate a potential cause. (D) Equalizing middle ear pressure will not prevent hearing loss.

16. **(C)** Client need: physiological integrity; subcategory: reduction of risk potential; content area: med/surg

    RATIONALE

    (A) TENS units do not have this effect, but whirlpool therapy does. (B) TENS units do not produce endogenous opioids, only the body can do that. (C) TENS units do work based on the gate-control theory of pain control. (D) TENS units do not have this effect, but possibly changing the client's position would.

17. **(B)** Client need: physiological integrity; subcategory: physiological adaptation; content area: med/surg

    RATIONALE

    (A) This statement is entirely false. (B) Phantom pain may be caused by nerves continuing to carry sensation to the brain even though the limb is removed. It is real, intense, and should be treated as ordinary pain would. (C) Although the cause of phantom pain is still unknown, these measures may promote the relief of any type of pain, not just phantom pain. (D) Phantom pain is not caused by trauma, spasms, and edema and will not be relieved by decreasing edema.

18. **(C)** Client need: physiological integrity; subcategory: reduction of risk potential; content area: med/surg

    RATIONALE

    (A) Dressing changes are done as necessary for bleeding. However, frequently, post-thyroidectomy bleeding may not be visible on the dressing, but blood may drain down the back of the neck by gravity. (B) Narcotics are administered for acute pain as necessary. They are not necessarily given on return of the client to her room. (C) The most serious postthyroidectomy complication is ineffective airway and breathing pattern related to tracheal compression and edema. A tracheostomy set, O_2, and suction should be available at bedside for at least the first 24 hours postoperatively. (D) Impaired verbal communication may occur due to laryngeal edema or nerve damage, but most commonly, it occurs due to endotracheal intubation. The client is usually able to communicate but is hoarse.

19. **(A)** Client need: physiological integrity; subcategory: physiological adaptation; content area: med/surg

    RATIONALE

    (A) Assessment should focus on detection of tetany, which is the most common symptom of hypoparathyroidism. Left undetected and untreated, tetany resulting from hypocalcemia can progress to seizures. (B) Hypocalcemia is difficult to detect on nursing assessment alone. Abdominal cramping may be an indication of hypocalcemia, but laboratory data are required to confirm diagnosis. (C) Depression can be a symptom of hypoparathyroidism, but it is not definitive. (D) Premature cataract formation can occur, but it also is not specific to parathyroidism and poses no immediate danger to the client.

20. **(C)** Client need: psychosocial integrity; subcategory: coping and adaptation; content area: med/surg

    RATIONALE

    (A) Depression may be an underlying feature, but it is not evident from limited data presented here. (B) Anger is not exhibited in his response. (C) Denial is evident in the client's actions; through the years, he has had a casual approach to his illness. He only becomes concerned when bodily changes affect his present lifestyle, when in fact he should have been concerned all along.

His verbal response also reflects denial. (D) There is no evidence of bargaining in the client's actions or verbal response.

21. **(D)** Client need: health promotion and maintenance; subcategory: prevention and early detection of disease; content area: med/surg

    RATIONALE

    (A) Monthly blood transfusions are not indicated postgastrectomy. (B) Increasing iron in the client's diet may cause irritation and will not alleviate pernicious anemia. (C) It may be necessary that the client eat small meals several times per day, but this measure has no relevance to prevention of pernicious anemia. (D) Pernicious anemia is caused by lack of Vitamin B_{12}, and replacement therapy will be necessary because the client's stomach has been removed.

22. **(B)** Client need: health promotion and maintenance; subcategory: prevention and early detection of disease; content area: med/surg

    RATIONALE

    (A) Isolation is not necessary, even in the acute phase. (B) Separate bathroom facilities are recommended. If unavailable, daily cleansing with a chloride solution is recommended. (C) Precautions continue to be necessary while the client is in the active phase of hepatitis. (D) Clothes are to be laundered separately in hot water with a chloride solution.

23. **(A)** Client need: physiological integrity; subcategory: physiological adaptation; content area: med/surg

    RATIONALE

    (A) Relief of pain is the primary goal of nursing intervention because this client is experiencing acute pain. (B) Fluid volume deficit is being treated with IV fluid replacement. (C) Knowledge deficit will not be addressed at this time because a client in acute pain is not ready to learn. (D) Alteration in nutrition is the third priority after relief of pain and fluid volume deficit.

24. **(D)** Client need: psychosocial integrity; subcategory: coping and adaptation; content area: med/surg

    RATIONALE

    (A) A regimented schedule, allowing no flexibility, will not foster the client's self-esteem. (B) Isolating the client may only enhance his feelings of social isolation due to his disfigurement. (C) Standardized care plans must be personalized and adapted to each client's situation. (D) Allowing the client control over his care will foster his self-esteem and prepare him for life outside of the hospital.

25. **(C)** Client need: health promotion and maintenance; subcategory: growth and development through the life span; content area: maternity

    RATIONALE

    (A) At 10 weeks, the fundus is located slightly above the symphysis pubis. (B) At 16 weeks, the fundus is halfway between the symphysis pubis and the umbilicus. (C) At 20 weeks, the fundus is located approximately at the umbilicus. (D) At 30 weeks, the fundal height is about 30 cm, or 10 cm above the umbilicus.

26. **(A)** Client need: health promotion and maintenance; subcategory: growth and development through the life span: content area: maternity

    RATIONALE

    (A) According to Nägele's rule, the estimated date of delivery is calculated by adding 7 days to the date of the first day of the normal menstrual period (December 10 + 7 days = December 17), and then by counting back 3 months (December 17 − 3 mo = September 17). (B, C, D) These answers are incorrect.

27. **(D)** Client need: health promotion and maintenance; subcategory: prevention and early detection of disease; content area: maternity

RATIONALE

(A) Rh immune globulin is given to Rh-negative mothers to prevent the maternal Rh immune response. (B) Rh immune globulin is given to Rh-negative mothers to prevent the maternal Rh immune response. (C) The rubella vaccine is not given during pregnancy because of its teratogenicity. (D) Nonimmune mothers are vaccinated early in the postpartum period to prevent future infection with the rubella virus.

28. **(B)** Client need: physiological integrity; subcategory: reduction of risk potential; content area: maternity

    RATIONALE

    (A) A contraction stress test is unnecessary following a reactive (normal) nonstress test. (B) The results are considered reactive, indicating that the fetus is not showing distress. Therefore, a contraction stress test, which is a more in-depth test for fetal distress, is unnecessary. (C) A nonreactive test would show fewer than two fetal movements or a failure of the FHR to increase at least 15 bpm with the movements in a 20-minute period. (D) A contraction stress test should follow a nonreactive nonstress test to validate fetal distress.

29. **(D)** Client need: physiological integrity; subcategory: reduction of risk potential; content area: maternity

    RATIONALE

    (A) Placental maturity is assessed by a biophysical profile. (B) L/S ratio and presence of phosphatidylglycerol are not used to determine fetal asphyxia. A biophysical profile score of ≤ 6 may indicate this condition. (C) Cord compression is not reflected by the L/S ratio or presence of phosphatidylglycerol. Variable decelerations observed through electronic fetal monitoring could reflect umbilical cord compression. (D) An L/S ratio ≥ 2 and the presence of phosphatidylglycerol in amniotic fluid indicate fetal lung maturity.

30. **(A)** Client need: health promotion and maintenance; subcategory: prevention and early detection of disease; content area: maternity

    RATIONALE

    (A) RhoGAM is given to Rh-negative mothers to prevent the maternal Rh immune response to fetal Rh-positive antigens. (B) If the infant is Rh positive, the mother will receive another dose postdelivery to prevent maternal sensitization. (C) Prevention of maternal sensitization will protect future pregnancies because the mother's blood will be free of antibodies against her fetus. (D) RhoGAM prevents maternal sensitization to Rh-positive blood.

31. **(C)** Client need: physiological integrity; subcategory: physiological adaptation; content area: maternity

    RATIONALE

    (A) At least eight glasses of fluid per day are encouraged to help dilute stomach contents, thereby decreasing irritation. (B) Alka Seltzer contains aspirin, which is irritating to gastric mucosa, and therefore should be avoided. (C) Small, frequent bland meals help to decrease gastric pressure and to prevent reflux. (D) Lying down after meals may cause gastric reflux and prevents optimal gastric emptying.

32. **(A)** Client need: psychosocial integrity; subcategory: coping and adaptation; content area: maternity

    RATIONALE

    (A) During the transition phase, the mother may become frustrated and unclear in her communication owing to severe pain and fear of loss of control. (B) These behaviors are common in the active phase of labor. (C) These behavioral clues are seen in the latent phase of labor. (D) These characteristics are observed in the latent phase of labor.

33. **(C)** Client need: health promotion and maintenance; subcategory: growth and development through the life span; content area: maternity

RATIONALE

(A) Early decelerations are reassuring and do not warrant notification of the physician. (B) Because early decelerations is a reassuring pattern, it would not be necessary to change the client's position. (C) Early decelerations warrant the continuation of close FHR monitoring to distinguish them from more ominous signs. (D) O_2 is not warranted in this situation, but it is warranted in situations involving variable and/or late decelerations.

34. **(B)** Client need: physiological integrity; subcategory: physiological adaptation; content area: maternity

RATIONALE

(A) The embryo itself may develop normally in the first several weeks of an ectopic pregnancy. (B) An ectopic pregnancy in the fallopian tube causes severe pain owing to the size of the growing embryo within the narrow lumen of the tube, causing distention and finally rupture within the first 12 weeks of pregnancy. (C) The Fallopian tube may either be normal or contain adhesions caused by a history of pelvic inflammatory disease or tubal surgeries, neither of which are congenital causes. (D) An ectopic pregnancy does not involve a dysfunctional placenta, but the implantation of the blastocyst outside the uterus.

35. **(B)** Client need: physiological integrity; subcategory: physiological adaptation; content area: maternity

RATIONALE

(A) An inevitable abortion includes the signs of cervical dilation and effacement as well as pain and bleeding. (B) A threatened abortion is a condition in which intrauterine bleeding occurs early in pregnancy, the cervix remains undilated, and the uterine contents are not necessarily expelled. (C) An incomplete abortion occurs when some portions of the products of conception are expelled from the uterus. (D) A missed abortion occurs when the embryo dies in utero and is retained in the uterus.

36. **(C)** Client need: health promotion and maintenance; subcategory: prevention and early detection of disease; content area: maternity

RATIONALE

(A) Respiratory distress syndrome occurs in the newborn, not the fetus. It may be treated postnatally with surfactant therapy. (B) Betamethasone is a corticosteroid, not an anti-infective drug; therefore, its use would not prevent uterine infection. (C) Betamethasone binds with glucocorticoid receptors in alveolar cells to increase production of surfactant, thus increasing lung maturity in the preterm fetus. (D) Betamethasone does not affect uteroplacental circulatory exchange.

37. **(A)** Client need: physiological integrity; subcategory: physiological adaptation; content area: maternity

RATIONALE

(A) Abruptio placentae, the complete or partial separation of the placenta from the uterine wall, can be caused by external trauma. When hemorrhage is concealed, one sign is a rapid increase in uterine size with rigidity. (B) Ectopic pregnancy occurs when the embryo implants itself outside the uterine cavity. (C) Massive uterine rupture occurs during labor when the uterine contents are extruded through the uterine wall. It is usually due to weakness from a pre-existing uterine scar and trauma from instruments or an obstetrical intervention. (D) Placenta previa is the condition in which the placenta is implanted in the lower uterine segment and either completely or partially covers the cervical os.

38. **(C)** Client need: health promotion and maintenance; subcategory: growth and development through the life span; content area: maternity

RATIONALE

(A) Lochia rubra is bloody with clots and occurs 1–3 days postpartum. (B) There is no such term as lochia rosa. (C) Lochia serosa is a pink-brown discharge with a serosanguineous consistency that occurs 4–9 days postpartum. (D) Lochia alba is yellow to white in color and occurs approximately 10 days postpartum.

39. **(D)** Client need: health promotion and maintenance; subcategory: growth and development through the life span; content area: maternity

RATIONALE

(A) The nurse should first implement independent and dependent measures to achieve uterine tone before calling the physician. (B) Assessment of vital signs will not help to restore uterine atony, which is the priority need. (C) Giving a prescribed oxytocic drug would be necessary if the uterus did not maintain tone with massage. (D) Fundal massage generally restores uterine tone within a few moments and should be attempted first.

40. **(D)** Client need: physiological integrity; subcategory: pharmacological and parenteral therapies; content area: maternity

RATIONALE

(A) Bromocriptine inhibits the secretion of prolactin. (B) Hypotension is a side effect of this drug; hypertension is not. (C) Bromocriptine is generally taken for 14 days. (D) The administration of bromocriptine is delayed at least 4 hours postpartum and given only when the client's blood pressure is stable, because it can cause hypotension and syncope.

41. **(C)** Client need: health promotion and maintenance; subcategory: growth and development through the life span; content area: maternity

RATIONALE

(A) Limiting initial feeding times will only delay nipple soreness as well as the establishment of the letdown reflex, thus encouraging engorgement from clogged ducts and ductules. (B) Soap should be avoided because it may be excessively drying, predisposing nipples to cracking. (C) For optimal milk production, an additional 500 kcal over maintenance levels are needed daily. (D) Lipase, not lactose, emulsifies the fat in breast milk, making it almost totally digestible by infants.

42. **(B)** Client need: health promotion and maintenance; subcategory: prevention and early detection of disease; content area: maternity

RATIONALE

(A) Bradycardia of 50–70 bpm may be considered normal post-partally because the heart compensates for the decreased resistance in the pelvis. (B) The uterus is displaced from the midline by a full bladder. This condition could lead to a boggy uterus and increased risk of postpartal hemorrhage; therefore, the bladder should be kept empty. (C) Re-establishment of normal bowel function is delayed into the first postpartum week. (D) A postpartum woman's oral temperature may go as high as 100.4°F within 24 hours of delivery resulting from muscular exertion, dehydration, and hormonal changes.

43. **(B)** Client need: psychosocial integrity; subcategory: coping and adaptation; content area: maternity

RATIONALE

(A) This response is nontherapeutic because it belittles the client's response and gives a meaningless rationalization. (B) This response acknowledges the client's feelings and demonstrates the therapeutic offering of self by the nurse. (C) This response is nontherapeutic because it does not focus on the client's feelings and offers false reassurance. (D) This response is nontherapeutic because it belittles the client's feelings and offers her advice.

44. **(C)** Client need: physiological integrity; subcategory: reduction of risk potential; content area: maternity

RATIONALE

(A) The instillation of erythromycin ophthalmic preparation, not phototherapy, prevents ophthalmia neonatorum. (B) The administration of vitamin K (AquaMEPHYTON) assists the infant's clotting mechanism. (C) Excessive bilirubin accumulates when the infant's liver cannot handle the increased load caused by the breakdown of red blood cells postnatally. This excessive bilirubin seeps out of the blood and into the tissues, staining them yellow. Phototherapy accelerates the removal of bilirubin from the skin by breaking it down into substances that can be excreted in stool or urine. (D) Phototherapy decreases levels of unconjugated bilirubin, thereby preventing kernicterus.

45. **(A)** Client need: health promotion and maintenance; subcategory: prevention and early detection of disease; content area: maternity

RATIONALE

(A) Before petrolatum gauze is removed, it should be soaked with warm water to prevent trauma to adherent tissues. (B) A yellow exudate often forms normally over the surgical site. Only if it becomes foul-smelling and purulent would it need to be reported. (C) Alcohol should never be used on the site; this would be extremely painful to the infant. (D) Special care and observance should continue until the site is completely covered with clean, pink granulation tissue, which could take 7–10 days.

46. **(C)** Client need: health promotion and maintenance; subcategory: growth and development through the life span; content area: maternity

RATIONALE

(A) The umbilical area should be kept dry for healing to occur. Moisture is conducive to bacterial growth and therefore could lead to infection at the site. (B) The diaper should be folded below the cord to allow the cord stump to be exposed to the air for healing. (C) The umbilical cord should be swabbed with alcohol at each diaper change to remove urine and stool and to facilitate the desiccation process through drying. (D) Soap and water should not be used to clean the umbilical area because the area could retain moisture, thus making it susceptible to bacterial growth and infection.

47. **(C)** Client need: health promotion and maintenance; subcategory: prevention and early detection of disease; content area: maternity

RATIONALE

(A) This practice is the proper use of the bulb syringe to clear the infant's airway in case of regurgitation. (B) Placing the infant on either side or on the stomach prevents aspiration of regurgitated milk. (C) "Bottle propping" is an unsafe practice because it increases the likelihood of aspiration. (D) This practice is one correct way of burping an infant.

48. **(B)** Client need: health promotion and maintenance; subcategory: prevention and early detection of disease; content area: maternity

RATIONALE

(A) The infant has not ingested any protein immediately after birth, which is necessary to detect excessive serum phenylalanine. (B) It is important that the infant take in 2–3 full days of milk or formula feedings to preclude a false-negative reading. (C) At 2–3 days of age, inadequate milk could have been ingested owing to a delay in the initial feeding. (D) The biochemical buildup of serum phenylalanine is detectable after 2–3 days of milk or formula ingestion.

49. **(A)** Client need: health promotion and maintenance; subcategory: prevention and early detection of disease; content area: pediatrics

RATIONALE

(A) Aspirin should never be given to children with influenza because of the possibility of causing Reye's syndrome. Pepto-Bismol is also classified as a salicylate and should be avoided. (B) Depending on the severity of symptoms, the child may be receiving IV therapy or clear liquids. (C) The disease has a 1–3 day incubation period and affected children are most infectious 24 hours before and after the onset of symptoms. (D) Although viral pneumonia can be a complication of influenza, this would not be an initial priority.

50. **(B)** Client need: health promotion and maintenance; subcategory: prevention and early detection of disease; content area: pediatrics

RATIONALE

(A) This condition causes aseptic necrosis of the head of the femur in the acetabulum. Drinking large quantities of milk at this time cannot hasten recovery. (B) The aim of treatment is to keep the head of the femur in the acetabulum. Non–weight-bearing is essential. Activity causes microfractures of the epiphysis. (C) In addition to non–weight-bearing, clients are often placed on bedrest, which helps to reduce inflammation. Later, active motion is encouraged. (D) Weight is not generally an issue with this disease. Slipped femoral capital epiphysis, which is most frequently observed in obese pubescent children, usually requires a weight reduction diet.

51. **(B)** Client need: health promotion and maintenance; subcategory: prevention and early detection of disease; content area: pediatrics

RATIONALE

(A) Aspirin should not be given on an empty stomach because it is irritating to the mucosa. (B) Bleeding from decreased clotting capacity may be caused by aspirin toxicity. (C) A regular schedule of aspirin administration is important to maintain a satisfactory drug level in the body. (D) Aspirin toxicity may affect cranial nerve VIII, leading to tinnitus (ringing in the ears).

52. **(A)** Client need: physiological integrity; subcategory: reduction of risk potential; content area: pediatrics

RATIONALE

(A) Because the extremity may continue to swell and the cast could constrict circulation, the nurse should elevate the limb and observe for capillary refill, warmth, mobility of toes and circulation. (B) Although muscle tone may diminish over time in the affected limb, this is not the immediate concern. (C) The limb has been immobilized already by the cast, and therefore immobilization is not a concern. (D) Heated fans and dryers are discouraged because the outside cast will dry quickly, yet the area beneath the cast remains wet and could cause burns.

53. **(D)** Client need: physiological integrity; subcategory: pharmacological and parenteral therapies; content area: pediatrics

RATIONALE

(A) Giving the drug with or after meals may allay gastrointestinal discomfort. Giving the drug with a fatty meal (ice cream or milk) increases absorption rate. (B) Griseofulvin may alter taste sensations and thereby decrease the appetite. Monitoring of food intake is important, and inadequate nutrient intake should be reported to the physician. (C) The child may experience symptomatic relief after 48–96 hours of therapy. It is important to stress continuing the drug therapy to prevent relapse (usually about 6 weeks). (D) The incidence of side effects is low; however, headaches are common. Nausea, vomiting, diarrhea, and anorexia may occur. Dizziness, although uncommon, should be reported to the physician.

54. **(C)** Client need: health promotion and maintenance; subcategory: prevention and early detection of disease; content area: pediatrics

RATIONALE

(A) Concentrated sweets are eliminated from diet planning. Complex carbohydrates may be taken at the time of increased activity. (B) Food restriction is not used for diabetic control of growing children. Caloric restriction may be imposed for weight control if necessary. (C) Total caloric intake and proportions of basic nutrients should be consistent from day to day. Distribution of these calories should fit the activity pattern. Extra food is needed for increased activity. A balance of food, exercise, and insulin should be maintained. (D) Because of the increased risk of atherosclerosis, the fat percentage of the total caloric intake is reduced.

55. **(D)** Client need: physiological integrity; subcategory: reduction of risk potential; content area: pediatrics

RATIONALE

(A) The nurse should discourage the child from coughing, clearing the throat, or putting objects in his mouth. These may induce bleeding. (B) Cool, clear liquids may be given when child is fully alert. Warm liquids may dislodge a blood clot. The nurse should avoid red- or brown-colored liquids to distinguish fresh or old blood from ingested liquid should the child vomit. (C) Gargles and vigorous toothbrushing could initiate bleeding. (D) Postoperative hemorrhage, though unusual, may occur. The nurse should observe for bleeding by looking directly into the throat and for vomiting of bright red blood, continuous swallowing, and changes in vital signs.

56. **(A)** Client need: physiological integrity; subcategory: physiological adaptation; content area: pediatrics

RATIONALE

(A) The airway in children is much smaller than it is in adults. The diameter of the trachea in the newborn is 4 mm and that of the adult is 20 mm. A small change in the diameter of the airway can make a major difference in the pediatric client. (B) The tongue is proportionally larger in children and fills most of the oral cavity, thereby decreasing air space. (C) The entire pediatric airway is elastic. Elasticity diminishes with age, however. (D) The distances between respiratory structures are shorter than that of adults, and therefore organisms are able to move more rapidly down the throat, leading to more extensive respiratory involvement.

57. **(B)** Client need: physiological integrity; subcategory: reduction of risk potential; content area: pediatrics

RATIONALE

(A) A high-protein diet is usually indicated because protein is excreted in urine. Protein restriction is usually prescribed with severe azotemia. (B) The kidneys usually enlarge in these children, and sodium and water are retained. (C) Fluid restriction may be ordered to help reduce edema; however, monitoring for dehydration is indicated. (D) A high-cholesterol diet would not be indicated for any child, especially one with elevated blood pressure.

58. **(C)** Client need: physiological integrity; subcategory: physiological adaptation; content area: pediatrics

RATIONALE

(A) Wiping from front to back is wiping from an area of lesser contamination (urethra) to an area of greater contamination (rectum). (B) Generous fluid intake reduces the concentration of urine. (C) Cotton is a natural, absorbent fabric. Nylon often predisposes the client to urinary tract infections. Dark, warm, moist areas are excellent media for bacterial growth. (D) With vesicoureteral reflux, urine refluxes into the ureter(s) during voiding and then returns to the bladder (residual), which becomes a source for future infection.

59. **(B)** Client need: physiological integrity; subcategory: pharmacological and parenteral therapies; content area: pediatrics

RATIONALE

(A) If awakened first, the child will know that nothing painful will be done without the child being alerted. (B) The ventrogluteal site is a safe site for children because it is a large muscle free of major nerves and blood vessels. (C) The dorsogluteal site is not recommended in children who have not been walking for at least 1 year because the muscle is not fully developed. (D) The parent will be able to offer support and comfort during and after the injection.

60. **(A)** Client need: physiological integrity; subcategory: pharmacological and parenteral therapies; content area: pediatrics

RATIONALE

(A) The volume to be infused should be diluted medication volume added to the volume control chamber (10 mL) plus the tubing volume (12 mL). The general formula for calculating IV medications for children is: Rate = Volume to Be Infused × Administration Set Drop Factor (microdrop: 60 gtts/min) ÷ Desired Time to Infuse in Minutes Rate = (10 + 12)22 × 60 ÷ 30 = 44 mL/hr. (B, C, D) These values are incorrect.

61. **(B)** Client need: physiological integrity; subcategory: basic care and comfort; content area: pediatrics

RATIONALE

(A, C, D) These answers are incorrect. (B) Normal fluid requirement for this pediatric client is based on the fact that 0–10 kg of weight equals 100 mL/kg per day. This infant weighs 15 pounds (6.8 kg). Thus, 100 mL × 6.8 = 680 mL/day.

62. **(A)** Client need: physiological integrity; subcategory: reduction of risk potential; content area: pediatrics

RATIONALE

(A) The nurse should emphasize what is required to elicit cooperation and help to develop a sense of autonomy. (B) The child may express discomfort verbally and should be encouraged to express his feelings. (C) Selecting nonthreatening words to explain a procedure will prevent misinterpretation. (D) When explaining the procedure to the parent with the child present, the nurse should use words that the child can understand to avoid misunderstanding.

63. **(B)** Client need: psychosocial integrity; subcategory: coping and adaptation; content area: pediatrics

RATIONALE

(A) The 6 month old should be examined first. If several children will be examined, begin with the most cooperative and less anxious child to provide modeling. (B) Providing time for play and getting acquainted minimizes stress and anxiety associated with assessment of body parts. (C) Children generally cooperate best when their mother remains with them. (D) Painful areas are best examined last and will permit maximum accuracy of assessment.

64. **(D)** Client need: physiological integrity; subcategory: physiological adaptation; content area: pediatrics

RATIONALE

(A) There is no evidence of pain in infants with pyloric stenosis whether eating or not. (B) There are both good appetite and feeding habits in these children. (C) Because of regurgitation, there is usually decreased frequency and quantity of stools and also signs of dehydration and weight loss. (D) Along with upper abdominal distention, there is a characteristic palpable olive-shaped mass located to the right of the umbilicus.

65. **(B)** Client need: physiological integrity; subcategory: physiological adaptation; content area: pediatrics

RATIONALE

(A) With the slight and mild hard of hearing, auditory training is beneficial. (B) Speech is the most difficult task because it is

learned by visual and auditory stimulation, imitation, and reinforcement. (C, D) Lip reading and signing are aimed at establishing communicative skills, but they are learned more easily by
visual stimulation.

66. **(C)** Client need: health promotion and maintenance; subcategory: prevention and early detection of disease; content area:
pediatrics

RATIONALE
(A) Oral iron supplements are contraindicated in thalassemia. (B)
Although heart failure may be an end result of this disease, this
action is unnecessary. (C) Iron overload is a potential complication of frequent blood transfusions of children with thalassemia.
(D) Children should be encouraged to pursue activities related to
their exercise tolerance.

67. **(A)** Client need: health promotion and maintenance; subcategory: prevention and early detection of disease; content area:
pediatrics

RATIONALE
(A) Partial thromboplastic time measures activity of thromboplastin, which depends on the intrinsic clotting factors deficient
in children who are hemophiliacs. (B) Platelet counts are normal
in hemophilia. (C) Hemophilia does not affect the complete
blood count. (D) Bleeding times are normal in hemophiliacs.
They measure the time interval for the bleeding from small superficial wounds to cease.

68. **(B)** Client need: physiological integrity; subcategory: physiological adaptation; content area: pediatrics

RATIONALE
(A) Because the left atrial pressure is greater than right atrial pressure, oxygenated blood flows from the left to the right atria. (B)
Because of the risk of pulmonary obstructive diseases and congestive heart failure later in life, surgery is usually performed between age 4 and 6 years, with essentially no operative mortality
or postoperative complications. (C) Many ventricular septal defects close spontaneously (20–60%) as a result of growth and
proliferation of the muscular septum or formation of a membrane across the opening. (D) This management is usually recommended with children with mild pulmonary stenosis.

69. **(D)** Client need: physiological integrity; subcategory: pharmacological and parenteral therapies; content area: psychiatric

RATIONALE
(A) When alcohol is ingested with disulfiram therapy, the client
experiences nausea, vomiting, and a potentially serious drop in
blood pressure. (B) Disulfiram is most successful when used
early in the recovery process while the individual makes major
lifestyle changes necessary for long-term recovery. (C) Disulfiram works on the classical conditioning principle. (D) The effects
of disulfiram can be felt when alcohol is ingested 1–2 weeks after disulfiram is discontinued.

70. **(C)** Client need: psychosocial integrity; subcategory: coping
and adaptation; content area: psychiatric

RATIONALE
(A) This response cuts off communication with the client. It does
not address her feelings. (B) Reality orientation frequently does
not work alone. Feelings must be addressed. Telling a client to
calm down is frequently ineffective. (C) Reminiscence is used
here to reorient and recall past pleasant events. Talking about the
restaurant will allay anxiety. (D) This response may confirm to
the client that she indeed does still own a restaurant, buying into
her confusion. Her feelings and anxiety require nursing intervention.

71. **(A)** Client need: psychosocial integrity; subcategory: coping
and adaptation; content area: psychiatric

RATIONALE
(A) This statement acknowledges that it is difficult but is not
threatening or punitive. (B) This statement is threatening and describes specific punishment for further deviant behavior. (C)
This response elicits shame by blaming her for involving others.
(D) This response gives her permission to break the rules but indicates that getting caught is wrong.

72. **(D)** Client need: psychosocial integrity; subcategory: coping
and adaptation; content area: psychiatric

RATIONALE
(A) Identity versus role confusion is experienced by adolescents
making the transition from childhood to adulthood as they attempt to develop a sense of identity. (B) Integrity versus despair
is experienced by the elderly as they reflect on their life in an attempt to find meaning. (C) Intimacy versus isolation is experienced by young adults as they establish intimate bonds of love
and friendship. (D) Generativity versus self-absorption is experienced by middle-aged adults as they fulfill life goals that involve
family, career, and society. The client is experiencing this crisis.

73. **(D)** Client need: psychosocial integrity; subcategory: coping
and adaptation; content area: psychiatric

RATIONALE
(A) Asking the client to provide an explanation for her feelings is
often intimidating. (B) This response is probing and may make the
client feel used and valued only for the information she can provide. (C) This underrates the client's feelings and belittles her concerns. It may cause the client to stop sharing feelings for fear that
they will be ridiculed. (D) The emphasis is on working with the
client. It shows that there is hope for change through collaboration.

74. **(C)** Client need: physiological integrity; subcategory; pharmacological and parenteral therapies; content area: psychiatric

RATIONALE
(A) A daily dose of fluoxetine should be taken in the morning.
Afternoon doses may cause nervousness and insomnia. (B) Although fluoxetine is less sedating than other antidepressants, it
may still cause dizziness or drowsiness in some clients. The nurse
should caution clients to avoid driving or hazardous activities
until the central nervous system effects of the drug are demonstrated. (C) Rashes or pruritus do commonly occur early in therapy and respond to antihistamines or topical corticosteroids. (D)
Advise the client not to take over-the-counter or other prescription drugs without consulting with the physician. Fluoxetine
does interact with other common drugs such as monoamine oxidase inhibitors, diazepam, insulin, oral antidiabetic agents, tricyclic antidepressants, and tryptophan.

75. **(D)** Client need: psychosocial integrity; subcategory: coping
and adaptation; content area: psychiatric

RATIONALE
(A) Repression is blocking a desire from conscious expression.
The client is conscious of his desires. (B) Regression is returning
to an earlier form of expression, which is not demonstrated here.
(C) Reaction formation is acting out the opposite of true feelings.
The client felt anger concerning his wife's cooking and acted out
his feelings. (D) Rationalization is unconsciously falsifying an experience by giving a "rational" explanation. The client is attempting to justify his behavior by giving an explanation.

76. **(D)** Client need; psychosocial integrity; subcategory: psychosocial adaptation; content area: psychiatric

RATIONALE
(A) To the client, suicide may be a reasonable action and the only
one he can cope with at this time. (B) This response indicates to
the client that his intention to commit suicide is not important to
the nurse at this time. (C) The client is so depressed that he is not
able to see the positive aspects of his life. At no time should the

nurse discuss another client's problems in conversation. (D) This statement tells the client that the nurse recognizes his problem is of a serious nature and will take all steps necessary to help him.

77. **(A)** Client need: physiological integrity; subcategory: physiological adaptation; content area: psychiatric

    RATIONALE

    (A) The client is demonstrating dyskinesia, which is involuntary muscular activity, such as tic, spasm, or myoclonus. (B) Akathisia is regular rhythmic movements usually of the lower limbs, such as constant motor restlessness. (C) Echopraxia is mimicking the movements of another person. (D) Echolalia is mimicking the speech of another person.

78. **(D)** Client need: psychosocial integrity; subcategory: coping and adaptation; content area: psychiatric

    RATIONALE

    (A) This statement is an example of adaptive rationalization. She is coping with her disappointment by rationalizing. This is adaptive because no harm is done to self or others. It is used to protect her ego. (B) This is an example of maladaptive suppression. She is suppressing the seriousness of the lump. It is maladaptive because delaying treatment will cause harm to her. (C) The client's actions are an example of maladaptive denial. She is denying her son's death by not facing his possessions. Until she faces his death, she cannot face reality. (D) This is an example of adaptive suppression. She realizes the impact of her husband's statement but delays discussion until she can devote her full attention to the matter.

79. **(A)** Client need: psychosocial integrity; subcategory: psychosocial adaptation; content area: psychiatric

    RATIONALE

    (A) The nurse must be honest, direct, professional, and attentive in her interview to gain the parent's trust. (B) The nurse should approach the parents in private, away from the child. (C) Asking them to relive and evaluate the situation may be looked at as placing blame on the parents for the child's "accident." At this point, the parents may get defensive and stop communicating. (D) Although you may call child protective services, the nurse should inform the parents of their responsibility to do this and explain the process to them.

80. **(D)** Client need: psychosocial integrity; subcategory: psychosocial adaptation; content area: psychiatric

    RATIONALE

    (A) There is no evidence of fear as the child is unable to communicate. (B) There is actual injury, but the parents have not yet admitted causing the child's injuries. (C) This diagnosis is incomplete. There is no specific ineffective coping behavior identified in this nursing diagnosis. (D) Altered family process best describes the family dynamics in this situation. The parents have admitted severe disciplinary action.

81. **(C)** Client need: psychosocial integrity; subcategory: psychosocial adaptation; content area: psychiatric

    RATIONALE

    (A) Assessing the level of anxiety, coping responses, and support systems is very important, but not of highest priority at this time. (B) A history of physical abuse is an important part of assessment. The nurses must also always ask if there is abuse of the children. (C) Although all of these answers are very important in assessment, the highest priority is assessment of suicide potential, because this could cause the greatest harm to the client. Feeling there is no other way out, abused spouses may consider suicide. (D) The spouse may be self-medicating herself with alcohol or drugs to escape an awful situation. The abuser may also be abusing drugs or alcohol. If this is so, the nurse should encourage the spouse to seek counseling and not to return to the home.

82. **(A)** Client need: psychosocial integrity; subcategory: psychosocial adaptation; content area: psychiatric

    RATIONALE

    (A) Providing the victim with these instructions will aid in the determination of physical evidence of rape. Victims frequently feel "dirty" after rape, and their first instinct is to take care of personal hygiene before facing anyone. (B) This action is of lesser importance at this time. (C) Although this is a nursing measure appropriate in this situation, contacting a counselor can be done once the victim enters the hospital. Frequently victims call but do not follow up with the visit. (D) Once the victim enters the emergency room, it is important not to leave her alone.

83. **(B)** Client need: psychosocial integrity; subcategory: coping and adaptation; content area: psychiatric

    RATIONALE

    (A) Dissociation is separating a group of mental processes from consciousness or identity, such as multiple personalities. That is not evident in this situation. (B) Intellectualization is excessive use of reasoning, logic, or words usually without experiencing associated feelings. This is the defense mechanism that this client is using. (C) Rationalization is giving a socially acceptable reason for behavior rather than the actual reason. She is discussing events, not reasons. (D) Displacement is a shift of emotion associated with an anxiety-producing person, object, or situation to a less threatening object.

84. **(C)** Client need: psychosocial integrity; subcategory: coping and adaptation; content area: psychiatric

    RATIONALE

    (A) The nurse should not ask him to sit down. Pacing is the activity he has chosen to deal with his anxiety. The nurse dealing with this client should speak slowly and with short, simple sentences. (B) The client may already recognize the anxiety and is attempting to deal with it. (C) Walk with the client as he paces. This gives support while he uses anxiety-generated energy. (D) Increasing the level of supervision may be appropriate after he stops pacing. It would minimize self-injury and/or loss of control.

85. **(A)** Client need: psychosocial integrity; subcategory: coping and adaptation; content area: psychiatric

    RATIONALE

    (A) This situation provides specific evidence that the client is able to integrate muscle relaxation technique into his lifestyle to alleviate anxiety. (B) The client may not experience anxiety at the concert, but there is no evidence regarding the technique that he used to alleviate anxiety. (C) The client may state he no longer experiences anxiety, but there is no evidence demonstrating this. He may be denying anxiety to discontinue therapy prematurely. (D) Does he experience anxiety in the darkroom? He may have taken this job to force himself to deal with the phobia directly.

86. **(D)** Client need: psychosocial integrity; subcategory: coping and adaptation; content area: psychiatric

    RATIONALE

    (A) It is rare that a hospital has a specific policy addressing this particular issue. If the statement is true, the nurse should show evidence of the policy to the family and suggest alternatives, such as the hospital chapel. (B) Refusal to leave the room demonstrates a lack of understanding related to the family's need to grieve in their own manner. (C) The nurse should leave the room and allow the family privacy in their grief. (D) The family's wish to conduct a religious ceremony in the client's room is part of the grief process. The request is based on specific cultural and religious differences dictating social customs.

87. **(C)** Client need: physiological integrity; subcategory: pharmacological and parenteral therapies; content area: psychiatric

RATIONALE

(A) The client should maintain a normal diet including normal salt intake. A low-sodium diet can cause lithium retention, leading to toxicity. (B) Lithium must be taken with meals because it is irritating to the gastric mucosa. (C) Diarrhea, vomiting, or diaphoresis can cause dehydration, which will increase lithium blood levels. If these symptoms occur, the nurse should instruct the client to withhold lithium. (D) Lithium is not to be taken with over-the-counter drugs without specific instruction. Some drugs raise lithium levels, whereas others lower lithium levels.

88. **(A)** Client need: physiological integrity; subcategory: pharmacological and parenteral therapies; content area: psychiatric

RATIONALE

(A) Tardive dyskinesia is a common side effect of antipsychotic medications such as haloperidol. Discontinuing the medication can alleviate symptoms. (B) Although mild tremors are an early sign of Parkinson's disease, haloperidol must be discontinued first and the client further evaluated. (C) These symptoms do not necessarily indicate a more advanced stage of Alzheimer's disease. (D) Most antipsychotic drugs are chemically similar and will produce the same side effects.

89. **(D)** Client need: psychosocial integrity; subcategory: psychosocial adaptation; content area: psychiatric

RATIONALE

(A) This expected outcome is specific as related to attendance, but not specific as related to outcome criteria. (B) Stating activities does not guarantee involvement. (C) This goal may help the recovery process, but postcounseling behavior is not addressed. (D) This statement best describes the expected outcome. The client will be attending group therapy sessions and through them he will deal with his feelings.

TEST 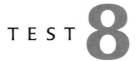 8

East Carolina University School of Nursing Test

MOCK NCLEX-RN BOARD REVIEW TEST QUESTIONS

1. A client has been instructed in how to take her nitroglycerin tablets. The nurse giving her instructions knows the client understands the information when she tells her:

   A. "I should contact my physician if I have headaches after I take this medicine."
   B. "I should keep the tablets in the refrigerator."
   C. "I should call the doctor if three doses of the medicine do not relieve my pain."
   D. "I should take these with water but not with milk."

2. A client has renal failure. Today's lab values indicate he has an elevated serum potassium. What additional priority information does the nurse need to obtain?

   A. Evaluation of his level of consciousness
   B. Evaluation of an electrocardiogram
   C. Measurement of his urine output for the past 8 hours
   D. Serum potassium lab values for the last several days

3. A client's wife is concerned over his behavior in recent months. He has been diagnosed with Parkinson's disease, and she is telling his nurse that he has been doing "strange things." The nurse reassures the wife that the following behavior is normal with Parkinson's disease:

   A. "Your husband will experience some periods of muscle flaccidity. Be sure to make him sit down during these periods."
   B. "Your husband may move his hands in motions that look like he is rolling a pill between his fingers."
   C. "Twitching of the muscles is to be expected and can occur at any time during the day."
   D. "Parkinson's disease causes severe pain in the joints. You should give your husband Tylenol at those times."

4. A male client tells his nurse that he has had an ulcer in the past and is afraid it is "flaring up again." The nurse begins to ask him specific questions about his symptoms. The nurse knows that a symptom that might indicate a serious complication of an ulcer is:

   A. Pain in the middle of the night
   B. A bowel movement every 3–5 days
   C. Melena
   D. Episodes of nausea and vomiting

5. A client has chronic obstructive pulmonary disease. She is slowly losing weight, and her daughter is very concerned about increasing her nutrition. The nurse helps the daughter devise a plan of care for her mother. The plan of care should include which of the following interventions to promote nutrition?

   A. Offer her oral hygiene before and after meals.
   B. Encourage her to consume milk products.
   C. Encourage her to engage in an activity before a meal to stimulate her appetite.
   D. Restrict her fluid intake to three glasses of water a day.

6. A female client is concerned that she is in a "high-risk" group for the development of acquired immunodeficiency syndrome (AIDS). She wants to know about the advisability of donating blood. Which of the following responses is correct?

   A. "Individuals who donate blood are at risk of getting the AIDS virus. You should not donate."
   B. "It's OK for you to donate because the blood bank has a test that is 100% effective."
   C. "You should not donate since it takes time to develop antibodies to the AIDS virus. If you donate blood before you develop the antibody, you could pass it on in the blood."
   D. "It is not a good idea for you to donate. If you have AIDS, the information is made public and could destroy your personal life."

7. A 50-year-old male client is to receive chemotherapy. The physician's orders include antiemetics. When planning his care, the nurse should take into consideration

that antiemetics are best administered in the following way:

A. Give antiemetics when nausea is experienced and continue on a regular schedule for 12–24 hours.
B. Give antiemetics prior to the client receiving chemotherapy and continue on a regular basis for at least 24–48 hours after chemotherapy.
C. Give antiemetics one at a time because combinations of antiemetics cause overwhelming side effects.
D. Give antiemetics intermittently during the entire course of chemotherapy.

8. A 30-year-old female client is receiving antineoplastic chemotherapy. Which of the following symptoms should especially concern the nurse when caring for her?

A. Respiratory rate of 16 breaths/min
B. Pulse rate of 80 bpm
C. Complaints of muscle aches
D. A sore throat

9. Seven days ago, a 45-year-old female client had an ileostomy. She is self-sufficient and well otherwise. Which of the following long-term objectives would be unrealistic?

A. She should be able to control evacuation of her bowels.
B. She should be able to return to a regular diet.
C. She should be able to resume sexual activity.
D. She should be able to manage her own care.

10. A 26-year-old client has no children. She has had an abdominal hysterectomy. In the first 24 hours postoperatively, the nurse would be concerned if the client:

A. Cries easily and says she is having abdominal pain
B. Develops a temperature of 102°F
C. Has no bowel sounds
D. Has a urine output of 200 mL for 4 hours

11. A 44-year-old female client is receiving external radiation to her scapula for metastasis of breast cancer. Teaching related to skin care for the client would include which of the following?

A. Teach her to completely clean the skin to remove all ointments and markings after each treatment.
B. Teach her to cover broken skin in the treated area with a medicated ointment.
C. Encourage her to wear a tight-fitting vest to support her scapula.
D. Encourage her to avoid direct sunlight on the area being treated.

12. A male client is being treated in the burn unit for third-degree burns on his head, neck, and upper chest received in the last 24 hours. The nurse is evaluating the effectiveness of fluid resuscitation. Which of the following indicates effective fluid balance?

A. His weight increases from 165 to 175 lb.
B. His urine output is equal to his total fluid intake.
C. His urine output has been >35 mL/hr for the past 12 hours.
D. His blood pressure is 94/62.

13. A 24-year-old male client is admitted with a diagnosis of sickle cell anemia. The nurse discusses his disease with him and emphasizes the following information:

A. He should monitor his sputum, stools, and urine for signs of bleeding.
B. His daily diet should include a large amount of fluid.
C. He should not be concerned about having to fly on a commuter airplane on a weekly basis.
D. He should not worry about having children because this disease is passed on only by female carriers.

14. A female client has been diagnosed with chronic renal failure. She is a candidate for either peritoneal dialysis or hemodialysis and must make a choice between the two. Which information should the nurse give her to help her decide?

A. Hemodialysis involves less time to filter the blood; but the client must consider travel time, distance, and inconvenience.
B. Hemodialysis involves more time to filter the blood than does peritoneal dialysis.
C. Peritoneal dialysis has almost no complications and is less time consuming than hemodialysis. Therefore it is preferred.
D. Peritoneal dialysis requires that a home health nurse prepare and administer the treatments.

15. A female client decides on hemodialysis. She has an internal vascular access device placed. To ensure patency of the device, the nurse must:

A. Assess the site for leakage of blood or fluids
B. Auscultate the site for a bruit
C. Assess the site for bruising or hematoma
D. Inspect the site for color, warmth, and sensation

16. A client is receiving peritoneal dialysis. He has been taught to warm the dialyzing fluid prior to instilling it because:

A. Warmed solution helps keep the body temperature maintained within a normal range during instillation
B. Warmed solution helps dilate the peritoneal blood vessels
C. Warmed solution decreases the risk of peritoneal infection
D. Warmed solution promotes a relaxed abdominal muscle

17. A female client is exhibiting signs of respiratory distress. Which of the following signs indicate a possible pneumothorax?

A. Crackles or rales on the affected side
B. Bradypnea and bradycardia
C. Shortness of breath and sharp pain on the affected side
D. Increased breath sounds on the affected side

18. A female client has a chest tube placed. It is accidentally pulled out of the intrapleural space when she is ambulating. The first action the nurse should take is to:

A. Instruct the client to cough deeply to re-expand her lung
B. Put on sterile gloves and replace the tube
C. Apply a petrolatum dressing over the site

D. Auscultate the lung to determine if she needs the tube replaced

19. A male client has heart failure. He has been instructed to gradually increase his activities. Which signs and symptoms of worsening heart failure should the nurse tell him to watch for that would indicate a need for him to lower his activity level?
    A. Pain in his legs when he walks
    B. Thirst, weight loss, and polyuria
    C. Drowsiness and lethargy after his activities
    D. Weight gain, edema in his lower extremities, and shortness of breath

20. A male client is undergoing cardiac tests. He has been instructed to wear a Holter monitor. The nurse knows she has included the appropriate information in her teaching when the client tells her:
    A. "He should remove the electrodes for bathing."
    B. "Damage to his heart muscle will be recorded by the monitor."
    C. "He is to keep a record of everything he does during the day."
    D. "He is to refrain from activities that cause chest pain."

21. To prevent thrombophlebitis in a client on complete bed rest, the nursing care plan should include:
    A. Dangle the client's legs over the edge of the bed every shift.
    B. Massage the client's calves briskly every shift.
    C. Keep the client's legs extended and discourage any movement.
    D. Have the client tighten and relax leg muscles several times daily.

22. A 78-year-old female client has a total hip arthroplasty. Her nurse should know that which of the following is contraindicated?
    A. Encourage exercises in the unaffected extremities.
    B. Encourage her to cross and uncross her legs.
    C. Check neurological and circulatory status of the affected leg hourly.
    D. Place a trochanter roll along the upper thigh of the affected leg.

23. A male client has a history of diverticulosis. He has questions about the foods that he should eat. His nurse gives him the following information:
    A. He should be on a high-fiber diet.
    B. He should eat a low-residue diet.
    C. He should drink minimal amounts of fluids.
    D. He does not need to make any modifications.

24. A term neonate has experienced no distress at birth and has an Apgar score of 9. Her mother has asked to breast-feed her following delivery. Immediately after birth, the neonate was most susceptible to heat loss. The most appropriate intervention to conserve heat loss and promote bonding is to:
    A. Place her under the radiant warmer
    B. Dry her with blankets

C. Place her to her mother's breast
D. Place her on a heated pad

25. A client who is gravida 1 para 1 vaginally delivered a 7-lb girl. She received a midline episiotomy at delivery. When assessing the level of her uterus immediately following delivery, the nurse would expect the fundus to be located:
    A. At the umbilicus
    B. At the symphysis pubis
    C. Midway between the umbilicus and the xiphoid process
    D. Midway between the umbilicus and the symphysis pubis

26. A 19-year-old primigravida is admitted to the labor and delivery suite of the hospital. Her husband is accompanying her. The couple tells the nurse that this is the first hospital admission for her. The client's vaginal exam indicates she is 3 cm dilated, 80% effaced, and at −0 station. Based on the vaginal exam, she is in:
    A. Stage 2, latent phase
    B. Stage 1, active phase
    C. Stage 3, transition phase
    D. Stage 1, latent phase

27. A client is pregnant for the fourth time and has had three normal vaginal deliveries. She is in active labor and fully dilated. Suddenly she calls, "Nurse, the baby is coming." As the nurse responds to her call, which one of the following observations should the nurse make first?
    A. Inspect the perineum.
    B. Time the contractions.
    C. Prepare a sterile area for delivery.
    D. Auscultate for fetal heart rate (FHR).

28. A client has just received an epidural block. She is laboring on her right side. The nurse notes that her blood pressure has dropped from 132/68 to 78/42 mm Hg. The nurse's first action would be to:
    A. Call the physician immediately and give dopamine IM
    B. Turn her on her left side and recheck her blood pressure in 5 minutes
    C. Administer oxytocin (Pitocin) immediately and increase the rate of IV fluids
    D. Increase the rate of IV fluids and start O_2 by mask

29. A 28-year-old client comes to the clinic for her first prenatal examination. In relating her obstetrical history, she tells the nurse that she has been pregnant twice before. She had a "miscarriage" with the first pregnancy after 6 weeks. With the second pregnancy, she delivered twin girls at 31 weeks' gestation. One of the twins was stillborn and the other twin died at 4 days of age. Using a five-digit system, the nurse records her as being:
    A. 2-0-2-1-0
    B. 2-2-2-1-2
    C. 3-0-1-1-0
    D. 2-1-1-0-0

30. A 22-year-old client is 16 weeks pregnant. She and her husband are expecting their first baby. The client tells

the nurse that her last normal menstrual period was February 16, with 3 days of spotting on February 17, 18, and 19. The nurse calculates her expected date of delivery to be:

A. November 23rd
B. December 26th
C. September 14th
D. December 9th

31. On the third postpartum day, a client complains of extremely tender breasts. On palpation, the nurse notes a very firm, shiny appearance to the breasts and some milk leakage. She is bottle feeding. The nurse should initially recommend to her to:

A. Take 2 ibuprofen (Motrin) tablets by mouth now because the baby will be returning for feeding in 20 minutes
B. Allow the infant to breast-feed at the next feeding time to empty the breasts
C. Apply ice packs to the breasts and wear a supportive, well-fitting bra
D. Take a warm shower and express milk from both breasts until empty

32. A registered nurse is trying to determine the appropriate care that she should provide for her obstetrical clients. Which of the following documents is considered the legal standard of practice?

A. State nursing practice act
B. AWHONN Standards for the Nursing Care of Women and Newborns
C. American Nurses' Association Standards of Maternal-Child Health Nursing
D. International Council of Nurses' Code

33. A female client admitted to the labor and delivery unit thinks her bag of water "broke" approximately 2 hours ago. She is having mild contractions 5 minutes apart. The *most* immediate nursing intervention would be to:

A. Note the color and amount of fluid on her clothes.
B. Assess the FHR.
C. Notify the physician.
D. Place the nitrazine test paper at the cervical os and note the color change.

34. A new mother experiences strong uterine contractions while breast-feeding her baby. She excitedly rings for the nurse. When the nurse arrives the mother tells her, "Something is wrong. This is like my labor." Which reply by the nurse identifies the physiological response of the client?

A. "Your breasts are secreting a hormone that enters your bloodstream and causes your abdominal muscles to contract."
B. "Prolactin increases the blood supply to your uterus, and you are feeling the effects of this blood vessel engorgement."
C. "The same hormone that is released in response to the baby's sucking, causing milk to flow, also causes the uterus to contract."
D. "There is probably a small blood clot or placental fragment in your uterus, and your uterus is contracting to expel it."

35. A 20-year-old female client delivers a stillborn infant. Following the delivery, an appropriate response by the labor nurse to the question, "Why did this happen to my baby?" is:

A. "It's God's will. It was probably for the best. There was something probably wrong with your baby."
B. "You're young. You can have other children later."
C. "I know your other children will be a great comfort to you."
D. "I can see you're upset. Would you like to see and hold your baby?"

36. A client's prenatal screening indicated that she has no immunity to rubella. She is now 10 weeks pregnant. The *best* time to immunize her is:

A. In the immediate postpartum period
B. After the first trimester
C. At 28 weeks' gestation
D. Within 72 hours postpartum

37. A 24-year-old woman who is gravida 1 reports, "I can't take iron pills because they make me sick." She continues, "My bowels aren't moving either." In counseling her based on these complaints, the nurse's *most* appropriate response would be, "It would be beneficial for you to eat . . .

A. prunes."
B. green leafy vegetables."
C. red meat."
D. eggs."

38. A 26-year-old female client presents at 10 weeks' gestation. She currently is a G_3 1-0-1-1. Her mother and grandmother have heart disease. Her grandmother also has insulin-dependent diabetes. The client's previous delivery was a term female infant weighing 9 lb 13 oz. The client is 5 ft 6 inches tall and her current weight is 130 lb. Based on her history, she is at risk for developing diabetes in pregnancy. Which of the following factors places her at risk for gestational diabetes?

A. Age >25 years
B. Maternal weight
C. Previous birth of an infant weighing >9 lb
D. Family history of heart disease

39. The nurse assesses a client's monitor strip and finds the following: uterine contractions every 3–4 minutes, lasting 60–70 seconds; FHR baseline 134–146 bpm, with accelerations to 158 bpm with fetal movement. Which nursing intervention is appropriate?

A. Notify physician of nonreassuring FHR pattern.
B. Turn the client to her left side.
C. Start IV for fetal distress and administer O_2 at 6–8 liters by mask.
D. Evaluate to see if the monitor strip is reassuring.

40. Early in her ninth month of pregnancy, a client has been diagnosed as having mild preeclampsia. In counseling her about her diet, the nurse must emphasize the importance of:

A. Decreasing her sodium intake
B. Decreasing her fluids

C. Increasing her carbohydrate intake

D. Eating a moderate to high-protein diet

41. A 30-year-old client in the third trimester of her pregnancy asks the nurse for advice about upper respiratory discomforts. She complains of nasal stuffiness and epistaxis, most noticeable on the left side. Which reply by the nurse is correct?

A. "It sounds as though you are coming down with a bad cold. I'll ask the doctor to prescribe a decongestant for relief of symptoms."

B. "A good vaporizer will help; avoid the cool air kind. Also, try saline nose drops, and spend less time on your left side."

C. "These discomforts are all a result of increased blood supply; one of the pregnancy hormones, estrogen, causes them."

D. "This is most unusual. I'm sure your obstetrician will want you to see an ENT (ear, nose, throat) specialist."

42. A newborn girl's father expresses concern that the newborn does not have good control of her hands and arms. It is important for the father to realize certain neurological patterns that characterize the newborn:

A. Mild hypotonia is expected in the upper extremities.

B. Purposeless, uncoordinated movements of the arms are indicative of neurological dysfunction.

C. Function progresses in a head-to-toe, proximal-distal fashion.

D. Asymmetrical movement of the extremities is not unusual and will disappear with maturation of the central nervous system.

43. A client delivered a term infant 1 hour ago. Her uterus on assessment is boggy and is U +1 in contrast to the previous assessment of U −2. The immediate nursing response is to:

A. Administer methergine IM

B. Remove the retained placental fragments

C. Assist the client to the bathroom and provide cues to stimulate urination

D. Massage the fundus until firm

44. A 35-year-old primigravida comes to the clinic for her first prenatal visit. The midwife, on examining the client, suspects that she is approximately 11 weeks pregnant. The pregnancy is positively confirmed by finding:

A. Chadwick's sign

B. FHR by ultrasound

C. Enlargement of the uterus

D. Breast tenderness and enlargement

45. A female client has been treated since childhood for mitral valve prolapse. The antibiotic of choice for her during pregnancy would be:

A. Sulfa

B. Tetracycline

C. Hydralazine

D. Erythromycin

46. A pregnant client complains of varicosities in the third trimester. Which of the following activities should she be advised to avoid?

A. Sitting with legs crossed at ankles

B. Wearing thromboembolic disease (TED) stockings

C. Wearing support pantyhose

D. Wearing knee-high stockings

47. A client at 9 weeks' gestation comes for an initial prenatal visit. On assessment, the nurse discovers this is her second pregnancy. Her first pregnancy resulted in a spontaneous abortion. She is 28 years old, in good health, and works full-time as an elementary school teacher. This information alerts the nurse to which of the following:

A. An increased risk in maternal adaptation to pregnancy

B. The need for anticipatory guidance regarding the pregnancy

C. The need for teaching regarding family planning

D. An increased risk for subsequent abortions

48. A client is pleased about being pregnant, yet states, "It is really not the best time, but I guess it will be OK." The nurse's assessment of this response is:

A. Initial maternal-infant bonding may be poor.

B. Client may have a poor relationship with her husband.

C. This response is normal in the first trimester.

D. This response is abnormal, to be re-evaluated at the next visit.

49. A client at 6 months' gestation complains of tiredness and dizziness. Her hemoglobin level is 10 g/dL, and her hematocrit value is 32%. Her nutritional intake is assessed as sufficient. The most likely diagnosis is:

A. Iron-deficiency anemia

B. Physiological anemia

C. Fatigue due to stress

D. No problem indicated

50. In counseling a client, the nurse emphasizes the danger signals during pregnancy. On the next visit, the client identifies which of the following as a danger signal that should be reported immediately?

A. Backache

B. Leaking of clear yellow fluid from breasts

C. Constipation with hemorrhoids

D. Visual changes

51. The client will be more comfortable and the results more accurate when the nurse prepares the client for Leopold's maneuvers by having her:

A. Empty her bladder

B. Lie on her left side

C. Place her arms over her head

D. Force fluids 1 hour prior to procedure

52. Before giving methergine postpartum, the nurse should assess the client for:

A. Decreased amount of lochial flow

B. Elevated blood pressure

C. Flushing

D. Afterpains

53. When assessing the client 6 hours postpartum, the fundus is found to be U +3, displaced to the right of midline, and slightly boggy. The nurse would first:

    A. Increase the IV oxytocin drip rate
    B. Give methergine IM
    C. Assess for a full bladder
    D. Grasp the uterus and massage vigorously

54. A 24-hours' postpartum client complains of discomfort at the episiotomy site. On assessment, the nurse notes the episiotomy is without signs of infection. To relieve the discomfort, the nurse should first:

    A. Assist her with a sitz bath
    B. Administer the prescribed medication for pain
    C. Teach her Kegel exercises
    D. Apply an ice pack

55. The nurse explains perineal hygiene self-care postpartum to the client. She should be instructed to:

    A. Wear gloves for the procedure
    B. Place and adjust the pad from back to front
    C. Cleanse and wipe the perineum from front to back
    D. Protect the outer surface of the pad from contamination

56. In teaching the client about proper umbilical cord care, the nurse recommends that:

    A. Petrolatum be placed around the cord after the sponge bath
    B. A belly binder be applied to prevent umbilical hernia
    C. The area be cleansed at diaper changes with alcohol and inspected for redness or drainage
    D. The cord clamp be left on until the cord stump separates

57. A baby is circumcised. Immediate postoperative care should include:

    A. Applying a loose diaper
    B. Keeping the baby NPO for 4 hours to avoid vomiting
    C. Changing the dressing frequently using dry, sterile gauze
    D. Taking the baby to his mother for cuddling

58. A 28-year-old multigravida has class II heart disease. At her prenatal visit at 34 weeks' gestation, all of the following observations are made. Which would require intervention?

    A. Weight gain of 2 kg in 4 weeks
    B. Blood pressure of 128/78
    C. Subjective data: shortness of breath after showering
    D. Ankle edema reported present in late afternoon and evenings

59. A client is admitted to the labor room. She is dilated 4 cm. She is placed on electric fetal monitoring. Which of the following observations necessitates notifying the physician?

    A. Contractions every 2 minutes, lasting 100 seconds
    B. Fetal heart decelerations during a contraction
    C. Beat-to-beat variability between contractions
    D. Fetal heart decelerations at the beginning of contractions

60. A client has been in labor 10 hours and is becoming very tired. She has dilated to 7 cm and is at 0 station with the fetus in a right occipitoposterior position. She is complaining of severe backache with each contraction. One comfort measure the nurse can employ is to:

    A. Place her in knee-chest position during the contraction
    B. Use effleurage during the contraction
    C. Apply strong sacral pressure during the contraction
    D. Have her push with each contraction

61. The nurse in the mental health center is instructing a depressed client about the dietary restrictions necessary in taking her medication, which is a monoamine oxidase (MAO) inhibitor. Which of the following is she restricting from the client's diet?

    A. Cream cheese
    B. Fresh fruits
    C. Aged cheese
    D. Yeast bread

62. A client suffering from schizophrenia has been taking chlorpromazine (Thorazine) for 6 months. On one of his follow-up visits to the mental health center, the nurse reports to the physician that he has developed tardive dyskinesia. Which of the following symptoms might she have observed in the client to support this conclusion?

    A. High fever, tachycardia, stupor, renal failure
    B. Lip smacking, chewing, blinking, lateral jaw movements
    C. Photosensitivity, orthostatic hypotension, dry mouth
    D. Constipation, blurred vision, drowsiness

63. On morning rounds, the nurse found a manic-depressive client who is taking lithium in a confused mental state, vomiting, twitching, and exhibiting a coarse hand tremor. Which one of the following nursing actions is essential at this time?

    A. Administer her next dosage of lithium, and then call the physician.
    B. Withhold her lithium, and report her symptoms to the physician.
    C. Place her on NPO to decrease the excretion of lithium from her body, and call the physician.
    D. Contact the lab and request a lithium level in 30 minutes, and call the physician.

64. In acute episodes of mania, lithium is effective in 1–2 weeks, but it may take up to 4 weeks, or even a few months, to treat symptoms fully. Sometimes an antipsychotic agent is prescribed during the first few days or weeks of an acute episode to manage severe behavioral excitement and acute psychotic symptoms. In addition to the lithium, which one of the following medications might the physician prescribe?

    A. Diazepam (Valium)
    B. Haloperidol (Haldol)
    C. Sertraline (Zoloft)
    D. Alprazolam (Xanax)

65. The healthcare team determines that an elderly client has had progressive changes in memory over the last 2 years

that have interfered with her personal, social, or occupational functioning. Her memory, learning, attention, and judgment have all been affected in some way. These symptoms describe which of the following conditions?

A. Dementia
B. Parkinsonism
C. Delirium
D. Mania

66. A husband and wife and their two children, age 9 and age 5, are requesting family therapy. Which of the following strategies is most therapeutic for the nurse to use during the initial interaction with a family?

A. Always allow the most vocal person to state the problem first.
B. Encourage the mother to speak for the children.
C. Interpret immediately what seems to be going on within the family.
D. Allow family members to assume the seats as they choose.

67. In healthcare settings, nurses must be familiar with primary, secondary, and tertiary levels of care. As a nurse in the community, which of the following interventions might be a primary prevention strategy?

A. Crisis intervention with an intoxicated teenager whose mother just committed suicide
B. Referring a client who has been on a detoxification unit to a rehabilitation center
C. Teaching fifth-grade children the harmful effects of substance abuse
D. Counseling a client with post-traumatic stress disorder

68. While the nurse is taking a male client's blood pressure, he makes flirtatious remarks to her. The nurse will handle this effectively if she:

A. Politely tells the client, "Keep your hands off"
B. Ignores the remarks and hopes he will not try it again
C. Confronts the remarks but attempts not to reject the client
D. Leaves the room in order to compose herself

69. A client is a victim of domestic violence. She is now receiving assistance at a shelter for battered women. She tells the nurse about the cycle of violence that she has been experiencing in her relationship with her husband of 5 years. In the "tension-building phase," the nurse might expect the client to describe which of the following?

A. Promises of gifts that her husband made to her
B. Acute battering of the client, characterized by his volatile discharge of tension
C. Minor battering incidents, such as the throwing of food or dishes at her
D. A period of tenderness between the couple

70. Which of the following symptoms might the nurse observe in a client with a lithium blood level over 2.0?

A. Fine hand tremor, headache, mental dullness
B. Vomiting, impaired consciousness, decreased blood pressure
C. Polyuria, polydipsia, edema
D. Gastric irritation, nausea, diarrhea

71. A psychiatric nurse is providing an orientation to a new staff nurse. She reminds the nurse that psychiatrists often use categories of medications and that it is important that she recall that some categories of medications have synonyms. Another name used to describe minor tranquilizers is which of the following?

A. Antipsychotic medications
B. Antidepressant medications
C. Antianxiety medications
D. Antimania medication

72. The nurse has been caring for a 16-year-old female who recently experienced date rape. After having had crisis intervention and been hospitalized for 2 weeks, the nurse knows that the client is effectively coping with the rape when she tells the nurse:

A. "I know it was my fault that it happened, because I shouldn't have been out so late."
B. "If I had not worn that sexy dress that night, he wouldn't have raped me."
C. "I know my date just had so much passion he couldn't handle me saying 'no.' "
D. "I know now that it was not my fault, but I want to continue counseling after my discharge."

73. A 42-year-old male client has been treated at an alcoholic rehabilitation center for physiological alcohol dependence. The nurse will be able to determine that he is preparing for discharge and is effectively coping with his problem when he shares with her the following information:

A. "I know that I will not ever be able to socially drink alcohol again and will need the support of the AA group."
B. "I know that I can only drink one or two drinks at social gatherings in the future, but at least I don't have to continue AA."
C. "I really wasn't addicted to alcohol when I came here, I just needed some help dealing with my divorce."
D. "It really wasn't my fault that I had to come here. If my wife hadn't left, I wouldn't have needed those drinks."

74. Degenerative disorders are attributed to many factors. As a nurse assigned to a convalescent home, one must often educate families about how such conditions occur. Which of the following statements might the nurse need to explore when a daughter tries to explain to her mother what caused her degenerative disorder?

A. "Some folks believe that aging causes this, Mother."
B. "Perhaps, it's the way your parents used those double-bind messages, Mother."
C. "I know some people who are having this problem and they were exposed to chemicals at work, Mother."
D. "It can be caused by lots of things, toxic agents and even alcohol, Mother."

75. A family is experiencing changes in their lifestyle in many ways. The invalid grandmother has moved in with them. The couple have a 2-year-old son by their marriage, and the wife has two children by her previous marriage. The older children are in high school. In applying systems

theory to this family, it is important for the nurse to remember which of the following principles?

A. The parts of a system are only minimally related.
B. Dysfunction in one part affects every other part.
C. A family system has no boundaries.
D. Healthy families are enmeshed.

76. The nurse is trying to help a mother understand what is happening with her son who has recently been diagnosed with paranoid schizophrenia. At present, he is experiencing hallucinations and delusions of persecution and suffers from poor hygiene. The nurse can best help her understand her son's condition by which of the following statements?

A. "Sometimes these symptoms are caused by an overstimulation of a chemical called dopamine in the brain."
B. "Has anyone in your family ever had schizophrenia?"
C. "If your son has a twin, he probably will eventually develop schizophrenia, too."
D. "Some of his symptoms may be a result of his lack of a strong mother-child bonding relationship."

77. A male client is experiencing auditory hallucinations. His nurse enters the room and he tells her that his mother is talking to him, and he will take his medicine after she leaves. The nurse looks around the room and sees that she and the client are the only ones in the room. The nurse's most therapeutic response will be:

A. "I don't see your mother in the room. Let's talk about how you're feeling."
B. "OK, I'll come back later when you're feeling more like taking your medicine."
C. "She may be here, but I can't see her."
D. "Why don't you finish talking to her, and I'll wait."

78. A female client with major depression stated that "life is hopeless and not worth living." The nurse should place *highest* priority on which of the following questions?

A. "How has your appetite been recently?"
B. "Have you thought about hurting yourself?"
C. "How is your relationship with your husband?"
D. "How has your depression affected your daily living activities?"

79. A client presented herself to the mental health center, describing the following symptoms: a weight loss of 20 lb in the past 2 months, difficulty concentrating, repeated absences from work due to "fatigue," and not wanting to get dressed in the morning. She leaves her recorded message on her telephone and has lost interest in answering the phone or doorbell. The nurse's assessment of her behavior would most likely be:

A. Deep depression
B. Psychotic depression
C. Severe anxiety
D. Severe depression

MOCK NCLEX-RN BOARD REVIEW TEST ANSWERS

1. **(C)** Client need: physiological integrity; subcategory: pharmacological and parenteral therapies; content area: med/surg

   RATIONALE

   (A) Headaches may occur after taking nitroglycerin because of vasodilation. (B) The tablets do not need to be refrigerated. The client should carry them with her. (C) The client should contact the physician if repeated doses of nitroglycerin do not relieve the discomfort. (D) Nitroglycerin tablets should be dissolved under the tongue, not swallowed.

2. **(B)** Client need: physiological integrity; subcategory: reduction of risk potential; content area: med/surg

   RATIONALE

   (A) The level of consciousness is not affected by elevated potassium levels. (B) An electrocardiogram (EKG) can tell the nurse whether this client is experiencing any cardiac dysfunction or arrhythmias related to the elevated potassium level. (C) Measurement of the urine output is not a priority nursing action at this time. (D) The client's serum potassium values for the past several days may provide information about his renal function, but they are not a priority at this time.

3. **(B)** Client need: physiological integrity; subcategory: physiological adaptation; content area: med/surg

   RATIONALE

   (A) Clients with Parkinson's disease generally experience stiffness and rigid movement. (B) Pill-rolling movements are a symptom experienced by the Parkinson client. (C) Twitching of the muscles is not an expected symptom of Parkinson's disease. (D) Parkinson's disease does not cause joint pain. Mild muscular pain may be present.

4. **(C)** Client need: physiological integrity; subcategory: physiological adaptation; content area: med/surg

   RATIONALE

   (A) Clients with ulcers generally experience abdominal pain. It is common to have pain in the early morning hours with an ulcer. (B) Constipation is not a symptom associated with ulcers and would indicate a need to look at other factors. (C) Melena is blood in the stools. This could indicate a slow bleeding ulcer, which could result in significant amounts of blood loss over time. (D) Nausea and vomiting may be present as a result of the ulcer, especially if it is a gastric ulcer. This does not indicate an immediate life-threatening complication.

5. **(A)** Client need: physiological integrity; subcategory: basic care and comfort; content area: med/surg

   RATIONALE

   (A) Clients with respiratory diseases are generally mouth breathers. Cleaning the oral cavity may improve the client's appetite, increase her feelings of well-being, and remove the taste and odor of sputum. (B) Milk causes thick sputum; therefore, milk products would not be beneficial for this client. (C) Exercise prior to a meal would require increased O_2 consumption and most likely would decrease the client's ability to eat. (D) Clients with respiratory diseases need increased fluid to liquefy secretions.

6. **(C)** Client need: physiological integrity; subcategory: reduction of risk potential; content area: med/surg

   RATIONALE

   (A) The AIDS virus cannot be transmitted to the donor through the blood donation procedure. (B) The test for the AIDS virus is not absolutely foolproof; therefore, it is not wise for a person with known risk factors to donate blood. (C) It takes time for antibodies to the AIDS virus to develop. An infected individual could donate contaminated blood without it testing positive for the virus. (D) For reasons of confidentiality, information about individuals infected with AIDS is not made public.

7. **(B)** Client need: physiological integrity; subcategory: pharmacological and parenteral therapies; content area: med/surg

   RATIONALE

   (A) Nausea is more difficult to control if antiemetics are withheld until nausea is experienced. (B) Antiemetics should be given prophylactically at the beginning of chemotherapy and continued on an around-the-clock basis to prevent nausea. (C) Combinations of antiemetics give the best control for nausea by blocking various causes of nausea induced by chemotherapy. (D) Antiemetics should be given around the clock during the course of chemotherapy. This prevents nausea from developing and prevents anticipatory nausea during subsequent chemotherapy administrations.

8. **(D)** Client need: physiological integrity; subcategory: reduction of risk potential; content area: med/surg

   RATIONALE

   (A) A respiratory rate of 16 breaths/min is normal and is not a cause for alarm. (B) A pulse rate of 80 bpm is normal and is not a cause for alarm. (C) Complaints of muscle aches are unrelated to her receiving chemotherapy. There may be other causes related to her hospital stay or the disease process. (D) A sore throat is an indication of a possible infection. A client receiving chemotherapy is at risk of neutropenia. An infection in the presence of neutropenia can result in a life-threatening situation.

9. **(A)** Client need: physiological integrity; subcategory: physiological adaptation; content area: med/surg

   RATIONALE

   (A) Because of the location of an ileostomy, the client will not be able to control the evacuation of her bowels. The ileostomy will drain liquid stool continuously. (B) The client should be able to return to a normal, well-balanced diet. She should avoid foods that cause diarrhea or excessive gas production, and she should eat small meals. (C) The client should be able to resume sexual activity. She will be able to wear a pouch. (D) The client has no other health or mental problems and should be able to manage her own ileostomy.

10. **(B)** Client need: physiological integrity; subcategory: reduction of risk potential; content area: med/surg

    RATIONALE

    (A) The client may be more tearful than normal due to the stress of the surgery and its implications for her future life. She would be expected to have pain following surgery. (B) A temperature of 102°F indicates an infectious process. This is not a normal sequence to surgery and indicates a need for further assessment. (C) The client is expected to have no bowel sounds for 24–48 hours after surgery because of the trauma to the bowel. (D) Normal urine output is 30 mL/hr. This represents an output of 50 mL/hr, which is greater than normal.

11. **(D)** Client need: health promotion and maintenance; subcategory: prevention and early detection of disease; content area: med/surg

    RATIONALE

    (A) The skin in a treatment area should be rinsed with water and patted dry. Markings should be left intact, and the skin should not be scrubbed. (B) Clients should avoid putting any creams or lotions on the treated area. This could interfere with treatment. (C) Radiation therapy clients should wear loose-fitting clothes and avoid tight, irritating fabrics. (D) The area of skin being treated is sensitive to sunlight, and the client should take care to prevent sun damage by avoiding direct sunlight and covering the area when she is in the sun.

12. **(C)** Client need: physiological integrity; subcategory: physiological adaptation; content area: med/surg

    RATIONALE

    (A) A weight gain of 10 lb represents a state of overhydration. (B) He is losing fluids through insensible losses; a urine output equal to his intake indicates that he is receiving too little fluids. (C) A urine output greater than his intake indicates that he is receiving adequate fluid resuscitation to account for urinary and insensible losses. (D) A blood pressure of 94/62 indicates a state of underhydration and inadequate circulatory volume.

13. **(B)** Client need: health promotion and maintenance; subcategory: prevention and early detection of disease; content area: med/surg

    RATIONALE

    (A) Bleeding is not a symptom of sickle cell anemia or sickle cell crisis. (B) Decreased blood viscosity leads to sickling of red blood cells. Increased fluid intake maintains adequate circulating blood volume and decreases the chance of sickling. (C) Hypoxia leads to sickling of cells. Flying in nonpressurized planes places the client in a situation of low O_2 tension, which can lead to sickling. (D) Male and female clients with sickle cell disease can pass the trait on to their offspring. Therefore, this client should receive genetic counseling prior to having children.

14. **(A)** Client need: health promotion and maintenance; subcategory: prevention and early detection of disease; content area: med/surg

    RATIONALE

    (A) Hemodialysis is faster in clearing the blood of toxins than peritoneal dialysis. However, clients must consider the time that they spend traveling to the dialysis center and the disruption in their daily lives. (B) Peritoneal dialysis requires several exchanges with dwelling time for the dialysate and therefore takes longer than hemodialysis. (C) Several serious complications of peritoneal dialysis include peritonitis, catheter displacement and/or plugging, or pain during dialysis. (D) A client can be taught to self-administer peritoneal dialysis without the aid of a professional.

15. **(B)** Client need: physiological integrity; subcategory: reduction of risk potential; content area: med/surg

    RATIONALE

    (A) This is an internal device. Assessment of the site should include assessing for swelling, pain, warmth, and discoloration. This measure does not assess patency. (B) The presence of a bruit indicates good blood flow through the device. (C) The nurse should inspect the site for bruising or hematoma; however, this measure does not assure patency of the device. (D) The nurse should inspect the vascular access site frequently for signs of infection. However, this does not assure patency.

16. **(B)** Client need: physiological integrity; subcategory: reduction of risk potential; content area: med/surg

    RATIONALE

    (A) Instilling a cool solution does not significantly lower the body temperature during peritoneal dialysis. (B) Warmed solution does help dilate the peritoneal blood vessels, facilitating the exchange of fluids. (C) Warming the dialysate does not decrease the risk of peritoneal infection. Sterile technique decreases this risk. (D) Relaxing the abdominal muscles does not facilitate peritoneal dialysis.

17. **(C)** Client need: physiological integrity; subcategory: physiological adaptation; content area: med/surg

RATIONALE

(A) With a pneumothorax, air occupies the pleural space. Crackles or rales are heard with increased fluid or secretions and would not be present with air in the space. (B) With a pneumothorax, the client would experience tachypnea and tachycardia to compensate for the decrease in oxygenation. (C) Symptoms of pneumothorax include shortness of breath, sharp pain on the affected side with movement or coughing, asymmetrical chest expansion, and diminished or absent breath sounds on the affected side. (D) With a pneumothorax, breath sounds would be decreased on the affected side (indicates air in the pleural space).

18. **(C)** Client need: physiological integrity; subcategory: physiological adaptation; content area: med/surg

    RATIONALE

    (A) This action is inappropriate. Coughing will not re-expand the lung and could result in further harm. (B) This action is a medical procedure, not a nursing procedure. (C) An occlusive dressing will prevent further air leak until the physician institutes further treatment. (D) The decision to reinsert the tube is a medical decision, not a nursing one.

19. **(D)** Client need: health promotion and maintenance; subcategory: prevention and early detection of disease; content area: med/surg

    RATIONALE

    (A) Pain in the legs could be indicative of doing too much too quickly, but not of worsening heart failure. The client should be cautioned to increase his activities slowly. (B) Thirst, weight loss, and frequent urination are not indicative of heart failure. The client should report these symptoms to his physician. (C) Drowsiness and lethargy are not indicative of worsening heart failure. The client should report these symptoms to his physician. (D) All of these symptoms indicate a worsening cardiac condition possibly associated with too much activity. The client's activity level should be evaluated.

20. **(C)** Client need: health promotion and maintenance; subcategory: prevention and early detection of disease; content area: med/surg

    RATIONALE

    (A) The client should leave the electrodes in place during the entire time the test is ordered. He should not even remove the electrodes for bathing. (B) The Holter monitor will record cardiac electrical activity but will not record damage to his myocardium. (C) The client should keep a record of all of his activities so the physician can correlate the ECG findings with his activities. (D) The client should continue doing his regular activities. The purpose of the Holter monitor is to record heart activity during routine activities.

21. **(D)** Client need: health promotion and maintenance; subcategory: prevention and early detection of disease; content area: med/surg

    RATIONALE

    (A) Dangling the client's legs over the edge of the bed will contribute to stasis and pooling of blood and increases the risk of thrombus formation. (B) Massaging the client's calves could result in dislodging an embolus. (C) Decreased movement will contribute to pooling of blood and increased risk of venous thrombosis. (D) Tightening and relaxing leg muscles increases circulation and decreases the risk of venous thrombosis.

22. **(B)** Client need: physiological integrity; subcategory: reduction of risk potential; content area: med/surg

    RATIONALE

    (A) Exercising the unaffected extremities will prevent contractures and emboli. (B) Crossing and uncrossing the affected leg after surgery can dislocate the joint. (C) Neurological and circulatory status of the affected leg has been compromised by surgery. Hourly checks are needed to monitor the status of the leg. (D) A trochanter roll will prevent the upper thigh from rolling outward, increasing the chances of dislocation.

23. **(A)** Client need: physiological integrity; subcategory: basic care and comfort; content area: med/surg

    RATIONALE

    (A) Clients with diverticulosis should maintain a high-fiber diet and prevent constipation with bran or bulk laxatives. (B) Low-residue diets lead to constipation and are contraindicated in clients with diverticulosis. (C) Clients with diverticulosis should drink at least eight glasses of water each day to prevent constipation. (D) Clients with diverticulosis should modify their diet to include high-fiber foods and bulk laxatives.

24. **(C)** Client need: health promotion and maintenance; subcategory: growth and development through the life span; content area: maternity

    RATIONALE

    (A) A radiant warmer maintains an optimal thermal environment by use of a thermal skin sensor taped to the infant. The warmer limits parental attachment, so, although appropriate, it is not an intervention that promotes infant attachment. (B) Warmed blankets prevent heat loss in the neonate by conduction. In addition, tactile stimuli promote crying and lung expansion. This intervention does not promote attachment, however. (C) Skin-to-skin contact is an effective way to conserve heat after delivery and promotes parental attachment following birth in the healthy term infant. The first period of reactivity lasts approximately 30 minutes following birth. A strong sucking reflex and an active, awake newborn characterize this period. (D) Surfaces of objects warmer than the infant promote overheating by conduction, and neonatal hyperthermia may result.

25. **(D)** Client need: health promotion and maintenance; subcategory: growth and development through the life span; content area: maternity

    RATIONALE

    (A) Within 12 hours of delivery, the fundus of the uterus rises to, or slightly above or below, the umbilicus. Fundal height generally decreases 1 fingerbreadth, or 1 cm/day. (B) The uterus descends into the pelvic cavity at approximately 10–12 postpartal days and can no longer be palpated abdominally. (C) Within 12 hours of delivery, the fundus of the uterus rises to, or slightly above or below, the umbilicus. Fundal height generally decreases 1 fingerbreadth, or 1 cm/day. An enlarged uterus may indicate subinvolution or postpartal hemorrhage. (D) Immediately following delivery, the uterus lies midline, about midway between the umbilicus and the symphysis pubis.

26. **(D)** Client need: health promotion and maintenance; subcategory: growth and development through the life span; content area: maternity

    RATIONALE

    (A) The second stage of labor is from full cervical dilation through birth of the baby. The three phases of this stage include latency or resting, descent, and final transition. The client is less than fully dilated so she is not in stage 2. (B) The first stage of labor begins with regular uterine contractions and continues until the woman is 10 cm dilated. The three phases of this stage include the early or latent phase (0–3 cm), the active phase (4–7 cm), and the transitional phase (7–10 cm). The client is <4 cm dilated so she is in the latent phase of the first stage of labor. (C) The third stage of labor is from the birth of the baby until the delivery of the placenta. The client is less than fully dilated. (D) The first stage of labor begins with regular uterine contractions and continues until the woman is 10 cm dilated. The three phases of this stage include the early or latent phase (0–3 cm), the active

phase (4–7 cm), and the transitional phase (7–10 cm). The client is <4 cm dilated so she is in the latent phase of the first stage of labor.

27. **(A)** Client need: health promotion and maintenance; subcategory: growth and development through the life span; content area: maternity

    RATIONALE

    (A) The nurse must assess the labor status to determine if birth is imminent. The nurse may note perineal bulging, crowning, or birth of the head to ascertain labor status. (B) Assessing uterine contractions is one intervention to ascertain labor status. Based on the client's cry, it is not the intervention of choice. (C) If delivery of the infant is imminent, preparing a clean or sterile area for delivery is appropriate, but labor status must be established, whether delivery is imminent, by perineal assessment. (D) Assessing FHR is one intervention to ascertain fetal well-being. Based on the client's cry, this is not the intervention of choice.

28. **(D)** Client need: physiological integrity; subcategory: physiological adaptation; content area: maternity

    RATIONALE

    (A) Nursing measures to support fetal oxygenation and promote maternal blood pressure would precede calling the physician. (B) Systolic pressures below 100 mm Hg or a reduction in the systolic pressure of ≥30% necessitate treatment. Assessing the blood pressure in 5 minutes may allow for further fetal and/or maternal compromise. Turning the client on her left side will promote uteroplacental perfusion and is appropriate. (C) Oxytocin (Pitocin) increases the strength of uterine contractions and may cause maternal hypotension; thus it is an inappropriate drug for use in this clinical situation. IV fluids would be increased to expand the circulating blood volume and promote increased blood pressure. (D) Turning the mother to her left lateral side promotes uteroplacental perfusion. IV fluids are administered to increase the circulating blood volume, and O_2 is administered to promote fetal oxygenation and decrease the nausea accompanying the hypotension.

29. **(C)** Client need: health promotion and maintenance; subcategory: growth and development through the life span; content area: maternity

    RATIONALE

    (A) The first digit represents the total number of pregnancies. This client has been pregnant 3 times including this pregnancy. The twin pregnancy counts as only one pregnancy, and because she delivered prior to 37 weeks' gestation, the third digit is recorded as 1. (B) The first digit represents the total number of pregnancies. This client has been pregnant 3 times including this pregnancy. The second digit represents the total number of full-term deliveries; she has lost two pregnancies before 37 weeks' gestation. At present, she has no living children, so the fifth digit is noted as 0. (C) The client is pregnant for the third time, and the first digit reflects the total number of pregnancies. She has had no full-term deliveries, because she delivered prior to 37 gestational weeks, so the second digit is recorded as 0. The third digit represents the number of preterm deliveries, and a twin pregnancy counts as only one delivery. She lost an earlier pregnancy prior to 20 gestational weeks, and the fourth digit reflects spontaneous or elective abortions. Lastly, the fifth digit indicates the number of children currently living, and she has no living children. (D) She is pregnant for the third time, and the first digit reflects the total number of pregnancies. In the previous two pregnancies, she delivered prior to 37 gestational weeks, thus having no full-term deliveries, which is indicated by the second digit. The fourth digit represents the total number of abortions, spontaneous or elective, and she reported a spontaneous abortion with her first pregnancy.

30. **(A)** Client need: health promotion and maintenance; subcategory: growth and development through the life span; content area: maternity

    RATIONALE

    (A) Nägele's rule is as follows: add 7 days to the 1st day of the last menstrual period, subtract 3 months, and then add 1 year. (B) Nägele's rule presumes that the woman has a 28-day menstrual cycle, with conception occurring on the 14th day of the cycle. Slight vaginal spotting may occur in early gestation for unknown reasons but is insignificant in the calculation of Nägele's rule. (C) Nägele's rule presumes that the woman has a 28-day menstrual cycle, with conception occurring on the 14th day of the cycle. Slight vaginal spotting may occur in early gestation for unknown reasons but is insignificant in the calculation of Nägele's rule. (D) Nägele's rule presumes that the woman has a 28-day menstrual cycle, with conception occurring on the 14th day of the cycle. Slight vaginal spotting may occur in early gestation for unknown reasons but is insignificant in the calculation of Nägele's rule.

31. **(C)** Client need: health promotion and maintenance; subcategory: prevention and early detection of disease; content area: maternity

    RATIONALE

    (A) Judicious use of analgesics is appropriate with breast engorgement; however, mechanical suppression would be the initial recommendation. (B) Breast-feeding every 1½–3 hours will reduce and/or prevent breast engorgement. Breast-feeding will promote milk production, which will compound the distention and stasis of the venous circulation of engorgement in a bottle-feeding mother. (C) Ice packs reduce milk flow while the snug, supportive bra provides mechanical suppression and decreases pulling on Cooper's ligament. In addition, breast binders or ace bandages may be used for some women. (D) Warmth promotes milk production and may stimulate the let-down reflex. These measures would contribute to the venous congestion of engorgement.

32. **(A)** Client need: safe, effective care environment; subcategory: management of care; content area: all nursing

    RATIONALE

    (A) The state nursing practice act determines the standard of care for the professional nurse. (B) AWHONN Standards are published as recommendations and guidelines for maternal-newborn nursing. (C) American Nurses' Association Standards are published as recommendations and guidelines for maternal-child health nursing. (D) The International Council of Nurses' Code emphasizes the nurse's obligations to the client rather than to the physician. It is published as recommendations and guidelines by the international organization for professional nursing.

33. **(B)** Client need: health promotion and maintenance; subcategory: prevention and early detection of disease; content area: maternity

    RATIONALE

    (A) Amniotic fluid is generally pale and straw colored. Meconium-stained amniotic fluid would indicate a previous hypoxic episode. This intervention, though appropriate, is not the immediate priority. (B) With rupture of the membranes, the umbilical cord may prolapse if the presenting part does not fill the pelvis. Assessing FHR ascertains fetal well-being. (C) More information regarding fetal status and assessing for membrane rupture is needed prior to contacting the physician. (D) Nitrazine test paper differentiates amniotic fluid from urine. Amniotic fluid is normally alkaline in contrast to urine, which is acidic. This intervention, though appropriate, is not the immediate priority.

34. **(C)** Client need: health promotion and maintenance; subcategory: growth and development through the life span; content area: maternity

    RATIONALE

    (A) Mammary growth as well as milk production and maintenance in the breast occur in response to hormones produced primarily by the hypothalamus and the pituitary gland. (B) Prolactin stimulates the alveolar cells of the breast to produce milk. It is important in the initiation of breast-feeding. (C) Oxytocin, which is released by the posterior pituitary, stimulates the let-down reflex by contraction of the myoepithelial cells surrounding the alveoli. In addition, it causes contractions of the uterus and uterine involution. (D) Afterpains may occur with retained placental fragments. A boggy uterus and continued bleeding are other symptoms that occur in response to retained placental fragments.

35. **(D)** Client need: psychosocial integrity; subcategory: coping and adaptation; content area: maternity

    RATIONALE

    (A) The mother and the father require support; the nurse should not minimize their grief in this situation. (B) Attachment to this infant occurs during the pregnancy for both the mother and father. Another child cannot replace this child. (C) Attachment to this infant occurs during the pregnancy for both the mother and father. Siblings will not replace their feelings or minimize their loss of this infant. (D) Holding and viewing the infant decreases denial and may facilitate the grief process. The nurse should prepare family members for how the infant appears ("she is bruised") and provide support.

36. **(A)** Client need: health promotion and maintenance; subcategory: prevention and early detection of disease; content area: maternity

    RATIONALE

    (A) The rubella vaccine is made with attenuated virus and is given in the immediate postpartal period to prevent infection during pregnancy and subsequent adverse fetal and neonatal sequelae. Mothers are advised to prevent pregnancy for 3 months following immunization. (B) Rubella infection during the second trimester may result in permanent hearing loss for the fetus. (C) RhoGam is the drug generally administered at 28 weeks' gestation to Rh-negative women. It is contraindicated to administer rubella vaccine during pregnancy. (D) RhoGam is the drug administered within 72 hours postpartum to Rh-negative women to prevent the development of antibodies to fetal cells.

37. **(A)** Client need: physiological integrity; subcategory: basic care and comfort; content area: maternity

    RATIONALE

    (A) Prunes provide fiber to decrease constipation and are an excellent source of dietary iron, as the prenatal client is not taking her supplemental iron and iron-deficiency anemia is common during pregnancy. (B) Green leafy vegetables provide a source of fiber and iron; however, prunes are a better source of both. (C) Red meat is a good iron source but will not address the constipation problem. (D) Eggs are a good iron source but do not address the constipation problem.

38. **(C)** Client need: health promotion and maintenance; subcategory: prevention and early detection of disease; content area: maternity

    RATIONALE

    (A) Maternal age older than 30 years is an identified risk factor for diabetes. Age younger than 30 years is insignificant for diabetes unless there is a familial history of diabetes. (B) The client's weight is appropriate for her height. Obesity or pregnancy weight >20% of the ideal weight is a contributing factor to the development of gestational diabetes. (C) The birth of an infant weighing >9 lb (4000 g) is an identified risk factor for gestational diabetes. (D) A familial history of heart disease is insignificant in the development of diabetes. However, a familial history of type II diabetes mellitus is identified as a risk factor in the development of diabetes during pregnancy.

39. **(D)** Client need: health promotion and maintenance; subcategory: growth and development through the life span; content area: maternity

RATIONALE

(A) These indices are within normal parameters; therefore, the nurse does not need to contact the physician. (B) The purpose of turning a client to her left side is to maximize uteroplacental blood flow. Based on the above assessment, there is no indication that blood flow is compromised. (C) These interventions are appropriate nursing interventions for late and prolonged decelerations. Following these interventions, the nurse should notify the physician. These indices are within normal parameters; therefore, the nurse does not need to start an IV and administer O_2. (D) Variations of 20 bpm above or below the baseline FHR is considered normal. Normal FHRs range from 120–160 bpm. As the fetus moves, the FHR increases, and accelerations often occur in concert with contractions. During the active phase of labor, the frequency of uterine contractions is every 2–4 minutes, with an appropriate duration of 60 sec.

40. **(D)** Client need: health promotion and maintenance; subcategory: prevention and early detection of disease; content area: maternity

RATIONALE

(A) Women with pregnancy-induced hypertension have a reduced plasma volume secondary to venous vessel constriction, not hypovolemia; therefore, sodium restriction is not recommended. It is suggested that these women avoid extremely salty foods. (B) Drinking six to eight glasses of water per day facilitates optimal fluid volume and renal perfusion, but it will not decrease the venous vessel constriction of pregnancy-induced hypertension. (C) Carbohydrate needs increase during pregnancy, specifically during the second and third trimesters, but they have not been linked to pregnancy-induced hypertension. (D) Loss of urinary protein (proteinuria) is associated with increased permeability of the large protein molecules with pregnancy-induced hypertension. Additional dietary protein also helps increase the plasma colloidal osmotic pressure. Diets deficient in protein have been linked to pregnancy-induced hypertension.

41. **(C)** Client need: health promotion and maintenance; subcategory: prevention and early detection of disease; content area: maternity

RATIONALE

(A) Decongestants may exaggerate the nasal stuffiness associated with pregnancy. Judicious use of decongestants and nasal sprays is advocated during pregnancy. (B) Cool air vaporizers and saline drops may help to relieve the nasal stuffiness. Positioning on either lateral side does not decrease nasal stuffiness or prevent epistaxis. (C) Increased estrogen levels result in nasal mucosa edema with subsequent nasal stuffiness. Estrogen also promotes vasodilation, which contributes to epistaxis. The nurse may recommend cool air vaporizers and saline drops to help with the nasal stuffiness. (D) Increased estrogen levels result in nasal mucosa edema with subsequent nasal stuffiness. Estrogen also promotes vasodilation discomforts associated with pregnancy.

42. **(C)** Client need: health promotion and maintenance; subcategory: prevention and early detection of disease; content area: maternity

RATIONALE

(A) Term neonates are predominantly in a flexed position with strong active muscle tone that increases. Newborns are slightly hypertonic. (B) Neonatal movements may be jerky and uncoordinated as the neonate works against gravity in contrast to the buoyancy of the amniotic fluid. Jerky movements must be differentiated from the tremors of hypoglycemia, hypocalcemia, and neurological dysfunction. (C) Growth of the newborn progresses in a cephalocaudal, proximal-distal fashion. Knowledge regarding infant development may facilitate parental involve-

ment and infant stimulation. (D) Asymmetrical movements of the extremities are indicative of neurological dysfunction.

43. **(D)** Client need: health promotion and maintenance; subcategory: growth and development through the life span; content area: maternity

RATIONALE

(A) Methergine is given following placental delivery to promote uterine contractions and prevent hemorrhage. Methergine may be administered in this clinical situation, but fundal massage would be the first response. (B) Removal of retained placental fragments is done by the physician and is not the first response. (C) If the fundus rises and is deviated, particularly to the right, the nurse should suspect bladder distention secondary to bladder and urethral trauma associated with birth and decreased bladder tone following delivery. Therefore, women have a diminished sensation to void. (D) A boggy fundus rises and is indicative of blood pooling, predisposing the woman to clot formation. Massage the uterus until firm. Too vigorous massage will result in atonia. Clots may be expelled by a kneading motion of the uterus by the nurse.

44. **(B)** Client need: physiological integrity; subcategory: reduction of risk potential; content area: maternity

RATIONALE

(A) Chadwick's sign is a presumptive sign of pregnancy. The coloration may not subside from past pregnancy or could be caused by other situations that create vasocongestion. (B) FHR (movement) observed on ultrasound is a positive diagnosis of pregnancy. (C) Enlargement of the uterus may be due to fibroids or infection. It is considered a probable sign. (D) Breast tenderness and enlargement is a presumptive sign because it may be due to other conditions, such as premenstrual changes.

45. **(D)** Client need: physiological integrity; subcategory: pharmacological and parenteral therapies; content area: maternity

RATIONALE

(A) Sulfa is a teratogen and will cause kernicterus. (B) Tetracycline is a teratogen and will effect tooth development. (C) Hydralazine is not an antibiotic but a calcium channel blocker. (D) Erythromycin is safe during pregnancy and can be used when the client is allergic to penicillin.

46. **(D)** Client need: health promotion and maintenance; subcategory: prevention and early detection of disease; content area: maternity

RATIONALE

(A) Sitting with the legs crossed at the ankles does not interfere with circulation or create pressure points. (B) TED stockings will help to reduce the varicosity by supporting the vein. Stockings must be applied with legs elevated. (C) Support pantyhose help to reduce the varicosity by supporting the vein. They also provide support to the uterus and allow for better return circulation. Hose must be applied like TED stockings. (D) Knee-high stockings create constriction and pressure points that interfere with circulation in the lower extremities.

47. **(B)** Client need: health promotion and maintenance; subcategory: prevention and early detection of disease; content area: maternity

RATIONALE

(A, D) There are no data to support this. (B) Anticipatory guidance and health maintenance is a first-line defense in the promotion of healthy mothers and healthy babies. (C) There are no data to support this at this time. This will be a concern later.

48. **(C)** Client need: psychosocial integrity; subcategory: coping and adaptation; content area: maternity

RATIONALE

(A) Ambivalence is normal during the first trimester. Reva Rubin addresses the issue of "not now" in the first trimester. The statement still leaves room for exploration. (B) There are no data to support this. This statement by the mother still leaves room for exploration. (C) Ambivalence is normal during the first trimester. Reva Rubin addresses the issue of "not now." This fact should be shared with the mother during further exploration of the comment. (D) It is not abnormal. If it were, another month would also be too long to wait.

49. **(A)** Client need: physiological integrity; subcategory: physiological adaptation; content area: maternity

RATIONALE

(A) This clinical situation is indicative of iron-deficiency anemia because the client has inadequate nutritional intake. Her blood volume is increasing faster than her red blood cell volume. Anemia is present in the second trimester when the hemoglobin level is <10.5 and the hematocrit value falls below 35%. She needs increased iron supplements with follow-up. (B) The client's values are below levels for physiological anemia. (C) The client is fatigued because of a low hemoglobin level. (D) Her hemoglobin level is low and will probably decrease even more when the blood volume peaks at 28 weeks.

50. **(D)** Client need: health promotion and maintenance; subcategory: prevention and early detection of disease; content area: maternity

RATIONALE

(A) Backache is a common complaint during pregnancy. Proper body mechanics, pelvic rock, back rubs, and other comfort measures should relieve the discomfort. In the presence of uterine contractions, the backache would radiate to the lower abdomen. (B) Colostrum is normal and can be present anytime in the second half of pregnancy. (C) Constipation and hemorrhoids are common and do need attention, but they do not constitute a dangerous situation. (D) Visual changes are possibly related to PIH. The client should be assessed immediately to rule out or prevent worsening of PIH.

51. **(A)** Client need: physiological integrity; subcategory: physiological adaptation; content area: maternity

RATIONALE

(A) A full bladder would cause discomfort and possible urinary incontinence during the exam. (B) The left side-lying position would not accommodate the exam. The head of the exam table or bed can be slightly elevated to prevent supine hypotension. (C) Arms extended over the head would cause the abdomen to be tighter and less easily palpable. (D) Forcing fluids would encourage a full bladder, which is not desired for the exam.

52. **(B)** Client need: physiological integrity; subcategory: reduction of risk potential; content area: maternity

RATIONALE

(A) Methergine is given to contract the uterus and to control postpartal hemorrhage; therefore, lochial flow should decrease. (B) Methergine may elevate the blood pressure. A client with an elevated blood pressure should not receive methergine, but she could be given oxytocin if necessary. (C) Flushing is not a side effect of methergine. (D) Afterpains are increased with methergine usage. The client should be informed that this is a normal response.

53. **(C)** Client need: health promotion and maintenance; subcategory: growth and development through the life span; content area: maternity

RATIONALE

(A) Oxytocin may not be necessary if the bladder is emptied and if the uterus remains firm, midline, and at about U11 after massage. (B) The same rationale as for answer "A" applies. (C) A full bladder is the most common cause of uterine atony. If the bladder is full, it should be emptied and the uterus reassessed before further intervention. (D) If the bladder is full, the uterus will not

stay contracted or return to a normal position. Overly vigorous massage also encourages uterine atony.

54. **(A)** Client need: physiological integrity; subcategory: physiological adaptation; content area: maternity

RATIONALE

(A) Warm, moist heat will promote circulation and provide comfort. A sitz bath should be tried before medication is given. (B) Pain medication can be given when other comfort measures such as a sitz bath and topical applications are ineffective. (C) Kegel exercises facilitate sitting by decreasing tension on the episiotomy. They will not be effective for pain control or sustained comfort level. (D) Ice packs are appropriate to apply in the first 12 hours postdelivery to produce vasoconstriction and to reduce edema to the area.

55. **(C)** Client need: physiological integrity; subcategory: reduction of risk potential; content area: maternity

RATIONALE

(A) Perineal hygiene is a clean procedure and does not require the client to wear gloves. A care provider should wear gloves to adhere to universal precautions. (B) The pad should be applied from front to back to prevent contamination of the birth canal or urinary tract from rectal bacteria. (C) Wiping from front to back and discarding the wipe prevents contamination of the urinary tract and birth canal from rectal bacteria. (D) The inner surface of the pad should not be touched to maintain asepsis.

56. **(C)** Client need: health promotion and maintenance; subcategory: growth and development through the life span; content area: maternity

RATIONALE

(A) Petrolatum does not allow the cord to dry and will encourage infection. (B) Belly binders do not facilitate drying of the cord and will encourage abdominal relaxation. (C) Frequent applications of alcohol will facilitate drying and discourage infection. (D) The cord clamp can be removed in 24 hours. Leaving it on is cumbersome and could pull on the cord unnecessarily.

57. **(D)** Client need: physiological integrity; subcategory: reduction of risk potential; content area: maternity

RATIONALE

(A) A pressure diaper should be applied to discourage hemorrhage. (B) The baby can be fed by his mother soon after the procedure, once it is assessed that he is not in any distress and is stable. (C) Dressing changes should not be dry. Dry dressing will stick. (D) Cuddling after the procedure will hopefully quiet the baby. Feeding is also important if his feeding was withheld prior to the procedure or it is time for a feeding.

58. **(C)** Client need: physiological integrity; subcategory: physiological adaptation; content area: maternity

RATIONALE

(A) This is not an excessive weight gain indicative of fluid retention. (B) The blood pressure is within normal range. (C) Showering should not cause shortness of breath. This could be a sign of cardiac decompensation. (D) Dependent ankle edema is normal late in the day among pregnant women. Progressive edema would be a dangerous development.

59. **(A)** Client need: health promotion and maintenance; subcategory: prevention and early detection of disease; content area: maternity

RATIONALE

(A) These are tetanic in nature and can cause rupture of the uterus. (B) The FHR decreases during contractions owing to vasoconstriction and should recover after the contraction. (C) Beat-to-beat variability is a normal finding and demonstrates fetal well-being. (D) The FHR may decrease at the beginning of a contraction owing to head compression.

60. **(C)** Client need: health promotion and maintenance; subcategory: growth and development through the life span; content area: maternity

    RATIONALE

    (A) This measure is inappropriate. The knee-chest position is employed to take pressure off the cord. (B) Effleurage is a comfort measure but not the one that will contribute most to the relief of backache caused by a posterior position. (C) Sacral pressure will counteract the pressure created by the position of the fetal head. (D) The client is not completely dilated. Pushing is contraindicated until the second stage of labor.

61. **(C)** Client need: health promotion and maintenance; subcategory: prevention and early detection of disease; content area: psychiatric

    RATIONALE

    (A) Cream cheese does not contain tyramine, which might cause a hypertensive crisis. (B) Fresh fruits do not contain tyramine, which might cause a hypertensive crisis. (C) Aged or matured cheese combined with a monoamine oxidase predisposes the client to a hypertensive crisis. (D) Bread products raised with yeast do not contain tyramine.

62. **(B)** Client need: physiological integrity; subcategory: pharmacological and parenteral therapies; content area: psychiatric

    RATIONALE

    (A) These symptoms are found in clients with neuroleptic malignant syndrome. (B) These symptoms are found in clients with tardive dyskinesia. (C) These are normal side effects found in clients taking antipsychotic medications. (D) These are also normal side effects found in clients taking antipsychotic medications.

63. **(B)** Client need: physiological integrity; subcategory: pharmacological and parenteral therapies; content area: psychiatric

    RATIONALE

    (A) The client has lithium toxicity, and the nurse must withhold further dosages. (B) Because of her level of toxicity, further lithium could cause coma and death. The nurse needs further orders from the physician to stabilize the client's lithium level. (C) Ensuring adequate intake of sodium chloride will promote excretion of lithium and will assist in managing the client's lithium toxicity. (D) A lithium blood level must be drawn immediately to determine the seriousness of the toxicity and to provide the physician with data for medical orders.

64. **(B)** Client need: physiological integrity; subcategory: pharmacological and parenteral therapies; content area: psychiatric

    RATIONALE

    (A) Diazepam is an antianxiety medication and is not designed to reduce psychotic symptoms. (B) Haloperidol is an antipsychotic medication and may be used until the lithium takes effect. (C) Sertraline is an antidepressant and is used primarily to reduce symptoms of depression. (D) Alprazolam is an antianxiety medication and is not designed to reduce psychotic symptoms.

65. **(A)** Client need: physiological integrity; subcategory: physiological adaptation; content area: psychiatric

    RATIONALE

    (A) These changes are common characteristics of dementia. (B) Parkinson's disease affects the muscular system. Progressive memory changes are not presenting symptoms. (C) Delirium includes an altered level of consciousness, which is not found in dementia. (D) Mania includes symptoms of hyperactivity, flight of ideas, and delusions of grandeur.

66. **(D)** Client need: psychosocial integrity; subcategory: coping and adaptation; content area: psychiatric

    RATIONALE

    (A) One will always hear what the most vocal person has to say. It is best to start with the quietest family member to encourage that person to express emotions. (B) All family members are encouraged to speak for themselves. (C) In the initial family assessment, only data collection occurs; interpretations are made later. (D) Allowing family members to choose their own seats will assist the nurse in assessing the family system and in determining who feels closer to whom.

67. **(C)** Client need: health promotion and maintenance; subcategory: prevention and early detection of disease; content area: psychiatric

    RATIONALE

    (A) The teenager is already coping ineffectively and requires early detection and treatment, which is secondary prevention. (B) The client must be sent to a rehabilitation unit, which requires tertiary prevention. (C) Reducing the incidence of disease through education supports primary prevention. (D) A client with identified symptoms of post-traumatic stress disorder requires intervention by treatment.

68. **(C)** Client need: psychosocial integrity; subcategory: coping and adaptation; content area: psychiatric

    RATIONALE

    (A) This response does not recognize normal feelings of attraction and rejects the client. (B) By ignoring the situation, the nurse has not set limits to discourage other remarks or perhaps more sexually aggressive behavior. (C) By confronting the remarks, she can recognize that his feelings of attraction may be normal but are not appropriate within the context of their nurse-client relationship. (D) Leaving the room does not deal with setting limits for future interactions.

69. **(C)** Client need: psychosocial integrity; subcategory: psychosocial adaptation; content area: psychiatric

    RATIONALE

    (A) This description is characteristic of the "honeymoon" or "respite" phase. (B) This description is characteristic of the "battering" phase. (C) This description is characteristic of the "tension-building" phase prior to the volatile discharge of tension found in the battering phase. (D) This description is characteristic of the "honeymoon" or "respite" phase.

70. **(B)** Client need: physiological integrity; subcategory: pharmacological and parenteral therapies; content area: psychiatric

    RATIONALE

    (A) These symptoms are acute, common, and usually harmless central nervous system side effects of lithium. (B) These symptoms of lithium toxicity are usually dose related. (C) These symptoms are acute, common, and usually harmless renal side effects of lithium. (D) These symptoms are acute, common, and usually harmless gastrointestinal side effects of lithium.

71. **(C)** Client need: physiological integrity; subcategory: pharmacological and parenteral therapies; content area: psychiatric

    RATIONALE

    (A) Antipsychotic medications are also known as major tranquilizers. (B) Antidepressants fall into different categories, such as the tricyclics or the MAO inhibitors. (C) Antianxiety medications are also known as minor tranquilizers. (D) Antimania medications are those such as lithium and lithium carbonate (Lithobid).

72. **(D)** Client need: health promotion and maintenance, subcategory: prevention and early detection of disease; content area: psychiatric

    RATIONALE

    (A) This response does not show any insight; the client falsely assumes that she is responsible for the rape. (B) The client continues to falsely assume responsibility for the rapist's behavior. (C) The client believes falsely that rape is an act of passion, rather than one of violence, control, and domination. (D) The client has insight into the rape; she does not believe it was her fault and shows good judgment in deciding to continue with counseling after discharge.

73. **(A)** Client need: psychosocial integrity; subcategory: coping and adaptation; content area: psychiatric

RATIONALE

(A) The client has insight into the severity of his alcohol addiction and has chosen one of the most effective treatment strategies to support him—Alcoholics Anonymous. (B) The client is still using denial and is not dealing with his alcohol addiction. (C) The client is exhibiting denial about his alcohol addiction and projecting blame on his divorce. (D) The client is projecting blame onto his wife for being in the hospital while still denying his alcohol addiction.

74. **(B)** Client need: psychosocial integrity; subcategory: psychosocial adaptation; content area: psychiatric

RATIONALE

(A) Aging is a factor in the cause of degenerative disorders. (B) Double-bind messages may be found in the histories of families of individuals who develop schizophrenia, but they are not related to degenerative disorders. (C) Chemicals (toxic agents) in work environments are predisposing factors to degenerative disorders. (D) Alcohol causes some degenerative disorders, such as Wernicke's syndrome.

75. **(B)** Client need: health promotion and maintenance; subcategory: prevention and early detection of disease; content area: psychiatric

RATIONALE

(A) The parts of a system are interrelated. (B) Any change in any part of the system affects all other parts. (C) A family system, like any other system, has boundaries. (D) Healthy families are neither enmeshed nor disengaged.

76. **(A)** Client need: psychosocial integrity; subcategory: psychosocial adaptation; content area: psychiatric

RATIONALE

(A) The most plausible theory to date is that dopamine causes an overstimulation in the brain, which results in the psychotic symptoms. (B) This statement will only create anxiety in the mother, and the genetic theory is only one of the etiological factors. (C) This statement will cause the mother much alarm, and nothing was mentioned about any other child. (D) The mother-child relationship is one of the previous theories examined, but it is not one to be emphasized, thereby causing a lot of anxiety for the mother.

77. **(A)** Client need: psychosocial integrity; subcategory: psychosocial adaptation; content area: psychiatric

RATIONALE

(A) This response uses the principle of reality orientation by the nurse telling the client that he or she does not see anything, but it does recognize his feelings. (B) This response does not make it clear that the nurse does not see anyone else in the room, and the nurse leaves the client alone to continue hallucinating. (C) This response leaves room for doubt; the nurse is further confusing the client by this statement. (D) This response reinforces the hallucination and implies that the nurse sees his mother, too.

78. **(B)** Client need: psychosocial integrity; subcategory: psychosocial adaptation; content area: psychiatric

RATIONALE

(A) Although eating habits are important to assess, they are less important than suicidal intent. (B) Maintenance of the client's life is the priority; assessment of suicidal intent is imperative. (C) Relationships and support systems are an important part of assessment, but they are less important than suicidal intent. (D) Daily living activities will give additional information about the level of depression, and are less significant than suicidal intent, although this information may give additional information about the actual plan for a suicidal attempt.

79. **(D)** Client need: psychosocial integrity; subcategory: psychosocial adaptation; content area: psychiatric

RATIONALE

(A) A client in deep depression would have been brought to the mental health center and would not be physically able to seek help for herself. (B) She is not manifesting psychotic symptoms in her behaviors. (C) The client's symptoms are more indicative of depression than anxiety. (D) Although the client was able to bring herself to the mental health center, the extent of her weight loss and the interference of symptoms with activities of daily living indicate that she is severely depressed.

TEST 9

Baton Rouge General Medical Center School of Nursing Test

MOCK NCLEX-RN BOARD REVIEW TEST QUESTIONS

1. A 48-year-old male client is hospitalized with mild ascites, bruising, and jaundice. He has a 20-year history of alcohol abuse. The client is diagnosed with cirrhosis. His serum ammonia level is high, indicating hepatic encephalopathy. He has esophageal varices. Which of the following may cause the varices to rupture?

   A. Lifting heavy objects
   B. Walking briskly
   C. Ingestion of barbiturates
   D. Ingestion of antacids

2. Due to his prolonged history of alcohol abuse, an alcoholic client will most likely have deficiencies of which of the following nutrients?

   A. Vitamin C and zinc
   B. Folic acid and niacin
   C. Vitamin A and biotin
   D. Thiamine and pyroxidine

3. The physician of an alcoholic client places him on a low-protein, high-carbohydrate diet. When choosing his menu, the client's best choice from the items below would be:

   A. Liver and onions, macaroni and cheese, tea with sugar
   B. Baked chicken, baked potato with bacon bits, milk
   C. Waffles with butter and honey, orange juice
   D. Cheese omelette with ham and mushrooms, milk

4. A chronic alcoholic client's condition deteriorates, and he begins to exhibit signs of hepatic coma. Which of the following is an early sign of impending hepatic coma?

   A. Hiccups
   B. Anorexia
   C. Mental confusion
   D. Fetor hepaticus

5. The physician of a client diagnosed with alcoholism orders neomycin 0.5 g q6h to prevent hepatic coma. Neomycin decreases serum ammonia levels by:

   A. Decreasing nitrogen-forming bacteria in the intestines
   B. Acidifying colon contents by causing ammonia retention in the colon
   C. Decreasing the uptake of vitamin D, thereby drawing more water into the colon
   D. Irritating the bowel and promoting evacuation of stool

6. A 26-year-old male client is brought by his wife to the emergency department (ED) unconscious. Blood is drawn for a stat blood count (CBC), fasting blood sugar level, and electrolytes. An indwelling urinary catheter is inserted. He has a history of type 1 diabetes (insulin-dependent diabetes mellitus [IDDM]). A diagnosis of ketoacidosis is made. Stat lab values reveal a blood sugar level of 520 mg/dL. Which of the following should the nurse expect to administer in the ER?

   A. $D_{50}W$ by IV push
   B. NPH insulin SC
   C. Regular insulin by IV infusion
   D. Sweetened grape juice by mouth

7. A client with IDDM is given IV insulin for a blood glucose level of 520 mg/dL. Life-threatening complications may occur initially, so the nurse will monitor him closely for serum:

   A. Chloride level of 99 mEq/L
   B. Sodium level of 136 mEq/L
   C. Potassium level of 3.1 mEq/L
   D. Potassium level of 6.3 mEq/L

8. An IDDM client's condition stabilizes. He begins to receive a daily injection of NPH insulin at 6:30 AM. The nurse can most likely expect a hypoglycemic reaction to occur that same day at:

   A. 8:30 AM–10:30 AM
   B. 2:30 PM–4:30 PM

C. 7:30 PM–9:30 PM
D. 10:30 PM–11:30 PM

9. After several days, an IDDM client's serum glucose stabilizes, and the registered nurse continues client teaching in preparation for his discharge. The nurse helps him plan an American Diabetes Association diet and explains how foods can be substituted on the exchange list. He can substitute 1 oz of poultry for:

A. One frankfurter
B. One ounce of ham
C. Two slices of bacon
D. One-fourth cup dry cottage cheese

10. When discussing the relationship between exercise and insulin requirements, a 26-year-old client with IDDM should be instructed that:

A. When exercise is increased, insulin needs are increased
B. When exercise is increased, insulin needs are decreased
C. When exercise is increased, there is no change in insulin needs
D. When exercise is decreased, insulin needs are decreased

11. A 64-year-old client is admitted to the hospital with benign prostatic hypertrophy (BPH). He has a history of adult-onset diabetes and hypertension and is scheduled to undergo a resection of the prostate. When recording his health history, the nurse asks about his chief complaint. The most serious symptom that may accompany BPH is:

A. Acute urinary retention
B. Hesitancy in starting urination
C. Increased frequency of urination
D. Decreased force of the urinary stream

12. A client undergoes a transurethral resection, prostate (TURP). He returns from surgery with a three-way continuous Foley irrigation of normal saline in progress. The purpose of this bladder irrigation is to prevent:

A. Bladder spasms
B. Clot formation
C. Scrotal edema
D. Prostatic infection

13. Following TURP, which of the following instructions would be appropriate to prevent or alleviate anxiety concerning the client's sexual functioning?

A. "You may resume sexual intercourse in 2 weeks."
B. "Many men experience impotence following TURP."
C. "A transurethral resection does not usually cause impotence."
D. "Check with your doctor about resuming sexual activity."

14. A client is having an amniocentesis. Prior to the procedure, an ultrasound is performed. In preparing the client, the nurse explains the reason for a sonogram in this situation to be:

A. Determination of multiple gestations
B. Determination of gross anomalies

C. Determination of placental location
D. Determination of fetal age

15. A client is resting comfortably after delivering her first child. When assessing her pulse rate, the nurse would recognize the following finding to be typical:

A. Thready pulse
B. Irregular pulse
C. Tachycardia
D. Bradycardia

16. A client is being admitted to the labor and delivery unit. She has had previous admissions for "false labor." Which clinical manifestation would be most indicative of true labor?

A. Increased bloody show
B. Progressive dilatation and effacement of the cervix
C. Uterine contractions
D. Decreased discomfort with ambulation

17. In evaluating the effectiveness of magnesium sulfate ($MgSO_4$), which of the following might indicate that the client was developing $MgSO_4$ toxicity?

A. A 31 patellar tendon reflex
B. Respirations of 12 breaths/min
C. Urine output of 40 mL/hr
D. A 21 proteinuria value

18. A client has had amniocentesis. One of the tests performed on the amniotic fluid is a lecithin/sphingomyelin (L/S) ratio. The results show a ratio of 1:1. This is indicative of:

A. Lung immaturity
B. Intrauterine growth retardation (IUGR)
C. Intrauterine infection
D. Neural tube defect

19. On admission to the postpartal unit, the nurse's assessment identifies the client's fundus to be soft, 2 fingerbreadths above the umbilicus, and deviated to the right. This is most likely an indication of:

A. Normal involution
B. A full bladder
C. An infection pain
D. A hemorrhage

20. A client's membranes have just ruptured spontaneously. Which of the following nursing actions should take priority?

A. Assess quantity of fluid.
B. Assess color and odor of fluid.
C. Document on fetal monitor strip and chart.
D. Assess fetal heart rate (FHR).

21. The nurse and prenatal client discuss the effects of cigarette smoking on pregnancy. It would be correct for the nurse to explain that with cigarette smoking there is increased risk that the baby will have:

A. A low birth weight
B. A birth defect
C. Anemia
D. Nicotine withdrawal

22. Which of the following blood values would require further nursing action in a newborn who is 4 hours old?

    A. Hemoglobin 17.2 g/dL
    B. Platelets 250,000/mm^3
    C. Serum glucose 30 mg/dL
    D. White blood cells 18,000/mm^3

23. A client is admitted to the psychiatric unit after lavage and stabilization in the emergency room for an overdose of antidepressants. This is her third attempt in 2 years. The highest priority intervention at this time is to:

    A. Assess level of consciousness
    B. Assess suicide potential
    C. Observe for sedation and hypotension
    D. Orient to her room and unit rules

24. A client's record from the ED indicates that she overdosed on phenelzine sulfate (Nardil), a monoamine oxidase (MAO) inhibitor. Which diet would be the *most* appropriate at this time?

    A. High carbohydrate, low cholesterol
    B. High protein, high carbohydrate
    C. 1 g sodium
    D. Tyramine-free

25. Two weeks after a client's admission for depression, the physician orders a consult for electroconvulsive therapy (ECT). Which of the following conditions, if present, would be a contraindication for ECT?

    A. Brain tumor or other space-occupying lesion
    B. History of mitral valve prolapse
    C. Surgically repaired herniated lumbar disk
    D. History of frequent urinary tract infections

26. A client is medically cleared for ECT and is tentatively scheduled for six treatments over a 2-week period. Her husband asks, "Isn't that a lot?" The nurse's best response is:

    A. "Yes, that does seem like a lot."
    B. "You'll have to talk to the doctor about that. The physician knows what's best for the client."
    C. "Six to 10 treatments are common. Are you concerned about permanent effects?"
    D. "Don't worry. Some clients have lots more than that."

27. A husband asks if he can visit with his wife on her ECT treatment days and what to expect after the initial treatment. The nurse's *best* response is:

    A. "You'll have to get permission from the physician to visit. Clients are pretty sick after the first treatment."
    B. "Visitors are not allowed. We will telephone you to inform you of her progress."
    C. "There's really no need to stay with her. She's going to sleep for several hours after the treatment."
    D. "Yes, you may visit. She may experience temporary drowsiness, confusion, or memory loss after each treatment."

28. A client is placed in five-point restraints after exhibiting sudden violence after illegal drug use, and haloperidol (Haldol) 5 mg IM is administered. After 1 hour, his behavior is more subdued, but he tells the nurse, "The devil followed me into this room, I see him standing in the corner with a big knife. When you leave the room, he's going to cut out my heart." The nurse's best response is:

    A. "I know you're feeling frightened right now, but I want you to know that I don't see anyone in the corner."
    B. "You'll probably see strange things for a while until the PCP wears off."
    C. "Try to sleep. When you wake up, the devil will be gone."
    D. "You're probably feeling guilty because you used illegal drugs tonight."

29. A violent client remains in restraints for several hours. Which of the following interventions is *most* appropriate while he is in restraints?

    A. Give fluids if the client requests them.
    B. Assess skin integrity and circulation of extremities before applying restraints and as they are removed.
    C. Measure vital signs at least every 4 hours.
    D. Release restraints every 2 hours for client to exercise.

30. After 7 hours in restraints and a total of 30-mg haloperidol in divided doses, a client complains of stiffness in his neck and his tongue "pulling to one side." These extrapyramidal symptoms (EPS) will *most* likely be relieved by the administration of:

    A. Lorazepam (Ativan)
    B. Benztropine (Cogentin)
    C. Thiothixene (Navane)
    D. Flurazepan (Dalmane)

31. Medication is administered to a client who has been placed in restraints after a sudden violent episode, and his EPSs subside. Restraints can be removed when:

    A. The physician orders it
    B. A therapeutic alliance has been established, and violent behavior subsides
    C. The violent behavior subsides, and the client agrees to behave
    D. The nurse deems that removal of restraints is necessary

32. A 16-year-old female client is admitted to the hospital because she collapsed at home while exercising with videotaped workout instructions. Her mother reports that she has been obsessed with losing weight and staying slim since cheerleader try-outs 6 months ago, when she lost out to two of her best friends. The client is 5'4'' and weighs 92 lb, which represents a weight loss of 28 lb over the last 4 months. The *most* important initial intervention on admission is to:

    A. Obtain an accurate weight
    B. Search the client's purse for pills
    C. Assess vital signs
    D. Assign her to a room with someone her own age

33. Assessment of a client reveals a 30% loss of preillness weight, lanugo, and cessation of menses for 3 months. Her vital signs are BP 90/50, P 96 bpm, respirations 30, and temperature 97°F. She admits to the nurse that she has induced vomiting 3 times this morning, but she had to continue exercising to lose "just 5 more lb." Her symptoms are consistent with:

A. Pregnancy
B. Bulimia
C. Gastritis
D. Anorexia nervosa

34. Blood work reveals the following lab values for a client who has been diagnosed with anorexia nervosa: hemoglobin 9.6 g/dL, hemocrit 27%, potassium 2.7 mEq/L, sodium 126 mEq/L. The greatest danger to her at this time is:

A. Hypoglycemia from low-carbohydrate intake
B. Possible cardiac dysrhythmias secondary to hypokalemia
C. Dehydration from vomiting
D. Anoxia secondary to anemia

35. A client suspected of having anorexia nervosa is placed on bed rest with an IV infusion and a high-carbohydrate liquid diet. Within 72 hours, the results of her lab work show a return to normal limits. She is transferred to the psychiatric service for further treatment. A behavior modification plan is initiated. Three days after her transfer, the client tells the nurse, "I haven't exercised in 6 days. I won't be eating lunch today." This statement by her most likely reflects:

A. Her lack of internal awareness about the outcome of the behavior
B. Increased knowledge about personal exercise plans
C. A manipulative technique to trick the nurse into allowing her to miss a meal
D. A true desire to stay fit while in the hospital

36. A client who has been diagnosed with anorexia nervosa refuses to eat lunch. The most therapeutic response by the nurse to her refusal is:

A. "Okay, missing one meal won't hurt."
B. "You'll have to eat lunch, or we'll force-feed you."
C. "It's not appropriate for you to try to manipulate the staff into granting your wishes."
D. "We will not allow you to starve yourself. You may choose to eat voluntarily or be fed."

37. A client who has been diagnosed with anorexia nervosa reluctantly agrees to eat all prescribed meals. The *most* important intervention in monitoring her dietary compliance would be to:

A. Allow her privacy at mealtimes
B. Praise her for eating everything
C. Observe behavior for 1–2 hours after meals to prevent vomiting
D. Encourage her to eat in moderation, choose foods that she likes, and avoid foods that she dislikes

38. A 2-year-old boy fell out of bed and has a subdural hematoma. When his mother leaves him for the first time, you will expect the child to:

A. Be comforted when he is held
B. Cry
C. Not notice that his mother has left
D. Withdraw and become listless

39. The doctor has ordered a restricted fluid intake for a 2-year-old child with a head injury. Normal fluid intake for a child of 2 years is:

A. 900 mL/24 hr
B. 1300 mL/24 hr
C. 1600 mL/24 hr
D. 2000 mL/24 hr

40. A 2-year-old child with a scalp laceration and subdural hematoma of the temporal area as a result of falling out of bed should be prevented from:

A. Crying
B. Falling asleep
C. Rolling from his back to his tummy
D. Sucking his thumb

41. A seventh grader lost consciousness after being hit in the head with a basketball. In the emergency room his vital signs are stable, and he demonstrates no neurologic deficit. He will not be admitted to the hospital. It is *most* important that you advise his mother to:

A. Encourage him to drink plenty of fluids
B. Expect him to have nausea with vomiting
C. Keep him awake for the next 12 hours
D. Wake him up every 1–2 hours during the night

42. A 14-year-old boy fell off his bike while "popping a wheelie" on the dirt trails. He has sustained a head injury with laceration of his scalp over his temporal lobe. If he were to complain of headache during the first 24 hours of his hospitalization, the nurse would:

A. Ask the physician to order a sedative
B. Have the client describe his headache every 15 minutes
C. Increase his fluid intake to 3000 mL/24 hr
D. Offer diversionary activities

43. An 18-year-old girl is admitted to the hospital with a depressed skull fracture as a result of a car accident. If the nurse were to observe a rising pulse rate and lowering blood pressure, the nurse would suspect that the client:

A. Has a sudden and severe increase in intracranial pressure
B. Has sustained an internal injury in addition to the head injury
C. Is beginning to experience a dangerously high level of anxiety
D. Is having intracranial bleeding

44. The nurse is caring for a 2-year-old girl with a subdural hematoma of the temporal area as a result of falling out of bed and notices that she has a runny nose. The nurse should:

A. Call the doctor immediately
B. Help her to blow her nose carefully
C. Test the discharge for sugar
D. Turn her to her side

45. A 2-year-old boy is in the hospital outpatient department for observation after falling out of his crib and hitting his head. The nurse calls the physician to report:

A. Evidence of perineal irritation
B. Pulse fell from 102 to 96
C. Pulse increased from 96 to 102
D. Temperature rose to 102°F rectally

46. The nurse is caring for a 3-month-old girl with meningitis. She has a positive Kernig's sign. The nurse expects her to react to discomfort if she:

    A. Dorsiflexes her ankle
    B. Flexes her spine
    C. Plantiflexes her wrist
    D. Turns her head to the side

47. The nurse is admitting an infant with bacterial meningitis and is prepared to manage the following possible effects of meningitis:

    A. Constipation
    B. Hypothermia
    C. Seizure
    D. Sunken fontanelles

48. The nurse is caring for a 6-week-old girl with meningitis. To help her develop a sense of trust, the nurse should:

    A. Give her a small soft blanket to hold
    B. Give her good perineal care after each diaper change
    C. Leave the door open to her room
    D. Pick her up when she cries

49. A 6-year-old girl is visiting the outpatient clinic because she has a fever and a rash. The doctor diagnoses chickenpox. Her mother asks the nurse how many baby aspirins her daughter can have for fever. The nurse should:

    A. Advise the mother not to give her aspirin
    B. Ask if the client is allergic to aspirin before giving further information
    C. Assess the function of the client's cranial nerve VIII
    D. Check the aspirin bottle label to determine milligrams per tablet

50. A 2-year-old child is recovering from surgery. Considering growth and development according to Erikson, the nurse identifies which of the following play activities as most appropriate?

    A. Assembling a puzzle with large pieces
    B. Being taken for a wheelchair ride
    C. Listening to a story about the Muppets
    D. Watching Sesame Street on television

51. A 14-year-old boy has a head injury with laceration of his scalp over his ear. The nurse should call the physician to report:

    A. Blood pressure increase from 100/80 to 115/85 after lunch
    B. Headache that is unresponsive to acetaminophen (Tylenol)
    C. Pulse rate ranges between 68 bpm and 76 bpm
    D. Temperature rise to 102°F rectally

52. The nurse is teaching a child's parents how to protect the child from lead poisoning. The nurse knows that a common source of lead poisoning in children is:

    A. Dandelion leaves
    B. Pencils
    C. Old paint
    D. Stuffing from toy animals

53. A woman diagnosed with multiple sclerosis is disturbed with diplopia. The nurse will teach her to:

    A. Limit activities which require focusing (close vision)
    B. Take more frequent naps
    C. Use artificial tears
    D. Wear a patch over one eye

54. In planning daily care for a client with multiple sclerosis, the nurse would take into consideration that multiple sclerosis:

    A. Becomes progressively debilitating without remission
    B. Has unpredictable remissions and exacerbations
    C. Is rapidly fatal
    D. Responds quickly to antimicrobial therapy

55. A client with a head injury asks why he cannot have something for his headache. The nurse's response is based on the understanding that analgesics could:

    A. Counteract the effects of antibiotics
    B. Elevate the blood pressure
    C. Mask symptoms of increasing intracranial pressure
    D. Stimulate the central nervous system

56. To prevent transmission of bacterial meningitis, the nurse would instruct an infected baby's mother to:

    A. Avoid touching the baby while in the room.
    B. Stay outside of the baby's room.
    C. Wear a gown and gloves and wash her hands before and after leaving the room.
    D. Wear a mask while in the room.

57. A client is scheduled for a magnetic resonance imaging (MRI) to locate a cerebral lesion. It is important for the nurse to find out if he has a(n):

    A. Allergy to seafood
    B. History of seizures
    C. Movable metal implant
    D. Pin or screw in any bone

58. A child is admitted with severe headache, fever, vomiting, photophobia, drowsiness, and stiff neck associated with viral meningitis. She will be more comfortable if the nurse:

    A. Dims the lights in her room
    B. Encourages her to breathe slowly and deeply
    C. Offers sips of warm liquids
    D. Places a large, soft pillow under her head

59. A 30-year-old client has been admitted to the psychiatric service with the diagnosis of schizophrenia. He tells the nurse that when the woman he had been dating broke up with him, the CIA had replaced her with an identical twin. The client is experiencing:

    A. Grandiose delusions
    B. Paranoid delusions
    C. Auditory hallucinations
    D. Visual hallucinations

60. A client tells the nurse that he has been hearing voices that tell him to kill his girlfriend because she is a spy. He further states that he is having difficulty not obeying the voices because, if he does not, his house will be burned

down. The highest priority nursing diagnosis for him at this time is:

- A. Sensory-perceptual alteration: auditory command hallucinations
- B. Alteration in thought processes: paranoid delusions
- C. Potential for violence directed at others
- D. Impaired verbal communication: loose associations

61. A client reports to the nurse that the voices are practically nonstop and that he needs to leave the hospital immediately to find his girlfriend and kill her. The best verbal response to the client by the nurse at this time is:

- A. "I understand that the voices are real to you, but I want you to know I don't hear them. They are a symptom of your illness."
- B. "Just don't pay attention to the voices. They'll go away after some medication."
- C. "You can't leave here. This unit is locked and the doctor has not ordered your discharge."
- D. "We will have to put you in seclusion and restraints for a while. You could hurt someone with thoughts like that."

62. The physician orders haloperidol 5 mg IM stat for a client and tells the nurse that the dose can be repeated in 1–2 hours if needed. The most likely rationale for this order is:

- A. The client will settle down more quickly if he thinks the staff is medicating him
- B. The medication will sedate the client until the physician arrives
- C. Haloperidol is a minor tranquilizer and will not oversedate the client

D. Rapid neuroleptization is the most effective approach to care for the violent or potentially violent client

63. Two hours after the second injection of haloperidol, a client complains to the nurse of a stiff neck and inability to sit still. He is experiencing symptoms consistent with:

- A. Parkinsonism and dystonia
- B. Dystonia and akathisia
- C. Akathisia and parkinsonism
- D. Neuroleptic malignant syndrome

64. The physician orders medication for a client's unpleasant side effects from the haloperidol. The *most* appropriate drug at this time is:

- A. Lorazepam
- B. Triazolam (Halcion)
- C. Benztropine
- D. Thiothixene

65. A psychiatric client has been stabilized and is to be discharged. The nurse will recognize client insight and behavioral change by which of the following client statements?

- A. "When I get home, I will need to take my medicines and call my therapist if I have any side effects or begin to hear voices."
- B. "If I have any side effects from my medicines, I will take an extra dose of Cogentin."
- C. "When I get home, I should be able to taper myself off the Haldol because the voices are gone now."
- D. "As soon as I leave here, I'm throwing away my medicines. I never thought I needed them anyway."

MOCK NCLEX-RN BOARD REVIEW TEST ANSWERS

1. **(A)** Client need: physiological integrity; subcategory: physiological adaptation; content area: med/surg
   RATIONALE
   (A) Lifting heavy objects will increase intrathoracic pressure, thus placing the client at risk for rupturing esophageal varices. (B, C, D) This activity will not cause an increase in intrathoracic pressure.

2. **(D)** Client need: physiological integrity; subcategory: physiological adaptation; content area: med/surg
   RATIONALE
   (A) Chronic alcoholism can lead to deficiencies of B complex vitamins including thiamine and pyroxidine. (B) Chronic alcoholism can lead to deficiencies of vitamins A, D, K, and B complex. (C) Chronic alcoholism can lead to deficiencies of vitamins A, D, K, and B complex. (D) Vitamins A, D, K, and B require bile salts to be absorbed from the gastrointestinal tract. A damaged liver does not form bile salts.

3. **(C)** Client need: physiological integrity; subcategory: basic care and comfort; content area: med/surg
   RATIONALE
   (A, B, D) These foods are high in protein, which needs to be restricted. (C) Serum ammonia levels can be decreased by restricting dietary protein intake. Waffles, honey, and orange juice are high in carbohydrate and low or completely lacking in protein. Butter, a concentrated fat, will provide extra calories.

4. **(C)** Client need: physiological integrity; subcategory: physiological adaptation; content area: med/surg
   RATIONALE
   (A) Hiccups are not a sign of impending hepatic coma. (B) Anorexia is not a sign of impending hepatic coma. (C) One of the earliest symptoms of hepatic coma is mental confusion. Asterixis, a flapping tremor of the hand, may also be seen. (D) This sign is associated with the later stages of hepatic coma. Fetor hepaticus, a characteristic odor on the breath that smells like acetone, may sometimes be noted when the liver fails.

5. **(A)** Client need: physiological integrity; subcategory: pharmacological and parenteral therapies; content area: med/surg
   RATIONALE
   (A) Neomycin interferes with protein synthesis in the bacterial cell, causing bacterial death. Neomycin reduces the growth of the ammonia-producing bacteria in the intestines and is used for the treatment of hepatic coma. (B) This choice describes the action of lactulose, another drug commonly used to decrease systemic ammonia levels. (C) Neomycin's action does *not* decrease uptake of vitamin D to reduce serum ammonia levels. (D) Bowel irritation with diarrhea is more likely to occur with administration of lactulose rather than of neomycin. Besides, diarrhea is a side effect of a drug, not the action of the drug.

6. **(C)** Client need: physiological integrity; subcategory: reduction of risk potential; content area: med/surg
   RATIONALE
   (A) This action would further increase the client's blood sugar. (B) NPH insulin is an intermediate-acting insulin, with an average of 4–6 hours before onset of action. The client needs insulin that will act immediately. During a ketoacidotic state, the client is dehydrated, so any insulin administered SC will be poorly absorbed. (C) Regular insulin is the fastest acting-insulin; when given IV, it will immediately act to decrease blood sugar. Regular insulin is given to decrease blood glucose levels by promot-

ing metabolism of glucose, inhibiting lipolysis and formation of ketone bodies. (D) This action would further increase the client's blood sugar.

7. **(D)** Client need: physiological integrity; subcategory: reduction of risk potential; content area: med/surg
   RATIONALE
   (A) The chloride level is within acceptable limits. (B) The sodium level is within acceptable limits. (C) This value indicates hypokalemia, rather than the hyperkalemia that occurs during diabetic ketoacidosis. (D) When diabetic ketoacidosis exists, intracellular dehydration occurs and potassium leaves the cells and enters the vascular system, thus increasing the serum level beyond an acceptable range. When insulin and fluids are administered, cell walls are repaired and potassium is transported back into the cells. Normal serum potassium levels range from 3.5–5.0 mEq/L.

8. **(B)** Client need: physiological integrity; subcategory: pharmacological and parenteral therapies; content area: med/surg
   RATIONALE
   (A) This time describes the time of onset of NPH insulin's action, rather than its peak effect. (B) NPH insulin, an intermediate-acting insulin, usually begins to lower serum glucose levels about 2 hours after administration. The action of NPH insulin peaks 8–14 hours after administration. It has a 20–30 hour duration. (C) The time stated is not the time of peak action for NPH insulin administered at 6:30 AM. (D) The time stated is not the time of peak action for NPH insulin administered at 6:30 AM.

9. **(D)** Client need: physiological integrity; subcategory: basic care and comfort; content area: med/surg
   RATIONALE
   (A) A frankfurter is a high-fat meat on the diabetic exchange list. (B) Ham is a medium-fat meat on the diabetic exchange list, unless it is a center-cut slice. (C) One strip of bacon equals one *fat* exchange rather than a *meat* exchange. Dietary substitutions should occur within exchange lists and not between exchange lists. (D) Diabetic meat-exchange lists are categorized into lean-meat foods, medium-fat meats, and high-fat meats. Cottage cheese (dry, 2% butterfat), one-fourth cup, can substitute for one lean-meat exchange.

10. **(B)** Client need: health promotion and maintenance; subcategory: prevention and early detection of disease; content area: med/surg
    RATIONALE
    (A) If the client's insulin is increased when activity level is increased, hypoglycemia may result. (B) Exercise decreased the blood sugar by promoting uptake of glucose by the muscles. Consequently, less insulin is needed to metabolize ingested carbohydrates. Extra food may be required for extra activity. (C) This statement directly contradicts the correct answer and is inaccurate. (D) When exercise is decreased, the client's insulin dose does not need to be altered unless the blood sugar becomes unstable.

11. **(A)** Client need: physiological integrity; subcategory: physiological adaptation; content area: med/surg
    RATIONALE
    (A) Acute urinary retention requires urgent medical attention. If measures such as a warm tub bath or warm tea do not occur after 6 hours, the client should go to the ED for catheterization. (B, C, D) This choice is a symptom of BPH, but it is not serious or life threatening.

12. **(B)** Client need: physiological integrity; subcategory: reduction of risk potential; content area: med/surg

RATIONALE

(A) The purpose of bladder irrigation is not to prevent bladder spasms, but to drain the bladder and decrease clot formation and obstruction. (B) A three-way system of bladder irrigation will cleanse the bladder and prevent formation of blood clots. A catheter obstructed by clots or other debris will cause prostatic distention and hemorrhage. (C) Scrotal edema seldom occurs after TURP. Bladder irrigation will not prevent this complication. (D) Prostatic infection seldom occurs after TURP. Bladder irrigation will not prevent this complication.

13. **(C)** Client need: psychosocial integrity; subcategory: coping and adaptation; content area: med/surg

RATIONALE

(A) Sexual activity should be delayed until cleared by the client's physician. (B) Although many men experience retrograde ejaculation following prostate surgery, potency is seldom affected. (C) Although the client may experience retrograde ejaculation, it will not limit his ability to engage in sexual intercourse. (D) Although the client should obtain clearance from his physician before resuming sexual activity, this statement does not give the client any information or reassurance about future sexual activity or potency that could decrease his anxiety.

14. **(C)** Client need: psychosocial integrity; subcategory: coping and adaptation; content area: maternity

RATIONALE

(A) Sonography can be used to determine the presence of multiple gestation. In this question, the sonogram is used as a preparatory step for a specific invasive procedure. (B) Sonography can be used to determine the presence of gross anomalies. In this question, the sonogram is used as a preparatory step for a specific invasive procedure. (C) Prior to amniocentesis, the abdomen is scanned by ultrasound to locate the placenta, thus reducing the possibility of penetrating it with the spinal needle used to obtain amniotic fluid. (D) Sonography can be used to determine fetal age. In this question, the sonogram is used as a preparatory step for a specific invasive procedure.

15. **(D)** Client need: physiological integrity; subcategory: physiological adaptation; content area: maternity

RATIONALE

(A) A thready pulse is indicative of hypotension and excessive blood loss and is often rapid. (B) Pulse irregularities or dysrhythmias do not occur in the normal postpartum woman. (C) Tachycardia occurs less frequently than bradycardia and is related to increased blood loss or prolonged difficult labor and/or birth. (D) Puerperal bradycardia with rates of 50–70 bpm commonly occurs during the first 6–10 days of the postpartal period. It may be related to decreased cardiac strain, decreased blood volume, contraction of the uterus, and increased stroke volume.

16. **(B)** Client need: health promotion and maintenance; subcategory: growth and development through the life span; content area: maternity

RATIONALE

(A) Bloody show is considered a sign of imminent labor, which usually begins in 24–48 hours. An increase in bloody show is an indication that the cervix is changing. (B) Contractions of true labor produce progressive cervical effacement and dilatation. (C) Contractions of false labor may mimic those of true labor. However, the contractions of false labor do not produce progressive effacement and dilatation of the cervix. (D) In true labor, the discomfort is not relieved by ambulation; walking may intensify the discomfort.

17. **(B)** Client need: physiological integrity; subcategory: pharmacological and parenteral therapies; content area: maternity

RATIONALE

(A) Diminished (not accentuated) patellar tendon reflex is a sign of developing $MgSO_4$ toxicity. A value of 21 is considered a normal tendon reflex; 3+ is considered brisker than normal. (B) $MgSO_4$ is a central nervous system (CNS) depressant. It also relaxes smooth muscle. If the respiratory rate is <16 bpm magnesium toxicity may be developing. (C) Urine output of 40 mL/hr is enough to allow elimination of toxic levels of magnesium. Urinary output of <100 mL in a 4-hour period may result in toxic levels of magnesium. (D) Presence of protein in the urine is a symptom of pregnancy-induced hypertension (PIH), a clinical syndrome for which magnesium sulfate is frequently used in medical management. Protein in the urine is not induced by magnesium sulfate intake.

18. **(A)** Client need: physiological integrity; subcategory: physiological adaptation; content area: maternity

RATIONALE

(A) At about 30–32 weeks' gestation, the amounts of the surfactants, lecithin, and sphingomyelin become equal. As the fetal lungs mature, the concentration of lecithin begins to exceed that of sphingomyelin. At 35 weeks, the L/S ratio is 2:1. Respiratory distress syndrome is unlikely if birth occurs at this time. (B) IUGR is associated with compromised uteroplacental perfusion or with viral infections, chromosomal disorders, congenital malformations, and maternal malnutrition. IUGR is not specifically assessed by analysis of the L/S ratio. (C) Analysis of the L/S ratio is not an assessment used to confirm intrauterine infection. (D) Elevated levels of α-fetoprotein in maternal serum or in amniotic fluid have been found to reflect open neural tube defects, such as spina bifida and anencephaly.

19. **(B)** Client need: health promotion and maintenance; subcategory: growth and development through the life span; content area: maternity

RATIONALE

(A) Immediately after expulsion of the placenta, the fundus should be in the midline and remain firm. (B) A boggy displaced uterus in the immediate postpartum period is a sign of urinary distention. Because uterine ligaments are stretched, a full bladder can displace the uterus. (C) Symptoms of infection may include unusual uterine discomfort, temperature elevation, and foul-smelling lochia. The stem of this question does not address any of these factors. (D) While excessive bleeding is associated with a soft, boggy uterus, the stem of this question includes displacement of the uterus, which is more commonly associated with bladder distention.

20. **(D)** Client need: physiological integrity; subcategory: reduction of risk potential; content area: maternity

RATIONALE

(A) Assessing the quantity of amniotic fluid is important as an indication of maternal fetal well-being, but it does not take priority over assessment of FHR. (B) Greenish-brown discoloration of amniotic fluid indicates presence of meconium. Foul odor may indicate presence of infection. Both of these are important assessment data, but they do not take priority over possible life-threatening compression of the umbilical cord. (C) Documentation is important, but it does not take priority over the possible life-threatening compression of the umbilical cord. (D) If changes in the FHR are noted, the nurse should check for umbilical cord prolapse. This intervention has priority over the other actions. The danger of a prolapsed cord is increased once membranes have ruptured, especially if the presenting part of the fetus does not fit firmly against the cervix.

21. **(A)** Client need: health promotion and maintenance; subcategory: prevention and early detection of disease; content area: maternity

    RATIONALE

    (A) Women who smoke during pregnancy are at increased risk for miscarriage, preterm labor, and IUGR in the fetus. (B) Although smoking produces harmful effects on the maternal vascular system and the developing fetus, it has not been directly linked to fetal anomalies. (C) Smoking during pregnancy has not been directly linked to anemia in the fetus. (D) Smoking during pregnancy has not been linked to nicotine withdrawal symptoms in the newborn.

22. **(C)** Client need: physiological integrity; subcategory: reduction of risk potential; content area: maternity

    RATIONALE

    (A) The normal range for hemoglobin in the newborn is 17–19 g/dL; 17.2 g/dL is within normal limits. (B) A normal value range for platelets in the newborn is 150,000–400,000 mm^3; 250,000/mm^3 is within normal range. (C) A serum glucose of 30 mg/dL in the first 72 hours of life is indicative of hypoglycemia and warrants further intervention. (D) On the day of birth, a white blood cell count of 18,000–40,000/mm^3 is normal in the newborn.

23. **(B)** Client need: psychosocial integrity; subcategory: psychosocial adaptation; content area: psychiatric

    RATIONALE

    (A) The client was stabilized in the ED and consequently would not be sent to the psychiatric unit if comatose. (B) Suicide assessment is always appropriate for clients with a history of previous attempts or depression, because either of these factors places the client at high risk. (C) The admission assessment should include observation for sedation and hypotension, but this is not in priority over suicide assessment. (D) Orientation to room and unit rules is of low priority at this time.

24. **(D)** Client need: physiological integrity; subcategory: basic care and comfort; content area: psychiatric

    RATIONALE

    (A) There are no data to support the need for increased carbohydrates or decreased cholesterol in the diet. (B) There is no data to support the need for increased protein or increased carbohydrates in the diet. (C) There is no assessment or laboratory data indicating that sodium should be restricted in the diet. (D) Tyramine is an amino acid activated by MAO in the liver and intestinal wall. It is released as proteins are hydrolyzed through aging, pickling, smoking, or spoilage of foods. When MAO is inhibited, tyramine levels rise, stimulating the adrenergic system to release large amounts of norepinephrine, which can produce a hypertensive crisis.

25. **(A)** Client need: physiological integrity; subcategory: reduction of risk potential; content area: psychiatric

    RATIONALE

    (A) A contraindication for ECT is a space-occupying lesion such as a brain tumor. During ECT, intracranial pressure increases. Therefore, ECT would not be prescribed for a client whose intracranial pressure is already elevated. (B) Any cardiac dysrhythmias or complications that arise during ECT are usually attributed to the IV anesthetics used, not to preexisting cardiac structural conditions. (C) Musculoskeletal injuries during ECT are extremely rare because of the IV use of centrally acting muscle relaxers. (D) A history of any kind of infection would not contraindicate the use of ECT. In fact, concurrent treatment of infections with ECT is not uncommon.

26. **(C)** Client need: psychosocial integrity; subcategory: coping and adaptation; content area: psychiatric

    RATIONALE

    (A) This response indicates that the nurse is unsure of herself and not knowledgeable about ECT. It also reinforces the husband's fears. (B) This response is "passing the buck" unnecessarily. The information needed to appropriately answer the husband's question is well within the nurse's knowledge base. (C) The most common range for affective disorders is 6–10 treatments. This response confirms and reinforces the physician's plan for treatment. It also opens communication with the husband to identify underlying fears and knowledge deficits. (D) This response offers false reassurance and dismisses the husband's underlying concerns about his wife.

27. **(D)** Client need: psychosocial integrity; subcategory: coping and adaptation; content area: psychiatric

    RATIONALE

    (A) It is within the nurse's realm of practice to grant visiting privileges according to hospital policy. ECT treatments do not make clients sick. (B) Visitors are allowed and encouraged, particularly family members. (C) Clients are usually awake within 1 hour posttreatment. Drowsiness wanes as the anesthetic wears off. (D) A family member is encouraged to stay with the client after return to the unit. The nurse has used an opportunity to do family teaching and allay fears by explaining temporary side effects of the treatment.

28. **(A)** Client need: psychosocial integrity; subcategory: psychosocial adaptation; content area: psychiatric

    RATIONALE

    (A) The nurse is the client's link to reality. This response validates the authenticity of the client's experience by casting doubt on his belief and reinforcing reality. (B) Although this statement may be literally correct, it is nontherapeutic because it lacks validation. (C) This response encourages the client to attempt to do something that may be impossible at this time, offers false reassurance, and reinforces delusional content. (D) The nurse is making an incorrect assumption about the client's feelings by offering a nontherapeutic interpretation of the motivation for the client's actions.

29. **(D)** Client need: psychosocial integrity; subcategory: psychosocial adaptation; content area: psychiatric

    RATIONALE

    (A) Fluids (nourishment) should be offered at regular intervals whether the client requests (or refuses) them or not. (B) Skin integrity and circulation of the extremities should be checked regularly while the client is restrained, not only before restraints are applied and after they are removed. (C) Vital signs should be checked at least every 2 hours. If the client remains agitated in restraints, vital signs should be monitored even more closely, perhaps every 1–2 hours. (D) Restraints should be released every 2 hours for exercise, one extremity at a time, to maintain muscle tone, skin and joint integrity, and circulation.

30. **(B)** Client need: physiological integrity; subcategory: pharmacological and parenteral therapies; content area: psychiatric

    RATIONALE

    (A) Lorazepam is an antianxiety agent that produces muscle relaxation and inhibits cortical and limbic arousal. It has no action in the basal ganglia of the brain. (B) Benztropine acts to reduce EPS by blocking excess CNS cholinergic activity associated with dopamine deficiency in the basal ganglia by displacing acetylcholine at the receptor site. (C) Thiothixene is an antipsychotic known to block dopamine in the limbic system, thereby causing EPS. (D) Flurazepan is a hypnotic that acts in the limbic system, thalamus, and hypothalamus of the CNS to produce sleep. It has no known action in the vasal ganglia.

31. **(B)** Client need: psychosocial integrity; subcategory: psychosocial adaptation; content area: psychiatric

RATIONALE

(A) The physician *may* order release of restraints, but prior to that, the client must meet criteria for release. (B) While the client is still restrained, but after violent behavior has subsided, a therapeutic bridge is built. This alliance encourages dialogue between nurse and client, allowing the client to determine causative factors, feelings prior to loss of control, and adaptive alternatives to violence. (C) If the client only "agrees to behave" after violent behavior subsides, he has developed no insight into cause and effect of violence or his response to stress. (D) Removal of restraints occurs only when the client meets the criteria for release, not just because the nurse says it is necessary.

32. **(C)** Client need: psychosocial integrity; subcategory: coping and adaptation; content area: psychiatric

    RATIONALE

    (A) On admission, vital signs are the highest priority. Weight is not a vital sign. (B) Belongings are routinely searched on admission to a psychiatric unit, but this search is not a high priority. (C) Vital signs are a high priority when working with self-destructive clients. (D) Room assignment is of low priority.

33. **(D)** Client need: psychosocial integrity; subcategory: psychosocial adaptation; content area: psychiatric

    RATIONALE

    (A) Presenting behaviors collectively are inconsistent with depression. (B) A preillness weight loss of 30%, lanugo, and cessation of menses are inconsistent with bulimia. (C) Symptoms and vital signs do not indicate the presence of infection. (D) All symptoms and vital signs are consistent with anorexia nervosa.

34. **(B)** Client need: physiological integrity; subcategory: physiological adaptation; content area: psychiatric

    RATIONALE

    (A) There is no lab data to support hypoglycemia. (B) Hypokalemia, caused by vomiting and decreased dietary intake of potassium, can result in life-threatening dysrhythmias. (C) Evidence of dehydration is not life threatening at this time, although fluid volume deficit does need to be addressed. (D) The client's hemoglobin does not reflect a life-threatening value sufficient to render the client anoxic.

35. **(A)** Client need: psychosocial integrity; subcategory: psychosocial adaptation; content area: psychiatric

    RATIONALE

    (A) Indirect self-destructive behavior such as that seen in anorexia nervosa is characterized by the client's lack of insight and the awareness that the outcome of the dieting, exercising, and weight loss will ultimately result in death if uninterrupted. (B) Although the client is knowledgeable about exercise, knowledge about the balance between nutrition, exercise, and rest is absent. (C) The client's level of denial and lack of awareness disallow this behavior as a manipulative trick. (D) The client's illness-maintaining behaviors are inconsistent with fitness.

36. **(D)** Client need: psychosocial integrity; subcategory: psychosocial adaptation; content area: psychiatric

    RATIONALE

    (A) This response reinforces the client's maladaptive behavior, thereby contributing to the client's risk. (B) Ultimatums are not therapeutic. (C) This comment invites an argument because it puts the client on the defensive and stabs at her self-esteem, which is already compromised. (D) Setting limits assures the client that staff has genuine concern for her safety and well-being. Giving her an actual choice will give the client an increased sense of control over her life and avoid an argument or power struggle.

37. **(C)** Client need: psychosocial integrity; subcategory: psychosocial adaptation; content area: psychiatric

RATIONALE

(A) Eating alone is not recommended for anorexic clients because they tend to hoard food instead of eating it. (B) The client should be praised for whatever she eats, which is usually a small portion or percentage of what is served. Praise should not be withheld until she eats everything. (C) The client should be observed eye-to-eye for at least 1 hour following meals to prevent discarding food stashed in her clothing at mealtime or engaging in self-induced vomiting. (D) If offered these choices, the client would choose low-caloric foods, not a nutritious diet.

38. **(B)** Client need: health promotion and maintenance; subcategory: growth and development through the life span; content area: pediatrics

    RATIONALE

    (A) It will be difficult to comfort a 2 year old with a headache without his mother. (B) This baby probably will cry, which should be prevented because it will increase his intracranial pressure (ICP). Asking the mother to wait until the baby is asleep may help. (C) An awake 2 year old will notice when his mother leaves. (D) An older child may withdraw when feeling afraid, but a 2 year old will probably show more aggressive behavior.

39. **(C)** Client need: physiological integrity; subcategory: basic care and comfort; content area: pediatrics

    RATIONALE

    (A, B, D) These values are incorrect. Normal intake for a child of 2 years is about 1600 mL in 24 hours. (C) This value is correct. Normal intake for a child of 2 years is about 1600 mL in 24 hours.

40. **(A)** Client need: physiological integrity; subcategory: reduction of risk potential; content area: pediatrics

    RATIONALE

    (A) A child with a subdural hematoma has increased ICP. Crying may significantly increase this pressure. (B) Adequate sleep is essential, but it is important that the child can be aroused from sleep after head injury. (C) This child is free to roll from his back to his abdomen. (D) Thumb-sucking serves to reduce anxiety and should not be prevented at this time.

41. **(D)** Client need: physiological integrity; subcategory: physiological adaptation; content area: pediatrics

    RATIONALE

    (A) Fluid intake should be normal. Fluid intake may be restricted when there is a risk for increased ICP in a hospitalized client. (B) Nausea is possible, but vomiting without nausea is more likely with increased ICP. Neither one should be expected, but the mother should know to notify the physician or hospital if they occur. (C) The child does not need to be kept awake. It is important that he can be aroused from sleep. (D) If the child cannot be awakened from sleep after head injury, it is an indication of serious increase in ICP. The mother should call an ambulance right away.

42. **(D)** Client need: physiological integrity; subcategory: physiological adaptation; content area: pediatrics

    RATIONALE

    (A) CNS depressants are not given for headache due to head injury because they would mask changes in neurological status and because they could further depress the CNS. (B) The client should not be asked to think about his headache every 15 minutes. (C) Fluid intake should be normal or restricted for a client with a head injury. Normal fluid intake for a 14 year old is about 2000–2400 mL daily. (D) Diversion may help the child to focus on a pleasant activity instead of on his headache.

43. **(B)** Client need: physiological integrity; subcategory: physiological adaptation; content area: pediatrics

RATIONALE

(A) Widening pulse pressure (high systolic and low diastolic) with compensatory slowing of pulse rate are late signs of increasing ICP. (B) Rising pulse rate and lowering blood pressure are indicative of hypovolemia due to hemorrhage. (C) High anxiety, in the absence of hemorrhage, would result in a high pulse rate and a high blood pressure. (D) Intracranial bleeding results in increased ICP. A change in level of consciousness is an early sign of increasing ICP, and vital sign changes are late signs of increasing ICP.

44. **(C)** Client need: physiological integrity; subcategory: physiological adaptation; content area: pediatrics

RATIONALE

(A) The nasal discharge could be due to a cold. It is necessary to gather additional assessment data to identify a possible cerebrospinal fluid leak. (B) If the discharge is cerebrospinal fluid, it would not be safe to encourage the girl to blow her nose. (C) Cerebrospinal fluid is positive for sugar; mucus is not. (D) Turning her to her side will have no effect on her "runny nose." It is necessary to gather further assessment data.

45. **(D)** Client need: physiological integrity; subcategory: physiological adaptation; content area: pediatrics

RATIONALE

(A) Perineal irritation needs to be addressed, but it is probably not necessary to call the physician. (B) This fall in pulse rate remains within normal limits and is probably insignificant. It is important to monitor for continued change. (C) This rise in pulse rate is probably not significant, but it is important to monitor for continued change. (D) This temperature is above normal limits and needs medical investigation. It may or may not be related to the head injury.

46. **(B)** Client need: physiological integrity; subcategory: physiological adaptation; content area: pediatrics

RATIONALE

(A) Discomfort with ankle dorsiflexion is not expected with meningitis. (B) Spinal flexion, flexing the neck or the hips with legs extended, causes discomfort if the meninges are irritated. (C) Discomfort with wrist flexion is not expected with meningitis. (D) Rotating the cervical spine may cause discomfort with meningitis, but pain with flexion is more indicative of meningeal irritation.

47. **(C)** Client need: physiological integrity; subcategory: physiological adaptation; content area: pediatrics

RATIONALE

(A) Constipation may occur if the child is dehydrated, but it is not directly associated with meningitis. (B) It is more likely the child will have fever. (C) Seizure is often the initial sign of meningitis in children and could become frequent. (D) It is more likely the child will have bulging fontanelles.

48. **(D)** Client need: psychosocial integrity; subcategory: coping and adaptation; content area: pediatrics

RATIONALE

(A) A soft blanket may be comforting, but it is not directed toward developing a sense of trust. (B) Good perineal care is important, but it is not directed toward developing a sense of trust. (C) An infant with meningitis needs frequent attention, but leaving the door open does not foster trust. (D) Consistently picking her up when she cries will help the child feel trust in her caregivers.

49. **(A)** Client need: health promotion and maintenance; subcategory: prevention and early detection of disease; content area: pediatrics

RATIONALE

(A) Aspirin taken during a viral infection has been implicated as a predisposing factor to Reye's syndrome in children and adoles-

cents. Children and adolescents should not be given aspirin. (B) Allergy to aspirin is not related to Reye's syndrome. (C) Tinnitus, caused by damage to the acoustic nerve, occurs with aspirin toxicity, but this is not related to Reye's syndrome. (D) A 6-year-old child should not be given any baby aspirin.

50. **(A)** Client need: health promotion and maintenance; subcategory: growth and development through the life span; content area: pediatrics

RATIONALE

(A) A 2-year-old child is in the stage of autonomy, according to Erikson. Assembling a puzzle with large pieces enables her to "do it herself." (B) A wheelchair ride would probably be fun, but it is not directed toward helping the child to achieve autonomy. (C) Listening to a story may be fun and educational, but it is not directed toward helping the child to achieve autonomy. (D) Watching television may be a favorite activity, but it does not foster autonomy.

51. **(D)** Client need: physiological integrity; subcategory: physiological adaptation; content area: pediatrics

RATIONALE

(A) This change in blood pressure may not be significant and does not indicate a widening pulse pressure, a late sign of increased ICP. It is important to continue to monitor for change in blood pressure. (B) Acetaminophen may be ineffective in relieving headache after head injury. Stronger analgesics are contraindicated because they mask neurological signs and may depress the CNS. (C) Pulse rates between 68 bpm and 76 bpm are within normal limits for a 14-year-old child. It is important to monitor for a consistent drop in pulse rate, which is a late sign of increasing ICP. (D) An elevated temperature is abnormal and requires further assessment and medical intervention. The temperature may be unrelated to the head injury, but CNS infection is serious and difficult to control.

52. **(C)** Client need: health promotion and maintenance; subcategory: prevention and early detection of disease; content area: pediatrics

RATIONALE

(A) Dandelion leaves are not a source of lead. (B) Pencils are not a source of lead poisoning. (C) Chewing on objects painted before 1960 is a common source of lead poisoning in children. Gasoline is another source. (D) Stuffed animals are not a source of lead.

53. **(D)** Client need: health promotion and maintenance; subcategory: prevention and early detection of disease; content area: med/surg

RATIONALE

(A) Limiting activities requiring close vision will not alleviate the discomfort of double vision. (B) Frequent naps may be comforting, but they will not prevent double vision. (C) Artificial tears are necessary in the absence of a corneal reflex, but they have no effect on diplopia. (D) An eye patch over either eye will eliminate the effects of double vision during the time the eye patch is worn. An eye patch is safe for a person with an intact corneal reflex.

54. **(B)** Client need: health promotion and maintenance; subcategory: prevention and early detection of disease; content area: med/surg

RATIONALE

(A) Multiple sclerosis eventually becomes debilitating, but it is characterized by remission of symptoms. (B) Remissions and exacerbations are unpredictable with multiple sclerosis. The client experiences progressive dysfunction after each exacerbation episode. (C) Multiple sclerosis is usually slowly progressive. (D) Multiple sclerosis is an autoimmune disease. Antimicrobial therapy has no effect on its course.

55. **(C)** Client need: physiological integrity; subcategory: pharmacological and parenteral therapies; content area: med/surg

RATIONALE

(A) Analgesic medication does not counteract the effects of antibiotics. (B) Analgesic medication may lower blood pressure elevated due to anxiety. (C) Analgesic medication, especially CNS depressants, is not given if there is danger of increasing ICP, because neurological changes may not be apparent. Also, further depression of the CNS is contraindicated. (D) Analgesics do not stimulate the CNS.

56. **(C)** Client need: health promotion and maintenance; subcategory: prevention and early detection of disease; content area: pediatrics

RATIONALE

(A) The mother should be allowed and encouraged to touch her baby. (B) With care, transmission can be prevented. There is no need for the mother to stay outside the room. (C) Everyone entering the baby's room should take appropriate measures to prevent transmission of pathogens. (D) Wearing a mask will not protect against transmission of pathogens.

57. **(C)** Client need: physiological integrity; subcategory: reduction of risk potential; content area: med/surg

RATIONALE

(A) Iodine is not used as a contrast medium for MRI. It is important to inquire about allergy to seafood if the client is to have an arteriogram or enhanced computer tomography. (B) MRI is safe if seizures are under control. It is more important to inquire about movable metal implants. (C) Clients with movable metal implants such as shrapnel or aneurysm clips or clients with permanent pacemakers or implanted pumps can be traumatized during an MRI. (D) Nonmovable metal prostheses or hardware will not cause trauma during an MRI.

58. **(A)** Client need: physiological integrity; subcategory: physiological adaptation; content area: pediatrics

RATIONALE

(A) The discomfort of photophobia is alleviated by dimming the lights. (B) Helping the child to breathe slowly and deeply may help to reduce anxiety, but it will not alleviate other discomforts of viral meningitis. (C) It is important to maintain fluid balance, but sips of warm liquids do not alleviate the discomforts of meningitis. (D) A large, soft pillow under her head causing neck flexion is likely to increase her discomfort owing to stretching of the meninges.

59. **(B)** Client need: psychosocial integrity; subcategory: psychosocial adaptation; content area: psychiatric

RATIONALE

(A) There are no indications that the client's thoughts reflect special powers or talents characteristic of grandiosity. (B) The client's thought content is fixed, false, persecutory, and suspicious in nature, which is characteristic of paranoid delusions. (C, D) The client is not demonstrating a sensory experience.

60. **(C)** Client need: psychosocial integrity; subcategory: psychosocial adaptation; content area: psychiatric

RATIONALE

(A) Although the client is having command hallucinations, this is second in priority to real or potential violence, which can be a threat to life itself. (B) Although the client is experiencing delusions, this is also a lower priority than his potential or actual loss of control. (C) Whether real or potential, violence directed at self or others is always high priority. (D) There is no evidence of loosening of associations.

61. **(A)** Client need: psychosocial integrity; subcategory: psychosocial adaptation; content area: psychiatric

RATIONALE

(A) This response validates the client's experience and presents reality to him. (B) This nontherapeutic response minimizes and dismisses the client's verbalized experience. (C) This response can be interpreted by a paranoid client as a threat, thereby increasing the client's potential for violence and loss of control. (D) This response is also threatening. The client's behavior does not call for restraints because he has not lost control or hurt anyone. If seclusion or restraints were indicated, the nurse should never confront the client alone.

62. **(D)** Client need: physiological integrity; subcategory: pharmacological and parenteral therapies; content area: psychiatric

RATIONALE

(A) If the client could think logically, he would not be paranoid. In fact, he is probably suspicious of the staff, too. Newly admitted clients frequently experience high levels of anxiety, which can contribute to delusions. (B) The goal of pharmacological intervention is to calm the client and assist with reality-based thinking, not to sedate him. (C) Haloperidol is a neuroleptic and antipsychotic drug, not a minor tranquilizer. (D) Haloperidol is a high-potency neuroleptic and first-line choice for rapid neuroleptization, with low potential for sedation.

63. **(B)** Client need: physiological integrity; subcategory: pharmacological and parenteral therapies; content area: psychiatric

RATIONALE

(A) Stiff neck is consistent with a dystonic reaction, but the client has no symptoms of drooling, shuffling gait, or pill-rolling movements characteristic of parkinsonism. (B) Stiff neck is consistent with a dystonic reaction, and inability to sit still with varying degrees of psychomotor agitation is characteristic of akathisia. (C) The client has symptoms of dystonia but not of parkinsonism. (D) The client has none of the characteristic symptoms of neuroleptic malignant syndrome: hyperpyrexia, generalized muscle rigidity, mutism, obtundation, agitation, sweating, increased blood pressure and pulse.

64. **(C)** Client need: physiological integrity; subcategory: pharmacological and parenteral therapies; content area: psychiatric

RATIONALE

(A) Lorazepam is a benzodiazepine, or antianxiety agent, that potentiates the effects of γ-aminobutyric acid in the CNS, which is not the CNS neurotransmitter EPS. (B) Triazolam is a benzodiazepine sedative-hypnotic whose action is mediated in the limbic, thalamic, and hypothalamic levels of the CNS by γ-aminobutyric acid. (C) Benztropine is an anticholinergic agent, and the drug of choice for blocking CNS synaptic response, which causes EPS. (D) Thiothixene is an antipsychotic and neuroleptic drug that blocks dopamine neurotransmission at the CNS synapses, thereby causing EPS.

65. **(A)** Client need: psychosocial integrity; subcategory: coping and adaptation; content area: psychiatric

RATIONALE

(A) The client verbalizes that he is responsible for compliance and keeping the treatment team member informed of progress. This behavior puts him at the lowest risk for relapse. (B) Noncompliance is a major cause of relapse. This statement reflects lack of responsibility for his own health maintenance. (C) This statement reflects lack of insight into the importance of compliance. (D) This statement reflects no insight into his illness or his responsibility in health maintenance.

TEST 10

University of South Alabama College of Nursing Test

MOCK NCLEX-RN BOARD REVIEW TEST QUESTIONS

1. The nurse is developing a plan of care for a client with an electrolyte imbalance and identifies a nursing diagnosis of decreased physical mobility. Which alteration is *most* likely the etiology?

   A. Hypernatremia
   B. Hypocalcemia
   C. Hypokalemia
   D. Hypomagnesemia

2. The nurse is assessing breath sounds in a bronchovesicular client. She should expect that:

   A. Inspiration is longer than expiration
   B. Breath sounds are high pitched
   C. Breath sounds are slightly muffled
   D. Inspiration and expiration are equal

3. Discharge teaching for the client who has a total gastrectomy should include which of the following?

   A. Need for the client to increase fluid intake to 3000 mL/day
   B. Follow-up visits every 3 weeks for the first 6 months
   C. B_{12} injections needed for the rest of the client's life
   D. Need to eat three full meals with plenty of fiber per day

4. Which of the following findings would necessitate discontinuing an IV potassium infusion in an adult with ketoacidosis?

   A. Urine output 22 mL/hr for 2 hours
   B. Serum potassium level of 3.7
   C. Small T wave of ECG
   D. Serum glucose level of 180

5. A client is receiving IV morphine 2 days after colorectal surgery. Which of the following observations indicate that he may be becoming drug dependent?

   A. The client requests pain medicine every 4 hours.

   B. He is asleep 30 minutes after receiving the IV morphine.
   C. He asks for pain medication although his blood pressure and pulse rate are normal.
   D. He is euphoric for about an hour after each injection.

6. The nurse assesses a postoperative mastectomy client and notes that breath sounds are diminished in both posterior bases. The nurse's action should be to:

   A. Encourage coughing and deep breathing each hour
   B. Obtain arterial blood gases
   C. Increase O_2 from 2–3 L/min
   D. Remove the postoperative dressing to check for bleeding

7. Which of the following should the nurse anticipate receiving as an as-needed order for a postoperative carotid endarterectomy client?

   A. Nifedipine 10 mg SL for B/P 140/90
   B. Furosemide 20 mg/PO for decreased urine output
   C. Magnesium salicylate to decrease inflammation
   D. Nitroglycerin gr 1/150 for chest pain

8. Three hours postoperatively, a 27-year-old client complains of right leg pain after knee reduction. The first action by the nurse will be to:

   A. Assess vital signs
   B. Elevate the extremity
   C. Perform a lower extremity neurovascular check
   D. Remind the client that he has a client-controlled analgesic pump, and reinstruct him on its use

9. Goal setting for a client with Meniere's disease should include which of the following?

   A. Frequent ambulation
   B. Prevention of a fall injury
   C. Consumption of three meals per day
   D. Prevention of infection

10. Which of the following physician's orders would the nurse question on a client with chronic arterial insufficiency?

    A. Neurovascular checks every 2 hours
    B. Elevate legs on pillows
    C. Arteriogram in the morning
    D. No smoking

11. A client is admitted to the hospital with a diagnosis of aplastic anemia and placed on isolation. The nurse notices a family member entering the room without applying the appropriate apparel. The nurse will approach the family member using the following information as a basis for discussion:

    A. The risks of exposure of the visitor to infectious organisms is great.
    B. Hospital regulations mandate that everyone in the facility adhere to appropriate codes.
    C. The client is at extreme risk of acquiring infections.
    D. Adherence to the guidelines are the latest Centers for Disease Control and Prevention recommendations on use of protective apparel.

12. The nurse enters the room of a client on which a "do not resuscitate" order has been written and discovers that she is not breathing. Once the husband realizes what has occurred he yells, "please save her!" The nurse's action would be:

    A. Call the physician and inform him that the client has expired.
    B. Remind the husband that the physician wrote an order not to resuscitate.
    C. Discuss with the husband that these orders are written only on clients who are not likely to recover with resuscitative efforts.
    D. Call a code and proceed with cardiopulmonary resuscitation.

13. The nurse is in the hallway and one of the visitors faints. The nurse should:

    A. Sit the victim up and lightly slap his face
    B. Elevate the victim's legs
    C. Apply a cool cloth to the victim's neck and forehead until he recovers
    D. Sit the victim up and place the head between the knees

14. The nurse is teaching a client how to perform monthly testicular self-examination (TSE) and states that it is best to perform the procedure right after showering. This statement is made by the nurse based on the knowledge that:

    A. The client is more likely to remember to perform the TSE when in the nude
    B. When the scrotum is exposed to cool temperatures, the testicles become large and bulky
    C. The scrotum will be softer and more relaxed after a warm shower, making the testicles easier to palpate
    D. The examination will be less painful at this time

15. The nurse discovers that a 78-year-old client who received hydralazine (Apresoline) 20 mg 45 minutes ago has a blood pressure of 70/40 mm Hg. The client has been on this dose of the medication for 3 years. Which of the following data is most likely significant in relation to the cause of the low blood pressure?

    A. Pedal pulses 11 (weak)
    B. Twenty-four-hour intake 1000 mL/day for past 2 days
    C. Serum potassium 3.3
    D. Pulse rate 150 bpm

16. A client admitted with a diagnosis of possible myocardial infarction is admitted to the unit from the emergency room. The nurse's first action when admitting the client will be to:

    A. Obtain vital signs
    B. Connect the client to the cardiac monitor
    C. Ask the client if he is still having chest pain
    D. Complete the history profile

17. The nurse is interviewing a client with a diagnosis of possible abdominal aortic aneurysm. Which of the following statements will be reflected in the client's chief complaint?

    A. "I've been having a dull pain at the upper left shoulder."
    B. "My legs have been numb for three months."
    C. "I've only been urinating three times a day lately."
    D. "I don't remember anything in particular, I just haven't felt well."

18. The nurse is collecting a nutritional history on a 28-year-old female client with iron-deficiency anemia and learns that the client likes to eat white chalk. When implementing a teaching plan, the nurse should explain that this practice:

    A. Will bind calcium and therefore interfere with its metabolism
    B. Will cause more premenstrual cramping
    C. Interferes with iron absorption because the iron precipitates as an insoluble substance
    D. Causes competition at iron-receptor sites between iron and vitamin B_1

19. Which of the following lab data is representative of a client with aplastic anemia?

    A. Hemoglobin 9.2, hematocrit 27, red blood cells 3.2 million
    B. White blood cells 4000, erythrocytes 2.5 million, thrombocytes 100,000
    C. White blood cells 3000, hematocrit 27, red blood cells 2.8 million
    D. Red blood cells 1 million, white blood cells 1500, thrombocytes 16,000

20. A 20-year-old male client is being treated for protein deficiency. If he likes all of the following foods, which one would the nurse recommend to increase in the diet?

    A. Cantaloupe
    B. Rice
    C. Chicken
    D. Green beans

21. A male client is considering having laser abdominal surgery and asks the nurse if there is any advantage in having this type of surgery? The nurse will respond based on the knowledge that laser surgery:

    A. Has a smaller postoperative infection rate than routine surgery
    B. Will eliminate the need for preoperative sedation
    C. Will result in less operating time
    D. Generally eliminates problems with complications

22. A client states to his nurse that "I was told by the doctor not to take one of my drugs because it seems to have caused decreasing blood cells." Based on this information, which drug might the nurse expect to be discontinued?

    A. Prednisone
    B. Timolol maleate (Blocadren)
    C. Garamycin (Genticin)
    D. Phenytoin (Dilantin)

23. Forty-eight hours after a thyroidectomy, a female client complains of numbness and tingling of the toes and fingers. The nurse notes upper arm and facial twitching. The nurse needs to:

    A. Report the findings to the physician
    B. Assist the client to do range of motion exercises
    C. Check the client's potassium level
    D. Administer the as-needed dose of phenytoin (Dilantin)

24. The nurse is admitting a client with folic acid deficiency anemia. Which of the following questions is most important for the nurse to ask the client?

    A. "Do you take aspirin on a regular basis?"
    B. "Do you drink alcohol on a regular basis?"
    C. "Do you eat red meat?"
    D. "Have your stools been normal?"

25. An 18-month-old child has been playing in the garage. His mother brings him to a nurse's home complaining of his mouth being sore. His lips and mouth are soapy and white, with small ulcerated areas beginning to form. The child begins to vomit. His pulse is rapid and weak. The nurse suspects that the child has:

    A. Inhaled gasoline fumes
    B. Ingested a caustic alkali
    C. Eaten construction chalk
    D. Lead poisoning

26. In discussing the plan of care for a child with chronic nephrosis with the mother, the nurse identifies that the purpose of weighing the child is to:

    A. Measure adequacy of nutritional management
    B. Check the accuracy of the fluid intake record
    C. Impress the child with the importance of eating well
    D. Determine changes in the amount of edema

27. The parents of a 9-year-old child with acute lymphocytic leukemia expressed concern about his alopecia from cranial irradiation. The nurse explains that:

    A. Alopecia is an unavoidable side effect.
    B. There are several wig makers for children.

C. Most children select a favorite hat to protect their heads.
D. His hair will grow back in a few months.

28. Loss of appetite for a child with leukemia is a major recurrent problem. The plan of care should be designed to:

    A. Reinforce attempts to eat
    B. Help the child gain weight
    C. Increase his appetite
    D. Make mealtimes pleasant

29. The mother of a child taking phenytoin will need to plan appropriate mouth care and gingival stimulation. When tooth-brushing is contraindicated, the next most effective cleansing and gingival stimulation technique would be:

    A. Using a water pik
    B. Rinsing with water
    C. Rinsing with hydrogen peroxide
    D. Rinsing with baking soda

30. When planning care for a 9-year-old client, the nurse uses which of the most effective means of helping siblings cope with their feelings about a brother who is terminally ill?

    A. Open discussion and understanding
    B. Play-acting out feelings in different roles
    C. Storytelling
    D. Drawing pictures

31. During the active phase of rheumatic fever, the nurse teaches parents of a child with acute rheumatic fever to assist in minimizing joint pain and promoting healing by:

    A. Putting all joints through full range-of-motion twice daily
    B. Massaging the joints briskly with lotion or liniment after bath
    C. Immobilizing the joints in functional position using splints, rolls, and pillows
    D. Applying warm water bottle or heating pads over involved joints

32. The initial focus when providing nursing care for a child with rheumatic fever during the acute phase of the illness should be to:

    A. Maintain contact with her parents
    B. Provide for physical and psychological rest
    C. Provide a nutritious diet
    D. Maintain her interest in school

33. During discharge planning, parents of a child with rheumatic fever should be able to identify which of the following as toxic symptoms of sodium salicylate?

    A. Tinnitus and nausea
    B. Dermatitis and blurred vision
    C. Unconsciousness and acetone odor of the breath
    D. Chills and an elevation of temperature

34. Parents of a child with rheumatic fever express concern that she will always be arthritic. The nurse discusses their concerns and tells them the joint pain usually:

    A. Subsides in ≤3 weeks
    B. Is relieved by aspirin

C. Is responsive to ibuprofen (Motrin)
D. Subsides in 3–6 days

35. In caring at home for a child who just ingested a caustic alkali, the nurse would immediately tell the mother to:

    A. Give vinegar, lemon juice, or orange juice
    B. Phone the doctor
    C. Take the child to the emergency room
    D. Induce vomiting

36. The most important goal in the care plan for a child who was hospitalized with an accidental overdose would be to:

    A. Determine child's activity pattern
    B. Reduce mother's sense of guilt
    C. Instruct parents in use of ipecac
    D. Teach parents appropriate safety precautions

37. A 4 year old has an imaginary playmate, which concerns the mother. The nurse's best response would be:

    A. "I understand your concern and will assist you with a referral."
    B. "Try not to worry because you will just upset your child."
    C. "Just ignore the behavior and it should disappear by age 8."
    D. "This is appropriate behavior for a preschooler and should not be a concern."

38. Parents should be taught not to prop the bottle when feeding their infants. In addition to the risk of choking, it puts the infant at risk for:

    A. Otitis media
    B. Asthma
    C. Conjunctivitis
    D. Tonsillitis

39. When assessing a female child for Turner's syndrome, the nurse observes for which of the following symptoms?

    A. Tall stature
    B. Amenorrhea
    C. Secondary sex characteristics
    D. Gynecomastia

40. The mother of a client is apprehensive about taking home her 2 year old who was diagnosed with asthma after being admitted to the emergency room with difficulty breathing and cyanosis. She asks the nurse what symptoms she should look for so that this problem will not happen again. The nurse instructs her to watch for the following early symptoms:

    A. Fever, runny nose, and hyperactivity
    B. Changes in breathing pattern, moodiness, fatigue, and edema of eyes
    C. Fatigue, dark circles under the eyes, changes in breathing pattern, glassy eyes, and moodiness
    D. Fever, cough, paleness, and wheezing

41. A 3-year-old female client is brought into the pediatric clinic because she limps. She has not been to the clinic since she was 9 months old. The nurse practitioner describes the limp as a "Trendelenburg gait." This gait is characteristic of:

    A. Scoliosis
    B. Dislocated hip

C. Fractured femur
D. Fractured pelvis

42. A child has a nursing diagnosis of fluid volume excess related to compromised regulatory mechanisms. Which of the following nursing interventions is the most accurate measure to include in his care?

    A. Weigh the child twice daily on the same scale.
    B. Monitor intake and output.
    C. Check urine specific gravity of each voiding.
    D. Observe for edema.

43. The pediatric nurse charts that the parents of a 4-year-old child are very anxious. Which observation would indicate to the nurse unhealthy coping by these parents:

    A. Discussing their needs with the nursing staff
    B. Discussing their needs with other family members
    C. Seeking support from their minister
    D. Refusing to participate in the child's care

44. A 9-week-old female infant has a diagnosis of bilateral cleft lip and cleft palate. She has been admitted to the pediatric unit after surgical repair of the cleft lip. Which of the following nursing interventions would be appropriate during the first 24 hours?

    A. Position on side or abdomen.
    B. Maintain elbow restraints in place unless she is being directly supervised.
    C. Clean suture line every shift.
    D. Offer pacifier when she cries.

45. A 6-month-old infant who was diagnosed at 4 weeks of age with a ventricular septal defect, was admitted today with a diagnosis of failure to thrive. His mother stated that he had not been eating well for the past month. A cardiac catheterization reveals congestive heart failure. All of the following nursing diagnoses are appropriate. Which nursing diagnosis should have priority?

    A. Altered nutrition: less than body requirements related to inability to take in adequate calories
    B. Altered growth and development related to decreased intake of food
    C. Activity intolerance related to imbalance between oxygen supply and demand
    D. Decreased cardiac output related to ineffective pumping action of the heart

46. A 9-year-old child was in the garage with his father, who was repairing a lawnmower. Some gasoline ignited and caused an explosion. His father was killed, and the child has split-thickness and full-thickness burns over 40% of his upper body, face, neck, and arms. All of the following nursing diagnoses are included on his care plan. Which of these nursing diagnoses should have top priority during the first 24–48 hours postburn?

    A. Pain related to tissue damage from burns
    B. Potential for infection related to contamination of wounds
    C. Fluid volume deficit related to increased capillary permeability
    D. Potential for impaired gas exchange related to edema of respiratory tract

47. A female baby was born with talipes equinovarus. Her mother has requested that the nurse assigned to the baby come to her room to discuss the baby's condition. The nurse knows that the pediatrician has discussed the baby's condition with her mother and that an orthopedist has been consulted but has not yet seen the baby. What should the nurse do first?

    A. Call the orthopedist and request that he come to see the baby now.
    B. Question the mother and find out what the pediatrician has told her about the baby's condition.
    C. Tell the mother that this is not a serious condition.
    D. Tell the mother that this condition has been successfully treated with exercises, casts, and/or braces.

48. Cystic fibrosis is transmitted as an autosomal recessive trait. This means that:

    A. Mothers carry the gene and pass it to their sons
    B. Fathers carry the gene and pass it to their daughters
    C. Both parents must have the disease for a child to have the disease
    D. Both parents must be carriers for a child to have the disease

49. Diabetes mellitus is a disorder that affects 3.1 out of every 1000 children younger than 20 years old. It is characterized by an absence of, or marked decrease in, circulating insulin. When teaching a newly diagnosed diabetes client, the nurse includes information on the functions of insulin:

    A. Transport of glucose into body cells and storage of glycogen in the liver
    B. Glycogenolysis and facilitation of glucose use for energy
    C. Glycogenolysis and catabolism
    D. Catabolism and hyperglycemia

50. A 14-year-old boy has had diabetes for 7 years. He takes 30 U of NPH insulin and 10 U of regular insulin every morning at 7 AM. He eats breakfast at 7:30 AM and lunch at noon. What time should he expect the greatest risk for hypoglycemia?

    A. 9 AM
    B. 1 PM
    C. 11 AM
    D. 3 PM

51. A 16-year-old diabetic girl has been selected as a cheerleader at her school. She asks the nurse whether she should increase her insulin when she is planning to attend cheerleading practice sessions lasting from 8 to 11 AM. The most appropriate answer would be:

    A. "You should ask your doctor about this."
    B. "Yes, increase your insulin by 1 U for each hour of practice because exercise causes the body to need more insulin."
    C. "No, do not increase your insulin. Exercise will not affect your insulin needs."
    D. "No, do not increase your insulin, but eating a snack prior to practice exercise will make insulin more effective and move more glucose into the cells."

52. The physician decides to prescribe both a short-acting insulin and an intermediate-acting insulin for a newly diagnosed 8-year-old diabetic client. An example of a short-acting insulin is:

    A. Novolin Regular
    B. Humulin NPH
    C. Lente Beef
    D. Protamine zinc insulin

53. When preparing insulin for IV administration, the nurse identifies which kind of insulin to use?

    A. NPH
    B. Human or pork
    C. Regular
    D. Long acting

1. **(C)** Client need: physiological integrity; subcategory: physiological adaptation; content area: med/surg

   RATIONALE
   (A) A deficit in sodium concentration results in muscular weakness and lethargy. (B) Muscle fatigue and hypotonia are caused by hypercalcemia. (C) Muscle weakness and fatigue are classic signs of hypokalemia. (D) Hypermagnesemia can cause muscle weakness, paralysis, and coma.

2. **(D)** Client need: physiological integrity; subcategory: physiological adaptation; content area: med/surg

   RATIONALE
   (A) Inspiration is normally longer in vesicular areas. (B) High-pitched sounds are normal in bronchial area. (C) Muffled sounds are considered abnormal. (D) Inspiration and expiration are equal normally in this area, and sounds are medium pitched.

3. **(C)** Client need: health promotion and maintenance; subcategory: prevention and early detection of disease; content area: med/surg .

   RATIONALE
   (A) There will be no need to increase fluid intake excessively, because dumping syndrome could present a problem. (B) Follow-up visits every 3 weeks are not a standard recommendation. Follow-up visits will be highly individualized. (C) With removal of the stomach, intrinsic factor will no longer be produced. Intrinsic factor is necessary for vitamin B_{12} absorption. Parenteral injections of B_{12} will be needed on a monthly basis for the rest of the person's life. (D) Smaller, more frequent meals, rather than large, bulky meals, are recommended to prevent problems with dumping syndrome.

4. **(A)** Client need: physiological integrity; subcategory: reduction of risk potential; content area: med/surg

   RATIONALE
   (A) Adequate renal flow of 30 mL/hr is a necessity with potassium infusions because potassium is excreted renally. (B) Because potassium level will decrease during correction of diabetic ketoacidosis, potassium will be infused even if plasma levels of potassium are normal. (C) A small T wave is normal and desired on the electrocardiogram. A tall, peaked T-wave could indicate overinfusion of potassium and hyperkalemia. (D) Glucose levels of <200 are desirable.

5. **(D)** Client need: physiological integrity; subcategory: pharmacological and parenteral therapies; content area: med/surg

   RATIONALE
   (A) Frequent requests for pain medication do not necessarily indicate drug dependence after complex surgeries such as colorectal surgery. (B) Sleeping after receiving IV morphine is not an unexpected effect because the pain is relieved. (C) A person may be in pain even with normal vital signs. (D) A subtle sign of drug dependency is the tendency for the person to appear more euphoric than relieved of pain.

6. **(A)** Client need: physiological integrity; subcategory: reduction of risk potential; content area: med/surg

   RATIONALE
   (A) Decreased or absent breath sounds are frequently indicators of postoperative atelectasis. (B) Arterial blood gases are not indicated because there is no other information indicating impending danger. (C) Increasing O_2 rate is not indicated without additional information. (D) Removing the dressing is not indicated without additional information.

7. **(A)** Client need: physiological integrity; subcategory: reduction of risk potential; content area: med/surg

   RATIONALE
   (A) It is important to maintain a normal to slightly lower pressure to prevent the graft from blowing and excessive pressure to surgical vascular areas. (B, C, D) None of these drugs is related to managing the problem at hand. Also, none of the problems for which these drugs would be indicated is expected with this type of surgery, except if there is a prior history.

8. **(C)** Client need: physiological integrity; subcategory: reduction of risk potential; content area: med/surg

   RATIONALE
   (A) Vital signs may be altered if there is acute pain or complications related to bleeding or swelling, but they should not be assessed before checking the affected extremity. (B) The extremity will be elevated if ordered by the doctor. (C) Assessment of the postoperative area is important to determine if bleeding, swelling, or decreased circulation is occurring. (D) Reinforcement of teaching on use of the client-controlled analgesic pump is important, but not the first action.

9. **(B)** Client need: physiological integrity; subcategory: reduction of risk potential; content area: med/surg

   RATIONALE
   (A) Although not contraindicated, initially ambulation may be difficult because of vertigo and is recommended only with assistance. (B) Vertigo resulting in balance problems is one of the most common manifestations of Meniere's disease. (C) Adequate nutrition is important, but the emphasis in Meniere's disease is not the number of meals per day but a decrease in intake of sodium. (D) Infection is not an anticipated problem.

10. **(B)** Client need: physiological integrity; subcategory: reduction of risk potential; content area: med/surg

    RATIONALE
    (A) Neurovascular checks are a routine part of assessment with clients having this diagnosis. (B) Elevation of the legs is contraindicated because it reduces blood flow to areas already compromised. (C) Arteriogram is a routine diagnostic order. (D) Smoking is highly correlated with this disorder.

11. **(C)** Client need: psychosocial integrity; subcategory: coping and adaptation; content area: med/surg

    RATIONALE
    (A) Although clients with a compromised immune system may acquire infections, the primary emphasis is on protecting the client. (B, D) Most people are aware of the guidelines once they see posted signs, so quoting regulations is not likely to result in consistent adherence to regulations. (C) Clients with aplastic anemia have white cell counts of 2000 or lower, making them more vulnerable to infections from others.

12. **(D)** Client need: safe, effective care environment; subcategory: management of care; content area: med/surg

    RATIONALE
    (A, B, C) The last request from the husband overrides the decision not to initiate resuscitation efforts. (D) The nurse should begin cardiopulmonary resuscitation unless a living will and durable power of attorney are in force. In the meantime, the nurse should talk with the husband and notify the doctor.

13. **(B)** Client need: physiological integrity; subcategory: physiological adaptation; content area: med/surg

RATIONALE

(A) Sitting the client up defeats the goal of re-establishing cerebral blood flow. (B) Elevating the legs anatomically redirects blood flow to the cerebral area. (C) This strategy is a nice general comfort measure after the victim has regained consciousness. (D) This strategy is not as effective a strategy in helping the client to regain consciousness as elevating the legs.

14. **(C)** Client need: health promotion and maintenance; subcategory: prevention and early detection of disease; content area: med/surg

RATIONALE

(A) Nudity is not a trigger for reminding males to perform TSE. (B) Testicles become more firm when exposed to cool temperatures, but not large and bulky. (C) The testicles will be lower and more easily palpated with warmer temperatures. A protective mechanism of the body to protect sperm production is for the scrotum to pull closer to the body when exposed to cooler temperatures. (D) The examination should not be painful.

15. **(B)** Client need: physiological integrity; subcategory: physiological adaptation; content area: med/surg

RATIONALE

(A, D) Decreased pulse volume and increased pulse rate are signs of an acute hypotensive episode. (B) Inadequate fluid volume when taking vasodilators can result in a drop in blood pressure when vasodilation starts to physiologically occur as an action of the drug. (C) A potassium level of 3.3 would not be associated with a significant drop in blood pressure.

16. **(B)** Client need: physiological integrity; subcategory: reduction of risk potential; content area: med/surg

RATIONALE

(A) Obtaining vital signs is important after connecting the client to the monitor because vital signs should be stable before the client is discharged from the emergency room. (B) All are important, but the first priority is to monitor the client's rhythm. (C) If the client is in severe pain, pain medication should be given after connecting him to the monitor and obtaining vital signs. (D) Completion of the history profile is the least important of the nursing actions.

17. **(D)** Client need: physiological integrity; subcategory: physiological adaptation; content area: med/surg

RATIONALE

(A, B, C) These complaints are not specific signs and symptoms associated with abdominal aortic aneurysm. If symptoms are present, the aneurysm is expanding or rupture is imminent. (D) Many clients may experience no symptoms. The only symptom may be a pulsation noted in the abdomen in the reclining position.

18. **(C)** Client need: health promotion and maintenance; subcategory: prevention and early detection of disease; content area: med/surg

RATIONALE

(A) Eating chalk is not related to calcium and its absorption. (B) Poor nutritional habits may result in increased discomfort during premenstrual days, but this is not a primary reason for the client to stop eating chalk. Premenstrual discomfort has not been mentioned. (C) Iron is rendered insoluble and is excreted through the gastrointestinal tract. (D) There is no competition between the two nutrients.

19. **(D)** Client need: physiological integrity; subcategory: reduction of risk potential; content area: med/surg

RATIONALE

(A, B, C) Although all of the lab data are abnormal and although these values are decreased in aplastic anemia, the disorder is defined by severe deficits in red cell, white cell, and platelet counts.

(D) Aplastic anemia is typically defined in terms of abnormalities of red blood cell count, usually <1 million, white cell count <2,000, and thrombocytes <20,000.

20. **(C)** Client need: physiological integrity; subcategory: basic care and comfort; content area: med/surg

RATIONALE

(A) Cantaloupe is a good source of carbohydrates, vitamin C, and vitamin A. (B) Rice contains about 4 g of protein per 200 g. (C) Chicken contains 35 g protein per breast. Chicken is a rich source of vitamin B_6 (pyridoxine), which is needed for adequate protein synthesis. As protein intake increases, vitamin B_6 intake must also be increased. Vitamin B_6 is a coenzyme in amino acid metabolism. (D) Green beans only contain 2 g of protein per cup.

21. **(A)** Client need: physiological integrity; subcategory: reduction of risk potential; content area: med/surg

RATIONALE

(A) A lower postoperative infection has been documented as a result of laser therapy versus routine surgery. (B) Clients will still need preoperative sedation to facilitate anxiety reduction. (C) Operating time may actually increase in some laser surgeries. (D) The client must still be observed for postoperative complications.

22. **(D)** Client need: health promotion and maintenance; subcategory: prevention and early detection of disease; content area: med/surg

RATIONALE

(A) Prednisone is not linked with hematological side effects. (B) Timolol, a β-adrenergic blocker is metabolized by the liver. It has not been linked to blood dyscrasia. (C) Gentamicin is ototoxic and nephrotoxic. (D) Phenytoin usage has been linked to blood dyscrasias such as aplastic anemia. The drug most commonly linked to aplastic anemia is chloramphenicol (Chlormycetin).

23. **(A)** Client need: physiological integrity; subcategory: physiological adaptation; content area: med/surg

RATIONALE

(A) Muscular hyperactivity and parasthesias may indicate hypocalcemic tetany and require immediate administration of calcium gluconate. Tetany can occur if the parathyroid glands were erroneously excised during surgery. (B) Range of motion exercises are not appropriate to presenting symptoms. (C) These characteristics are not usual signs of potassium imbalance, but of calcium imbalance. (D) Phenytoin is indicated for seizure activity mainly of neurological origin.

24. **(B)** Client need: health promotion and maintenance; subcategory: prevention and early detection of disease; content area: med/surg

RATIONALE

(A) Aspirin does not affect folic acid absorption. (B) Folic acid deficiency is strongly associated with alcohol abuse. (C) Because folic acid is a coenzyme for single carbon transfer purines, calves liver or other purines are the meat sources. (D) Folic acid does not affect stool character.

25. **(B)** Client need: physiological integrity; subcategory: physiological adaptation; content area: pediatrics

RATIONALE

(A, C, D) These agents would not cause ulcerations on mouth and lips. (B) Strong alkali or acids will cause burns and ulcerations on the mucous membranes.

26. **(D)** Client need: health promotion and maintenance; subcategory: prevention and early detection of disease; content area: pediatrics

RATIONALE

(A) Weighing a child with nephrosis is to assess for edema, not nutrition. (B, C) This is not the purpose for weighing the child.

(D) Weight and measurement are the primary ways of evaluating edema and fluid shifts.

27. **(D)** Client need: physiological integrity; subcategory: reduction of risk potential; content area: pediatrics

RATIONALE

(A) Alopecia has occurred, and knowing it is a side effect does not address their concern. (B) Although true, it does not give them hope for the future. (C) Although true, it does not provide them with information of the temporary nature of the situation. (D) Knowing the hair will grow back provides comfort that the alopecia is temporary.

28. **(A)** Client need: physiological integrity; subcategory: basic care and comfort; content area: pediatrics

RATIONALE

(A) Ignoring refusals to eat and rewarding eating attempts are the most successful means of increasing intake. (B) This goal is not specific enough or related to the loss of appetite. (C) This goal is not possible at this time based on his illness. (D) This goal is helpful, but alone will not address his loss of appetite.

29. **(A)** Client need: health promotion and maintenance; subcategory: prevention and early detection of disease; content area: pediatrics

RATIONALE

(A) This technique provides effective rinsing and gingival stimulation. (B) This technique does not provide gingival stimulation. (C) This technique provides effective rinsing but not gingival stimulation. Using peroxide is not pleasant for the child. (D) This technique provides effective rinsing but not gingival stimulation.

30. **(B)** Client need: psychosocial integrity; subcategory: coping and adaptation; content area: pediatrics

RATIONALE

(A) When dealing with grief, siblings are usually most comfortable initially with open discussion. (B) Assuming different roles allows children to act out their feelings without fear of reprisals and to gain insight and control. (C) This method may be helpful, but having the child take an active part through role playing is more effective. (D) This technique may be helpful, but being an active participant through role playing is more effective.

31. **(C)** Client need: health promotion and maintenance; subcategory: prevention and early detection of disease; content area: pediatrics

RATIONALE

(A) Any movement of the joint causes severe pain. (B) Touching or moving the joint causes severe pain. (C) Immobilization in a functional position allows the joint to rest and heal. (D) Pressure from the warm water bottle or pads can cause severe pain or burning of the skin.

32. **(B)** Client need: health promotion and maintenance; subcategory: prevention and early detection of disease; content area: pediatrics

RATIONALE

(A) This goal is helpful, but rest is essential during the acute phase. (B) Rest is essential for healing to occur and for pain to be relieved. (C) This goal is important, but rest is essential. (D) This goal should be part of the plan of care, but it is not the priority during the acute phase.

33. **(A)** Client need: health promotion and maintenance; subcategory: prevention and early detection of disease; content area: pediatrics

RATIONALE

(A) These are toxic symptoms of sodium salicylate. (B, C, D) These are not symptoms associated with sodium salicylate.

34. **(A)** Client need: physiological integrity; subcategory: physiological adaptation; content area: pediatrics

RATIONALE

(A) Joints usually remain inflamed and tender until the disease runs its course in ≤3 weeks. (B) This response does not answer the question of whether she will always be arthritic. (C) This response does not answer the question asked. (D) The disease takes ≤3 weeks to run its course.

35. **(A)** Client need: health promotion and maintenance; subcategory: prevention and early detection of disease; content area: pediatrics

RATIONALE

(A) The immediate action is to neutralize the action of the chemical before further damage takes place. (B) This action should be done after neutralizing the chemical. (C) This action should be done after neutralizing the chemical. (D) Never induce vomiting with a strong alkali or acid. Additional damage will be done when the child vomits the chemical.

36. **(D)** Client need: health promotion and maintenance; subcategory: prevention and early detection of disease; content area: pediatrics

RATIONALE

(A) This goal is not the most important. (B) There is always some guilt when an accident occurs; however, the priority is to be sure future accidents are prevented. (C) Ipecac is not used for caustic alkali and acid ingestions. (D) Determining the parent's knowledge about safety hazards and teaching appropriate preventive measures are likely to prevent recurrence of accidents.

37. **(D)** Client need: psychosocial integrity; subcategory: coping and adaptation; content area: pediatrics

RATIONALE

(A) This is normal for a preschooler, and a referral is not appropriate. (B) Telling a parent not to worry is unhelpful. This response does not address the mother's concern. (C) This response is incorrect. The behavior is normal and will usually disappear by the time the child enters school. (D) This behavior is normal development for a preschooler.

38. **(A)** Client need: health promotion and maintenance; subcategory: prevention and early detection of disease; content area: pediatrics

RATIONALE

(A) Because the eustachian tube is short and straight in the infant, formula that pools in the back of the throat attacks bacteria which can enter the middle ear and cause an infection. (B) Asthma is not associated with propping the bottle. (C) Conjunctivitis is an eye infection and not associated with propping the bottle. (D) Tonsillitis is usually a result of pharyngitis and not propping the bottle.

39. **(B)** Client need: physiological integrity; subcategory: physiological adaptation; content area: pediatrics

RATIONALE

(A) This syndrome is caused by absence of one of the X chromosomes. These children are short in stature. (B) Amenorrhea is a symptom of Turner's syndrome, which appears at puberty. (C) Sexual infantilism is characteristic of this syndrome. (D) Gynecomastia is a symptom in Klinefelter's syndrome.

40. **(C)** Client need: health promotion and maintenance; subcategory: prevention and early detection of disease; content area: pediatrics

RATIONALE

(A) The child with asthma may not have fever unless there is an underlying infection. (B) Edema of the eyes will not be present because the child with asthma is more likely to have dehydration related to excessive water loss during the work of breathing. (C) All of these symptoms indicate decreased oxygenation and are early symptoms of asthma. (D) Coughing and wheezing are not early signs of difficulty.

41. **(B)** Client need: physiological integrity; subcategory: physiological adaptation; content area: pediatrics

RATIONALE

(A, C, D) A Trendelenburg gait is not characteristic of any of these disorders. (B) The downward slant of one hip is a positive sign of dislocation in the weight-bearing hip. If one hip is dislocated, the child walks with a characteristic limp known as the Trendelenburg gait.

42. **(A)** Client need: health promotion and maintenance; subcategory: prevention and early detection of disease; content area: pediatrics

RATIONALE

(A) Although all of these interventions are important aspects of care, weight is the most sensitive indicator of fluid balance. (B) Although monitoring intake and output is important, weight is a more accurate indicator of fluid status. (C) Urine specific gravity does not necessarily indicate fluid volume excess. (D) Edema may not be apparent, yet the client may have fluid volume excess.

43. **(D)** Client need: psychosocial integrity; subcategory: coping and adaptation; content area: pediatrics

RATIONALE

(A, B, C) These methods are healthy ways of dealing with anxiety. (D) Participation minimizes feelings of helplessness and powerlessness. It is important that parents have accurate information and that they seek support from sources available to them.

44. **(B)** Client need: physiological integrity; subcategory: reduction of risk potential; content area: pediatrics

RATIONALE

(A) Placing the infant on her abdomen may allow for injury to the suture line. (B) Elbow restraints prevent the infant from touching the suture line and yet leaves hands free. (C) The suture line is cleaned as often as every hour to prevent crusting and scarring. (D) Sucking of a bottle or pacifier places pressure on the suture line and may delay healing and cause scarring.

45. **(D)** Client need: physiological integrity; subcategory: physiological adaptation; content area: pediatrics

RATIONALE

(A) Altered nutrition occurs owing to the fatigue from decreased cardiac output associated with congestive heart failure. (B) The decreased intake occurs due to fatigue from the altered cardiac output. (C) Fatigue occurs due to the decreased cardiac output. (D) The ineffective action of the myocardium leads to inadequate O_2 to the tissues, which produces activity intolerance, altered nutrition, and altered growth and development.

46. **(D)** Client need: physiological integrity; subcategory: reduction of risk potential; content area: pediatrics

RATIONALE

(A, B, C) These answers are all correct; however, maintenance of airway is the top priority. (D) Persons burned about the face and neck during an explosion are also likely to suffer burns of the respiratory tract, which can lead to edema and respiratory arrest.

47. **(B)** Client need: psychosocial integrity; subcategory: coping and adaptation; content area: pediatrics

RATIONALE

(A) The nurse should call the orthopedist after assessing the mother's knowledge. (B) The nurse must first assess the knowledge of the parent before attempting any explanation. (C) The nurse should assess the mother's knowledge of the baby's condition as the first priority. (D) This answer is correct, but the priority is B.

48. **(D)** Client need: physiological integrity; subcategory: physiological adaptation; content area: pediatrics

RATIONALE

(A) Cystic fibrosis is not an X-linked or sex-linked disease. (B) The only characteristic on the Y chromosome is the trait for hairy ears. (C) Both parents do not need to have the disease but must be carriers. (D) If a trait is recessive, two genes (one from each parent) are necessary to produce an affected child.

49. **(A)** Client need: physiological integrity; subcategory: pharmacological and parenteral therapies; content area: pediatrics

RATIONALE

(A) Lack of insulin causes glycogenolysis, catabolism, and hyperglycemia. (B) Insulin promotes the conversion of glucose to glycogen for storage and regulates the rate at which carbohydrates are used by cells for energy. (C) Insulin is anabolic in nature. (D) Glucose stimulates protein synthesis within the tissue and inhibits the breakdown of protein into amino acids.

50. **(C)** Client need: physiological integrity; subcategory: reduction of risk potential; content area: pediatrics

RATIONALE

(A) This time is incorrect because regular insulin would peak after the teenager has eaten breakfast. (B) This time is incorrect because it is after lunch when the NPH peaks. (C) Regular insulin peaks in 2–3 hours and has a duration of 4–6 hours. NPH insulin's onset is 4–6 hours and peaks in 8–16 hours. Blood sugar would peak after meals and be lowest before meals and during the night. (D) This time is incorrect because it is before the NPH and after the regular insulin peak times.

51. **(D)** Client need: physiological integrity; subcategory: reduction of risk potential; content area: pediatrics

RATIONALE

(A) A nurse can give this information to a client. (B) Exercise makes insulin more efficient in moving more glucose into the cells. No more insulin is needed. (C) Exercise makes insulin more efficient unless the diabetes is poorly controlled. (D) Exercise makes insulin more efficient in moving more glucose into the cells.

52. **(A)** Client need: physiological integrity; subcategory: pharmacological and parenteral therapies; content area: pediatrics

RATIONALE

(A) Novolin is a short-acting insulin. (B, C) NPH and Lente are intermediate-acting insulins. (D) Protamine zinc insulin is a long-acting insulin preparation.

53. **(C)** Client need: physiological integrity; subcategory: pharmacological and parenteral therapies; content area: pediatrics

RATIONALE

(A, B, D) Intermediate-acting and long-acting preparations contain materials that increase length of absorption time from the subcutaneous tissues but cause the preparation to be cloudy and unsuitable for IV use. Human insulin must be given SC. (C) Only regular insulin can be given IV.

Texas Tech University Health Sciences Center Test

MOCK NCLEX-RN BOARD REVIEW TEST QUESTIONS

1. A 33-year-old client is diagnosed with bipolar disorder, acute phase. This is her first psychiatric hospitalization, and she is being evaluated for treatment with lithium. Which of the following diagnostic tests are essential prior to the initiation of lithium therapy with this client?

   A. Hematocrit, hemoglobin, and white blood cell (WBC) count
   B. Blood urea nitrogen, electrolytes, and creatinine
   C. Glucose, glucose tolerance test, and random blood sugar
   D. X-rays, electroencephalogram, and electrocardiogram (ECG)

2. A client has been taking lithium 300 mg po bid for the past two weeks. This morning her lithium level was 1 mEq/L. The nurse should:

   A. Notify the physician immediately
   B. Hold the morning lithium dose and continue to observe the client
   C. Administer the morning lithium dose as scheduled
   D. Obtain an order for benztropine (Cogentin)

3. A 23-year-old male client is admitted to the chemical dependency unit with a medical diagnosis of alcoholism. He reports that the last time he drank was 3 days ago, and that now he is starting to "feel kind of shaky." Based on the information given above, nursing care goals for this client will initially focus on:

   A. Self-concept problems
   B. Interpersonal issues
   C. Ineffective coping skills
   D. Physiological stabilization

4. One afternoon 3 weeks into his alcohol treatment program, a client says to the nurse, "It's really not all my fault that I have a drinking problem. Alcoholism runs in my family. Both my grandfather and father were heavy drinkers." The nurse's *best* response would be:

   A. "That might be a problem. Tell me more about them."
   B. "Risk factors can often be controlled by self-responsibility."
   C. "It sounds like you're intellectualizing your drinking problem."
   D. "Your grandfather and father were both alcoholics?"

5. A 14-year-old teenager is hospitalized for anorexia nervosa. She is admitted to the adolescent mental health unit and placed on a behavior modification program. Nursing interventions for the teenager will most likely include:

   A. Establishing routine tasks and activities around mealtimes
   B. Administering medications such as lithium
   C. Requiring the client to eat more during meals
   D. Checking the client's room frequently

6. A measurable outcome criterion in the nursing care of an adolescent with anorexia nervosa would be:

   A. Accepting her present body image
   B. Verbalizing realistic feelings about her body
   C. Having an improved perception of her body image
   D. Exhibiting increased self-esteem

7. A 23-year-old female client is brought to the emergency room by her roommate for repeatedly making superficial cuts on her wrists and experiencing wide mood swings. She is very angry and hostile. Her medical diagnosis is adjustment disorder versus borderline personality disorder. The client comments to the nurse, "Nobody in here seems to really care about the clients. I thought nurses cared about people!" The client is exhibiting the ego defense mechanism:

   A. Reaction formation
   B. Rationalization
   C. Splitting
   D. Sublimation

8. A client hospitalized with a medical diagnosis of adjustment disorder versus personality disorder states, "Nobody cares about the clients." The nurse's most effective response would be:

   A. "How can you say that I don't care? We just met."
   B. "What makes you think the nurses don't care?"
   C. "You will feel differently about us in a few days."
   D. "You seem angry. Tell me more about how you feel."

9. A 45-year-old client diagnosed with major depression is scheduled for electroconvulsive therapy (ECT) in the morning. Which of the following medications are routinely administered either before or during ECT?

   A. Thioridazine (Mellaril), lithium, and benztropine
   B. Atropine, sodium brevitol, and succinylcholine chloride (Anectine)
   C. Sodium, potassium, and magnesium
   D. Carbamazepine (Tegretol), haloperidol, and trihexyphenidyl (Artane)

10. A 35-year-old client is receiving psychopharmacological treatment of his major depression with tranylcypromine sulfate (Parnate), a monoamine oxidase (MAO) inhibitor. The nurse teaches the client that while he is taking this type of antidepressant, he needs to restrict his dietary intake of:

    A. Potassium-rich foods
    B. Tryptophan
    C. Tyramine
    D. Saturated fats

11. The nurse will be alert to the most potentially life-threatening side effect associated with the administration of monoamine oxidase (MAO) inhibitor. This is:

    A. Oculogyric crisis
    B. Hypertensive crisis
    C. Orthostatic hypotension
    D. Tardive dyskinesia

12. A 38-year-old female client with a history of chronic schizophrenia, paranoid type, is currently an outpatient at the local mental health and mental retardation clinic. The client comes in once a week for medication evaluation and/or refills. She self-administers haloperidol 5 mg twice a day and benztropine 1 mg once a day. During a recent clinic visit, she says to the nurse, "I can't stay still at night. I toss and turn and can't fall asleep." The nurse suspects that she may be experiencing:

    A. Akathisia
    B. Akinesia
    C. Dystonia
    D. Opisthotonos

13. On assessment, the nurse learns that a chronic paranoid schizophrenic has been taking "the blue pill" (haloperidol) in the morning and evening, and "the white pill" (benztropine) right before bedtime. The nurse might suggest to the client that she try:

    A. Doubling the daily dose of benztropine
    B. Decreasing the haloperidol dosage for a few days
    C. Taking the benztropine in the morning
    D. Taking her medication with food or milk

14. A 27-year-old male client is admitted to the acute care mental health unit for observation. He has recently lost his job, and his wife told him yesterday that she wants a divorce. The client is placed on suicide precautions. In assessing suicide potential, the nurse should pay close attention to the client's:

    A. Level of insight
    B. Thought processes
    C. Mood and affect
    D. Abstracting abilities

15. The nurse knows that children are more susceptible to respiratory tract infections owing to physiological differences. These childhood differences, when compared to an adult, include:

    A. Fewer alveoli, slower respiratory rate
    B. Diaphragmatic breathing, larger volume of air
    C. Larger number of alveoli, diaphragmatic breathing
    D. Rounded shape of chest, smaller volume of air

16. A 2-year-old toddler is hospitalized with epiglottitis. In assessing the toddler, the nurse would expect to find:

    A. A productive cough
    B. Expiratory stridor
    C. Drooling
    D. Crackles in the lower lobes

17. Which of the following nursing care goals has the *highest* priority for a child with epiglottitis?

    A. Sleep or lie quietly 10 hr/day.
    B. Consume foods from all four food groups.
    C. Be afebrile throughout her hospital stay.
    D. Participate in play activities 4 hr/day.

18. Which of the following nursing orders has the highest priority for a child with epiglottitis?

    A. Vital signs every shift
    B. Tracheostomy set at bedside
    C. Intake and output
    D. Specific gravity every shift

19. Often children are monitored with pulse oximeter. The pulse oximeter measures the:

    A. O_2 content of the blood
    B. Oxygen saturation of arterial blood
    C. Po_2
    D. Affinity of hemoglobin for O_2

20. A 4-year-old boy is brought to the emergency room with bruises on his head, face, arms, and legs. His mother states that he fell down some steps. The nurse suspects that he may have been physically abused. In accordance with the law, the nurse must:

    A. Tell the physician her concerns
    B. Report her suspicions to the authorities
    C. Talk to the child's father
    D. Confront the child's mother

21. The mother of a preschooler reports to the nurse that he frequently tells lies. The admission assessment of the child indicates possible child abuse. The nurse knows that his:

A. Behavior is not normal, and a child psychiatrist should be consulted.
B. Mother is lying to protect herself.
C. Lying is normal behavior for a preschool child who is learning to separate fantasy from reality.
D. Behavior indicates a developmental delay, because preschoolers should be able to tell right from wrong.

22. A family by court order undergoes treatment by a family therapist for child abuse. The nurse, who is the child's case manager knows that treatment has been effective when:

A. The child is removed from the home and placed in foster care
B. The child's parents identify the ways in which he is different from the rest of the family
C. The child's father is arrested for child abuse
D. The child's parents can identify appropriate behaviors for children in his age group

23. Nursing assessment of early evidence of septic shock in children at risk includes:

A. Fever, tachycardia, and tachypnea
B. Respiratory distress, cold skin, and pale extremities
C. Elevated blood pressure, hyperventilation, and thready pulses
D. Normal pulses, hypotension, and oliguria

24. A 3-year-old child is in the burn unit following a home accident. The first sign of sepsis in burned children is:

A. Disorientation
B. Low-grade fever
C. Diarrhea
D. Hypertension

25. One of the most reliable assessment tools for adequacy of fluid resuscitation in burned children is:

A. Blood pressure
B. Level of consciousness
C. Skin turgor
D. Fluid intake

26. A child with celiac disease is being discharged from the hospital. The mother demonstrates knowledge of nutritional needs of her child when she is able to state the foods which are included in a:

A. Lactose-restricted diet
B. Gluten-restricted diet
C. Phenylalanine-restricted diet
D. Fat-restricted diet

27. An 80-year-old male client with a history of arteriosclerosis is experiencing severe pain in his left leg that started approximately 20 minutes ago. When performing the admission assessment, the nurse would expect to observe which of the following:

A. Both lower extremities warm to touch with 2+ pedal pulses
B. Both lower extremities cyanotic when placed in a dependent position
C. Decreased or absent pedal pulse in the left leg
D. The left leg warmer to touch than the right leg

28. A male client is scheduled to have angiography of his left leg. The nurse needs to include which of the following when preparing the client for this procedure?

A. Validate that he is not allergic to iodine or shellfish.
B. Instruct him to start active range of motion of his left leg immediately following the procedure.
C. Inform him that he will not be able to eat or drink anything for 4 hours after the procedure.
D. Inform him that vital signs will be taken every hour for 4 hours after the procedure.

29. A female client is started on warfarin (Coumadin) 5 mg po bid. To adequately evaluate the effectiveness of the warfarin therapy, the nurse must know that this medication:

A. Dissolves any clots already formed in the arteries
B. Prevents the conversion of prothrombin to thrombin
C. Interferes with the synthesis of vitamin K-dependent clotting factors
D. Stimulates the manufacturing of platelets

30. A client is to be discharged from the hospital and is to continue taking warfarin 2.5 mg po bid. Which of the following should be included in her discharge teaching concerning the warfarin therapy?

A. "If you forget to take your morning dose, double the night time dose."
B. "You should take aspirin instead of acetaminophen (Tylenol) for headaches."
C. "Carry a medications alert card with you at all times."
D. "You should use a straight-edge razor when shaving your arms and legs."

31. A 40-year-old client has been admitted to the hospital with severe substernal chest pain radiating down his left arm. The nurse caring for the client establishes the following priority nursing diagnosis—Alteration in comfort, pain related to:

A. Increased excretion of lactic acid due to myocardial hypoxia
B. Increased blood flow through the coronary arteries
C. Decreased stimulation of the sympathetic nervous system
D. Decreased secretion of catecholamines secondary to anxiety

32. Morphine sulfate 4 mg IV push q2h prn for chest pain was ordered for a client in the emergency room with severe chest pain. The nurse administering the morphine sulfate knows which of the following therapeutic actions is related to the morphine sulfate?

A. Increased level of consciousness
B. Increased rate and depth of respirations
C. Increased peripheral vasodilation
D. Increased perception of pain

33. A client had a cardiac catheterization with angiography and thrombolytic therapy with streptokinase. The nurse should initiate which of the following interventions immediately after he returns to his room?

A. Place him on NPO restriction for 4 hours.
B. Monitor the catheterization site every 15 minutes.

C. Place him in a high Fowler position.

D. Ambulate him to the bathroom to void.

34. The nurse notes scattered crackles in both lungs and 1+ pitting edema when assessing a cardiac client. The physician is notified and orders furosemide (Lasix) 80 mg IV push stat. Which of the following diagnostic studies is monitored to assess for a major complication of this therapy?

    A. Serum electrolytes
    B. Arterial blood gases
    C. Complete blood count
    D. 12-Lead ECG

35. Prior to his discharge from the hospital, a cardiac client is started on digoxin (Lanoxin) 25 mg po qd. The nurse initiates discharge teaching. Which of the following statements by the client would validate an understanding of his medication?

    A. "I would notify my physician immediately if I experience nausea, vomiting, and double vision."
    B. "I could stop taking this medication when I begin to feel better."
    C. "I should only take the medication if my heart rate is greater than 100 bpm."
    D. "I should always take this medication with an antacid."

36. When assessing a client, the nurse notes the typical skin rash seen with systemic lupus erythematosus. Which of the following descriptions correctly describes this rash?

    A. Small round or oval reddish brown macules scattered over the entire body
    B. Scattered clusters of macules, papules, and vesicles over the body
    C. Bright red appearance of the palmar surface of the hands
    D. Reddened butterfly shaped rash over the cheeks and nose

37. The nurse notes multiple bruises on the arms and legs of a newly admitted client with lupus. The client states, "I get them whenever I bump into anything." The nurse would expect to note a decrease in which of the following laboratory tests?

    A. Number of platelets
    B. WBC count
    C. Hemoglobin level
    D. Number of lymphocytes

38. A client is started on prednisone 2.5 mg po bid. Which of the following instructions should be included in her discharge teaching specific to this medication?

    A. Increase your oral intake of fluids to at least 4000 mL every day.
    B. Avoid contact with people who have contagious illnesses.
    C. Brush your teeth at least 4 times a day with a firm toothbrush.
    D. Immediately stop taking the prednisone if you feel depressed.

39. During the assessment, the nurse observes a client scratching his skin. He has been admitted to rule out Laennec's cirrhosis of the liver. The nurse knows the pruritus is directly related to:

    A. A loss of phagocytic activity
    B. Faulty processing of bilirubin
    C. Enhanced detoxification of drugs
    D. The formation of collateral circulation

40. Four days after admission for cirrhosis of the liver, the nurse observes the following when assessing a male client: increased irritability, asterixis, and changes in his speech pattern. Which of the following foods would be appropriate for his bedtime snack?

    A. Fresh fruit
    B. A milkshake
    C. Saltine crackers and peanut butter
    D. A ham and cheese sandwich

41. A client with cirrhosis of the liver is to receive 50 mL of salt-poor albumin. The nurse infusing the albumin should assess for which of the following therapeutic responses to this therapy?

    A. Decreased heart rate and blood pressure
    B. Increased urinary output
    C. Adventitious breath sounds
    D. Hyperthermia

42. A client with cirrhosis of the liver becomes comatose and is started on neomycin 300 mg q6h via nasogastric tube. The rationale for this therapy is to:

    A. Prevent systemic infection
    B. Promote diuresis
    C. Decrease ammonia formation
    D. Acidify the small bowel

43. The following nursing diagnosis is written for a comatose client with cirrhosis of the liver and secondary splenomegaly—High risk for injury: Increased susceptibility to bleeding related to:

    A. Increased absorption of vitamin K
    B. Thrombocytopenia due to hypersplenism
    C. Diminished function of the Kupffer cells
    D. Increased synthesis of the clotting factors

44. A 52-year-old female client is admitted to the hospital in acute renal failure. She has been on hemodialysis for the past 2 years. Stat arterial blood gases are drawn on the client yielding the following results: pH 7.30, PCO_2 51 mm Hg, HCO_3, 18 mEq/L, PaO_2, 84 mm Hg. The nurse would interpret these results as:

    A. Compensated metabolic alkalosis
    B. Respiratory acidosis
    C. Partially compensated metabolic alkalosis
    D. Combined respiratory and metabolic acidosis

45. Stat serum electrolytes ordered for a client in acute renal failure revealed a serum potassium level of 6.4. The physician is immediately notified and orders 50 mL of dextrose and 10 U of regular insulin IV push. The nurse administering these drugs knows the Rationale for this therapy is to:

A. Remove the potassium from the body by renin exchange
B. Protect the myocardium from the effects of hypokalemia
C. Promote rapid protein catabolism
D. Drive potassium from the serum back into the cells

46. The nurse writes the following nursing diagnosis for a client in acute renal failure—Impaired gas exchange related to:

A. Decreased red blood cell production
B. Increased levels of vitamin D
C. Increased red blood cell production
D. Decreased production of renin

47. A 6-year-old child returned to the surgical floor 20 hours ago after an appendectomy for a gangrenous appendix. His mother tells the nurse that he is becoming more restless and is anxious. Assessment findings indicate that the child has atelectasis. Appropriate nursing actions would include:

A. Allowing the child to remain in the position of comfort, preferably semi-or high-Fowler position
B. Administering analgesics as ordered
C. Having the child turn, cough, and deep breathe every 1–2 hours
D. Remaining with the child and keeping as calm and quiet as possible

48. A client develops an intestinal obstruction postoperatively. A nasogastric tube is attached to low, intermittent suction with orders to "Irrigate NG tube with sterile saline q1h and prn." The rationale for using sterile saline, as opposed to using sterile water to irrigate the NG tube is:

A. Water will deplete electrolytes resulting in metabolic acidosis.
B. Saline will reduce the risk of severe, colicky abdominal pain during NG irrigation.
C. Water is not isotonic and will increase restlessness and insomnia in the immediate postoperative period.
D. Saline will increase peristalsis in the bowel.

49. A 35-year-old client has returned to her room following surgery on her right femur. She has an IV of D5 in one-half normal saline infusing at 125 mL/hr and is receiving morphine sulfate 10–15 mg IM q4h prn for pain. She last voided 5½ hours ago when she was given her preoperative medication. In monitoring and promoting return of urinary function after surgery, the nurse would:

A. Provide food and fluids at the client's request
B. Maintain IV, increasing the rate hourly until the client voids
C. Report to the surgeon if the client is unable to void within 8 hours of surgery
D. Hold morphine sulfate injections for pain until the client voids, explaining to her that morphine sulfate can cause urinary retention

50. A 47-year-old male client is admitted for colon surgery. Intravenous antibiotics are begun 2 hours prior to surgery. He has no known infection. The rationale for giving antibiotics prior to surgery is to:

A. Provide cathartic action within the colon
B. Reduce the risk of wound infection from anaerobic bacteria
C. Relieve the client's concern regarding possible infection
D. Reduce the risk of intraoperative fever

51. A 19-month-old child is admitted to the hospital for surgical repair of patent ductus arteriosus. The child is being given digoxin. Prior to administering the medication, the nurse should:

A. Not give the digoxin if the pulse is <60
B. Not give the digoxin if the pulse is >100
C. Take the apical pulse for a full minute
D. Monitor for visual disturbances, a side effect of digoxin

52. The family member of a child scheduled for heart surgery states, "I just don't understand this open-heart or closed-heart business. I'm so confused! Can you help me understand it?" The nurse explains that patent ductus arteriosus repair is:

A. Open-heart surgery. The child will be placed on a heart-lung machine while the surgery is being performed.
B. Closed-heart surgery. It does not require that the child be placed on the heart-lung machine while the surgery is being performed.
C. A pediatric version of the coronary artery bypass graft surgery performed on adults. It is an open-heart surgery.
D. A pediatric version of percutaneous transluminal coronary angioplasty performed on adults. It is a closed-heart surgery.

53. A child is to receive atropine 0.15 mg (1/400 g) as part of his preoperative medication. A vial containing atropine 0.4 mg (1/150 g)/mL is on hand. How much atropine should be given?

A. 0.06 mL
B. 0.38 mL
C. 2.7 mL
D. Information given insufficient to determine the amount of atropine to be administered

54. Following a gastric resection, a 70-year-old client is admitted to the postanesthesia care unit. He was extubated prior to leaving the suite. On arrival at the postanesthesia care unit, the nurse should:

A. Check airway, feeling for amount of air exchange noting rate, depth, and quality of respirations
B. Obtain pulse and blood pressure readings noting rate and quality of pulse
C. Reassure the client that his surgery is over and that he is in the recovery room
D. Review physician's orders, administering medications as ordered

55. A 25-year-old client is admitted for a tonsillectomy. She tells the nurse that she has had episodes of muscle cramps, weakness, and unexplained temperature elevation. Many years ago her father died shortly after

surgery after developing a high fever. She further tells the nurse that her surgeon is having her take dantrolene sodium (Dantrium) prophylactically prior to her tonsillectomy. Dantrolene sodium is ordered preoperatively to reduce the risk or prevent:

A. Infection postoperatively
B. Malignant hyperthermia
C. Neuroleptic malignant syndrome
D. Fever postoperatively

56. A 44-year-old client had an emergency cholecystectomy 3 days ago for a ruptured gallbladder. She complains of severe abdominal pain. Assessment reveals abdominal rigidity and distention, increased temperature, and tachycardia. Diagnostic testing reveals an elevated WBC count. The nurse suspects that the client has developed:

A. Gastritis
B. Evisceration
C. Peritonitis
D. Pulmonary embolism

57. A 35-year-old client is admitted to the hospital for elective tubal ligation. While the nurse is doing preoperative teaching, the client says, "The anesthesiologist said she was going to give me balanced anesthesia. What exactly is that?" The best explanation for the nurse to give the client would be that balanced anesthesia:

A. Is a type of regional anesthesia
B. Uses equal amounts of inhalation agents and liquid agents
C. Does not depress the central nervous system
D. Is a combination of several anesthetic agents or drugs producing a smooth induction and minimal complications

58. A 29-year-old client is admitted for a hysterectomy. She has repeatedly told the nurses that she is worried about having this surgery, has not slept well lately, and is afraid that her husband will not find her desirable after the surgery. Shortly into the preoperative teaching, she complains of a tightness in her chest, a feeling of suffocation, lightheadedness, and tingling in her hands. Her respirations are rapid and deep. Assessment reveals that the client is:

A. Having a heart attack
B. Wanting attention from the nurses
C. Suffering from complete upper airway obstruction
D. Hyperventilating

59. A client develops complications following a hysterectomy. Blood cultures reveal *Pseudomonas aeruginosa.* The nurse expects that the physician would order an appropriate antibiotic to treat *P. aeruginosa* such as:

A. Cefoperazone (Cefobid)
B. Clindamycin (Cleocin)

C. Dicloxacillin (Dycill)
D. Erythromycin (Erythrocin)

60. A couple is experiencing difficulties conceiving a baby. The nurse explains basal body temperature (BBT) by instructing the female client to take her temperature:

A. Orally in the morning and at bedtime
B. Only one time during the day as long as it is always at the same time of day
C. Rectally at bedtime
D. As soon as she awakens, prior to any activity

61. A client is having episodes of hyperventilation related to her surgery that is scheduled tomorrow. Appropriate nursing actions to help control hyperventilating include:

A. Administering diazepam (Valium) 10–15 mg po q4h and q1h prn for hyperventilating episode
B. Keeping the temperature in the client's room at a high level to reduce respiratory stimulation
C. Having the client hold her breath or breathe into a paper bag when hyperventilation episodes occur
D. Using distraction to help control the client's hyperventilation episodes

62. A client delivered a stillborn male at term. An appropriate action of the nurse would be to:

A. State, "You have an angel in heaven."
B. Discourage the parents from seeing the baby.
C. Provide an opportunity for the parents to see and hold the baby for an undetermined amount of time.
D. Reassure the parents that they can have other children.

63. A pregnant client is having a nonstress test (NST). It is noted that the fetal heart beat rises 20 bpm, lasting 20 seconds, every time the fetus moves. The nurse explains that:

A. The test is inconclusive and should be repeated
B. Further testing is needed
C. The test is normal and the fetus is reacting appropriately
D. The fetus is distressed

64. Which stage of labor lasts from delivery of the baby to delivery of the placenta?

A. Second
B. Third
C. Fourth
D. Fifth

65. On the third postpartum day, the nurse would expect the lochia to be:

A. Rubra
B. Serosa
C. Alba
D. Scant

1. **(B)** Client need: physiological integrity; subcategory: pharmacological and parenteral therapies; content area: psychiatric

   RATIONALE

   (A) These are general diagnostic blood studies (usually done on admission), but they are not reliable indicators of lithium therapy clearance. (B) These are the primary diagnostic tests to determine kidney functioning. Because lithium is excreted through the kidneys and because it can be very toxic, adequate renal function must be ascertained before therapy begins. (C) These are diagnostic blood tests used to determine the presence of endocrine (not renal) dysfunction. (D) These are other types of diagnostic procedures used to determine musculoskeletal, neural, and cardiac (rather than renal) functioning.

2. **(C)** Client need: physiological integrity; subcategory: pharmacological and parenteral therapies; content area: psychiatric

   RATIONALE

   (A) There is no need to phone the physician because the lithium level is within therapeutic range and because there are no indications of toxicity present. (B) There is no reason to withhold the lithium because the blood level is within therapeutic range. Also, it is necessary to give the medication as scheduled to maintain adequate blood levels. (C) The lab results indicate that the client's lithium level is within therapeutic range (0.2–1.4 mEq/L), so the medication should be given as ordered. (D) Benztropine is an antiparkinsonism drug frequently given to counteract extrapyramidal symptoms associated with the administration of antipsychotic drugs (not lithium).

3. **(D)** Client need: physiological integrity; subcategory: physiological adaptation; content area: psychiatric

   RATIONALE

   (A) Self-concept and self-esteem problems may emerge during the client's treatment, but these are not immediate concerns. (B) Interpersonal issues may become evident during the course of the client's treatment, but these are also not immediate areas of concern. (C) Improving individual coping skills is generally a primary focus in the treatment and nursing care of persons with substance abuse problems. However, this is still not the immediate concern in this client situation. (D) Correction of fluid and electrolyte status and vitamin deficiencies, as well as prevention of delirium, is the immediate concern in the care of this client.

4. **(B)** Client need: psychosocial integrity; subcategory: coping and adaptation; content area: psychiatric

   RATIONALE

   (A) Focusing is an effective therapeutic strategy. This response, however, allows the client to "defocus" off the topic of learning how to accept responsibility for his behavior and future growth. (B) The nurse can educate the client about both the "genetic risk" for the development of alcoholism and ways to make long-term healthy lifestyle changes. (C) This response is inappropriately confrontational and condescending to the client. (D) Reflection of content can be an effective verbal therapeutic technique. It is used inappropriately here.

5. **(A)** Client need: psychosocial integrity; subcategory: psychosocial adaptation; content area: pediatrics

   RATIONALE

   (A) Providing a more structured, supportive environment addresses safety and comfort needs, thereby helping the anorexic client develop more internal control. (B) Medications (commonly antidepressants) are frequently ordered for the anorexic client. However, lithium (used primarily with bipolar disorder) is not commonly used to treat the anorexic client. (C) Requiring and/or demanding that the anorexic client "eat more" at mealtimes increases the client's feelings of powerlessness. (D) Like the previous strategy, checking the client's room frequently contributes to the client's feelings of powerlessness.

6. **(B)** Client need: psychosocial integrity; subcategory: coping and adaptation; content area: pediatrics

   RATIONALE

   (A) This outcome criterion is inadequate because the term "accepts" is not directly measurable. (B) This outcome criterion is directly measurable because specific goal-related verbalizations can be heard and verified by the nurse. (C) "Improved perception of body image" is not directly measurable and is therefore open to many interpretations. (D) Although long-term goals for the anorexic client should focus on increased self-esteem, this outcome criterion (as stated) does not include specific indicators or behaviors for which to observe.

7. **(C)** Client need: psychosocial integrity; subcategory: coping and adaptation; content area: psychiatric

   RATIONALE

   (A) Reaction formation is the development and demonstration of attitudes and/or behaviors opposite to what an individual actually feels. The client's comment does reveal her anger and hostility. (B) Rationalization, another ego defense mechanism, is offering a socially acceptable or seemingly logical explanation to justify one's feelings, behaviors, or motives. The client's comment does not reflect rationalization. (C) Splitting, the viewing of people or situations as either all good or all bad, is frequently used by persons experiencing a disruption in self-concept. This ego defense mechanism is reflective of the individual's inability to integrate the positive and negative aspects of self. (D) Sublimation, the channeling of socially unacceptable impulses and behaviors into more acceptable patterns of behavior, is another ego defense mechanism. The client's comment reveals that she is not engaging in sublimation.

8. **(D)** Client need: psychosocial integrity; subcategory: coping and adaptation; content area: psychiatric

   RATIONALE

   (A) This statement is a defensive response that places the nurse in a vulnerable countertransference position, and at the same time, fails to challenge the client's "splitting" behavior. (B) This statement is a defensive response by the nurse. In addition, this type of nontherapeutic statement requests that the client explain the reasons for her behavior, a difficult task for an individual with limited insight. (C) This statement is a nontherapeutic response that both ignores the intensity of the client's emotions and the dynamics underlying "splitting" behavior. (D) By simultaneously acknowledging the client's emotional intensity and gently challenging her "splitting" behavior, the nurse addresses the client's current distortions and prepares for further interventions with angry or ambivalent feelings.

9. **(B)** Client need: physiological integrity; subcategory: pharmacological and parenteral therapies; content area: psychiatric

   RATIONALE

   (A) Thioridazine (an antipsychotic drug), lithium (an antimanic drug), and benztropine (an antiparkinsonism agent) are generally administered to treat schizophrenic and bipolar disorders. (B) Atropine (a cholinergic blocker), sodium brevitol (a short-acting anesthetic), and succinylcholine (a neuromuscular blocker) are administered either before or during ECT to counteract bradycardia and to provide anesthesia and total muscle relaxation. (C) These are electrolyte substances administered to correct fluid and electrolyte imbalances in the body. (D) Carbamazepine (an anticonvulsant), haloperidol (an antipsychotic), and trihexyphenydyl (an antiparkinsonism agent) are usually administered in psychiatric settings to control problems associated with psychotic behavior.

10. **(C)** Client need: physiological integrity; subcategory: pharmacological and parenteral therapies; content area: psychiatric

RATIONALE

(A) The client may need to avoid some potassium-rich foods (such as bananas, raisins, etc.). However, this is not because of the potassium content of these foods. (B) Tryptophan is an essential amino acid that is present in high concentrations in animal and fish protein. (C) The client will need to watch his dietary intake of tyramine. Tyramine is a by-product of the conversion of tyrosine to epinephrine. Tyramine is found in a variety of foods and beverages, ranging from aged cheese to caffeine drinks. Ingestion of tyramine-rich foods while taking a MAO inhibitor may lead to an increase in blood pressure and/or a life-threatening hypertensive crisis. (D) To maintain a healthy lifestyle, restriction of dietary saturated fats is advisable.

11. **(B)** Client need: physiological integrity; subcategory: pharmacological and parenteral therapies; content area: psychiatric

RATIONALE

(A) Oculogyric crisis, involuntary upward deviation and fixation of the eyeballs, is usually associated with either postencephalitic parkinsonian or drug-induced extrapyramidal symptoms (EPS). (B) Hypertensive crisis is a potentially life-threatening side effect. This may occur if the client ingests foods, beverages, or medications containing tyramine. (C) Orthostatic hypotension, a drop in blood pressure resulting from a rapid change of body position, can occur with the administration of antidepressants. (D) Tardive dyskinesia, characterized by slow, rhythmical, automatic or stereotyped muscular movements, usually is associated with the administration of certain antipsychotic medications.

12. **(A)** Client need: physiological integrity; subcategory: pharmacological and parenteral therapies; content area: psychiatric

RATIONALE

(A) Akathisia, or motor restlessness, is a reversible EPS frequently associated with the administration of antipsychotic drugs such as haloperidol. (B) Akinesia, or muscular or motor retardation, is an example of reversible EPS frequently associated with the administration of major tranquilizers such as haloperidol. (C) Acute dystonic reactions, bizarre and severe muscle contractions usually of the tongue, face, neck or extraocular muscles, are examples of EPS. (D) Opisthotonos, a severe type of whole-body dystonic reaction in which the head and heels are bent backward while the body is bowed forward, is an example of EPS.

13. **(C)** Client need: physiological integrity; subcategory: pharmacological and parenteral therapies; content area: psychiatric

RATIONALE

(A) Suggesting that a client increase a medication dosage is an inappropriate (and illegal) nursing action. This action requires a physician's order. (B) To suggest that a client decrease a medication dosage is an inappropriate (and illegal) nursing action. This action requires a physician's order. (C) This response is an appropriate independent nursing action. Because motor restlessness can also be a side effect of cogentin, the nurse may suggest that the client try taking the drug early in the day rather than at bedtime. (D) Certain medications can cause gastric irritation and may be taken with food or milk to prevent this side effect.

14. **(C)** Client need: psychosocial integrity; subcategory: coping and adaptation; content area: psychiatric

RATIONALE

(A) Assessing the client's level of insight is an important part of the mental status exam (MSE), but it does not reflect suicide potential. (B) Assessing the client's thought processes is an important part of the MSE, but it does not reflect suicide potential. (C) Assessing the client's mood and affect is an important part of the MSE, and it can be a very valuable indicator of suicide potential. Frequently a client who has decided to proceed with suicide plans will exhibit a suddenly improved mood and affect. (D) Assessing a client's abstracting abilities is an important part of the MSE, but it does not reflect suicide potential.

15. **(D)** Client need: health promotion and maintenance; subcategory: growth and development through the life span; content area: pediatrics

RATIONALE

(A) Although a child has fewer alveoli than an adult, the child's respiratory rate is faster. (B) Although a child may use diaphragmatic breathing, the adult exchanges a larger volume of air. (C) The adult has a larger number of alveoli than a child. (D) The child's chest is rounded whereas the adult chest is more of an oval shape, and the child does exchange a smaller volume of air than an adult.

16. **(C)** Client need: health promotion and maintenance; subcategory: prevention and early detection of disease; content area: pediatrics

RATIONALE

(A) A productive cough is not associated with epiglottitis. (B) Children with epiglottitis seldom have expiratory stridor. Inspiratory stridor is more common due to edema of the supraglottic tissues. (C) Because of difficulty with swallowing, drooling often accompanies epiglottitis. (D) Crackles are not heard in the lower lobes with epiglottitis because the infection is usually confined to the supraglottic structures.

17. **(A)** Client need: physiological integrity; subcategory: physiological adaptation; content area: pediatrics

RATIONALE

(A) Of these four goals, maintenance of a calm, quiet atmosphere to reduce anxiety and to allow for rest is the most important. (B) Although nutrition is important, the child needs fluids to maintain fluid and electrolyte balance more than solid foods. In addition, the child may not be able to swallow solid foods owing to epiglottic swelling. (C) This goal is unrealistic because fever is a common symptom of the infection associated with epiglottitis. (D) If overexerted, the child will need more O_2 and energy than available, and these requirements may exacerbate the condition.

18. **(B)** Client need: physiological integrity; subcategory: physiological adaptation; content area: pediatrics

RATIONALE

(A) Because of the possibility of fever or respiratory failure, vital signs should be done more often than every eight hours. (B) If the epiglottitis worsens, the edema and laryngospasm may close the airway and an emergency tracheostomy may be necessary. (C) Although intake and output are a part of the nursing care of a child with epiglottitis, it is not as important as the safety measure of keeping the tracheostomy set at the bedside. (D) Specific gravity will indicate hydration status, but it is not as important as keeping the tracheostomy set at the bedside.

19. **(B)** Client need: physiological integrity; subcategory: physiological adaptation; content area: pediatrics

RATIONALE

(A) The O_2 content of whole blood is determined by the partial pressure of oxygen (PO_2) and the oxygen saturation. The pulse oximeter does not measure the PO_2. (B) The pulse oximeter is a noninvasive method of measuring the arterial oxygen saturation.

(C) The PO_2 is the amount of O_2 dissolved in plasma, which the pulse oximeter does not measure. (D) The affinity of hemoglobin for O_2 is the relationship between oxygen saturation and PO_2 and is not measured by the pulse oximeter.

20. **(B)** Client need: health promotion and maintenance; subcategory: growth and development through the life span; content area: pediatrics

RATIONALE

(A) Although the nurse probably would talk to the physician about these concerns, the nurse is not required by law to do so. (B) All healthcare workers are required by the Federal Child Abuse Prevention and Treatment Act of 1974 to report suspected and actual cases of child abuse and/or neglect. (C) Talking to the child's father may or may not help the child, and the nurse is not required by law to do so. (D) Confrontation may not be indicated; the nurse is not required by law to confront the child's mother with these suspicions.

21. **(C)** Client need: psychosocial integrity; subcategory: psychosocial adaptation; content area: pediatrics

RATIONALE

(A) Because preschoolers often tell "stories" as they learn to differentiate fantasy from reality, the child's behavior is normal. (B) The nurse has no reason to believe the child's mother is lying, because children of his age often tell lies. (C) The child's lying is actually "storytelling" as he learns to separate fantasy from reality, a normal developmental task for his age group. (D) The child's behavior is consistent with his age and does not indicate a developmental delay.

22. **(D)** Client need: psychosocial integrity; subcategory: psychosocial adaptation; content area: pediatrics

RATIONALE

(A) Removing an abused child from the home and placement in a foster home are not the desired outcome of treatment. (B) Children who are perceived as "different" from the rest of the family are more likely to be abused. (C) Although legal action may be taken against abusive parents, it is not an indicator of an effective treatment program. (D) Identification of age-appropriate behaviors is essential to the role of parents, because misunderstanding children's normal developmental needs often contributes to abuse or neglect.

23. **(A)** Client need: physiological integrity; subcategory: physiological adaptation; content area: pediatrics

RATIONALE

(A) Fever, tachycardia, and tachypnea are the classic early signs of septic shock in children. (B) Respiratory distress, cold skin, and pale extremities are later signs of septic shock. (C) Elevated blood pressure, hyperventilation, and thready pulses are later signs of septic shock. (D) Normal pulses, hypotension, and oliguria are not early signs of septic shock.

24. **(A)** Client need: physiological integrity; subcategory: reduction of risk potential; content area: pediatrics

RATIONALE

(A) Disorientation is the first sign of sepsis in burn children. (B) Low-grade fever is not indicative of sepsis. (C) Diarrhea is not indicative of sepsis. (D) Hypertension is not indicative of sepsis.

25. **(B)** Client need: physiological integrity; subcategory: physiological adaptation; content area: pediatrics

RATIONALE

(A) Blood pressure can remain normotensive in a state of hypovolemia. (B) Capillary refill, alterations in sensorium, and urine output are the most reliable indicators for assessing hydration.

(C) Skin turgor is not a reliable indicator for assessing hydration in a burn client. (D) Fluid intake does not indicate adequacy of fluid resuscitation in a burn client.

26. **(B)** Client need: physiological integrity; subcategory: basic care and comfort; content area: pediatrics

RATIONALE

(A) A lactose-restricted diet is prescribed for children with lactose intolerance or diarrhea. (B) A gluten-restricted diet is the diet for children with celiac disease. (C) A phenylalanine-restricted diet is prescribed for children with phenylketonuria. (D) A fat-restricted diet is prescribed for children with disorders of the liver, gallbladder, or pancreas.

27. **(C)** Client need: health promotion and maintenance; subcategory: prevention and early detection of disease; content area: med/surg

RATIONALE

(A) This statement describes a normal assessment finding of the lower extremities. (B) This assessment finding reflects problems caused by venous insufficiency. (C) Decreased or absent pedal pulses reflect a problem caused by arterial insufficiency. (D) The leg that is experiencing arterial insufficiency would be cool to touch due to the decreased circulation.

28. **(A)** Client need: physiological integrity; subcategory: reduction of risk potential; content area: med/surg

RATIONALE

(A) Angiography, an invasive radiographic examination, involves the injection of a contrast solution (iodine) through a catheter that has been inserted into an artery. (B) The client is kept on complete bed rest for 6–12 hours after the procedure. The extremity in which the catheter was inserted must be immobilized and kept straight during this time. (C) The contrast dye, iodine, is nephrotoxic. The client must be instructed to drink a large quantity of fluids to assist the kidneys in excreting this contrast media. (D) The major complication of this procedure is hemorrhage. Vital signs are assessed every 15 minutes initially for signs of bleeding.

29. **(C)** Client need: physiological integrity; subcategory: pharmacological and parenteral therapies; content area: med/surg

RATIONALE

(A) Thrombolytic agents (e.g., streptokinase) directly activate plasminogen, dissolving fibrin deposits, which in turn dissolves clots that have already formed. (B) Heparin prevents the formation of clots by potentiating the effects of antithrombin III and the conversion of prothrombin to thrombin. (C) Warfarin prevents the formation of clots by interfering with the hepatic synthesis of the vitamin K-dependent clotting factors. (D) Platelets initiate the coagulation of blood by adhering to each other and the site of injury to form platelet plugs.

30. **(C)** Client need: physiological integrity; subcategory: pharmacological and parenteral therapies; content area: med/surg

RATIONALE

(A) Warfarin must always be taken exactly as directed. Clients should be instructed never to skip or double up on their dosage. (B) Aspirin decreases platelet aggregation, which would potentiate the effects of the coumadin. (C) Healthcare providers need to be aware of persons on warfarin therapy prior to the initiation of any diagnostic tests and/or surgery to help prevent bleeding complications. (D) An electric razor should be used to prevent accidental cutting, which can lead to bleeding.

31. **(A)** Client need: physiological integrity; subcategory: physiological adaptation; content area: med/surg

RATIONALE

(A) Anaerobic metabolism results because the decreased blood supply to the myocardium causes a release of lactic acid. Lactic acid is an irritant to the myocardial neural receptors, producing chest pain. (B) Chest pain is caused by a decrease in the O_2 supply to the myocardial cells. Treatment modalities for chest pain are aimed toward increasing the blood flow through coronary arteries. (C) Chest pain causes an increase in the stimulation of the sympathetic nervous system. This stimulation increases the heart rate and blood pressure, causing an increase in myocardial workload aggravating the chest pain. (D) Chest pain and anxiety cause increased secretion of catecholamines by stimulating the sympathetic nervous system. This stimulation increases chest pain by increasing the workload of the heart.

32. **(C)** Client need: physiological integrity; subcategory: pharmacological and parenteral therapies; content area: med/surg

RATIONALE

(A) Morphine sulfate, a narcotic analgesic, causes sedation and a decrease in level of consciousness. (B) The side effects of morphine sulfate include respiratory depression. (C) Morphine sulfate causes peripheral vasodilation, which decreases afterload, producing a decrease in the myocardial workload. (D) Morphine sulfate alters the perception of pain through an unclear mechanism. This alteration promotes pain relief.

33. **(B)** Client need: physiological integrity; subcategory: reduction of risk potential; content area: med/surg

RATIONALE

(A) A contrast dye, iodine, is used in this procedure. This dye is nephrotoxic. The client must be encouraged to drink plenty of liquids to assist the kidneys in eliminating the dye. (B) Streptokinase activates plasminogen, dissolving fibrin deposits. To prevent bleeding, pressure is applied at the insertion site. The client is assessed for both internal and external bleeding. (C) The extremity used for the insertion site must be kept straight and be immobilized because of the potential for bleeding. (D) The client is kept on bed rest for 8–12 hours following the procedure because of the potential for bleeding.

34. **(A)** Client need: physiological integrity; subcategory: pharmacological and parenteral therapies; content area: med/surg

RATIONALE

(A) Furosemide, a potassium-depleting diuretic, inhibits the reabsorption of sodium and chloride from the loop of Henle and the distal renal tubules. Serum electrolytes are monitored for hypokalemia. (B) Severe acid-base imbalances influence the movement of potassium into and out of the cells, but arterial blood gases to not measure the serum potassium level. (C) Furosemide is a potassium-depleting diuretic. A complete blood count does not reflect potassium levels. (D) Abnormalities in potassium (both hyperkalemia and hypokalemia) are reflected in ECG changes, but these changes do not occur until the abnormality is severe.

35. **(A)** Client need: physiological integrity; subcategory: pharmacological and parenteral therapies; content area: med/surg

RATIONALE

(A) The first signs of digoxin toxicity include abdominal pain, anorexia, nausea, vomiting, and visual disturbances. The physician should be notified if any of these symptoms are experienced. (B) The positive inotropic effects of digoxin increase cardiac output and result in an enhanced activity tolerance. "Feeling better" indicates the drug is working and medication therapy must be continued. (C) Clients should be taught to take their pulse prior to taking the digoxin. If their pulse rate becomes irregular, slows significantly, or is >100 bpm the physician should be notified. (D) Antacids decrease the effectiveness of digoxin.

36. **(D)** Client need: health promotion and maintenance; subcategory: prevention and early detection of disease; content area: med/surg

RATIONALE

(A) The appearance of small, round or oval reddish brown macules scattered over the entire body is characteristic of rubeola. (B) The appearance of scattered clusters of macules, papules, and vesicles throughout the body is characteristic of chickenpox. (C) Palmar redness is seen in clients with cirrhosis of the liver. (D) The characteristic butterfly rash over the cheek and nose and into the scalp is seen with systemic lupus erythematosus.

37. **(A)** Client need: health promotion and maintenance; subcategory: prevention and early detection of disease; content area: med/surg

RATIONALE

(A) Thrombocytopenia, a decrease in platelets, occurs in lupus and causes a decrease in blood coagulation and thrombus formation. (B) Clients with lupus will have a decrease in the WBC count decreasing their resistance to infection. (C) Clients with lupus may have a decrease in the hemoglobin level causing anemia. (D) Leukopenia, a decrease in white blood cells, is seen in lupus and decreases resistance to infection.

38. **(B)** Client need: physiological integrity; subcategory: pharmacological and parenteral therapies; content area: med/surg

RATIONALE

(A) Fluid retention is a side effect of prednisone. The nurse should teach clients to weigh themselves daily and to observe for signs of edema. If these signs of fluid retention occur, they should notify the physician. (B) Prednisone, a glucocorticoid, suppresses the normal immune response making the client more susceptible to infections. (C) An increase in bleeding tendencies is a side effect of prednisone therapy. The nurse should teach clients to use preventive measures (i.e., electric razors and soft toothbrushes). (D) Depression and personality changes are side effects of prednisone therapy. Prednisone should never be discontinued abruptly.

39. **(B)** Client need: physiological integrity; subcategory: physiological adaptation; content area: med/surg

RATIONALE

(A) A loss in the phagocytic activity of the Kupffer cells occurs with cirrhosis of the liver, which increases the susceptibility to infections. (B) The faulty processing of bilirubin produces bile salts, which are irritating to the skin. (C) The detoxification of drugs is impaired with cirrhosis of the liver. (D) Collateral circulation develops due to portal hypertension. This is manifest through the development of esophageal varices, hemorrhoids, and caput medusae.

40. **(A)** Client need: physiological integrity; subcategory: reduction of risk potential; content area: med/surg

RATIONALE

(A) High levels of ammonia, a by-product of protein metabolism, can precipitate metabolic encephalopathy. These clients need a diet high in carbohydrates and bulk. (B) Metabolic encephalopathy of the brain associated with liver failure is precipitated by elevated ammonia levels. Ammonia is a by-product of protein metabolism. (C, D) Metabolic encephalopathy in liver failure is precipitated by elevated ammonia levels. Ammonia is a by-product of protein metabolism.

41. **(B)** Client need: physiological integrity; subcategory: pharmacological and parenteral therapies; content area: med/surg

RATIONALE

(A) Albumin, a blood volume expander, increases the circulating blood volume by exerting an osmotic pull on tissue fluids, pulling them into the vascular system. This fluid shift causes an increase in the heart rate and blood pressure. (B) Albumin, a blood volume expander, exerts an osmotic pull on fluids in the interstitial spaces, pulling the fluid back into the circulatory system. This fluid shift causes an increase in the urinary output. (C) Adventitious breath sounds and dyspnea can occur due to circulatory overload if the albumin is infused too rapidly. (D) Chills, fever, itching, and rashes are signs of a hypersensitivity reaction to albumin.

42. **(C)** Client need: physiological integrity; subcategory: pharmacological and parenteral therapies; content area: med/surg

    RATIONALE
    (A) Neomycin is an antibiotic, but this is not the Rationale for administering it to a client in hepatic coma. (B) Diuretics and salt-free albumin are used to promote diuresis in clients with cirrhosis of the liver. (C) Neomycin destroys the bacteria in the intestines. It is the bacteria in the bowel that break down protein into ammonia. (D) Lactulose is administered to create an acid environment in the bowel. Ammonia leaves the blood and migrates to this acidic environment where it is trapped and excreted.

43. **(B)** Client need: physiological integrity; subcategory: physiological adaptation; content area: med/surg

    RATIONALE
    (A) There is a decreased absorption of vitamin K with cirrhosis of the liver. This decrease impairs blood coagulation and the formation of prothrombin. (B) Thrombocytopenia, an increased destruction of platelets, occurs secondary to hypersplenism. (C) A diminished function of the Kupffer cells occurs with cirrhosis of the liver, causing the client to become more susceptible to infections. (D) A decrease in the synthesis of fibrinogen and clotting factors VII, IX, and X occurs with cirrhosis of the liver and increases the susceptibility to bleeding.

44. **(D)** Client need: physiological integrity; subcategory: physiological adaptation; content area: med/surg

    RATIONALE
    (A) Compensated metabolic alkalosis would be reflected by the following: pH within normal limit (7.35–7.45), $P_{CO_2} > 45$ mm Hg, $HCO_3 > 26$ mEq/L. (B) Respiratory acidosis would be reflected by the following: pH < 7.35, $P_{CO_2} > 45$ mm Hg, HCO_3 within normal limits (22–26 mEq/L). (C) Partially compensated metabolic alkalosis would be reflected by the following: pH > 7.45, $P_{CO_2} > 45$ mm Hg, $HCO_3 > 26$ mEq/L. (D) Combined respiratory and metabolic acidosis would be reflected by the following: pH < 7.35, $P_{CO_2} > 45$ mm Hg, $HCO_3 < 22$ mEq/L.

45. **(D)** Client need: physiological integrity; subcategory: physiological adaptation; content area: med/surg

    RATIONALE
    (A) Sodium polystyrene sulfonate (Kayexalate), a cation exchange resin, exchanges sodium ions for potassium ions in the large intestine reducing the serum potassium. (B) Calcium is administered to protect the myocardium from the adverse effects of hyperkalemia. Serum levels reflect hyperkalemia. (C) Rapid catabolism releases potassium from the body tissue into the bloodstream. Infection and hyperthermia increase the process of catabolism. (D) The administration of dextrose and regular insulin IV forces potassium back into the cells decreasing the potassium in the serum.

46. **(A)** Client need: physiological integrity; subcategory: physiological adaptation; content area: med/surg

    RATIONALE
    (A) Red blood cell production is impaired in renal failure owing to impaired erythropoietin production. This causes a decrease in

the delivery of oxygen to the tissue and impairs gas exchange. (B) The conversion of vitamin D to its physiologically active form is impaired in renal failure. (C) In renal failure, a decrease in red blood cell production occurs owing to an impaired production of erythropoietin, leading to impaired gas exchange at the cellular level. (D) The decreased production of renin in renal failure causes an increased production of aldosterone causing sodium and water retention.

47. **(C)** Client need: physiological integrity; subcategory: reduction of risk potential; content area: med/surg

    RATIONALE
    (A) Allowing the client to remain in the position of comfort will not resolve the atelectasis. This position, if left unchanged, over time may actually increase the atelectasis. (B) Analgesics will not resolve the atelectasis and may contribute to it if proper nursing actions are not taken to help resolve the atelectasis. (C) Having the client turn, cough, and deep breathe every 1–2 hours will aid in resolving the atelectasis. Surgery clients are at risk for postoperative respiratory complications because pulmonary function is reduced as a result of anesthesia and surgery. (D) Remaining with the client and keeping him calm and quiet will not affect the client's anxiety, restlessness, or help to resolve the atelectasis. The cause (atelectasis) needs to be treated, not the symptoms (anxiety and restlessness).

48. **(A)** Client need: physiological integrity; subcategory: reduction of risk potential; content area: med/surg

    RATIONALE
    (A) Water is a hypotonic solution and will deplete electrolytes and cause metabolic acidosis when used for nasogastric irrigation. (B) Irrigating with saline does not cause abdominal discomfort. Severe, colicky abdominal pain is a symptom of intestinal obstruction. (C) Irrigating with water will not cause restlessness or insomnia in the postoperative client. Restlessness and insomnia can be emotional complications of surgery. (D) A nasogastric tube placed in the stomach is used to decompress the bowel. Irrigating with saline ensures a patent, well-functioning tube. Irrigating with saline will not increase peristalsis.

49. **(C)** Client need: physiological integrity; subcategory: pharmacological and parenteral therapies; content area: med/surg

    RATIONALE
    (A) Provision of food and fluid promotes bowel elimination. Nutritional needs postoperatively are determined by the physician, not the client. (B) Increasing IV fluids postoperatively will not cause a client to void. Any change in rate of administration of IV fluids should be determined by the physician. (C) The postoperative client with normal kidney function who cannot void 8 hours after surgery is retaining urine. The client may need catheterization or medication. The physician must provide orders for both as necessary. (D) Although morphine sulfate can cause urinary retention, withholding pain medication will not ensure that the client will void. The client with uncontrolled pain will probably not be able to void.

50. **(B)** Client need: physiological integrity; subcategory: pharmacological and parenteral therapies; content area: med/surg

    RATIONALE
    (A) Cathartic drugs promote evacuation of intestinal contents. (B) The client undergoing intestinal surgery is at increased risk for infection from large numbers of anaerobic bacteria that inhabit the intestines. Administering antibiotics prophylactically can reduce the client's risk for infection. (C) Antibiotics are indicated in the treatment of infections and have no effect on emotions. (D) Antipyretics are useful in the treatment of elevated temperatures. Antibiotics would have an effect on infection, which causes temperature elevation, but would not directly affect such an elevation.

51. **(C)** Client need: physiological integrity; subcategory: pharmacological and parenteral therapies; content area: pediatrics

RATIONALE

(A) Digoxin should not be given to adults with an apical pulse < 60 bpm. (B) Digoxin should be given to children with an apical pulse > 100 bpm. With a pulse < 100 bpm, the medication should be withheld and the physician notified. (C) Prior to digoxin administration in both children and adults, an apical pulse should be taken for 1 full minute. Aside from the rate per minute, the nurse should note any sudden increase or decrease in heart rate, irregular rhythm, or regularization of a chronic irregular heart rhythm. (D) Early indications of digoxin toxicity, such as visual disturbances, occur rarely as initial signs in children.

52. **(B)** Client need: physiological integrity; subcategory: physiological adaptation; content area: pediatrics

RATIONALE

(A) Patent ductus arteriosus repair is a closed-heart procedure. The client is not placed on a heart-lung machine. (B) Patent ductus arteriosus is a ductus arteriosus that does not close shortly after birth but remains patent. Repair is a closed-heart procedure involving ligation of the patent ductus arteriosus. (C) Coronary artery bypass graft surgery is an open-heart surgical procedure in which blocked coronary arteries are bypassed using vessel grafts. (D) Percutaneous transluminal coronary angioplasty is a closed-heart procedure that improves coronary blood flow by increasing the lumen size of narrowed vessels.

53. **(B)** Client need: physiological integrity; subcategory: pharmacological and parenteral therapies; content area: med/surg

RATIONALE

(A, C) Information was incorrectly placed in the formula, resulting in an incorrect answer. (B) The answer is correct.
0.4 mg = 1 mL:0.15 mg 5 = mL
   0.4 x = 0.15
       x = 0.15/0.4
       x = 0.375 or 0.38 mL
(D) Sufficient information is provided to determine the amount of atropine to administer. The amount of atropine available and the amount of atropine ordered is required to determine the amount of atropine to be given.

54. **(A)** Client need: physiological integrity; subcategory: reduction of risk potential; content area: med/surg

RATIONALE

(A) Adequate air exchange and tissue oxygenation depend on competent respiratory function. Checking the airway is the nurse's priority action. (B) Obtaining the vital signs is an important action, but it is secondary to airway management. (C) Reorienting a client to time, place, and person after surgery is important, but it is secondary to airway and vital signs. (D) Airway management takes precedence over physician's orders unless they specifically relate to airway management.

55. **(B)** Client need: physiological integrity; subcategory: reduction of risk potential; content area: med/surg

RATIONALE

(A, D) Dantrolene sodium is a peripheral skeletal muscle relaxant and would have no effect on a postoperative infection. (B) Dantrolene sodium is indicated prophylactically for clients with malignant hyperthermia or with a family history of the disorder. The mortality rate for malignant hyperthermia is high. (C) Neuroleptic malignant syndrome is an exercise-induced muscle pain and spasm and is unrelated to malignant hyperthermia.

56. **(C)** Client need: physiological integrity; subcategory: reduction of risk potential; content area: med/surg

RATIONALE

(A) Assessment findings for gastritis would reveal anorexia, nausea and vomiting, epigastric fullness and tenderness, and discomfort. (B) Evisceration is the extrusion of abdominal viscera as a result of trauma or sutures failing in a surgical incision. (C) Peritonitis, inflammation of the peritoneum, can occur when an abdominal organ, such as the gallbladder, perforates and leaks blood and fluid into the abdominal cavity. This causes infection and irritation. (D) Assessment findings of pulmonary embolism would reveal severe substernal chest pain, tachycardia, tachypnea, shortness of breath, anxiety or panic, and wheezing and coughing often accompanied by blood-tinged sputum.

57. **(D)** Client need: physiological integrity; subcategory: pharmacological and parenteral therapies; content area: med/surg

RATIONALE

(A) Regional anesthesia does not produce loss of consciousness and is indicated for excision of moles, cysts, and endoscopic surgeries. (B) Varying amounts of anesthetic agents are used when employing balanced anesthesia. Amounts depend on age, weight, condition of the client, and surgical procedure. (C) General anesthesia is a drug-induced depression of the central nervous system that produces loss of consciousness and decreased muscle activity. (D) Balanced anesthesia is a combination of a number of anesthetic agents that produce a smooth induction, appropriate depth of anesthesia, and appropriate muscle relaxation with minimal complications.

58. **(D)** Client need: physiological integrity; subcategory: reduction of risk potential; content area: med/surg

RATIONALE

(A) Classic symptoms of a heart attack include heaviness or squeezing pain in the chest, pain spreading to the jaw, neck, and arm. Nausea and vomiting, sweating, and shortness of breath may be present. The client does not exhibit these symptoms. (B) Clients suffering from anxiety or fear prior to surgical procedures may develop hyperventilation. This client is not seeking attention. (C) Symptoms of complete airway obstruction include not being able to speak, and no airflow between the nose and mouth. Breath sounds are absent. (D) Tightness in the chest; a feeling of suffocation; lightheadedness; tingling in the hands; and rapid, deep respirations are signs and symptoms of hyperventilation. This is almost always a manifestation of anxiety.

59. **(A)** Client need: physiological integrity; subcategory: pharmacological and parenteral therapies; content area: med/surg

RATIONALE

(A) Cefoperazone is indicated in the treatment of infection with *Pseudomonas aeruginosa*. (B) Clindamycin is not indicated in the treatment of infection with *P. aeruginosa*. (C) Dicloxacillin is not indicated in the treatment of infection with *P. aeruginosa*. (D) Erythromycin is not indicated in the treatment of infection with *P. aeruginosa*.

60. **(D)** Client need: health promotion and maintenance; subcategory: growth and development through the life span; content area: maternity

RATIONALE

(A) Monitoring temperature twice a day predicts the biphasic pattern of ovulation. (B) Prediction of ovulation relies on consistency in taking temperature. (C) Nightly rectal temperatures are more accurate in predicting ovulation. (D) Activity changes the accuracy of basal body temperature and ability to detect the luteinizing hormone surge.

61. **(C)** Client need: health promotion and maintenance; subcategory: prevention and early detection of disease; content area: med/surg

RATIONALE

(A) An adult diazepam dosage for treatment of anxiety is 2–10 mg PO 2–4 times daily. The order as written would place a client at risk for overdose. (B) A high room temperature could increase hyperventilating episodes by stimulating the respiratory system. (C) Breath holding and breathing into a paper bag may be useful in controlling hyperventilation. Both measures increase CO_2 retention. (D) Distraction will not prevent or control hyperventilation caused by anxiety or fear.

62. **(C)** Client need: psychosocial integrity; subcategory: coping and adaptation; content area: maternity

    RATIONALE

    (A) This is not a supportive statement. There are also no data to indicate the family's religious beliefs. (B) Seeing their baby assists the parents in the grieving process. This gives them the opportunity to say "good-bye." (C) Parents need time to get to know their baby. (D) This is not a comforting statement when a baby has died. There are also no guarantees that the couple will be able to have another child.

63. **(C)** Client need: health promotion and maintenance; subcategory: prevention and early detection of disease; content area: maternity

    RATIONALE

    (A) The test results were normal, so there would be no need to repeat to determine results. (B) There are no data to indicate further tests are needed, because the result of the NST was normal. (C) An NST is reported as reactive if there are two to three increases in the fetal heart rate of 15 bpm, lasting at least 15 seconds during a 15-minute period. (D) The NST results were normal, so there was no fetal distress.

64. **(B)** Client need: health promotion and maintenance; subcategory: growth and development through the life span; content area: maternity

    RATIONALE

    (A) This stage is from complete dilatation of the cervix to delivery of the fetus. (B) This is the correct stage for the definition. (C) This stage lasts for about 2 hours after the delivery of the placenta. (D) There is no fifth stage of labor.

65. **(A)** Client need: health promotion and maintenance; subcategory: growth and development through the life span; content area: maternity

    RATIONALE

    (A) This discharge occurs from delivery through the 3rd day. There is dark red blood, placental debris, and clots. (B) This discharge occurs from days 4–10. The lochia is brownish, serous, and thin. (C) This discharge occurs from day 10 through the 6th week. The lochia is yellowish white. (D) This is not a classification of lochia but relates to the amount of discharge.

APPENDIX A

Abbreviations

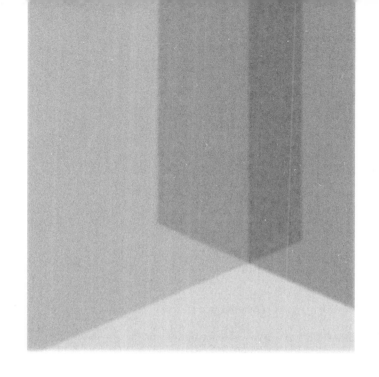

AA	Alcoholics Anonymous
ABG	arterial blood gas
ACTH	corticotropic hormone
ADH	antidiuretic hormone
ADHD	attention-deficit hyperactivity disorder
ADL	activities of daily living
AFP	α-fetoprotein
AIDS	acquired immunodeficiency syndrome
ALL	acute lymphocytic leukemia
ARDS	adult respiratory distress syndrome
ARF	acute respiratory failure
AROM	artificial rupture of membranes
AST	aspartate transaminase
BHCG	Bacille Calmette-Guérin (TB vaccine)
BPH	benign prostatic hypertrophy
BSA	body surface area
BUN	blood urea nitrogen
CAT	computerized adaptive testing
CBC	complete blood count
CGFNS	Commission on Graduates of Foreign Nursing Schools
CHF	congestive heart failure
CLL	chronic lymphocytic leukemia
CMM	chronic myelogenous leukemia
CNS	central nervous system
COPD	chronic obstructive pulmonary disease
CPD	cephalopelvic disproportion
CPK	creatinine phosphokinase
CRH	corticotropin-releasing hormone
CSF	cerebrospinal fluid
CST	contraction stress test
CT	computed tomography
CVA	cerebrovascular accident
CVP	central venous pressure
D & C	dilatation and curettage
DIC	disseminated intravascular coagulation
DPT	diphtheria-pertussis-tetanus
DTR	deep tendon reflex
ECG	electrocardiogram, electrocardiography
ECMO	extracorporeal membrane oxygenation
ECT	electroconvulsive therapy
ED	emergency department
EDB	expected date of birth
EDC	expected date of confinement
EEG	electroencephalogram, electroencephalography
EFM	electronic fetal monitor
EGD	esophagogastroduodenoscopy
ELISA	enzyme-linked immunosorbent assay
EPS	extrapyramidal symptoms
ER	emergency room
ERCP	endoscopic retrograde cholangiopancreatogram
ESR	erythrocyte sedimentation rate
ETS	Educational Testing Services
FB	fingerbreadth
FHR	fetal heart rate
FHT	fetal heart tone
FSH	follicle-stimulating hormone
FTT	failure to thrive
GFR	glomerular filtration rate
GH	growth hormone
GI	gastrointestinal
GTPAL	G = gravida, T = term birth, P = preterm birth, A = abortions, L = living children
GTT	glucose tolerance test
GU	genitourinary
HbA, HbS	hemoglobin A, hemoglobin S
HCG	human chorionic gonadotropin
HCT	hematocrit
HGH	human growth hormone
HIB	Haemophilus influenzae type B
HIV	human immunodeficiency virus
HNP	herniated nucleus pulposus
HPL	human chorionic gonadotropin
HPV	human papilloma virus

ICP	intracranial pressure	PGE$_2$	prostaglandin E$_2$
ICU	intensive care unit	PID	pelvic inflammatory disease
IDDM	insulin-dependent diabetes mellitus	PIH	pregnancy-induced hypertension
IDM	infant of diabetic mother	PKU	phenylketonuria
ITP	idiopathic thrombocytopenic purpura	PMI	point of maximum impulse
IUGR	intrauterine growth retardation	PROM	premature rupture of membranes
IVP	intravenous pyelogram	PT	prothrombin time
JVD	jugular venous distention	PTC	percutaneous transhepatic cholangiogram
17-KS	17-ketosteroid	PTH	parathyroid hormone
KUB	kidney, blood, ureter	PTSD	posttraumatic stress disorder
LDH	lactic dehydrogenase	PTT	partial thromboplastin time
LE	lupus erythematosus	RBC	red blood cell
LH	luteinizing hormone	RDS	respiratory distress syndrome
LMP	last menstrual period	REM	rapid eye movement
LOA	left occipitoanterior	RF	rheumatoid factor
L/S	lecithin/sphingomyelin	RN	registered nurse
MAO	monoamine oxidase	ROM	range of motion
MgSO$_4$	magnesium sulfate	RPR	rapid plasma reagin
MI	myocardial infarction	S/D	systolic-to-diastolic
MMR	measles, mumps, rubella	SIDS	sudden infant death syndrome
MRI	magnetic resonance imaging	T$_3$	triiodothyronine
MSE	mental status examination	T$_4$	thyroxine
NCLEX-RN	National Council Licensure Examination for Registered Nurses	TB	tuberculosis
NCSBN	National Council of State Boards of Nursing	TED	thromboembolic disease
		TIA	transient ischemic attack
NG	nasogastric	TPN	total parenteral nutrition
NIDDM	non–insulin-dependent diabetes mellitus	TRF	thyroid-releasing factor
NST	nonstress test	TSE	testicular self-examination
OCT	oxytocin challenge test	TSH	thyroid-stimulating hormone
17-OCHS	17-hydroxycorticosteroid	TURP	transurethral resection, prostate
OPV	oral poliovirus vaccine	URI	upper respiratory infection
PAP	pulmonary artery pressure	UTI	urinary tract infection
PEEP	positive end-expiratory pressure	VBAC	vaginal birth after cesarean
PEFR	positive expiratory flow rate	VDRL	Venereal Disease Research Laboratory
PG	prostaglandin	VSD	ventricular septal defect
		WBC	white blood cell

APPENDIX B

State Boards of Nursing

ALABAMA Board of Nursing
RSA Plaza, Suite 250
770 Washington Ave.
Montgomery, AL 36130-3900
Lynn Norman, RN, MSN, *Contact Person*
Phone: (334) 242-4060
Fax: (334) 242-4360

ALASKA Board of Nursing
Department of Commerce and Economic
    Development
Division of Occupational Licensing
3601 C Street, Suite 722
Anchorage, AK 99503
Dorothy Fulton, RN, MA, *Executive Director*
Phone: (907) 269-8161
Fax: (907) 269-8196

ALASKA Board of Nursing—Juneau
P.O. Box 110806
Juneau, AK 99811
Phone: (907) 465-2544
Fax: (907) 465-2974

AMERICAN SAMOA Health Services
Regulatory Board
LBJ Tropical Medical Center
Pago Pago, AS 96799
Etenauga Lutu, RN, *Executive Secretary*
Phone: (684) 633-1222
Fax: (684) 633-1869

ARIZONA State Board of Nursing
1651 E. Morten Ave., Suite 150
Phoenix, AZ 85020
Joey Ridenour, RN, MN,
    Executive Director
Phone: (602) 331-8111
Fax: (602) 906-9365

ARKANSAS State Board of Nursing
University Tower Building
1123 S. University, Suite 800
Little Rock, AR 72204
Faith Fields, RN, MSN, *Executive Director*
Phone: (501) 686-2700
Fax: (501) 686-2714

CALIFORNIA Board of Registered Nursing
400 R Street, Suite 4030
P.O. Box 944210
Sacramento, CA 95814
Ruth Ann Terry, RN, MPH, *Executive Officer*
Phone: (916) 322-3350
Fax: (916) 327-4402

CALIFORNIA Board of Vocational
    Nursing and Psychiatric Technicians
2535 Capitol Oaks Drive, Suite 205
Sacramento, CA 95833
Teresa Bello-Jones, RN, MS, JD, *Executive Officer*
Phone: (916) 263-7800
Fax: (916) 263-7859

COLORADO Board of Nursing
1560 Broadway, Suite 670
Denver, CO 80202
Jan Zubieni, RN, MS, BSN, *Interim Program Administrator*
Phone: (303) 894-2430
Fax: (303) 894-2821

CONNECTICUT Board of Examiners for Nursing
Division of Health Systems Regulation
410 Capitol Ave., MS#12HSR
P.O. Box 340308
Hartford, CT 06134-0328
Wendy Furniss, RNC, MS, *Public Health Services Manager*
Phone: (860) 509-7624
Fax: (860) 509-7286

DELAWARE Board of Nursing
861 Silver Lake Blvd.
Cannon Building, Suite 203
Dover, DE 19904
Iva Boardman, RN, MSN, *Executive Director*
Phone: (302) 739-4522
Fax: (302) 739-2711

DC Board of Nursing
614 H Street, NW
Washington, DC 20001
Barbara Hagans, *Contact Person*
Phone: (202) 727-7468
Fax: (202) 727-7662

FLORIDA Board of Nursing
4080 Woodcock Drive, Suite 202
Jacksonville, FL 32207
Ruth R. Stiehl, RN, PhD, MN, MA, BS,
   Executive Director
Phone: (904) 858-6940
Fax: (904) 858-6964

**GEORGIA State Board of Licensed Practical
   Nurses**
166 Pryor Street, SW
Atlanta, GA 30303
Jacqueline Hightower, *Executive Director*
Phone: (404) 656-3921
Fax: (404) 651-9532

GEORGIA Board of Nursing
166 Pryor Street, SW
Atlanta, GA 30303
Shirley Camp, RN, BSN, JD, *Executive Director*
Phone: (404) 656-3943
Fax: (404) 657-7489

GUAM Board of Nurse Examiners
P.O. Box 2816
Agana, GU 96910
Teofila Cruz, RN, *Nurse Examiner Administrator*
Phone: (671) 475-0251
Fax: (671) 477-4733

HAWAII Board of Nursing
Professional and Vocational Licensing Division
P.O. Box 3469
Honolulu, HI 96801
Kathleen Yokouchi, *Executive Officer*
Phone: (808) 586-3000
Fax: (808) 586-2689

IDAHO Board of Nursing
280 N. 8th Street, Suite 210
P.O. Box 83720
Boise, ID 83720
Sandra Evans, RN, MA, Ed, *Executive Director*
Phone: (208) 334-3110
Fax: (208) 334-3262

ILLINOIS Department of Professional Regulation
James R. Thompson Center
100 W. Randolph, Suite 9-300
Chicago, IL 60601
Jacqueline Waggoner, RN, MSN, *Nursing Act Coordinator*
Phone: (312) 814-2715
Fax: (312) 814-3145

INDIANA State Board of Nursing
Health Professions Bureau
402 W. Washington St., Suite 041
Indianapolis, IN 46204
Laura Langford, RN, *Executive Director*
Phone: (317) 232-2960
Fax: (317) 233-4236

IOWA Board of Nursing
State Capitol Complex
1223 E. Court Ave.
Des Moines, IA 50319
Lorinda Inman, RN, MSN, *Executive Director*
Phone: (515) 281-3255
Fax: (515) 281-4825

KANSAS State Board of Nursing
Landon State Office Building
900 SW Jackson, Suite 551-S
Topeka, KS 66612
Patsy Johnson, RN, MN, *Executive Administrator*
Phone: (785) 296-4929
Fax: (785) 296-3929

KENTUCKY Board of Nursing
312 Whittington Parkway, Suite 300
Louisville, KY 40222
Sharon Weisenbeck, RN, MS, *Executive Director*
Phone: (502) 329-7000
Fax: (502) 329-7011

**LOUISIANA State Board of Practical Nurse
   Examiners**
3421 N. Causeway Blvd., Suite 203
Metairie, LA 70002
Dennis Stewart Mann, JD, *Executive Director*
Phone: (504) 838-5791
Fax: (504) 838-5279

LOUISIANA State Board of Nursing
3510 N. Causeway Blvd., Suite 501
Metairie, LA 70002
Barbara Morvant, MN, RN, *Executive Director*
Phone: (504) 838-5332
Fax: (504) 838-5349

MAINE State Board of Nursing
158 State House Station
Augusta, ME 04333
Myra Broadway, JD, MS, RN, *Executive Director*
Phone: (207) 287-1133
Fax: (207) 287-1149

MARYLAND Board of Nursing
4140 Patterson Avenue
Baltimore, MD 21215
Donna Dorsey, RN, MS, *Executive Director*
Phone: (410) 585-1900
Fax: (410) 358-3530

MASSACHUSETTS Board of Registration in Nursing
Levertt Saltonstall Building
100 Cambridge Street, Room 1519
Boston, MA 02202
Theresa Bonanno, MSN, RN, *Executive Director*
Phone: (617) 727-9961
Fax: (617) 727-1630

MICHIGAN CIS/Office of Health Services
611 W. Ottawa, 1st Floor
Lansing, MI 48933
Carol Engle, *Licensing Director*
Phone: (517) 373-9102
Fax: (517) 373-2179

MICHIGAN Testing Services Division
P.O. Box 30018
Lansing, MI 48909
Kara Schmitt, PhD, *Director*
Phone: (517) 241-9289
Fax: (517) 241-7539

MINNESOTA Board of Nursing
2829 University Avenue, SE
Suite 500
Minneapolis, MN 55414
Joyce Schowalter, RN, MNAd, Med, *Executive Director*
Phone: (612) 617-2270
Fax: (612) 617-2190

MISSISSIPPI Board of Nursing
1935 Lakeland Drive, Suite B
Jackson, MS 39216
Marcia Rachel, PhD, RN, *Executive Director*
Phone: (601) 987-4188
Fax: (601) 364-2352

MISSOURI State Board of Nursing
3605 Missouri Blvd.
P.O. Box 656
Jefferson City, MO 65102-0656
Marcia K. Flesner, RN, MSN, MHCA, CNAA, *Executive
  Director*
Phone: (573) 751-0681
Fax: (573) 751-0075

MONTANA State Board of Nursing
Arcade Building, Suite 4C
111 North Jackson
Helena, MT 59620-0513
Dianne Wickham, RN, MN, *Executive Director*
Phone: (406) 444-2071
Fax: (406) 444-7759

**NEBRASKA Department of Health and Human
  Services Regulation and Licensure**
Credentialing Division–Nursing/Nursing Support Section
301 Centennial Mall South
P.O. Box 94986
Lincoln, NE 68509-4986
Charlene Kelly, PhD, RN, *Executive Director*
Phone: (402) 471-4376
Fax: (402) 471-3577

NEVADA State Board of Nursing
4330 S. Valley View, Suite 106
Las Vegas, NV 89103
Phone: (702) 486-5800
Fax: (702) 486-5803

NEVADA State Board of Nursing
1755 East Plumb Lane, Suite 260
Reno, NV 89502
Kathy Apple, RN, MS, *Executive Director*
Phone: (702) 688-2620
Fax: (702) 688-2628

NEW HAMPSHIRE Board of Nursing
78 Regional Drive
P.O. Box 3898
Concord, NH 03302
Doris Nuttelman, RN, EdD, *Executive Director*
Phone: (603) 271-2323
Fax: (603) 271-6605

NEW JERSEY Board of Nursing
124 Halsey Street, 6th Floor
P.O. Box 45010
Newark, NJ 0710
Patricia Lynch Polansky, RN, MS, *Executive Director*
Phone: (973) 504-6586
Fax: (973) 648-3481

NEW MEXICO Board of Nursing
4206 Louisiana Blvd., NE, Suite A
Albuquerque, NM 87109
Debra Brady, PhD, RN, *Executive Director*
Phone: (505) 841-8340
Fax: (505) 841-8347

NEW YORK State Board of Nursing
State Education Department
Cultural Education Center, Room 3023
Albany, NY 12230
Milene Sower, RN, PhD, *Executive Secretary*
Phone: (518) 474-3845
Fax: (518) 473-0578

**NORTHERN MARIANA ISLAND Commonwealth Board
  of Nurse Examiners Public Health Center**
P.O. Box 1458
Saipan, MP 96950
Elizabeth Torres-Untalan, RN, *Chairperson*
Phone: (670) 234-8950
Fax: (670) 234-8930

NORTH CAROLINA Board of Nursing
3724 National Drive
Raleigh, NC 27602
Polly Johnson, RN, MSN, *Executive Director*
Phone: (919) 782-3211
Fax: (919) 781-9461

NORTH DAKOTA Board of Nursing
919 South 7th Street, Suite 504
Bismark, ND 58504
Constance Kalanek, RN, *Executive Director*
Phone: (701) 328-9777
Fax: (701) 328-9785

OHIO Board of Nursing
77 South High Street, 17th Floor
Columbus, OH 43266-0316
Dorothy Fiorino, RN, MS, *Executive Director*
Phone: (614) 466-3947
Fax: (614) 466-0388

OKLAHOMA Board of Nursing
2915 N. Classen Blvd., Suite 524
Oklahoma City, OK 73106
Sulinda Moffett, RN, MSN, *Executive Director*
Phone: (405) 962-1800
Fax: (405) 962-1821

OREGON State Board of Nursing
800 NE Oregon Street, Box 25
Suite 465
Portland, OR 97232
Joan Bouchard, RN, MN, *Executive Director*
Phone: (503) 731-4745
Fax: (503) 731-4755

PENNSYLVANIA State Board of Nursing
124 Pine Street
P.O. Box 2649
Harrisburg, PA 17101
Miriam Limo, RN, MS, MSN, *Executive Secretary*
Phone: (717) 783-7142
Fax: (717) 783-0822

Commonwealth of PUERTO RICO
Board of Nurse Examiners
800 Roberto H. Todd Ave.
Room 202, Stop 18
Santurce, PR 00908
Beverly Davila, *Executive Director*
Phone: (787) 725-8161
Fax: (787) 725-7903

RHODE ISLAND Board of Nursing
  Registration and Nursing Education
Cannon Health Building
Three Capitol Hill, Room 104
Providence, RI 02908
Nikki Deary, *Chief, Health Services Regulation*
Phone: (401) 222-3855
Fax: (401) 222-2158

SOUTH CAROLINA State Board of Nursing
110 Centerview Drive, Suite 202
Columbia, SC 29210
Patricia Durgin, BS, MSN, *Executive
  Administrator*
Phone: (803) 896-4550
Fax: (803) 896-4525

SOUTH DAKOTA Board of Nursing
4300 South Louise Ave., Suite C-1
Sioux Falls, SC 57106-3124
Diana Vander Woude, RN, MS, *Executive Secretary*
Phone: (605) 362-2760
Fax: (605) 362-2768

TENNESSEE State Board of Nursing
426 Fifth Avenue North
1st Floor–Cordell Hull Building
Nashville, TN 37247
Elizabeth Lund, RN, MSN, *Executive Director*
Phone: (615) 532-5166
Fax: (615) 741-7899

TEXAS Board of Nurse Examiners
333 Guadalupe, Suite 3-460
Austin, TX 78701
Katherine Thomas, MN, RN, *Executive Director*
Phone: (512) 305-7400
Fax: (512) 305-7401

TEXAS Board of Vocational Nurse Examiners
William P. Hobby Building, Tower 3
333 Guadalupe, Suite 3-400
Austin, TX 78701
Mary Strange, RN, *Executive Director*
Phone: (512) 305-8100
Fax: (512) 305-8101

UTAH State Board of Nursing
Heber M. Wells Bldg., 4th Floor
160 East 300 South
Salt Lake City, UT 84111
Laura Poe, RN, MS, *Executive Administrator*
Phone: (801) 530-6628
Fax: (801) 530-6511

VERMONT State Board of Nursing
109 State Street
Montpelier, VT 05609-1106
Anita Ristau, RN, MS,
  Executive Director
Phone: (802) 828-2396
Fax: (802) 828-2484

VIRGIN ISLANDS Board of Nurse Licensure
Veterans Drive Station
St. Thomas, VI 00803
Winifred Garfield, RN, CRNA,
  Executive Secretary
Phone: (340) 776-7397
Fax: (340) 777-4003

VIRGINIA Board of Nursing
6606 W. Broad Street, 4th Floor
Richmond, VA 23230
Nancy Durrett, RN, MSN, *Executive Director*
Phone: (804) 662-9909
Fax: (804) 662-9512

**WASHINGTON State Nursing Care Quality
  Assurance Commission**
Department of Health
1300 Quince Street, SE
Olympia, WA 98504-7864
Paula Meyer, RN, MSN, *Executive Director*
Phone: (360) 236-4713
Fax: (360) 586-2165

**WEST VIRGINIA State Board of Examiners for
  Practical Nurses**
101 Dee Drive
Charleston, WV 25311
Nancy Wilson, RN, *Executive Secretary*
Phone: (304) 558-3572
Fax: (304) 558-4367

**WEST VIRGINIA State Board of Examiners for
  Registered Professional Nurses**
101 Dee Drive
Charleston, WV 25311
Laura Rhodes, RN, MSN, *Executive Secretary*
Phone: (304) 558-3596
Fax: (304) 558-3666

WISCONSIN Department of Regulation and Licensing
1400 E. Washington Avenue
P.O. Box 8935
Madison, WI 53708
Thomas Neumann, RN, MSN,
  Regulatory Education Officer
Phone: (608) 266-2112
Fax: (608) 267-0644

WYOMING State Board of Nursing
2020 Carey Avenue, Suite 110
Cheyenne, WY 82002
Mary Schaper, RN, MS, *Interim Executive Director*
Phone: (307) 777-7601
Fax: (307) 777-3519

INDEX

Page numbers followed by an "*f*" signify figures; page numbers followed by a "*t*" signify tables.